Coronary C

Aaron Nash-Davis

For Churchill Livingstone
Commissioning Editor: Gavin Smith
Project Controller: Anita Sekhri
Copy Editor: Alison Bowers
Cover Design: Andrew Jones

Coronary Care Manual

Peter L Thompson MD MBBS FRACP FACP FACC
Clinical Professor of Medicine, University of Western Australia
Head of Cardiovascular Medicine and Director of Coronary Care
Sir Charles Gairdner Hospital, Perth
Western Australia, Australia

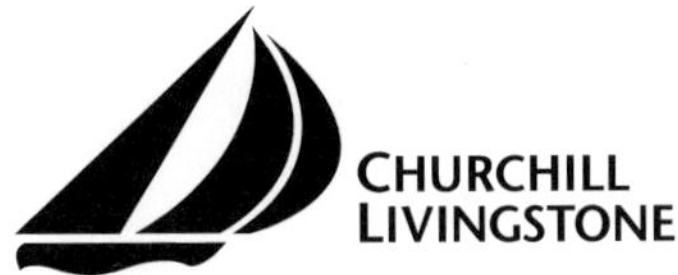

NEW YORK • EDINBURGH • LONDON • MADRID • MELBOURNE • SAN FRANCISCO AND TOKYO 1997

CHURCHILL LIVINGSTONE
Medical Division of Pearson Professional Limited

Distributed in the United States of America by Churchill Livingstone Inc., 650 Avenue of the Americas, New York, N.Y. 10011, and by associated companies, branches and representatives throughout the world.

First Published 1997

ISBN 0 443 052 328

British Library Cataloguing in Publication Data
A catalogue record for this book is available from the British Library.

Library of Congress Cataloguing in Publication Data
A catalogue record for this book is available from the library of Congress.

Printed in Hong Kong

The publisher's policy is to use **paper manufactured from sustainable forests**

Contents

Contents

Part 6 Non-drug therapies 331

Part 7 Acute myocardial infarction 427

Part 8 Other cardiac problems 491

Part 9 Special problems in the CCU patient 583

Part 10 Post-CCU management 601

Part 11 Other CCU issues 655

Appendices 669

Index 677

List of contributors

Kevin C Allman MBBS, FRACP
Director of Nuclear Cardiology Laboratory
Concord Hospital, Sydney, NSW
Australia

Philip EG Aylward MA, BMBCh, PhD, MRCP, FRACP
Director of Cardiovascular Medicine
Flinders Medical Centre, Adelaide, SA
Australia

Lillian J Barrie RN, Crit. Care Cert., BHSc(Nursing)
Nurse Manager
Intensive Care and Coronary Care Unit
St John of God Hospital, Perth, WA
Australia

George J Bautovich MBBS, BSc (Med), PhD, FRACP
Head of Department
Department of Nuclear Medicine
Royal Prince Alfred Hospital, Sydney, NSW
Australia

JH Nick Bett MBBS, MRACP, FRACP, DDU
Director of Cardiology
The Prince Charles Hospital, Chermside, Brisbane, QLD
Australia

Pamela J Bradshaw RN, BA, Grad. Dip.(Nsg.Ed), MSc
Clinical Trials Co-ordinator
Department of Cardiovascular Medicine and Heart Research Institute
Sir Charles Gairdner Hospital, Perth, WA
Australia

Tom G Briffa BPE, MPE
Exercise Physiologist
Department of Cardiovascular Medicine
Sir Charles Gairdner Hospital, Perth, WA
Australia

Wendy L Bryson RN, Dip Adv Nursing (NZ), BAppSc.
Clinical Nurse Specialist
Department of Cardiovascular Medicine
Sir Charles Gairdner Hospital, Perth, WA
Australia

Terence J Campbell MD, DPhil, FRACP, FACC
Associate Professor of Medicine, The University of New South Wales
Director of Coronary Care
Deputy Director, Department of Clinical Pharmacology
St Vincent's Hospital, Sydney, NSW
Australia

Philip A Cooke MBBS
Electrophysiology/Pacing Fellow, Royal Perth Hospital
Advanced Trainee Cardiologist
Department of Cardiovascular Medicine
Sir Charles Gairdner Hospital, Perth, WA
Australia

Gregory B Cranney MBBS, FRACP
Senior Lecturer, University of New South Wales
Director of Cardiac Imaging
Prince Henry Hospital, Sydney, NSW
Australia

Michael JE Davis MBBS, FRACP
Cardiologist
Department of Cardiology, Royal Perth Hospital
Director of Cardiology,
Hollywood Private Hospital,
Perth, WA
Australia

Timothy J Day MBBS, FRACP
Head of Department
Department of Neurology and Clinical Neurophysiology
Sir Charles Gairdner Hospital,
Perth, WA
Australia

John T Dowling MBBS, FRACP
Assistant Director of Cardiology
Royal Melbourne Hospital
Cardiologist
Epworth Medical Centre,
Melbourne, VIC
Australia

Peter J Fletcher MBBS, BSc(Med), PhD, FRACP
Professor of Cardiovascular Medicine,
University of Newcastle
Director, Department of Cardiovascular Medicine
John Hunter Hospital, Newcastle, NSW
Australia

S Ben Freedman MBBS, BSc(Med), PhD, FRACP, FACC
Head, Department of Cardiology
Concord Repatriation Hospital,
Sydney, NSW
Australia

Alexander S Gallus MBBS, FRACP, FRCPA
Chairman, Division of Laboratory Medicine
Department of Haematology
Flinders Medical Centre,
Adelaide, SA
Australia

Clay L Golledge MBBS, BSc(Med), MRCP, FRCPA, FACTM, DTM&H
Consultant in Clinical Microbiology and Infectious Diseases
The Western Australian Centre for Pathology and Medical Research
Queen Elizabeth II Medical Centre, Perth, WA
Australia

Stephen PF Gordon MBBS, FRACP
Consultant Cardiologist
Department of Cardiovascular Medicine
Sir Charles Gairdner Hospital,
Perth, WA
Australia

Geoffrey Groom MBBS, FRACP
Nuclear Medicine Physician
Department of Nuclear Medicine
Sir Charles Gairdner Hospital,
Perth, WA
Australia

Ian Hamilton Craig MBBS, PhD(McMaster), FRACP
Director, Preventive Cardiology and Lipid Management Clinic
North Adelaide, SA
Australia

Mark E Hands MBBS, FRACP
Consultant Cardiologist
Department of Cardiovascular Medicine
Sir Charles Gairdner Hospital,
Perth, WA
Australia

Phillip J Harris MBBS, D Phil, FRACP, FACC
Clinical Professor, Department of Medicine, University of Sydney
Head, Department of Cardiology
Royal Prince Alfred Hospital,
Sydney, NSW
Australia

Barry E Hopkins MBBS (Hons), PhD, FRACP, FACC
Cardiologist
St John of God Hospital, Perth, WA
Australia

John D Horowitz MBBS, BMedSci(Hons), PhD, FRACP
Professor of Cardiology,
University of Adelaide
Director of Cardiology
Queen Elizabeth Hospital,
Adelaide, SA
Australia

Joseph Hung MBBS(Hons), FRACP, FACC
Senior Lecturer in Cardiology,
University of Western Australia
Consultant Cardiologist
Department of Cardiovascular Medicine
Sir Charles Gairdner Hospital,
Perth, WA
Australia

David Hunt MBBS, MD, FRACP, FACC, DDU
Senior Cardiologist
Department of Cardiology
Royal Melbourne Hospital,
Melbourne, VIC
Australia

Marcus K Ilton MBBS, FRACP
Research Fellow in Cardiology,
Heart Research Institute
Senior Medical Registrar
Sir Charles Gairdner Hospital,
Perth, WA
Australia

Konrad Jamrozik MBBS, Dphil, FAFPHM
Associate Professor
Department of Public Health
University of Western Australia,
Perth, WA
Australia

Michael V Jelinek MD, FRACP, FACC
Director of Cardiology
St Vincent's Hospital, Melbourne,
VIC
Australia

Desmond Julian MD, FRCP, FRACP
Emeritus Professor of Cardiology
University of Newcastle upon
Tyne
Formerly Director of the British
Heart Foundation, London
UK

David T Kelly AM, MB, ChB, FRACP, FACC, FRCP
Professor of Cardiology,
University of Sydney
Director, Hallstrom Institute of
Cardiology
Royal Prince Alfred Hospital,
Sydney, NSW
Australia

Anne M Keogh MBBS, MD, FRACP
Senior Transplant Cardiologist
St Vincent's Hospital, Sydney
Senior Lecturer in Medicine,
University of NSW
Australia

Leonard Kritharides MBBS, PhD, FRACP
Senior Clinical Scientist and Co-
Group Leader, Clinical Research
Group
The Heart Research Institute
Associate Cardiologist
Royal Prince Alfred Hospital,
Sydney, NSW
Australia

Ashok B Kumar MBBS, FRCR, FRACR
Consultant Radiologist
Sir Charles Gairdner Hospital,
Perth, WA
Australia

Paul E Langton BSc, MBBS(Hons)
Cardiology Fellow, Heart
Research Institute and
Department of Cardiovascular
Medicine
Sir Charles Gairdner Hospital,
Perth, WA
Australia

Bernard H Laurence MBBS, B Med Sci(Hon), FRACP
Gastroenterologist
The Mount Hospital, Perth, WA
Australia

Brian L Lloyd MBBS, PhD, FRACP, FACC
Consultant Cardiologist
Department of Cardiovascular
Medicine
Sir Charles Gairdner Hospital,
Perth, WA
Australia

Peter Macdonald MBBS, FRACP, PhD
Staff Cardiologist
Heart and Lung Transplant Unit
St Vincent's Hospital, Sydney,
NSW
Australia

Harry G Mond MD, FRACP, FACC
Physician to Pacemaker Clinic
The Royal Melbourne Hospital,
Melbourne, VIC
Australia

John E Morgan MBBS, FACEM
Deputy Head, Department of
Emergency Medicine,
Royal North Shore Hospital,
Sydney, NSW
Australia

Mark AJ Newman MBBS(Hons), DS, FRACS
Director of Cardiothoracic
Surgery
Sir Charles Gairdner Hospital,
Perth, WA
Australia

List of contributors

S Mark Nidorf MD, MBBS, FRACP, FACC
Consultant Cardiologist
Department of Cardiovascular Medicine
Sir Charles Gairdner Hospital, Perth, WA
Australia

Robin M Norris MD, FRCP, FRACP
Honorary Consultant Cardiologist and Senior Visiting Fellow
Cardiac Research Department
Royal Sussex County Hospital, Brighton
UK

Michael F O'Rourke AM, MD BS, FRACP, FACC, FESC
Medical Professorial Unit
The University of New South Wales
St Vincent's Hospital, Sydney, NSW
Australia

Donna M O'Shannessy Reg.Comp.N.,BAppSc(N), PGradDipHlth Admin, MRCNA
Transplant Nurse Consultant
Heart Transplant Unit
Royal Perth Hospital, Perth, WA
Australia

Bradley M Power MBBS, FRACP
Intensive Care Specialist
Intensive Care Unit
Sir Charles Gairdner Hospital, Perth, WA
Australia

David AB Richards BSc(Med), MD, FRACP, FACC
Consultant Cardiologist
Westmead Hospital, Sydney, NSW
Australia

JG (Dick) Richards MBBS, FRCP, FRACP, FACC
Consultant Cardiologist
Royal Prince Alfred Hospital
Ex-chief M.O. of Australian Mutual Provident Society, Sydney, NSW
Australia

James S Robinson MBBS, FRACP
Consultant Cardiologist
Department of Cardiovascular Medicine
Sir Charles Gairdner Hospital, Perth, WA
Australia

David Ross MBBS, FRACP, FACC
Clinical Professor of Medicine
Director of Cardiology
Westmead Hospital, Sydney, NSW
Australia

D Norman Sharpe MD, FRACP, FACC
Professor of Medicine, University of Auckland School of Medicine
Cardiologist, Auckland Hospital, Auckland
New Zealand

Jonathan S Silberberg MB BCh, MSc, FRACP
Senior Lecturer in Medicine, University of Newcastle
Consultant Cardiologist
John Hunter Hospital, Newcastle, NSW
Australia

I Nigel Sinclair MA, MB, B.Chir, FRACP
Consultant Cardiologist
Mount Hospital, Perth, WA
Australia

J Graeme Sloman AM, ED, BSc, FRCP, FRCPE, FRACP, FACC
Consultant Cardiologist
Cardiovascular Unit
Epworth Hospital, Melbourne, VIC
Australia

Anthony C Thomas MBBS, PhD, FRCPA, FRCPath
Associate Professor
Senior Specialist in Histopathology
Flinders Medical Centre, Adelaide, SA
Australia

Peter L Thompson MD, MBBS, FRACP, FACC, FACP
Clinical Professor of Medicine, University of Western Australia
Head of Cardiovascular Medicine and Director of Coronary Care
Sir Charles Gairdner Hospital, Perth, WA
Australia

Andrew Thomson MBBS, PhD, MRCP, FRACP
Cardiologist
Cardiology Department
Royal Hobart Hospital, Hobart, TAS
Australia

Andrew M Tonkin MBBS, MD, FRACP
Directory of Cardiology
Austin and Repatriation Medical Centre, Melbourne, VIC
Australia

John B Uther AO, BSc(Med), MD, FRACP
Clinical Professor of Medicine
Chairman, Division of Medicine
Westmead Hospital, Sydney, NSW
Australia

P Vernon van Heerden MBBCh, MMed(Anaes), DA(SA), FFARCSI, FFICANZCA, FCCP
Staff Specialist
Department of Intensive Care
Sir Charles Gairdner Hospital,
Perth, WA
Australia

Jitu K Vohra MD, FRCP, FRACP, FACC
Cardiologist
Department of Cardiology
The Royal Melbourne Hospital,
Melbourne, VIC
Australia

Timothy A Welborn PhD, MBBS, FRCP, FRACP
Clinical Professor of Medicine,
University of Western Australia
Department of Endocrinology
Sir Charles Gairdner Hospital,
Perth, WA
Australia

Harvey D White MBChB, DSc, FRACP, FACC, FESC
Director of Coronary Care
Department of Cardiology
Green Lane Hospital, Auckland
New Zealand

Eric G Whitford MBBS, FRACP
Consultant Cardiologist
Department of Cardiovascular Medicine
Sir Charles Gairdner Hospital,
Perth, WA
Australia

Foreword

Two decades ago, it would have been extremely difficult to predict where acute care of patients with evolving myocardial infarction would be headed. What started out as a technique to dissolve coronary blood clot in the cardiac catheterization laboratory setting has been transformed to standard therapy administered intravenously, on an empirical basis, in emergency centres or even a patient's home. With the widespread acceptance of myocardial reperfusion therapy for acute myocardial infarction, there has indeed been a revolution in our approach and considerable opportunity for further refinement in the years ahead.

The whole book of acute myocardial infarction has had to be rewritten. Rather than the supportive care that was available until the early 1980s, a very aggressive approach has become state-of-the-art. This includes timely diagnosis of a patient in the emergency centre with an acute coronary syndrome, given the potential to prevent the event or markedly attenuate the myocardial damage that may occur. Once diagnosed, patients are considered for intravenous thrombolytic therapy along with aspirin, heparin, beta blockers, nitro-glycerine, and angiotensin converting enzyme inhibitors. The goal of treatment is the rapid, complete, and sustained restoration of infarct artery blood flow. In certain situations this can be more efficiently or safely achieved with the quick transfer of a patient into the cardiac catheterization laboratory for performance of balloon angioplasty. If a patient fails to reperfuse, as may be detected by significant clinical deterioration, or has evidence of haemodynamic compromise at the time of admission, an emergency coronary angiogram with an eye towards coronary revascularization is routine. Similarly, post-infarction ischaemia will typically prompt an angiogram to determine the extent and severity of underlying disease. Careful screening and provocative testing is performed before hospital discharge to determine whether there is substantive risk ahead.

This whole strategy represents a major frameshift in philosophy from where we were in the early 1980s. This is an active approach, with unwillingness to accept the natural course of myocardial necrosis and all of its potential complications and unfortunate sequelae. Opiates, once the main approach to make a patient more comfortable while myocardial necrosis was ensuing, are moving towards obsolescence. Nowadays the attitude is to establish reperfusion – whatever it takes – and maintain it in order to provide the affected patient the best chance of not only surviving, but enjoying the best possible quality of life. This requires a comprehensive strategy that incorporates clot dissolution or mechanical dilatation within the infarct vessel and the medication to prevent re-thrombosis, unfavourable remodelling, arrhythmias, or excessive cardiac demand. Chest pain is a medical emergency roughly equivalent to a cardiac arrest which requires the active participation of the emergency room staff to facilitate fast diagnosis and treatment initiation. Furthermore, the interventional cardiologist must be available on a continuous basis to take a patient to the catheterization laboratory. All of this bespeaks a remarkably deliberate and assertive approach.

The outgrowth of this revolution in treatment has been a striking difference in the profile of patients whom we see with acute myocardial infarction. Not only has the fatality rate for patients eligible for reperfusion dipped below double-digits, but the likelihood of early hospital discharge and early return to work and society has dramatically improved. In parallel, efforts to achieve a better outcome for the full gamut of patients with acute coronary syndromes, including those with unstable angina, non-Q wave myocardial infarction, and those ineligible for thrombolytic therapy, are being actively pursued.

The spirit of the total revamping of our approach to patients with acute coronary syndromes has been fully captured in this book. Thompson and all of the authors are to be congratulated on providing the most comprehensive approach to coronary care in the modern era that has yet been presented. Virtually every aspect has been addressed that bears relevance to the coronary care unit of the next millennium. Following the historical perspective and review of the epidemiology and pathophysiology, each diagnostic, drug, and procedural intervention is fully reviewed. Related co-morbidities and other key diagnostic subgroups of patients are systematically presented, along with long-term follow-up considerations. By pulling so much of the contemporary era of coronary care together, this book will undoubtedly be well received by the cardiology community and serve as a vital reference tool for years to come.

As we go forward to the next era of coronary care, the need for the database at each centre to track risk-adjusted outcomes and actual costs will become paramount. While new therapies will be developed that build upon our current knowledge base, and ultimately coronary plaque rupture will be a largely preventable event, as presaged by the remarkable success of lipid-lowering agents, the issues of cost and effectiveness will be centre stage. Faced with technological advances which lack affordability, the challenge that lies ahead will be to provide even better care for our patients with acute manifestations of coronary artery disease, but to do so with heightened awareness of economic restraint.

Eric J. Topol
Cleveland, Ohio

Preface

This book aims to provide a readable summary of the scientific background, clinical trial evidence and practical management of patients with acute cardiac disease. Since the establishment of Coronary Care Units in the late 1960's, hospitals have generally encouraged the management of acute cardiac patients in a specialised area, usually separate from but often adjacent to the Intensive Care Unit. This specialised cardiac care area has expanded its role from the management of acute myocardial infarction to the management of other coronary syndromes, cardiac arrhythmias, cardiac decompensation and the support of patients undergoing interventional cardiology procedures. Although 'coronary care' is a misnomer for the modern acute cardiac care area, the term CCU is well entrenched. For this reason the title 'Coronary Care Manual' has been chosen, as the term 'Coronary Care' succinctly, though somewhat inaccurately, describes a well established and rapidly expanding area of medical practice.

The original model for this book was the 'Intensive Care Manual' now in its fourth edition and for the past decade a standard reference for intensive care. It was edited by Professor Teik Oh, previously of Sir Charles Gairdner Hospital. The success of Teik Oh's book demonstrated that an Antipodean text book will be internationally successful if it is succinct, authoritative, readable and well referenced. On this basis the contributors to the 'Coronary Care Manual' have been carefully chosen from this region based on their international contributions to the field of coronary care.

The first half of the book (Parts 1 to 6) aims to describe in an accurate and readable fashion the scientific and clinical trial basis for coronary care practice. Parts 1, 2 and 3 of the manual describe the background to coronary care and the scientific knowledge base required for acute cardiac care management. Part 4 describes the clinical investigative tools available for evaluation of the patient and Parts 5 and 6 describe the drug and non-drug therapies available.

The second half of the book (Parts 7 to 11) presents practical advice on the management of the wide variety of clinical problems which are treated in the modern coronary care unit and associated facilities. Part 7 describes the pre-hospital emergency department and CCU management of acute myocardial infarction. Part 8 describes the in-hospital management of other cardiac problems. Part 9 describes special problems in the coronary care patient and Part 10 the post-coronary care management. Part 11 details other coronary care issues. The Appendices are included as references for single dose and infusion of cardiac drugs.

The practical management is based firmly on the scientific and clinical trial data presented in the first part of the book. The aim is to transcend national and regional idiosyncrasies. Where possible, management plans are based on randomised clinical trial evidence. Where this is not possible, management plans are based on 'usual practice'. Those which are solely opinion-based have been discouraged or excluded in the editorial process. Nevertheless, the book is intended primarily as a 'Manual' and I trust that the reader will find that the management advice presented is clear and unequivocal.

The book is designed to meet the needs of medical and nursing staff in the coronary care unit, as well as in related hospital areas such as intensive care, emergency department, operating theatre and medical wards. The book should also be of assistance to allied health staff involved in the pre-hospital, in-hospital and post hospital management of acutely ill cardiac patients.

I consider myself fortunate that my mentors in cardiology include some of the great pioneers of coronary care including Bernard Lown of Boston, Graeme Sloman and Alan Goble of Melbourne and Jim Robinson of Perth. I hope that their analytical approach, high standards in management of patients with heart disease and their perception of the patient as the focus of all medical endeavour, are reflected in this book.

PETER L THOMPSON
Perth 1996

Acknowledgements

I wish to acknowledge the support of the many colleagues who contributed to the completion of this book. The enthusiastic support of the contributing authors and their forbearance with the editorial process is greatly appreciated. The efforts of the skilled typists who drafted the early versions of many chapters including Jenny Levy, Lesley Gant and Judith Guest, is much appreciated. The entire text was proof read in detail by Deb Fitzpatrick, Georgia Richter and Pamela Bradshaw. I have received great assistance from the editorial team at Churchill Livingstone including Geoffrey Nuttall who suggested the project, Gavin Smith who supervised it throughout and whose editorial and design experience was invaluable. I am particularly indebted to Anita Sekhri at Churchill Livingstone for her meticulous attention to layout and proof reading of the final manuscript.

The most important person in the production of the book has been Maxine Croot who worked tirelessly over two years in liaising between contributors and the publisher and managing each task with unfailing tact, good humour and attention to detail.

I would also like to acknowledge the support of my friend and colleague, Eric Topol, for his generous Foreword.

Finally, I would like to acknowledge the forbearance of my family in their acceptance and support in the completion of the task.

PETER L THOMPSON

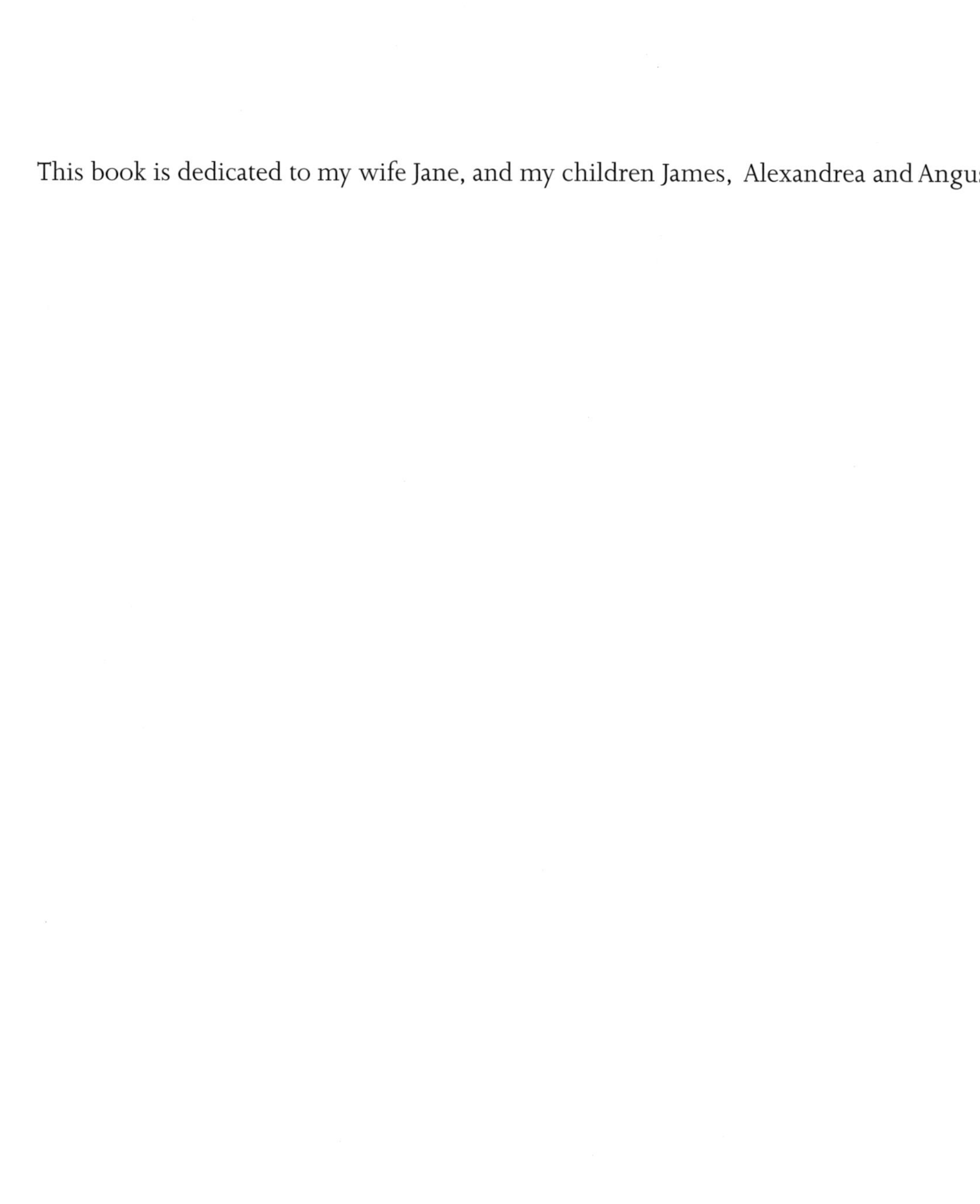

This book is dedicated to my wife Jane, and my children James, Alexandrea and Angus.

Part 1
Background to coronary care

1 History and future of the coronary care unit

J Graeme Sloman and Desmond Julian

Introduction

Prior to 1960, physicians may have done more harm than good to patients with myocardial infarction (MI). Certainly symptoms were alleviated by opiates and nitrates, and anticoagulants helped to combat the tendency to thromboembolic complications because of the prolonged bed-rest then fashionable. But enthusiasm for inotropes (especially digitalis and noradrenaline) may have been responsible for many of the deaths of hospitalized patients with myocardial infarction at that time: 30% died.

The turning point was undoubtedly the development of closed-chest cardiopulmonary resuscitation by Kouwenhoven, Jude and Knickerbocker in 1960.[1] Although the technique was clearly effective if instituted quickly by trained personnel, the organization of most hospitals meant that patients with heart attacks were accommodated in general wards with no special supervision. It soon became apparent that good results could only be obtained if patients at high risk were closely observed by skilled staff, equipped with electrocardiographic monitoring and defibrillators. It was proposed in 1961 that intensive care units for this purpose should be developed,[2] and in the next two years what Day[3] christened 'coronary care units' were created in Kansas, Philadelphia, New York, Toronto, Sydney and Melbourne. Initially the results were not impressive, but by 1964 it was possible to report that ventricular fibrillation had been successfully corrected in six of 15 cases.[4] Subsequently it was found that most cases of primary ventricular fibrillation (i.e. without complicating heart failure or shock) could be treated successfully.

Focus on arrhythmias

The next stage was one of intense interest in the detection and treatment of lesser ventricular arrhythmias and the vigorous use of pacemaking for heart block. It was claimed that if ventricular ectopic beats were treated with lignocaine, ventricular fibrillation would not occur.[5] Subsequent clinical trials have confirmed that lignocaine can reduce the incidence of ventricular fibrillation, but at the risk of increasing the incidence of asystole.[6] Furthermore, there is little evidence that ventricular ectopic beats are of prognostic value in this context. Pacemaking was used aggressively in some units not only for heart block but also for sinus bradycardia—in one hospital for one third of all infarction patients.[7] In retrospect, one can conclude that disorders of rhythm and conduction received more attention than they deserved, but CCUs at this time improved knowledge of the natural history of MI that played an important role in later advances. Furthermore, the excellent nursing and more enlightened medical care to which patients were exposed undoubtedly contributed to the fall in mortality to about 15–20%. Correction of ventricular fibrillation alone was probably responsible for about a 5% fall.

Mobile coronary care

In 1966 Pantridge[8] in Belfast first developed pre-hospital coronary care, a very important initiative in drawing attention to the fact that most deaths from acute heart attacks occur outside hospital. The Belfast units were doctor-staffed, as they continue to be there and in some countries. But it is now widely accepted that paramedics can carry out most of the emergency care, including defibrillation and drug administration, very successfully.

Pump failure and infarct size limitation

By the late 1960s it became apparent that ventricular fibrillation was no longer the single greatest cause of death in the hospitalized patient, and pump failure became the focus of attention. The introduction of the Swan–Ganz catheter permitted the study of heart failure in all well-equipped units and unquestionably provided a better understanding of the different haemodynamic syndromes. In the United States, the massive Myocardial Infarction Research Unit programme greatly expanded our knowledge of the pathophysiology of infarction and promoted the concept of infarct size limitation. The latter was largely based on animal experiments and many agents were thought to have a beneficial effect in this regard. Subsequent clinical trials were disappointing and it was only with the development of reperfusion with thrombolytic agents and angioplasty that the concept of infarct size limitation has been established in man. It is true that intravenous beta blockade, which was originally promoted as limiting infarct size, reduces mortality but it is doubtful if this is the mechanism involved.[9]

Thrombolysis and aspirin

Undoubtedly, the most important advance in the care of MI in the last two decades had been the introduction of aspirin (see Ch. 36) and the thrombolytic agents (see Ch. 34). Thrombolysis has received more attention, and the fact that it is most effective if given early has put pressure on physicians to accelerate the care of patients with suspected MI. Overall, fibrinolytic trials have demonstrated a 16% reduction in 35 day mortality (from 11.5% to 9.6%) although there are major differences between the various subgroups.[10] Thus there is a 25% reduction in those with anterior ST elevation, and little benefit or even harm in those with ST depression or normal electrocardiographs (ECGs). Thrombolytic treatment is probably appropriate for about 50% of all infarct patients, whereas aspirin treatment is suitable for some 90%. In the 'Aspirin papers' it is reported that antiplatelet therapy in a meta-analysis of trials reduced mortality from 14.6% to 10.6%—a reduction by 26%.[11] The two agents are synergistic in their effects.

Coronary angioplasty

The effectiveness of percutaneous coronary angioplasty (PTCA)[12,13] has added a new dimension to coronary care (see Ch. 45), as it implies that appropriate radiological screening facilities (and staff qualified to use them) should be available. Although there seems little to choose between primary angioplasty and thrombolysis, there is no doubt that PTCA has a place in the significant proportion of patients for whom thrombolysis is inadvisable or unsuccessful.

Prevention of infarct expansion and extension

Currently, particular attention is being paid to the prevention of infarct expansion and extension and to the prevention of reinfarction. Trials with angiotensin-converting enzyme (ACE) inhibitors have shown that when started a few days after infarction in patients who have experienced heart failure or who have impaired left ventricular function, they reduce mortality in the succeeding months and years (see Ch. 33).[14,15] Although there was a reduction in 35 day mortality in the GISSI-III[16] and ISIS-4[17] trials, in which the ACE inhibitor was given on the first day to all patients for whom it was not contraindicated, it is not clear that this would be superior to a policy giving the agent to selected patients a day or two later.

The impact of coronary care on mortality

It is difficult to know what the effect of CCUs has been on the mortality of MI patients. The in-hospital mortality 35 years ago, before they were developed, was 25–35%, but the case mix was different then, as were the criteria for diagnosis. Initially CCUs tended to exclude older patients, but this is less common now. Mortality is strongly related to age, and death is now uncommon under the age of 60 (certainly less than 5%). It is probably reasonable now to quote an in-hospital mortality of 10–15%, but there are great variations in this figure. In a recent report from centres involved in the MONICA study,[18] the 28 day mortality in those hospitalized was surprisingly high, ranging from 13% to 27% in men and 20% to 35% for women. A recent survey of Ontario hospitals[19] showed that the mortality had fallen from 22.3% in 1981 to 21.4% in 1985, to 16.3% in 1991.

Has the coronary care unit a future?

The term 'coronary care unit' was always a misnomer, as from the earliest days the units admitted many patients who were not suffering from MI. This trend has increased over the years and by the early 1980s, hospitals such as Epworth Hospital in Melbourne were admitting patients with many different cardiac problems such as recurrent ventricular tachycardia, unstable angina, severe heart failure requiring inotropic drugs and/or the intra-aortic balloon pump, following angioplasty and coronary bypass surgery, out-of-hospital resuscitation and other haemodynamically complex cardiovascular conditions, as well as patients awaiting urgent angioplasty or pacemakers. The modern unit is, therefore, not truly a 'coronary care unit' but a 'cardiac care unit' (still allowing one to use the popular acronym CCU) or an 'acute cardiovascular unit', as preferred at Epworth and elsewhere.

In considering the design, operation and location of such a unit, there are several factors to be taken into account:

- The urgency of diagnosis and treatment of MI means that patients should either be admitted directly to the CCU or be evaluated and treated by suitably trained personnel in the accident and emergency department. In the former case, space and facilities for assessment are necessary, as are arrangements for the rapid transfer or discharge of the patient if a cardiac diagnosis is disproved.
- In centres performing angioplasty and/or cardiac surgery, 24-hour access to a catheter laboratory and open-heart surgery facilities is essential.
- A variety of complications may arise in cardiac patients that necessitate other forms of intensive care. It used to be argued this implied that a CCU should be integral with or adjacent to an intensive care unit. On the whole this has not proved popular because the 'cultures' of the two environments are so different. Nevertheless, ready access to ventilatory support and renal dialysis is essential.
- Patients are now often discharged from the unit quickly, sometimes within hours and usually within a day or two. Yet it is important that there is continuity of care as the patient moves into the convalescent phase. It is, therefore, best if patients during this progressive period are accommodated in wards close to the CCU. This is particularly so if arrhythmias continue to give concern. Fortunately, the development and use of more reliable telemetry has enabled monitoring of the ECG to be more widely and more efficiently used. The telemetered ECG is now technically at least as reliable as the hard wired bedside monitor.

It is not easy to reconcile all these requirements. The acute cardiovascular unit, accommodating a wide variety of patients in the acute and post-acute phases of cardiac illness, is perhaps the best model, although it requires a large pool of highly trained nursing and medical staff. In hospitals with cardiac surgical units, there is a strong case for integration between the medical and surgical departments, and excellent liaisons between cardiologists and cardiac surgeons are essential. In smaller hospitals, it may be advantageous to keep the concept of the small specialized CCU. Unpredictable developments will occur over the next few years but one may be confident that there will be an increasing justification for the amalgamation of all aspects of the management of patients with acute cardiovascular illness.

References

1. Kouwenhoven WB, Jude JR, Knickerbocker GG. Closed-chest cardiac massage. JAMA 1960; 178: 1064
2. Julian DG. Treatment of cardiac arrest in acute myocardial ischaemia and infarction. Lancet 1961; ii: 840–4
3. Day HW. An intensive coronary care area. Dis Chest 1963; 44: 423–7
4. Julian DG, Valentine PA, Miller GG. Disturbances of rate, rhythm and conduction in acute myocardial infarction. Am J Med 1964; 37: 915–27
5. Lown B, Vassaux C. Lidocaine in acute myocardial infarction. Am Heart J 1968; 76: 586–7
6. MacMahon S, Collins R, Peto R et al. Effects of prophylactic lidocaine in suspected acute myocardial infarction. JAMA 1988; 260: 1910–16
7. Meltzer LE, Kitchell JR. The development and current status of coronary care. In: Meltzer LE, Dunning AJ, eds. Textbook of

coronary care. Amsterdam: Excerpta Medica, 1975: 3–25
8. Pantridge JF, Geddes JS. A mobile intensive care unit in the management of myocardial infarction. Lancet 1967: ii: 271–3
9. ISIS-1 Collaborative Group. Mechanisms for the early mortality reduction produced by beta-blockade started early in myocardial infarction. Lancet 1988; i: 921–3
10. Fibrinolytic Therapy Trialists' (FTT) Collaborative Group. Indications for fibrinolytic therapy in suspected myocardial infarction. Lancet 1994; 343: 311–22
11. Antiplatelet Trialists' Collaboration. Collaborative overview of randomised trials of antiplatelet therapy (Pt. 1): Prevention of death, myocardial infarction and stroke by prolonged antiplatelet therapy in various categories of patients. Br Med J 1994; 308: 81–106
12. Grines CL, Browne KF, Marco J et al. A comparison of immediate angioplasty with thrombolytic therapy for acute myocardial infarction. N Engl J Med 1993; 328: 673–9
13. Zijlstra F, de Boer MJ, Hoorntje JC et al. A comparison of immediate angioplasty with intravenous streptokinase in acute myocardial infarction. N Engl J Med 1993; 328: 685–91
14. Pfeffer MA, Braunwald E, Moyé LA, Basta L, Brown EJ, Cuddy TE et al. Effect of captopril on mortality and morbidity in patients with left ventricular dysfunction after myocardial infarction. N Engl J Med 1988; 319: 80–6
15. Acute Infarction Ramipril Efficacy (AIRE) Investigators. Effect of ramipril on mortality and morbidity of survivors of acute myocardial infarction with clinical evidence of heart failure. Lancet 1993; 342: 821–8
16. Gruppo Italiano per lo studio della supravvivenza nell'infarcto miocardico. GISSI-III: effects of lisinopril and transdermal glyceryl trinitrate singly and together on 6-week mortality and ventricular function after acute myocardial infarction. Lancet 1994; 334: 1115–21
17. ISIS 4 Collaborative Group. ISIS 4. A randomised factorial trial assessing early oral captopril, oral mono-nitrate and intravenous magnesium sulphate in 58,000 patients with suspected acute myocardial infarction. Lancet 1995; 345: 669–85
19. Naylor CD, Chen E. Population-wide mortality trends among patients hospitalized for acute myocardial infarction: the Ontario experience, 1981 to 1991. J Am Coll Cardiol 1994; 24: 1431–8

2 Design and management of the coronary care unit

Peter L Thompson

Introduction

Early versions of the coronary care unit (CCU) were designed to manage and prevent complications from acute myocardial infarction (AMI) (see Ch. 1). The essential resources to achieve this were continuous electrocardiographic monitoring around the clock, availability of dedicated nursing staff to observe arrhythmias at a 'central station', and the immediate availability of a defibrillator and medical and nursing staff skilled in resuscitation and defibrillation. In the modern CCU, most of these elements are still present but the emphasis on the role of 'warning arrhythmias' and increasing sophistication of monitoring devices has de-emphasized the arrhythmia control aspects of coronary care and redirected efforts towards early coronary reperfusion and salvage of infarcting myocardium in coronary occlusion. In addition, there is a widening role of the CCU as a specialized cardiac care unit for other acute cardiac problems. While the CCU in the past has primarily had links to the intensive care unit, there is now an increasing need for the CCU to establish wider links with other community and hospital cardiac care services.

Relationships with other cardiac care services

Each hospital needs to make its own decisions about positioning the CCU in the community's range of cardiac care services. In the design and management of the CCU, relationships with the following cardiac care services need to be considered:

- **Community cardiac care services.** A CCU should be available as a resource to the local and referring medical community for advice on cardiac management.[1–4] Communication technology, including the use of facsimile machines and other data transferring methods, should be in place for advice on management of cardiac problems at remote locations, on air and road transport of patients critically ill with acute cardiac emergencies,[5,6] and to contribute to high quality pre-coronary care services in the community. Post coronary care management requires team-work and a detailed understanding of medical and nursing and community support facilities, particularly in the current era where hospital stays are shortened and much of the post coronary management is conducted by the primary care physician or community nursing services.
- **Emergency department.** Several important aspects of cardiac care require close collaboration between the emergency department and CCU.[1–4] These include the joint development of protocols for acute arrhythmia management, circulatory support and reperfusion strategies.[7–9] Joint protocol development and regular review and joint staff development programmes are essential strategies for maintaining high quality acute cardiac care. The success of these strategies needs to be monitored and continually improved by the monitoring of outcomes such as 'door to needle' time.
- **Intensive care unit.** Whether there is an integrated coronary and intensive care unit (ICU) or separate units, there should ideally be close understanding of the facilities and expertise available in each unit. Clear-cut definition of responsibilities needs to be established for the maintenance of expertise and equipment for the more advanced life support procedures, such as haemodynamic monitoring, circulatory assist

devices and assisted ventilation, and for the more specialized cardiologic procedures such as pacemaker technology and echocardiography.

- **Cardiac catheterization laboratory.** The integration of coronary angiography and coronary interventional procedures into the management of acute coronary syndromes has been a feature of cardiologic practice in the past decade.[10–13] Understanding by the coronary care staff of the principles of cardiac catheterization and interventional procedures, such as angioplasty and stent implantation, is now required in the modern CCU. Similarly, an understanding of electrophysiology, catheter ablation, pacing and inflatable defibrillator techniques is required for the modern management of cardiac arrhythmias.
- **Cardiac surgical service.** A CCU needs close relationships either with on-site cardiac surgical facilities or with an efficient cardiac surgical team in a nearby hospital[14] to ensure that options for management of ischaemia, arrhythmias and cardiac failure are well understood and readily available to patients being treated in the CCU.

A well-directed CCU will ensure that these inter-relationships between the various units involved in the management of cardiac patients are encouraged, with informal communication and regular formal inter-unit meeting and discussion forums.

Models of coronary care

A variety of models of coronary care exist, ranging from the simplest bedside or telemetry arrhythmia monitor through to the sophisticated unit providing the full range of circulatory support, cardiac catheterization, cardiac surgery and transplantation.

Bedside arrhythmia monitoring in a general medical ward – not recommended

The provision of bedside or telemetry-based monitoring in a general medical ward is the simplest form of coronary care. Although it has the virtue of economy, and may occasionally alert the staff to the development of a lethal arrhythmia, there is little to support this form of cardiac monitoring in modern medical practice.[15] This form of surveillance will provide little additional safety for a patient unless backed up with clearly defined management protocols, medical and nursing staff trained in cardiac emergencies and subject to regular staff development programmes, and ready access to resuscitative drugs and facilities including defibrillator and external pacemaker. To meet these requirements, it is usually more economical to provide a specialized monitoring facility in a clearly defined coronary care area, rather than attempting to provide ad hoc facilities in an open ward. Experience with this form of monitoring has frequently led to misunderstanding (or turning off) the arrhythmia alarms, misinterpretation of arrhythmia patterns and inappropriate management.

Limited coronary care in a specialized nursing unit

Coronary care provided in a specially equipped area with bedside or telemetry monitoring, ready access to resuscitative facilities, dedicated nursing staff trained in cardiac care and medical staff on call, is the common model of coronary care in small community hospitals. It can be highly effective in the management of acute coronary syndromes and some cardiac arrhythmias,[16] but to be effective, there are certain essential requirements. The equipment, management protocols and staff expertise must be capable of delivering a high quality of care. The resources to ensure this may not be available in every community hospital, and affiliation or linkage with a larger hospital CCU is essential. While this model of coronary care is capable of delivering high standards of care, including arrhythmia management and thrombolysis for the majority of patients, the limitations should be recognized and efficient channels of communication and referral to a tertiary centre should be established, to ensure that patients receive the benefits of coronary angiography, coronary intervention and cardiac surgery.

Combined coronary intensive care

There are clear-cut advantages in terms of physical and human resources in combining coronary and intensive care in the same hospital area (see Ch. 1). Much of the monitoring and resuscitative equipment is common to coronary and intensive care and the combining of nursing resources into 'critical care nursing' provides flexibility in rostering staff development and career opportunities. For this reason, this model of providing coronary care or acute cardiac care has proven popular in medium sized hospitals. However, the exposure of relatively well, fully conscious and alert patients with acute cardiac conditions to desperately ill patients requiring full scale intensive care and artificial respiration can be traumatic and exacerbate the coronary patient's nascent anxiety. Furthermore, the increasing dependence of acute cardiac patients on cardiac investigative facilities means that much of the medical decision-making is done by the cardiology team rather than the intensive care team. Without careful delineation of responsibility, conflicts may arise.

Dedicated coronary care (cardiac care) unit

The preferred model for modern coronary care in a tertiary hospital is the dedicated coronary or cardiac care unit.[17,18] In this unit the full range of cardiac monitoring and support is provided, from electrocardiographic monitoring to haemodynamic monitoring and circulatory support devices. Usually short-term assisted ventilation is provided, but if more prolonged respiratory support is deemed necessary, this is usually provided by transfer to an intensive care area.

Increasingly the coronary care area has expanded into a cardiac care area, providing a full range of support, not only for patients with acute coronary syndromes but also those with cardiac arrhythmias, and for patients before and after cardiac investigative procedures and cardiac interventions such as angioplasty and stent implantations. Patients who have undergone open heart surgery or cardiac transplantation may be managed in such a CCU or in specialized post-operative facilities. In reaching a decision about combining these facilities into a single unit or keeping them separate, the same arguments apply in balancing the economics of scale of building, equipment and staff versus provoking unnecessary anxiety and distress in the lower-risk patients.

The features of these four levels of coronary (cardiac) care units are summarized in Table 2.1.

Role of the 'step-down' unit

The provision of a 'step down' facility to provide a bridge between the more intensive coronary care and management in the open ward or at home allows most efficient utilization of the more intensive coronary care beds.[19] Furthermore, there are benefits in maintaining continuity of care and the capability to re-admit the patient rapidly to the CCU, as well as arranging pre-discharge investigations including cardiac catheterization. Patients with lower-risk chest pain or coronary syndromes may be admitted directly to such a unit.

Staffing

Nursing staff ratios will depend on local conditions and on the acuity of the patients, which is determined by admission policy. If assisted ventilation is required, more intensive nursing will be necessary than in units which are designed not to treat patients requiring assisted ventilation.

The nursing ratio is usually about 1.5 times that required for general ward nursing. In hospitals which provide coronary care in a specialized nursing care unit or a combined coronary and intensive care unit, there are advantages in pooling nursing staff with other critical care areas, but in hospitals with a dedicated CCU, it is more logical to pool nursing staff with the cardiac catheterization laboratory and cardiac step-down ward, and possibly the cardiac surgical ward and other critical care areas.

The level and direction of nursing expertise will vary with each model of coronary care. Minimum standards for all staff include a clinical assessment of the cardiac patient, basic and advanced cardiac life support skills including an understanding of modern cardiac drugs and procedures including coronary thrombolysis and revascularization, resuscitation and defibrillation. It may not be possible to provide this level of nursing and medical staff development in a small hospital, and linkages with larger hospitals should be considered mandatory if coronary care facilities are to be provided in small community hospitals.

In all coronary care facilities, immediate medical assistance should be available. In hospitals with combined ICU/CCU or dedicated CCU, 24-hour junior medical staff coverage should be regarded as mandatory. At the Sir Charles Gairdner Hospital, CCU junior medical staff are available

Table 2.1 Four models of coronary care

Model	Staffing	Equipment	Comments
ECG monitoring in a medical ward	No additional staff required	Bedside or telemetry ECG monitor	Not recommended
ECG monitoring in a specialized nursing unit	Specialized full time nursing cover. Part time medical cover. Staff development links with larger centre essential	1. Bedside or telemetry ECG monitor. 2. Defibrillator and resuscitation equipment	Preferred model in small community hospital. Referral for selected cases must be readily available
Combined coronary and intensive care	Specialized full time nursing cover with critical care staff development. Full time junior medical cover. Senior medical cover shared with intensivists and cardiologists	1. Bedside or telemetry ECG monitor 2. Defibrillator and resuscitation equipment. 3. Haemodynamic monitoring. 4. Assisted ventilation	Preferred model in medium sized community hospital
Dedicated coronary (cardiac) care unit	Specialized full time nursing cover with cardiac nursing staff development. Full time medical director. Invasive cardiologists readily available	1. Bedside or telemetry ECG monitor. 2. Defibrillator and resuscitation equipment. 3. Haemodynamic monitoring. 4. May or may not provide assisted ventilation. 5. Intra-aortic balloon pump and other cardiac assist devices. 6. Access to non-invasive and (preferably) invasive cardiology facilities	Preferred model for tertiary hospital. May be combined with a 'step-down' unit for lower risk patients

on a 24-hour basis, with strict instructions not to leave the area during their shift of duty.

To provide continuity and medical decision-making, a more experienced cardiac fellow or cardiology registrar, preferably with training in cardiac catheterization, cardiac pacing and haemodynamic monitoring, should be readily available. A medical director is necessary for development, in conjunction with senior nursing staff, of the policies and procedures, supervision of quality improvement, monitoring of outcomes, database supervision, maintenance and updating of equipment and supervision of clinical research.

In hospitals with cardiac invasive laboratories, a cardiologist skilled in and regularly performing cardiac catheterization should be available for urgent consultation.[20] If a primary angioplasty programme is to be provided, this should be performed in a laboratory performing over 1000 catheterizations and 400 angioplasties per year and restricted to highly trained operators whose total angioplasty workload exceeds 200 cases per year.[20–22]

Equipment

The minimum level of equipment for a CCU includes the following:

- **Bedside electrocardiographic monitor with central station.** Monitoring equipment should display trends in heart rate and analysis of arrhythmias. The minimum of beds equipped for monitoring is largely determined by the capacity to provide round-the-clock nursing staff, and four monitored beds is usually regarded as the minimum number for an economically viable unit.
- **Automated blood pressure recording**. Non-invasive blood pressure recording with automatic cuff inflation is necessary. The capability to display trends should be included in the monitoring device to allow continuous display of trends in heart rate and blood pressure.
- **Defibrillator.** The unit should have a dedicated defibrillator for emergency defibrillation. The equipment should include synchronized cardioversion and external pacing capability.
- **Resuscitation equipment.** Resuscitation equipment should include a full range of cardiac drugs required for emergency resuscitation, including lignocaine (lidocaine), amiodarone, metoprolol or atenolol, atropine, adrenaline (epinephrine), dopamine, dobutamine, isoprenaline, and hydrocortisone. Equipment for airway maintenance should include oropharyngeal airways, endotracheal tubes and a bag-valve-mask device for temporary manual assisted respiration and oxygen delivery. Each bed should be equipped with oxygen, humidifier and suction equipment.
- **Image intensifier.** For emergency pacemaker wire insertion, there should be ready access to an image intensifier or preferably a C-arm image intensifier available at the bedside, with radiolucent beds.
- **Bed design.** The CCU bed should be equipped with removable bed ends to allow ready access for resuscitation. They should also be adjustable for height and position.
- **Diagnostic support.** There should be ready access to 24-hour biochemistry and haematology laboratory, and portable chest X-ray. An exercise testing facility should be adjacent to the CCU.
- **Communication facilities.** A facsimile machine for sending and receiving ECG tracings and other data should be available within the CCU.

The above minimum requirements demand a modest investment, but should be within the reach of most community hospitals. As previously stated, the cheaper option of providing a bedside or telemetry electrocardiographic monitor does not reach a minimum standard for modern acute cardiac care.

A larger hospital providing a wider range of cardiac services would include the following options:

- **Bedside echocardiography.** Although two-dimensional echocardiography can provide useful information about left ventricular function and undiagnosed low output state such as pericardial compression, detailed evaluation of valvular function and bedside assessment of ventricular septal defect (VSD) or acute mitral regurgitation requires colour Doppler flow studies and this should be regarded as the standard (see Ch. 16).
- **Haemodynamic monitoring.** Provision of haemodynamic monitoring will require the provision of pressure transducers, pre-amplifiers and monitoring equipment which can document trends in pulmonary artery pressures. With increasing sophistication of non-invasive blood pressure monitoring, there is now less need than previously to provide for arterial pressure monitoring, although this is essential in units which provide cardiac catheterization and angioplasty which may require the use of indwelling arterial sheaths (see Ch. 24).
- **Radionuclide facility.** Bedside echocardiography has tended to replace radionuclide studies for evaluation of ventricular function. Although bedside radionuclide studies are a useful option to the CCU, a high throughput is required for economic viability and reliable studies. Most hospitals provide this service in a separate nuclear medicine facility. Ideally, this should be located adjacent to the CCU (see Ch. 18).
- **Circulatory support.** Intra-aortic balloon pumping should be available in CCUs which are dealing with patients with pump failure, especially to provide circulatory assistance as a bridge to coronary angioplasty or cardiac surgery (see Ch. 47).

- **Cardiac catheterization laboratory.** Ideally, the modern management of acute coronary syndromes includes the ability to visualize the coronary artery anatomy, localize the obstruction and make decisions of suitability for revascularization with angioplasty or bypass surgery. Although there have been published studies which demonstrate that the availability of on-site cardiac catheterization facilities increases the number of complex procedures without any improvement in outcome,[12] there are many persuasive arguments in favour of catheterization and consideration of revascularization in patients with acute coronary syndromes[11] (see Chs 21 and 78). The availability of a catheterization laboratory also facilitates pacemaker implantation and provision of diagnostic and interventional electrophysiology procedures. While it is not economically feasible to provide a catheterization laboratory in every hospital providing a CCU, established routines for consideration of catheterization and rapid and safe transport[6] to a catheterization facility need to be established in every hospital providing acute coronary care.
- **Interventional cardiology.** While the role of coronary angioplasty in the asymptomatic post-coronary patient remains to be clarified, there is a clear-cut role for angioplasty in patients with continuing symptoms post-infarction or unstable angina (see Chs 45 and 78). The arguments in favour of primary angioplasty as an alternative to coronary thrombolysis have gathered strength in recent years.[23] Provision of a full round-the-clock angioplasty service and maintenance of adequate levels of skill for dealing with acute coronary occlusion, together with continuing arguments about the need for on-site cardiac surgical backup, to date have limited the provision of this facility to selected tertiary referral centres.
- **Cardiac surgery and cardiac transplantation.** Modern high quality coronary care does not require the provision of on-site cardiac surgery or transplantation, but established links and capability for rapid transfer to these facilities is essential.[6]

Design

The CCU should preferably be allocated its own space so that it is a recognizable physical entity within the hospital complex. Individual patient rooms should be available for privacy, but should be arranged to allow ready observation and access by nursing and medical staff. Ideally, there should be a natural flow of patients through the area, with sicker patients requiring haemodynamic monitoring separated from stable bed-bound patients, separated from ambulant patients. A variety of circular, U-shaped longitudinal and more complex designs have all been proposed and used without any consensus on the ideal design. An essential component is that there should be a central station to allow display of trends in heart rate, arrhythmias and other parameters and an alarm system to alert staff to arrhythmias requiring urgent treatment.

There are obvious advantages in locating the CCU adjacent to other critical care areas such as the intensive care unit and other cardiology services such as echocardiography and exercise testing, and invasive cardiac services such as cardiac catheterization and electrophysiology laboratories.

Management and practice guidelines

At the very least, there need to be clearly defined policies and procedures for admission and discharge and management of major diagnostic categories such as MI, unstable angina pectoris, ventricular tachycardia, atrial fibrillation, and for procedures such as pain relief, coronary thrombolysis, resuscitation, cardioversion, temporary and permanent pacemaking, cardiac catheterization and revascularization.

Joint development of these protocols between medical and nursing staff and other staff as appropriate is essential and they should be updated regularly to incorporate recent developments. As a minimum standard they should be revised each 3 years. The policies and procedures manual should be kept clearly displayed in the CCU and staff encouraged to know the procedures, as well as highlighting areas which do not reflect the latest developments in coronary care. While many units will prefer to devise their own protocols and procedures, adherence to accepted practice guidelines, as published from time to time by various expert committees, helps in ensuring that best practice is followed. Such guidelines are available for the management of unstable angina,[24] AMI[2–4] and thrombolytic therapy.[2–4,25,26]

Quality management

The principles of continuous quality improvement and total quality management have been outlined in the considerable literature on quality improvement and health care.[27–29] The principles of Kaizen,[30,31] the continuous search for opportunities for improvement, are readily applicable to coronary care. Central to the process is the perception of the patient as a customer who deserves not only excellence in medical care, but in all aspects of their care as a person. This is a far more wide-ranging challenge than the traditional processes of quality assurance (QA). While QA is essential and needs resources allocated to it, it represents only a narrow part of the spectrum of total quality management.[32]

The CCU needs to have a focus on total quality management which includes clear direction from the director of the unit, a team responsible for overseeing the quality assurance activities as well as continuous data collection (see Ch. 84) for review of outcomes and regular staff meeting to allow continuous resetting of goals and targets.

The importance of 'closing the loop' in quality improvement activities,[33] that is, defining the problem, monitoring the outcomes, reviewing the results, creating a plan for improvement, implementing it and monitoring the outcome with a view to continuous improvement, needs to be a part of the philosophy of all members of the coronary care staff. Examples of readily monitored outcomes include delays in administration of thrombolytic therapy (door to needle time), delays in initiating resuscitation, outcomes such as major arrhythmias and mortality, rates of phlebitis from intravenous cannula, unplanned re-admission to the CCU during hospital stay and unplanned hospital re-admissions within 30 days. These activities extend the concept of traditional peer-review, but as far as possible, integration into the routine work of the unit should be attempted.

Experience with quality improvement programmes has shown that a combination of regular monitoring of readily identifiable outcomes, together with intermittent surveys of other processes, produces consistent results and quality improvement.[34]

Critical pathways

The use of critical clinical pathways in the CCU is a further outgrowth of quality management principles and their application to patient care.[35] The CCU lends itself to the development of critical pathways in acute coronary syndromes such as AMI[36] with or without haemodynamic compromise, unstable angina pectoris, and certain cardiac arrhythmias such as recent onset atrial fibrillation and bradyarrhythmias requiring pacemaker implantation. Development of these pathways has been reported to be associated with improved patient outcomes and satisfaction and shortened hospital stays. Predefined pathways are available for a variety of acute cardiac care categories but will usually require local modification. An example of the critical care pathways in use in the coronary care unit at Sir Charles Gairdner Hospital is shown in Figure 2.1.

Staff development

Highly trained and dedicated nursing staff are a major resource for the CCU and every effort should be made to attract and retain the services of medical and nursing staff who have specialized in this aspect of patient care. As well as regular in-service staff development programmes, peer review activities and involvement in clinical trial and quality improvement activities, regular attendance at regional and national cardiology and critical care courses and involvement in community education and health promotion activities are all helpful in ensuring that a core of dedicated medical and nursing staff is maintained.

In addition, a coordinated orientation and training programme for new staff is essential for maintaining standards and ensuring continuous improvement in patient care.

Infection control

An understanding of and close adherence to infection control guidelines is essential (see Ch. 83). Intravenous (IV) site

CLINICAL PATHWAY:
ACUTE CARDIAC ADMISSION
Ward:

VIA **G42**

ATTACH PATIENT ADDRESSOGRAPH LABEL

PRESENTING PROBLEM (Indicate as appropriate)

Suspected Angina
- Unstable

Suspected AMI
- Anterior
- Non-anterior
- Unspecified

Consultant: ____________

Risk Assessment for AMI

On Admission
- Age >60
- Past AMI
- Diabetes
- P/oedema
- Shock
- OOHCA
- LBBB
- Q wave

@ 24 hours
- VF
- CHB
- Pulmonary Oedema
- Shock
- Score >0 on admission

Thrombolysis
- Probable AMI
- ST elevation or LBBB
- Onset ≤ 12hrs
- SBP <200mm Hg
- Surgery >4 week
- No recent bleeding
- No past stroke

This is the expected Clinical Pathway for patients with uncomplicated AMI and Angina. The 4 day path for Angina and the 7 day path for AMI should be achievable in >50% of pts.

1: Each day the Doctor MUST indicate the minimum goals to be achieved over the next 24hrs.

2: If a patient is NOT to be moved up the Pathway, the reason MUST BE STATED OVERLEAF.

3: A patient whose course has not been complicated by Angina or LVF can be moved through Stages 4, 5 and 6 by the primary/associate nurse.

PATHWAY TRACK — CURRENT STATUS (Angina, AMI)

Stage:		
VII	Discharge	Telephone GP
		Discharge letter written
		Prescriptions written
		Follow up appointments made
VI		Ambulate fully in ward
		Book OPD Stress Test, Echo, Cath and Clinic appt
		Review medications and home programme with patient
		Re-affirm discharge transport for next morning
V		Hygiene independent
		Complete education
		Contact Silver Chain / Social Work if needed
		Notify family re-discharge plan
IV	Ambulation &Education	Ambulate in room
		Remove IV if not needed
		Continue background education and reading
		Contact physiotherapist and dietitian
III		Cease GTN
		Re-assess need for Heparin - resite IV if needed
		Plan transfer to G41
		- Review diagnosis and medications
		- Alert G41 staff re-special requirements
II		Re-assess the need for GTN
		Continue Heparin and start Warfarin if indicated
		Consider ACE inhibitor - Ant MI, LVF
		Book Stress Test, Echo or Cath as indicated
		Commence Education
I	Admission to G42	Administer Aspirin and Consider ThrombolyticTherapy
		Start Beta-blocker unless contra-indicated
		Start GTN for Angina, Anterior MI or Pulm. Oedema
		Start Heparin unless contra-indicated

Date of Admission: ____________
Time of Admission: ____________

Hospital Day:	1	2	3	4	5	6	7	8	9	10	11	12	13	14
Date:														

INITIAL REGISTER Please Print Name Clearly

Initial	Printed Name	Desig.	Initial	Printed Name	Desig.	Initial	Printed Name	Desig

VERSION 2
DRAFT 4
NSL
6/6/95

CLINICAL PATHWAY FOR ACUTE CARDIAC ADMISSION

710

Fig. 2.1 Example of a critical pathway in use in the coronary care unit, Sir Charles Gairdner Hospital, Perth. Reproduced by permission of Board of Management, SCGH.

phlebitis can be a serious but largely preventable complication of CCU admission and on occasions can overshadow the coronary event or arrhythmia which required admission.[37] Protection of staff from transmissible blood borne diseases is a continuing challenge which requires close monitoring of developments in prevention of cross infection.

Electrical safety

The potential hazards of electric shock with the development of ventricular fibrillation from intracardiac catheters and pacing electrodes requires an awareness by staff in the CCU of the potential hazards, adherences to standard protocols for avoidance of alternating current to the heart, and meticulous maintenance of equipment to recognized standards.[38] Medical and nursing staff are unlikely to have the appropriate expertise in this area, and regular biophysics and bio-engineering liaison and backup is essential.

References

1. National Heart Attack Alert Programme (NHAAP). Staffing and equipping emergency medical services systems. Rapid identification and treatment of acute myocardial infarction. US Department of Health and Human Services NIH Publication No 93–3304, Washington, DC, 1993
2. Weston CFM, Penny WJ, Julian DG, on behalf of the British Heart Foundation Working Group. Guidelines for the early management of patients with myocardial infarction. Br Med J 1994;308:767–71
3. National Heart Foundation of Australia Heart Attack Committee. Emergency coronary care. Guidelines for the emergency management of the patients with suspected coronary occlusion. Canberra: National Heart Foundation of Australia, 1995
4. ACC/AHA Task Force. Guidelines for the early management of patients with acute myocardial infarction. J Am Coll Cardiol 1990;16:249–92
5. Aufderheide TP, Hendley GE, Thakur RK et al. The diagnostic impact of prehospital 12-lead electrocardiography. Am Emerg Med 1990;19:1280–7
6. Cummins RO. Interhospital transfer of acutely ill patients. JAMA 1988;159:1707–8
7. American Heart Association Emergency Cardiac Care Committee and Subcommittees. Guidelines for cardiopulmonary resuscitation and emergency cardiac care. JAMA 1992;268:2171–302
8. European Resuscitation Council. Guidelines for basic and advanced life support. Resuscitation 1992;24:103–22
9. Australian Resuscitation Council Advanced Life Support Committee. Adult advanced life support. The Australian Resuscitation Council guidelines. Med J Aust 1993;159:616–21
10. Kulick DL, Rahimtoola SH. Is non-invasive risk stratification sufficient, or should all patients undergo cardiac catheterization and angiography after a myocardial infarction? Cardiovasc Clin 1990;21:3–25
11. Nicod P, Gilpin EA, Dittrich H et al. Trends in use of coronary angiography in subacute phase of myocardial infarction. Circulation 1991;84:1004–15
12. Every NR, Larson EB, Litwin PE et al. The association between on-site cardiac catheterization facilities and the use of coronary angiography after acute myocardial infarction. N Engl J Med 1993;329:546–51
13. Czarn AOS, Jamrozik K, Hobbs MST, Thompson PL. Follow-up care after myocardial infarction in Perth, Western Australia. Med J Aust 1992;157:302–5
14. Kennedy JW, Ivey TD, Misbach G et al. Coronary artery bypass surgery early after acute myocardial infarction. Circulation 1989;79(suppl 1):73–8
15. Romhilt DW, Bloomfield SS, Chou TC, Fowler NO. Unreliability of conventional electrocardiographic monitoring for arrhythmias in coronary care units. Am J Cardiol 973;31:457–61
16. Stross JK, Willis PW, Reynolds EW et al. Effectiveness of coronary care in small community hospitals. Am Int Med 1976;85:709–13
17. Lee TH, Goldman L. The coronary care unit turns 25. Trends and future directions. Am Int Med 1988;108:887
18. O'Rourke MF, Walsh B, Fletcher M, Crowley A. Impact of the new generation coronary care unit. Br Med J 1976; ii: 837–9
19. Weinberg SL. Intermediate coronary care—observations on the validity of the concept. Chest 1978; 73: 154
20. ACC/AHA Task Force on Assessment of Diagnostic and Therapeutic Cardiovascular Procedures (Subcommittee on Coronary Angiography). Guidelines for coronary angiography. J Am Coll Cardiol 1987;10:935–50
21. Ryan TJ, Faxon DP, Gunnar RF et al. Guidelines for percutaneous transluminal coronary angioplasty: a report of the ACC/AHA Task Force on Assessment of Diagnostic and Therapeutic Cardiovascular Procedures (Subcommittee on Percutaneous Transluminal Coronary

Angioplasty). J Am Coll Cardiol 1988;12:529–45
22. Australian Health Technology Advisory Committee. Superspecialty service guidelines for acute cardiac interventions. Canberra: Dept of Human Services and Health 1995
23. International Roundup. Primary angioplasty in myocardial infarction. Br Heart J 1995;76:403–16
24. Braunwald E, Jones RH, Mark DB et al. Diagnosing and managing unstable angina. Circulation 1994;90:613–22
25. Thompson PL, Tonkin AM, Aylward P, White H. Thrombolysis '93—is there a consensus? Aust NZ J Med 1993;23:778
26. National Heart Foundation of Australia Heart Attack Advisory Committee. Guidelines for thrombolytic therapy. Canberra: National Heart Foundation of Australia, 1995
27. Berwick DM. Continuous improvement as an ideal in health care. N Engl J Med 1989;320:53–6
28. Berwick DM, Enthoven A, Bunker JP. Quality management in the NHS: the doctor's role (Pt I). Br Med J 1992;304:235–9
29. Berwick DM, Enthoven A, Bunker JP. Quality management in the NHS: the doctor's role (Pt II). Br Med J 1992;304:304–8
30. Kaizen Imal M. The key to Japan's competitive success. New York: McGraw Hill, 1986.
31. Smith R. Medicine's need for Kaizen: putting quality first. Br Med J 1990;302:53–6
32. Eastman CJ. Total quality management: the challenge for hospitals in the 1990s. Med J Aust 1992;157:219–20.
33. Australian Council of Healthcare Standards. ACHS accreditation guide. Standards for Australian healthcare facilities. 13th ed. Sydney: Australian Council of Healthcare Standards, 1995
34. Blumenthal D. Total quality management and physicians' clinical decisions. JAMA 1993;269:2775–8
35. Hofmann PA. Critical path method: an important tool for coordinating clinical care. Journal of Quality Improvement 1993;19:233–46
36. Reinhart SI. Uncomplicated acute myocardial infarction: a critical path. Cardiovascular Nursing 1995;31:1–7
37. Schendorf WA, Brown RB, Sands M, Hosman D. Infections in a coronary care unit. Am J Cardiol 1985;56:757–9
38. Whalen RE, Starmer CF, McIntosh HD. Electric shock hazards in cardiology. Mod Concepts Cardiovasc Dis 1967;36:2

Part 2

Epidemiology, genetics and risk factors

3 Clinical epidemiology of acute myocardial infarction and coronary heart disease

Konrad Jamrozik and Peter L Thompson

Introduction

Despite rapidly advancing understanding of coronary heart disease, our knowledge of the natural history is based on studies of selected sub-groups of cases.

Acute myocardial infarction (AMI) is the best documented syndrome of coronary heart disease. It represents a major but nevertheless limited portion of the spectrum of myocardial ischaemia which includes silent ischaemia, exertional angina, unstable angina, cardiac failure, cardiac dysrhythmias and sudden death. Furthermore, patients with clinically-recognized AMI form a subset of all patients with AMI since electrocardiographic surveys suggest that up to 20% of patients surviving an infarction have not sought medical advice.[1] Similarly, patients who die in hospital from AMI may not be representative of all coronary deaths because epidemiologic studies show that 66–75% of the fatalities from an acute coronary event occur outside hospital[2] (see Fig. 3.1).

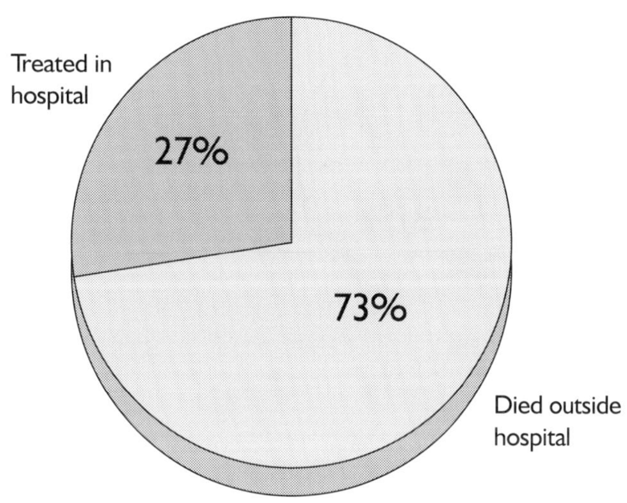

Fig. 3.1 1234 deaths within 28 days after 3421 acute coronary events in Perth 1985–1989. 73% of the deaths occurred out of hospital, only 27% after hospital treatment. Some of the 2–28 day deaths also occurred outside hospital following discharge. Data from the Perth MONICA project.[5]

It is not clear from the available data how many of the coronary sudden deaths that occur out of hospital are due to dysrhythmias complicating the earliest stages of AMI, which might have benefited from modern coronary care, as opposed to sudden deaths due to inevitably fatal dysrhythmias or asystole. Pathologic studies show that fatal coronary heart disease is not necessarily synonymous with fatal AMI, many cases dying without evidence of coronary thrombosis or myocardial necrosis.[3,4] From these comments, it is clear that AMI treated in the CCU represents a somewhat biased sample of the spectrum of patients with acute coronary events. It is self-evident that trends in case fatality from AMI managed in hospital may not necessarily parallel trends in mortality from coronary heart disease in the wider community. Nevertheless, the majority of deaths occur on day 1, and this is when the combined efforts of emergency services and CCUs will have their major impact (see Fig. 3.2).

Differences between 'incidence' and 'event', 'mortality' and 'case fatality' rates

The *incidence* of coronary events, including AMI, refers to the rate of occurrence of the totality of fatal and non-fatal events. In its purest

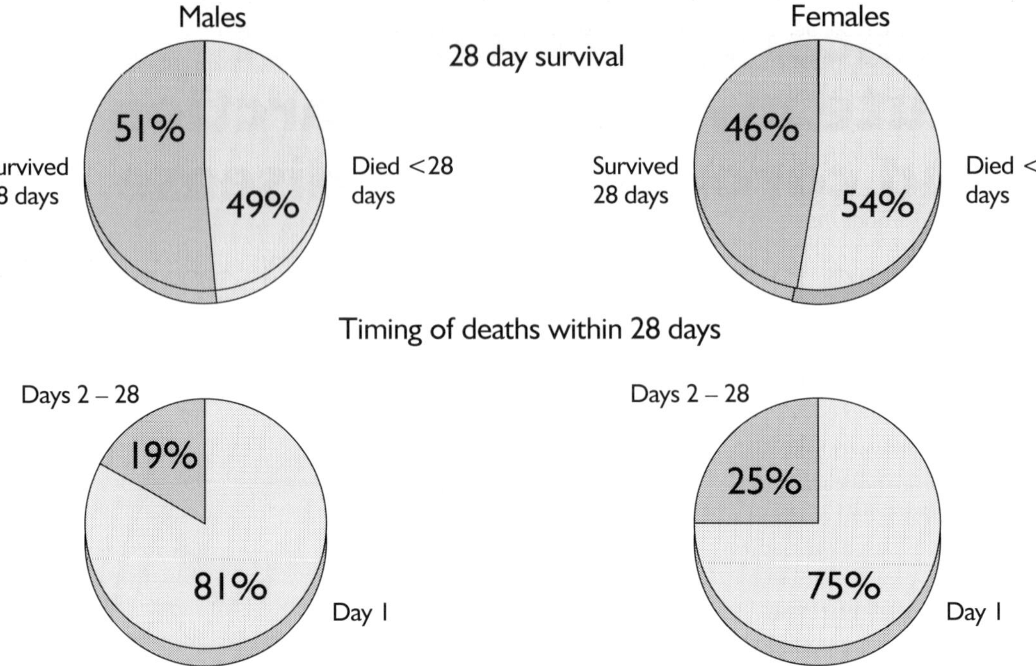

Fig. 3.2 28 day survival and timing of deaths within 28 days following an acute coronary event. Data from the WHO MONICA project in 38 populations from 21 countries.[2] Note the higher case fatality overall but lesser proportion of early deaths in females.

form, incidence refers to occurrence of first-ever-in-a-lifetime events, with subsequent events recorded as recurrences. In practice, initial and recurrent events are difficult to distinguish and may be lumped together and their combined frequency referred to as *event rates*. Incidence and event rates are difficult to document as they have to be obtained by exhaustive analysis of hospital admission data and other sources.

Mortality from coronary heart disease (CHD) is usually measured as the annual number of deaths occurring per 100 000 population. In clinical usage 'mortality' is often used to describe the risk of death after an event, but more correctly this should be termed the 'case fatality'.

Case fatality refers to the proportion of patients who die within a set period, such as 24 hours, 28 days, 1 year or 5 years after the occurrence of a coronary event such as AMI. Strictly speaking, case fatality is not a rate at all, since the denominator is measured in persons, not person-time.

The term *hospital mortality* is widely used but can be confusing not only because the 'mortality' is actually 'case fatality', but also because the duration of stay in hospital varies widely from one institution to another and over different historical periods.

Interpreting event and mortality rates and case fatality

CHD mortality rates are collected routinely in most countries but regional variations in diagnostic coding may produce anomalies when compared with standardized definitions of the causes of death,[3] particularly in countries with low CHD mortality.[2] Collection of data on event rates including non-fatal events is a far more laborious task, and for this reason data are not so readily available.

Because event rates are difficult to obtain and mortality data are collected routinely, there is a temptation to infer (or even to misinterpret) differences in mortality as representing differences in event rates. To do so denies the possibility that better treatment of cases after an event, as well as fewer events, may be having an impact on mortality.

Community-wide data on event rates are available from 21 countries in the WHO MONICA Project[2] and are a valuable source of data but these include only persons up to age 65, and reliable information on event rates in the elderly is not available.

Case fatality varies according to whether deaths out of hospital as well as those occurring in hospital are included. If all deaths occurring after the onset of major acute coronary events are included, 28 day case fatality can be as high as 50% (see Table 3.1) – a figure that is unfamiliar and puzzling for clinicians but that underlines the lethal nature of CHD. Similarly, case fatality based on cases managed in hospital, but which includes patients who reach hospital alive only to die shortly after admission to the emergency department, will also be relatively high. Case fatality in patients with AMI who survive until the morning hand-over round is much lower since the period of highest risk of a fatal dysrhythmia has already passed. These differences are readily apparent in data from the Perth MONICA Register[5] shown in Table 3.1.

Data from clinical trials are an alternative source of benchmarks for case fatality, but with the obvious flaw that selection of patients for a clinical trial will produce lower figures because of exclusion of patients who have already died or are moribund.

International differences in incidence, mortality and case fatality

Comparisons between countries of mortality rates from CHD are normally based on official data from death registrations. Such comparisons have been published since the 1960s (see Fig. 3.3). Over the last 30 years, there have been consistently high rates in Scotland, Finland and northern Europe, intermediate rates for the USA, Australia, New Zealand and southern Europe, and low rates for France, Japan and China.[7] These official statistics may be influenced by national diagnostic habits and recent comparisons in MONICA communities have shown discrepancies between official rates and those using stricter definitions, especially in populations with relatively low mortality from CHD.[2]

The first concerted attempt at comparing the incidence of AMI between countries was a World Health Organization Collaborative Study in 1970 which encouraged the development of population-based registers of AMI.[6] These demonstrated a sevenfold difference in event rates between communities. More recently the MONICA Project has shown even wider inter-country differences (see Table 3.2). There is a twelvefold difference in annual incidence for males from North Karelia, Finland compared with Beijing, China (915 versus 76 per 100 000). In comparison, for women, an eightfold difference has been demonstrated between Glasgow, UK and Catalonia, Spain (256 versus 30 per 100 000).

Because of the expense and complexity of registering non-fatal events, there have been attempts to extrapolate from official mortality rates to estimate the rate of non-fatal MI in a community.[2,8] Data from the MONICA Project show that, between 1985 and 1989, 1.5 non-fatal definite

Table 3.1 28 day case fatality (%) for men and women age 25–64 in Perth 1985–1989. Note that the case fatality can vary dramatically, depending on the group being studied. Based on data from Lowel H, Dobson A, Keil U et al 1993.[5]

	28 Day Case Fatality %		
	Total	Hospital cases	Hospital 24-hour survivors
MALE	36.9	13.1	8.2
FEMALE	43.6	20.3	13.4

Table 3.2 Event rates (per 100 000 population) and 28 day case fatality (%) for eight communities participating in the WHO MONICA Project showing the wide range of event rates from North Karelia (highest) to Beijing (lowest). Based on data from Tunstall-Pedoe H, Kuulasmaa K, Amouyel P et al 1994[2]

		Total*		First event**	
		Event rate (/100 000)	Case fatality (%)	Event rate (/100 000)	Case fatality (%)
Australia	Newcastle	561	43	363	37
	Perth	422	38	259	25
New Zealand	Auckland	466	49	325	44
Finland	North Karelia	915	48	586	44
France	Toulouse	240	45	183	38
UK	Glasgow	823	49	557	47
USA	Stanford	508	50	299	41
China	Beijing	76	53	58	51

* Definite, possible and unclassifiable fatal events and definite non-fatal MI.
** Total without previous MI.

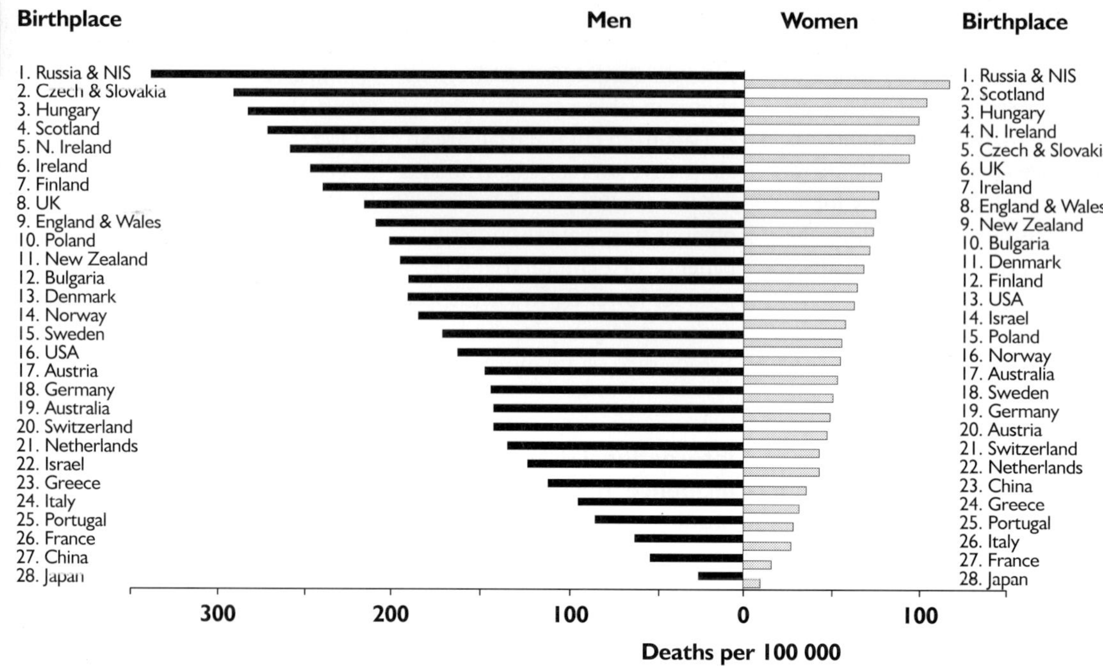

Fig. 3.3 Comparison of death rates from coronary heart disease in 28 countries. Source: National Heart Foundation of Australia. Heart and stroke facts 1995.

AMIs occurred per coronary death in communities with low coronary mortality (of the order of 100 per 100 000 per annum), dropping to 1.0 case of non-fatal definite AMI per coronary death in populations with high coronary mortality (around 500 per 100 000).[2] These rates are only for persons aged 25–64 years and there may be a lower ratio of non-fatal infarctions to fatal events in older individuals.

Case fatality after AMI varies widely between countries (see Table 3.2). The MONICA data for 1985 to 1989 show a case fatality at 28 days for all coronary events of 49% (range 37 to 81%) for males and 54% (range 31 to 91%) for females.[2] For first coronary events the corresponding figures were 37% and 43%, with equally wide ranges. There was no correlation between rates of events and case fatality in men and only a weak correlation in women.

Trends in incidence, mortality and case fatality

Variations in mortality from CHD and AMI over time or between populations may reflect differences in the incidence of major coronary events, or differences in the case fatality of AMI, or a combination of these. The incidence of AMI will reflect several aspects of medical care including detection and management of asymptomatic individuals at high risk and the follow-up care received by those in whom ischaemic heart disease (IHD) is already clinically evident. The case fatality of AMI will also be influenced by medical care but this influence is necessarily limited when at least 66% of fatalities occur before the patient reaches hospital.

Trends in mortality from CHD showed an inexorable rise in most countries during the 1950s and 1960s. In 1967 to 1968 a flattening and then a downturn in mortality was noted in several countries.

The timing of the WHO Collaborative Study in 1970[6] was fortunate in that it occurred very soon after trends in mortality from CHD began to diverge. By 1980 it was possible to discern a number of distinct trends over the preceding decade. In general, the fastest rates of decrease were observed in Australia, Canada, New Zealand and the United States, all of which had previously experienced steadily increasing mortality from CHD since World War II to reach very high levels by the late 1960s. The UK, along with a number of other countries in western Europe, continued to experience an upward trend for almost another decade before mortality from CHD began to decrease, the rate of fall being slower than in the non-European nations. Certain other countries including some with very low initial mortality from CHD, such as Japan, experienced modest increases throughout the 1970s whilst most countries in eastern Europe observed sharp upward trends (see Fig. 3.4).

All of these trends appear to have continued throughout the 1980s although evidence is emerging from the MONICA Registers in eastern Europe that mortality from CHD may have stabilized from the mid 1980s onwards.

By 1992 in Australia, mortality from CHD was less than half of what it had been in 1968, with a parallel decline in total mortality indicating that changes in diagnostic fashion alone do not explain the trends (see Fig. 3.5).

Data from record linkage techniques available for Perth, Western Australia,[8] have shown that the fall in mortality from CHD has been accompanied by decreases in rates of non-fatal events and of deaths both out of and in hospital.

The explanation for these trends remains unclear, most analyses attributing the declines approximately equally to changes in risk factors in the community and to changes in medical treatment.[9,10,11] Most data are available from the USA[12] and Australia.[13] In both countries there have been steady declines in smoking. In the USA there have been clear declines in average serum cholesterol but this has not been recognized in Australia. The prevalence of untreated hypertension in both countries continued to fall during the 1980s. One should not forget that small changes in risk factors that are

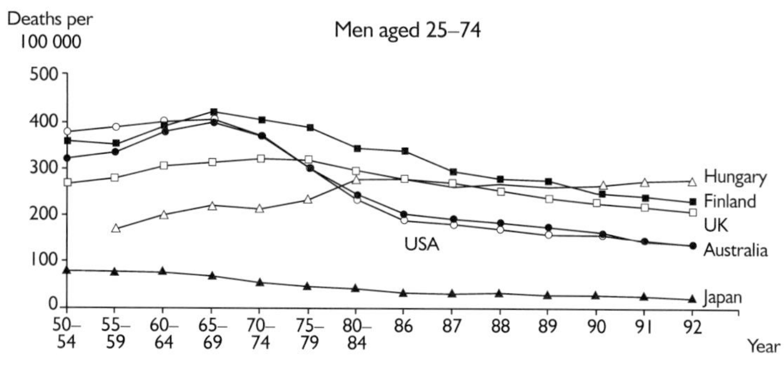

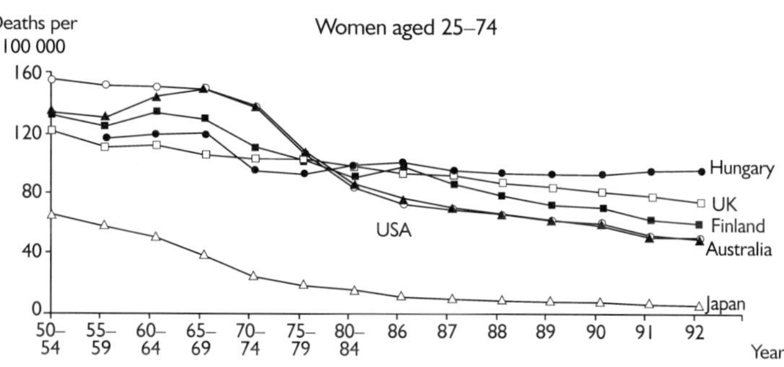

Fig. 3.4 Trends in CHD deaths over 40 years in five countries. Source: National Heart Foundation of Australia. Heart and stroke facts 1995.

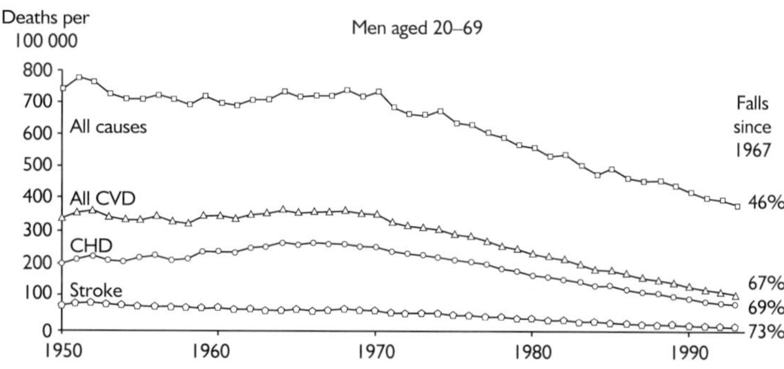

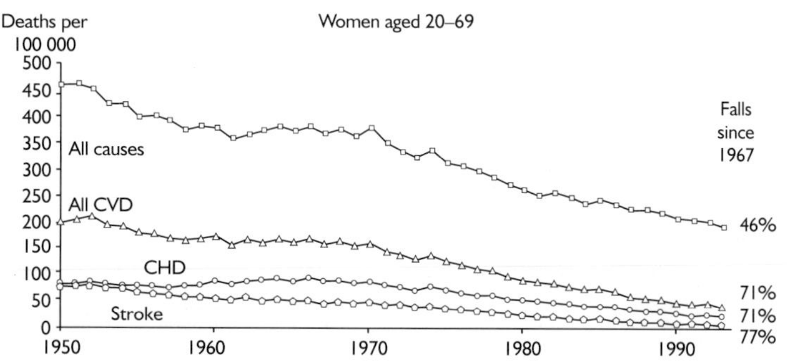

Fig. 3.5 Trends in cardiovascular disease (CVD), coronary heart disease (CHD), stroke and all-cause mortality in Australia over 40 years. The downward trend in CHD deaths matches the trend in all-cause mortality, and is not due to changing classification of the cause of death. Source: National Heart Foundation of Australia. Heart and stroke facts 1995.

spread widely in a population have the potential for major effects on coronary disease. For example, MacMahon et al[14] have estimated that a decrease in average systolic blood pressure of just 2.5 mmHg might produce a saving in coronary mortality of 6.9%, while the Lipids Research Clinics Coronary Primary Prevention Trial[15] indicated that a reduction of 1% in average serum cholesterol would yield a fall of 2% in the incidence of coronary events. Nevertheless, the relatively modest changes in coronary risk factors that have been observed in countries that have also experienced the most dramatic declines in fatal and non-fatal MI suggest that changes in other unrecognized coronary risk factors and in medical care are also contributing factors.[16] These questions are being studied in more detail in the MONICA Project.[2]

When it first appeared in Australia, the fall in mortality from IHD occurred in both sexes and in all age groups simultaneously, arguing against a cohort effect. Data from the Perth MONICA Register indicate that the rate of decrease may have now slowed in women relative to men but the absolute changes that have already occurred in both sexes have clear implications for future planning for coronary care resources.

Despite the improvements, coronary heart disease remains the largest single cause of total and premature (age < 70) death in most western communities (see Fig. 3.6A, B).

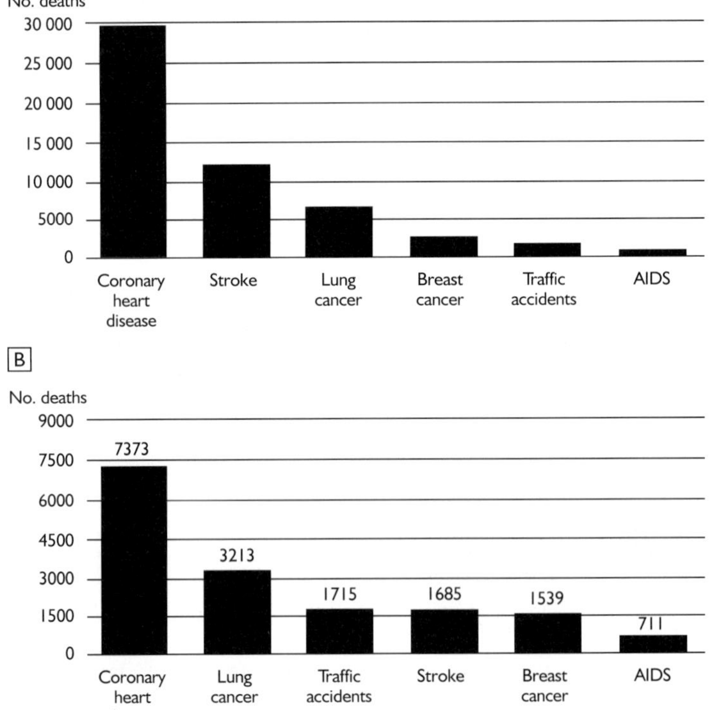

Fig. 3.6 Single cause of A death and B premature death before age 70 in Australia 1993. Source: National Heart Foundation of Australia. Heart and stroke facts 1995.

Trends in case fatality of acute myocardial infarction

Reports of series of patients with AMI from the 1950s and 1960s describe in-hospital case fatalities as high as 35%. However, the type of patients being treated and the reporting of 'hospital mortality' from an era when the duration of stay in hospital was several weeks make comparisons of these data with modern figures invalid because the introduction of CCUs has encouraged the admission of patients with milder infarctions and the duration of stay in hospital has shortened dramatically.

To reduce bias in comparisons of survival it is important to match patients with regard to severity of infarction and to study the outcome over a fixed interval from the onset of AMI such as 28 days. This has been done in a meta-analysis of 36 studies published between the 1960s and 1987 that shows case fatalities at 28 days of 31% in the 1960s, 25% in the 1970s and 18% in the 1980s.[17] However, as clinical series even of consecutive patients are subject to differences in case-mix and in patterns of referral, population-wide studies are required to determine whether survival after AMI really has improved. Very few communities have the necessary data available. Those that do include Perth in Western Australia,[8] Auckland in New Zealand,[18] Worcester, Massachusetts[19] and Minnesota[20] in the USA. In each of these communities there is evidence of improvements between the 1960s and 1970s, predominantly due to a decline in deaths due to dysrhythmias, stable case fatality during the 1970s and early 1980s, followed by a clear improvement from the mid-1980s onwards. A recent detailed analysis from Canada[21] has demonstrated a similar trend of an improving case fatality from 1985 onwards that is independent of changes in length of stay in hospital.

The trends for coronary care treated patients in Perth over the past decade are shown in Figure 3.7 indicating a 30% decline in case fatality.

Changes in the management of AMI and their impact on mortality and case fatality of CHD

What has been the role of the CCU in determining these trends?

Of all the techniques that have now become part of routine care of the patient with AMI, only the development of CCUs in the mid 1960s precedes the downturn in coronary mortality which occurred in Australia, Canada, New Zealand and the United States in the late 1960s.[22] It was already well known that most deaths from AMI occurred very early after the onset of symptoms and that most of these events were electrical in nature. Thus the adoption of the CCU was not preceded by randomized controlled trials to test whether the approach was effective, as it seemed self-evident that close monitoring of patients with AMI and rapid defibrillation of any who had a 'cardiac arrest' would significantly alter the known natural history of fatal coronary events. Evidence has since been presented, particularly from CCUs in Australia[23–25] and New Zealand[26] that the introduction of the CCU was followed by improvements in survival. Although patients in these studies were matched to exclude a dilution effect from admission to CCUs of cases with less severe infarctions, the observations were not derived from randomized studies and are therefore not conclusive. Belatedly, randomized trials of coronary care compared with care at home of cases of suspected AMI were conducted in Britain.[27,28] However, because the patients treated at home and entering these studies were believed to be highly selected and at low risk, these trials have been largely discounted in assessing the impact of the CCU. There is evidence even now that patients who do reach the CCU form a selected subset of all patients with potentially life-threatening acute coronary events and a subset that is destined to do well. Thus, the scope of CCUs to contribute to a downward trend in mortality from CHD is distinctly limited.[29] The broader significance of CCUs may lie not in their direct contribution to saving lives but that their development heralded the beginning of much more active clinical management of acute coronary events.

Mobile coronary care ambulances were a logical response to a situation where numbers of patients were dying of treatable dysrhythmias before reaching a CCU. The concept of taking the CCU to the patient, pioneered by Pantridge and Geddes in Belfast in 1969, has subsequently evolved into a number of different types of ambulance services (see Ch. 52).

None of these innovations was preceded by an adequately controlled trial and most retrospective evaluations have been limited to small, highly selected series of patients and have used the patient reaching hospital alive as the principal end point. A true population-based assessment of the impact of ambulance services on coronary mortality in Perth, Western Australia, revealed that an increasing proportion of patients with acute coronary symptoms travelled to hospital by ambulance over the period 1978 to 1990.[30] Each year less than 1% of all patients with AMI suffered a cardiac arrest in the presence of an ambulance crew and few of these patients survived to 28 days

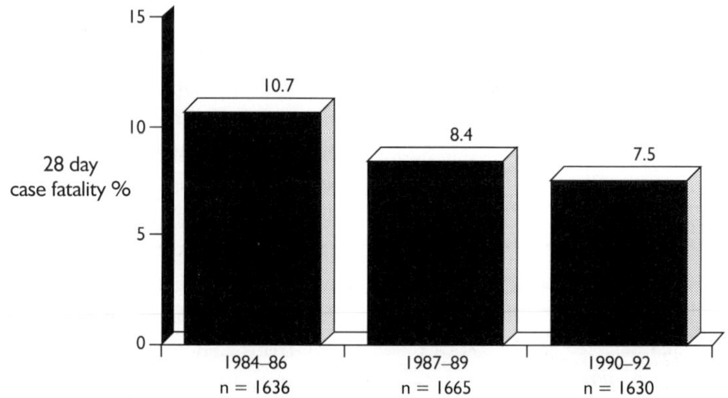

Fig. 3.7 Trends in 28 day case fatality for patients under age 65 treated with definite myocardial infarction in coronary care units in Perth, 1984–1992. Source: Dobson SK, Penman AG and 82 others. Clinical health goals and targets for Western Australia 1994. Health Department of Western Australia, 1994.

after the onset of their symptoms. It therefore appears highly improbable that the ability to defibrillate patients at the scene of their arrest has contributed to the steady fall in mortality from AMI observed in this community over the period of the study.

Dramatic changes in the medical care of patients with AMI have been documented over the past decade.[31]

Trends in AMI treatment

The significant impact of new treatments demonstrated in clinical trials and their widespread use suggest that they may have contributed to the recent improvement in case fatality and hence to maintenance of the downward trend in population-wide mortality from CHD. The trends in medical treatments are summarized in Figure 3.8.

Beta adrenergic blocking drugs were first used for treatment of patients surviving an AMI in the late 1970s. The efficacy of this approach was confirmed in randomized controlled trials in the early- to mid-1980s (see Ch. 28). A further series of trials in the mid- to late 1980s demonstrated the efficacy of beta blockade in the acute stage of infarction but these drugs are still not used as frequently in the acute stage as they are in the post-coronary period. The trends for prescription of oral beta blockers following AMI in the Perth MONICA Project showed an increase from 50% to over 70% in the 10-year period from 1984.[31,31a]

Aspirin and other antiplatelet agents were first tested in clinical trials for post-coronary patients in the mid-1970s. By the mid-1980s numerous small studies had been completed and, in systematic overview, they suggested an improvement in long term survival of 25–30% (see Ch. 36). Cardiological practice has been influenced swiftly and profoundly by this finding and that of the ISIS-2 trial which showed a benefit on survival to 35 days from aspirin administered to patients with suspected AMI from soon after their admission to hospital. The proportion of patients with AMI in Perth who received aspirin whilst in hospital has increased from less than 20% in 1984 to over 90% in 1992 with more than 80% of patients now being prescribed aspirin on discharge from hospital.[31,31a] These changes in use of aspirin are likely to have had a major impact on case fatality of AMI and possibly on trends in mortality from CHD in the community as a whole.

Thrombolytic therapy has become so widespread that the 1990s have been referred to as the thrombolytic era of treatment of AMI (see Ch. 34). This trend is firmly based on the results of several very large and numerous smaller randomized controlled trials. The proportion of patients receiving thrombolytic therapy in Perth has increased from 3% in 1984 to over 30% in 1992.[31,31a] This trend has undoubtedly had an influence on case fatality but the less than universal application of thrombolytic therapy suggests that aspirin and beta blockers may have had a greater overall impact on case fatality and possibly on trends in mortality from CHD.

Calcium channel blockers were used increasingly frequently during the 1980s but by the early 1990s reports began to appear of adverse effects of such treatment in AMI (see Ch. 29). It is generally accepted now that these agents need to be used more selectively. On balance, calcium channel blockers are unlikely to have had any effect on the trends in case fatality of AMI or mortality from CHD.

Coronary artery bypass graft surgery (CABG) and *coronary angioplasty* have been used progressively more frequently for the treatment of CHD[32,33,34] (Figure 3.9 shows the

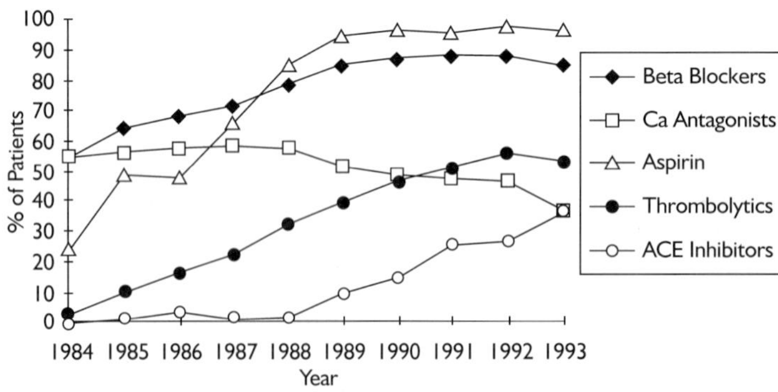

Fig. 3.8 Trends in drug therapy in myocardial infarction 1984–1993 in hospitals in the Perth metropolitan area. Source: Jamrozik et al.[31a]

trends for Australia) but their proper role in the acute phase of infarction remains to be clarified by randomized controlled trials. By contrast, both procedures demonstrably relieve ischaemic symptoms and controlled trials have demonstrated that CABG improves survival in patients with 3-vessel disease plus left ventricular dysfunction or with left main disease. Currently neither technique is used widely in the acute phase of infarction but follow-up of survivors from the Perth MONICA Register for the years 1984 to 1988 showed that 73% underwent an exercise stress test, 61% a coronary angiogram and approximately one third had either percutaneous transluminal coronary angioplasty (PTCA) or CABG or both in the 6 months after their AMI.[34] The quantitative effects on survival of CABG following AMI have not been estimated directly from randomized controlled trials. Similarly, PTCA is widely used, but in the absence of clinical trials, the benefits on overall mortality from CHD cannot be estimated.

Overall impact of trends in management of AMI on mortality from CHD

Using a population-based register of major coronary events, it is possible to estimate the impact of the changes in clinical practice described above on overall mortality from CHD in the relevant community. In Perth the case fatality of clinically defined AMI managed in hospital has fallen by one third over the 10 years from 1984. During the same period the incidence of AMI fell by 22% and overall mortality from IHD decreased by 31%.

The improvements in short-term survival represent a significant reduction in the total number of deaths in the acute phase of infarction. Thus, the adoption of new practices based on the results of the randomized clinical trials has had a significant impact on coronary mortality in the community.

In the cohort of patients with AMI from 1984 to 1988 who survived to 28 days after the onset of symptoms, a multivariate analysis suggested that each of antiplatelet therapy, treatment with beta blockers and either CABG or PTCA within 6 months of the index episode was associated with a significant improvement in long term survival.[34] Overall, follow-up care alone of these survivors of AMI probably contributed one sixth of the decrease in coronary mortality observed in this population between 1984 and 1990 inclusive. Further contributions would be expected from continuing care of survivors of AMI from earlier years and from the management of other coronary syndromes.

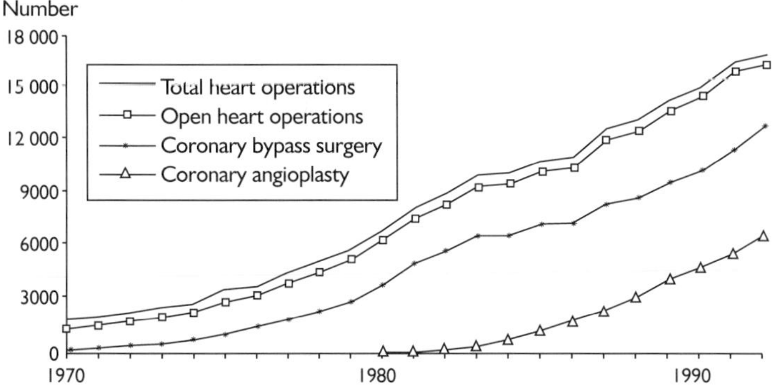

Fig. 3.9 Trends in revascularization procedures, Australia 1970–1992. Source: National Heart Foundation of Australia. Heart and stroke facts 1995.

References

1. Margolis JR, Kannel WS, Feinleib M. Clinical features of unrecognized myocardial infarction—silent and symptomatic. Eighteen year follow up: the Framingham study. Am J Cardiol 1973; 32:1–7
2. Tunstall-Pedoe H, Kuulasmaa K, Amouyel P, Arveiler D, Rajakangas A-M, Pajak A. Myocardial infarctions and coronary deaths in the World Health Organization MONICA Project. Registration procedures, event rates and case fatality rates in 38 populations from 21 countries in four continents. Circulation 1994; 90: 583–612
3. Davies MJ, Thomas A. Thrombosis and acute coronary lesions in sudden cardiac ischaemic death. N Engl J Med 1984; 310: 1137–40
4. Lovegrove T, Thompson PL. The role of acute myocardial infarction in sudden cardiac death: a statistician's nightmare. (Editorial). Am Heart J 1978; 96: 711–14
5. Lowel H, Dobson A, Keil U et al. Coronary heart disease case fatality in four countries. A community study. Circulation 1993; 88: 2524–31

6. World Health Organization Regional Office for Europe. Myocardial infarction community registers (results of a WHO International Collaborative Study co-ordinated by the Regional Office for Europe) (Public Health in Europe No. 5). Copenhagen: WHO European Office, 1976
7. Uemura K, Pisa Z. Recent trends in cardiovascular disease mortality in 27 industrialized countries. World Health Stat Q 1985; 38: 142–62
8. Martin CA, Hobbs MST, Armstrong BK et al. Trends in the incidence of myocardial infarction in Western Australia between 1971 and 1982. Am J Epidemiol 1989; 129: 655–68
9. Goldman L, Cook EF. The decline in ischemic heart disease mortality rates. An analysis of the comparative effects of medical interventions and changes in lifestyle. Ann Intern Med 1984; 101: 825–36
10. Thompson PL, Hobbs MST, Martin CA. The rise and fall of ischaemic heart disease in Australia. Aust NZ J Med 1988; 18: 327–37
11. Beaglehole R. International trends in coronary heart disease mortality, morbidity and risk factors. Epidemiol Rev 1990; 12: 1–15.
12. Gillum RF. Trends in acute myocardial infarction and coronary heart disease deaths in the United States. J Am Coll Cardiol 1994; 23: 73–7
13. Bennett SA, Magnus P. Trends in cardiovascular risk factors in Australia. Results from the National Heart Foundation's Risk Factor Prevalence Study 1980–1989. Med J Aust 1994; 161: 519–28
14. MacMahon SW, Peto R, Cutler J et al. Blood pressure, stroke and coronary heart disease (Pt I). Prolonged differences in blood pressure: prospective observational studies corrected for the regression dilution bias. Lancet 1990; 335: 765–74
15. Lipid Research Clinics Program. The Lipid Research Clinics Coronary Primary Prevention Trial II. The relationship of reduction of incidence of coronary heart disease to cholesterol lowering. JAMA 1984; 251: 365–74
16. Lloyd BL. Declining cardiovascular disease incidence and environmental components. Aust NZ J Med 1994; 24: 124–32
17. De Vreede JJM, Gorgels AP, Verstraaten GMP, Vermeer F, Dassen WRM, Wellens HJ. Did prognosis after acute myocardial infarction change during the past 30 years? J Am Coll Cardiol 1991; 18: 698–706
18. Stewart AW, Fraser J, Norris RM, Beaglehole R. Changes in severity of myocardial infarction and 3 year survival rates after myocardial infarction in Auckland 1966–67 and 1981–82. Br Med J 1988; 297: 517–19
19. Goldberg RJ, Gorak EJ, Varzebski J et al. A community wide perspective of sex differences and temporal trends in the incidence and survival rates after acute myocardial infarction and out-of-hospital deaths caused by coronary heart disease. Circulation 1993; 87: 1947–53
20. McGovern PG, Folsom AR, Sprafra JM et al. Trends in survival of hospitalized patients between 1970 and 1985: the Minnesota Heart Survey. Circulation 1992; 85: 172–9
21. Naylor CD, Chen E. Population-wide mortality trends among patients hospitalised for acute myocardial infarction: the Ontario experience 1981 to 1991. J Am Coll Cardiol 1994; 24: 1431–8
22. Lee TH, Goldman L. The coronary care unit turns 25: trends and future directions. Ann Intern Med 1988; 108: 887
23. Hunt D, Sloman G, Christie D, Penington C. Changing patterns and mortality of acute myocardial infarction in a coronary care unit. Br Med J 1977; i: 795–8
24. O'Rourke MF, Walsh B, Fletcher M, Crowley A. Impact of the new generation coronary care unit. Br Med J 1976; ii: 837–9
25. Thompson PL, Hudson M, Solar M, Robinson JS. Analysis of mortality trends by matching of patients with comparative risk. Aust NZ J Med 1979; 9: 755
26. Norris RM. Myocardial infarction: its presentation, pathogenesis and treatment. Edinburgh: Churchill Livingstone, 1982: 41
27. Mather HG, Morgan DC, Pearson NG et al. Myocardial infarction: a comparison between home and hospital care for patients. Br Med J 1976; i: 925–9
28. Hill JD, Hampton JR, Mitchell JR. A randomised trial of home versus hospital management for patients with suspected myocardial infarction. Lancet 1978; i: 837–41
29. Higgins MW, Luepker RV (eds). Trends in coronary heart disease mortality: the influence of medical care. Oxford: Oxford University Press, 1988
30. Jacobs IG. The contribution of ambulance services to falling mortality from ischaemic heart disease in Perth, Western Australia. Unpublished PhD thesis, University of Western Australia, 1993
31. Thompson PL, Parsons RW, Jamrozik K, Hockey RL, Hobbs MST, Broadhurst RJ. Changing patterns of medical treatment in acute myocardial infarction: observations from the Perth MONICA study 1984–1990. Med J Aust 1992; 157: 87–92
31a. Jamrozik K, Broadhurst R, Parsons RW, Hobbs MST, Thompson PL. Ten year trends in medical management and case fatality in acute myocardial infarction. J Am Coll Cardiol 1996; 27: 278A

32. National Heart Foundation of Australia. Cardiac surgery Report No 30. Canberra: National Heart Foundation, 1994
33. National Heart Foundation of Australia. Coronary angioplasty 1993. Canberra: National Heart Foundation, 1995
34. Czarn AOS, Jamrozik K, Hobbs MST, Thompson PL. Follow-up care after myocardial infarction in Perth, Western Australia. Med J Aust 1992; 157: 302–5

4 Molecular genetics of coronary heart disease

Jonathan S Silberberg

The impact of molecular biology on medicine has been so significant that it is now necessary for all clinicians involved in the treatment of heart disease to have some understanding of molecular genetics. Application of this knowledge at the bedside will be a feature of future coronary care practice.

Advances in molecular genetic technology have now made possible direct studies of genotype in persons with coronary heart disease (CHD). While we may hope for rapid answers, finding a genetic marker linked to CHD does not itself prove that the link is causal: additional metabolic and molecular studies will be needed before the role of any marker in disease is established.

As will be discussed below, it is usually simpler to study the pattern of inheritance of an intermediate phenotype known to contribute to CHD. From these individual building blocks it is hoped that models of disease expression will evolve. This chapter will discuss the role of several candidate genes in the development of intermediate phenotypes which lead to CHD, as well as putative associations between genetic markers and myocardial infarction (MI). For those unfamiliar with these terms, a brief glossary is provided (see information box).

Glossary of terms in molecular genetics

allele	alternative form of a gene; one allele is inherited from each parent
candidate gene	a likely gene to begin a search for the genetic basis of disease; usually selected by awareness of a protein's role
deletion	loss of a segment of DNA
exon	a segment in a gene coding for protein synthesis
frameshift mutation	a DNA mutation which interferes with the normal reading frame; usually leads to premature termination of protein synthesis
gene	a sequence of DNA which codes for a polypeptide; includes protein coding and regulatory elements
genome	the total genetic complement of an individual
genotype	the genetic make-up at a specific locus
homozygous	two alleles the same at a particular locus
heterozygous	two different alleles at a particular locus
intron	DNA segment which is transcribed but spliced out of mRNA; does not lead to a protein product
linkage	tendency to inherit two or more characteristics together, more often than by chance alone
linkage disequilibrium	tendency for some alleles to be found together
phenotype	the outward appearance of an organism
polymorphism	variation in DNA; usually identified by fragment length after digestion by cutting enzyme

CHD: A 'complex' trait

What we recognize as clinical CHD results from the expression of several different metabolic pathways acting in concert in the individual. All actions of genes are molecular; ultimately all gene functions can be described in terms of the kind and amount of protein synthesized in cells. The observed biochemical phenotype is the consequence of these varied protein products interacting with each other and with the environment. When this does not correspond to variation at a genetic marker, we speak of *complexity*. This is usually a euphemism to conceal our lack of understanding of the individual elements that contribute to the phenotype.

There may be several reasons for apparent complexity. First, the definition of phenotype is usually imprecise. The factors underlying acute coronary occlusion are different from those leading to lipid accumulation in the arterial wall; these are unlikely to have the same genetic basis, and studies which do not recognize such differing forms of CHD may provide conflicting results. Second, most genetic studies focus on variation in a single gene region rather than the combination of DNA sequences which defines the genome type of the individual. Expression may require specific combinations of alleles at several loci and unless we recognize variation at another locus, it may be difficult to understand why a gene appears to be expressed sometimes and sometimes not. Third, exposure to a particular environment may be necessary for a gene to be expressed; this may be difficult to measure or to identify in the first instance.

Genetic markers and CHD

Until the advent of recombinant DNA technology there were no means to detect variant genes unless variant proteins were produced. Genetic markers can now be studied directly, for example using restriction fragment length polymorphisms (RFLPs) or variable number of tandem repeats (VNTRs). All genetic markers identify DNA sequences of one form or another, but these may not be causal: the marker may be in linkage disequilibrium with a nearby causal gene, it may alter the activity of a protein product itself, or it may be a linkage marker of a gene elsewhere that affects protein activity.

In some instances, studies of cell biology have better defined the link between genotype, intermediate phenotype and CHD. An example is the low density lipoprotein (LDL) receptor defect in familial hypercholesterolaemia.

Genes associated with CHD, with well-defined phenotypes

Familial hypercholesterolaemia (FH)

FH is the best-studied example of a familial disorder leading to CHD. With a prevalence of the heterozygous state of 1/500 in most populations, it underlies only a few cases of CHD in daily practice. The abnormality arises from impaired function of the LDL receptor, leading to accumulation of LDL particles in plasma. Over 150 mutant alleles have been identified, most of which have been cloned at the DNA level.[1] These mutants code for protein receptors whose function ranges from null to defective, which in turn affects the LDL cholesterol level and the propensity to CHD.

Although it is considered a monogenic disorder, other genes may modulate the LDL-C level in FH. Another LDL receptor-related protein, $apoC_{III}$, or hepatic lipase may also be involved. In some individuals with FH, the presence of the $apoE_2$ allele increases levels of both VLDL cholesterol and triglyceride; the X_2 allele at the apoB gene has also been associated with higher levels of LDL cholesterol. There is also evidence for a major locus which suppresses LDL levels, although this has yet to be characterized.

In addition to influencing the lipoprotein phenotype, gene–gene interaction has been shown to affect the expression of CHD. Apo(a) isoforms of higher molecular weight lead to CHD at an earlier age, at any level of LDL-C.

Familial defective ApoB (FDB)

Individuals with this abnormality display abnormal clearance of LDL particles due to defective binding of apoB to the LDL receptor.[2] Several mutations in the apoB gene are under investigation. Not all affected individuals have high levels of LDL cholesterol, and expression of CHD is variable. The interactions underlying these phenomena are still being elucidated.

Type III hyperlipoproteinaemia

Characterized by raised levels of both cholesterol and triglyceride, tendon and palmar xanthomata and both peripheral and coronary atherosclerosis, this syndrome accounts for relatively few cases of CHD. Affected individuals display impaired clearance of triglyceride-rich remnant particles via the hepatic apoE receptor. In the 'recessive' form, affected individuals are homozygous for the E_2/E_2 phenotype, and a second abnormality (such as hypothyroidism or diabetes) is required for the lipoprotein abnormality to be expressed. In 'dominant' forms, variants of the more common E_3 isoform lead to defective binding and hyperlipoproteinaemia.

Familial combined hyperlipidaemia (FCH)

Although inconsistently defined, this syndrome is characterized by the finding of raised cholesterol, triglyceride or both along with CHD in family members.[3] Most individuals have small, dense LDL particles (so-called 'pattern B' LDL), raised levels of apoB, and low HDL-C. Complex segregation analysis has suggested a monogenic inheritance, with reduced expression before the age of 20 in males and before the menopause in females.[4] Given the many factors influencing lipid and protein transfer between particles, it is unlikely that a single gene accounts for LDL particle size in most cases. It is likely that FCH includes the heterozygous expression of several well-characterized recessive disorders, each of which would be more easily recognized in the homozygous state. A subset of FCH patients appears to be heterozygous for lipoprotein lipase deficiency, and linkage to several other genetic markers has been proposed.

Homocyst(e)inaemia

In this condition homocyst(e)ine levels are mildly elevated, either fasting or following a methionine load. The condition is present in approximately 10% of individuals with 'unexplained' CHD. Abnormalities are being investigated at the genes for cystathionine-b-synthase and methyltetrahydrofolate reductase, key enzymes involved in homocyst(e)ine metabolism.

Clotting factors

A common polymorphism of the Factor VII gene, leading to substitution of arginine for glutamine in the amino acid sequence, leads to a 25% lowering of Factor VII coagulant activity (FVIIc) and also lesser tendency for FVIIc to rise with triglyceride levels. This is likely to be clinically important because higher FVIIc has been associated with an increased risk of coronary events.[5] A similar genotype-specific effect of triglyceride has been shown for a polymorphism at the plasminogen activator inhibitor (PAI-1) gene.

Genes associated with CHD, phenotype not fully defined

ACE gene

An insertion/deletion polymorphism at intron 16 of the angiotensin-converting enzyme gene has been reported to be associated with familial CHD in populations from France[6] as well as Australia.[7] Odds ratios reported for the DD allele range from 1.3 to 3.0, being higher in those at low conventional risk and possibly confined to those with the C allele at the angiotensin II AT_1 receptor gene.[8] However the effects of these genotypes on tissue systems remain to be determined: the restriction site for the ACE I/D polymorphism is located on an intron, from which no protein product is expected, so it is likely that the marker is in linkage disequilibrium with a causative gene. Caution is due against assigning too much importance to the DD allele since the finding has not been confirmed in all populations and a study in French centenarians[9] surprisingly found the DD allele to have a high prevalence.

$ApoA_I/C_{III}/A_{IV}$ cluster

It is possible that these genes lead to CHD through the HDL cholesterol level. A polymorphism defined by four restriction enzymes was found to explain 80% of the excess risk associated with a family history of CHD in a Scottish study. Statistics such as these must be interpreted with regard to the selection of the study sample and the ethnic homogeneity of the population from which it was drawn, since both these will influence the frequency of any observed trait.

Other candidate genes for atherosclerosis

All biologic processes implicated in the pathogenesis of atherosclerosis are likely to have genetic determinants. Thus, genes which influence blood pressure, the response of the endothelium to shear stress, cellular cholesterol homeostasis, interactions with the arterial wall, lipoprotein oxidation, immune responses, angiogenesis, etc., are likely to assume greater significance in the future. Some candidate genes being explored are listed in Table 4.1.

Family history: a window on disease mechanisms

Identification of familial factors can influence management of subjects with CHD and their relatives. In either case, the question is reduced to that posed by Acheson

Table 4.1 Candidate genes for atherosclerosis

Phenotype	Protein	Chromosomal location
Apolipoproteins	AI-CIII-AIV	11q23–24
	AII	1q21–q23
	E-CI-CII	19q13
	B	2q24–p23
	(a)	6q26–q27
Receptors	LDL receptor	19p13.3
	Insulin receptor	19q13.3–p13.2
Enzymes	Lecithin cholesterol acyltransferase	16q22.1
	Lipoprotein lipase	8p22
	Hepatic lipase	15q21–q23
	Cholesterol ester transfer protein	16q13
	ACE-1	17q23
	Cystathionine-β-synthase	21q22.3
Vessel wall proteins	Fibronectin	2q34–36
	Collagen	17q21–22
	Endothelial leucocyte adhesion molecule	1q22–25
Growth factors	Platelet derived growth factor β	22q12–13
	Insulin-like factor	12q23
Coagulation factors	Fibrinogen A,B	4q28
	PAI-1	18q21–q22
	Thrombin	11p11–p12
	Factor VII	13q34

How to take a family history

Consider:
- The number of relatives at risk, and their sex
- Their age, and the age at which they developed disease
- Whether another explanation for coronary disease—such as smoking or diabetes—exists

When is a 'positive' family history really STRONG?
- When several of the first degree relatives have been affected (the precise number depends on how many relatives there are!)
- When disease developed at a young age
- When cases have included females
- When the affected persons did not smoke

When is a 'negative' family history really PROTECTIVE?
- When the family is large, yet few have developed disease
- When most members have lived to a ripe old age
- When no disease develops despite a large number of smokers

(attributed to his teachers at the Oxford Clinical School): why did this person (or this family) develop this disease at this time?

Family history as a predictive tool

Most studies have been hampered by imprecise definitions of 'positive family history'. Usual definitions, such as a parent or first degree relative with the disease, do not take into account the number of at-risk relatives, the age at which the disease occurred, or whether the affected family member smoked. Similarly, 'negative family history' sometimes means a small family, one which is very young, or one about which little is known. Such families are uninformative, rather than negative. A suggested guide to taking a family history is given in the information box.

Future direction

The Human Genome Project offers the exciting possibility of a map of the entire human genome. While it may seem that the genetics of CHD will be rapidly understood, several major hurdles will remain. Not least of these are limitations of the statistical models available for analysis, and misclassification of CHD status. Innovative approaches,[10] such as cladistic analysis and the selection of healthy elderly as controls, offer the prospect of enlightened studies of the genetics of CHD.

References

1. Hobbs HH et al. Molecular genetics of the LDL receptor in

familial hypercholesterolaemia. Hum Nutr 1992; 1:445–66
2. Myant NB. Familial defective apoprotein B-100: a review, including some comparisons with familial hypercholesterolaemia. Atherosclerosis 1993; 104:1–18
3. Goldstein J et al. Hyperlipidaemia in coronary disease (Pt II). Genetic analysis of lipid levels in 176 families and delineation of a new inherited disorder, combined hyperlipidaemia. J Clin Invest 1973; 52:1544–68
4. Austin MA et al. Inheritance of LDL subclass patterns: results of complex segregation analysis. Am J Hum Genet 1988; 43:838–46
5. Hamsten A et al. Relationships of thrombosis and fibrinolysis to atherosclerosis. Curr Opin Lipidol 1994; 5:382–9
6. Cambien F, Poirier O, Lecerf L et al. Deletion polymorphism in the gene for angiotensin-converting enzyme is a potent risk factor for myocardial infarction. Nature 1992; 359: 641–4
7. Badenop R et al. Angiotensin-converting enzyme genotype in children and coronary events in their grandparents. Circulation 1995; 91: 1655–8
8. Tiret L et al. Synergistic effects of angiotensin-converting enzyme and angiotensin-II type 1 receptor gene polymorphisms on risk of myocardial infarction. Lancet 1994; 344: 910–913
9. Schachter F et al. Genetic associations with human longevity at the *apoE* and *ACE* loci. Nature Genetics 1994; 6:29–32
10. Zerba K, Sing C. The role of genome type-environment interaction and time in understanding the impact of genetic polymorphisms on lipid metabolism. Curr Opin Lipidol 1993; 4:152–162

Further Reading

Trent RJ. Molecular Medicine: an introductory text for students. Edinburgh: Churchill Livingstone, 1993

Sutton HE. An introduction to human genetics. Florida: Harcourt Brace Jovanovich, 1988

5 Coronary risk factors

Ian Hamilton Craig

Knowledge of risk factors for coronary heart disease (CHD) is essential for the appropriate management of patients presenting to the coronary care unit (CCU). Risk factor modification may significantly improve prognosis in many individuals.

This chapter will provide useful information for the assessment of patients in the CCU and for planning their future management.

Many patients with premature CHD have familial conditions, and family screening is an important but often neglected area of patient management which can detect asymptomatic risk factors in relatives.[1] In other patients, environmental and lifestyle factors are of major importance in determining their current CHD status and their future prognosis.

Age and gender

For each 5-year increase in age, CHD death rates almost double in both men and women; see Figure 5.1.[2]

According to the Framingham study,[3] angina is more often the first presenting symptom of CHD in women, while for men it is MI (myocardial infarction). A second MI is more frequent in women (40%) than in men (13%). Sudden death is rare in women until old age, but is a frequent event in middle-aged and older men.

Age is the major non-modifiable risk factor which affects prognosis after MI.[4]

Post-menopausal women

Mortality rates for CHD in women increase after the menopause, approaching that of men of the same age (see Fig. 5.1). Lack of the protective effects of oestrogens may be responsible for this post-menopausal increase in CHD mortality.[5,6]

Family history

A history of parental death from CHD is an independent risk factor for CHD, showing a similar strength of association to blood pressure, smoking and cholesterol.[7]

Blood pressure

There are continuous, linear, positive relationships between systolic blood pressure (SBP) and diastolic blood pressure (DBP) and the incidence of MI.[8] Overall, hypertension is associated with a two- to threefold increase in CHD mortality rates.[9]

The risk of CHD varies over an eightfold range depending on the presence of coexisting risk factors.[9] There does not appear to be a blood pressure threshold below which CHD does not occur, and most MIs occur at 'normal' levels of blood pressure.[8] Among hypertensive patients, CHD is the most frequent cause of death.[9]

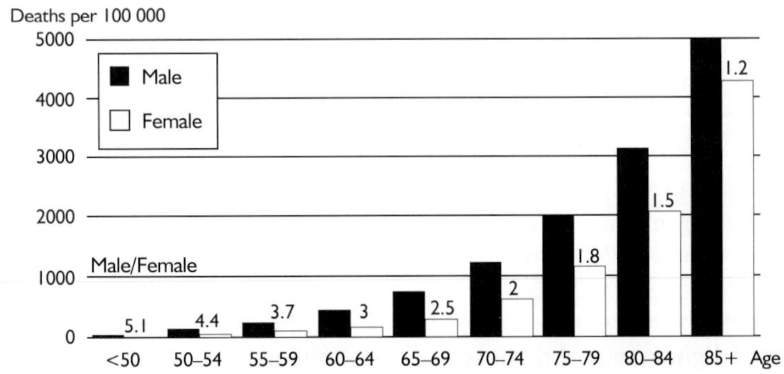

Fig. 5.1 Increasing coronary heart disease mortality (per 100 000) with each decade of age. Males in black bars, females in white bars. Male/female ratio is given above white bars for each decade of age.
Source: National Heart Foundation of Australia Heart and Stroke Facts, 1995.

About half of patients with hypertension also have abnormal plasma lipids.[10]

Left ventricular hypertrophy

Left ventricular hypertrophy (LVH) reflects either pressure and/or volume overload of the left ventricle, and its incidence has declined markedly over the last 30 years with more effective blood pressure control.[11]

The appearance of LVH on the electrocardiogram (ECG) is associated with increased risk for CHD and total mortality as well as for sudden death.[11,12]

More recently, echocardiographic criteria for LVH have been developed, and also predict increased risk for CHD and total mortality.[13] The prevalence of LVH defined by echocardiographic criteria is about seven times greater than that for LVH on ECG criteria.[13]

Cigarette smoking

Smoking one packet of cigarettes a day increases CHD risk about twofold.[14] Long-term smoking habits correlate with the severity of atherosclerosis, and activation of atherosclerotic lesions may lead to acute CHD events.[15] Cigarette smoking also lowers high density lipoprotein (HDL) cholesterol levels, and remains a powerful predictor of increased CHD risk after acute myocardial infarction (AMI).[15]

Passive smoking is associated with increased CHD risk.[16]

Blood glucose and diabetes mellitus

Both insulin-dependent diabetes mellitus (IDDM) and non-insulin-dependent diabetes mellitus (NIDDM) increase CHD risk independently of other risk factors, but the influence of diabetes is greatly dependent on coexistent risk factors which occur frequently. These include increased levels of triglycerides, blood pressure, fibrinogen, cigarette smoking, cholesterol and insulin, in addition to obesity and low levels of HDL cholesterol.[17] Diabetes also increases CHD risk after MI.[4]

Non-fasting glucose levels have also been related to cardiovascular disease in non-diabetic women but not in men.[18]

Exercise

Regular physical exercise is associated with reduced CHD risk and reduces the rate of recurrent AMI and total mortality after previous AMI.[19] Plaque rupture, however, may be triggered by strenuous physical exercise as well as emotional stress, presumably on the basis of coronary spasm and/or haemodynamic changes.[20]

Obesity

Young obese adults have several markers for atherosclerosis, including dyslipidaemias, and increased levels of insulin, endothelin, catecholamines and prothrombotic factors.[21]

According to the Framingham Study, abdominal obesity has an independent effect increasing cardiovascular and all-cause mortality in men, indicating that abdominal obesity is as closely linked to cardiovascular risk as general obesity.[22] In women, only one indicator of central obesity (subscapular to triceps skinfold ratio) was independently associated with CHD, cardiovascular and all-cause mortality.[22]

Other studies in Framingham associated a 2.3 kg weight gain (one body mass index unit) with a 5% reduction in HDL cholesterol, as well as increased levels of low density lipoprotein (LDL) and very low density lipoprotein (VLDL) cholesterol.[23]

Obesity appears to be a strong determinant of coexisting risk factors, and weight loss may reverse the above lipid changes, lower blood pressure and lower the risk of developing NIDDM.[24,25]

Cholesterol and cholesterol fractions

Total cholesterol (TC) and low density lipoprotein cholesterol (LDL) are strongly positively associated with increased CHD risk in numerous prospective studies in both men and women. A lower threshold has not been observed; in China, a gradient in CHD risk still occurs with TC levels below 3.5 mmol/L.[26]

There is a fivefold difference in CHD risk between countries with high and low average cholesterol levels. Risk of CHD almost doubles between average cholesterol levels of 5.5 mmol/L and 6.5 mmol/L.

An increase of 1% in LDL levels is associated in medium-term follow-up with a 2% increased risk of CHD.[27] A stronger relationship probably occurs in the longer term, with 1% increase in TC and LDL levels having a 3%–4% increased risk of CHD.[28]

Familial disorders of LDL

The central role of LDL in increasing CHD risk is illustrated by the inherited disorders of lipid metabolism in which levels of LDL are elevated. These include familial hypercholesterolaemia, familial defective apo B, familial combined hyperlipidaemia and polygenic hypercholesterolaemia.[29]

Cholesterol in the elderly

The strength of TC as a risk factor for CHD falls with increasing age between 40 and 60 years, after which it remains stable. Correction for regression-dilution bias may increase the strength of this association, however.[30]

HDL cholesterol

Levels of HDL cholesterol are strongly and inversely correlated with CHD risk in both men and women, a 1% decrease in HDL C being associated with a 3–5% increased risk of CHD.[31–33] Low levels of HDL C below 0.9 mmol/L also predict increased CHD risk at all blood triglyceride levels.[27]

Low levels of HDL cholesterol are frequently observed in those with premature CHD,[34] as is the '*isolated low HDL syndrome*' in which levels of TC are normal but HDL cholesterol levels are below 0.9 mmol/L.[35,36] Low HDL levels also predict future CHD in those with normal levels of TC and previous CHD.[37]

Ratio of total cholesterol/HDL cholesterol

The ratio of total cholesterol/HDL cholesterol is the single most powerful lipid predictor of CHD risk.[38] Problems remain in interpreting ratios in patients with normal TC levels and low HDL C levels: these patients have high TC/HDL C ratios and may represent the 'isolated low HDL syndrome' which occurs frequently in patients with CHD.[35,36]

Triglycerides

Blood triglyceride (TG) levels appear to be more strongly correlated with CHD risk in women than in men.[39,40] Elevated TG levels are generally associated with reduced HDL levels. On multivariate analysis, TG levels generally fail to correlate independently with increased CHD risk, unlike HDL.[39,40] Elevated TG, however, may causally reduce HDL. The importance of TG and TG-rich lipoproteins as risk factors for CHD is demonstrated by the increased risk of CHD in familial lipid disorders with elevated TG levels, which include familial hypertriglyceridaemia, type III hyperlipidaemia and hyperapobetalipoproteinaemia.[41]

Apolipoproteins

Apo A-I and apo B

Apo A-1 and apo B are the major apolipoproteins of HDL and LDL respectively. They may be more powerful predictors of CHD risk than either HDL or LDL alone, as may hyperapobetalipoproteinaemia, a condition which may be a variant of familial combined hyperlipoproteinaemia.[42–44]

Apo E

An increased frequency of the E4 allele has been described in patients with CHD and in those with restenosis after coronary angioplasty.[45]

Lp(a)

Increased levels of Lp(a) have been associated with increased CHD.[46] Lp(a) is an LDL-like lipoprotein containing apo B-100, with a structural similarity to plasminogen. It may affect CHD risk through promotion of thrombosis as well as through lipid-mediated mechanisms.[47]

Blood coagulation and fibrinolytic risk factors

Many factors involved in blood coagulation and fibrinolysis have been implicated as risk factors for CHD, as would be expected by the role of thrombosis in acute CHD events and in atherogenesis. These factors include fibrinogen, plasminogen activator inhibitor-1, Factor VII, von Willebrand factor and Lp(a).[47–51]

Lipoprotein oxidation

The results of prospective epidemiological studies have confirmed a role for antioxidants in CHD, and several large clinical trials of antioxidant therapy are now in progress.[52]

The susceptibility of LDL to oxidation is modified by its content of vitamin E and beta carotene, which protect core polyunsaturated fatty acids from oxidation.[53] Lipid peroxidation of polyunsaturated fatty acids may damage cellular organelles and cell membranes and impair cell function.[54]

Dietary flavenoids (including those in red wine) also act as antioxidants and have been correlated inversely with CHD incidence in elderly men.[53–55]

Dietary cholesterol versus saturated fats

In spite of a great deal of publicity regarding the dangers of excessive consumption of saturated fats and cholesterol, many health professionals as well as members of the public are confused about the relative importance of dietary cholesterol versus dietary saturated fats (SFA).

For many years it has been recognized that plasma cholesterol levels are predominantly influenced by the intake of SFA, and that the major fraction affected is LDL C.[56] SFA, furthermore, are about twice as potent as polyunsaturated fats (PUFA) with regard to changes in plasma cholesterol and LDL cholesterol levels, and more recently monounsaturated fats (MUFA) have been shown to be similar in effect to PUFA in lowering TC and LDL cholesterol levels.[56]

Many commercially-available foods labelled as 'cholesterol-free' may not have any cholesterol, but may be rich in SFA and therefore have an adverse effect on TC and LDL C. Such products contain either coconut and/or palm oils, which are rich in SFA rather than PUFA or MUFA.

Dietary trans-fatty acids

Trans-fatty acids (TFA) appear to increase plasma levels of TC and LDL, and crude estimates of dietary TFA intake have suggested a positive correlation with CHD risk. The Nurses' Health Study observed a 50% increase in CHD incidence in those consuming more than 5.7 g/d of TFA compared with those consuming less than 2.4 g/d.[57] The intake of trans-fatty acids in Australia is low and unlikely to affect lipid levels, however.

Dietary fish oils (omega-3 fatty acids)

Consumption of more than two fish meals per week has been associated with a 50% reduction in CHD incidence, although this reduction occurred for fatty as well as non-fatty fish consumption.[58] Increased fish intake after MI was also associated with a 30% reduction in reinfarction rate and mortality from MI and all causes.[59]

Alcohol

A large amount of epidemiological evidence supports alcohol as a negative risk factor for CHD; moderate alcohol intake is associated with about a 20% reduction in CHD.[60–63] Alcohol consumption is associated with increased HDL levels, reduction in levels of LDL and fibrinogen, inhibition of platelet aggregation, increased levels of plasminogen activator and increased prostacyclin synthesis.[64]

Other coronary heart disease risk factors

Homocysteine

Elevated homocysteine levels have been associated with increased CHD risk through several mechanisms, including endothelial injury, disruption of the internal elastic lamina, precipitation of glycosaminoglycan-lipoprotein complexes within the arterial intima, increased thromboxane A_2 synthesis and reduced platelet survival.[65]

Uric acid and gout

The relationship between gout, hyperuricaemia and CHD is controversial. Increased CHD risk may be mediated through coexistent risk factors including hypertension, obesity and hyperlipidaemia.[66]

Occupation and education

Lower socio-economic groups with lower educational levels have significantly higher CHD rates, which have been attributed to an increased prevalence of risk factors for CHD.[2]

Ethnicity

Australian Aboriginals have CHD rates which are 2.7 times greater than the national average in men and 2.5 times greater in women. For the young and middle-aged, CHD rates are 10–20 times greater, largely as a result of increased levels of blood pressure, smoking habits, diabetes mellitus, obesity and excessive alcohol consumption.[2] New Zealand Maoris have similar risk factor profiles and increased CHD risk.[67]

Regional variation

In Europe, CHD mortality rates are highest in Scotland and Northern Ireland and lowest in Italy and France, suggesting a north-south gradation in CHD risk. In the USA, CHD mortality rates are higher in the east and lower in the mid-west, and in Australia CHD mortality rates are highest in the Northern Territory (20% above the national average in men and 47% above in women), and lowest in the Australian Capital Territory (25% below the national average). Australian CHD mortality rates generally decline from northeast to southwest.[2]

Psychological factors in coronary heart disease

A vast literature has suggested a link between certain psychological factors and CHD risk. Perhaps the best-known is the 'Type A personality', for which conflicting data occur.[68] Emotional stress may act as a trigger event for plaque rupture.[20] Psychological factors have also been implicated as risk factors for sudden death.[69]

Endothelial dysfunction

Primary endothelial dysfunction has yet to be described as a risk factor for CHD. There is increasing evidence, however, that secondary endothelial dysfunction may play an important role in the pathogenesis of CHD. Risk factors that may adversely affect endothelial function include hypertension, hypercholesterolaemia and cigarette smoking.[70–71] Atherosclerosis is associated with impaired flow-mediated vasodilatation due to endothelial dysfunction.[72]

Diurnal variation

Rates of CHD are increased in the morning, a diurnal variation which may be related to increased platelet aggregation and decreased fibrinolytic activity.[74]

Lipids post myocardial infarction

Total cholesterol after myocardial infarction

Elevated TC levels increase the long-term risk of reinfarction, CHD mortality and all-cause mortality according to the Framingham Study.[73] The association was stronger in men, and correlation for CHD mortality and all-cause mortality strongest in those aged over 65 years.[73]

HDL cholesterol after myocardial infarction

Levels of HDL cholesterol are also predictive of recurrent CHD in patients after MI with normal or 'desirable' levels of TC,[37] and levels of HDL C predict long-term outcome after 10 years of follow-up in patients after MI.[73]

Changes in serum lipid levels after myocardial infarction

Following MI there are changes in lipids and apolipoproteins which generally return to baseline within 3 months. Of particular importance is the rapid fall in TC and rise in TG levels within 24–48 hours after MI, TC levels falling by up to 40% in the succeeding 2 months and TG increasing by up to 60%.[41]

Lipid levels may be reliably measured on presentation to the CCU (immediately after the onset of symptoms), but confirmation of dyslipidaemia should be made by comparison with previous lipid levels and/or by repeat measurements 2–3 months after hospital discharge.

Risk factors for different manifestations of CHD

Silent myocardial ischaemia

Silent myocardial ischaemia on exertion increases the risk of CHD by three to five times, and occurs in 0.5–15% of patients with CHD depending on diagnostic criteria.[75] Independent risk factors for silent ischaemia in men include age, waist/hip ratio and low HDL levels.[75]

Sudden death

Similar risk factors have been described for sudden death (SD) as for CHD, in those with and without previous CHD. Left ventricular hypertrophy (LVH) is a particularly powerful predictor of SD,[12] especially in women.[76]

Trends in coronary risk factors

Recent data for the US and Australia show that there have been significant changes in the prevalence of CHD risk factors over the last several decades, partly accounting for observed reductions in CHD mortality rates. In the US, the age-adjusted prevalence of smoking decreased by 1.1% per year between 1987 and 1990, and only 28.8% of adult Americans were smokers in 1987.[77]

Improvement in the prevalence of hypertension was documented in the US between 1976 and 1980, the percentage of hypertensives, the percentage of hypertensives aware of their condition, the percentage receiving medication and the control rate of hypertension improving from 30%, 54%, 33% and 33% respectively to 26%, 65%, 49% and

43% respectively.[77] Serum cholesterol levels in the US have also improved significantly from the 1971–74 period to 1988–91, the prevalence of cholesterol levels at or above 240 mg/dl (6.2 mmol/L) falling from 26% to 20% overall.[77]

Similar data have been published for Australia from the National Heart Foundation Risk Factor Prevalence Studies.[78]

Conclusion

Each of the major risk factors should be assessed in every individual presenting to the CCU. A management plan, formulating target values for risk factors that are present, should be made prior to hospital discharge. This plan should be discussed fully with the patient and communicated to his or her family doctor. As a result, each patient should be provided with as reliable a prognosis as possible, and intervention undertaken when reasonable data for benefit are available.

Figure 5.2 is provided as a guide to multiple risk assessment, based on Framingham data for men and women with one or more CHD risk factors.[79]

References

1. Williams R, Hunt SC, Schumacher C et al. Diagnosing heterozygous familial hypercholesterolemia using new practical criteria validated by molecular genetics Am J Cardiol 1993; 72:171–6
2. National Heart Foundation of Australia. Heart facts report 1992. National Heart Foundation of Australia, 1994
3. Wilson PW, Evans JC. Coronary artery disease prediction. Am J Hypert 1993; 6:309S–313S
4. Kannel WB, Wolf PA. Pulling it all together: changing the cardiovascular outlook. Am Heart J 1992; 123:264–7
5. Nabulsi AA, Folsom AR, White A et al. Association of hormone-replacement therapy with various cardiovascular risk factors in postmenopausal women. N Engl J Med 1993; 328:1069–75
6. Stampfer MJ, Colditz GA, Willett WC et al. Postmenopausal estrogen therapy and cardiovascular disease. N Engl J Med 1991; 325:756–62
7. Myers RH, Kiely DK, Cupples LA, Kannel WB. Parental history is an independent risk factor for coronary artery disease: the Framingham study. Am Heart J 1990; 120:963–9
8. Onrot J. Hypertension and the J-curve. How low should you go? Canad Fam Phys 1993; 39:1939–43
9. Alderman MH. Blood pressure management: individualized treatment based on absolute risk and the potential for benefit. Ann Intern Med 1993; 119:329–351
10. Castelli WP. Cardiovascular disease and multifactorial risk: challenge of the 1980s. Am Heart J 1983; 106:1191–200
11. Levy D. Clinical significance of left ventricular hypertrophy: insights from the Framingham study. J Cardiovasc Pharmacol 1991; 17 Suppl 2: S1–6
12. Messerli FH. Left ventricular hypertrophy, arterial hypertension and sudden death. J Hypertens 1990; 8: S181–6
13. De Simone G, Ganau A, Verdecchia P, Devereux RB. Echocardiography in arterial hypertension: when, why and how? J Hypert 1994;12:1129–36

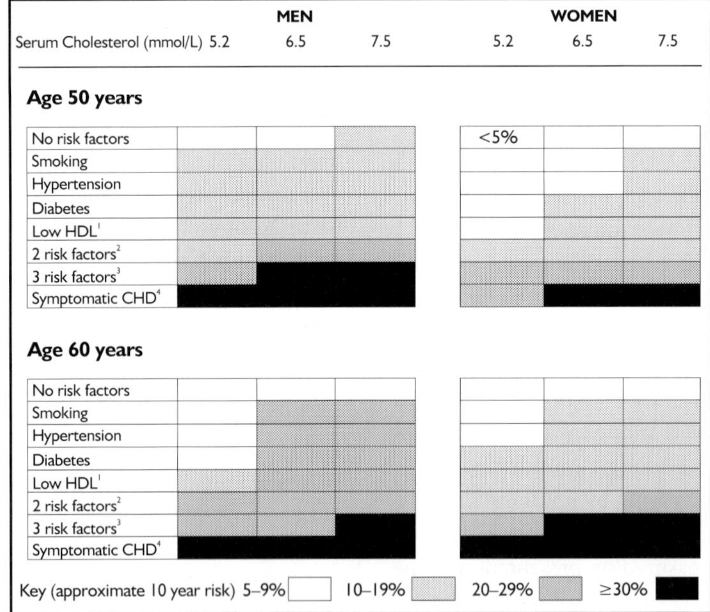

Fig. 5.2 Risk of developing coronary heart disease in 10 years according to age, gender and presence of risk factors. Each vertical bar represents CHD risk for serum total cholesterol levels of 5.2, 6.5 and 7.5 mmol/L in men (LHS) and women (RHS), according to age 50 (upper figure) and 60 years (lower figure). Estimates are irrespective of other CHD risk factors and are based on the Framingham Study, adapted from Mann et al.[79]
[1] HDL cholesterol (<0.9 mmol/L); [2] smoking and hypertension (>160/95 mmHg; [3] smoking, hypertension and low HDL

14. Weintraub WS. Cigarette smoking as a risk factor for coronary heart disease. Adv Exp Med Biol 1990;273:27–37
15. Freund KM, Belanger AJ, D'Agostino RB, Kannel WB. The health risks of smoking. The Framingham study: 34 years of follow-up. Ann Epidemiol 1993;3:417–24
16. Moskowitz WB, Mosteller M, Schieken RM et al. Lipoprotein and oxygen transport alterations in passive smoking preadolescent children. The MCV twin study. Circulation 1991;81:586–92
17. Kannel WB, D'Agostino RB, Wilson PW, Gagnon DR. Diabetes, fibrinogen and risk of cardiovascular disease: the Framingham experience. Am Heart J 1990;120:672–6
18. Wilson PW, Cupples LA, Kannel WB. Is hyperglycemia associated with cardiovascular disease? The Framingham study. Am Heart J 1991;121:586–90
19. Chandrasheckhar Y, Anand IS. Exercise as a coronary protective factor. Am Heart J 1991;122:1723–39
20. MacIsaac AI, Thomas JD, Topol EJ. Toward the quiescent plaque. J Am Coll Cardiol 1993;22:1228–41
21. Licata G, Scaglione R, Avellone G, Parinello G, Merlino G, Corrao S. Obesity, hypertension and atherosclerosis. Int Angiol 1993;12:326–30
22. Kannel WB, Cupples LA, Ramaswami R et al. Regional obesity and risk of cardiovascular disease; the Framingham study. J Clin Epidemiol 1991;44:183–90
23. Hubert HB, Feinleib M, McNamara MP et al. Obesity as an independent risk factor for cardiovascular disease: a 26-year follow-up of participants in the Framingham heart study. Circulation 1983;67:968–77
24. Wolf RN, Grundy SM. Influence of weight reduction on plasma lipoproteins in obese patients. Arteriosclerosis 1983;3:160–9
25. Bantle JP. The dietary treatment of diabetes mellitus. Med Clin North Am 1988;72:1285–99
26. Chen Z, Peta R, Collins R, MacMahon S, Lu J, Li W. Serum cholesterol concentration and coronary heart disease in a population with low cholesterol concentrations. BMJ 1991;303:276–82
27. Assmann G, Schulte H. Results and conclusions of the Prospective Cardiovascular Munster (PROCAM) study. In: Assmann G (ed). Lipid metabolism disorders and coronary heart disease. 2nd ed. Munchen: MMV Medizin Verlag, 1993:19–67.
28. Kannel WB, Wilson PW. Efficacy of lipid profiles in prediction of coronary disease. Am Heart J 1992;124:768–74
29. Genest J Jr, Martin-Munley SS, McNamara JR et al. Familial lipoprotein disorders in patients with premature coronary artery disease. Circulation 1992;85:2025–33
30. Hulley SB, Newman TB. Cholesterol in the elderly. Is it important? JAMA 1994;272:1372–3
31. Gordon DJ, Probstfield JL, Garrison RJ et al. High-density lipoprotein cholesterol and cardiovascular disease: four prospective American studies. Circulation 1989;79:8–15
32. Bass KM, Newschaffer CJ, Klag MJ, Bush TL. Plasma lipoprotein levels as predictors of cardiovascular death in women. Arch Intern Med 1993;153:2209–16
33. Barrett-Connor E, Khan KT, Wingard DL. A ten-year prospective study of coronary heart disease mortality among Rancho Bernardo women. In: Eaker ED, Packard B, Wender NK (eds). Coronary heart disease in women. New York: Haymarket Doyma, 1987:117–21
34. Jacobs DR Jr, Mebane IL, Bandiwala SI, Criqui MH, Tyroler HA. High density lipoprotein cholesterol as a predictor of cardiac disease mortality in men and women: the follow-up study of the Lipid Research Clinics' Prevalence Study. Am J Epidemiol 1990;131:32–47
35. Ginsburg GG, Safran C, Pasternak RC. Frequency of low serum high-density lipoprotein cholesterol levels in hospitalized patients with 'desirable' total cholesterol levels. Am J Cardiol 1991;68:187–92
36. Rosenson RS. Low levels of high-density lipoprotein cholesterol (hypoalphalipoproteinemia): an approach to management. Arch Intern Med 1993;153:1528–38
37. Miller M, Seidler A, Kwiterovich PO, Pearson TA. Long-term predictors of subsequent cardiovascular events with coronary artery disease and 'desirable' levels of plasma total cholesterol. Circulation 1992;86:1165–70
38. Wilson PW. High-density lipoprotein, low-density lipoprotein and coronary artery disease. Am J Cardiol 1990;66:7A–10A
39. Austin MA. Plasma triglyceride and coronary heart disease. Arterioscler Thromb 1991; 11: 2–14
40. Grundy SM, Vega GL. Two different views of the relationship of hypertriglyceridemia to coronary heart disease: implications for treatment. Arch Intern Med 1992; 152: 28–34
41. Rosenson RS, Fraunheim WA, Tangney CC. Dyslipidemias and the secondary prevention of coronary heart disease. Disease-a-month 1994; 40: 380
42. Avogaro P, Bon GB, Cazzolato G, Quinci GB. Are apolipoproteins better discriminations than lipids for atherosclerosis? Lancet 1979; 1: 901–3
43. Genest J Jr, McNamara JR, Ordovas JM et al. Lipoprotein cholesterol, apolipoproteins A-1 and B, and lipoprotein abnormalities in men with premature coronary artery disease. J Am Coll Cardiol 1992; 19: 792–802

44. Kwiterovich PO, Coresh J, Bachorik PS. Prevalence of hyperapobetalipoproteinemia and other lipoprotein phenotypes in men (aged < 50 years) and women (< 60 years) with coronary artery disease. Am J Cardiol 1993; 72: 631–9
45. Wilson PWF, Myers RH, Larson MG et al. Apolipoprotein E alleles, dyslipidemia and coronary heart disease. The Framingham offspring study. JAMA 1994; 272: 1666–71
46. Seed M, Hoppichler F, Reaveley D et al. Relation of serum lipoprotein(a) concentration and apolipoprotein(a) phenotype to coronary heart disease in patients with familial hypercholesterolemia. N Engl J Med 1990; 322: 1494–9
47. Loscalzo J, Weinfeld M, Fless GM et al. Lipoprotein(a), fibrin binding, and plasminogen activation. Arteriosclerosis 1990; 10: 240–5
48. Kannel WB, D'Agostino RB, Belanger AJ. Update of fibrinogen as a cardiovascular risk factor. Ann Epidemiol 1992; 2: 457–66
49. Heinrich J, Balleisen L, Schulte H, Assmann G, van de Loo J. Fibrinogen and factor VII in the prediction of coronary risk. Results from the PROCAM study in healthy men. Arterioscler Thromb 1994; 14: 54–9
50. Etingin OR, Hajjar DP, Hajjar KA et al. Lipoprotein(a), fibrin binding, and plasminogen activator inhibitor-1 expression in endothelial cells. J Biol Chem 1991; 266: 2459–65
51. Meade TW, Brozovic M, Chakabarati RR et al. Haemostatic function and ischaemic heart disease: principal results of the Northwick Park Heart Study. Lancet 1986; 2: 533–7
52. Hankinson SE, Stampfer MJ. All that glitters is not beta carotene. JAMA 1994; 272: 1455–6
53. Manson JE, Gaziano JM, Jonas MA, Hennekens CH. Antioxidants and cardiovascular disease: a review. J Am Coll Nutr 1993; 12: 426–32
54. Kendall MJ, Rajman I, Maxwell SRJ. Cardioprotective therapeutics—drugs used in hypertension, hyperlipidaemia, thromboembolism, arrhythmias, the post-menopausal state and as anti-oxidants. Postgrad Med J 1994; 70: 329–43
55. Criqui MH, Ringel BL. Does diet or alcohol explain the French paradox? Lancet 1994; 344: 1719–23
56. Posner BM, Cobb JL, Belanger AJ, Cupples LA, D'Agostino RB, Stokes J III. Dietary lipid predictors of coronary heart disease in men. The Framingham study. Arch Intern Med 1991; 151: 1181–7
57. Willett WC, Stampfer MJ, Manson JE et al. Intake of trans fatty acids and risk of coronary heart disease among women. Lancet 1993; 341: 581–5
58. Kromhout D, Bosschieter EB, De Lesenne Coulander C. The inverse relation between fish consumption and 20-year mortality from coronary heart disease. N Engl J Med 1985; 312: 1205–9
59. Burr ML, Fehily AM, Gilbert JF et al. Effects of changes in fat, fish, and fibre intakes on death and myocardial reinfarction: diet and reinfarction trial (DART). Lancet 1989; 2: 757–61
60. Steinberg D, Pearson TA, Kuller LH. Alcohol and atherosclerosis. Ann Intern Med 1991; 114: 967–76
61. Blackwelder WC; Yano K, Rhoads GG et al. Alcohol and mortality. The Honolulu Heart Study. Am J Med 1980; 68: 164–9
62. Stampfer MH, Colditz GA, Willett WC et al. A prospective study of moderate alcohol consumption and the risk of coronary disease and stroke in women. N Engl J Med 1988; 319: 1829–34
63. Gaziano JM, Buring JE, Breslow JL et al. Moderate alcohol intake, increased levels of high-density lipoprotein and its subfractions, and decreased risk of myocardial infarction. N Engl J Med 1993; 329: 1829–34
64. Langer RD, Criqui MH, Reed DM. Lipoproteins and blood pressure as biological pathways for effect of moderate alcohol consumption on coronary heart disease. Circulation 1992; 85: 910–5
65. Murphy-Chutorian D, Alderman EL. The case that homocysteinemia is a risk factor for coronary artery disease. Am J Cardiol 1994; 73: 705–7
66. Roubenoff R. Gout and hyperuricemia. Rheum Dis Clin N Am 1990; 16: 539–50
67. Hay DR. Heart facts: recent statistical information on cardiovascular disease in New Zealand. Auckland: National Heart Foundation of New Zealand, 1992: Technical Report no. 58
68. Schwalbe FC. Relationship between Type A personality and coronary heart disease. Analysis of five cohort studies. J Flor Med Assoc 1990; 77: 803–5
69. Frank C, Smith S. Stress and the heart: biobehavioural aspects of sudden cardiac death. Psychosomatics 1990; 31: 255–64
70. Panza JA, Quyyumi AA, Brush JE Jr, Epstein SE. Abnormal endothelium-dependent vascular relaxation in patients with essential hypertension. N Engl J Med 1990; 323: 22–7
71. Celermajer DS, Sorensen KE, Gooch VM et al. Non-invasive detection of endothelial dysfunction in children and adults at risk of atherosclerosis. Lancet 1992; 340: 1111–5
72. Cox DA, Vita VI, Krantz DS et al. Atherosclerosis impairs flow-mediated dilation of coronary arteries in humans. Circulation 1989; 80: 458–65
73. Wong ND, Wilson PW, Kannel WB. Serum cholesterol as a prognostic factor after myocardial infarction: the Framingham

study. Ann Internal Med 1991; 115: 687–93
74. Muller JE, Stone PH, Turi TG et al. Circadian variation in the frequency of the onset of acute myocardial infarction. N Engl J Med 1985; 313: 1315–22
75. Katzel LI, Sorkin JD, Colman E et al. Risk factors for exercise-induced silent myocardial ischemia in healthy volunteers. Am J Cardiol 1994; 74: 869–74
76. Dahlbert ST. Gender differences in the risk factors for sudden cardiac death. Cardiol 1990; 77(Suppl 2): 31–40.
77. Gillum RF. Trends in acute myocardial infarction and coronary heart disease death in the United States. J Am Coll Cardiol 1993; 23: 1273–7
78. Bennett S, Magnus P. Trends in cardiovascular risk factors in Australia. Results from the National Heart Foundation's Risk Factor Prevalence Study, 1980–1959. Med J Aust 1994; 161: 519–27
79. Mann JI, Crooke M, Fear H et al. Guidelines for detection and management of dyslipidaemia. NZ Med J 1993; 106: 133–42

Part 3
Pathophysiology

6 Pathophysiology of atherosclerosis

Leonard Kritharides

Introduction

Coronary care clinicians are accommodating rapidly changing concepts in the initiation and development of acute coronary syndromes, and recognize the potential such concepts offer for controlling the progression of atherosclerotic vascular disease after a coronary event.

Atherosclerosis is a complex disease involving the infiltration and proliferation of various cell types including monocytes, smooth muscle cells, and T-lymphocytes in the vascular intima. Its component processes include the progressive intracellular and extracellular deposition of lipid (principally cholesterol and cholesteryl ester), the deposition of extracellular matrix, the dysfunction of endothelial cells, and, of particular importance in the clinical management of ischaemic heart disease, thrombotic occlusion of coronary vessels. While our knowledge of this disease process and its causes is far from complete, key elements of its pathogenesis have been elucidated by complementary human, animal and in vitro studies.

Lipoproteins and atherosclerosis

Atherogenic lipoproteins

Elevated total plasma cholesterol, low density lipoprotein (LDL) cholesterol, remnants of triglyceride-rich lipoproteins, and low levels of HDL cholesterol are established risk factors for atherosclerosis (reviewed in detail in Chapter 5). Numerous studies have isolated apo B-containing lipoproteins from normal and atherosclerotic aorta.[1,2] Very low density lipoprotein (VLDL), intermediate density lipoprotein (IDL) and LDL can enter the arterial intima in vivo.[3,4] Certain arterial locations, such as arterial branch points, are predisposed to develop pre-atherosclerotic eccentric and diffuse endothelial intimal thickening, and are more susceptible to atherosclerosis than neighbouring arterial segments.[5] This appears attributable to the combination of increased turbulence, increased endothelial cell turnover and endothelial permeability to LDL, decreased wall shear stress, and increased wall tensile stress at these sites.[5–7] Patients homozygous for familial hypercholesterolaemia (FH), who have impaired hepatic LDL clearance because of a deficiency of LDL receptors, have elevated circulating LDL levels and develop very premature atherosclerosis.[8,9] The presence of extracellular, cholesterol-rich lipid protein complexes containing apo B in the vessel wall appears to precede fatty streak lesion formation.[10,11] This suggests that LDL deposited in the arterial intima could be responsible for the recruitment of monocytes and the initiation of atherosclerosis.

High density lipoprotein

Serum HDL levels correlate negatively with the development of premature coronary heart disease.[12] It has been postulated that HDL may exert its protective effect against the development of atherosclerosis by removing cholesterol from arterial cells and transporting it to the liver for catabolism and excretion,[13,14] so-called 'reverse cholesterol transport'. Alternatively, HDL may be a marker of other more important, unidentified lipoprotein interactions, its concentration inversely related to concentrations of potentially atherogenic lipoprotein remnant particles.[15,16] A direct anti-atherogenic effect of HDL, possibly via the reverse cholesterol transport pathway, is supported by the demonstration of direct cholesterol-removing effects of HDL and apo A-I, A-II, A-IV and apo E particles in vitro, and the demonstration that mice transgenic for human apo A-I or apo E were protected from developing atherosclerotic lesions.[17–19b] These observations raise the possibility that HDL-mediated removal of cholesterol from the vessel wall may be important for the regression of atherosclerotic lesions, and that impaired efflux of cholesterol could be a critical component of foam cell formation and atherogenesis.

Oxidized and other forms of modified LDL

Initial attempts to generate foam-cells in vitro by incubating macrophages with LDL were unsuccessful.[20] This suggested that macrophages possess an alternative route for the accumulation of LDL-cholesterol.

Certain chemical modifications were found to enhance net negative charge on the LDL particle and promote uptake of modified LDL via the so-called 'scavenger' receptor.[13] Acetylation was the first effective modification described;[20] a number of other modifications were subsequently demonstrated to result in LDL which was taken up via this receptor.[13,21] In each case, binding to the scavenger receptor was followed by endocytosis, lysosomal degradation of protein and cholesteryl ester components of the modified LDL, and eventual cholesteryl ester deposition in the macrophage cytoplasm.[20] Importantly, unlike the case of LDL-receptor, expression of the scavenger receptor was not down-regulated by cellular cholesterol levels. Consequently, uptake of modified LDL was not restricted as cellular cholesterol accumulation occurred. This scavenger receptor has now been cloned, and has been found to exist in two forms, both of which share high affinity for certain polyanions and mediate endocytosis of chemically-modified LDL.[22,23] The receptor is differentially expressed during monocyte-macrophage differentiation and foam cell formation, and is expressed by macrophages but not smooth muscle cells in atherosclerotic plaque.[24]

It is unlikely that acetylated LDL can be generated in vivo, but other forms of modified LDL may be generated. Oxidation is a biologically plausible LDL modification which has been shown to result in high uptake of LDL by macrophages.[25] A number of cells, including endothelial cells (EC), smooth muscle cells (SMC), monocytes and macrophages are capable of oxidizing LDL (OxLDL) in vitro.[25,26]

Several lines of evidence have been interpreted as supporting a role for lipoprotein oxidation in atherogenesis (see information box).

Cellular pathology of atherosclerosis

Sequential histologic changes

Atherogenesis involves lipid deposition, cellular infiltration, cellular proliferation, and fibrosis within the arterial intima (Figure 6.1).[31] Fatty streaks arise from the endothelial adherence and intimal penetration of blood-borne monocytes which subsequently transform into cells which are hypertrophied, laden with lipid droplets and consequently possess a 'foamy' appearance (Fig. 6.1 A, B).[33,34] As plaques progress, they become increasingly 'fibrous' with a dense cap of connective tissue and smooth muscle cells overlying a lipid core (Fig. 6.1 C).[31,34–36] The synthesis and deposition of

Selected evidence indicating a potential role for LDL oxidation in atherogenesis

Evidence suggesting a role for LDL oxidation in atherogenesis
- Lipid peroxidation products present in atherosclerotic plaque
- Inverse relation between plasma antioxidant levels and rates of coronary disease
- Isolation of subpopulations of oxidized LDL from human plasma
- Prevention of atherosclerosis in animals by administration of antioxidants
- Positive staining of antibodies to epitopes of oxidized LDL in human atherosclerotic lesions

Potentially atherogenic properties of oxidized LDL
- Induces monocyte migration, differentiation and adhesion
- Promotes expression of adhesion molecules and growth factors by cells
- Oxidized LDL is endocytosed by cells more readily than unmodified LDL
- May promote vessel occlusion; promotes vessel constriction, platelet aggregation and macrophage tissue factor expression
- Impaired efflux of sterols from cells loaded with oxidized LDL

Box derived from several references including 25–30

matrix and connective tissue is ascribed to smooth muscle cells.[37] The relative proportions of cells within atherosclerotic lesions may vary between vessels, with a greater proportion of smooth muscle cells in coronary lesions and a greater proportion of macrophages in aortic lesions.[38] Pathogenic processes should not be considered complete or static at any stage; there is ongoing adherence of platelets, monocytes and penetration of LDL throughout lesion development.

Progression of atherosclerosis as a consequence of plaque disruption, thrombosis and platelet adhesion

It has been proposed that while earlier stages of atherosclerosis may be characterized by gradual evolution of histological changes described above, rapid progression of atherosclerosis, with or without clinical manifestations, may be attributable to fissuring and subsequent intraluminal thrombosis of an advanced fatty or fibrous plaque (Fig. 6.1D).[39] Small degrees of plaque fissuring causing intraplaque haemorrhage could manifest as increased angiographic stenosis without necessarily causing luminal thrombosis and occlusion, while deep fissuring is more likely to be associated with vessel occlusion (discussed in more detail in Ch. 7).[40]

As the thrombus formed undergoes fibrosis and organization, smooth muscle cell hypertrophy, proliferation, activation and extracellular matrix secretion could be stimulated by the release of growth factors and cytokines from adherent platelets.[31] Although this mecha-

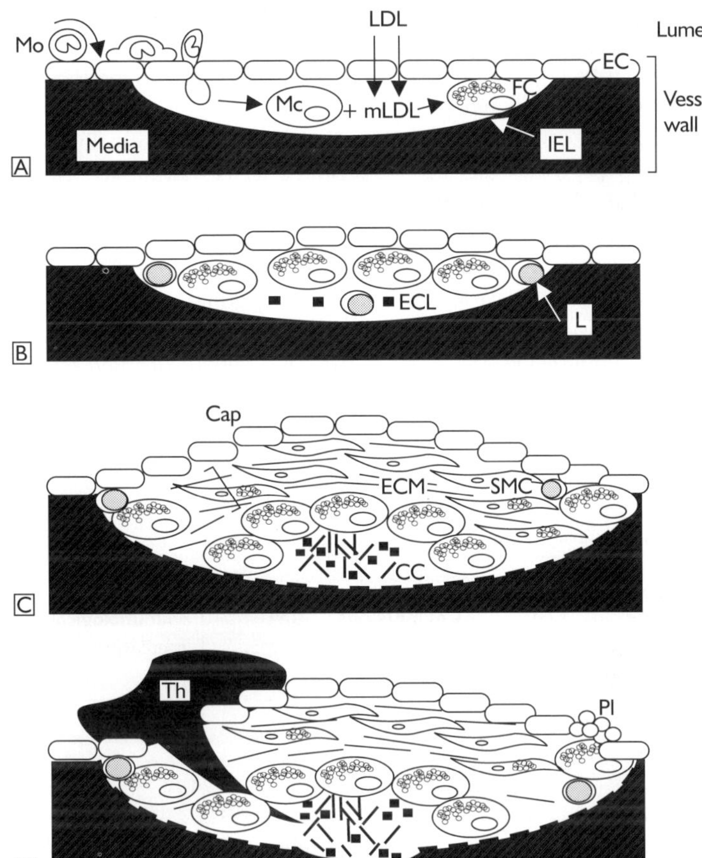

Fig. 6.1 Simplified schematic representation of atherosclerotic plaque evolution. Derived from references 31, 32, 34–36, 40, 42. [A] Microscopic changes: Monocytes (Mo) attach to endothelium, roll (arrow), then adhere firmly upon activation prior to penetrating the endothelial layer (EC) and migrating across the subendothelial space. LDL penetrates into the subendothelium either by passing through or between endothelial cells. Once modified (mLDL), LDL is more readily endocytosed by macrophages (Mc) to generate foam cells (FC) containing cytoplasmic lipid droplets. Additionally, various mLDL can be chemotactic for monocytes. The early stages of atherosclerotic pathology are restricted to the tunica intima and its internal elastic lamina (IEL). [B] Fatty streak: This earliest macroscopic lesion of atherosclerosis consists of macroscopically flat or slightly raised, lipid-rich lesions containing very small numbers of smooth muscle cells, some T-lymphocytes (L) and relatively large numbers of lipid-filled macrophages and some extracellular lipid (ECL). [C] Advanced, fibrous or fibrofatty plaque: As plaques progress, they become in turn 'fibrous' and finally 'advanced', with a dense cap ('cap') of connective tissue, matrix (ECM) and large numbers of embedded smooth muscle cells (SMC) overlying a core of lipid, cholesterol crystals (CC), necrotic debris and macrophages. Concurrently, the internal elastic lamina is often seen to become discontinuous. Some macrophages and lymphocytes are located in the shoulder region of such plaques. [D] Complex plaques: Platelets (P1) can adhere to collagen and macrophages exposed after endothelial denudation. Such plaques often extend to the tunica media. Fissuring of an advanced plaque results in intramural thrombus (Th) formation, which in some cases can extend to form intraluminal thrombus and cause acute ischaemic syndromes. The possible relevance of such fissuring to plaque progression is discussed in the text.

nism attractively links acute coronary syndrome pathogenesis with atherosclerotic progression, it is clear that platelet adherence to plaque does not necessarily require plaque fissuring. Endothelial cell separation and denudation can permit platelet adhesion to exposed subendothelium and foam cell macrophages within lesions. This typically occurs at the shoulders of advanced plaques.[40,41]

Cellular interactions

Endothelial cells and monocytes

The endothelium normally provides a vessel wall surface which is non-thrombogenic and non-adherent for leukocytes. Changes in endothelial morphology, permeability, adhesiveness to leukocytes and vasodilator release are characteristic of atherosclerosis.[43] The accumulation of subendothelial monocytes during the early stages of atherosclerosis does not require endothelial denudation as monocytes penetrate between endothelial cells to enter the arterial wall. This attachment and penetration is markedly accelerated by placing animals on a high fat and high cholesterol diet.[31] The expression of adhesion molecules by endothelial cells is critical for the initial rolling (reversible), firm adhesion and subsequent diapedesis (irreversible) by monocytes of the endothelial layer (see Table 6.1). Cytokines can potently augment leukocyte-endothelial cell adhe-

Table 6.1 Summary of cytokines, chemotaxins and cell adhesion molecules relevant to atherosclerosis.

Promote cell proliferation	Cell source	Chemotaxins	Cell source	Immunological mediators	Cell source	Cell adhesion molecules	Leukocyte function regulated
IL-1	S,E,**M**,TL	*for monocytes*		IL-1	S,E,M,TL	*on endothelium*	
IL-6	S,E,M,TL	M-CSF	S,E,M	TNFα	S,E,M,TL	**Selectins**	
IGF-1	S,E,M,P	GM-CSF	S,E,M	IFNγ	TL	E-selectin	rolling
HB-EGF	S,E,M,TL	MCP-1	S,E,M	IL-2	TL	P-selectin	rolling
bFGF	S,E,M,TL	TGFβ	S,E,M,**TL**,P			**IgG family**	
PDGF	S,E,M,P	OxLDL	S,E,M,L*			VCAM-1	firm adhesion
TGFβ	S,E,M,**TL**,P						and diapedesis
TNFα	S,E,**M**,TL	*for smooth*				ICAM-1,2	"
TGFα	M	*muscle cells*				PECAM-1	"
VEGF	S,M	PDGF	S,E,M,P			MadCAM-1	"
Thrombin	P	IGF-1	S,E,M,P				
		TGFβ	S,E,M,TL,P			*on leukocytes*	
						L-selectin	rolling
						Integrins	firm adhesion
						(e.g. β1, β2)	and diapedesis

Most of the above data have been derived from *in vitro* studies. Those derived from *ex vivo* studies have usually localized the factor without necessarily indicating its site of origin. Many factors have multiple actions (e.g. CSFs maintain cell viability and prevent apoptosis, and MCP-1 has important roles in monocyte adhesion as well as chemotaxis) but only major biological functions have been described. In addition, the relative importance of individual factors can be difficult to assess because of the potential for interplay. Most of the observations of cell proliferation relate to smooth muscle cells, however, other cells in atherosclerotic tissue may be stimulated to proliferate. TGFβ, thrombin and OxLDL are also chemotactic for neutrophils, but the quantitative importance of these cells in atherosclerosis is unclear. Many cells are capable of oxidizing LDL *in vitro*, however, their relative importance in generating OxLDL *in vivo* is unclear. Only major cell adhesion molecules are described.
IL-1/2, interleukin-1/2; IFG-1, insulin-like growth factor-1; HB-EGF, heparin binding epidermal growth factor-like growth factor; bFGF, basic fibroblast growth factor, PDGF, platelet derived growth factor; TGFβ/α, transforming growth factor β/α; TNFα, tumour necrosis factor α; M/GM-CSF, monocyte/granulocyte-monocyte-colony stimulating factor; MCP-1, monocyte chemotactic protein 1; OxLDL, oxidized LDL; IFNγ, interferon γ; VEGF, vascular endothelial growth factor; CAM, cell adhesion molecule(s); S, smooth muscle cell; E, endothelial cell; M, monocyte-derived macrophage; TL, T-lymphocyte; P, platelet; L, lymphocyte; E-, P-, and L-selectin represent endothelial-, platelet- and leukocyte- selectin respectively; VCAM, ICAM, PECAM, and MadCAM respectively represent vascular-, intercellular-, platelet-endothelial-, and mucosal addressin- Cell Adhesion Molecules. Where one particular cell type is especially important in the release of a particular cytokine, this is indicated by the larger bold font. Derived from references 31, 39, 42, 50, 51, 55, 56.

sion by promoting the expression of such endothelial adhesion molecules.[42] In addition, activation of monocytes promotes the expression of a range of ligand molecules which facilitate such attachment.

Endothelial dysfunction, nitric oxide release and atherosclerosis

In addition to many complex inflammatory and biochemical functions, the endothelium plays a critical role in maintaining vascular tone by releasing prostacyclin (PGI_2), endothelin (ET) and endothelium-derived relaxing factor (EDRF, which appears to be nitric oxide, NO, or NO bound to a carrier molecule).[44] NO is synthesized by a number of different cell types from the amino acid L-arginine by a family of enzymes known as the nitric oxide synthases (NOS) and mediates its effect on target cells via the activation of soluble guanylate cyclase and the consequent increase in cyclic guanosine monophosphate (cGMP) (see Fig. 6.2). It is possible that NO release by endothelial cells may be directly anti-atherogenic.[45]

Although NO exerts 'physiological' effects such as regulating vascular tone and acting as a neuronal messenger, it also mediates 'pathological' processes such as the microbicidal effects of macrophages and endotoxic shock.[46] The different effects are likely to be attributable to different concentrations of NO, which are in turn determined by the activity of two classes of NOS. Endothelial cells, for example, express NOS constitutively (cNOS) in the 'physiological' states. Such cNOS activity is modulated by calmodulin and calcium, resulting in the generation of small quantities of NO for short periods of time. In contrast, macrophage NOS activity is induced (iNOS) by the action of cytokines and bacteria, and, once activated, demonstrates a sustained activity which apparently cannot be modulated.

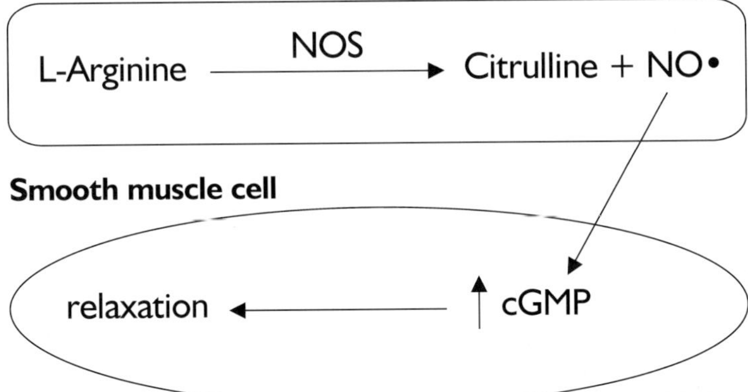

Fig. 6.2 Nitric oxide synthesis. Intact endothelium synthesizes nitric oxide (NO·) from L-arginine via the enzyme nitric oxide synthase (NOS). In response to stimuli such as shear stress and acetylcholine, NO· is released from endothelial cells and diffuses to underlying smooth muscle cells either as unbound NO· or bound to a carrier molecule. NO· activates the enzyme guanylate cyclase, generating an increase in cGMP, and thereby stimulates smooth muscle cell relaxation.

Additionally, some 'toxic' effects of NO may be attributable to the formation of peroxynitrite by the reaction of NO with superoxide anion, both of which can be produced by cells of the vessel wall.

Endothelium-dependent arterial dilatation can be clinically distinguished from direct smooth muscle cell-dependent dilatation by pharmacological and physiological means. For example, low dose acetylcholine induces endothelial cell-mediated dilatation in normal vessels (by stimulating the release of NO from endothelial cells), but causes constriction in atherosclerotic vessels (because of its unopposed smooth muscle constrictor effect).[44] In addition, impaired endothelial function can be detected by the loss of flow-mediated, endothelium-dependent vessel dilatation in the peripheral circulation.[47] Restoration of endothelial cell-mediated dilatation has been demonstrated in angiographically normal human coronary arteries of hypercholesterolaemic patients following lowering of serum cholesterol,[48] indicating that such dysfunction is an early feature of atherosclerosis. However, while impaired endothelium-dependent dilatation may precede angiographically detectable atherosclerosis, it is not yet established whether such dysfunction precedes macrophage foam cell formation and fatty streak development or arises after the appearance of subendothelial foam cell macrophages and foam cell smooth muscle cells.

Lymphocytes and immune activation in atherosclerosis

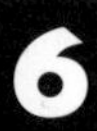

Large numbers of T-lymphocytes, but not B- or natural killer (NK) lymphocytes, have been identified in all stages of atherosclerosis including fatty streaks and advanced plaques. Among T-lymphocytes, it appears that CD8+ve cells (cytotoxic/suppressor cells) predominate in early lesions, while CD4+ve cells (inducers of antibody production and regulators of cell-mediated immmunity) predominate in more advanced lesions.[36] The T-lymphocytes present are immunologically active and are not trapped passive bystander cells.[49,50]

Additional evidence for an involvement of humoral immunity in atherogenesis is afforded by the detection of immunoglobulins, terminal C5b-9 complement complex and complement receptors in human atheromatous tissue.[36,50] This could represent complement activation following the deposition of antibodies to antigens such as OxLDL, adducts to apolipoprotein B, glycosylated lipoproteins, or even infectious agents, or could represent a direct activation of complement by extracellular lipid fractions such as those present in the necrotic core of atherosclerotic plaque.

Smooth muscle cells

The origin of smooth muscle cells (SMC) found in atherosclerotic plaque has been controversial, with some investigators inferring a medial origin of atherosclerotic SMC,[51] while others have concluded that they arise, at least in part, from the proliferation of intimal SMC and not from migratory medial SMC.[43] This situation may be different from the induction of SMC proliferation seen in re-stenosis following percutaneous coronary angioplasty and in experimental models involving endothelial denudation, which clearly involve medial SMC migration and proliferation.[51]

At least two different SMC phenotypes have been described: 'contractile' or 'actin-rich'; 'synthetic' or 'rough endoplasmic reticulum-rich'.[43,51,52] Growth factors and vaso-active compounds released from cells present in atherosclerotic lesions can induce both the change in the SMC phenotype and the subsequent release of cytokines, growth factors, and extracellular matrix from SMC. The localization of platelet-derived growth factor (PDGF) in association with SMC at all stages of atheroma development suggests a role for this factor in particular in smooth cell growth in vivo.[31] Conversely, some components of extracellular matrix (e.g. heparan sulphate) can act upon SMC cell surface receptors to inhibit cell phenotype transformation, proliferation and migration.[43,53] More recently, vascular SMC have also been found to express cell adhesion molecules (CAMs),[54] and these may influence the migration of SMC in the vessel wall.

Growth factors and cytokines

Many growth factors and cytokines are implicated in atheroma formation. In addition, other vaso-active agents (such as NO) can inhibit or promote cell proliferation. Growth factors such as platelet-derived growth factor, insulin-like growth factor-1 (IGF-1), interleukin-1 (IL-1) and tumour necrosis factor-α (TNF-α) are expressed at low concentrations in normal vessels and require cellular activation to promote expression. Such growth factors are potential targets for immunomodulation of atherosclerosis.[55,56]

Specific aspects of atherosclerosis and related conditions

Re-stenosis after percutaneous transluminal coronary angioplasty (PTCA)

Pathology

The incidence of re-stenosis following percutaneous balloon angioplasty remains 30–50% at 6 months after the procedure regardless of the angioplasty procedure used.[57] Although vessel wall recoil and thrombus formation contribute to early re-stenosis, the primary pathology underlying later re-stenosis is generally interpreted as an exaggerated response of SMC to injury.[31,57] Medial SMC migrate into the intima, proliferate and secrete extracellular matrix resulting in the expansion and encroachment of the intima upon the vessel lumen. Following arterial trauma such as angioplasty, intimal histology matures from initial proliferative intimal hyperplasia to differentiated fibrocellular hypertrophy.[58] The degree of the proliferative response, the time required for the arterial segment to transform from the proliferative to the differentiated histology, and the diameter of the artery lumen determine whether haemodynamically significant re-stenosis occurs, and may in part be determined by complex effects of mechanical forces upon cell growth.[58]

Mediators of re-stenosis

Heparan sulphate, NO and prostacyclin inhibit SMC growth and platelet activity and are normally released by endothelial cells. Angioplasty removes these inhibitory influences by damaging the endothelium, and also directly induces smooth muscle proliferation and platelet activity. Cell activation and proliferation are mediated by the combination of:

- platelet adhesion to the endothelially damaged vessel wall and cytokine release
- thrombin
- PDGF and other cytokines released from stimulated atheroma cells such as endothelial cells, macrophages, lymphocytes and SMC
- induction of endothelial adhesion molecules.[57]

Pressure, shear stress and vascular injury are known to induce a range of specific pro-inflammatory and proliferative cell effects in the vessel wall including DNA synthesis, endothelin expression, and activation of the renin-angiotensin system.

Future approaches to re-stenosis

Agents successful in animal studies such as angiotensin-converting enzyme inhibitors and heparin have been unsuccessful so far in preventing re-stenosis in humans. Therapies aimed at the maintenance of flow, thus increasing wall shear stress, may help stabilize the degree of neointimal response.[58] Future prevention of the promigratory and proliferative effects of the aforementioned cytokines and growth factors may involve:

- the local or systemic application of inhibitors of the various growth factors and cytokines (for example, antibodies to PDGF, TGFβ, bFGF, IL-1 and TNFα, and endothelin receptor antagonists)
- the inhibition of signal transduction pathways by which cytokines and growth factors act upon SMC
- topical intimal application of toxins specifically targeting replicating cells
- interference with the expression of cell proliferation, migration or secreted cytokine genes (for example, by the incorporation of antisense DNA for a specific protein or cytokine).[57] Topical applications of anti-inflammatory agents,[59] transfection of vascular SMC and endothelial cells with genes for growth-inhibitory agents such as atrial natriuretic peptide (ANP)[60] and NOS [60b], and blocking expression of proto-oncogenes such as *c-myc* and *c-myb*[61,62] have shown promise in animal studies. The much higher SMC replication rates associated with vessel injury than with atherosclerotic plaque[31] may mean such strategies are more likely to be successful in the treatment of re-stenosis than in the treatment of atherosclerosis.

Atheroma regression and plaque stabilization

Lesions from long-term, low cholesterol-fed, non-human primate models resemble more closely the lesion of human atheroma than do those of high cholesterol-fed rabbit models.[41] Regression of atherosclerotic lesions in such non-human primate models occurred far more readily in fatty streaks than in raised fibrous lesions, was associated with an increase in lesion calcification and collagen deposition, and a decrease in lesion cholesteryl ester content.[63] However, arteries did not return to their prediseased state even after more than 3 years of low serum cholesterol levels. These observations confirm that lowering serum cholesterol may preferentially induce regression of foam cell-rich fatty streaks and perhaps reduce the cellularity and lipid content of macrophage and lipid-rich lesions of advanced plaque, while only producing mild changes in angiographically apparent coronary stenosis.[64]

The impressive reduction in rates of cardiac events following effective lowering of serum LDL cholesterol in human studies may be due to improved mechanical stability of plaques.[65] Most atherosclerotic plaque fissuring occurs at the shoulder of an eccentric lipid-rich plaque which is a site of high foam cell macrophage density and circumferential shear stress,[66] and the vast majority of cap fissures which lead to infarction extend into an unstructured pool of extracellular lipid.[40,67] Improved mechanical stability following cholesterol-lowering therapy may derive from reduction in the size of the soft lipid core of advanced lesions, increased plaque fibrosis, and decreased macrophage-derived proteolytic enzyme secretion due to reduced numbers of macrophages and decreased lipid content of these cells.[40]

Saphenous vein graft stenosis

Approximately 50% of saphenous vein grafts (SVG) are occluded within 10 years of coronary artery bypass graft surgery.[68] The pathology underlying occlusion or stenosis of SVG varies according to the length of time after surgery at which graft occlusion occurs. Following anastomosis, SVG endothelial cells experience severe stretching, which leads to cell damage, and within 24 hours endothelial cells are surrounded by luminal and subendothelial polymorphonuclear cells and subendothelial oedema.[69] Increased endothelial permeability, endothelial cell loss, intimal fibrin deposition, and smooth muscle cell necrosis in the media are common in vein grafts examined within 24 hours of anastomosis.[69] Early occlusion prior to hospital discharge is usually acutely related to platelet aggregation and thrombosis in the vein graft which in turn may be precipitated by mechanical closure, narrowing, or kinking of the vessel. Pre-existing phlebitic saphenous vein disease, mechanical factors reducing blood flow and promoting turbulence, and damage to vein graft endothelium during handling may affect vein graft patency.

Fibro-intimal hyperplasia of the SVG first appears within 2 weeks of grafting. This is characterized by the proliferation of SMC, the synthesis of a mucopolysaccharide matrix and a lack of intimal fat deposition. While such hyperplasia is usually self-limiting, it underlies most vein graft occlusions occurring in 1–12 months after surgery, with or without superimposed thrombosis.[70] Subsequent replacement of SMC by collagen results in fibrous scarring and thinning of the graft wall, and is also commonly seen at this time. The prevention of occlusions within 1 year of surgery by aspirin supports a role for platelets in such early events.[71,72]

Beyond the first year, vein graft atherosclerotic lesions become more prevalent, with progressive replacement of SMC by fibrous tissue and loss and disruption of vein graft elastic fibres. Grafts greater than 3 years of age commonly show lipid-laden foam cells in the intima, and beyond 5 years rupture of atherosclerotic plaque predominates as a cause of stenosis and occlusion of vein grafts. Conventional risk factors for atherosclerosis such as smoking, hypertension and hyperlipidaemia are generally acknowledged to contribute to later atherosclerotic vein graft stenoses.[70] The lack of effect of antiplatelet agents on the development of occlusions between 1 and 3 years after surgery suggests that platelet activation is not essential to this stage of graft stenosis.[73]

Internal mammary arteries are much more resistant to late occlusion than vein grafts.[68] Veins are relatively inelastic compared to arteries when exposed to normal arterial pressures, vein endothelial cells are more permeable and more rapidly take up lipid than those of arteries, and the endothelium of the internal mammary artery is less prone to damage than that of the saphenous vein. Veins also produce lesser quantities of prostacyclin and nitric oxide which may contribute to platelet aggregation in the vein, and veins are more sensitive to vasoconstrictors such as endothelin-1 than are arteries.[70,74] Such differences may underlie the different rates of graft occlusion seen using arterial and vein graft conduits.

Conclusions

Increased understanding of the pathobiology of atherosclerosis has generated exciting prospects for the prevention and treatment of this disease. Envisaged interventions could be directed at a number of component processes of atherogenesis. These range from reducing circulating plasma lipoprotein concentrations, preventing lipoprotein oxidation or other lipoprotein modification, interfering with cellular lipoprotein uptake, and selective inhibition of certain inflammatory, immunological and proliferative components of this disease. Further elucidation of the relative importance of these processes is crucial for the development of specific and effective interventions.

Acknowledgements

Professor Roger T Dean and Dr Wendy Jessup (Group Leaders, Cell Biology Group, Heart Research Institute, Sydney, Australia) and Dr Carolyn Geczy (Group Leader, Immunology Group, Heart Research Institute, Sydney, Australia) are thanked for their constructive comments.

References

1. Hoff H, Gaubatz JW, Gotto AM. Apo B concentration in the normal human aorta. Biochem Biophys Res Commun 1978; 85: 1424–30
2. Stender S, Hjelms E. *In vivo* influx of free and esterified cholesterol into human aortic tissue without atherosclerotic lesions. J Clin Invest 1984; 74: 1871–81
3. Stender S, Zilversmit DB. Arterial influx of esterified cholesterol from two plasma lipoprotein fractions and its hydrolysis *in vivo* in hypercholesterolemic rabbits. Atherosclerosis 1981; 39: 97–109
4. Nordestgaard BG, Tybjaerg-Hansen A, Lewis B. Influx in vivo of low density, intermediate density, and very low density lipoproteins into aortic intimas of genetically hyperlipidemic rabbits. Arterioscler Thromb 1992; 12: 6–18
5. Stary HC, Blankenhorn DH, Chandler AB et al. A definition of the intima of human arteries and of its atherosclerosis-prone lesions. Circulation 1992; 85: 391–405
6. Caplan BA, Schwartz CJ. Increased endothelial cell turnover in areas of *in vivo* Evans blue uptake in the pig aorta. Atherosclerosis 1973; 17: 401–17
7. Packham MA, Rowsell HC, Jorgensen L, Mustard JF. Localized protein accumulation in the wall of the aorta. Exp Mol Pathol 1967; 7: 214–32
8. Goldstein JL, Brown MS. Regulation of low-density lipoprotein receptors: implications for pathogenesis and therapy of hypercholesterolemia and atherosclerosis. Circulation 1987; 76: 504–7
9. Thompson GR. A handbook of hyperlipidaemia. London: Current Science, 1990: 187
10. Simionescu N, Vasile E, Lupu F, Popescu G, Simionescu M. Prelesional events in atherogenesis-accumulation of cholesterol-rich liposomes in the arterial intima and cardiac valves of the hyperlipidemic rabbit. Am J Pathol 1986; 123: 109–25
11. Mora R, Lupu F, Simionescu N. Prelesional events in atherogenesis-colocalisation of apolipoprotein B, unesterified cholesterol and extracellular phospholipid liposomes in the aorta of hyperlipidemic rabbit. Atherosclerosis 1987; 67: 143–54
12. Miller GJ, Miller NE. Plasma high density lipoprotein concentration and the development of ischaemic heart disease. Lancet 1975; 16–19
13. Brown MS, Goldstein JL. Lipoprotein metabolism in the macrophage: implications for cholesterol deposition in atherosclerosis. Ann Review Biochem 1983; 52: 223–61
14. Johnson WJ, Mahlberg FH, Rothblat GH, Phillips MC. Cholesterol transport between cells and high density lipoproteins. Biochem Biophys Acta 1991; 1085: 273–98
15. Eisenberg S. High density lipoprotein metabolism. J Lipid Res 1984; 25: 1017–58
16. Barter PJ. High density lipoproteins and coronary heart disease. Aust NZ J Med 1991; 21: 299–301
17. Ho YK, Brown MS, Goldstein JL. Hydrolysis and excretion of cytoplasmic cholesteryl esters by macrophages: stimulation by high density lipoprotein and other agents. J Lipid Res 1980; 21: 391–8
18. Hara H, Yokoyama S. Interaction of free apolipoproteins with macrophages. J Biol Chem 1991; 266: 3080–6
19. Rubin EM, Krauss RM, Spangler EA, Verstuyft JG, Clift SM. Inhibition of early atherogenesis in transgenic mice by human apolipoprotein A-I. Nature 1991; 353: 265–7
19b. Bellosta S, Manley RW et al. Macrophage-specific expression of human apolipoprotein E reduces atherosclerosis in hypercholesterolemic apolipoprotein E-null mice. J. Clin. Invest. 1995; 96: 2170–9
20. Goldstein JL, Ho YK, Basu SK, Brown MS. Binding site on macrophages that mediates uptake and degradation of acetylated low density lipoprotein producing massive cholesterol deposition. Proc Natl Acad Sci USA 1979; 76: 333–7
21. Haberland ME, Olch CL, Fogelman AM. Role of lysines in mediating interaction of modified low density lipoproteins with the scavenger receptor of human monocyte macrophages. J Biol Chem 1984; 259: 11305–11
22. Rohrer L, Freeman M, Kodama T, Penman M, Krieger M. Coiled-coil fibrous domains mediate ligand binding by macrophage scavenger receptor type II. Nature 1990; 343: 570–2
23. Kodama T, Freeman M, Rohrer L, Zabrecky J, Matsudaira P, Krieger M. Type I macrophage scavenger receptor contains a-helical and collagen-like coiled coils. Nature 1990; 343: 531–5
24. Luoma J, Hiltunen T, Sarkioja T et al. Expression of a_2-macroglobulin receptor/low density lipoprotein receptor-related protein and scavenger receptor in human atherosclerotic lesions. J Clin Invest 1994; 93: 2014–21
25. Steinberg D, Parthasarathy S, Carew TE, Khoo JC, Witztum JL. Beyond cholesterol: modifications of low density lipoprotein that increase its atherogenicity. N Eng J Med 1989; 320: 915–24
26. Steinbrecher UP, Zhang H, Lougheed M. Role of oxidatively modified LDL in atherosclerosis. Free Rad Biol Med 1990; 9: 155–68
27. Berliner J, Territo MC, Sevanian A et al. Minimally modified low

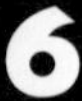

density lipoprotein stimulates monocyte endothelial interactions. J Clin Invest 1990; 85: 1260–6
28. Gey KF, Puska P, Jordan P, Moser UK. Inverse correlation between plasma vitamin E and mortality from ischaemic heart disease in cross-cultural epidemiology. Am J Clin Nutr 1991; 53: 326s–334s
29. Haberland ME, Fong D, Cheng L. Malondialdehyde-altered protein occurs in atheroma of Watanabe heritable hyperlipidemic rabbits. Science 1988; 241: 215–8
30. Kritharides L, Jessup W, Mander E, Dean RT. Impaired efflux of lipids from macrophages loaded with oxidized low density lipoprotein. Arterioscler Thromb Vasc Biol 1995; 15: 276–89
31. Ross R. The pathogenesis of atherosclerosis: a perspective for the 1990s. Nature 1993; 362: 801–9
32. Ross R. The pathogenesis of atherosclerosis—an update. New Engl J Med 1986; 314: 488–500
33. Gerrity RG. The role of the monocyte in atherogenesis 1—Transition of blood-borne monocytes into foam cells in fatty lesions. Am J Pathol 1981, 103: 181–90
34. Gown AM, Tsukada T, Ross R. Human atherosclerosis 2—Immunocytochemical analysis of the cellular composition of human atherosclerotic lesions. Am J Pathol 1986; 125: 191–207
35. Jonasson L, Holm J, Bondjers G, Hansson GK. Regional accumulations of T cells, macrophages, and smooth muscle cells in the human atherosclerotic plaque. Arteriosclerosis 1986; 6: 131–8
36. Hansson G, Jonasson L, Seifert PS, Stemme S. Immune mechanisms in atherosclerosis. Arteriosclerosis 1989; 9: 567–78
37. Ross R. The smooth muscle cell: growth of smooth muscle in culture and formation of elastic fibres. J Cell Biol 1971; 50: 172–180
38. Shiomi M, Ito T, Tsukada T, Yata T, Ueda M. Cell compositions of coronary and aortic atherosclerotic lesions in WHHL rabbits differ. Arterioscler Thromb 1994; 14: 931–7
39. Fuster V, Badimon L, Badimon JJ, Chesebro JH. The pathogenesis of coronary artery disease and the acute coronary syndromes (Pt 1). N Engl J Med 1992; 326: 242–50
40. Davies MJ, Woolf N. Atherosclerosis: what is it and why does it occur? Br Heart J 1993; 69: 3–11
41. Masuda J, Ross R. Atherogenesis during low level hypercholesterolemia in the nonhuman primate: fatty streak conversion to fibrous plaque. Arteriosclerosis 1990; 10: 178–87
42. Carlos TM, Harian JM. Leukocyte-endothelial adhesion molecules. Blood 1994; 84: 2068–101.
43. Stary HC, Chandler AB, Glagov S et al. A definition of initial, fatty streak, and intermediate lesions of atherosclerosis. Circulation 1994; 89: 2462–78
44. Moncada S, Higgs A. The L-arginine-nitric oxide pathway. N Engl J Med 1993; 329: 2002–12
45. Cooke JP, Tsao PS. Is NO an endogenous antiatherogenic molecule? Arterioscler Thromb 1994; 14: 653–5
46. Prince RC, Gunson DE. Rising interest in nitric oxide synthase. Trends Biochem Sci 1993; 18: 35–6
47. Celermajer DS, Sorensen KE, Gooch VM et al. Non-invasive detection of endothelial dysfunction in children and adults at risk of atherosclerosis. Lancet 1992; 340: 1111–5
48. Leung W-H, Lau C-P, Wong C-K. Beneficial effect of cholesterol-lowering therapy on coronary endothelium-dependent relaxation in hypercholesterolaemic patients. Lancet 1993; 341: 1496–500
49. Hansson GK, Holm J, Jonasson L. Detection of activated T lymphocytes in the human atherosclerotic plaque. Am J Pathol 1989; 135: 169–75
50. Libby P, Hansson GK. Involvement of the immune system in human atherogenesis: current knowledge and unanswered questions. Lab Invest 1991; 64: 5–15
51. Raines EW, Ross R. Smooth muscle cells and the pathogenesis of the lesions of atherosclerosis. Br Heart J 1993; 69(S): s30–s37
52. Campbell GR, Campbell JH. The phenotypes of smooth muscle expressed in human atheroma. Ann NY Acad Sci 1990; 598: 143–58
53. Campbell JH, Kalevitch SG, Rennick RE, Campbell GR. Extracellular matrix-smooth muscle phenotype modulation by macrophages. Ann NY Acad Sci 1990; 598: 159–66
54. Skinner MP, Raines EW, Ross R. Dynamic expression of a_1b_1 and a_2b_1 integrin receptors by human vascular smooth muscle cells. Am J Pathol 1994; 145: 1070–81
55. Silverman DI. Atherogenesis. In: Waters DD (ed). Stabilization of atherosclerosis. London: Science Press, 1994: 15–43
56. Blotnick S, Peoples GE, Freeman MR, Eberlein TJ, Klagsburn M. T lymphocytes synthesize and export heparin-binding epidermal growth factor and basic fibroblast growth factor, mitogens for vascular cells and fibroblasts: differential production and release by CD4+ and CD8+ T cells. Proc Natl Acad Sci USA 1994; 91: 2890–4.
57. Epstein SE, Speir E, Unger EF, Guzman RJ, Finkel T. The basis of molecular strategies for treating coronary restenosis after angio-

plasty. J Am Coll Cardiol 1994; 23: 1278–88

58. Glagov S. Intimal hyperplasia, vascular modeling, and the restenosis problem. Circulation 1994; 89: 2888–91

59. Villa AE, Guzman LA, Chen W, Golomb G, Levy RJ, Topol EJ. Local delivery of dexamethasone for prevention of neointimal proliferation in a rat model of balloon angioplasty. J Clin Invest 1994; 93: 1243–9

60. Morishita R, Gibbons GH, Pratt RE et al. Autocrine and paracrine effects of atrial natriuretic peptide gene transfer on vascular smooth muscle and endothelial cellular growth. J Clin Invest 1994; 94: 824–9

60b. von der Leyen HE, Gibbons GH, et al. Gene therapy inhibiting neointimal vascular lesion: In vivo transfer of endothelial cell nitric oxide synthase gene. Proc. Natl. Acad. Sci. USA 1995; 92: 1137–41

61. Simons M, Edelman ER, DeKeyser J, Langer R, Rosenberg R. Antisense *c-myb* oligonucleotides inhibit arterial smooth muscle cell accumulation *in vivo*. Nature 1992; 359: 67–70

62. Bennett MR, Anglin S, McEwan JR, Jagoe R, Newby AC, Evan GI. Inhibition of vascular smooth muscle cell proliferation *in vitro* and *in vivo* by *c-myc* antisense oligonucleotides. J Clin Invest 1994; 93: 820–8

63. Strong JP, Bhattacharyya AK, Egen DA, Malcolm GT, Newman WP, Restrepo C. Long-term induction and regression of diet-induced atherosclerotic lesions in Rhesus monkeys (Pt I). Morphological and chemical evidence for regression of lesions in the aorta and carotid and peripheral arteries. Arterioscler Thromb 1994; 14: 958–65

64. Brown BG, Zhao X-Q, Sacco DE, Albers JJ. Arteriographic view of treatment to achieve regression of coronary atherosclerosis and to prevent plaque disruption and clinical cardiovascular events. Br Heart J 1993; 69(S): s48–s53

65. Simvastatin Study Group. Randomised trial of cholesterol lowering in 4444 patients with coronary heart disease: the Scandinavian Simvastatin Survival Study (4S). Lancet 1994; 344: 1383–9

66. Lendon CL, Davies MJ, Born GVR, Richardson PD. Atherosclerotic plaque caps are locally weakened when macrophage density is increased. Atherosclerosis 1991; 87: 87–90

67. Richardson PD, Davies MJ, Born GVR. Influence of plaque configuration and stress distribution on fissuring of coronary atherosclerotic plaques. Lancet 1989; ii: 941–4

68. Rutherford JD, Braunwald E. Chronic ischemic heart disease. In: Braunwald E (ed). Heart disease—a textbook of cardiovascular medicine. 4th ed. Philadelphia: Harcourt Brace Jovanovich, 1992: 1293–352

69. Davies MG, Hagen P-O. Structural and functional consequences of bypass grafting with autologous vein. Cryobiology 1994; 31: 63–70

70. Cox JL, Chiasson DA, Gotlieb AI. Stranger in a strange land: the pathogenesis of saphenous vein graft stenosis with emphasis on structural and functional differences between veins and arteries. Prog Cardiovasc Dis 1991; 34: 45–68

71. Gavaghan TP, Gebski V, Baron DW. Immediate postoperative aspirin improves vein graft patency early and late after coronary bypass surgery: a placebo-controlled, randomized study. Circulation 1991; 83: 1526–33

72. van der Meer J, Hillege HL, Kootstra GJ et al. Prevention of 1 year vein-graft occlusion after aorto-coronary bypass surgery: a comparison of low-dose aspirin, low-dose aspirin plus dipyridamole, and oral anticoagulants. Lancet 1993; 342: 257–64

73. Goldman S, Copeland J, Moritz T et al. Long-term graft patency (3 years) after coronary artery surgery. Effects of aspirin: results of a VA cooperative study. Circulation 1994; 89: 1138–43

74. Chua YL, Pearson PJ, Evora PRB, Schaff HV. Detection of intraluminal release of endothelium-derived relaxing factor from human saphenous veins. Circulation 1993; 88 (pt.2): 128–32

7 Pathophysiology of coronary occlusion

Anthony C Thomas

Introduction

Although a few coronary arterial occlusions are due to non-atherosclerotic disease, the vast majority are related to coronary atherosclerosis and its complications. This chapter deals predominantly with the pathophysiology of atherosclerotic occlusion and concludes with a brief description of the non-atheroma-related causes.

Atherosclerotic coronary arterial occlusion

Historical background

The association between coronary thrombosis and myocardial infarction (MI) was first described by Malmsten in 1861[1] and later substantiated by Herrick in 1912.[2] Since that time, and until recently, the role of coronary thrombosis complicating atherosclerosis in the pathogenesis of acute myocardial infarction has repeatedly been in and out of favour. Following a number of reports describing AMI without thrombotic occlusion, Branwood and Montgomery in 1956[3] tentatively put forward a proposal that the infarct might antedate the thrombosis. This view was shared by Spain and Bradess who, in 1960[4] in their necropsy series, found that the incidence of thrombi in cases of death from myocardial ischaemia increased progressively with the duration of the final episode. This they interpreted as supporting the view that coronary thrombosis was almost an entirely secondary phenomenon. Such controversy was, in part, due to the inclusion of cases dying suddenly of ischaemic heart disease and *assumed* to be the result of early infarction and, in part, due to the inclusion of all types of myocardial necrosis and infarction in the study groups. Following the work of Fulton and Sumner,[5] Davies, Woolf and Robertson[6] in 1976 and Davies, Fulton and Robertson in 1979,[7] involving detailed histological examination of occluded coronary arteries at necropsy, the pendulum again swung towards thrombosis being the cause of regional transmural infarction in atherosclerotic coronary artery disease, rather than the effect. More recently, clinical studies[8–12] have shown that during the early hours after the onset of MI, a thrombus is usually present within the subtending coronary artery.

Morphological patterns of myocardial infarction

In assessing the role of occlusive thrombosis in MI, it is necessary to distinguish between the different patterns of infarction as described by Davies in 1977.[13] In regional MI, the necrosis is confined to the myocardium supplied by one major epicardial artery. In diffuse infarction, the necrosis involves two or often the three main regions of supply, and is typically subendocardial and often circumferential in distribution. The pathogenesis of these two basic patterns of infarction is quite different. In regional infarction, coronary thrombosis complicating atheroma is the usual finding and it is this pattern that is normally seen in clinical practice. Such infarcts may be transmural involving the endocardium through to pericardium, or subendocardial only, if limited by collateral supply or thrombolysis of the occluded vessel. Diffuse subendocardial infarction is not infrequently seen as a terminal event in autopsy cases. Here the incidence of coronary thrombi is low. Infarction is due to underperfusion of the subendocardial zone, usually as a consequence of severe triple vessel disease or severe left ventricular hypertrophy complicated by a low cardiac output.

The morphology of 'occlusive' coronary thrombosis

In the majority of cases, occlusive thrombi are associated with underlying plaque fissuring or rupture of the atheromatous plaque. This was recognized as early as 1926 by Benson[14] and later emphasized by Constantinides in 1966[15] and Ridolfi and Hutchins in 1977.[16] More recently, detailed histological reconstructions of occlusive coronary thrombi[17,18] have confirmed the presence of plaque fissuring and have revealed a thrombotic component within the plaque in direct continuity with the luminal thrombus (see Fig. 7.1). It is important to realize that the histological picture obtained differs according to the plane of section taken through the thrombosis,[19] and that serial sectioning is required to demonstrate some fissures and even some thrombi (Fig. 7.2). Failure to recognize this point has compounded the controversy over the role of thrombosis in coronary occlusion. Furthermore, we now realize that coronary thrombosis is a very dynamic process that waxes and wanes, and what the pathologist observes at necropsy might not represent the situation that was present some 2–3 hours prior to death. Falk,[20] in a post mortem study of coronary thrombosis, clearly demonstrated identifiable layers of differing ages within the occluding thrombus, confirming the dynamic nature of the process. Thus, many 'occlusive' coronary thrombi that have led to regional MI during life may no longer be completely occlusive as judged by post mortem coronary angiography.

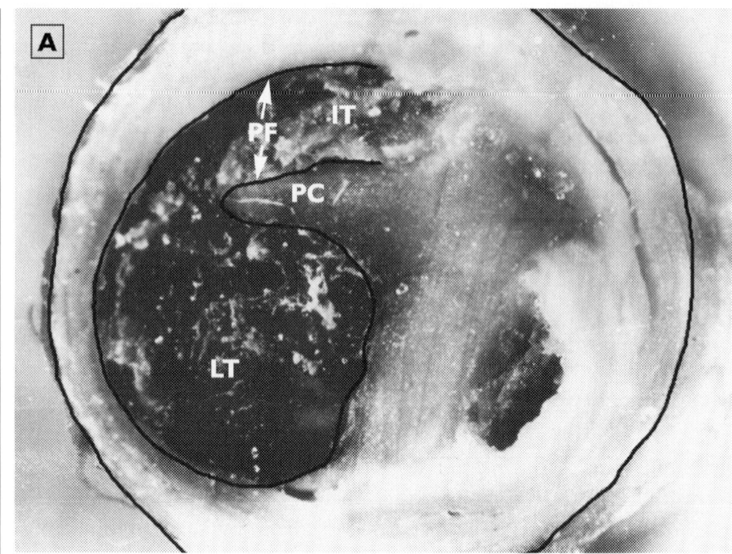

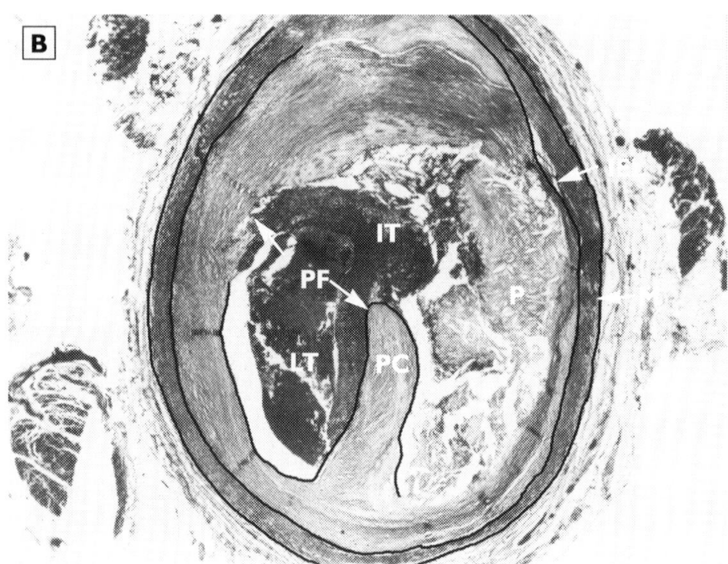

Fig. 7.1 A Dissecting microscope appearance (× 25) and B corresponding histological appearance (Elastic Haematoxylin and Eosin × 25) of an occlusive coronary thrombosis complicating coronary atherosclerosis. The intraluminal thrombus (LT) is in continuity with intra-intimal thrombus (IT) and eccentric lipid-rich plaque contents (P) via a plaque fissure (PF) which has occurred at the junction of the adjacent intima with the fibrous plaque cap (PC). Retraction artefact during tissue processing often leads to apparent retraction of 'occlusive' thrombus from the surrounding wall. IEL – internal elastic lamina, M – vessel media.

The morphology of the coronary arteries in sudden ischaemic death

Until 1984, it was thought that there were two clear-cut groups of patients presenting with sudden ischaemic coronary death: those in whom there was acute occlusive coronary thrombosis and a second much larger group in whom there was severe atherosclerotic narrowing of the coronary arteries without throm-

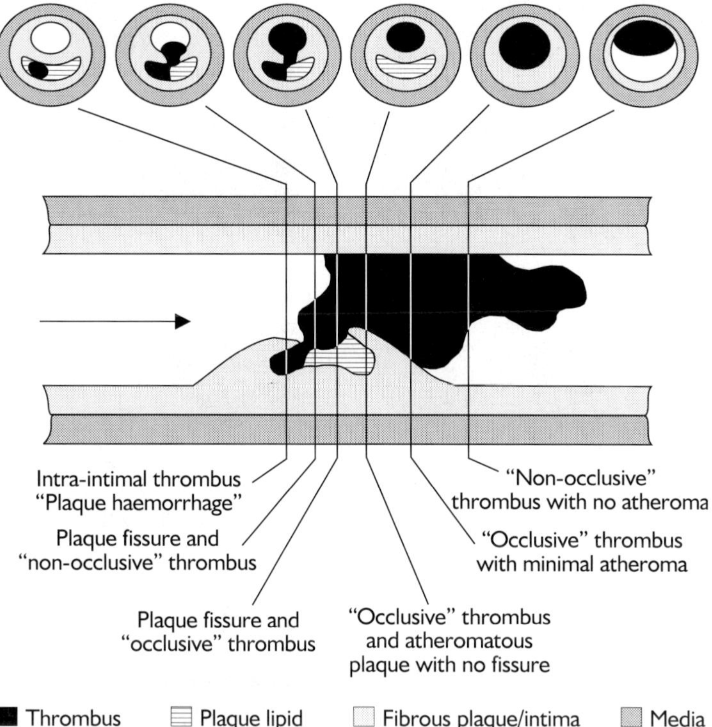

Fig. 7.2 Diagrammatic representation of an occlusive coronary thrombus showing the histological appearances that might be expected as serial sections are taken through the lesion. Arrow indicates direction of flow. (Modified from Thomas and Pazios 1992.)[19]

bosis. The factors determining the moment of death in this second group, compared with controls having a similar degree of coronary artery narrowing but dying suddenly of non-coronary causes, were poorly understood. Subsequently, detailed histological examination of the coronary artery morphology in these cases showed that, in fact, the vast majority had complicated atheromatous plaques characterized by plaque disruption or fissuring and lesser degrees of mural non-occlusive thrombosis.[21–23]

The morphology of the coronary arteries in unstable angina

Recent angiographic studies of patients presenting with unstable angina have revealed coronary artery stenoses with irregular borders and intraluminal lucencies when compared to the smooth stenoses of patients with stable angina.[24,25] The interpretation is that such lesions represent ruptured plaques with, or without, non-occlusive mural thrombosis and are seen in those cases more likely to progress to MI or sudden death. Pathological studies of cases of unstable angina culminating in sudden death or MI also support this view.[20,26]

Plaque rupture and the acute coronary syndromes

Thus the concept of plaque disruption or fissuring, recognized since the beginning of the century, assumed an overwhelming importance in the understanding of the acute coronary artery syndromes. Davies and Thomas[26] put forward a unifying concept for the evolution of advanced atherosclerotic plaques with clinico-pathological correlation between the different morphological appearances and the various clinical presentations of coronary artery disease (see Figs. 7.3 and 7.4). Since then, there has been a spate of publications supporting the concept of plaque fissuring and thrombosis in MI, unstable angina and the majority of cases of sudden ischaemic coronary death.[27–29]

The causation of plaque rupture

The acceptance of atherosclerotic plaque rupture as a precursor of coronary thrombosis has led to a search for the cause. Many factors have been implicated and some are open to therapeutic intervention.

The morphology of plaques liable to rupture

Plaque fissuring is most often seen in eccentric plaques that contain an intimal lipid-rich pool separated from the vessel lumen by a thinned fibrous cap, and often occurs at the point where the fibrous cap joins the relatively normal adjacent intima[26] (see Fig. 7.1). The extent of pre-existing stenosis associated with plaque fissuring and subsequent thrombosis is often severe,[18,30] but up to 35% of major intraluminal thrombi are associated with less than 75% stenosis by area (50% by diameter),[21] and some clinical

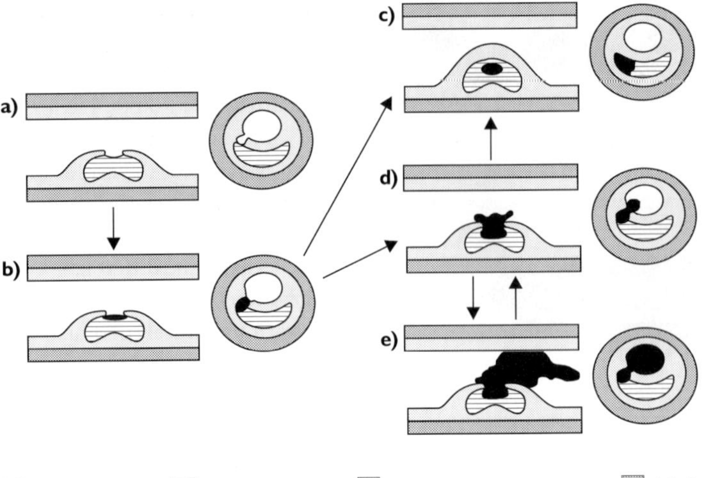

Fig. 7.3 Diagrammatic representation of the evolution of plaque fissuring. (a) Represents the initial phase which is then complicated by intra-intimal thrombosis (b). The 'unstable' plaque may reseal (c) with resultant increasing severity of 'stable' stenosis, or may progress with the formation of intraluminal thrombus (d) which is in direct continuity with the intra-intimal thrombus and plaque contents via the fissure. Thrombolysis with resealing results in a 'stable' lesion (c) whilst progression of thrombosis leads to vessel occlusion (e). Thrombolysis of the occlusive thrombus leads to reperfusion (d) with the potential for stabilization (c). Alternatively, with time, the occlusive thrombus may organize and remain occlusive or show later recanalization with subsequent partial reperfusion. (Modified from Davies and Thomas 1985.)[26]

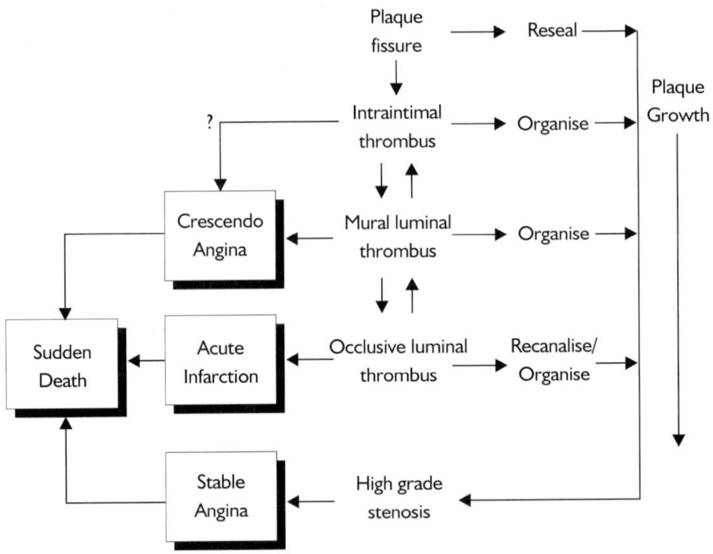

Fig. 7.4 Relationship between the clinical expressions of atherosclerotic ischaemic heart disease and the stages of plaque fissuring. (Modified from Davies and Thomas 1985.)[26]

studies suggest that occlusive thrombosis associated with plaque fissuring often occurs at sites of only mild to moderate pre-existing stenosis.[31] This suggests that there are other factors responsible for triggering plaque rupture besides the degree of stenosis. Eccentric lipid-rich plaques that have undergone recent angioplasty also often show plaque disruption at a similar point, implicating mechanical forces.[32] In a recent study of fissured plaques,[33] 49% of plaques were eccentric and lipid-rich with deep fissuring at the periphery of the plaque, 29% were eccentric and lipid-rich with deep fissuring in the centre of the plaque, 5% were concentric and lipid-rich with deep fissuring, 13% were concentric and fibrous with superficial fissuring and 4% were eccentric and fibrous with fissuring occurring at the junction of the fibrous tissue and a plate of dystrophic calcification.

Arterial wall stresses in the causation of plaque rupture

Based on computer-assisted assessment of distribution of deformation and circumferential stress in the vessel wall, eccentric lipid-rich plaques concentrate stress on the plaque cap near the point of insertion into the adjacent normal intima during systole.[33] When the lipid pool is less than 15% of the vessel circumference and when the plaque cap is less stiff than the adjacent intima, the point of maximum stress is found to be over the centre of the plaque. Regions of high circumferential stress correlate well with the site of intimal tears but tears are also seen at points not computed to be under maximal stress. With a constant area stenosis, increasing the size of the lipid pool leads to a marked increase in maximum stress due to thinning of the overlying fibrous cap, but with a constant lipid pool an increasing severity of stenosis, or increase in fibrous cap thickness, results in a slightly decreased maximal stress.[34] It has also been suggested that turbulent pressure fluctuations play a role in fissuring when the stenosis is severe and due to an eccentric plaque.[35] Initiation of the atheromatous process classically occurs at points of low shear stress[36,37] and tends to occur on the myocardial aspect of the coronary artery.[38] Platelet deposition tends to occur at points of high shear stress,[39] which is always highest on the outside wall of a curved tube,[40] and yet is commonly seen in association with atheromatous plaques. This can be explained by the finding that even minimal atheromatous plaques significantly alter the arterial wall shear stress and that the entire blood flow pattern can change upon the formation of such a plaque.[41] Areas of high shear stress are observed on the wall opposite the plaque but also on both sides of the stenosis. There is often a reversal of wall shear stress with the flow field being markedly unsteady under excited conditions and shear stress peaking on the inside wall.[40] Thus it is likely that both circumferential tensile stress alterations and alterations in shear stress distribution play an important role in plaque fissuring and subsequent platelet deposition even when associated with only mild to moderate stenosis.

Plaque constituents in the causation of plaque rupture

Further studies of the constituents of plaque contents have helped to explain why some plaques fissure in the centre of the cap and not at the point of maximum computed stress. Hypocellular plaque caps are stiffer than cellular caps but not as stiff as calcified caps.[42] With increasing frequency of the stress, all plaque caps were found to increase in stiffness and become more resistant to deformation, leading to shifts in stress distribution within the plaque. It has long been known that plaques undergoing fissuring often possess a necrotic lipid-rich pool,[43] but now attention has been focussed on the inflammatory nature of atheroma in the genesis of fissuring. There is a significantly higher concentration of macrophages derived from blood monocytes in fissured or ulcerated plaque caps and this may be associated with a reduction in maximum stress required for fracture.[44] It appears that tearing of plaques is associated with a decreased resistance to mechanical deformation, a decrease in stress needed to result in fracture and an increase in plaque cap macrophage content. The accumulation of macrophages may directly weaken the collagenous structure of the plaque cap by infiltration, or lead to weakening through enzymic digestion of the cap itself.

Adventitial lymphocytes were first described as long ago as 1915 but more recently, their presence has been related to plaque severity and thrombosis.[45] T-cells are also often seen at the point of rupture and there is an abundant expression of HLA-DR antigens on inflammatory cells and adjacent smooth muscle cells suggesting an active inflammatory infiltrate.[46] The demonstrations of increased lipid peroxidation in atherosclerotic plaques with the potential for oxygen free radical formation,[47] circulating C-reactive protein in patients presenting with unstable angina[48] and the presence of VCAM-1 in atherosclerotic plaques[49] all point to the importance of inflammation and release of mediators in atherogenesis and plaque fissuring through weakening of the plaque cap. Although neutrophils are not usually conspicuous in uncomplicated plaques, they are occasionally seen in complicated plaques and have been implicated in the formation of thrombosis through their procoagulant effects.

Factors predisposing to increased arterial wall stress in the causation of plaque rupture

The realization that the acute coronary arterial syndromes are more prone to occur in the hours soon after awakening, and the understanding of the physiological variations brought about by this circadian rhythm, have shed further light on the causation of plaque rupture.[50–52] Peak occurrence of myocardial ischaemia in the morning after awakening closely parallels the temporal pattern of increase in heart rate, blood pressure, coronary arterial tone, platelet aggregability and a hypercoagulable state. The morning surge in blood pressure may lead to an increase in maximum stress on the plaque, with consequent rupture. Mental stress leading to elevations in blood pressure has also been postulated as a cause for plaque rupture,[53] as has vasospasm.[54,55] Similarly, an increase in heart rate and variations in the cardiac cycle with bending of the vessel wall may lead to repeated stress injury and 'fatigue' fracture analagous to fatigue fracture in metals.[34] There is now good evidence that atheromatous plaques behave quite differently with regard to vasomotor responses, for example, acetylcholine and the cold pressor test lead to constriction rather than dilatation in atheromatous arteries.[56] Furthermore, in atheromatous arteries, there appears to be widespread endothelial dysfunction resulting in decreased effects of endothelial-derived relaxing factor. Many segments of atheromatous arteries unassociated with significant obstruction show foci of endothelial denudation on scanning electron microscopy. It has been postulated that these foci may be due to endothelial cytotoxicity as a result of the generation of free radicals and may in turn lead to the formation of platelet aggregates and the liberation of powerful vasoconstrictors.[57] The finding that angioplasty triggers the release of intracoronary leukotrienes and lipoxin A_4[58] highlights the role of other mediators in the genesis of vasoconstriction and possible plaque rupture. Similar endothelial damage may result from the effects of smoking, hypertension, blood lipid levels and differences in shear wall stresses at varying sites throughout the coronary arterial tree.

Thrombogenesis following plaque rupture

Although fissured plaques not complicated by occlusive thrombosis may reseal with stabilization of the plaque, albeit with increased stenosis,[26] it has recently been suggested that irregular plaques (which are, by supposition, those showing plaque fissuring) identified on angiography remain irregular at repeated angiography some years later.[59,60] If this can be substantiated, then the question of why some fissured plaques undergo occlusive thrombosis and others do not becomes of vital importance. Certainly, many plaque fissures do not lead to significant thrombosis, and many fissures associated with a minor degree of mural thrombus do not show progression to occlusion. Three major factors contribute to arterial thrombosis:[39,61] local arterial changes, systemic factors and alterations in blood flow (Virchow's triad). Atheromatous plaques and medial tissue contain more thrombogenic collagens (Types I and III) than normal subendothelial tissue. Tissue thromboplastin is found within the fibrous plaque caps whilst lipid-rich necrotic plaque elements exposed to the circulation are powerful inducers of thrombosis, and mural thrombus itself is a potent thrombogenic substrate. Thus deep fissures involving the depths of a lipid-rich plaque are most susceptible to significant thrombus formation. There is now substantial evidence that inflammation within the plaque may be a factor in precipitating thrombosis. Increased thrombin formation in unstable angina may be related to expression of tissue factor-like activity by macrophages activated as part of a lymphocytic cell-instructed response.[62] Increased expression of granulocyte and monocyte CD11b/CD18 adhesion receptors indicating an inflammatory reaction in unstable angina may lead to vasoconstriction and/or thrombus formation.[63] Approximately 75% of angiographically recognizable intraluminal thrombi are associated with deep fissuring but a minority are associated with more superficial injury and endothelial loss.[56] Generally, however, thrombosis associated with more superficial injury is less major and tends not to cause occlusion. Local substrates such as high grade stenosis, small diameter vessels and diffuse infiltration by lipid-laden macrophages, systemic factors such as increased coagulability or decreased thrombolysis, and blood flow factors such as turbulence and platelet deposition due to high shear force associated with high grade stenosis may all contribute to progression to total occlusion.

Conclusions

With the general acceptance of the importance of plaque fissuring and subsequent thrombosis in the causation of acute coronary occlusion, attention has now been focused on the cause of plaque fissuring and mechanisms of thrombosis.

Pathological studies have clearly shown that eccentric lipid-rich plaques are the most susceptible to rupture but that other plaque constituents such as macrophage accumulation, inflammation and plaque cap thickness play an important role. Causes of endothelial cytotoxicity such as hypertension and smoking may be important in the more superficial fissuring of fibrous plaques. Computer modelling of eccentric lipid-rich plaques and finite element analysis of circumferential tensile stress have demonstrated that the maximum stress occurs at the edge of the plaque cap but that other variables may lead to fracture at points other than that of maximum computed stress. Rheological blood flow shear stresses and turbulence have also been implicated in the causation of plaque rupture. Factors postulated as leading to an increase in these stress loads include hypertension, increase in heart rate, mental stress, myocardial contractility and vasoconstriction, and may explain the increased morning prevalence in the presentation of the acute coronary syndromes. Repetitive stresses of low magnitude may lead to 'plaque fatigue' whilst a large sustained increase in stress may lead to a more abrupt fracture. Factors promoting thrombogenicity once fissuring has occurred include deep fissuring of lipid-rich plaques, liberation of thrombogenic mediators, hypercoagulability, reduced thrombolysis and rheological blood flow factors. Considerable progress in the treatment of the acute coronary syndromes has been made over the last decade but further understanding of the mechanisms of plaque rupture and thrombosis can only lead to the development of more efficacious therapy.

Non-atherosclerotic coronary arterial occlusion

Coronary artery dissection

Retrograde extension of aortic dissection from the aortic arch to the coronary arteries, particularly the right, may precipitate MI through compression of the true coronary arterial lumen by blood within the dissection track. Less common is isolated coronary artery dissection limited to the coronary artery itself and usually involving the left anterior descending artery of females in the third to fourth decade. The mechanism of isolated coronary dissection is poorly understood but is thought by many to differ from aortic dissection in that unlike aortic dissection, an intimal tear is seldom found despite serial sectioning.

Coronary arterial embolization

Thrombotic coronary artery emboli leading to arterial occlusion and MI may be due to left atrial appendage thrombosis, left ventricular wall thrombosis or valvular endocarditis. Increasing use of non-biological valve prostheses on which thrombus formation is inevitable, at least in small amounts, has led to their becoming the commonest source of coronary emboli, particularly in the Starr type prosthesis where flow is directed by the central ball around the aortic sinuses. Other sources of coronary emboli include calcific debris from calcified valve cusps and, occasionally, fragments of aortic wall traumatized by catheterization.

Coronary arteritis

Generalized polyarteritis involves the coronary arteries in up to 80% of fatal cases, although as a cause of MI it is rare. Kawasaki's disease or muco-cutaneous lymph node syndrome may lead to MI in young children through occlusive thrombosis complicating inflammation of the coronary arteries.

Coronary ostial stenosis

Pedunculated thrombi or small valve papillomata of the aortic cusps may prolapse into the coronary arteries and lead to coronary occlusion. Acquired coronary ostial stenosis classically occurred in syphilitic aortic root disease. Nowadays the majority of cases are related to atherosclerosis, which may lead to sudden death but rarely to MI.

Iatrogenic

Occlusion of a coronary ostium by the cage of a malaligned prosthetic valve, embolization of the coronary arteries by fragments of aortic wall or foreign bodies during catheterization, failure of perfusion of an artery during bypass surgery and failure to recognize anomalies of coronary artery origins during cardiac surgery are rare causes of intraoperative MI. More common is the thrombotic occlusion of the anastomosis of a vein graft despite adequate anticoagulation.

References

1. Malmsten. Dublin Med. Press 1861. Cited by Benson RL in Archives of Pathology 1926; 2:876–916
2. Herrick JB. Clinical features of sudden obstruction of the coronary arteries. JAMA 1912; 59:2015

3. Branwood AW, Montgomery GL. Observations on the morbid anatomy of coronary disease. Scott Med 1956; 1: 367–75
4. Spain DM, Bradess VA. The relationship of coronary thrombosis to coronary atherosclerosis and ischaemic heart disease. Am J Med Sci 1960; 240: 69/701–78/710
5. Fulton WFM, Sumner DJ. ^{125}I-labelled fibrinogen, autoradiography and stereo-arteriography in identification of coronary thrombotic occlusion in fatal myocardial infarction. Br Heart J 1976; 38: 880
6. Davies MJ, Woolf N, Robertson WB. Pathology of acute myocardial infarction with particular reference to occlusive coronary thrombi. Br Heart J 1976; 38: 659–64
7. Davies MJ, Fulton WFM, Robertson WB. The relation of coronary thrombosis to ischaemic myocardial necrosis. J Path 1979; 127: 99–110
8. Bertrand ME, Lefebvre JM, Laisne CL, Rousseau MF, Carre AG, Lekieffre JP. Coronary arteriography in acute transmural myocardial infarction. Am Heart J 1979; 97: 61–9
9. DeWood MA, Spores J, Notske R et al. Prevalence of total coronary occlusion during the early hours of transmural myocardial infarction. N Engl J Med 1980; 303: 897–902
10. Ganz W, Buchbinder N, Marcus H et al. Intracoronary thrombolysis in evolving myocardial infarction. Am Heart J 1981; 101: 4–13
11. Ganz W, Geft I, Maddahi J et al. Nonsurgical reperfusion in evolving myocardial infarction. J Am Coll Cardiol 1983; 1: 1247–53
12. Mandelkorn JB, Wolf NM, Singh S et al. Intracoronary thrombus in non transmural myocardial infarction and in unstable angina pectoris. Am J Cardiol 1983; 52: 1–6
13. Davies MJ. The pathology of myocardial ischaemia. J Clin Path 1977; 30(Suppl. II): 45–52
14. Benson RL. The present status of coronary arterial disease. Archives of Pathology and Laboratory Medicine 1926; 2: 876–916
15. Constantinides P. Plaque fissures in human coronary thrombosis. J Atheroscler Res 1966; 6: 1–17
16. Ridolfi RL, Hutchins GM. The relationship between coronary artery lesions and myocardial infarcts: ulceration of atherosclerotic plaques precipitating coronary thrombosis. Am Heart J 1977; 93: 468–86
17. Davies MJ, Thomas AC. The pathological basis and microanatomy of occlusive thrombus formation in human coronary arteries. Phil Trans Roy Soc London 1981; 274: 225–9
18. Falk E. Plaque rupture with severe pre-existing stenosis precipitating coronary thrombosis. Characteristics of coronary atherosclerotic plaques underlying fatal occlusive thrombi. Br Heart J 1983; 50: 127–34
19. Thomas AC, Pazios S. The postmortem detection of coronary artery lesions using coronary arteriography. Pathology 1992; 24: 5–11
20. Falk E. Unstable angina with fatal outcome: dynamic coronary thrombosis leading to infarction and/or sudden death. Circulation 1985; 71: 699–708
21. Davies MJ, Thomas AC. Thrombosis and acute coronary artery lesions in sudden cardiac ischaemic death. N Engl J Med 1984; 310: 1137–40
22. van Dantzig JM, Becker AE. Sudden cardiac death and acute pathology of coronary arteries. European Heart J 1986; 7: 987–91
23. El Fawal MA, Berg GA, Wheatley DJ, Harland WA. Sudden coronary death in Glasgow: nature and frequency of acute coronary lesions. Br Heart J 1987; 57: 329–35
24. Levin DC, Fallon JT. Significance of the angiographic morphology of localised coronary stenoses: histopathologic correlations. Circulation 1982; 66: 316–20
25. Ambrose JA, Winters SL, Stern A et al. Angiographic morphology and the pathogenesis of unstable angina pectoris. J Am Coll Cardiol 1985; 5: 609–16
26. Davies MJ, Thomas AC. Plaque fissuring—the cause of acute myocardial infarction, sudden ischaemic death, and crescendo angina. Br Heart J 1985; 53: 363–73
27 Davies MJ, Bland JM, Hangartner JRW, Angelini A, Thomas AC. Factors influencing the presence or absence of acute coronary artery thrombi in sudden ischaemic death. Eur Heart J 1989; 10: 203–8
28. Cohen M, Fuster V. Insights into the pathogenetic mechanisms of unstable angina. Haemostasis 1990; 20(Suppl I): 102–12
29. Chesebro JH, Zoldhelyi P, Fuster V. Pathogenesis of thrombosis in unstable angina. Am J Cardiol 1991; 68: 2B–10B
30. Horie T, Sekiguchi M, Hirosawa K. Coronary thrombosis in pathogenesis of acute myocardial infarction: histopathological studies of coronary arteries in 108 necropsied cases using serial section. Br Heart J 1978; 40: 153–61
31. Ambrose JA, Tannenbaum MA, Alexopoulos D et al. Angiographic progression of coronary artery disease and the development of myocardial infarction. J Am Coll Cardiol 1988; 12: 56–62
32. Thomas AC, Pazios S, Mahar L. Early morphological changes in the coronary arteries following angioplasty. Presentation to the 38th Annual Scientific Meeting of the Cardiac Society of Australia and New Zealand, Hobart, May 1990

33. Richardson PD, Davies MJ, Born GVR. Influence of plaque configuration and stress distribution on fissuring of coronary atherosclerotic plaques. Lancet 1989; 2: 941–4
34. Loree HM, Kamm RD, Stringfellow RG, Lee RT. Effects of fibrous cap thickness on peak circumferential stress in model atherosclerotic vessels. Circulation Research 1992; 71: 850–8
35. Loree HM, Kamm RD, Atkinson CM, Lee RT. Turbulent pressure fluctuations on surface of model vascular stenoses. Am J Physiol 1991; 261: H644–H650
36. Friedman MH, Hutchins GM, Bargeron CB, Deters OW, Mark FF. Correlation between intimal thickness and fluid shear in human arteries. Atherosclerosis 1981; 39: 425–36
37. Ku DN, Giddens DP, Zarins CK, Glagov S. Pulsatile flow and atherosclerosis in the human carotid bifurcation. Arteriosclerosis 1985; 5: 293–302
38. Fox B, Seed WA. Location of early atheroma in the human coronary arteries. J Biomech Engng 1981; 103: 208–12
39. Chesebro JH, Zoldhelyi P, Fuster V. Plaque disruption and thrombosis in unstable angina pectoris. Am J Cardiol 1991; 68: 9c–15c
40. Chang L-J, Tarbell JM. A numerical study of flow in curved tubes simulating coronary arteries. J Biomechanics 1988; 21: 927–37
41. Yamaguchi T, Hanai S. To what extent does a minimal atherosclerotic plaque alter the arterial wall shear stress distribution? Biorheology 1988; 25: 31–6
42. Lee RT, Grodzinsky AJ, Frank EH, Kamm RD, Schoen FJ. Structure-dependent dynamic mechanical behaviour of fibrous caps from human atherosclerotic plaques. Circulation 1991; 83: 1764–70
43. Friedman M. The coronary thrombus—its origin and fate. Hum Pathol 1971; 2: 81–128
44. Lendon CL, Davies MJ, Born GVR, Richardson PD. Atherosclerotic plaque caps are locally weakened when macrophages density is increased. Atherosclerosis 1991; 87: 87–90
45. Schwartz CJ, Mitchell JRA. Cellular infiltration of the human arterial adventitia associated with atheromatous plaques. Circulation 1962; 26: 73–8
46. van der Wal AC, Das PK, Tigges AJ, Becker AE. Macrophage differentiation in atherosclerosis. Am J Pathol 1992; 141: 161–8
47. Piotrowski JJ, Hunter GC, Eskelson CD, Dubick MA, Bernhard VM. Evidence for lipid peroxidation in atherosclerosis. Life Sciences 1990; 46: 715–21
48. Berk BC, Weintraub WS, Alexander RW. Elevation of C-reactive protein in 'active' coronary artery disease. Am J Cardiol 1990; 65: 168–72
49. O'Brien KD, Allen MD, McDonald TO et al. Vascular cell adhesion molecule-1 is expressed in human coronary atherosclerotic plaques. Implications for the mode of progression of advanced coronary atherosclerosis. J Clin Invest 1993; 92: 945–51
50. Muller JE. Morning increase of onset of myocardial infarction. Cardiology 1989; 76: 96–104
51. Willich SN, Jimenez AH, Tofler GH, DeSilva RA, Muller JE. Pathophysiology and triggers of acute myocardial infarction: clinical implications. Clin Investig 1992; 70: S73–S78
52. Stone PH. Triggers of transient myocardial ischaemia: circadian variation and relation to plaque rupture and coronary thrombosis in stable coronary artery disease. Am J Cardiol 1990; 66: 32G–36G
53. Bairey CN, Krantz DS, Rozanski A. Mental stress as an acute trigger of ischaemic left ventricular dysfunction and blood pressure elevation in coronary artery disease. Am J Cardiol 1990; 66: 28G–31G
54. Ciampricotti R, El Gamal M, Relik T et al. Clinical characteristics and coronary angiographic findings of patients with unstable angina, acute myocardial infarction, and survivors of sudden ischemic death occurring during and after sport. Am Heart J 1990; 120: 1267–78
55. Morimoto S, Shiga Y, Hiramitsu S et al. Plaque rupture possibly induced by coronary spasm. Jap Circ J 1988; 52: 1286–92
56. Davies MJ. The pathological basis of angina pectoris. Cardiovascular drugs and therapy 1989; 3: 249–55
57. Davies MJ, Woolf N, Rowles PM, Pepper J. Morphology of the endothelium over atherosclerotic plaques in human coronary arteries. Br Heart J 1988; 60: 459–64
58. Brezinski DA, Nesto RW, Serhan CN. Angioplasty triggers intracoronary leukotrienes and lipoxin A4. Impact of aspirin therapy. Circulation 1992; 86: 56–63
59. Haft JI, Al-Zarka AM. The origin and fate of complex coronary lesions. Am Heart J 1991; 121: 1050–61
60. Haft JI, Al-Zarka AM. Comparison of the natural history of irregular and smooth coronary lesions: insights into the pathogenesis, progression, and prognosis of coronary atherosclerosis. Am Heart J 1993; 126: 551–61
61. Ambrose JA. Plaque disruption and the acute coronary syndromes of unstable angina and myocardial infarction; if the substrate is similar, why is the clinical presentation different? J Am Coll Cardiol 1992; 19: 1653–8
62. Serneri GGN, Abbate R, Gori AM et al. Transient intermittent lymphocyte activation is responsible for the instability of angina. Circulation 1992; 86: 790–7

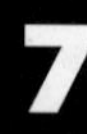

63. Mazzone A, De Servi S, Ricevuti G et al. Increased expression of neutrophil and monocyte adhesion molecules in unstable coronary artery disease. Circulation 1993; 88: 358–63

8 Pathophysiology of myocardial infarction

Peter J Fletcher

Introduction

The concept of the unstable plaque with plaque rupture,[1] described in detail in Chapters 6 and 7, is a unifying concept spanning all the clinical presentations of acute coronary disease. Sudden coronary death,[2] unstable angina, non-Q wave and Q wave infarction may all be different clinical consequences of an unstable plaque with superimposed thrombosis.[3] Sudden death occurs if a major ventricular arrhythmia occurs. The other presentations depend largely on the duration and severity of thrombotic coronary occlusion. Thus Q wave infarction occurs if occlusion persists in the absence of protective collateral circulation.[4,5] When the period of occlusion is shorter, either through spontaneous or drug-induced thrombolysis, the consequence is either non-Q wave infarction with only minor necrosis or even unstable angina with no evidence of necrosis.

The tissue response to coronary occlusion

Myocardium is critically dependent on its energy supply to maintain the cycle of contraction and relaxation.[6] In turn, myocardial energy supply is dependent on coronary blood flow, since myocardial oxygen extraction is near maximal even at rest in the normal coronary circulation. Thus, when coronary blood flow ceases, it causes severe myocardial ischaemia, and myocardial contraction virtually ceases within a few seconds.

The ultimate response of the myocardium depends on the severity and duration of ischaemia. All the components of the myocardium—myocytes, fibroblasts, blood vessels and autonomic nerves—have the potential to be damaged, either reversibly or irreversibly, by prolonged ischaemia, although the myocytes are most at risk because of their high oxygen consumption.

Several syndromes have been identified in relation to myocardial ischaemia.

Hibernating myocardium[7] refers to the situation of chronic low flow ischaemia, with flow too low to allow contraction, but just sufficient to prevent necrosis. Thus the myocytes are 'asleep' but viable. This may occur following myocardial infarction (MI) in the peri-infarctional zone. Efforts to identify viable but non-contractile myocardium which may benefit from revascularization have become a major focus of cardiology in the 1990s.

If blood flow is restored to ischaemic myocardium after a short period of occlusion, for example 10–15 minutes, contraction generally resumes and there is little evidence of damage. However longer and/or particularly repetitive periods of ischaemia produce progressively greater and cumulative functional and structural abnormalities.

Myocardial stunning[8] refers to the situation where blood flow is restored but myocardial contraction does not resume immediately, even though the myocytes appear viable and there is no evidence of necrosis.[9] It may take hours, days or even weeks for normal function to return completely. This is probably a major factor in the delayed return of left ventricular function weeks after successful thrombolysis for acute myocardial infarction (AMI), representing one facet of the complex spectrum of reperfusion injury.

If coronary occlusion persists and ischaemia is not ameliorated by collaterals, myocardial necrosis is inevitable. Necrosis generally begins after about 30–45 minutes of severe ischaemia. Necrosis starts in the centre of the ischaemic zone, since this area is completely inaccessible to collaterals and ischaemia is most severe. From the centre, a wavefront of necrosis spreads out to involve almost 80–90% of the ischaemic zone after a period of 4–6 hours.[10]

Ischaemia is also greatest in the subendocardium compared with the subepicardium. There are two reasons for this. Firstly, oxygen demand is higher in the subendocardium compared with the subepicardium because of higher wall tension. Secondly, subendocardial blood flow is most compromised, since it is derived from branches of epicardial coronary arteries penetrating the myocardium. For these reasons, necrosis also starts in the subendocardium,[10] with a wavefront spreading towards the epicardium at the same time as it spreads outwards from the centre of the ischaemic zone. Thus, during evolution, infarcts commonly have a larger area of subendocardial necrosis and a smaller amount of epicardial damage. This difference lessens once necrosis has progressed to involve most of the ischaemic zone, particularly in large areas of completed transmural infarction.

If reperfusion occurs in time to limit the amount of necrosis, the morphology of the infarct will be modified, not just its size. Thus, instead of infarction progressing to involve say 80% of the ischaemic zone, timely reperfusion may limit necrosis to only 40%. The preserved myocardium will be in the subepicardial region and at the border of the ischaemic zone, leaving predominantly subendocardial infarction with perhaps a much smaller central zone of transmural infarction. Preservation of an epicardial rim of myocardium is probably an important mechanism for preventing infarct expansion and remodelling.[11]

Serial electrocardiograms (ECGs) and cardiac enzymes during the evolution of AMI provide clinical correlates of this pathological process, specifically of the presence of reperfusion and limitation of infarct size. The correlations between ECG changes and underlying pathological processes are shown in Tables 8.1 and 8.2.

Peri-infarctional ischaemia and infarct extension

With any infarct there will be a surrounding or border zone with intermediate blood flow which has not undergone necrosis but is ischaemic or potentially so. This may occur even in the patient with single vessel disease. However it will be exacerbated in patients with multivessel disease where stenoses in the non-infarct-related arteries limit collateral blood flow.

Successful reperfusion will also increase the potential for peri-infarctional ischaemia.[12,13] Limitation of necrosis means that there is a segment of the previously ischaemic zone which remains viable and therefore at risk of further ischaemia if the infarct-related artery reoccludes. Re-occlusion is quite common following successful thrombolysis. It can be identified by recurrence of ischaemia clinically (chest pain) or on ECG (recurrence of ST elevation). Continuous ECG monitoring has demonstrated that ST segments are often quite unstable after thrombolysis.[14] Re-occlusion may require further attempts at revascularization, for example repeat administration of thrombolytic therapy. If not successfully treated, there may be extension of infarction which can be identified by ECG and enzymes.

Autonomic response to ischaemia/infarction

Activation of the autonomic nervous system is common in patients with acute MI.

The presence of myocardial ischaemia is sensed by 'receptors' in the myocardium and relayed to the central nervous system by visceral sympathetic afferents. This results in the awareness of classical ischaemic referred pain. In addition, many other symptoms and signs which accompany myocardial ischaemia—nausea, vomiting, burping, clamminess, sweating, etc.—are also reflex consequences of ischaemia. The thrombolytic era has provided support for this concept of pathogenesis, in that these autonomic manifestations generally disappear with successful reperfusion and relief of ischaemia. However, clinical improvement is not always a reliable sign of reperfusion.[15]

There are important differences between the autonomic response to anterior and inferior myocardial ischaemia. Thus the myocardial receptors activated by inferior ischaemia cause reflex bradycardia with vasodilatation and hypotension. By contrast, those activated by anterior wall ischaemia are more likely to cause reflex tachycardia with vasoconstriction.

However there are many other variables which determine the final autonomic response. For

Table 8.1 Correlation between ECG changes, enzyme changes and infarct morphology in anterior myocardial infarction

Initial ECG	Subsequent ECG	Creatine kinase levels	Pathological interpretation
Extensive anterior ST elevation	Persistent ST elevation with development of extensive Q waves in same leads	Large peak occurring more than 15 hours after onset of chest pain	Extensive anterior transmural infarction involving most of the ischaemic zone with persistent occlusion of the infarct-related artery
Extensive anterior ST elevation	Resolution of ST elevation but with development of extensive anterior Q waves in same leads	Large peak occurring more than 15 hours after onset of chest pain	Extensive anterior transmural infarction involving most of the ischaemic zone but with late opening of the infarct-related artery
Extensive anterior ST elevation	Resolution of ST elevation with Q waves in only 1 or 2 leads, minor loss of R wave in other leads and extensive T wave inversion	High peak occuring earlier than 15 hours after onset of chest pain	Successful reperfusion in time to limit infarct size resulting in a relatively small area of transmural infarction and a larger area of subendocardial infarction
Extensive anterior ST elevation	Resolution of ST elevation, no Q waves, no loss of R waves, extensive T wave inversion	Small peak occurring earlier than 15 hours	Even earlier reperfusion resulting in only a relatively small area of infarction, predominantly subendocardial
Extensive anterior ST elevation	Normal	No rise	Timely reperfusion with complete resolution of transmural ischaemia in time to completely prevent necrosis

Table 8.2 Interpretation of ECG changes post-infarction

ECG change	Interpretation
Extent and severity of ST elevation	Extent of transmural ischaemia
Resolution of ST elevation	Reperfusion due to opening of infarct-related artery
Development of Q waves or loss of R wave	Development of predominantly transmural infarction
Development of T wave inversion	Development of predominantly non-Q wave or subendocardial infarction
Extent of Q waves	Extent of transmural infarction
Extent of T wave inversion	Extent of subendocardial infarction

example, a large anterior infarct will be associated with severe haemodynamic changes and this will activate high pressure arterial baroreceptors in the carotid sinus and aortic arch, and low pressure baroreceptors in the ventricles, atria and great veins. The tachycardia with anterior infarction is primarily a reflex consequence of heart failure due to severe left ventricular (LV) dysfunction.

Likewise with inferior infarction, the right coronary artery frequently supplies the sino-atrial and atrioventricular nodes. Ischaemia of these structures is the major factor in the bradyarrhythmias which are characteristic of inferior infarction. Nevertheless, to the extent that reflex vagal bradycardia contributes to the bradycardia, there will be some response to atropine.

Neurally mediated changes in heart rate and blood pressure are only one consequence of reflex autonomic changes in MI, albeit one of the most easily detected. There are also extensive neurohumoral changes. Plasma noradrenaline levels rise, roughly in proportion to the level of activation of the sympathetic nervous system. Plasma vasopressin levels rise, probably in response to activation of low pressure receptors in the cardiac chambers and great veins. The renin-angiotensin system is also activated, probably by these same low-pressure receptors and also in response to reductions in renal blood flow. All three hormonal systems may contribute to vasoconstriction, reduced urine output and salt and water retention in acute infarction. In addition, atrial distension leads to release of atrial natriuretic peptide which tends to counteract the effect of the previous three hormones by causing vasodilatation and natriuresis.

Pathophysiology of heart failure post myocardial infarction

The development of heart failure is one of the most serious complications of AMI and carries a grave prognosis. The presence of various manifestations of left ventricular failure, such as basal crackles on auscultation, figure prominently in all the prognostic indices and classifications which have been developed for AMI.[16] It is essential to understand its pathogenesis, in order to provide rational investigation and treatment, both in the acute phase and subsequently.

Hypotension, bradycardia, poor urine output and signs of low cardiac output are common early manifestations particularly of acute inferior infarction. These patients generally respond to small doses of atropine and intravenous fluids. Severe bradyarrhythmias in inferior infarction may cause hypotension and heart failure. These are generally due to ischaemia of the atrioventricular node which will usually recover after several days of support from temporary ventricular pacing. Various tachyarrhythmias can cause profound haemodynamic deterioration and generally require urgent treatment which may involve DC cardioversion (see Ch. 55).

Patients who develop a *new systolic murmur* may have ventricular septal rupture or papillary muscle rupture. These are often associated with profound haemodynamic deterioration, and many patients will not survive. Corrective surgery is usually required, and its timing depends on the severity of the problem and the extent to which the patient can be stabilized by medical treatment (see Ch. 58). Acute cardiac tamponade is due to myocardial rupture and is most often rapidly fatal. Occasionally it is amenable to treatment.

Severe myocardial damage is the principal cause of heart failure in MI (see Ch. 56). This may be due to a single large infarct, or to the cumulative effects of a further small infarct in a patient with one or more previous infarcts. The left ventricle is most often involved, leading to acute left ventricular failure, often with overt acute pulmonary oedema. The latter patient would be classified as Killip III, which carries an in-hospital mortality in the range of 40–50%.

Systolic failure is the most important mechanism. MI leads to loss of contractile tissue. The practical consequence of this is a reduction in left ventricular ejection fraction, often to less than 30%, a rise in left ventricular filling pressure, often to above the threshold for pulmonary oedema, and a fall in stroke volume and cardiac output. Rational treatment[17,18] involves reducing intravascular volume, increasing venous compliance and reducing pre-load with loop diuretics and venodilating drugs, primarily glyceryl trinitrate. A small number of very sick patients will require additional treatment with parenteral afterload reduction (e.g. nitroprusside) and inotropic support (e.g. dobutamine).

Diastolic failure may also contribute to the pathogenesis of left ventricular failure. The pathology of myocardial necrosis involves early tissue oedema followed shortly by inflammatory cell infiltrate. As a consequence, the area of infarction initially becomes stiffer or less compliant than normal myocardium. This can lead to an elevation in filling pressure out of proportion to the reduction in systolic function and ejection fraction. This is the likely mechanism to account for the presence of crackles in patients with relative mild reduction in systolic function with ejection fraction often in the 40–50% range.

Fortunately, in most patients the left ventricular failure is only mild and does not require parenteral therapy. Early administration of diuretics and nitrates should be followed within 1–2 days by the introduction of an angiotensin-converting enzyme (ACE) inhibitor[19] (see Ch. 33).

The syndrome of *isolated right ventricular infarction* must be identified separately because it requires a different approach to therapy[20] (see Ch. 59). Pathologically, right ventricular free wall damage is common in inferior infarction due to right coronary artery occlusion. There are usually no clinical manifestations or consequences. Occasionally the right coronary artery supplies virtually all of the RV free wall, much of the inferior portion of the interventricular septum, but little of the left ventricular free wall. In these patients, isolated right ventricular failure develops, manifest by high jugular venous pressure and persistently clear lungs. Signs of low cardiac output are usually present, with hypotension, cool skin and poor urine output. In this case the right ventricle is the limiting part of the cardiac pump, and rational treatment involves increasing right ventricular pre-load further to improve right ventricular stroke volume. Thus, initial treatment involves cautious administration of intravenous fluid (providing the *absence* of left ventricular failure is confirmed on chest X-ray). Fortunately, the natural history is that right ventricular systolic function usually improves significantly over several days.

Infarct expansion and remodelling

The dual concepts of infarct expansion and ventricular remodelling following MI have become firmly established in the last few years.[11,21–26] The term basically refers to structural changes in the left ventricle following infarction. Both the infarcted segment and the non-infarcted residual myocardium participate in the remodelling process. During the process of infarct healing, the necrotic myocardium and inflammatory cellular infiltrate are gradually replaced by fibrous scar tissue formation. During this process the area of infarction becomes progressively thinner but at the same time it also expands. The most extreme example is a left ventricular aneurysm which can have a paper-thin fibrous wall.

At the same time as these changes are occurring in the infarcted segment, the residual non-infarcted myocardium is also undergoing important changes which involve a combination of lengthening and hypertrophy.[27] The hypertrophy is very similar to that which accompanies classical volume overload. It involves little increase in wall thickness but significant lengthening of myocytes with new sarcomeres laid down in series.

The consequence of lengthening of both the infarcted and non-infarcted segments is that left ventricular volume increases with a change in the shape of the ventricle.[28] This volume increase is generally much greater than occurs from distension during the acute phase of the infarct because it involves an actual rightward shift in the passive pressure-volume relationship of the left ventricle. As a result of this shift, filling pressure may actually decrease despite the larger volume. Thus the remodelling process confers short-term haemodynamic benefits on the infarcted ventricle with lower filling pressure and larger stroke volume generated for the same ejection fraction.

The time course of this process is very extensive. It probably starts almost immediately after coronary occlusion, and is certainly underway by 24 hours. Equally it is a progressive long-term process in many patients.[29] Thus, although the process of infarct healing is generally completed by 4–6 weeks, the process of remodelling and dilatation can continue for months or even years (see Fig. 8.1). Despite the short-term haemodynamic benefits, the presence of dilatation and remodelling carries a bad prognosis, with a high risk of the later development of left ventricular failure and of death.[30–32]

Determinants of remodelling

Not all myocardial infarcts undergo this overt process of ventricular dilatation.[29] There are two predictive factors:

- Infarct size is the most important. Small infarcts tend to heal without any dilatation. By contrast, large infarcts usually develop some degree of dilatation and remodelling. These are most commonly large anterior infarcts, although large inferior infarcts are also at risk. Size rather than site appears to be the important determinant. In general, dilatation is likely with infarcts associated with a left ventricular ejection fraction ≤40%.[23]
- The status of the infarct-related artery is the other determinant. Persistent occlusion of the infarct-related artery is highly predictive of the patient progressing to dilatation and remodelling, while patency seems to protect

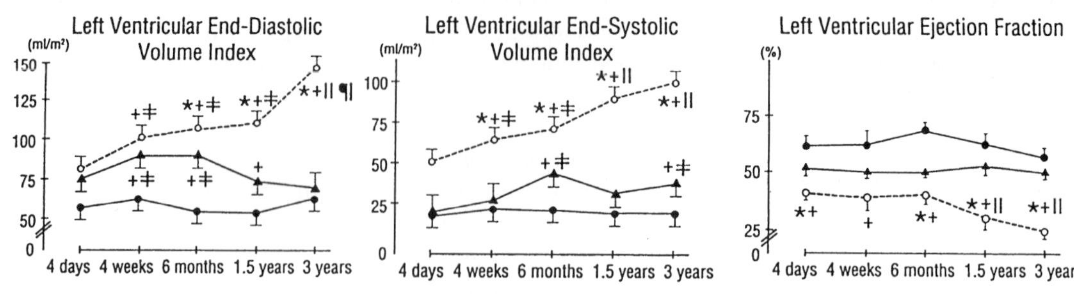

Fig. 8.1 Time course of changes in LV end-diastolic volume, end-systolic volume and ejection fraction in patients with progressive (○) limited (▲) and no (●) LV dilatation from 4 days until 3 years after acute myocardial infarction. Reprinted with permission from Gaudron P, Eilles C, Kugler I, et al 1993.[29]

the ventricle.[33–36] Potential mechanisms include preservation of myocardium by early reperfusion resulting in a smaller infarct less likely to undergo remodelling. However, later reperfusion, beyond the stage when there is much potential for myocardial salvage, also seems to protect against dilatation. The mechanism probably relates to improved infarct healing in the presence of a patent artery. Whatever the mechanism, attenuation of ventricular dilatation is a further benefit from a patent infarct-related artery, and underscores the importance of attempting to achieve reperfusion particularly in all large infarcts.

Prevention of infarct expansion and remodelling

The process of remodelling is probably largely a physical phenomenon related to the increased loads on the various segments of the heart. Reducing these loads by reducing both pre-load and afterload can attenuate the process. Thus, control of left ventricular failure and of systemic hypertension post-infarction are critical. In addition, research is only just starting to unravel the complex cellular processes associated with fibrosis and hypertrophy, but the renin-angiotensin system appears to play a major role. This involves both angiotensin II and probably aldosterone.

In keeping with these concepts, ACE inhibitors have been shown to attenuate the remodelling process. There have now been several studies documenting a lesser degree of ventricular enlargement post-infarction in patients treated with ACE inhibitors[37–41] (see Ch. 33). The effect is not restricted to ACE inhibitors, since nitrates can also attenuate the remodelling process and consequent volume expansion[42,43] (see Ch. 30). This suggests that favorable modification of the loading conditions by drugs may be the most important mechanism for this benefit.

Whatever the mechanism whereby ACE inhibitors influence remodelling, there are now demonstrated mortality benefits from ACE inhibitors post-infarction (see Ch. 33). The largest and most clear-cut benefits from a statistical viewpoint have occurred in those trials treating a small subset of post-infarct patients at high risk.[19,44] These trials have demonstrated a 20–30% reduction in mortality, persisting for several years. In the SAVE trial, which enrolled patients with LV dysfunction but without overt LV failure, the benefit became apparent only after around 12 months' therapy. The mortality benefit appeared to be mediated in large part through attenuation of volume expansion.[32] In the AIRE study, which enrolled patients with evidence of LV failure, the benefit was apparent somewhat earlier. Since remodelling starts early and ACE inhibitors can be safely introduced early, there seems little reason to delay their introduction in a patient likely to benefit.

References

1. Falk E. Atherogenesis and thrombosis. In: Califf RM, Mark DB, Wagner GS (eds). Acute coronary care. 2nd ed. St Louis: Mosby Press, 1995:3–13
2. Davies MJ, Bland JM, Hangartner JRW et al. Factors influencing the presence or absence of acute coronary artery thrombi in sudden ischaemic death. Eur Heart J 1989;10:203–8
3. Mizuno K, Miyamoto A, Satomura K et al. Angioscopic coronary macromorphology in

patients with acute coronary disorders. Lancet 1991;337:809–912
4. DeWood M, Spores J, Notske R et al. Prevalence of total coronary occlusion during the early hours of transmural myocardial infarction. N Engl J Med 1980; 303: 897–902
5. Sabia PJ, Powers ER, Ragosta M et al. An association between collateral blood flow and myocardial viability in patients with recent myocardial infarction. N Engl J Med 1992;327:1825–31
6. Marcus ML. The coronary circulation in health and disease. New York: McGraw-Hill, 1983
7. Braunwald E, Rutherford JD. Reversible ischemic left ventricular dysfunction: evidence for the 'hibernating myocardium'. J Am Coll Cardiol 1986;8:1467–70
8. Braunwald E, Kloner RA. The stunned myocardium: prolonged postischemic ventricular dysfunction. Circulation 1982;66:1146–9
9. Bolli R, Zhu WX, Thronby JL et al. Time-course and determinants of recovery of function after reversible ischemia in conscious dogs. Am J Physiol 1988; 254: H102–H104
10. Reimer KA, Jennings RB. The 'wavefront' phenomenon of myocardial ischemic cell death. Lab Invest 1979; 40: 633–44
11. Weisman HF, Healy B Myocardial infarct expansion, infarct extension, and reinfarction: pathophysiologic concepts. Prog Cardiovasc Dis 1987; 30: 73–110
12. Haber HL, Beller GA, Watson DD et al. Exercise thallium-201 scintigraphy after thrombolytic therapy with or without angioplasty for acute myocardial infarction. Am J Cardiol 1993; 71(15): 1257–61
13. Krucoff MW, Ohman EM, Trollinger KM et al. Noninvasive definition of failed reperfusion at the bedside: looking beyond the tip of the catheter. In: Califf RM, Mark DB, Wagner GS (eds). Acute coronary care. 2nd ed. St Louis: Mosby Press, 1995: 443–68
14. Veldkamp RF, Green CL, Wilkins ML et al. for the Thrombolysis and Angioplasty in Myocardial Infarction (TAMI)-7 Study Group: Comparison of continuous ST-segment recovery analysis with methods using static electrocardiograms for noninvasive patency assessment during acute myocardial infarction. Am J Cardiol 1994; 73: 1069–74
15. Califf RM, O'Neill W, Stack RS et al. and the TAMI Study Group: Failure of simple clinical measurements to predict perfusion status after intravenous thrombolysis. Ann Int Med 1988; 108: 658–62
16. Killip T, Kimbal JT. Treatment of myocardial infarction in a coronary care unit: a two year experience with 250 patients. Am J Cardiol 1967; 20: 457
17. Forrester JS, Diamond GA, Chatterjee K, Swan HJ. Medical therapy of acute myocardial infarction by application of hemodynamic subsets (Pt I). N Engl J Med 1976; 295: 1356–62
18. Forrester JS, Diamond GA, Chatterjee K, Swan HJ. Medical therapy of acute myocardial infarction by application of hemodynamic subsets (Pt II). N Engl J Med 1976; 295: 1404–23
19. The Acute Infarction Ramipril Efficacy (AIRE) Study Investigators. Effect of ramipril on mortality and morbidity of survivors of acute myocardial infarction with clinical evidence of heart failure. Lancet 1993; 342: 821–8
20. Wilson VE, Bates ER. Right ventricular myocardial infarction. In: Califf RM, Mark DB, Wagner GS (ed). Acute coronary care. 2nd ed. St Louis: Mosby Press, 1995: 741–53
21. Hutchins GM, Bulkley BH. Infarct expansion versus extension: two different complications of acute myocardial infarction. Am J Cardiol 1978; 41: 1127–32
22. Jeremy RW, Allman KC, Bautovich G, Harris PJ. Patterns of left ventricular dilatation during the six months after myocardial infarction. J Am Coll Cardiol 1989; 13: 304–10
23. Pfeffer MA, Braunwald E. Ventricular remodelling after myocardial infarction. Circulation 1990; 81: 1161–72
24. Pfeffer MA, Braunwald E (eds). Symposium. Ventricular remodelling and unloading following myocardial infarction. Am J Cardiol 1991; 68: 1D–131D
25. Zardini P, Marino P, Golia G et al. Ventricular remodelling and infarct expansion. Am J Cardiol 1993; 72: 98G–106G
26. Cohn JN. Structural basis for heart failure. Ventricular remodelling and its pharmacological inhibition. Circulation 1995; 91: 2504–7
27. McKay RG, Pfeffer MA, Pasternak RC et al. Left ventricular remodelling after myocardial infarction: a corollary to infarct expansion. Circulation 1986; 74: 693–702
28. Mitchell GF, Lamas GA, Vaughan DE et al. Left ventricular remodelling in the year after first anterior myocardial infarction: a quantitative analysis of contractile segment lengths and ventricular shape. J Am Coll Cardiol 1992; 19: 1136–44
29. Gaudron P, Eilles C, Kugler I et al. Progressive left ventricular dysfunction and remodelling after myocardial infarction: potential mechanisms and early predictors. Circulation 1993; 98: 755–63
30. Hammermeister KE, DeRouen TA, Dodge HT. Variables predictive of survival with coronary disease: selection by univariate and multivariate analyses from the clinical, electrocardiographic, exercise, arteriographic and quantitative angiographic evalua-

tions. Circulation 1979; 59: 421–50
31. White HD, Norris RM, Brown MA et al. Left ventricular end-systolic volume as the major determinant of survival after recovery from myocardial infarction. Circulation 1987; 76: 44–51
32. Sutton MSJ, Pfeffer MA, Plappert T et al., for the SAVE investigators. Quantitative two-dimensional echocardiographic measurements are major predictors of adverse cardiovascular events after acute myocardial infarction: the protective effects of captopril. Circulation 1994; 89: 68–75
33. Hochman JS, Choo H. Limitation of myocardial infarct expansion by reperfusion independent of myocardial salvage. Circulation 1987; 75: 299
34. Jeremy RW, Hackworthy RA, Bautovich G et al. Infarct artery perfusion and changes in left ventricular volume in the month after acute myocardial infarction. J Am Coll Cardiol 1987; 9: 989–95
35. Warren SE, Royal HD, Markis JE et al. Time course of left ventricular dilatation after myocardial infarction: Influence of infarct-related artery and success of coronary thrombolysis. J Am Coll Cardiol 1988; 11: 12
36. Shen WF, Lian QC, Gong LS et al. Beneficial effect of residual flow to the infarct region on left ventricular volume changes after acute myocardial infarction. Am Heart J 1990; 119: 525–9
37. Pfeffer MA, Lamas GA, Vaughan DE et al. Effect of captopril on progressive ventricular dilatation after anterior myocardial infarction. New Engl J Med 1988; 319: 80–6
38. Sharpe N, Smith H, Murphy J, Greaves S, Hart H, Gamble G. Early prevention of left ventricular dysfunction following myocardial infarction with angiotensin converting enzyme inhibition. Lancet 1991; 337: 872–6
39. Konstam MA, Rousseau MF, Kronenberg MW et al., for the SOLVD investigators. Effects of the angiotensin converting enzyme inhibitor enalapril on the long-term progression of left ventricular dysfunction in patients with heart failure. Circulation 1992; 86: 431–8
40. Pouleur H, Rousseau MF, van Eyll C et al., for the SOLVD investigators. Effects of long-term enalapril therapy on left ventricular diastolic properties in patients with depressed ejection fraction. Circulation 1993; 88: 481–91
41. Greenberg B, Quinones MA, Koilpillai C et al., for the SOLVD Investigators. Effects of long-term enalapril therapy on cardiac structure and function in patients with left ventricular dysfunction: results of the SOLVD echocardiography substudy. Circulation 1995; 91: 2573–81
42. Jugdutt BI, Warnica JW. Intravenous nitroglycerin therapy to limit myocardial infarct size, expansion and complications. Effect of timing, dosage and infarct location. Circulation 1988; 78: 906–19
43. Jugdutt BI. Effects of nitrate therapy on ventricular remodelling and function. Am J Cardiol 1993; 72: 161G–168G
44. Pfeffer MA, Braunwald E, Moye LA et al. Effect of captopril on mortality and morbidity in patients with left ventricular dysfunction after myocardial infarction: results of the Survival and Ventricular Enlargement Trial. N Engl J Med 1992; 327: 669–77

9 Pathophysiology of post-infarction ventricular arrhythmias

Andrew M Tonkin

Introduction

There has been appropriate emphasis recently upon the need for prompt presentation after the onset of myocardial infarction (MI) to maximize the beneficial effects of thrombolysis or coronary angioplasty in salvaging myocardial tissue. However, the major cause of early mortality after acute myocardial infarction (AMI) is still life-threatening ventricular arrhythmias. Although the immediate recognition and treatment of potentially lethal arrhythmias in CCUs has reduced mortality from such arrhythmias, many deaths still occur before the patient reaches hospital. In particular, the risk of ventricular fibrillation is highest in the early hours after the initial onset of infarction, necessitating adequate counselling about the need for early presentation of patients who are known to have coronary heart disease. Also, analysis of Holter monitor recordings has shown that out-of-hospital cardiac arrest and sudden death in the chronic phase after MI is usually due to sustained monomorphic ventricular tachycardia which often degenerates into ventricular fibrillation.[1]

Arrhythmias are often discussed within the framework of the underlying substrate (such as the functional changes resulting from acute ischaemia, or a pre-existing anatomical abnormality such as MI), the trigger (such as ventricular premature beats) and modulating factors (such as the autonomic nervous system, electrolyte abnormalities such as hypokalaemia, and drug effects).[2] However, the relative importance of these concepts has been reappraised after the disappointing results of a major recent trial of antiarrhythmic drugs aimed at suppression of ventricular premature beats.[3] More attention must be given to anatomical and functional abnormalities of the myocardium, and to the role of modulating factors.

This chapter discusses basic electrophysiological properties of the heart, and general and more specific mechanisms of arrhythmias following myocardial ischaemia and infarction. More detailed discussion will be restricted to ventricular arrhythmias.

Basic cardiac electrophysiology

The cardiac action potential has five phases: phase 0 (the upstroke due to rapid depolarization), phase 1 (early rapid depolarization), phase 2 (the plateau), phase 3 (rapid repolarization), and phase 4 (resting membrane potential and possible diastolic depolarization) (see Fig. 9.1).

These phases reflect many ion fluxes through specific channels in the cell membrane. These different protein or phospholipid channels are selective, favouring a particular ion. Some channels operate because of binding of transmitters to the extracellular site ('receptor-operated') while others respond to voltage change ('voltage-operated'). The following brief discussion is very simplified as these concepts are now recognized to be complex. They have been reviewed recently elsewhere.[4–7]

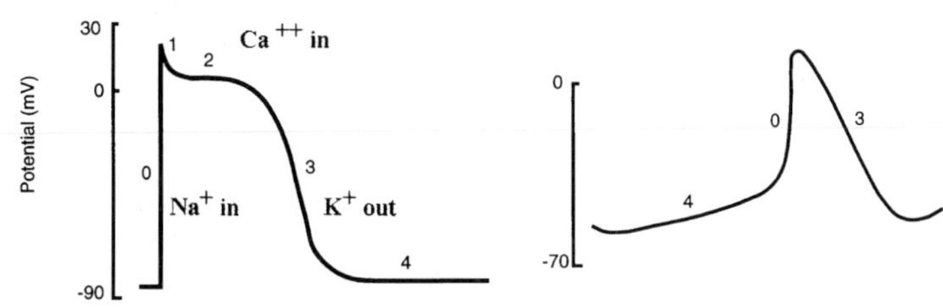

Fig. 9.1 Schematic representation of the 'fast' action potentials as found in working myocardial cells (left) and of 'slow' action potentials as found in nodal tissue (right).

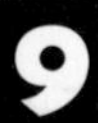

9 Pathophysiology

In normal atrial and ventricular myocardium and in His-Purkinje tissue, action potentials have a very rapid upstroke ('fast responses'). This is mediated by the fast inward sodium channel (I_{Na+}). Action potentials in the sinus and atrioventricular nodes have a slow upstroke ('slow responses'). The upstroke of the slow response is mediated by a slow inward current, carried principally by calcium (Ca^{++}). There are at least two types of Ca^{++} currents; a high threshold dihydropyridine-sensitive current which is slowly inactivating (slow or L-type) and a fast inactivating, low-threshold dihydropyridine-insensitive current (fast or T-type).

Phase 3 or final rapid repolarization depends on at least two currents: time-dependent inactivation of the slow inward current, and activation of an outward potassium (K) current (I_{K+}). I_{K+} itself has a number of components, including one which is rapidly activated and reaches a steady state during the course of the action potential, and is blocked by most antiarrhythmic drugs, and another which is slowly activated, increased by isoprenaline (and possibly the predominant K^+ current during conditions of increased sympathetic activity) and not blocked by most class III antiarrhythmic drugs. These different K^+ currents and their differential blockade may explain some variability between effects of class III antiarrhythmic agents.

General mechanisms of arrhythmias

General mechanisms of arrhythmias are indicated in the box below. These are now discussed.

Normal and abnormal automaticity

The sinus node is normally dominant among the hierarchy of pacemakers in the specific cardiac conduction system. This results from its greater rate of spontaneous phase 4 depolarization. However, the ionic mechanism(s) underlying spontaneous diastolic depolarization, the pacemaker potential of the sinus node, remain controversial. One view proposes that the decay in the outward current I_{K+} (activated during repolarization) and activation of inward T- and L-type Ca^{++} currents (during the later part of pacemaker depolarization) are operative.[8] In a contrasting view, I_f (an inward current activated upon hyperpolarization and carried by Na^+ and K^+) is considered to be the dominant current responsible for the pacemaker potential.[9]

Although the sinus node is normally the dominant pacemaker, pacemaker cells in the middle and lower regions of the AV node, the His bundle and Purkinje tissue can also demonstrate automaticity, although their effects are usually 'overdriven' by the sinus node, or because of electrotonic depolarization from adjacent fibres. Such subsidiary pacemakers can generate *automatic* impulses, not only because of slowing in the rate of discharge of the sinus node, but because entrance block may 'protect' these other pacemakers from activation by the sinus node. The rate of discharge of a latent subsidiary pacemaker can also increase inappropriately, particularly in cells with reduced maximum diastolic potential as may occur with ischaemia.

Triggered activity

Triggered activity refers to pacemaker activity that results consequent upon a preceding impulse or series of impulses; 'afterdepolarizations' are oscillations in the transmembrane

General mechanisms of arrhythmias

Disorders of impulse formation

- Automaticity
  - Normal, e.g. inappropriate sinus tachycardia, sinus bradycardia
  - Abnormal, e.g. accelerated idioventricular rhythm after MI
- Triggered activity
  - Early afterdepolarizations, e.g. torsades de pointes
  - Delayed afterdepolarizations, e.g. possibly some tachyarrhythmias associated with digitalis toxicity

Disorders of impulse conduction

- Unidirectional block with re-entry, e.g. ventricular fibrillation, ventricular tachycardia late after MI
- Without re-entry, e.g. atrioventricular block, bundle branch block

potential that are induced by the preceding action potential.

Early afterdepolarizations occur during phase 2 or 3 of the action potential, before or after full repolarization. During phase 2, they may be caused particularly by the effect of catecholamines in increasing the inward current related to L-type Ca^{++} channels:[10] in phase 3 (for example, in presence of class III antiarrhythmic drugs[11]) they relate to delayed repolarization because of decrease in I_{K+}. The amplitude of early afterdepolarization increases at *slow* stimulation rates and arrhythmias are more likely to arise during bradycardia or following a pause.

Late or delayed afterdepolarizations interrupt the normally quiescent transmembrane potential after full repolarization (phase 4). They are due to a transient inward current carried primarily by sodium (Na^+) that is normally small or absent (I_{Ti}), and intracellular Ca^{++} overload in conditions such as digitalis toxicity, increased catecholamine levels, ischaemia and myocardial stretch.[12] As stimulation rate *increases*, delayed afterdepolarizations increase in magnitude.

Triggered activity could be the mechanism of some cases of 'benign' ventricular ectopic activity, but particularly polymorphic ventricular tachycardia and possibly ventricular fibrillation.

Conduction abnormalities

Factors which may result in conduction delay or block can relate to both active and passive[13] membrane properties. Conduction velocity is slower and propagation may fail when repolarization is from a less negative transmembrane potential, possibly consequent upon ischaemia. Important determinants of conduction are the nature of the propagating impulse, and excitability and other properties of the tissue into which propagation is occurring.

Re-entry

Re-entry[14] is the mechanism of the great majority of arrhythmias which are clinically significant, including ventricular fibrillation and most cases of ventricular tachycardia. There are three major types of re-entry: anatomic, functional and anisotropic.

The anatomic model of re-entry involves a fixed abnormality such as previous MI. Following development of unidirectional block, and sufficiently delayed conduction and/or long conduction path through the remainder of the circuit, the area of initial block can recover excitability.[14] This can be followed by continued propagation about the re-entrant circuit, the size of which determines the rate of re-entry. In the anatomic model of re-entry, an excitable gap exists between the tail of refractoriness and the head of the propagating impulse.

However, re-entry without anatomical boundaries ('functional re-entry') can occur in relatively small areas of tissue in contiguous fibres that have functionally different and constantly changing electrophysiological properties. The 'leading circle' hypothesis,[15] applied particularly to fibrillation in which there are multiple wavelets, proposes that re-entry propagates around a functionally refractory centre, following a preferential course along fibres that have a shorter refractory period. The wavelength of a functional circuit is determined by the smallest circuit in which the leading wave front is able to excite tissue that is still relatively refractory. Shorter wavelength may predispose to fibrillation. It is considered that there is no excitable gap, with the head of the impulse always encroaching on the tail of refractoriness.

It is now appreciated that anisotropy may also be an important cause of re-entry.[16] There is a normal anisotropic structure in the heart. The cell membranes of many adjacent cells form close margins and may be in functional contact ('gap junctions'). These gap junctions allow low-resistance electrical coupling between cells at the longitudinal ends, but have higher resistance (and cell-to-cell connections are less and may not exist) in the transverse direction. Thus in the normal situation conduction is faster in myocardial tissue in the direction of the long axis of the myocardial fibre than perpendicular to this. However (and seemingly paradoxically) premature impulses may block more readily when propagating along the long axis than perpendicular to it.[17]

Following previous MI, fibrosis may make conduction even more difficult. The orientation of fibres becomes disarrayed as the muscle bands separate, and there are fewer connections between muscle bundles. In this situation, the myocardial fibres can have normal action potentials[16] but not propagate effectively, or follow a longer circuit between surviving

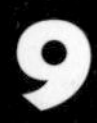

myocardial fibres surrounded by fibrotic tissue.

The mechanisms of the major clinical arrhythmias are now considered in the temporal sequence in which they usually occur.

Acute ischaemia: ventricular fibrillation

Ischaemia following coronary artery occlusion has a number of major effects on electrophysiological properties of myocardial cells which may lead to random re-entry and ventricular fibrillation.[18,19] Information is derived almost exclusively from studies in animals—a limitation, as no animal model is ideal because of differences in coronary anatomy from humans. The mechanisms have been reviewed extensively elsewhere.[20]

In experimental studies, within minutes of coronary occlusion, resting membrane potential falls from approximately −80 mV to −60 mV. This is related at least partly to net increase in extracellular K^+.[21] The accumulation of extracellular potassium occurs in two phases: the first rapidly reversible when reperfusion occurs within 15 minutes, the second after approximately 10–20 minutes during which resting potential remains relatively constant, most likely due to irreversible cell damage.[20] The cause of the net accumulation of extracellular K^+ is not completely understood, but may be multifactorial. Possible mechanisms include depression of Na^+-K^+ pump, the effects of (amphipathic) lipid metabolites with membrane disruption, and intracellular Ca^{++} overload.[20,22]

Within a few minutes of coronary artery occlusion the amplitude, conduction velocity and duration of ventricular myocardial action potentials also decrease. Theoretically, the decreased amplitude and velocity of depolarization in phase 0 could be caused either by reduction in I_{Na+} or be mediated by the slow inward Ca^{++} current. However, at least during the early period after ischaemia, there is reasonable evidence that the reduced upstroke of the action potential (and important slowing of conduction velocity) is caused by depressed inward flux through partially inactivated Na^+ channels. One line of supporting evidence is the finding that lignocaine[23] but not verapamil[24] depresses or abolishes action potentials recorded in experimental preparations from the centre of an ischaemic zone.

The decrease in amplitude and conduction velocity of myocardial action potentials cannot be attributed only to inactivation of Na^+ channels because of the decrease in resting potential. Other factors resulting from ischaemia which probably contribute include hypoxia, acidosis, high PCO_2 and accumulation of substances such as fatty acid metabolites and catecholamines.

Coronary occlusion results in a biphasic change in action potential duration. However, recordings have sometimes been from the epicardial surface and then the initial slight increase may be due to slight temperature reduction in the subepicardial muscle layers. Subsequently, the major effect is non-uniform shortening of action potential duration, particularly in epicardial tissues. This relates to a number of effects including that of ischaemia on ATP-sensitive K^+ channels. The refractory period of ventricular myocardial tissue also shortens, probably not only because of shortening in action potential duration. In normal tissue, recovery of excitability is primarily voltage-dependent. However, ischaemic fibres may be inexcitable even after complete repolarization ('post-repolarization refractoriness') probably related to decrease in resting maximum diastolic potential. Particularly in the chronic situation but also early following ischaemia, there has been interest in the analysis of QT dispersion as a measure of the dispersion of refractoriness.[25]

Inhomogeneity in extracellular K^+ (particularly in the 'border zone' between normal and ischaemic myocardium) may also contribute to the potential for arrhythmias following ischaemia. This leads to inhomogeneity in membrane potential, action potential duration and refractoriness.

Although in fibrillation the traditional thinking has been that there is no excitable gap, recently it has been shown in both atrial[26] and ventricular[27] fibrillation that it is possible to capture myocardial tissue with stimulation during a very short time window.

In summary, following myocardial ischaemia the changes underlying the development of multiple re-entrant circuits and ventricular fibrillation are membrane depolarization, reduced upstroke velocity and amplitude of the action potential with slow conduction, and shortening of refractoriness, particularly if inhomogeneous.

Reperfusion arrhythmias

Reperfusion arrhythmias could occur in patients following spontaneous or drug-induced thrombolysis or coronary angioplasty. Again relevant information is derived almost exclusively from experimental preparations. This may be a limitation because although accelerated idioventricular rhythm and non-sustained ventricular tachycardia are common in humans after presumed reperfusion, life-threatening arrhythmias such as ventricular fibrillation appear to be relatively rare and trials have shown no difference between those receiving thrombolytic agents and placebo.

In experimental studies, the occurrence of reperfusion arrhythmias is related to the length and severity of ischaemia, increasing as the duration of occlusion increases up to approximately 30 minutes, but then decreasing when reperfusion occurs after this. This is most likely because of irreversible cell damage, as some viability is necessary for re-entry to occur. Also, in animals there are two different periods of arrhythmias. The first, which often results in ventricular fibrillation, occurs immediately after reperfusion and is apparently due to re-entry. Reperfusion is accompanied by increased inhomogeneity of action potential duration in and around the previous ischaemic zone, and other changes which predispose to re-entry. The later phase is possibly related to triggered activity[28] or enhanced automaticity, resulting in ventricular premature beats or ventricular tachycardia. These mechanisms may relate to intracellular Ca^{++} overload, oxygen free radicals or other effects including changes in K^+ currents.[29]

Ventricular tachycardia in the chronic phase after myocardial infarction

Observations in experimental animals have been presented earlier in relation to other arrhythmias. However, it is in the clinical context of post-infarction ventricular tachycardia that the most information from patients is available. Findings have been obtained both during catheter electrophysiology study and arrhythmia surgery.

The mechanism is usually considered to be macro-re-entry about definite anatomical circuits related to previous infarction. Anisotropy may be important. Evidence supporting the role of re-entry is provided by the initiation and termination of ventricular tachycardia in patients using programmed electrical stimulation.[30] Other evidence has been obtained by recording of low voltage, fractionated electrograms during sinus rhythm at sites which are activated early during tachycardia,[31] implying marked local conduction delay and inhomogenous conduction properties. Also, recording of electrograms and the success of endocardial resection in preventing further episodes, suggests that ventricular tachycardia in this context usually originates in the subendocardial region at the border zone of scar tissue, with re-entry about tracts of surviving myocardial tissue within areas of fibrosis.[32]

Role of the sympathetic nervous system

There is very good evidence that increased sympathetic nervous activity contributes to ventricular arrhythmias, both in animals and patients. Ischaemia is associated with increased levels of catecholamines, and these have multiple effects both directly on electrophysiological properties of myocardial cells and also more generally by increased Na^+-K^+ pump activity which itself increases resting membrane potential. Also, infarction may cause denervation distal to the area of ischaemia, resulting in 'supersensitivity' of these tissues.

As a consequence of increased catecholamine levels, serum K^+ falls ('stress-induced' hypokalaemia) early after MI due to increased activity of Na^+-K^+-dependent ATPase activity and shift of K^+ from the vascular compartment to extravascular tissues, particularly in skeletal muscle.[33] The degree of hypokalaemia can be related to the prevalence of all ventricular arrhythmias following AMI, including ventricular fibrillation.[34]

Other 'indirect' effects contributing to arrhythmogenesis

Myocardial fibre stretch and increased ventricular volume,[35] and other morphologic characteristics such as hypertrophy,[36] can have important electrophysiological effects and are associated with a greatly increased risk of sudden death. This suggests that appropriate management of these other aspects such as left ventricular dysfunction (for example with vasodilators) could potentially have significant impact upon life-threatening ventricular arrhythmias and sudden death. The concept of the interplay between structural, functional and neural control elements and potential mechanisms of arrhythmias in coronary heart disease is summarized in Table 9.1.

Furthermore, 30-year follow-up data from the Framingham study[37] showed that the risk factors for sudden death were the same as those for coronary heart disease in general. Therefore, the global problem of sudden death ultimately may be most effectively addressed by measures directed towards primary as well as secondary prevention of coronary artery disease and myocardial infarction.

References

1. Nikolic G, Bishop RL, Singh JB. Sudden death during Holter monitoring. Circulation 1982; 66: 218–25
2. Coumel P. The management of clinical arrhythmias: an overview of invasive versus non-invasive electrophysiology. Eur Heart J 1987; 8: 92–9
3. Cardiac Arrhythmia Suppression Trial (CAST) Investigators. Preliminary report: effect of encainide and flecainide on mortality in a randomized trial of arrhythmia suppression after myocardial infarction. N Engl J Med 1989; 32: 406–12
4. Clapham D. Intracellular regulation of ion channels. In: Zipes DP, Jolife J (eds). Cardiac electrophysiology: from cell to bedside. Philadelphia: WB Saunders, 1990: 85–94
5. Zipes D. Genesis of cardiac arrhythmias: electrophysiological considerations. In: Braunwald E (ed). Heart disease: a textbook of cardiovascular medicine, 4th ed. Philadelphia: WB Saunders, 1992: 588–627
6. The Task Force of the Working Group on Arrhythmias of the European Society of Cardiology: The Sicilian Gambit. A new approach to the classification of antiarrhythmic drugs based on their actions on arrhythmogenic mechanisms. Eur Heart J 1991; 12(10): 1112–31
7. Noble D. The ionic basis of the heart beat and the cardiac arrythmias. In: Singh BN, Wellens HJJ, Hiraoka M (eds). Electropharmacological control of cardiac arrhythmias: to delay conduction or prolong refractoriness. New York: Futura, 1994: 1–20
8. Irisawa, H, Brown HCF, Giles W. Cardiac pacemaking in the sinoatrial node. Physiol Rev 1993; 73: 197–227
9. DiFrancesco D. Pacemaker mechanisms in cardiac tissue. Ann Rev Physiol 1993; 55: 455–72
10. January CT, Riddle JM, Salata JJ. A model for early afterdepolarisations: induction with the Ca^{++} channel agonist Bay K 8644. Circ Res 1988; 62: 563–70
11. Brachman J, Scherlag B, Rosenshkraukh IV, Lazzara R. Bradycardia—dependent triggered activity: relevance to drug-induced multiform ventricular tachycardia. Circulation 1983; 68: 846–53
12. Wit AL, Rosen MR. Afterdepolarisations and triggered activity. In: Fozzard HA, Haber E, Jenning RB et al. (eds). The heart and cardiovascular system. New York: Raven Press, 1986: 1449–90
13. Pressler ML. Passive electrical properties of cardiac tissue. In: Zipes DP, Jolife J (eds). Cardiac electrophysiology: from cell to bedside. Philadelphia: WB Saunders, 1990; 108–21
14. Mines GR. On dynamic equilibrium in the heart. J Physiol 1913; 46: 349–482
15. Allessie MA, Bonke FIM, Schopman FJG. Circus movement in rabbit atrial muscle as a mechanism of tachycardia (Pt III). The 'leading circle' concept: a new model of circus movement in cardiac tissue without the involvement of an anatomical obstacle. Circ Res 1977; 41: 9–18

Table 9.1 The interplay between structural, functional and sympathetic abnormalities and arrhythmia mechanisms

	Re-entry	EAD	DAD	ABN AUT
Structural	+			
Scar	+			
Fibrosis	+			
Dilatation	+		+	
Hypertrophy	+	+	+	
Ischaemia				+
Functional				
Increased wall stress			+	
Increased diastolic pressure			+	
Neural control				
Sympathetic activation	+	+	+	+

(EAD = early afterdepolarizations, DAD = delayed afterdepolarizations, ABN AUT = abnormal automaticity, + = effect).

16. Wit AL, Dillon S. Anisotropic reentry. In: Zipes DP, Jolife J (eds). Cardiac electrophysiology: from cell to bedside. Philadelphia: WB Saunders, 1990; 353–64
17. Spach MS, Miller WT, Dolber PC, Kootsey JM, Summer JR, Moscher CE. The functional role of structural complexities in the propagation of depolarisation in the atrium of the dog: cardiac conduction disturbances due to discontinuities of effective axial resistivity. Circ Res 1982; 50:175–91
18. Wit AL, Bigger JT Jr. Possible electrophysiological mechanisms for lethal arrhythmias accompanying ischaemia and infarction. Circulation 1975; 52 (6 Suppl.): III96–115
19. Janse MJ, Kleber AG. Electrophysiological changes and ventricular arrhythmias in the early phase of regional myocardial ischaemia. Circ Res 1981; 49: 1069–81
20. Janse MJ, Wit AL. Electrophysiological mechanisms of ventricular arrhythmias resulting from myocardial ischaemia and infarction. Physiol Rev 1989; 69: 1049–69
21. Weiss J, Shine KJ. Extracellular K^+ accumulation during myocardial ischaemia in isolated rabbit heart. Am J Physiol 1982; 242: H619–28
22. Creer MH, Dobmeyer DJ, Corr PB. Amphipathic lipid metabolites and arrhythmias during myocardial ischaemia. In: Zipes DP, Jolife J (eds.) Cardiac electrophysiology: from cell to bedside. Philadelphia: WB Saunders, 1990; 417–33
23. Brennan FJ, Cranefield PF, Wit AL. Effects of lidocaine on slow response and depressed fast fibers. J Pharmacol Exp Ther 1978; 204: 312–24
24. Gilmour RF, Zipes DP. Electrophysiological response of vascularized hamster cardiac transplants to ischaemia. Circ Res 1982; 50: 599–609
25. Surawicz B. Dispersion of refractoriness in ventricular arrhythmias. In: Zipes DP, Jolife J (eds.) Cardiac electrophysiology: from cell to bedside. Philadelphia: WB Saunders, 1990; 377–85
26. Allessie MA, Kirchhof C, Scheffer GJ et al. Regional control of atrial fibrillation by rapid pacing in conscious dogs. Circulation 1991; 84: 1689–97
27. Knight BH, Bayly PV, Gerstle RJ et al. Regional capture of fibrillating right ventricular myocardium: Evidence of an excitable gap in VF using high resolution cardiac mapping. J Am Coll Cardiol (in press)
28. Priori SG, Corr PB. Mechanisms underlying early and delayed afterdepolarisations induced by catecholamines. Am J Physiol 1990; 258: H1796–805
29. Hearse DJ, Tosaki A. Free radicals and calcium: simultaneous interacting triggers as determinants of vulnerability to reperfusion-induced arrhythmias in the rat heart. J Mol Cell Cardiol 1988; 20: 213–23
30. Wellens HJJ, Schuilenburg RM, Durrer D. Electrical stimulation of the heart in patients with ventricular tachycardia. Circulation 1972; 46: 216
31. Josephson ME, Horowitz LN, Farshidi A. Continuous local electrical activity: a mechanism of recurrent ventricular tachycardia. Circulation 1978; 57: 659–65
32. Harken AH, Horowitz LN, Josephson ME. Comparison of standard aneurysmectomy and aneurysmectomy with directed endocardial resection for the treatment of recurrent sustained ventricular tachycardia. J Thorac Cardiovasc Surg 1980; 80: 527–34
33. Brown MJ, Brown DC, Murphy MB. Hypokalaemia from beta 2-receptor stimulation by circulating epinephrines. N Engl J Med 1983; 309: 1414–9
34. Nordrehaug JE, Von der Lippe G. Hypokalaemia and ventricular fibrillation in acute myocardial infarction. Br Heart J 1983; 50: 525–9
35. Reiter MJ, Synhorst DP, Mann DE. Electrophysiological effects of acute ventricular dilatation in the isolated rabbit heart. Circ Res 1988; 62: 554–62
36. Kohya I, Kimura S, Myerburg RJ et al. Susceptibility of hypertrophied rat hearts to ventricular fibrillation during acute ischaemia. J Mol Cell Cardiol 1988; 20: 159–68
37. Kannel WB, Plehn JF, Couples LA. Cardiac failure and sudden death in the Framingham study. Am Heart J 1988; 870–5

10 Pathophysiology of cardiac failure

Peter Macdonald

Introduction

Heart failure is a common condition which has been estimated to affect between 1 and 2% of the population.[1] Many clinicians have the impression that heart failure is a relatively benign illness which runs a gradually progressive course over many years. The reality is in fact the opposite. Heart failure carries a prognosis which is worse than that of most cancers. The majority of heart failure sufferers will die within 5 years of diagnosis, with most patients dying suddenly or following an abrupt worsening of symptoms.[1] Apart from its impact on mortality, heart failure causes disabling symptoms and accounts for up to 5% of all admissions to a general hospital.[2] Heart failure is most prevalent in the elderly, in whom it markedly impairs quality of life and independence. The economic cost of heart failure in the USA has been calculated to be more than $8 billion per year.[3]

Definition

Heart failure may be defined as a syndrome in which the heart is unable to pump a sufficient cardiac output to meet the metabolic requirements of the body, or can only do so at an abnormally elevated filling pressure.

Acute versus chronic heart failure

Heart failure is a complex syndrome. The vast majority of patients with heart failure admitted to a coronary care unit (CCU) have myocardial dysfunction secondary to ischaemic heart disease as the underlying cause. In this context, heart failure may occur as an *acute* syndrome precipitated by extensive acute myocardial ischaemia or infarction which results in a sudden impairment of both systolic and diastolic function. In some patients, complications of acute myocardial infarction (AMI) such as cardiac arrhythmias, papillary muscle rupture or ventricular septal rupture may result in acute and often catastrophic heart failure.

Heart failure secondary to ischaemic heart disease or other causes may also present as a *chronic* syndrome. In these patients permanent structural changes have occurred in the heart resulting in ventricular dilatation and remodelling (see below) together with long term changes in the peripheral vasculature, other organs and skeletal muscle. Patients with chronic heart failure usually have stable symptoms while on appropriate treatment, but they may also present with acute deterioration. In such patients a number of acute precipitating factors should always be considered. These are summarized in the box.

Acute precipitants of heart failure

- Acute myocardial ischaemia/infarction
- New onset arrhythmia
- Intercurrent infection, particularly pulmonary
- Non-compliance—missed anti-failure medication, excess dietary salt
- New drug therapies including those with negative inotropic properties (e.g. beta blockers, some calcium antagonists, some antiarrhythmic drugs) or drugs that cause fluid retention (e.g. non-steroidal anti-inflammatory drugs)
- Acute pulmonary embolism

Structural changes within the failing heart

When the prevalence of heart failure is examined in the general community, the two most common antecedent cardiovascular diseases are ischaemic heart disease and systemic hypertension.[4] With both these diseases the brunt of the injury falls on the left ventricle, which usually fails before the right ventricle.

Ischaemic heart disease causes left ventricular dysfunction predominantly through the development of left ventricular infarction and dilatation. Following AMI the ventricle undergoes a process of healing with remodelling (see Ch.9). Within hours to days of the onset of the myocardial infarct, thinning and bulging of the infarct zone occurs, a process known as infarct expansion.[5] Over the subsequent weeks to months a process of ventricular remodelling occurs, accompanied by dilatation of the left ventricular cavity due to lengthening of both the infarcted and non-infarcted regions of the ventricle.[6] Thus a cycle of progressive left ventricular dilatation and dysfunction is established which may continue for years after the initial infarct and lead ultimately to terminal heart failure.

Whereas ischaemic heart disease produces heart failure predominantly through ventricular ischaemia and infarction, systemic hypertension produces heart failure through the development of pathological left ventricular hypertrophy (LVH). The mechanism whereby hypertension causes LVH is probably multifactorial. In addition to the direct effect of increased cardiac afterload, there is considerable experimental evidence that the sympathetic nervous system and renin-angiotensin system each play a key role.[7] Noradrenaline and angiotensin II have marked proto-oncogenic effects and stimulate growth of both cardiac myocytes and fibroblasts. The increased interstitial fibrosis produced by activated fibroblasts impairs microvascular perfusion, leading to myocyte ischaemia. Angiotensin II also stimulates intimal hyperplasia and smooth muscle growth, increasing coronary wall thickness, further impeding the diffusion of oxygen between the coronary circulation and the cardiac myocyte. Myocardial ischaemia in combination with interstitial fibrosis results in impaired systolic and diastolic function. Patients with electrocardiographic evidence of LVH are at particularly high risk of developing heart failure.[4]

Pathophysiology of heart failure

Changes in the heart

The structural changes in the failing heart result in impaired contractility and diastolic dysfunction.

Contractility

Contractility may be defined as the intrinsic contractile state of the myocardium independent of pre-load and afterload. It is determined by the number of contractile elements as well as the availability of essential co-factors required for excitation-contraction coupling, in particular cytosolic calcium. Interventions that increase contractility (such as sympathetic stimulation, administration of digitalis compounds) are known as *positive inotropic agents*. On the other hand, agents that reduce contractility (such as beta-blocking drugs and calcium-antagonist drugs) are known as *negative inotropic agents*.

In heart failure, reduced contractility may result from a loss of contractile elements, as occurs in MI or from impaired excitation-contraction coupling. Possible causes for the latter defect include reduced availability of cytosolic calcium,[8] reduced availability of high energy stores[9] or abnormalities in the contractile proteins themselves.[10] The relative importance of these factors in the failing heart is not known.

Diastolic dysfunction

Until recently, the major focus of heart failure management was directed towards the investigation and treatment of abnormal systolic function, i.e. cardiac emptying. It is now recognized that ventricular dysfunction may also be manifested as abnormal diastolic function, that is, cardiac filling. In general terms, diastolic dysfunction may be caused by myocardial ischaemia, hypertrophy, fibrosis or a combination of these processes.[11] Less commonly, diseases of the pericardium may impair cardiac filling and produce heart failure in the absence of ventricular systolic dysfunction. Heart failure due to 'pure' diastolic dysfunction may also be seen in diseases associated with left ventricular hypertrophy. More commonly, systolic and diastolic dysfunction coexist and both contribute to the development and clinical manifestations of heart failure.

Apart from the intrinsic changes in myocardial function just described, the overall performance of the heart as reflected by its cardiac output is critically dependent on the ventricular pre-load and afterload.

Pre-load

The ventricular pre-load may be defined as the intraventricular pressure that passively stretches the myocardium at the end of diastole, called the end-diastolic pressure. As ventricular end-diastolic pressure is progressively increased, there is a corresponding increase in the force of ventricular contraction (and stroke volume) up to an optimal end-diastolic pressure. Further increases in diastolic pressure lead to a fall in stroke volume, probably due to overstretching of the myocardial contractile elements. This relationship between ventricular pre-load and stroke volume is known as the Frank–Starling relationship and is illustrated in Figure 10.1.

The ventricular pre-load is determined by the venous return, which is in turn determined by the venous tone, blood volume and atrial contraction.

The failing heart has a reduced output at any given pre-load compared to the normal heart (point *b* versus point *a*). In a heart with a mild to moderate reduction in contractility, the cardiac output may be restored to normal simply by increasing the ventricular diastolic pressure (point *b* to point b_1, Curve B, Fig. 10.1). Retrograde transmission of the elevated diastolic pressure results in pulmonary venous congestion in the case of left ventricular failure and systemic venous congestion in the case of right ventricular failure. In a heart with severely impaired contractility, for example following massive MI, the cardiac output remains low despite maximal increases in ventricular diastolic pressure (Curve C, Fig. 10.1). Such patients will manifest features of pulmonary or systemic venous congestion and oedema (*backward failure*) as well as features of a reduced cardiac output (*forward failure*).

Cardiogenic shock

Cardiogenic shock is the most severe form of heart failure. In this syndrome, the reduction in cardiac output is so severe that perfusion of vital organs cannot

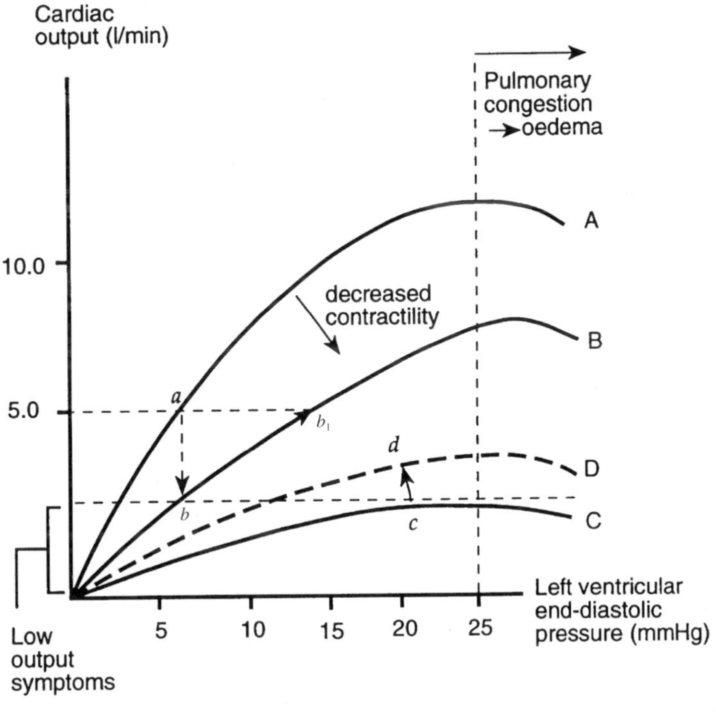

Fig. 10.1 The Frank–Starling relationship between pre-load and stroke volume in ventricular performance. Left ventricular pre-load is plotted as the left ventricular end-diastolic pressure (LVEDP) on the abscissa and ventricular performance as the cardiac output on the ordinate. Curve A shows the relationship for a heart of normal contractility. A reduction in contractility displaces the curve downwards and to the right: curves B and C show the Frank–Starling relationship in hearts with moderate and severe reductions in contractility, respectively. The failing heart has a reduced output at any given pre-load compared to the normal heart (point b versus point a). In a heart with a mild to moderate reduction in contractility, the cardiac output may be restored to normal simply by increasing the ventricular diastolic pressure (point b to point b_1, curve B). In a heart with severely impaired contractility, for example following massive myocardial infarction, the cardiac output remains low despite maximal increases in ventricular diastolic pressure (curve C). A positive inotropic intervention such as administration of a sympathomimetic agent may improve contractility (point c to point d) but at the expense of increased myocardial oxygen consumption. Elevation of the pre-load above a critical level leads to pulmonary and/or systemic congestion irrespective of the cardiac contractility. Conversely, reduction in pre-load below a critical level leads to symptoms and signs of a reduced cardiac output.

be maintained. Progressive hypotension, multiple organ failure and death is the inevitable consequence of cardiogenic shock in the absence of some intervention that is able to restore myocardial contractility within a critical time period.

Afterload

The ventricular afterload may be defined as the load that the ventricle must overcome before it is able to open its semi-lunar valve and eject blood. As the aortic pressure is normally much higher than the pulmonary arterial pressure, the left ventricle faces a higher afterload than the right ventricle and for this reason has a greater myocardial mass. The left ventricular afterload is determined primarily by the systemic vascular resistance which is set largely, but not entirely, by the arteriolar resistance vessels. Factors that increase arteriolar tone, for example alpha-adrenergic sympathetic stimulation, or administration of alpha-adrenergic agonist drugs such as metaraminol, increase afterload, while factors that reduce arteriolar tone such as beta-adrenergic sympathetic stimulation, or administration of the nitric oxide donor sodium nitroprusside, reduce afterload. In older patients, reduced compliance of the large elastic arteries may become an important contributor to the systemic vascular resistance. Other important determinants of afterload are blood viscosity and ventricular radius. The relationship between ventricular radius and afterload is described by La Place's Law, which is given by the equation: $T = P \times r$ where T is the tension developed in the wall of the ventricle, P is the intracavitary pressure and r is the radius. For example, if a ventricle doubles in radius, it will need to develop twice the wall tension to generate the same intracavitary pressure.

In heart failure due to left ventricular dysfunction, afterload is increased due to a combination of increased systemic vascular resistance (see below) and cardiac dilatation.

Neurohumoral changes

The essential abnormality in heart failure is an inadequate cardiac output to maintain normal perfusion pressure and blood flow to vital organs, in particular the brain, heart and kidney. This results in a complex activation of various neurohumoral systems, as summarized in the information box. Although the various systems activated have both additive and opposing actions, it is likely that the endogenous vasodilator/diuretic mechanisms are activated secondarily to the vasoconstrictor/fluid retentive mechanisms. The net effect is a state of vasoconstriction and sodium and fluid retention.

In general, each of the neurohumoral systems is activated in proportion to the severity of heart failure although some are more sensitive indicators of left ventricular dysfunction than others.[12] Activation of some of these systems (for example, plasma noradrenaline as a marker of sympathetic activity and plasma atrial natriuretic factor) has been shown to be an independent predictor of mortality in heart failure.[13,14]

Although activation of the vasoconstrictor/fluid retentive neurohumoral systems is an appropriate response to a reduced cardiac output due to volume depletion (for example, from haemorrhage or dehydration), it is now recognized that activation of these systems in heart failure represents a maladaptive response which contributes to the progressive nature of the syndrome. Systemic vasoconstriction increases left ventricular afterload, leading to a further reduction in cardiac output which in turn stimulates further systemic vasoconstriction. Sodium and fluid retention increases ventricular diastolic pressure which reduces subendocardial myocardial blood flow leading to further left ventricular dysfunction.[15] Other consequences of neurohumoral activation in heart failure include cardiac myocyte hypertrophy, myocardial fibrosis, coronary vasospasm, myocardial ischaemia and increased arrhythmogenesis. These latter effects undoubtedly contribute to the progression and mortality of heart failure.

The concept that the pattern of neurohumoral activation observed in heart failure is maladaptive is supported by the results of a number of recent clinical trials with drugs that block one or more of the neurohumoral systems. The vasodilator combination, hydralazine and isosorbide dinitrate, was the first drug treatment that was shown to reduce mortality in patients with heart failure.[16,17] The selective $alpha_1$-antagonist, prazosin, on the other hand was found to be no better than placebo, probably due to the rapid development of tolerance to this agent.[16]

Neurohumoral systems activated in heart failure

• **Vasoconstriction sodium, fluid retention**	• **Vasodilatation sodium, fluid excretion**
Sympathetic nervous system	Atrial natriuretic factor
Renin-angiotensin-aldosterone system	Prostacyclin, prostaglandin E_2
Vasopressin	Nitric oxide
Endothelin	

Angiotensin-converting enzyme (ACE) inhibitors have been shown to produce an even greater reduction in mortality in patients with mild to severe symptomatic heart failure.[17,18] ACE inhibitors also slow ventricular remodelling and dilatation in patients with asymptomatic left ventricular dysfunction.[19] Beta blockers have also been shown to partially reverse left ventricular dysfunction and dilatation in patients with moderate to severe symptomatic heart failure.[20]

On the other hand, more traditional heart failure therapies such as diuretics and some positive inotropic agents increase neurohumoral activation. While they often produce short-term symptomatic improvement, their long-term efficacy may be blunted by further activation of the above mentioned neurohumoral systems. Furthermore, there is evidence that inotropic drugs which act as sympathomimetic agents actually increase mortality in heart failure.[21,22]

Changes in the lung

Elevation of left ventricular diastolic pressure (pre-load) is a characteristic finding in left ventricular failure regardless of whether the failure is due to systolic or diastolic dysfunction. Retrograde transmission of the elevated LV diastolic pressure causes pulmonary venous congestion which increases lung stiffness and the work of breathing. Progressive elevation of the hydrostatic pressure at the venous end of the pulmonary capillary shifts the balance of forces acting across the capillary wall so that there is increased interstitial fluid formation. When hydrostatic intraluminal pressure rises above plasma oncotic pressure (normally about 25 mmHg) the rate of interstitial fluid accumulation from the pulmonary capillary bed exceeds the capacity of the pulmonary lymphatics to return the fluid to the systemic venous circulation and interstitial pulmonary oedema develops. This further increases lung stiffness and also impairs gas exchange. Further increases in intraluminal hydrostatic pressure cause alveolar pulmonary oedema and bronchial wall oedema. The former results in profound impairment of gas exchange and the latter causes large airway obstruction and is the basis for the wheeze which may mimic that seen in bronchogenic asthma, hence the term 'cardiac asthma'.

The consequences of increased pulmonary venous pressure depend to some extent on the rapidity with which the increase occurs. An abrupt rise in pulmonary venous pressure, as occurs in acute heart failure, may result in fulminant pulmonary oedema. In contrast, a more gradual and sustained rise in pulmonary venous pressure, as occurs in chronic left ventricular failure, permits adaptive changes to occur in the lungs that render them less prone to interstitial oedema formation. These changes include increased capacitance of the pulmonary lymphatics, reduced capillary permeability and pulmonary arteriolar vasoconstriction resulting in reduced pulmonary blood flow. In such individuals the symptom of dyspnoea becomes less troublesome but at a cost of increased fatigue and a further reduction in exercise tolerance.

Right heart failure—systemic venous congestion

Failure of the right ventricle most commonly occurs secondarily to left ventricular failure but may occur as an isolated entity in patients with primary lung or pulmonary vascular disease. Retrograde transmission of the elevated right ventricular diastolic pressure causes systemic venous congestion. This can be observed directly as elevation of the jugular venous pressure. As with pulmonary venous congestion, systemic venous congestion causes interstitial oedema to form. This is most obvious in the subcutaneous tissues in the dependent parts of the body. Other consequences of systemic venous congestion are hepatic congestion which produces hepatomegaly, hepatic pain and in severe cases hepatic dysfunction and ascites. Splanchnic congestion may be manifest as anorexia and indigestion. In severe cases marked weight loss occurs, due in part to reduced nutritional intake and in part to muscle atrophy and wasting. The combination of profound weight loss with abdominal bloating from ascites produces a characteristic clinical picture known as cardiac cachexia.

Changes in skeletal muscle

Pathophysiological changes in skeletal muscle are probably of minor importance in acute heart failure, but are thought to be a major source of fatigue and reduced exercise performance in patients with chronic heart failure. The changes in chronic heart failure are complex and are due in part to chronic reduction in skeletal muscle blood flow and in part to disuse atrophy. In addition, abnormal muscle metabolism possibly secondary to neurohumoral activation results in impaired oxidative metabolism and earlier onset of anaerobic metabolism.[23,24]

Conclusion

Heart failure is a syndrome characterized by complex pathophysiological changes not only in the heart but also in the vasculature and in other major organ systems. An improved understanding of these changes has led to a dramatic change in our approach to the treatment of heart failure. Patients with heart failure now face a better prognosis than a decade ago both with regard to quality of life and quantity of life. In spite of these advances, however, the overall prognosis remains poor and more effective treatment options and preventative strategies are urgently needed.

References

1. Parameshwar J, Shackell MM, Richardson A, Poole-Wilson PA, Sutton GC. Prevalence of heart failure in three general practices in north west London. J Gen Pract 1992; 42: 287–9
2. Parameshwar J, Poole-Wilson PA, Sutton GC. Heart failure in a district hospital. J R Coll Physicians Lond 1992; 26: 139–42
3. O'Connell JB, Bristow MR. Economic impact of heart failure in the United States: time for a different approach. J Heart Lung Transplant 1994; 13: S107–S112
4. Ho KL, Pinsky JL, Kannel WB, Levy D. The epidemiology of heart failure: the Framingham study. J Am Coll Cardiol 1993; 22(Suppl. A): 6A–13A
5. Hutchins GM, Bulkley BH. Infarct expansion versus extension: two different complications of acute myocardial infarction. Am J Cardiol 1978; 41: 1127–32
6. McKay RG, Pfeffer MA, Pasternak RC et al. Left ventricular remodelling after myocardial infarction: a corollary of infarct expansion. Circulation 1986; 74: 693–702
7. Dzau VJ. Implications of local angiotensin production in cardiovascular physiology and pharmacology. Am J Cardiol 1987; 59: 59A–65A
8. Beuckelmann DJ, Nabauer M, Erdmann E. Intracellular calcium handling in isolated ventricular myocytes from patients with terminal heart failure. Circulation 1992; 85: 1046–55
9. Conway MA, Allis J, Ouwerkerk R, Niioka T, Rajagopolan B, Radda GK. Detection of low phosphocreatine to ATP ratio in failing hypertrophied human myocardium by 31P magnetic resonance spectroscopy. Lancet 1991; 338: 973–6
10. Schwartz K, Chassagne C, Boheler KR. The molecular biology of heart failure. J Am Coll Cardiol 1993; 22: 30A–33A
11. Litwin SE, Grossman W. Diastolic dysfunction as a cause of heart failure. J Am Coll Cardiol 1993; 22(Suppl. A): 49A–55A
12. Francis GS, Goldsmith SR, Levine TB et al. The neurohumoral axis in congestive heart failure. Ann Intern Med 1984; 101: 370–7
13. Cohn JN, Levine TB, Olivari MT et al. Plasma norepinephrine as a guide to prognosis in patients with chronic congestive heart failure. N Engl J Med 1984; 311: 819–23
14. Gottlieb SS, Kukin ML, Ahern D, Packer M. Prognostic importance of atrial natriuretic peptide in patients with chronic heart failure. J Am Coll Cardiol 1989; 13: 1534–9
15. Hittinger L, Shannon R, Bishop SP, Gelpi R, Vatner SF. Subendomyocardial exhaustion of blood flow reserve and increased fibrosis in conscious dogs with heart failure. Circ Res 1989; 65: 971–80
16. Cohn JN, Archibald DG, Zeische S et al. Effect of vasodilator therapy on mortality in chronic congestive heart failure. N Engl J Med 1986; 314: 1547–52
17. Cohn JN, Johnson G, Zeische S et al. A comparison of enalapril with hydrallazine–isosorbide dinitrate in the treatment of chronic congestive heart failure. N Engl J Med 1991; 325: 303–10
18. The CONSENSUS Trial group. Effects of enalapril on mortality in severe congestive heart failure: results of the Cooperative North Scandinavian Enalapril Survival Study. N Engl J Med 1987; 316: 1429–35
19. Pfeffer MA, Braunwald E, Moye LA et al, on behalf of the SAVE Investigators. Effect of captopril

on mortality and morbidity in patients with left ventricular dysfunction after myocardial infarction. N Engl J Med 1992; 327: 669–77

20. Waagstein F, Bristow MR, Swedberg K et al. Beneficial effects of metoprolol in idiopathic dilated cardiomyopathy. Lancet 1993; 342: 1441–6
21. The Xamoterol in Severe Heart Failure study group. Xamoterol in severe heart failure. Lancet 1990; 336: 1–6
22. Packer M, Carver JR, Rodeheffer RJ et al. Effect of oral milrinone on mortality in severe chronic heart failure. New Engl J Med 1991; 325: 1468–75
23. Massie B, Conway M, Yonge R et al. Skeletal muscle metabolism in patients with congestive heart failure: relation to clinical severity and blood flow. Circulation 1987; 76: 1009–19
24. Drexler H, Reide U, Munzel T, Konig H, Funke E, Just H. Alterations of skeletal muscle in chronic heart failure. Circulation 1992; 85: 1751–9

Part 4
Evaluation of the patient

11 Patient history

Peter L Thompson

Introduction

Despite the almost universal availability of 12-lead electrocardiography, and the increasing availability of more sophisticated diagnostic techniques, a carefully taken history and meticulous physical examination remain the cornerstones of initial evaluation of the patient presenting with a possible coronary event.

On occasion it may be difficult to balance the need for a carefully conducted history and examination against the need for early and decisive action.[1] The overwhelming evidence that the efficacy of thrombolytic therapy is critically time-dependent imposes an urgency on the physician to consider the possibility of suspected acute myocardial infarction (AMI) if the clinical features are suggestive.

On the other hand, the potential for exposing the patient inappropriately to the risks of thrombolytic therapy in low risk infarction or unstable angina, or producing a catastrophic outcome in a patient with aortic dissection or gastrointestinal bleeding, emphasizes the need for achieving as accurate a diagnosis as possible within the shortest possible time.

The guiding principle in this situation is to obtain the appropriate information to initiate the correct course of action rather than finalizing the subtleties of diagnostic categorization.

Evaluation of chest discomfort and pain

The differential diagnosis of chest discomfort and pain can be a challenging clinical problem. The major causes are summarized in the information box.

Cardiac ischaemic causes

Acute myocardial infarction (AMI)

Approximately two thirds of patients with acute coronary occlusion present with chest discomfort or pain as their primary symptom. The patient presenting with the classical features of cardiac ischaemic chest pain will present little diagnostic challenge. The pain is typically described as retrosternal, gripping or tightening, sometimes as a heavy weight on the chest or as a burning sensation. Patients will frequently, without prompting, describe the pain in graphic terms such as a 'steel band tightening around my chest' or 'like an elephant standing on my chest', and 'like a red hot poker in the centre of my chest'. It is usually severe, distressing and associated with a sensation of severe apprehension and impending doom. Radiation of the pain is typically to the neck and lower jaw and to the left arm to the level of the elbow. On occasion the pain will radiate to the epigastrium, to the interscapular area, to the upper jaw, and into both arms, sometimes as far down as the wrists. Associated features include a sensation of weakness, light-headedness, nausea, sometimes vomiting and a sensation of shortness of breath.

Less typically, all of the above symptoms can occur in a milder form and it is not unusual for a patient to be relatively undisturbed by the chest discomfort, and attribute it to indigestion.[2–5] On occasion the location and character of the pain can be quite atypical, with lower jaw pain suggesting a dental cause, epigastric pain suggesting an upper gastrointestinal cause, or interscapular, shoulder, antecubital fossa, or wrist pains suggesting a musculo-skeletal cause. On occasion there may be no pain at all but a sensation of discomfort. It is important to elicit symptoms by means of open rather than closed questions. For example, the question 'Please describe what you are

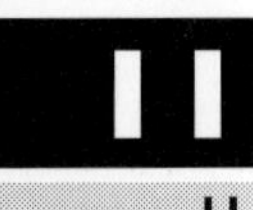

Classification of causes of chest discomfort/pain

Cardiac

- ISCHAEMIC
  Myocardial infarction
  Angina at rest
  Angina on exertion
  Prinzmetal's variant angina
  Angina with normal coronaries ('Syndrome X')
  Severe pulmonary hypertension
- NON-ISCHAEMIC
  Pericarditis
  Mitral valve prolapse

Non-cardiac

- AORTIC
  Aortic dissection
- PULMONARY
  Pulmonary embolism
  Pulmonary infarction
  Pleurisy
  Pneumothorax
- GASTROINTESTINAL
  Oesophageal spasm
  Oesophageal reflux
  Oesophageal rupture
  Peptic ulcer
  Biliary colic
- MUSCULOSKELETAL
  Costochondritis
  Cervical spondylosis
  Thoracic outlet syndromes
- NEUROLOGICAL
  Herpes zoster
  Cervical radiculopathy
- PSYCHOGENIC
  Hyperventilation
  Anxiety
  DaCosta's Syndrome

feeling', is preferable to 'Where is your chest pain?', which may elicit a response which overlooks significant retrosternal discomfort in the absence of pain or a pain which is recognizably ischaemic in origin but not in the chest.

It is sometimes useful to relate the symptom to a previously experienced anginal symptom. Questions such as 'Have you ever experienced this discomfort or pain before?', and 'Is it similar to the sensation you used to experience with exertion?', may be very useful.

Relief with nitroglycerin is a helpful diagnostic test but not entirely reliable as an indicator of myocardial ischaemia, partly because of the placebo effect and partly because nitroglycerine can sometimes partially relieve pain arising from the biliary tract or oesophageal spasm.

Angina

The symptoms of angina may be identical to those of MI apart from lesser intensity and duration. Prinzmetal's variant form of angina will reproduce identical pain but is characterized by transient, sometimes striking, ST segment elevation on ECG, spontaneous or nitroglycerine-induced relief after a few minutes, and absence of myocardial necrosis, and is due to transient spasm or thrombotic occlusion of a coronary artery. The clinical characteristics of angina pectoris with normal coronary arteries, sometimes referred to as syndrome X, may be indistinguishable from the myocardial ischaemic pain associated with coronary atherosclerosis. On occasion, severe pulmonary hypertension may produce an anginal syndrome indistinguishable from classical angina pectoris, but the diagnosis is usually obvious because the physical signs of advanced pulmonary hypertension are evident.

Cardiac non-ischaemic causes[3]

Pericarditis

The chest pain of pericarditis is typically sharp, and worsens with inspiration. The pain may radiate to the throat or jaw and on occasion to the left arm. Although the pain may be severe it is rarely associated with the dyspnoea, nausea and diaphoresis that characterizes myocardial ischaemic pain. The lack of response to nitrates and relief with anti-inflammatory drugs are helpful features in distinguishing pericardial from ischaemic pain.

Mitral valve prolapse

Mitral valve prolapse may be associated with chest pain. On occasion this can be typical anginal type pain, at other times it may be left infra-mammary pain. The mechanism of chest pain associated with mitral prolapse is poorly understood.

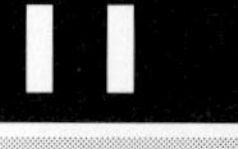

Non cardiac causes[3]

Aortic causes

Aortic dissection

The pain of aortic dissection is typically described as tearing in nature, although it may be a constant dull pain. In the typical case it is severe and distressing at the onset, in contrast to MI when the pain may start in mild form and become more severe. The pain may be mild, and aortic dissection without perceptible symptoms of chest pain is not rare. The pain is usually interscapular but may be located lower in the posterior chest. The pain syndrome may be complicated if there is proximal dissection with involvement of a coronary artery, producing myocardial ischaemic pain or leakage of blood into the pleural or pericardial cavities, producing pleuritic or pericardial pain.

There is the potential for a catastrophic outcome if a patient with aortic dissection is treated with thrombolytic therapy, so this diagnosis should be considered in every case if thrombolytic therapy is being considered. A history of severe untreated hypertension, or family history or clinical features of Marfan's syndrome, increase the likelihood that chest pain is due to aortic dissection.

Pulmonary causes

Pulmonary embolism

Massive pulmonary embolism with oppressive chest pain, dyspnoea and collapse may mimic MI but the features favoring pulmonary embolism are the intense dyspnoea and tachypnoea. There may be associated evidence of deep vein thrombosis such as unilateral leg swelling, calf tenderness and the known provoking factors for these such as long air or bus trips or recent surgery, especially in the presence of cardiac failure.

Lesser degrees of pulmonary embolism may produce pleuritic chest pain due to pulmonary infarction involving the pleural surface but this usually occurs several days after the pulmonary embolic event.

Other causes of pleuritic chest pain

Other causes include pleuritic involvement from pneumonitis of viral, rheumatic, traumatic or neoplastic involvement of the pleural cavity. The pain is usually localized, increases with inspiration, and may fluctuate in severity according to the patient's position or depth of respiration. The characteristic pleural friction rub confirms the clinical impression.

Pneumothorax

On occasion, pneumothorax due to a ruptured emphysematous bulla can produce a sharp pleuritic pain but usually less localized and more transient than other causes of pleuritic pain, and may be associated with symptoms of dyspnoea or signs of arterial desaturation.

Gastrointestinal causes

Oesophageal spasm and gastro-oesophageal reflux

Oesophageal spasm associated with gastro-oesophageal reflux can produce severe and distressing symptoms which can mimic those of myocardial ischaemia in character, severity and radiation. Relief with nitroglycerine does not rule out the possibility of oesophageal pain and recent reports have also indicated the possibility of associated electrocardiographic changes in the presence of oesophageal disease without known coronary artery disease.[5a]

A history of dietary indiscretion, known history of gastric or oesophageal disease, and relief with antacids and H_2 antagonists favour an oesophageal cause for chest pain. On occasion the distinction between myocardial ischaemic pain and oesophageal pain is impossible and coronary care admission and detailed evaluation is often necessary.

Oesophageal rupture

Oesophageal rupture following vomiting (the Mallory–Weiss syndrome) should be considered when chest pain comes on immediately after an episode of vomiting. This is in contrast to the pattern with myocardial ischaemic pain when the nausea and vomiting occurs after the chest pain has become well established. Oesophageal perforation due to trauma should be considered when there is a clear cut association with swallowing a fish or chop bone. A fever to suggest mediastinitis may be a helpful clue.

Peptic ulcer

On occasion gastric pain due to a penetrating or perforating peptic ulcer may cause retrosternal or

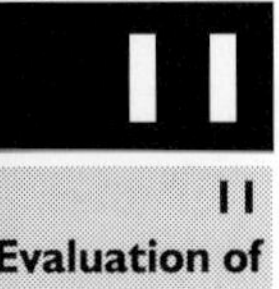

interscapular pain rather than the more typical epigastric pain.

Careful consideration of oesophageal and gastric causes for chest pain is now of even greater importance in the thrombolytic era of treatment of MI.

Biliary colic

Biliary colic can occasionally produce retrosternal or interscapular pain which may mimic myocardial ischaemia but the typical colicky pattern is not seen in myocardial ischaemia or infarction.

Musculo-skeletal causes

Costochondritis

Pain is usually localized over a costochondral junction, can be reproduced with pressure over the area and may be aggravated with movement or deep inspiration. It can be exacerbated by exertion. The worsening on exertion tends to occur after the exertion has been completed and may last for several hours thereafter. In this case, a poorly framed or casually asked question such as 'Is the chest pain brought on with exertion?' can lead to a confusing answer. Costochondritis may be part of a more generalized fibromyalgia syndrome, may occur after a recent viral illness, and is often associated with anxiety.

Cervical spondylosis and thoracic spine degenerative disease can produce pain in the upper chest with radiation to one or both arms. Pressure over the tender areas with reproduction of the symptoms may be a valuable diagnostic clue.

It is important to have a healthy respect for the variable nature of myocardial ischaemic pain. It is an important principle that *an area of tenderness on the chest wall does not rule out significant underlying ischaemic heart disease as the cause of chest pain symptoms.*

Neurological causes

On occasion a vague band-like pain across the upper chest may occur in the pre-vesicular phase of herpes zoster and has been an occasional cause for admission to the CCU in the author's experience. A sense of relief at finding an alternative diagnosis to myocardial ischaemia may rapidly dissipate when the patient has to face the pain and discomfort of shingles. Cervical radiculopathy may cause pain radiating down the left arm.

Psychogenic causes

Chest pain due to anxiety is a common problem which challenges the physician to focus all available diagnostic and management skills firstly to rule out significant underlying myocardial ischaemia and secondly to manage the patient's understandable anxiety.

Hyperventilation and anxiety can frequently produce chest pain. This is usually in the left inframammary region, may be associated with localized tenderness, and often can be reproduced with hyperventilation. Persistence of these symptoms has been referred to in the past as da Costa's Syndrome.

The physician's responsibility in the chest pain syndrome is to be alert to the possibility of underlying myocardial ischaemia and proceed conscientiously to rule out the possibility. A primary diagnosis of anxiety- or hyperventilation-induced chest pain on initial clinical contact is a potentially hazardous clinical choice and will often do little to reassure the patient. It may well guarantee their lack of cooperation in future management. It is sometimes necessary to arrange coronary care admission and subsequent diagnostic follow-up to manage this problem effectively.

Other symptoms

The modern CCU has become a 'clearing house' for patients presenting with symptoms and clinical problems other than chest pain and discomfort. The clinical presentations may include syncope or collapse, dyspnoea, and palpitations.

Syncope and collapse

The cause of an episode of syncope and collapse may elude initial evaluation in up to 40% of cases. Nevertheless, careful history taking is important to estimate cardiac causes which have a poor prognosis, with 1 year mortality as high as 20–30% compared with non-cardiac causes with a lower mortality of 5–10%. The search for a specific cause of syncope can be one of the most challenging clinical exercises facing the coronary care physician.[6,7] Some of the clues and the causes of syncope are summarized in Table 11.1.

A detailed history from the patient should include careful evaluation of prodromes such as

Table 11.1 Clues to the cause of syncope derived from the history

Clues	Likely cause
Precipitating event	
Emotional stress, pain	Vasovagal bradycardia and hypotension
Standing up from lying or sitting	Orthostatic hypotension
Looking up, turning head	Vertebro-basilar insufficiency
Exertion	Outflow tract obstruction (aortic or subaortic stenosis)
Insulin, missed meal	Hypoglycaemia
Preceding symptoms	
Confusion	Hypoglycaemia, hypotension
Palpitations	Tachyarrhythmia
Speech, motor or sensory abnormalities	Epileptiform or localized cerebral ischaemia
Rapidity of onset	
Gradual	Hypotension, hypoglycaemia, neuropsychiatric
Sudden	Vasovagal syncope, brady- or tachyarrhythmia, neurological

dizziness or light-headedness which may suggest a gradual onset; palpitations which may suggest a tachyarrhythmia; chest pain which may suggest a myocardial ischaemic cause; localized neurologic signs which may indicate localized cerebral ischaemia. The circumstances of the event are important. Onset on standing after sitting or lying suggests postural hypotension: a clear cut provocation such as the sight of blood, venepuncture, or other emotional triggers suggests neurocardiogenic syncope (vasovagal collapse). A relationship to head turning or looking up suggests vertebro-basilar insufficiency. A recent insulin injection in an unstable diabetic clearly indicates hypoglycaemia.

The pattern of the syncopal episodes is important, with a recurrent pattern suggesting epilepsy or recurrent cardiac arrhythmia. The duration of the event may give some clue as to the aetiology. Syncopal episodes due to cardiac arrhythmias are rarely prolonged and tend to suggest an obstructive cardiac cause, cerebral ischaemia or metabolic or psychogenic causes. Injury sustained during syncopal episodes is usually indicative of complete loss of consciousness and an indication for complete evaluation. Neuropsychiatric causes are rarely associated with injury and tend to be more controlled collapses, and often in full view of observers.

Finally, the detailed evaluation of an episode of syncope must include an accurate description from persons present at the event as well as family members, friends, or work mates who may have observed previous episodes.

Despite the importance of the history and evaluation of syncope, frequently the cause is not obvious on initial contact. A period of observation in the CCU may be helpful in establishing a cardiac arrhythmia as the cause. Alternatively, a cardiac cause can be ruled out if an episode occurs without disturbance of the cardiac rhythm. Prolonged observation in the CCU is no longer necessary with the availability of more definitive diagnostic tools including Holter monitoring, event related recording, electrophysiology study and tilt table testing.

Dyspnoea

Patients presenting to the CCU will often complain of dyspnoea. When dyspnoea occurs in the setting of chest pain it can be a valuable clue to indicate that the degree of myocardial ischaemia is sufficient to cause significant left ventricular dysfunction with pulmonary congestion.

Dyspnoea may be the primary reason for presentation. When this is associated with clinically obvious pulmonary oedema the cause is clear. Other causes of acute dyspnoea may be life-threatening, such as massive pulmonary embolism or spontaneous tension pneumothorax which require urgent evaluation and decisive action. The dyspnoea with massive pulmonary embolism is of sudden onset and associated with extreme apprehension, faintness and often an oppressive sensation of chest tightness.

The dyspnoea associated with pneumothorax is usually mild but can become severe with tension pneumothorax which should be obvious on clinical or chest X-ray examination.

Dyspnoea associated with pulmonary congestion may not necessarily be associated with clinical signs of râles or pulmonary oedema and may require

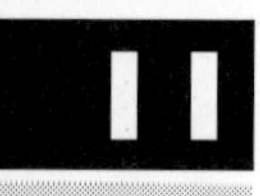

a chest X-ray for definite diagnosis.

The dyspnoea associated with acute bronchospasm is usually associated with widespread rhonchi and wheezes throughout the lung fields but in very severe cases these may be absent and may require measurement of peak flow or forced expiratory volume and response to inhaled bronchodilators for confirmation.

The dyspnoea associated with hyperventilation usually occurs in association with anxiety and may have the characteristic tingling and numbness of the extremities and peri-oral area.

Palpitation

With the widened role of the CCU, patients may be admitted with symptoms of palpitation. The likely causes of arrhythmia with different types of palpitations are summarized in Table 11.2.

Sudden onset of rapid, regular palpitations is typical of supraventricular tachycardia. The characteristic feature is the sudden cessation of the palpitations; however on occasion, the adrenergic drive accompanying the anxiety of the supraventricular tachycardia causes a sinus tachycardia following reversion of the supraventricular tachycardia, giving the sensation of a more gradual slowing. Sinus tachycardia usually produces a gradual increase and decrease in the heart rate and has a clear cut external cause. Sometimes the palpitations may have features of both supraventricular and sinus tachycardia, raising the possibility of the hybrid arrhythmia-sinus node re-entry tachycardia. Ventricular tachycardia can sometimes cause rapid, regular palpitations without syncope and this is more likely to be the diagnosis if there is a history of associated ischaemic heart disease. Rarely, atrial fibrillation can produce a sensation of rapid, regular tachycardia.

Rapid, irregular palpitations are usually due to paroxysmal atrial fibrillation. Occasionally, ventricular tachycardia produces a sensation of irregular palpitations because of the beat-to-beat variation in cardiac output resulting from the atrioventricular dyssynchrony. In some patients frequent atrial or ventricular premature beats can give a sensation of rapid, irregular palpitations.

Single, thumping palpitations are usually due to ventricular premature beats but on occasion can be caused by supraventricular premature beats. Frequently the sensation of palpitation is due to the strong beat which occurs after a compensatory pause and the patient will often describe a characteristic complex of a flutter followed by a pause and a thump in the chest.

Table 11.2 Likely cause of arrhythmia in relation to sensation of palpitation

Type of palpitation	Usual	Sometimes
Rapid regular	Sinus tachycardia	Sinus node re-entry tachycardia
	Supraventricular tachycardia	Ventricular tachycardia
Rapid irregular	Atrial fibrillation	Ventricular tachycardia, frequent ventricular or supraventricular premature beats
Single thumping	Ventricular premature beats, supraventricular premature beats	

Nausea and vomiting

Patients presenting for coronary care admission will often complain of nausea. This is usually a response to the pain of myocardial ischaemia but is often out of proportion to the severity of the pain, suggesting activation of vagal receptors via the Bezold–Jarisch reflex, especially in the presence of inferior MI.[8]

Sweating—diaphoresis

Myocardial ischaemia is often accompanied by sweating, sometimes quite profuse. This symptom is a valuable clue to myocardial ischaemia rather than other causes of chest pain.

Hiccups

Occasionally the patient with infarction will complain of persistent hiccups, usually thought to be due to diaphragmatic irritation from inferior myocardial infarction.

Silent ischaemia and infarction

Silent MI can occur.[9] By definition these patients do not present to the CCU but may on occasion be admitted some time after the silent event when the infarction is found incidentally on ECG, on biochemical testing or with a complication of the infarction such as pleuritic pain from post infarction pericarditis, stroke from thrombo-embolic complications, or dyspnoea from the late development of cardiac failure.

Associated medical problems

The history taking should be sufficiently detailed to elicit relevant coronary risk factors such as family history, hyperlipidaemia, smoking, hypertension, physical inactivity.

Associated medical problems need to be clearly identified on initial contact. Those which may increase the risk of thrombolytic therapy need special attention, e.g. a history of dyspepsia might indicate a risk of gastrointestinal bleeding, or a past history of cerebrovascular disease may indicate a risk of intracerebral haemorrhage. A history of wheezing or asthma is important in patients who are being considered for beta blocker therapy.

Conclusion

A carefully taken history is essential for the proper management of the patient presenting to a CCU and will usually provide sufficient clues to indicate a decisive course of action. If, however, the diagnosis and management are not clear on the initial evaluation, the correct course of action is admission to the CCU to allow a period of observation and the opportunity of further careful evaluation of the clinical problem. While there are often good reasons to abbreviate a detailed clinical history to allow decisive action, sloppy history taking technique in evaluating the coronary care patient can have fatal consequences, and at the least, can lead to inappropriate investigations and unnecessary anxiety for the patient.

References

1. Cummins RO (ed). Text book of advanced cardiac life support. Chapter: Acute myocardial infarctions. American Heart Association, Dallas, Texas, 1994
2. Levine SA. Coronary thrombosis—the variable clinical features. Medicine 1929; 8: 245
3. Sampson JJ, Cheitlin M. Pathophysiology and differential diagnosis of chest pain. Prog Cardiovasc Dis 1971; 13: 507–31
4. Uretsky BF, Farquhar DS, Borezin A, Hood WE. Symptomatic myocardial infarction without chest pain; prevalence and clinical course. Am J Cardiol 1977; 40: 498–503
5. Logan R, Wong F, Barclay J. Symptoms associated with myocardial infarction: are they of diagnostic value? NZ Med J 1986; 99: 276–8

5a. Davies HA, Rush EM, Lewis et al. Oesophageal stimulation lowers angina thresholds. Lancet 1985; 1: 1011–4

6. Manolis AS, Linzer M, Salem D, Estes NAM III. Syncope: current diagnostic evaluation and management. Ann Int Med 1990; 112: 850–63
7. Linzer M. Syncope 1991. Am J Med 1991; 90: 1–5
8. Wei JY, Markis JE, Malagold M, Braunwald E. Cardiovascular reflexes stimulated by reperfusion of ischaemic myocardium in acute myocardial infarction. Circulation 1983; 67: 796–801
9. Margolis JR, Kannel WB, Feinleib M et al. Clinical features of unrecognized myocardial infarction silent and symptomatic. Eighteen year follow up, the Framingham study. Am J Cardiol 1973; 32: 1

12 Physical examination

Peter L Thompson

Introduction

The detection of relevant findings in patients with ischaemic heart disease[1] and cardiac arrhythmias[2] is proportional to the care and skill exercised in the physical examination. Although it is true that on occasions there may be no abnormal physical signs, a perfunctory or incomplete examination can never be justified.[3,4]

Initial assessment

The initial assessment should target conscious state, degree of distress, extent of haemodynamic disturbances and cardiac arrhythmia. This determines the urgency of treatment such as pain relief, circulatory support and need for coronary reperfusion by thrombolysis or angioplasty, as well as the initial diagnostic categorization into suspected myocardial infarction (MI), other myocardial ischaemia, other cardiac problem or non-cardiac problem. The examination can be done during initiation of intranasal oxygen, continuous electrocardiogram (ECG) monitoring and performance of 12-lead electrocardiogram. Unless there are extenuating circumstances, this evaluation should be completed within minutes from the patient's initial presentation.

Complete physical examination

The more complete physical examination will involve a detailed assessment of the cardiovascular system and associated medical problems. All medical problems should be documented and included in a problem list. The degree of vigour in pursuing each medical problem will depend on hospital policy and the availability of facilities, but it is indefensible to ignore or overlook a major medical problem on the grounds that the patient was being admitted 'solely for coronary care'. It is the responsibility of the coronary care team to identify these problems and ensure that appropriate arrangements are made for treatment and follow-up.

During the period of coronary care unit (CCU) observation, regular evaluation of the cardiovascular system should be performed with each change in clinical status, and in the uncomplicated case at least three times in each 24 hour period.

General appearance

The patient complaining of cardiac chest pain usually prefers to sit and will often rub their chest with an open palm or closed fist (the Levine sign). Patients initially presenting with chest pain without pallor, cyanosis or clamminess tend to have a less complicated course and better long-term prognosis. The patient with more severe MI may be clammy and have a pale or grey mottled skin colour with central cyanosis and be in considerable distress. However, the patient's appearance at initial contact is not a reliable indicator of the extent of infarction or the risk of lethal arrhythmia and all patients suspected of myocardial ischaemia or infarction should be treated with the same degree of urgency.

A patient in cardiogenic shock may lie listless and lethargic, whereas the patient with acute pulmonary oedema will prefer to sit upright, gasping for air, coughing frothy, sometimes pink or blood-streaked sputum, sweating profusely, and mentally obtunded and confused.

The patient who has experienced a syncopal episode may be confused and irrational, especially if they have sustained a head injury in their fall, and additional information from family members or friends may be necessary to establish the details of the episode and the patient's usual mental state.

Pulse

If there is a tachycardia present it is important to establish whether this is sinus tachycardia indicative of an adrenergic response or a tachyarrhythmia which requires urgent management. Sinus tachycardia may have a slightly variable heart rate over several minutes and will usually slow on carotid sinus massage. Supraventricular tachycardia tends to retain the same rate throughout the episode and will either not respond or suddenly revert to sinus rhythm on carotid sinus massage. Ventricular tachycardia may manifest a variable pulse pressure depending on the degree of atrioventricular (AV) synchrony. This can sometimes be detected on palpation of the radial or carotid pulse but is better appreciated by evaluating the Korotkoff sounds by partial compression of the brachial pulse with the sphygmomanometer cuff.

When patients with abnormal tachyarrhythmia such as atrial fibrillation, supraventricular tachycardia or ventricular tachycardia are excluded, the pulse rate on admission is an important indicator of prognosis in AMI. In a series of 1000 patients with AMI admitted to the CCU at Sir Charles Gairdner Hospital[5] and followed up for 5 years, admission pulse rates of <70, 71–80, >80 identified groups of patients with significantly different survival patterns (see Fig. 12.1).

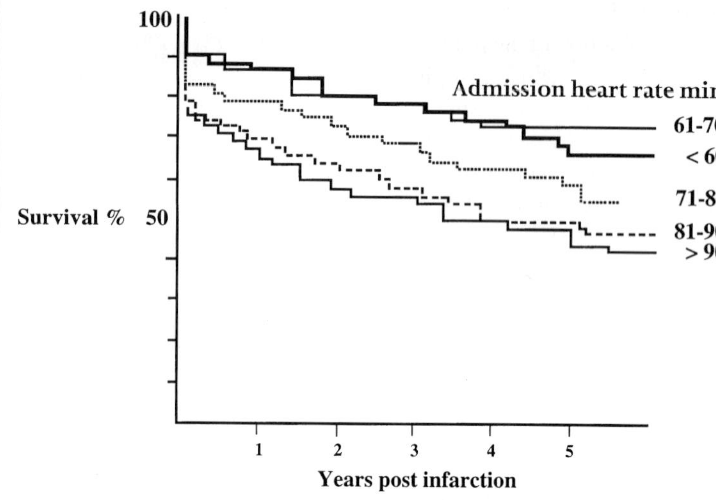

Fig. 12.1 Five year survival in relation to admission heart rate in acute myocardial infarction. Data from 1000 patients treated in a coronary care unit. Reproduced from Thompson PL. Prognosis of myocardial infarction with particular reference to infarct size. University of Western Australia: MD thesis, 1988.

A slow pulse rate may be seen in the presence of inferior MI either due to sinus bradycardia or complete atrioventricular block. On occasions a sudden profound bradycardia with hypotension can occur in inferior MI as part of the Bezold–Jarisch reflex or in healthy 'vagotonic' individuals with procedures such as venepuncture.

Pulsus alternans

Pulsus alternans is a sign of advanced left ventricular dysfunction and should be identifiable by the coronary care physician or nurse. Every second beat is of diminished amplitude. This can be detected either by palpation at the radial or carotid pulse or preferably by use of the sphygmomanometer cuff to partly occlude the brachial artery and gradually inflate above the pressure of the weaker pulse to produce a sudden halving of the apparent pulse rate.

Pulsus bigeminus

Pulsus bigeminus due to frequent ventricular ectopic beats in a coupled 'bigeminal' pattern, can produce a similar phenomenon to pulsus alternans, but this can be readily distinguished on the ECG monitor because the second beat is premature and it usually has the typical bizarre ectopic beat appearance.

Pulsus paradoxus

The coronary care physician should be familiar with the technique of detecting pulsus paradoxus as this is a crucial diagnostic clue in pericardial tamponade. The term 'paradoxus' refers to a decline of pulse amplitude of greater than 10 mmHg during inspiration. The normal decline is less than 3–4 mmHg. The patient should be sitting comfortably so that respiratory excursion is comfortable. The patient should be asked to breathe normally and comfortably and not increase the level of inspiratory effort. Diminution in the pulse amplitude is noted during inspiration. The degree of paradoxus must be severe to be detected by palpation and it is preferable to perform the procedure with a sphygmomanometer cuff over the brachial artery. The cuff is deflated very slowly until the systolic pressure during expiration is noted. The procedure is repeated carefully to determine the systolic pressure during peak (normal) inspiration. A greater drop than the normal 3–4 mmHg may be seen in some subjects, particularly in those with obstructive airways disease. A drop of 10 mmHg or greater is diagnostic of pulsus paradoxus. As long as the patient is not making visibly abnormal respiratory efforts such as during an acute attack of asthma, this observation is diagnostic of pericardial tamponade or constriction.

Blood pressure

Hypotension is usually an ominous sign in patients being admitted to the CCU. However, hypotension is not necessarily associated with a poor outcome.[9] Better understanding of vagally induced splanchnic vasodilatation in the Bezold–Jarisch reflex (responsive to atropine), hypovolaemia resulting from vigorous diuretic therapy (responsive to fluid infusion), and right ventricular dysfunction in right ventricular infarction (sometimes responsive to fluid infusion), has broadened our knowledge of the significance of hypotension.

On occasions patients with AMI or other acute myocardial ischaemia can have a hypertensive response. This may have greater significance in patients treated with thrombolytic therapy by increasing the risk of intracerebral haemorrhage and may have an adverse long-term effect because of the presence of associated hypertensive heart disease.

The level of diastolic blood pressure appears to have little effect on short- or long-term survival.

Jugular Venous pulse

Examination of the jugular venous pulse allows an estimate of the right heart pressures. The jugular venous pressure is often quite normal in the presence of severe left heart failure in AMI. Elevated venous pressure early after AMI suggests either that the right and left heart failure has preceded the development of the MI or indicates significant right ventricular involvement.[6,7] The management of right ventricular infarction requires special procedures (see Ch. 58).

Evaluation of the respiratory response to the venous pressure is an important part of assessing a patient with suspected pericardial tamponade or right ventricular infarction. Normally the venous pressure drops slightly during inspiration (although it is important not to be confused by the increased vigour of the jugular pulsation which also accompanies inspiration). In pericardial constriction or right ventricular infarction, venous pressure rises with inspiration (Kussmaul's sign).

The use of the jugular venous pulsations for diagnosis of cardiac arrythmias remains an elegant clinical skill but is of little additional value in the CCU patient whose ECG and cardiac rhythm are continuously monitored.

Pre-cordial inspection, palpation and percussion

Patients admitted to the CCU are primarily those with ischaemic heart disease or cardiac arrhythmias and the more prominent findings seen in congenital and valvular heart disease may not be present. However, there is still important information to be gained from inspection, palpation and percussion of the precordial area.

Muscular development of the upper chest may be associated with hypertrophic cardiomyopathy, and kyphoscoliosis may be associated with mitral valve prolapse and provides clues to a non-coronary cause of chest pain.

Careful palpation of the precordium in a patient with myocardial ischaemia may reveal an impulse lateral to the parasternal area but medial to the cardiac apex. This is best palpated with pressure of the flat of one hand accentuated by gentle pressure with the other, allowing the underlying cardiac pulsations to be more readily appreciated. On occasions a precordial bulge palpated in this manner may indicate abnormal wall motion or anterior wall dyskinesis in anterior MI. A pulsation immediately adjacent to the left parasternal area may indicate right ventricular enlargement.

Careful evaluation of the cardiac apex is an important component of the cardiovascular examination. The point of maximal impulse should be noted either by measuring in centimetres from the mid sternal line or by reference to the mid clavicular, anterior axillary or mid-axillary lines. In addition the intercostal space in which the impulse is most readily palpable should be noted. The characteristics of the apical pulsation are best appreciated with the patient in the left lateral decubitus position and this should be included in the evaluation of the coronary care patient whenever possible. A prominent presystolic pulsation (apical 'a' wave) may indicate reduced compliance which may be a feature of cardiac hypertrophy or myocardial ischaemia. A harsh systolic thrill may be palpated, indicative of mitral regurgitation or ventricular septal defect.

Percussion of the area of cardiac dullness is less rewarding but may occasionally be helpful. Clear-cut dullness to percussion, detected well clear of the lower right sternal border, may be an indication of a significant pericardial effusion.

Cardiac auscultation

A prominent fourth heart sound is frequently heard in patients admitted to the CCU. Although it has been stated that this is present in all cases of AMI,[8] this claim is based on phonocardiographic studies. Frequency of detection on auscultation will depend on the skill of the observer, the care taken to elicit the physical sign, and the characteristics of the patients being treated. It is conceivable that meticulous serial observation by a skilled observer, with careful auscultation in the left lateral decubitus position, will demonstrate a fourth heart sound in the majority of patients with AMI but the rate of detection in routine CCU practice is relatively low. In a series of 1000 patients admitted to the CCU at Sir Charles Gairdner Hospital observed as carefully as possible by junior house staff, a fourth heart sound was heard in only 30% of patients on the first hospital day, dropping to 20% by the fourth day.[5]

The controversy surrounding the frequency of detection of a fourth heart sound in AMI is out of proportion to its significance. It has little diagnostic value and in the author's experience has no prognostic significance (see Fig. 12.2).[5]

A fourth heart sound will not be heard in the presence of atrial fibrillation because of the absence of atrial contraction. On rare occasions a soft atrial contraction with features of a fourth heart sound can be heard asynchronous with the other heart sounds in the presence of complete atrioventricular block.

A first heart sound followed by a systolic click, splitting of the first heart sound or a presystolic murmur with a prominent first heart sound in mitral stenosis may all be confused with a fourth heart sound. The classic fourth heart sound is heard only at the cardiac apex, is of lower pitch than the first heart sound, and when the heart sounds are observed in conjunction with continuous ECG monitoring can be seen to precede ventricular contraction as evidenced by the ECG R wave. It can be made more prominent by isometric exercise such as handgrip.[10]

In contrast to the ubiquity and lack of predictive value of the fourth heart sound, a third heart sound is an important indicator of significant left ventricular dysfunction and a poor outcome.[9] It is strongly associated with a previous history of cardiac failure and can be detected on admission in 5–10% of patients with AMI. Patients with a third heart sound on admission will have a worse short-term survival and it is a useful indicator of a significantly worse long-term survival (see Fig. 12.2). It is important to seek a third heart sound with careful auscultatory technique including examining the patient in the left lateral decubitus position with the bell of the stethoscope applied lightly to detect the low pitched sound. Often the characteristic gallop cadence is more readily appreciated than the discrete third heart sound.

Abnormalities of first and second heart sounds

A prominent first heart sound of constant intensity is characteristically heard in supraventricular tachycardia. Variable pitch and amplitude of the first heart sound producing a characteristic 'water wheel' sound may be heard in ventricular tachycardia with atrioventricular dyssynchrony. Less obvious variations in pitch and amplitude of the first heart sound are heard in rapid atrial fibrillation. A cyclical variation in the amplitude of the first heart sound may be heard during Wenckebach atrioventricular block. It has been stated that diminution in the amplitude of the first heart sound is a typical feature of AMI. However, in the author's experience this is an unreliable indicator of MI because of lack of reference point to the amplitude of the first heart sound and because variations in adrenergic drive, heart rate and PR interval will all independently affect the amplitude of the first heart sound.

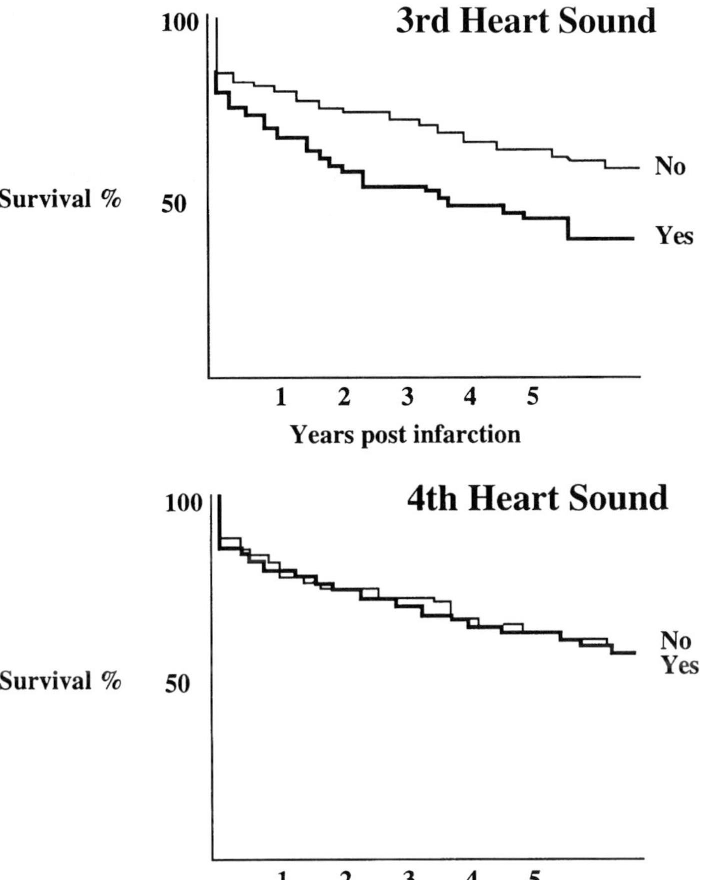

Fig. 12.2 Five year survival of third heart sound or fourth heart sound detected on admission with acute myocardial infarction. Data from 1000 patients treated in a coronary care unit. Reproduced from Thompson PL. Prognosis of myocardial infarction with particular reference to infarct size. University of Western Australia: MD thesis, 1988.

Inspiratory splitting of the second heart sound is usually well preserved in acute myocardial ischaemia or infarction. However, reverse splitting of the second heart sound has been documented.[11] It has been claimed that this is due to prolonged duration of left ventricular systole as a result of severe ischaemia but in the author's experience this physical finding in the CCU is invariably associated with left bundle branch block. Wide splitting of the second heart sound with minimal but preserved respiratory variation may be seen in right bundle branch block, complicating MI. Increased prominence of the pulmonary component of the second heart sound may be a feature of acute pulmonary embolism, with some patients showing quite striking diminution in the intensity of the accentuated sound over several days as the acute pulmonary hypertension reverses, or marked fluctuation over a period of months as the degree of pulmonary hypertension varies in recurrent pulmonary embolism.

Systolic bruits

An apical systolic bruit is a common accompaniment of ischaemic heart disease. It may be due to prior mitral valve disease or may represent mitral regurgitation due to papillary muscle dysfunction. This may vary according to the degree of myocardial ischaemia and the timing, character and amplitude of the systolic bruit may vary from examination to examination, or even during a single physical examination if the patient is experiencing an episode of severe myocardial ischaemia.

The sudden development of a harsh pan-systolic bruit during AMI may indicate the development of severe mitral regurgitation due to papillary muscle rupture or may be a first sign of post infarction ventricular septal defect. Although a variety of criteria have been proposed to distinguish these two possibilities,[12] in reality they may be indistinguishable and urgent bedside echo Doppler evaluation may be needed to establish the diagnosis.

Of course, the patient receiving acute coronary care may have valvular heart disease unrelated to their acute cardiac problem. This emphasizes the importance of careful documentation of the physical conditions on admission to the CCU to distinguish these murmurs from newly developing complications.

Diastolic bruits

Early diastolic bruits from mild aortic regurgitation are quite common in elderly persons and can vary in amplitude and duration with the level of blood pressure. The development of a new aortic bruit in a patient with atypical chest pain can indicate aortic root involvement in aortic dissection (see Ch. 70).[13]

Continuous bruits

A continuous bruit may indicate a congenital anomalous origin of the left coronary artery from the pulmonary trunk, or ruptured aneurysm of the sinus of Valsalva. These bruits are more subtle than the usual harsh 'machinery murmurs' of patent ductus. Occasionally a harsh systolic and diastolic precordial rub may mimic a continuous murmur—the characteristic feature is the changing pattern on serial auscultation.

Examination of the chest

In the patient with chest pain, non-cardiac causes should be considered in the examination of the chest. The clinical features of pneumothorax, costochondritis, or pneumonia/pleurisy may be evident. The patient with dyspnoea needs careful evaluation for respiratory causes such as bronchospasm, consolidation or pleural effusion before the clinician assumes that cardiac failure is the cause. In patients with known or suspected MI, the extent of clinical signs of pulmonary congestion must be sought and documented, as these will determine treatment as well as prognosis (see Fig. 12.3).

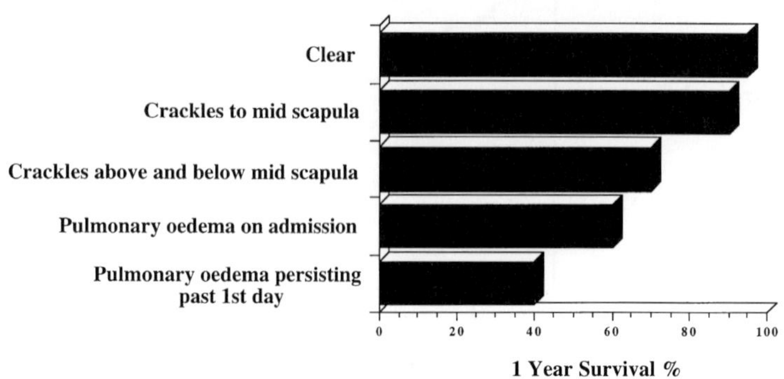

Fig. 12.3 One year survival in relation to the degree of pulmonary vascular congestion detected on clinical examination. Data from 1000 patients treated in a coronary care unit. Reproduced from Thompson PL. Prognosis of myocardial infarction with particular reference to infarct size. University of Western Australia: MD thesis, 1988.

References

1. Fowler NO. Physical signs in acute myocardial infarction and its complications. Prog Cardiovasc Dis 1968; 10: 287–97
2. Harvey WP, Ronan JA. Bedside diagnosis of arrhythmias. Prog Cardiovasc Dis 1966; 8: 419
3. Thompson PL. Physical examination in ischaemic heart disease. Med J Aust 1976; 1: 492–5
4. Perloff JK. Physical examination of the heart and circulation. Philadelphia: Saunders, 1982
5. Thompson PL. Prognosis of myocardial infarction with particular reference to infarct size. University of Western Australia: MD thesis, 1988
6. Cohn JN, Guiha NH, Broden MI, Limas CJ. Right ventricular infarction—clinical and haemodynamic features. Am J Cardiol 1974; 33: 209–14
7. Sharpe DN, Botvinick EH, Shames DM et al. The non-invasive diagnosis of right ventricular infarction. Circulation 1978; 57: 483–90
8. Hill JC, O'Rourke RA, Lewis RP, McGranahan GM. The diagnostic value of the atrial gallop in acute myocardial infarction. Am Heart J 1969; 78: 194–201
9. Riley CP, Russell RD, Rackley CO. Left ventricular gallop sound and acute myocardial infarction. Am Heart J 1973; 86: 598–602
10. Cohn PF, Thompson P, Strauss W, Todd J, Gorlin R. Diastolic heart sounds during static (handgrip) exercise in patients with chest pain. Circulation 1973; 47: 1217–21
11. Yurchak PM, Gorlin R. Paradoxic splitting of the second heart sound in coronary artery disease. N Engl J Med 1963; 269: 741–2
12. Meister SG, Helphant RH. Rapid bedside differentiation of ruptured intraventricular septum from acute mitral insufficiency. N Engl J Med 1972; 287: 1024–25
13. Heikkila J, Mitral incompetence complicating acute myocardial infarction. Br Heart J 1967; 29: 162–9
14. Slater EE, De Sanctis RS. The clinical recognition of dissecting aortic aneurysm. Am J Med 1976; 60: 625–33

13 Electrocardiography

Peter L Thompson and Marcus K Ilton

Introduction

The electrocardiograph (ECG) remains the only practical means of evaluation of the electrical behaviour of the heart and remains the most widely used diagnostic tool within coronary care units. The interpretation of alterations in the ECG wave form is complex, with different physiological or pathophysiological changes producing identical or similar changes in wave form. The ability to perform and interpret the ECG are essential skills for all nursing and medical staff in the CCU. The aim of this chapter is to further develop accuracy in interpretation of the ECG in the setting of acute coronary syndromes and related conditions, with emphasis on correct technique and assessment of common difficulties in interpretation. It is assumed that readers have basic training in electrocardiography or have access to one of the many excellent introductory texts in electrocardiography[1–4] and its application to diagnosis of myocardial infarction and other coronary syndromes.[5]

The ECG recording

Standardizing the recording

It is important to realize that the ECG is only standardized if the electrocardiogram is performed in a standard fashion. Common errors which complicate the interpretation of ECG and invalidate the markings and intervals include:

- **Recording at the wrong paper speeds**. Most machines are able to record at 50 mm/s, doubling the cardiac intervals including PR, QRS, QT, and RR interval, producing a false diagnosis of first degree atrioventricular (AV) block, bundle branch block, prolonged QT interval or bradycardia respectively. Some machines are also able to record at 10 mm/s giving the false appearance of tachycardia.
- **Recording at non-standard voltage**. Most ECG machines can record at normal voltage or half voltage. If the voltage is halved by manual setting, all voltages will be reduced by half. The 3-channel automatic machines will automatically reduce chest leads to half size if voltages are excessive and this can cause inaccuracy in formulas for the estimation of left ventricular hypertrophy or interpretation of sequential T wave changes.
- **Paper jamming**. Both single channel and multi-channel recorders are subject to paper jamming which can cause intermittent artefacts, rendering the 25 mm/s time standard for ECGs invalid.
- **Excessive dampening of ECG signal**. ECG machines which record in an excessively dampened fashion, due to electronic fault or excessive stylus pressure on the paper, can produce slurred and abnormal QRS and T wave contours. All machines should be checked regularly to ensure they meet industry standards of recording. Suspicion that the machine is recording incorrectly is often obtained from an abnormal standardization marker with rounded edges rather than sharp edges.

Lead placement

The standard 12-lead ECG provides an enormous amount of information with regard to myocardial ischaemia, infarction and hypertrophy but the accuracy of these interpretations is dependent on the leads being placed in the standardized positions.

- **Reversed limb leads placement**. Reversal of the right and left arm leads is the most common error in placement of the limb leads and can produce the false appearance of lateral infarction (see Figs 13.1A, B). The error in lead position is usually recognizable by reversal of the usual voltage appearance of lead AVR which is downwards and lead AVL which is usually upwards.
- **Incorrect placement of leads on limbs or trunk**. Standard ECG interpretation is based on recording the limb leads from the limbs, not the trunk. Placing the electrode on the proximal versus the distal portion of the limb has little effect. There can be significant effect on ECG appearance when the lower limb leads are recorded on the abdomen rather than on the lower limbs. This can confound and cause misinterpretation by automated ECG analysis systems. An example is shown in Figure 13.1C.
- **Misplacement of chest leads**. A common error is the recording of leads V1 and V2 in one or two intercostal spaces above the standard position of the fourth intercostal space, located between the fourth and fifth ribs. The angle of Louis (manubriosternal junction) marks the insertion of the second rib above the second intercostal space. Misplacement of leads V1 and V2 can not only cause misinterpretation of individual ECG tracings but confuse sequential recordings, particularly when there are subtle changes in leads V1, such as in true posterior infarction. An equally common error is misplacement of lead V6 which should be in the mid axillary line but is frequently recorded medially to this.

  Misplacement of leads V5 and V6 frequently causes confusion in interpretation of lateral T wave changes on serial ECGs. To overcome these problems a skin marker should be used so as to record in the same position when serial ECGs are recorded with a suction cup method, or disposable ECG electrodes should be left in position and when replaced, located in the same position (see Fig. 13.2). Examples of pseudo-abnormalities caused by misplacement of chest electrodes are shown in Figure 13.3.

- **Confluence effect**. If excessive ECG paste is used on the chest a confluence effect is produced, leading to confusion in interpretation of subtle anterolateral T wave changes. This can be overcome by using a small amount of ECG paste on each suction cup or ensuring that disposable electrodes are not overlapping each other.
- **The significance of respiratory variations**. The inferior ECG leads can be affected by respiratory variations with apparently significant T wave inversion or Q waves being a normal variant rather than indicative of inferior myocardial ischaemia. Serial ECG recordings should be recorded in inspiration and in expiration to attempt to separate these two possibilities. An example is shown in Figure 13.4.

Other ECG recording problems

- **Wandering baseline**. Wandering baseline is almost always due to poor electrode skin contact. Staff should check all leads to ensure that they are properly applied, that there is adequate ECG paste and the skin is not excessively moist. Some modern ECG machines with diagnostic capability will identify the culprit electrode. Sometimes a wandering baseline will stabilize when the electrodes have been left in position for a period of time allowing skin resistance to be lowered by the electrode gel, and therefore immediately repeating the tracing without moving electrodes can sometimes be successful.
- **Patient tremor**. Tremor can usually be overcome. It is frequently due to shivering, which can be overcome with reassurance and a warm blanket. Muscle tremor often arises from tensing of arm or leg muscles and this can be overcome by ensuring the limbs are resting comfortably. Sometimes the quality of the tracing can only be improved by recording the ECG tracing with the patient lying with the arms tucked under their back.
- **AC interference**. Alternating current interferences, usually due to detection of ambient electrical currents by poorly applied electrodes, can often be improved by improving

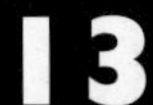

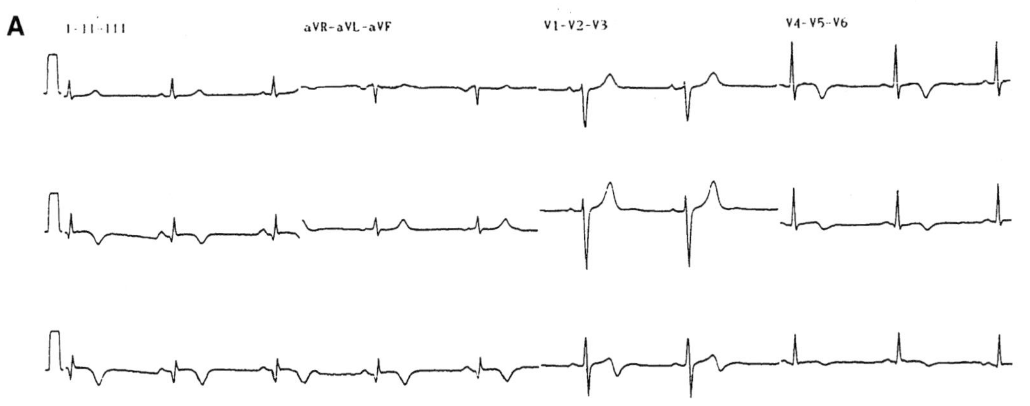

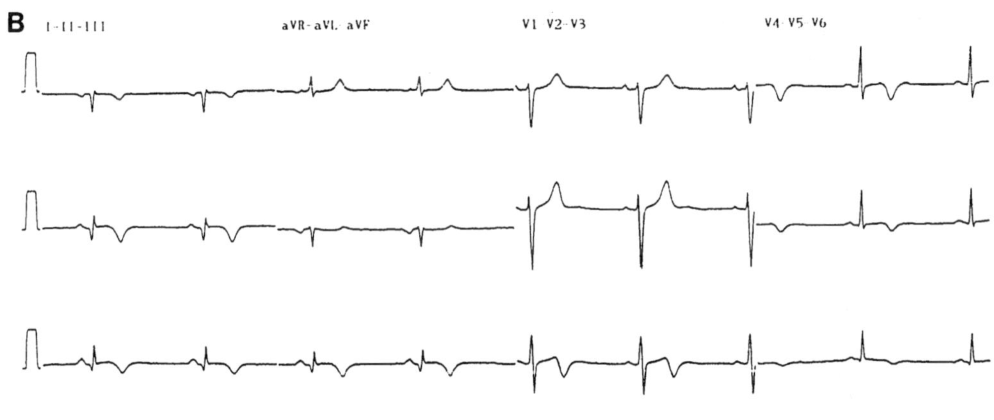

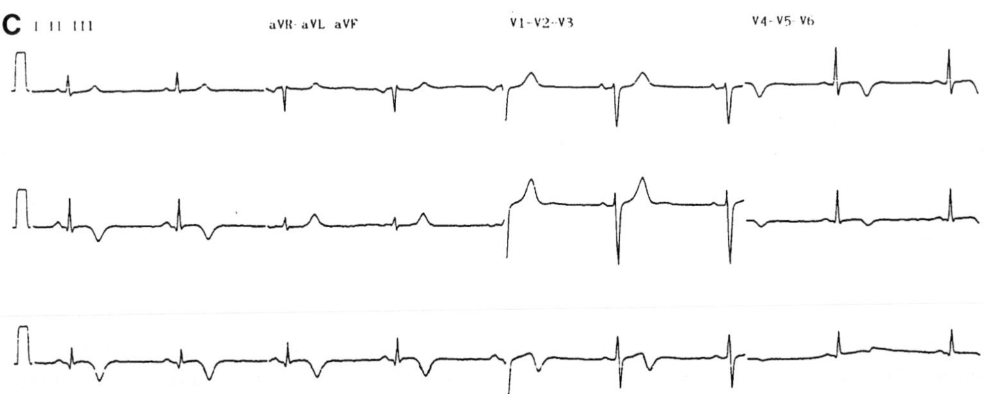

Fig. 13.1 Effect of incorrect limb lead placement on the ECGs of a patient with inferolateral myocardial infarction. A Correct limb lead placement. Note the upright AVL and downward AVR. B Reversed right and left arm leads which could lead to an inappropriate diagnosis of right axis deviation. Note the inappropriately downwards deflection of the AVL and upright AVR. C Placement of leg leads on the lower ribs. Note the significant diminution in amplitude of the inferior Q waves.

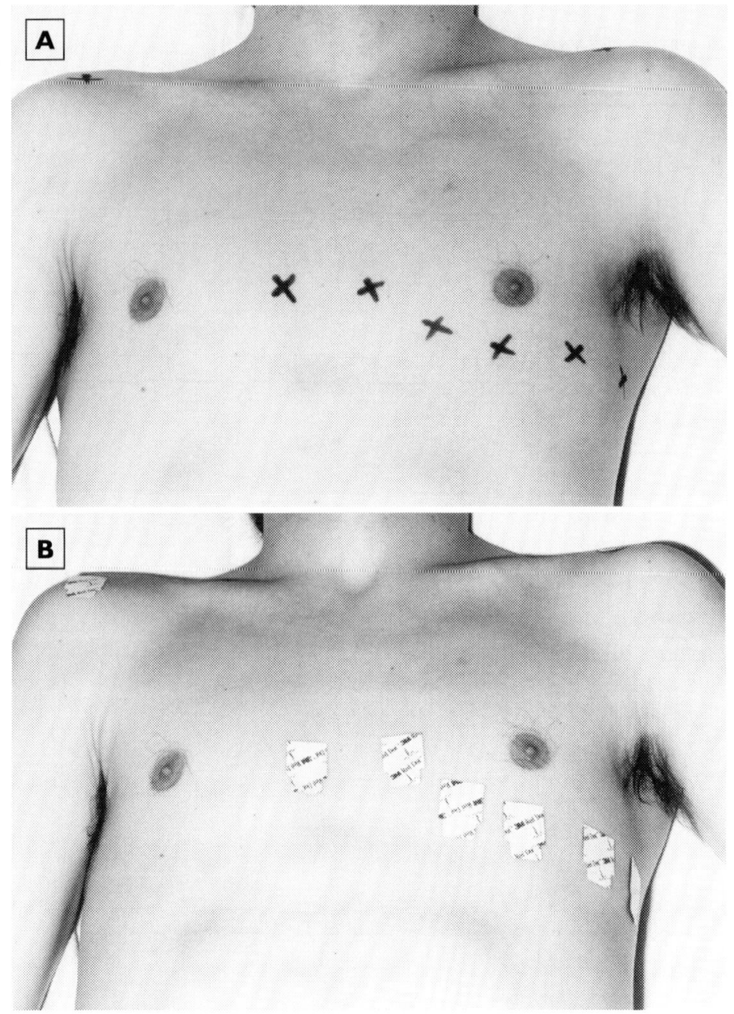

Fig. 13.2 Correct position of chest leads should be marked with a skin marker [A] or by leaving the disposable electrodes in situ [B].

skin contact. If this does not help there may be a faulty electrode which may be evident if the interference is located in a single lead. If AC interference persists despite these measures, the possibility of a significant AC leak should be considered and electrical safety standards should be reviewed. This is of particular importance if the patient has an intracardiac pacing wire or cannula. A check list for ensuring high quality ECG tracings is summarized in the information box.

Principles of ECG interpretation

All medical and nursing staff who work in the CCU should be capable of interpreting the usual electrocardiographic changes of acute myocardial ischaemia, infarction (AMI) and cardiac arrhythmias.[6,7] Computerized interpretation should serve as a useful aide-memoire to ensure that all aspects of ECG tracing have been analysed. On occasions the fastidious nature of the ECG analysis programme is of assistance in identifying an abnormality which may have been overlooked. However, the inadequacy of some computer analysis systems, and discrepancies between different programmes, mean that the final analysis and responsibility for clinical decisions must rest with the clinical rather than the automated interpretation of the ECG. To ensure that quality standards of ECG interpretation are maintained in the future, coronary care staff should discipline themselves to interpret the ECG first without reference to the automated analysis and only check the analysis to make sure that nothing has been overlooked.

ECG patterns of acute coronary syndromes and their complications

Myocardial ischaemia and infarction are reflected in the ECG by changes in the ST segments, T wave and the development of Q waves.

ST abnormalities

The earliest indicator of myocardial ischaemia is a deviation in the ST segment from the isoelectric line. Displacement of ST segment above or below the baseline of greater than 1 mm may be the only sign of myocardial ischaemia, although other conditions may produce similar changes.

ST segment depression

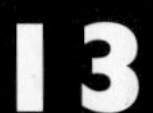

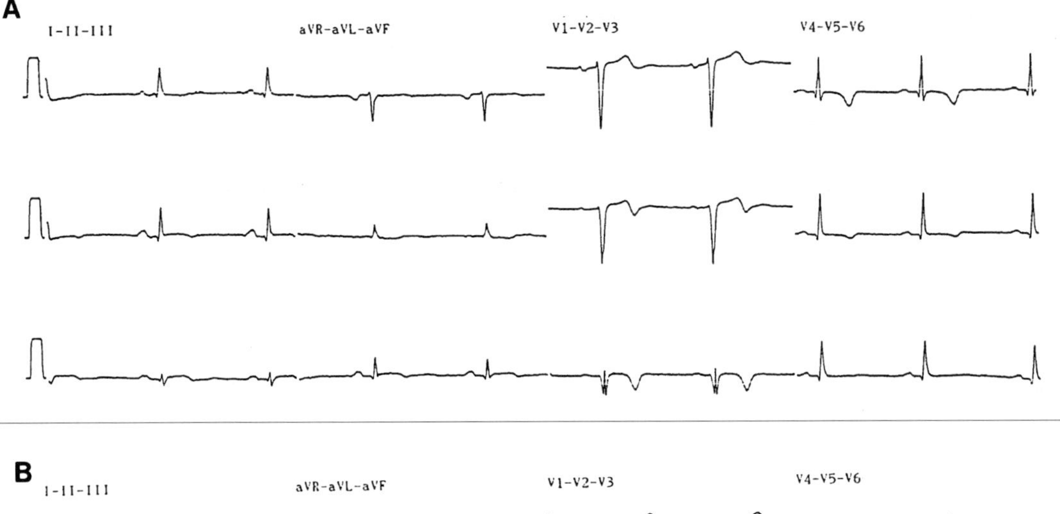

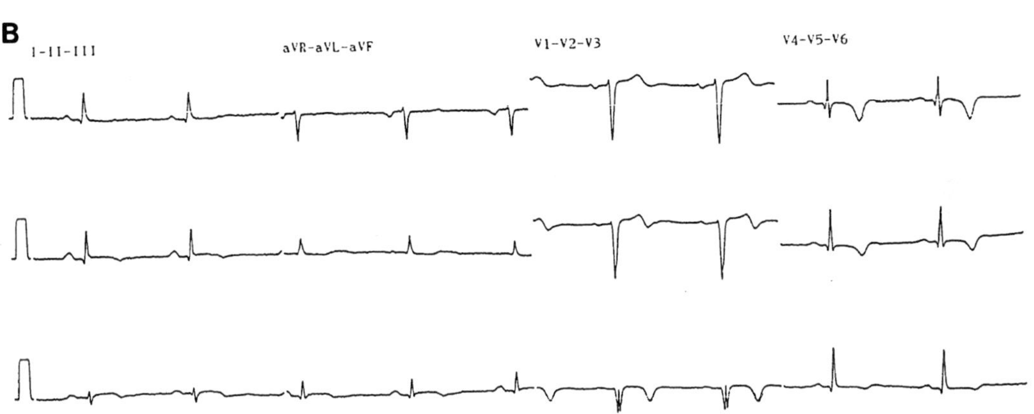

Fig. 13.3 Effect of incorrect chest lead placement in a patient with anterolateral myocardial infarction. A Correct chest lead placement. B Placement of V4, V5, V6 1 cm medial to their correct positions. Note the apparent deepening of the T wave inversion in lead V5, potentially leading to an incorrect diagnosis of extension of lateral ischaemia.

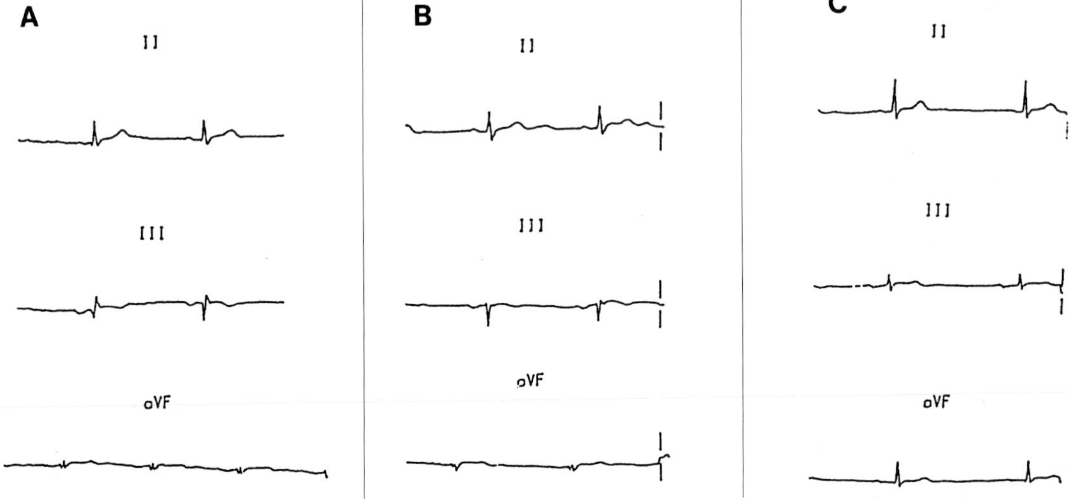

Fig. 13.4 Effect of respiratory variations on Q waves in inferior leads in a patient with a normal heart and no evidence of inferior infarction. A deep expiration; B normal; C deep inspiration.

CHECKLIST FOR HIGH QUALITY ECG RECORDING

- Ensure the recording is standardized at 25 mm/s and 10 mm/mv. If not, clearly mark the tracing.
- Ensure limb leads are correctly applied
  - — use limbs, not trunk
  - — check for reversed leads (AVL should be upright and AVR should be downwards)
- Ensure chest leads are correctly applied
  - — V1 and V2 should be in the fourth intercostal space, not second or third
  - — V4 should be in mid clavicular line
  - — V6 should be in mid axillary line
  - — chest lead positions should be marked clearly for serial ECGs
  - — avoid confluence effect
- Wandering baseline
  - — ensure adequate skin contact
  - — moisten dry skin
  - — wait for skin resistance to drop
- Trouble shoot muscle tremor
  - — reassurance
  - — warmth
  - — relax arms
  - — sit on hands
- Trouble shoot AC interference
  - — check electrodes application
  - — check electrode integrity
  - — if present in all leads, suspect a significant electrical leak and have the ECG machine and environment checked for electrical safety

The ST depression of myocardial ischaemia is associated with depression of the junction of the ST segment with the QRS complex (J point) and is typically flat and horizontal. Flat or down-sloping ST depression of greater than 1 mm is significant for ischaemic transient changes but needs to be distinguished from constant abnormalities as seen in left ventricular hypertrophy or digitalis effect. Up-sloping ST depression is not deemed significant for ischaemia unless the ST segment is 2 mm below the iso-electric line 80 ms (2 mm) after the J point. The presence of ST depression in two or more leads without ST elevation is suggestive of coronary ischaemia without infarction and would not routinely require thrombolytic therapy. On occasions ST segment depression can indicate infarction on the contralateral wall, so called 'reciprocal' change, as when anterior ST segment depression occurs with inferoposterior ischaemia.

ST segment elevation

Within a minute or two of coronary occlusion the ST segment becomes elevated, usually in a convex upwards pattern. In the early part of this phase the ischaemic process may still be reversible with coronary reperfusion but gradually specific QRS changes of local infarction begin to appear, and progress if coronary occlusion persists. The number of leads with ST elevation tends to indicate the extent of myocardial ischaemia and the height of the ST segment elevation tends to parallel the degree of ischaemia, although this may be affected by other factors. The usual sequence is progressive lowering of the extent of the ST segment elevation with T wave inversion (see Fig. 13.5). Persistence of the ST segment elevation for more than a week usually indicates extensive anterior wall motion abnormality.

Following successful reperfusion of the infarct-related artery, the ST segment may return to normal, followed by only minor T wave changes (see Fig. 13.6).

Non-infarction patterns of ST segment elevation include the following:

- **Prinzmetal's variant form of angina**. In 1959 Prinzmetal described a variant form of angina associated with ST segment elevation rather than ST depression. Increasing experience has shown that this pattern can be reproduced by coronary artery spasm, transient coronary thrombosis, as well as acute balloon occlusion during coronary angioplasty. In the typical pattern there is no progression to myocardial necrosis, as reperfusion, either by relief of spasm, lysis of coronary thrombus (or deflation of an occluding balloon catheter), allows the ECG to return to normal, similar to that seen after reperfusion with thrombolysis.
- **Acute pericarditis.** ST segment elevation of pericarditis is typically concave

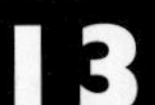

A

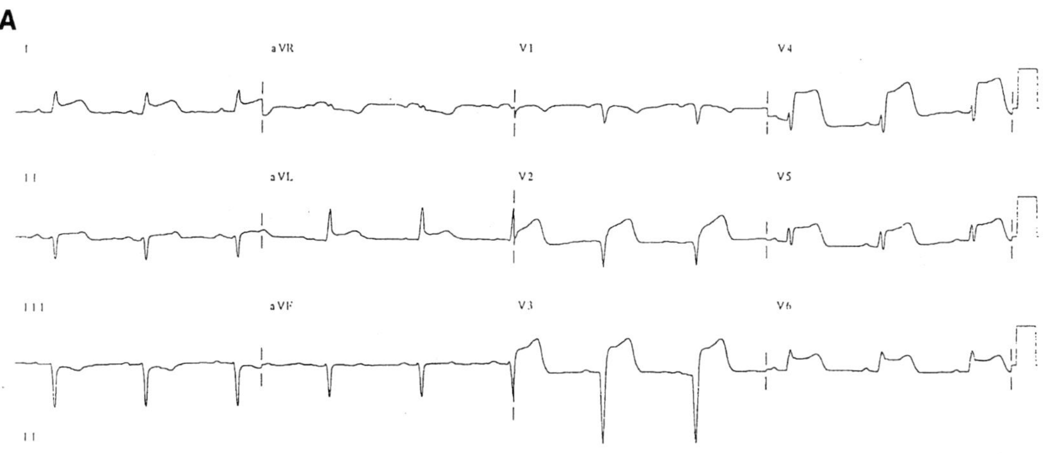

B

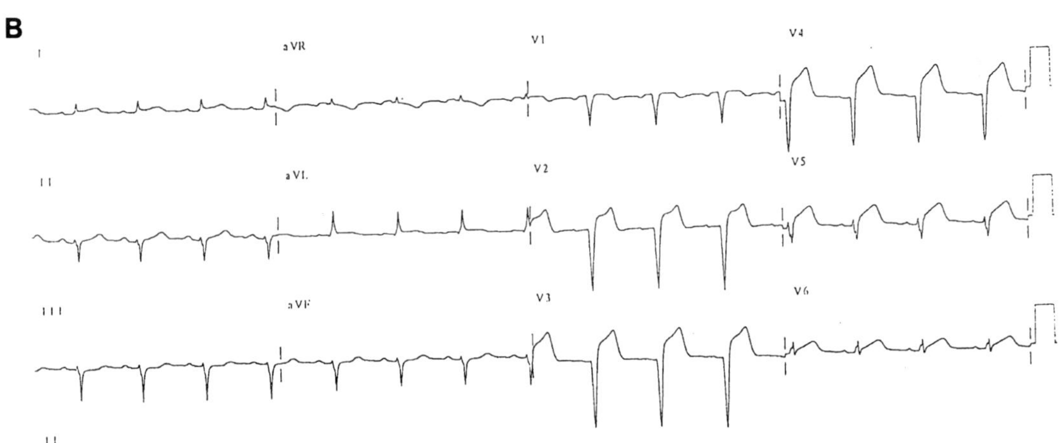

Fig. 13.5 Acute ST segment elevation in patient with extensive anterior MI showing only minimal lowering of the extent of ST elevation after 12 hours. Subsequent coronary angiography showed persisting occlusion of the left anterior descending coronary artery. Contrast with the example of successful reperfusion in Fig. 13.6.

upwards, is diffuse and is not localized to a particular set of leads. It is not associated with abnormal Q waves, is rarely greater than 5 mm, and takes off at the end of the QRS complex without any notching. A typical pattern is shown in Figure 13.7.

However, on occasions pericarditis can produce patterns more suggestive of myocardial infarction, particularly when associated with diffuse T wave changes. When this is associated with myopericarditis causing cardiac enzyme abnormalities a differential diagnosis may be challenging. On occasions detailed investigation for myocardial ischaemia may be justified. The typical pattern of ST segment elevation in acute pericarditis gradually settles and returns to normal within a few days. Differentiation from early repolarization abnormalities is based primarily on the absence of the characteristic notching of early repolarization and the transient nature of changes compared with the patterns of early repolarization (see Table 13.1).

- **Early repolarization.** Despite the widely accepted terminology, the mechanism of so-called early repolarization abnormalities is not fully understood. The typical

A

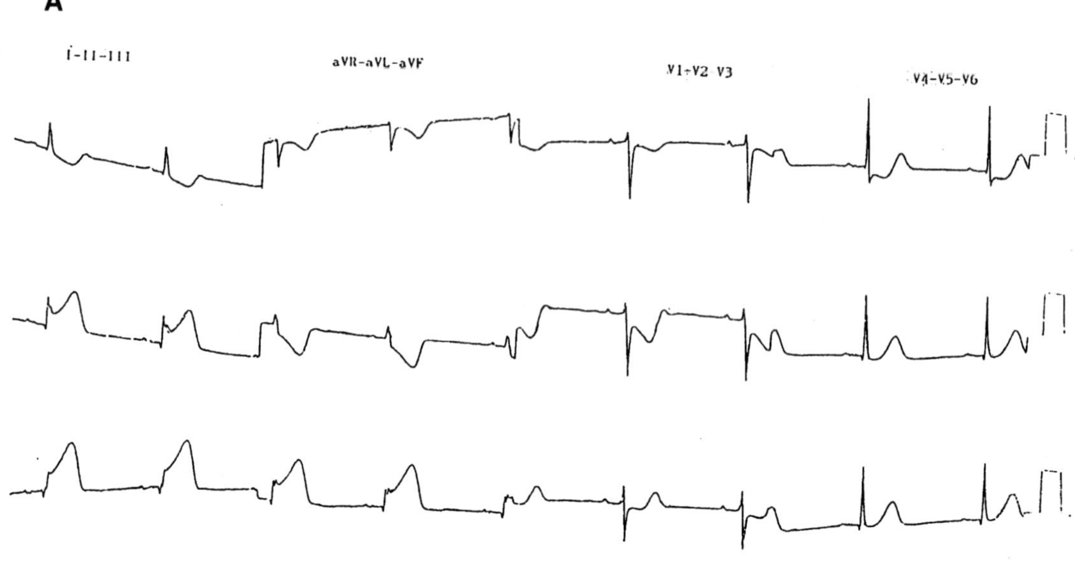

B

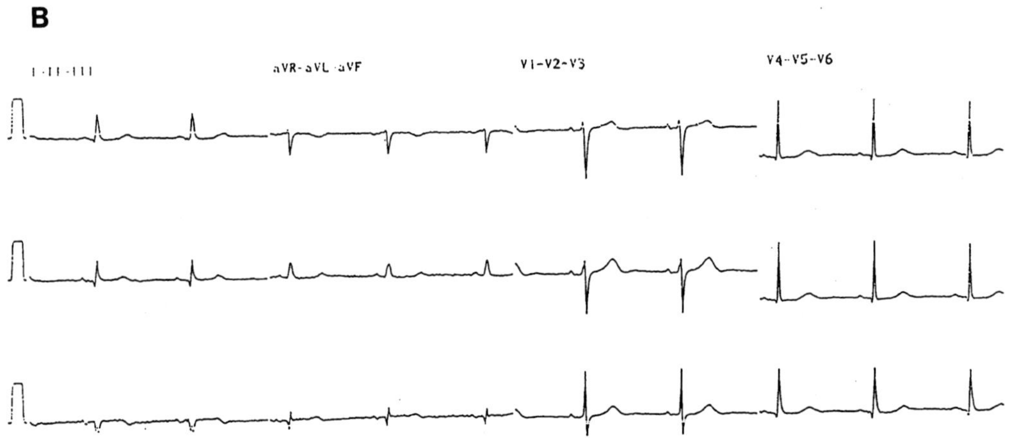

Fig. 13.6 Acute ST segment elevation in a patient with acute inferior myocardial infarction who was treated successfully with thrombolytic therapy; A pre-treatment and B post-treatment. Subsequent coronary angiography showed TIMI-III flow down the right coronary artery.

features of this normal variant are summarized in Table 13.1. Of these criteria, the most reliable for the diagnosis of early repolarization is its constancy on serial tracings.

When the variant shows marked ST elevation, confusion with acute infarction and pericarditis is common and a frequent cause for admission to the CCU.

- **ST elevation in leads V2 and V3.** This is a relatively common normal variant which may be confused with acute ST segment elevation of AMI. It does not have the typical notching appearance of early repolarization seen in the lateral precordial leads.
- **Hyperkalaemia.** Occasionally acute hyperkalaemia with marked T wave peaking can be associated with ST segment elevation.
- **Hypothermia.** Profound hypothermia can be associated with elevation of the J point associated with marked bradycardia and prolongation of the QT interval.
- **Bundle branch block.** Left bundle branch block is typically associated with ST segment elevation.

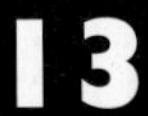

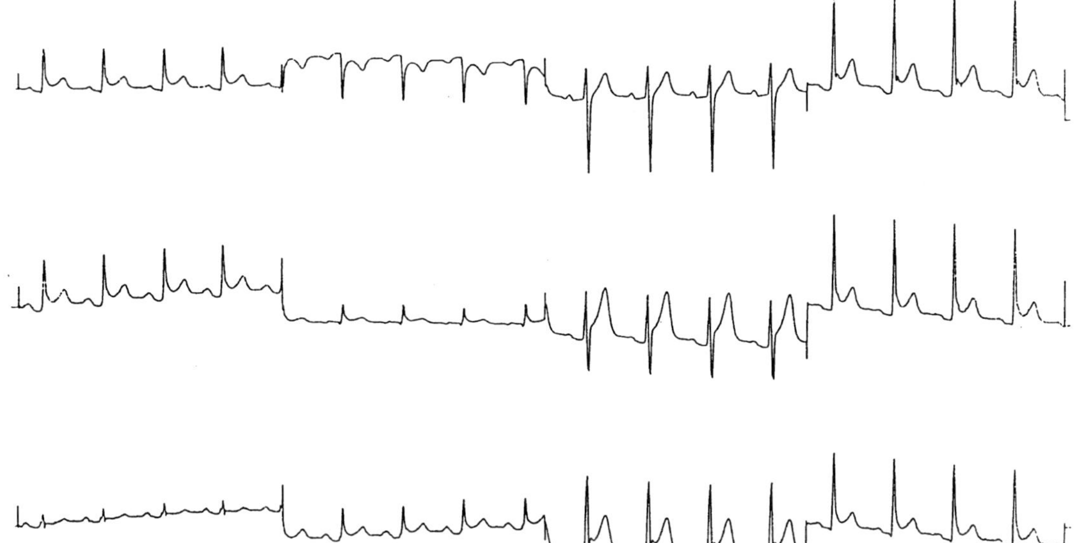

Fig. 13.7 Typical ST segment elevation in a patient with pericarditis. This may be difficult to distinguish from the normal variant of 'early repolarization'. (Note PR segment depression in the anterior leads. (see Table 13.1).

Table 13.1 Distinguishing the common types of ST segment elevation

	Acute myocardial infarction	Prinzmetal's variant angina	Pericarditis	Early repolarization
Pattern	Convex upwards highly variable	Convex upwards. Highly variable pattern from minute to minute	Concave upwards—ST usually comes straight off the QRS	Concave upwards—ST often has 'notch' at take off from QRS
Location	Localized to area of infarction	Localized to area of ischaemia	Widespread	Usually inferior or lateral leads
Extent	1–6 mm	1–6 mm	1–3 mm	1–2 mm
Time course	Constant, changes over hours or days (may change rapidly with reperfusion)	Variable, changes over minutes	Variable over days	Constant over days and weeks
Associated T wave changes	Typical T wave pattern of tall peaking followed by flattening and inversion	Usually no T wave change	T wave changes of flattening and inversion	No T wave change

T wave changes

Tall peaked T waves represent the hyperacute phase of AMI and can occur even before ST segment elevation or T wave change is seen (see Fig. 13.8). Patients with acute hyperkalaemia may have a similar appearance although serial ECGs should be able to confirm AMI.

Deep T wave inversion develops as part of the pattern of necrosis in the progression of AMI in either Q wave or non-Q wave MI but may occur without infarction (see Fig. 13.9). T wave inversion accompanying AMI is usually transient and resolves after several weeks or months, but on occasions can persist indefinitely.

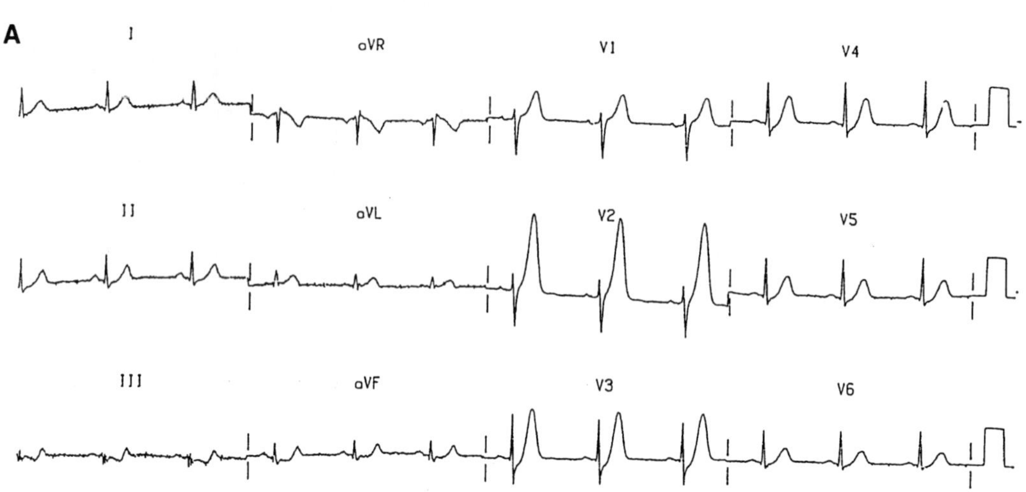

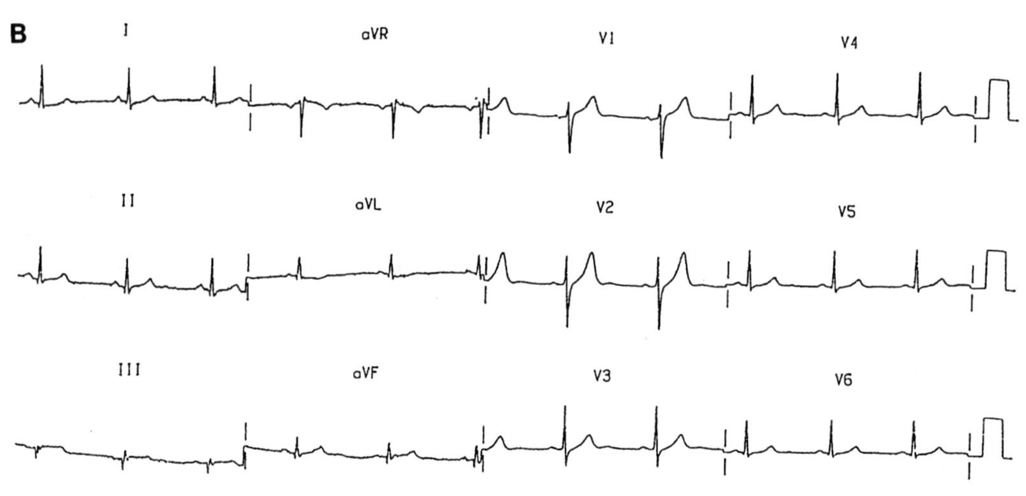

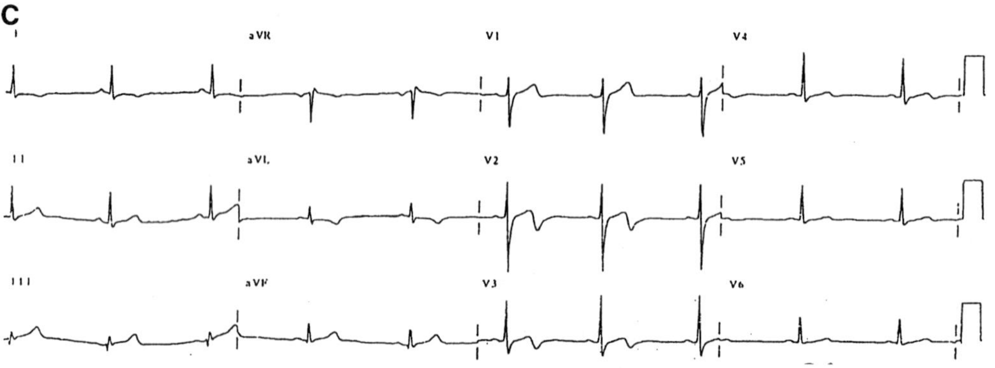

Fig. 13.8 Tall peaked precordial T waves in **A** the early stages of anterior MI, **B** progressing to a 'normal' ECG, and **C** subsequent anterior T wave inversion.

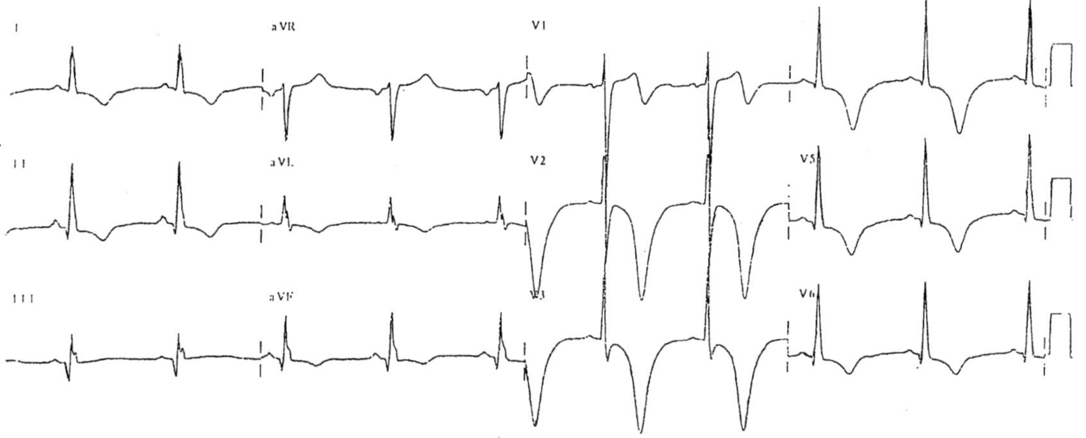

Fig. 13.9 Deep T wave inversion in a patient presenting with ischaemic chest pain, but without biochemical evidence of myocardial necrosis.

Other causes for T wave inversion

- **Juvenile T wave pattern.** Inverted T waves in the precordial leads are a normal finding in children. The pattern is localized to leads V2 to V4 and usually disappears by the age of 20 although in up to 25% of adults (more frequently in females) the childhood T wave pattern persists.
- **T wave inversion associated with early repolarization.** On occasions the normal variant of early repolarization is associated with biphasic T wave inversion particularly in the anterior ECG leads.
- **Intracerebral causes.** Intracranial haemorrhage, subarachnoid haemorrhage, or other intracerebral causes can be associated with diffuse deep T wave inversion often associated with prolongation at the QT interval. The pattern is usually localized over the anterior leads and is not associated with development of Q waves. T wave changes may be seen within hours of the initial cerebral event. The aetiology of this abnormality is not clear but may be associated with microscopic myocardial lesions as a result of intense neurogenic stimulation of the myocardium, possibly from catecholamines.
- **Post tachy/post pacemaker T wave inversions.** After cessation of tachyarrhythmias, there is occasionally diffuse T wave inversion which may last for up to 24 hours. Similarly, in a patient who has been pacemaker-dependent, and reverts to normal rhythm, T wave inversion may occur. The reason for these abnormalities is not clear but they are not thought to be associated with myocardial injury.
- **Mitral valve prolapse syndrome.** T wave inversion in the inferior leads is frequently seen in the mitral valve prolapse syndrome, with occasional T wave inversions seen also in the lateral leads.
- **Left ventricular hypertrophy.** Left ventricular hypertrophy may also be associated with T wave inversion in addition to the typical ST segment depression seen with myocardial strain. These changes usually do not indicate associated myocardial ischaemia.
- **Minor T wave inversion.** Minor T wave inversion may occur as a result of a variety of causes including electrolyte disturbance, drug therapy with antiarrhythmic drugs, tricyclic antidepressants, pentathiazines, hyperventilation or other causes. There is now increasing recognition that many of these T wave abnormalities which were described in the past as non-specific are possible indicators of myocardial ischaemia.

Q waves

Abnormal Q waves or QRS complexes may develop as early as 2 hours after the onset of pain and are usually fully developed within 12 hours with concurrent loss of R waves.[6] The presence of Q waves has been regarded an indicator for necrosis and was previously regarded as a marker of transmural MI. Patterns of Q wave development are quite variable[8] and the validity of the link of pathological Q waves with transmural infarction has been challenged repeatedly.[9,10]

It is now clear that both Q wave and non-Q wave infarctions are heterogeneous conditions.[10] Use of the terms Q wave and non-Q wave infarction is more appropriate terminology than transmural and subendocardial infarctions, and has specific prognostic significance.[11]

The ECG criteria for diagnosis of Q wave MI or non-Q wave MI would seem relatively straightforward. However, several studies have determined that a significant reduction in R wave amplitude is considered a Q wave MI although the definition of the amount of R wave reduction has not been standardized. There has also been some variation in the definition of pathological Q waves leading to some confusion in diagnosis of Q wave or non-Q wave MI.[12]

Another important dilemma is in true posterior infarct where most investigators regard an RS ratio of one or more in leads V1 and V2 as consistent with a Q wave infarct. Other anatomical sites where MI can be silent on the ECG, such as the lateral wall, may not be recognized as Q wave MI.

The baseline ECG with the presence of previous Q wave infarction, left bundle branch block, and underlying cardiomyopathies may also reduce the sensitivity of the Q wave in the diagnosis of MI.

Despite these difficulties there are significant differences in Q wave and non-Q wave MIs. Patients with non-Q wave infarctions are more likely to have had previous angina than the Q wave infarct group. They have smaller infarct size, more frequently have a patent infarct-related vessel and although the prognosis is better in the acute phase the 12 month prognosis is affected adversely by residual ischaemia.[12] In fact non-Q wave infarction represents an unstable state, with patients having twice the risk of recurrent angina or infarct extension compared with a patient with Q wave infarction. The ability to identify Q wave or non-Q wave infarction is therefore important so as to be able to identify this group of higher risk patients.

Q wave progression

Q waves usually persist following MI but up to 15% of Q waves following MI can regress within 18 months with a significant proportion of ECGs returning to normal after 3 years.[13]

Apart from regression of Q waves, the development of infarction in another location or development of a bundle branch block can be alternative explanations for disappearance of Q waves. It is important that coronary care staff comprehend the delayed development of Q waves after MI. If a patient presenting with clinical features of infarction has well developed Q waves on the ECG and is still experiencing chest pain, it is unlikely that these are due to the acute episode but more likely due to previous infarction or to non-infarctional causes of Q waves.

Non-infarctional Q waves

Q waves not related to MI can occur in the following situations:

- **Q waves in lateral leads.** Q waves in AVL can simulate the pattern of lateral infarction but may simply be due to septal depolarization and a vertical position of the heart. This will be evident from review of lead I which will tend to be isoelectric rather than upright. Septal Q waves due to septal hypertrophy in hypertrophic cardiomyopathy may also produce deep but narrow Q waves in leads I, AVL, V5 and V6. This is thought to be due to the initial septal depolarization being exaggerated in the presence of septal hypertrophy.[14] Sometimes these Q waves are indistinguishable from infarction Q waves and echocardiography is required for the differentiation between lateral infarction and septal hypertrophy.
- **QS waves in anterior leads.** On occasions deep QS complexes in V1 and V2 may be indistinguishable from anterior infarction. These may be due to the presence of left ventricular hypertrophy or to a hyperexpanded chest. They can be distinguished from infarctional Q waves by the lack of notching on the S wave, whereas infarction QS waves tend to show a notching pattern between the Q wave and the S wave. On occasions echocardiography may be necessary to distinguish these normal variants from old anterior MIs.
- **Q waves in inferior leads.** A Q wave may be present in lead III or in lead AVF as a normal variant. Q waves may be present in lead III in up to 15–20% of the normal population. 'Normal' nonpathologic Q waves are usually

less than 0.04 seconds in width and no deeper than 25% of the height of the R wave. These criteria are not always reliable, and diagnosis of inferior infarction cannot be confidently made on the basis of an abnormal Q wave in lead III if it is not supported by evidence of Q waves in the other inferior leads. This is particularly so if the Q wave normalizes with inspiration (see Fig. 13.4). Q waves in both leads III and AVF make the diagnosis of infarction more likely, particularly if they are abnormal Q waves. Nevertheless, these Q waves can also be normal variants and can be greatly influenced by the position of the patient or the location of the inferior limb recording electrodes, on ankle, thigh or trunk (see Fig. 13.2). An additional criterion which has been suggested is the appearance of the QRS complex in lead AVR.[6] The Q waves in leads III and AVF are likely to be normal if lead AVR shows an RS complex and abnormal if it shows a QS complex. On occasions septal hypertrophy can produce non-infarctional Q waves in leads II, III and AVF. These are usually narrow and are usually associated with Q waves in I, AVL, V5 and V6. Sometimes the delta wave associated with the Wolff–Parkinson–White anomaly can produce the appearance of deep Q waves in the inferior leads, and may be associated with repolarization abnormalities which mimic inferior MI (see Fig. 13.10).

- **Tall R wave in V1.** Tall R wave in V1 may indicate true posterior infarction which is of particular significance if it can be shown on serial ECGs to be increasing in size. However, it could be a normal variant due to counter-clockwise rotation of the heart as well as reflecting right ventricular hypertrophy, type A Wolff–Parkinson–White anomaly, and right bundle branch block. In addition true posterior infarction is usually associated with serial ECG changes in inferior leads (see Fig. 13.11), although this is not invariable.
- **Rare causes of non-infarctional Q waves.** These include left pneumothorax due to marked rightward shift of the heart. This may rarely need to be considered in a differential diagnosis of chest pain in a patient being admitted to the CCU. Other causes of abnormal QS pattern in the anterior leads, such as dextrocardia and pectus excavatum, would be evident on clinical examination. Duchenne muscular dystrophy and rarely dystrophia myotonica can be associated with tall R wave in V1 and deep and narrowed Q waves in the lateral leads because of posterolateral scarring with myocardial involvement in muscular dystrophies.

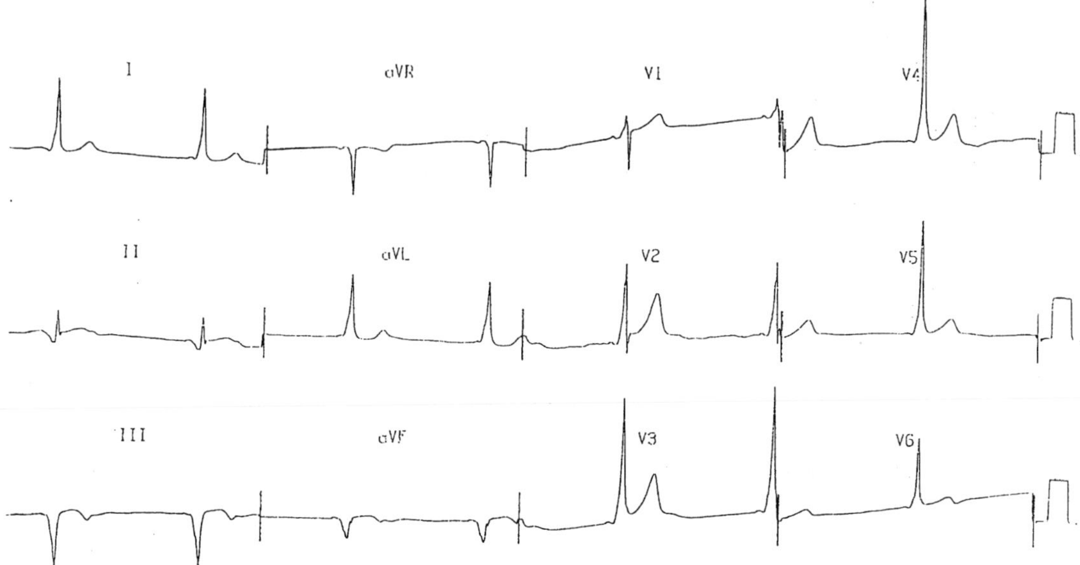

Fig. 13.10 Delta waves in the Wolff–Parkinson–White anomaly producing the appearance of inferior lead Q waves.

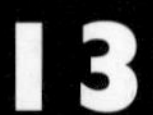

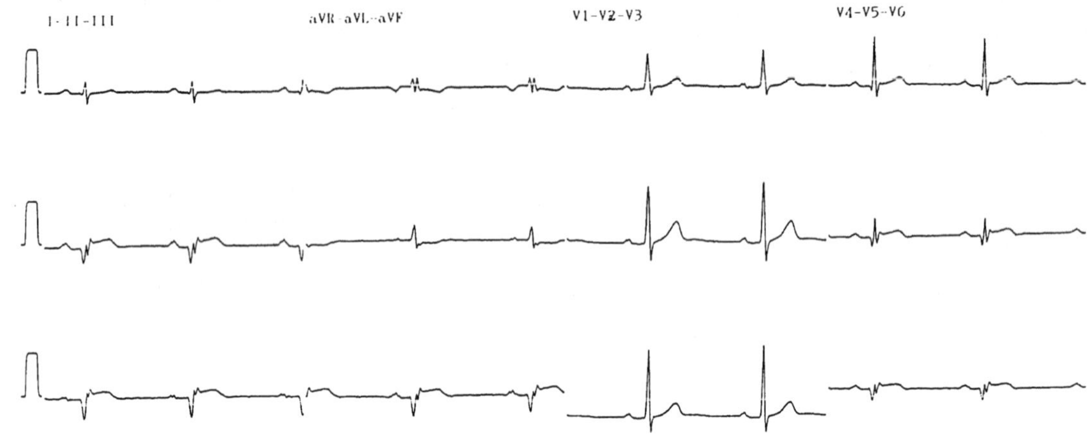

Fig. 13.11 Tall R wave in lead V1 in a patient with inferoposterior MI. Note the associated changes in leads II, III, AVF, V5 and V6.

Localizing site of infarction and infarct related artery from the electrocardiogram[6,15]

Accurate diagnosis of the site of infarction is important in targeting appropriate initial therapy in the treatment of MI as well as assessing prognostic significance with regard to morbidity and mortality. The lead groupings for location of ischaemia or infarction are summarized in Table 13.2. The culprit coronary vessel can often be determined from the 12-lead ECG, based on an understanding of the coronary anatomy (see Ch. 21).

Left anterior descending coronary artery

Anterior ECG changes almost invariably indicate occlusion of left anterior descending coronary artery. Coronary angiography performed early after the onset of infarction has shown that anterior electrocardiographic changes indicate LAD occlusion with a sensitivity of 90%, specificity of 95% and predictive value of 96%. However the localization within the LAD is less reliable, although associated ST segment depression in the inferior leads is an indication of more extensive anterior infarction.[7,15]

Right coronary artery

Inferior MI without posterior or lateral changes indicates right coronary artery occlusion with a sensitivity of 56%, specificity of 97% and predictive value of 88%.[15] Inferior ECG changes with ST elevation in V1 and V2 indicate very proximal right coronary artery occlusion and may indicate right ventricular infarction.[16] Inferior MI with anterior reciprocal ST segment depression in anterior leads V2 and V3 may indi-

Table 13.2 Localization of infarction from ECG leads and the usual corresponding infarct-related artery

Area of infarction	ECG Leads	Infarct-related artery
Inferior	II, III, AVF	Right or posterolateral of circumflex
Anterior	V_2, V_3, V_4	Mid left anterior descending or diagonal branch of LAD
Lateral	I, AVL, V_5, V_6	Circumflex or lateral ventricular branch of circumflex
True posterior	Tall R in V_1	Posterolateral of circumflex or posterior descending of right
Anterolateral	I, AVL, V_2–V_6	Proximal left anterior descending
Inferolateral	II, III, AVF, I, AVL, V_5, V_6	Proximal circumflex or large lateral ventricular in left dominant system
Right ventricular	V_3R, V_4R	Right coronary

cate proximal right coronary artery occlusion, whereas reciprocal changes in the more lateral leads may indicate more distal right coronary artery occlusion.[17,18]

Circumflex coronary artery

In contrast to the relative degree of accuracy diagnosing left anterior descending and right coronary artery occlusion, identification of circumflex coronary occlusion is more difficult. Posterior or lateral infarction without inferior ECG changes identified circumflex occlusion with a sensitivity of 24%, specificity of 98% and predictive value of 75%. In patients with known circumflex coronary artery occlusion ECG evidence of lateral infarction was seen in about 50%.[15,19] Occlusion of the circumflex coronary artery can be associated with inferolateral or true posterior infarction.

Variations in anatomy and responsible territory of the circumflex and right coronary artery systems make the differentiation of right coronary and circumflex coronary artery occlusions difficult although the direction of ST segment deviation in lead I may be a useful predictor, with elevation indicating circumflex occlusion and depression indicating right coronary artery occlusion.[19–21]

Recording of special leads on the right chest in the position V3 or V4 (V3R, V4R) may show ST–T changes indicating right ventricular infarction.[22]

Precordial ST segment depression in inferior myocardial infarction

The mechanism of anterior lead ST segment depression in the presence of inferior infarction can be due either to anterior myocardial ischaemia associated with critical left anterior descending coronary artery disease or to reciprocal change from the posterior or posterolateral walls. Whilst both explanations are conceivable and may indeed both contribute in the same patient, detailed studies of this ECG phenomenon have shown that reciprocal changes from the posterior wall are the predominant determinant.[17] The controversy about the mechanism of the phenomenon continues, but there is now general agreement that anterior ST segment depression in the presence of inferior MI indicates a more extensive infarct with a worse prognosis.[23,24] The extent, as well as the pressure, of the anterior ST segment depression correlate with the extent of left ventricular function and worse prognosis.[25] Left precordial ST segment depression may indicate a worse outcome than right precordial ST depression in inferior infarction.[26] Figure 13.12 shows a typical example.

Inferior ST segment depression in acute anterior infarction is less commonly recognized than anterior ST depression with inferior infarction (see Fig. 13.13). This phenomenon is usually less striking but also appears to be related to reciprocal change and is more likely to be associated with proximal rather than distal LAD occlusion especially when the LAD is a large vessel supplying the apex and part of the inferior wall.[27] It similarly predicts worse left ventricular function and prognosis.

The electrocardiogram in selection of patients for thrombolysis

Overview of the nine trials which included more than 1000 patients for thrombolytic therapy versus placebo included nearly 60 000 patients,[28] and showed quite clearly that the ECG on admission was an important indicator of the likely benefit from thrombolytic therapy. Patients in the trial whose entry ECG showed bundle branch block had the greatest benefit with an absolute benefit of 49 lives saved per 1000 patients treated.

Among patients with anterior ST segment elevation 37 lives were saved per 1000 treated, among those with inferior ST elevation 8 lives were saved per 1000 treated, and with ST elevation in other locations, 27 lives were saved per 1000 treated. These clear-cut benefits were in contrast to patients with ST segment depression on the ECG in whom thrombolytic therapy had a negative benefit of 14 lives per 1000 and patients with normal ECGs had a negative benefit of 7 lives per 1000 patients treated. This data clearly indicates the importance of the ECG in accurate selection of patients for thrombolytic therapy.

Diagnosis of infarction in the presence of left bundle branch block

Diagnosis of infarction in the presence of left bundle branch block (LBBB) presents considerable difficulties, because this conduction abnormality interferes with the initial QRS complex thus obscuring the pres-

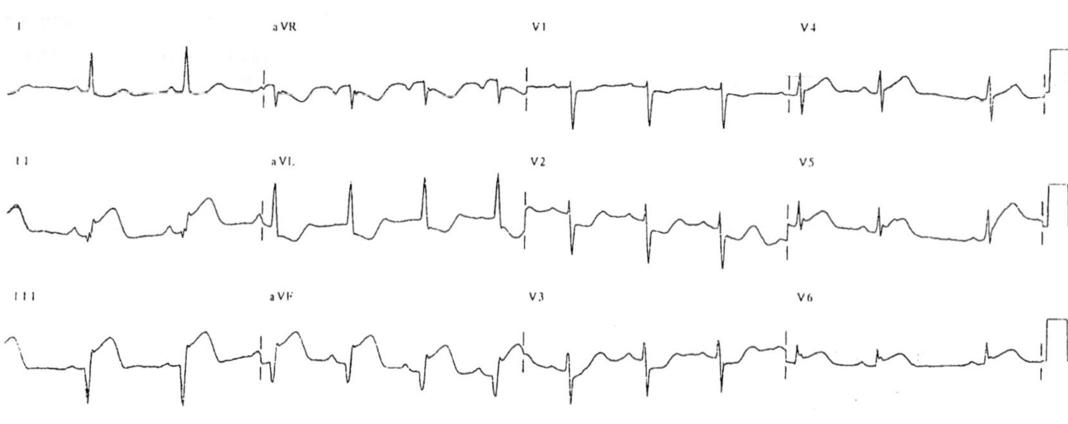

Fig. 13.12 Precordial ST segment depression in a patient with acute inferior MI.

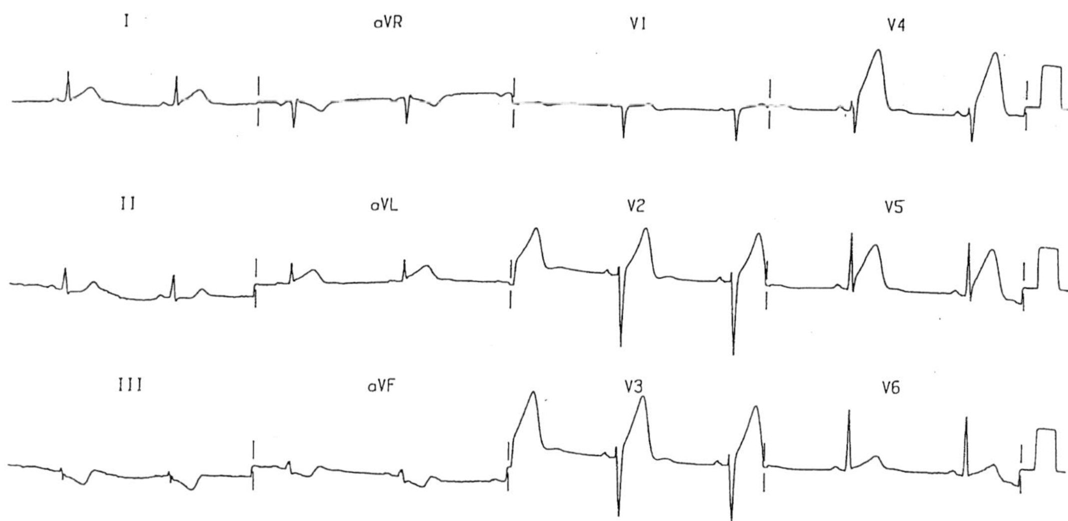

Fig. 13.13 Inferior ST segment depression in a patient with acute anterior MI.

ence of Q waves, as well as with the repolarization pattern thus obscuring the pattern of ST segment elevation and T wave inversion.[29] Nevertheless, criteria have been defined including Q waves in at least two lateral leads, R wave regression from lead V1 to V4, notching of the upstroke of the S wave in at least two anterior leads (Cabrerer's sign) and primary ST segment changes in two or more adjacent leads. These criteria are specific 90–100% but relatively insensitive (<40%) for the diagnosis of infarction.[30]

In contrast to the difficulty of diagnosis of infarction on a single tracing showing LBBB, the diagnosis may be relatively simplified when there is clear-cut sequential ST segment elevation on serial ECGs (see Fig. 13.14).

Diagnosis of infarction in the presence of right bundle branch block

Diagnosis of infarction in the presence of right bundle branch block (RBBB) is not as complex as in LBBB, as RBBB does not alter the initial deflection of the QRS complex and results only in a slurred S wave in the lateral leads.[23] The result is that Q waves and ST elevation are not obscured (see example in Fig. 13.15).

However, the presence of ischaemia with associated ST depression or T wave inversion may be difficult to interpret.

References

1. Marriott HJ. Practical electrocardiography. 8th ed. Baltimore: Williams and Wilkins, 1987
2. Schamroth L. An introduction to electrocardiography. 6th ed. Oxford: Alden Press, 1989
3. Schlant RC, Hurst JW et al. Advances in electrocardiography.

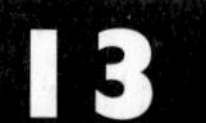

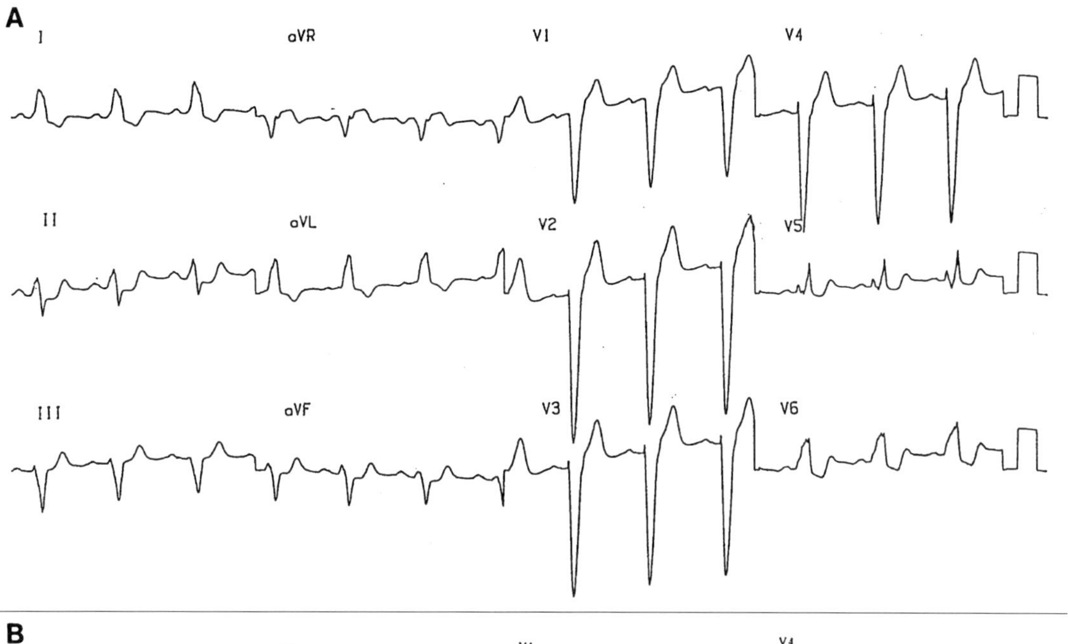

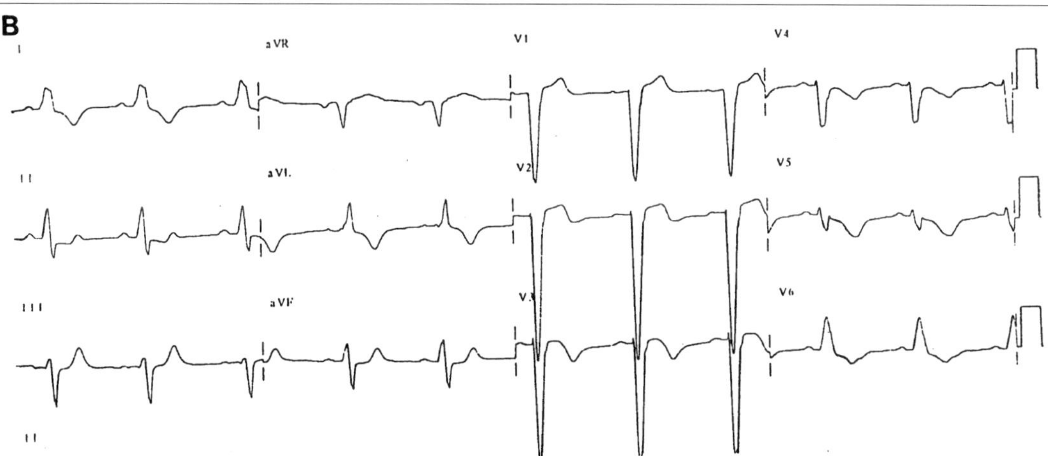

Fig. 13.14 Serial ECGs in a patient with left bundle branch block showing ST-T changes indicative of anterior MI. **A**. On admission. **B**. 24 hours later.

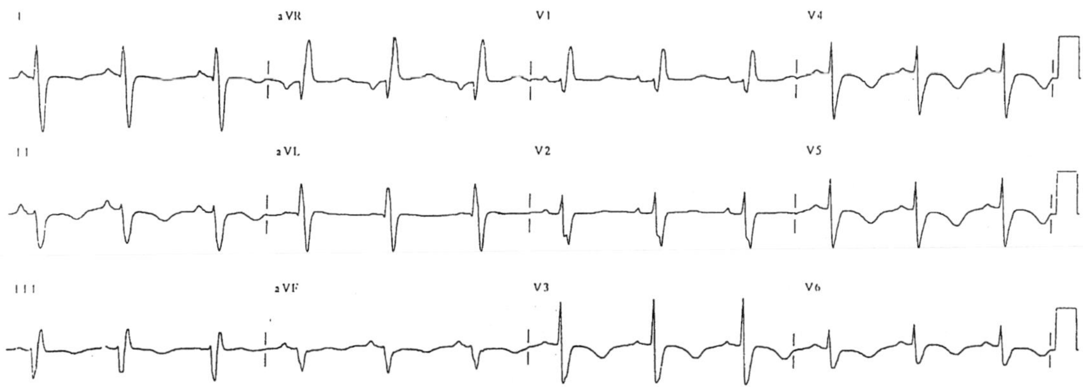

Fig. 13.15 Acute anterolateral MI in the presence of right bundle branch block. The ST–T changes in the anterolateral leads are obvious despite the conduction defect.

New York: Grune and Stratton, 1972
4. Macfarlane PW, Lawrie VTD. Comprehensive electrocardiology, vol 1. New York: Pergamon Press, 1989
5. Goldberger AL. Myocardial infarction: electrocardiographic differential diagnosis. Saint Louis: Mosby, 1975.
5a. Laks MM, Arzbaecher R, Bailey JJ, Geselowitz DB, Berson AS. Recommendations for safe current limits for electrocardiographs. Circulation 1996; 93: 837–9
6. Schweitzer P. The electrocardiographic diagnosis of acute myocardial infarction in the thrombolytic era. Am Heart J 1990; 119: 642–54
7. Bennett DH. Cardiac arrhythmias. 4th ed. Oxford: Butterworths 1993
8. Prinzmetal M et al. Angina pectoris. A variant form of angina pectoris. Am J Med 1959; 27: 375
9. Yusuf S, Lopez R, Maddison A, Sleight P. Variability of electrocardiographic and enzyme evolution of myocardial infarction in man. Brit Heart J 1981; 45: 271–80
10. Spodick, DH. Q Wave infarction versus ST infarction, non specificity of electrographic criteria for differentiating transmural and non transmural lesions. Am J Cardiol 1983; 51: 913–5
11. Phibbs B. 'Transmural' versus 'subendocardial' myocardial infarction: an electrocardiographic myth. J Am Coll Cardiol 1983; 1: 561–4
12. Maisel AS, Ahne S, Gilpin E et al. Prognosis after extension of myocardial infarct: the role of Q wave or non Q wave infarction. Circulation 1985; 71: 211–7
13. Surawicz B, Uhley H, Borun R et al. Task force 1. Standardisation of terminology and interpretation. Am J Cardiol 1978; 41: 130–45
14. Kaplan BM, Berkson DM. Serial electrocardiograms after myocardial infarctions. Ann Int Med 1964; 60: 430
15. Maron BJ. Q waves in hypertrophic cardiomyopathy: a reassessment. Editorial. J Am Coll Cardiol 1990; 16: 375
16. Blanke H, Cohen M, Schlueter G et al. Electrocardiographic and coronary angiographic correlation during acute myocardial infarction. Am J Cardiol 1984; 54: 249–55
17. Geft IL, Shah PK, Rodriguez L et al. ST elevation in leads V1–V5 may be caused by right coronary artery occlusion and acute right ventricular infarction. Am J Cardiol 1984; 53: 991–6
18. Lew AS, Maddahi J, Shah PK et al. Factors that determine the direction and magnitude of precordial ST-segment deviation during inferior wall acute myocardial infarction. Am J Cardiol 1985; 55: 883–8
19. Lew AS, Laramee P, Shah PK et al. Ratio of ST segment depression in lead V2 to ST segment elevation in lead AVF in evolving inferior myocardial infarction: an aid to the early recognition of right ventricular infarction. Am J Cardiol 1986; 57: 1047–51
20. Huey BL, Beller GA, Kaiser DL et al. A comprehensive analysis of myocardial infarction due to left circumflex artery occlusion: comparison with infarction due to right coronary artery and left anterior descending artery occlusion. J Am Coll Cardiol 1988; 12: 1156–66
21. Bairey CN, Shah PK, Lew AS et al. Electrocardiographic differentiation of occlusion of left circumflex versus the right coronary artery as a cause of inferior acute myocardial infarction. Am J Cardiol 1987; 60: 456–9
22. Erhardt LR, Sjogren A, Wahlberg J. Single right precordial lead in the diagnosis of right ventricular involvment in inferior myocardial infarction. Am Heart J 1976; 91: 571–6
23. Pichler M, Shah PK, Peter T et al. Wall motion abnormalities and electrocardiographic changes in acute myocardial infarction: implication of reciprocal ST depression. Am Heart J 1983; 106: 1003–9
24. Goldberg HL, Borer JS, Jacobstein JG et al. Anterior ST segment depression in acute inferior myocardial infarction: indicator of posterolateral or inferoseptal involvement. Am J Cardiol 1984; 54: 1009–15
25. Peterson ED, Hathway WR, Zabel M et al. The prognostic importance of anterior ST depression in inferior myocardial infarction: results in 16 185 patients. J Am Coll Cardiol 1995; 25: 342A
26. Birnbaum Y, Herz I, Sclarovsky S, Zlotikamien B, Chetrik A, Barbash G. Prognostic significance of different patterns of precordial segment depression in inferior wall acute myocardial infarction. J Am Coll Cardiol 1995; 25: 343A
27. Lew AS, Hod H, Cerce B et al. Inferior lead ST segment changes during acute anterior myocardial infarction: a marker of the presence or absence of concomitant inferior wall ischaemia. J Am Coll Cardiol 1987; 10: 519–26
28. Fibrinolytic Therapy Triallists (FTT) Collaborative Group. Indications for fibrinolytic therapy in suspected acute myocardial infarction. Collaborative overview of early mortality and major morbidity results from all randomised trials of more than 1000 patients. Lancet 1994; 343: 311–22
29. Sodi-Pallares D, Cisneros F et al. Electrocardiographic diagnosis of myocardial infarction in the presence of bundle branch block (right and left), ventricular premature beats and Wolff–Parkinson–White syndrome. Progr Cardiovasc Dis 1963; 6: 107
30. Hands ME, Cook F, Stone PH et al. Electrocardiographic diagnosis of myocardial infarction in the presence of complete left bundle branch block. Am Heart J 1988; 116: 23–31

14 Biochemical markers of myocardial necrosis

Peter L Thompson

Introduction

For many years, assays of cardiac enzymes have been used for the diagnosis of myocardial infarction (MI), detection of coronary reperfusion and detection of re-infarction.[1] The enzymes which have been used for this purpose have been total creatine kinase (CK), CK isoenzymes (CKMB), aspartate aminotransferase (AST) and lactic dehydrogenase (LD). Recently, more specific biochemical markers have been introduced including CKMM and CKMB isoforms, myoglobin and troponin I and troponin T.[2]

Creatine kinase, isoenzymes and isoforms

The use of creatine kinase as a serum marker of acute myocardial infarction (AMI) was first described in 1960.[3] Since then it has been widely used for diagnosis of AMI, but with increasing acceptance of the lack of specificity of total CK and the increased specificity of CKMB, the CKMB isoenzyme is now the most widely used standard for the diagnosis of myocardial necrosis.[2]

Skeletal muscle contains mostly the CKMM isoenzyme and contains less than 3% of CKMB. Cardiac muscle contains 15–20% CKMB.

Following irreversible ischaemic necrosis of myocardial cells there is a leakage of creatine kinase from the intracellular to the extracellular compartment. The enzyme in the interstitial space then passes into the lymphatic system before reaching the circulation.[4] During passage through the lymphatics there is a process of oxidation which breaks down the enzyme so that only 15–20% of the total myocardial CK release appears in the circulation. These factors account for a delay of 3–4 hours before the enzyme appears in blood samples in patients with AMI. The enzyme is widely distributed and is cleared by the reticuloendothelial system, a process which is remarkably consistent and appears to be free of the extent of infarction and haemodynamics.[5] The interplay between the rate of release, distribution volume and rate of degradation explains the typical plasma curves of CK with appearance in the plasma 3–4 hours post infarction, rising to a peak at 20–24 hours and gradually returning to normal over the subsequent 3–4 days. CKMB follows similar kinetics with a slightly earlier rise and earlier peak and slightly more rapid clearance[6].

When coronary reperfusion occurs before myocardial necrosis has been complete there is a 'shift to the left' of the curve with an early peaking and more rapid clearance as the lymphatic degradation processes are overwhelmed with the rapid washout of the enzyme from the necrotic cells.[7]

Although total CK is a sensitive marker of myocardial necrosis, it is relatively non-specific because of common causes of skeletal muscle release such as physical exercise, muscle trauma from surgery, defibrillation, resuscitation and limb ischaemia or less common causes such as muscular dystrophy, alcoholic muscle disease and myxoedema. The introduction of CKMB isoenzyme assays, initially with rather cumbersome electrophoretic methods and more recently with automated immunoassays, has overcome many of the difficulties of non-specificity with total CK assays (see Fig. 14.1).[2,6] It has always been recognized that despite the specificity of CKMB for myocardial injury, the small amount of CKMB in skeletal muscle can on occasions confound the results.[8] Therefore the concept of the ratio of CKMB to total CK[9] has been widely used to overcome this problem. On occasions, however, this may be misleading when myocardial necrosis is present in conjunction with

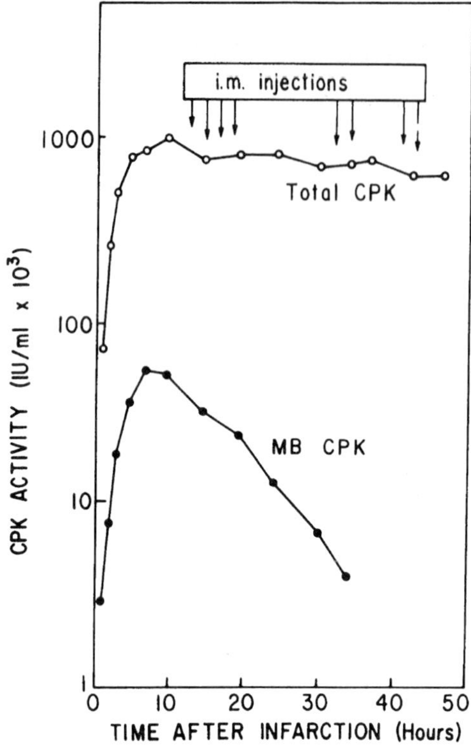

Fig. 14.1 Typical rise and fall of serum CK-MB after acute myocardial infarction in contrast to total CK which remains elevated, indicative of skeletal muscle injury from repeated intramuscular injections. Reproduced with permission. Roberts R, Serum enzyme determinations in the diagnosis of acute myocardial infaction. In: Karliner JS, Gregoratos G, eds. Coronary Care. Edinburgh: Churchill Livingstone, 1981.

massive skeletal muscle damage such as after major surgery or trauma. Conversely, in patients with chronic muscle diseases such as muscular dystrophy or polymyositis, there may be substantial release of CKMB from skeletal muscle. The latter group of patients are readily identified by a persistent CKMB pattern rather than the typical rise and fall seen with myocardial necrosis. Rarer causes of CKMB elevation include renal failure or some tumours. As with total CK, hypothyroidism may cause persistently abnormal CKMB because of delayed clearance.

In general the difficulties which non-cardiac sources of CKMB present in the diagnosis of MI can be overcome by serial measurements, a policy of caution in interpreting the CKMB/CK ratio and in not diagnosing infarction unless CKMB rises above the normal range.

Sensitivity and specificity of CKMB have been improved by the development of automated immunoinhibition assays using monocloncal anti-CKMB antibodies.[10] These techniques express the results as CK mass in micrograms per litre (μg/L) or nanograms per millilitre (ηg/ml) rather than the more familiar enzyme activity expressed as international units per litre (i.u./L). The correlation between the two methods appears to be excellent.[11] The particular advantages of these techniques are that they can provide the results within 30 minutes (rapid CKMB assay), and can be used to diagnose MI one hour earlier than conventional CKMB assays.[12]

Despite the high sensitivity and specificity of CKMB for diagnosis of MI, the minimum delay of 4–6 hours before abnormal levels appear in the serum and up to 12 hours may elapse before a diagnosis of MI can be accurately established.

More recently, assays of isoforms of CK have been described.[13,14] Early detection of CKMM isoforms is highly sensitive but not specific for the diagnosis of MI. In myocardial tissue there is a single form of CKMB (MB_2) which, on release into the serum, gets partially converted to an alternative subform ($CKMB_1$). The subforms of CKMB can be detected in the serum as early as 2 hours after the onset of MI. Levels of $CKMB_2$ greater than 1.0 units/L with a ratio of $CKMB_2$ to $CKMB_1$ greater than 1.5 are diagnostic of MI.[15] A rapid assay technique was over 90% specific and provided 56% sensitivity at 4 hours and 96% sensitivity at 6 hours for the diagnosis of MI[16] (see Fig. 14.2). However the specificity for MI has not been tested in the presence of skeletal muscle injury.

Lactic dehydrogenase (LD)

Lactic dehydrogenase consists of five isoenzymes.[17] The heart contains predominantly LD_1 and to a lesser extent LD_2. The isoenzymes can now be measured directly but previously hydroxybutyric dehydrogenase (HBDH) was measured as a surrogate for LD_1. Total lactic dehydrogenase rises to abnormal levels in the serum 24–48 hours after the onset of myocardial

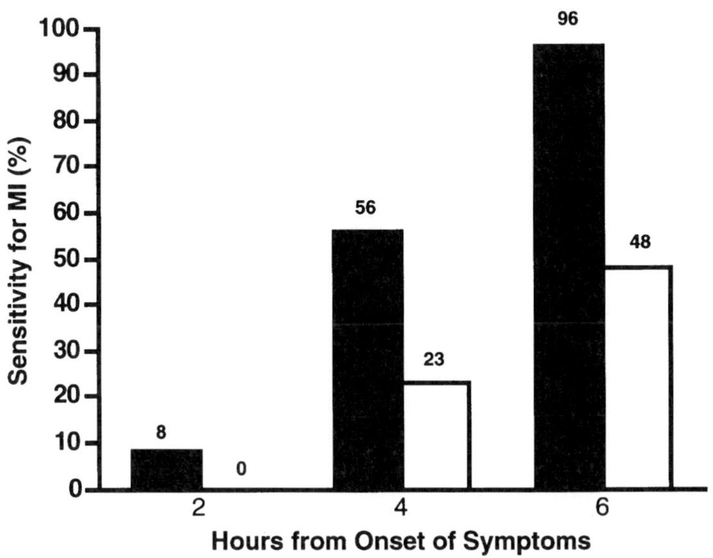

Fig. 14.2 Sensitivity of CKMB subforms (black bars) compared with CK-MB (white bars) (359 patients with confirmed MI) indicating 96% sensitivity at 6 hours after the onset of symptoms. Redrawn with permission from the New England Journal of Medicine. Puleo et al N Engl J Med 1994; 331: 961–6. Copyright 1994 Massachusetts Medical Society. All rights reserved.

necrosis, reaches a peak at 3–6 days and returns to normal at 7–14 days post infarction. Total LD may be abnormal in the presence of haemolysis, megaloblastic anaemia, hepatic congestion or pulmonary embolism. To improve the sensitivity of diagnosis, the ratio of LD_1 to LD_2 has been commonly used. The ratio of LD_1 to LD_2 greater than 0.76 has been reported to be 90% sensitive and specific for the diagnosis of MI. A ratio of 1.0 has less sensitivity but better specificity.[18] False positive increases in the LD_1:LD_2 ratio can occur in skeletal muscle injury or in the presence of severe haemolysis. Measurement of lactic dehydrogenase and isoenzymes is usually reserved for patients who have presented late after suspected MI.

Aspartate aminotransferase (AST)

AST has been used for nearly 50 years as a marker of myocardial necrosis[19] and is still used in many laboratories and CCUs. Its serum profile is intermediate between CK and LD, becoming abnormal at 8–12 hours and peaking at 24–36 hours and usually returning to normal within 3–4 days. The major limitation with AST is that it frequently has an hepatic origin and may be abnormally elevated in patients with liver disease. Transient rises and falls of AST have been seen as an indication of transient biliary obstruction in patients presenting with chest pain due to biliary colic. It may remain persistently elevated in patients whose MI is complicated by hepatic congestion.

Myoglobin

Myoglobin, being a relatively small molecule, is rapidly released from myocardium as a result of myocardial necrosis and will appear in the serum within 2 hours after the onset. Thus myoglobin can potentially fulfil the requirement for a marker of myocardial necrosis within a time span when intervention may be helpful.[20,21] A rapid assay which provides a semi-quantitative result within 10 minutes is available.[21a] However, myoglobin's abundance in skeletal muscle and its dependence on renal blood flow for clearance seriously impair its specificity, with some studies reporting false positive results as high as 50%.

Troponins

The troponin complex consists of three different protein subunits, T, I and C. Cardiac troponin I and T are antigenically distinct from the skeletal muscle troponins, a property which should confer 100% specificity for cardiac muscle injury.

Cardiac troponin I and T have been used for the diagnosis of myocardial infarction.[22,23] Both troponin I and T are available as rapid assays,[22a,24] and troponin is available as a semi-quantitative slide test for bedside application to detect levels above 0.2 μg/L.[25]

The sensitivity and specificity of troponin I and T have been shown to be comparable to CK MB for the diagnosis of myocardial infarction,[22,23] but the troponins have several properties which are attractive as biochemical markers for myocardial injury including an earlier rise to abnormal levels (median 3.8 hours for troponin T versus 4.8 hours for CK MB[23]) and elevated levels for up to two weeks post MI. Troponin I appears to be more specific than troponin T.[26a] The latter has shown false positives in some studies.[26b]

Myosin fragments

Myosin light chains (MLC) have been studied but are not widely used.[2]

Diagnosis of myocardial infarction

Serial quantitative CKMB levels are the most sensitive and specific biochemical marker in common use for AMI. Measurement each 12 hours is a reliable and cost-effective method for diagnosis of MI.[1,2] Abnormal plasma levels are seen at 6–10 hours, peak at 20–24 hours and return to normal by 36–72 hours (see Fig. 14.3).

If quantitative serial CKMB levels are not available, total CK measurements at the same intervals may be a satisfactory substitute in the absence of obvious skeletal muscle damage; however a confirmatory CKMB level should be obtained. AST levels are not sufficiently reliable for routine use. Total LD or $LD_1:LD_2$ ratio is a useful method of diagnosis of MI in patients who present late. Myoglobin does not have a place in the routine diagnosis of MI because of poor specificity. Of the newer markers serial quantitative troponin I or T levels appear to be the most promising, particularly for the detection of reinfarction and for the retrospective diagnosis of infarction with late presentation.

The high specificity of troponin I for myocardial necrosis makes it superior to CKMB for the diagnosis of perioperative myocardial infarction.[26c]

Early detection of myocardial infarction

Considerable effort has been expended in recent years on the development of rapid assay techniques for the earliest possible detection of myocardial necrosis. Rapid assay techniques are now available for CK MB,[10] CKMB subforms,[16] myoglobin,[21a] troponin I[22] and troponin T.[23,24] Unfortunately none of these markers can reliably exclude myocardial infarction at the time of admission to hospital.[26a] A combination of early, sensitive detection of muscle injury with myoglobin with a highly specific test for myocardial necrosis with troponin I may be the best approach to early and accurate diagnosis.

Estimation of troponin T has been shown to be helpful in the early prediction of subsequent coronary events in patients presenting with unstable angina.[25–27]

The semi-quantitative bedside assay may provide this information even before laboratory results are available.[25]

The precise role of these techniques in cardiac decision-making in the emergency room remains to be defined. At present, decisions about admission to the CCU are based on the likelihood of cardiac complications and the immediate need for more detailed cardiac investigation, reperfusion or revascularization. Patients who present with acute coronary syndromes may have critical and unstable coronary artery disease and require intensive treatment whether or not they have early evidence of myocardial necrosis. Decisions about coronary thrombolysis are based on the clinical history and ECG showing characteristic ST segment elevations or bundle branch block. Patients without these features do not benefit from thrombolysis. The role of early detection of myocardial necrosis in patients being considered for primary coronary angioplasty is yet to be defined.

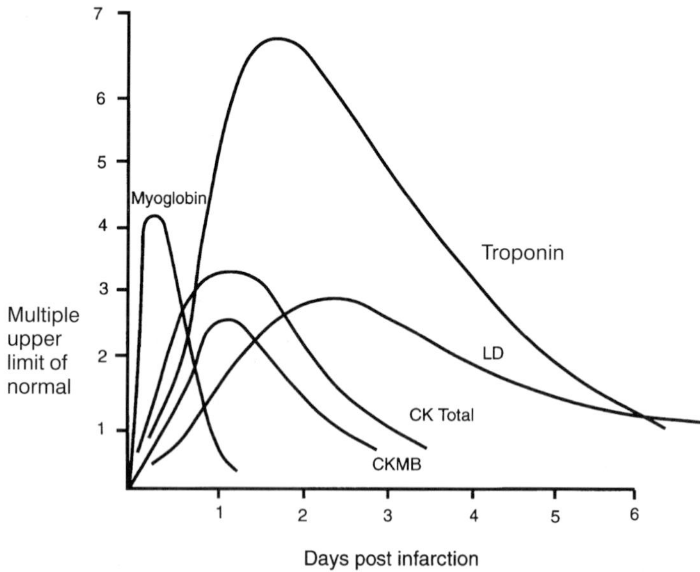

Fig. 14.3 Typical serum activity curves for biochemical markers after AMI. CK = creatine kinase; LD = lactic dehydrogenase; troponin refers to troponin I and troponin T.

Perhaps the most relevant use for early markers of myocardial necrosis is in the triage of the patient in whom the clinical features suggest a low risk of an acute coronary syndrome. The patient without evidence of myocardial necrosis may be considered for relatively low level coronary care such as an overnight chest pain observation unit. Unexpected early detection of MI would qualify such a patient for admission to a CCU and consideration of reperfusion therapy, rather than to a chest pain observation unit.[26]

Detection of recanalization after reperfusion therapy

Patients who have successful reperfusion, particularly with TIMI grade 3 flow in the infarct-related artery, have a low mortality, an uncomplicated course and may qualify for early hospital discharge. Patients with persistent occlusion have a higher short-term mortality and more complicated hospital course. It would be helpful to distinguish between these two groups of coronary occlusion patients particularly in helping to decide if the patient with failed reperfusion from thrombolysis may need to be considered for early 'rescue' angioplasty. Early peaking of the total CK or CKMB curve is well recognized as a marker of reperfusion; however a cut-off point for defining a reliable time for early peaking is problematic. An overview of 233 patients showed that a time to peak of less than 10 hours was 100% specific but only 27% sensitive for detection of reperfusion. A peak under 18 hours was 91% sensitive and 76% specific.[28] Specificity of 100% and sensitivity of 85% for reperfusion are possible by measuring the rate of increase of CKMB in the initial 2 hours of treatment.[28,29]

Serial measurement of CK isoforms has been claimed to improve accuracy but the lack of wide availability of serial quantitative assays is a limitation to this approach.[30] Myoglobin release has been studied and a rapid rise over the first 2 hours has been shown to have an accuracy comparable to the CK isoforms.[31]

Synchoronized CKMB and myoglobin serum activity curves can distinguish patients with successful (TIMI 3 flow) and unsuccessful (TIMI 0) thrombolysis by identifying the early peaking of both biochemical markers which accompanies coronary reperfusion.[36] Reperfusion is accompanied by a biphasic serum concentration wave of troponin T, with a sharp rise and fall followed by a secondary, more sustained curve.[37]

Measurement of infarct size

The classic studies of Shell and Sobel in the mid 1970s demonstrated that cumulative creatine kinase release (total CK or CKMB) correlated accurately with post mortem estimates of infarct size.[32] This was demonstrated to correlate well with short- and long-term prognosis. Other studies have shown that peak CK is a reasonable surrogate estimate of infarct size because of the constancy of creatine kinase clearance (Kd).[33] However, this work in the pre-thrombolysis era has been confounded by the effects of recanalization on CK curves, and accurate estimate of infarct size from CK serum curves in the patient undergoing reperfusion therapy has not been successful.[34]

Detection of reinfarction

Identification of reinfarction is possible with measurement of serum CKMB but because of the slowly declining curve and variation in the measurements, a 25% increase from previous values in two samples should be the criterion for reinfarction.[35] Re-elevation of troponin T or I may be a useful index of reinfarction, but experience with these markers is still limited.

Late detection of infarction

Recongition of recent myocardial infarction in a patient presenting several days after the onset is a relatively common clinical problem. Previously LD isoenzymes were used for this purpose, but the persistence of troponin T and I for more than a week post-infarction makes it likely that the troponins will become the method of choice for late recognition of infarction in the future.

Recommendations

The summary on the next page sets out the recommendations from an authoritative 1993 review on the clinical application of biochemical markers of myocardial injury. The wider availability of assays for CKMB isoforms and troponin I and T will undoubtedly lead to changes in these recommendations in the next few years.

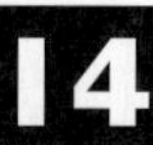

Acute myocardial infarction: summary of clinical applications of biochemical markers of myocardial injury. Reproduced with minor modification with permission from Adams et al. 1993.[2]

- **Routine diagnosis** The measurement of MBCK† remains the test of choice for the confirmation/exclusion of AMI and probably will remain so throughout the 1990s. Samples obtained 12-hourly provide adequate sensitivity and are cost-effective.
- **Retrospective diagnosis** LD is still useful, but probably will be replaced by more specific long-lived markers (e.g. the troponins) in the near future. Samples for these can be taken daily.
- **Diagnosis when skeletal muscle injury is present** More specific assays (e.g. cardiac troponin I) will in future be useful conjointly with MBCK. Because cardiac troponin I persists in plasma for prolonged periods, the troponins cannot replace the use of MBCK when timing of AMI is necessary.
- **Very early diagnosis*** Several approaches are possible. The conjoint use of MBCK isoforms and myoglobin or MMCK‡ isoforms could be a very sensitive approach and will compete with MBCK. Serial measurements over several hours are likely to be most useful; however, it is unclear how earlier diagnosis based on multiple samples would impact on patient care. The application of serial measurements to the large number of patients in whom one might wish to exclude AMI may not be cost-effective and would delay the initiation of early treatment. In addition, decisions on admission/discharge should not be based on the presence/absence of these markers of infarction alone. The most promising role at present for this approach is in distinguishing patients with possible AMI who may need admission to an ICU from those who can be treated in a less intensive facility. Whether use of markers other than MBCK to shorten the time to diagnosis to < 12 hours is clinically necessary and/or cost-effective remains to be shown.
- **Detection of coronary recanalization after thrombolysis** Criteria based on isoforms of MM and MBCK and myoglobin appear most promising. It is possible that conjoint use of two markers, e.g. myoglobin or MBCK isoforms combined with MMCK isoforms, will emerge as best strategy.
- **Estimation of infarct size** Longer-lived structural protein markers such as the troponins or MLC, whose release ratios are less affected by alterations in blood flow, probably will replace MBCK for this use. However, because of the prolonged release of these markers, blood samples will have to be obtained for an extended period for these studies. These techniques require further validation.

* The recent availability of rapid semi-quantitative assays for CKMB/subforms[16] and for troponin T[25] changes these 1993 recommendations for very early diagnosis. The kit form of the semiquantitatives tests makes them readily available as a test for early recognition of key myocardial necrosis. †MBCK = CKMB. ‡MMCK = CKMM.

References

1. Lee TH, Goldman L. Serum enzyme assays in the diagnosis of acute myocardial infarction. Ann Intern Med 1986; 105: 221–33
2. Adams JE III, Abendschein DR, Jaffe AS. Biochemical markers of myocardial injury. Is MB creatine kinase the choice for the 1990s? Circulation 1993; 88: 750–63
3. Dreyfus JC, Schapira G, Resnais J, Scebat L. Serum creatine kinase in the diagnosis of myocardial infarct. Rev Fr Etud Clin Biol 1960; 5: 386–90
4. Clark GL, Robinson AK, Gnepp DR, Roberts R, Sobel BE. Effects of lymphatic transport of enzyme on plasma creatine kinase time activity curves after myocardial infarction in dogs. Circ Res 1978; 43: 162–9
5. Sobel BE, Markham RP, Karlsberg RP, Roberts R. The nature of disappearance of creatine kinase from the circulation and its influence on enzymatic estimation of infarct size. Circ Res 1977; 41: 836–44
6. Roberts R, Gowda KS, Ludbrook PA, Sobel BE. Specificity of elevated serum MB creatine phosphokinase activity in the diagnosis of acute myocardial infarction. Am J Cardiol 1975; 36: 433–7
7. Vatner SF, Baig H, Manders WT, Maroko PR. Effects of coronary artery reperfusion on myocardial infarct size calculated from creatine kinase. J Clin Invest 1978; 61: 1048–56
8. Jaffe AS, Garfinkel BT, Ritter CS, Sobel BE. Plasma MB creatine kinase after vigorous exercise in professional atheletes. Am J Cardiol 1984; 53: 856–8
9. El Allaf M, Chapelle J, El Allaf D, Adam A, Faymonville M, Laurent P, Heugshem C. Differentiating muscle damage from myocardial injury by means of the serum creatine kinase (CK) isoenzyme MB mass measure/total CK activity ratio. Clin Chem 1986; 32: 291–5
10. Wu AH, Gornet TG, Harker CC, Chen HL. Role of rapid immunoassays for urgent ('stat') determinations of creatine kinase isoenzyme MB. Clin Chem 1989; 35: 1752–6
11. Eisenberg PR, Shaw D, Schaab C, Jaffe AS. Concordance of creatine

kinase–MB activity and mass. Clin Chem 1989; 35: 440–3
12. Mair J, Artner-Dworzak E, Dienstl A et al. Early detection of acute myocardial infarction by measurement of mass concentration of creatine kinase MB. Am J Cardiol 1991; 68: 1545–50
13. Jaffe AS, Serota H, Grace A, Sobel BE. Diagnostic changes in plasma creatine kinase isoforms early after the onset of acute myocardial infarction. Circulation 1986; 74: 105–9
14. Panteghini M, Cuccia C, Malchiodi A. Isoforms of creatine kinase MM and MB in acute myocardial infarction: a clinical evaluation. Clin Chim Acta 1986; 155: 1–10
15. Puleo PR, Gudagno PA, Roberts R, Scheel MV, Marion AJ, Churchill D, Perryman B. Early diagnosis of acute myocardial infarction based on assay for subforms of creatine kinase-MB. Circulation 1990; 82: 759–64
16. Puleo PR, Meyer C, Wathen CB et al. Use of a rapid assay of subforms of creatine kinase MB to diagnose or rule out acute myocardial infarction. N Engl J Med 1994; 331: 561–6
17. Vasudevan G, Mercer DW, Varat MA. Lactic dehydrogenase isoenzyme determination in the diagnosis of acute myocardial infarction. Circulation 1978; 57: 1055–7
18. Jablonsky G, Leung FY, Henderson AR. Changes in LD_1/LD_2 ratio during the first day after myocardial infarction. Clin Chem 1985; 31: 1960–5
19. La Due JS, Wroblewski F, Karmen A. Serum glutamine oxaloacetic transaminase in human acute transmural myocardial infarctions. Science 1954; 120: 497
20. Roberts R. Myoglobinemia as an index to myocardial infarction. Ann Intern Med 1977; 87: 788–9
21. Drexel H, Dworzak E, Kirchmair W, Milz MM, Puschendorf B, Diemstel F. Myoglobinemia in the early phase of acute myocardial infarction. Am Heart J 1983; 105: 642–50
21a. Bakker AT, Boymans DAG, Dijkstra D, Gorgels JPMC, Lerk R. Rapid determination of serum myoglobin with a routine chemistry analyzer. Clin Chem 1993; 39: 653–8
22. Cummins B, Auckland M, Cummins P. Cardiac-specific troponin-I radioimmunoassay in the diagnosis of acute myocardial infarction. Am Heart J 1987; 113: 1333–44
22a. Larue C, Calzolari C, Bertinchant JP, Lellerc QF, Grolleau R, Pau B. Cardiac-specific immunoenzymometric assay of troponin I in the early phase of acute myocardial infarction. Clin Chem 1993; 39: 972–9
23. Mair J, Artner-Dworzak E, Lechleitner P, Smidt J, Wagner I, Dienstl F, Puschendorf B. Cardiac troponin T in diagnosis of acute myocardial infarction. Clin Chem 1991; 37: 845–52
24. Katus HA, Muller-Bardorff M, Hallermayer K et al. Development and characterisation of an improved rapid enzyme immunoassay specific for cardiac troponin-T. J Am Coll Cardiol 1994; 77A
25. Antman EA, Grudzien C, Sacks DB. Evaluation of a rapid bedside assay for detection of serum cardiac troponin-T. JAMA 1995; 273: 1279–82
26. Editorial. Troponin-T and myocardial damage. Lancet 1991; 338: 23–4
26a. Adams JE, Bodor GS, Davila-Roman VG et al. Cardiac troponin I. A marker with high specificity for cardiac injury. Circulation 1993; 88: 101–6
26b. Bakker AJ, Koelemay MJW, Gorgels JPMC et al. Failure of new biochemical markers to exclude acute myocardial infarction at admission. Lancet 1993; 342: 1220–2
26c. Adams JE, Bicard GA, Allen BT et al. Diagnosis of perioperative myocardial infarction with measurement of cardiac troponin I. N Engl J Med 1994; 330: 670–4
27. Hamm C-W, Ravkilde J, Gerhardt W et al. The prognostic value of serum troponin-T in unstable angina. N Engl J Med 1992; 327: 146–50
28. Nidorf SM, Thompson PL, Byrne A, De Klerk NH and the National Heart Foundation of Australia Coronary Thrombolysis Group. The creatine kinase ratio: a useful means of detecting early peaking of the creatine kinase curve after acute myocardial infarctions. Am J Cardiol 1988; 62: 961–3
29. Grande P, Granborg J, Clemmensen P, Sevilla D, Wagner N, Wagner G. Indices of reperfusion in patients with acute myocardial infarction using characteristics of the CK-MB time-activity curve. Am Heart J 1991; 122: 400–8
30. Puleo PR, Perryman MB, Bresser MA et al. Creatine kinase isoform analysis in the detection and assessment of thrombolysis in man. Circulation 1987; 75: 1162–9
31. Gasser RNA, Hauptlorenz S, Dworzak E, Moll W, Puschendorf B, Dienstl F. The typical staccato phenomenon of myoglobin in acute myocardial infarction disappears under thrombolytic treatment. Fibrinolysis 1987; 1: 177–82
32. Sobel BE, Bresnahan GF, Shell WE, Yoder RD. Estimation of infarct size in man and its relation to prognosis. Circulation 1972; 46: 640–8
33. Thompson PL, Fletcher EE, Katavatis V. Enzymatic indices of myocardial necrosis: influence on short- and long-term prognosis after myocardial infarction. Circulation 1979; 59: 113–19
34. Roberts R. Enzymatic estimation of infarct size: thrombolysis induced its demise: will it now rekindle its renaissance? Circulation 1990; 81: 707–10

35. Muller JE, Rude RE, Braunwald E et al. Myocardial infarct extension: incidence, outcome and risk factors in the MILIS Study. Ann Intern Med 1988; 108: 1–6
36. Zabel M, Hohnloser SH, Koster W, Prinz M, Kasper W, Just H. Analysis of creatine kinase, CK-MB, myoglobin and troponin T timi-activity curves for early assessment of coronary artery reperfusion after intravenous thrombolysis Circulation. 1993; 87: 1542–50
37. Remppis A, Scheffold T, Karrer O et al. Assessment of reperfusion of the infarct zone after acute myocardial infarction by serial cardiac troponin T measurements in serum. Br Heart J 1994; 71: 242–8

15 Chest X-ray

Ashok B Kumar

Introduction

Almost every patient in a coronary care unit (CCU) has a chest X-ray at some time or another during their admission. Most of these X-rays are performed under sub-optimal conditions. These portable films have inherent limitations because of the projections used, position of the patient (usually supine or semi-erect) and other physical factors such as type of mobile X-ray machine, film/screen combinations and the geometrical unsharpness that results from low output X-ray machines using longer exposure times. The radiographs produced under these conditions are sub-optimal and this should be borne in mind when making comparisons with those taken in a radiology department or comparing previous portable films. Over-interpretation of subtle changes on chest X-rays due to a change in exposure or technique may lead to erroneous assumptions—for example, a diagnosis of pulmonary oedema in a supine patient.

As most of these films are taken in the frontal position, magnification of the heart is considerable and no reliance can be placed on the usual measurements for assessing cardiomegaly. Similarly, supine films appear to enlarge the mediastinum and hence false diagnosis of mediastinal pathology such as a dissecting aortic aneurysm or ruptured aorta has to be considered carefully. Notwithstanding the above, a systemic evaluation of the chest X-ray is necessary to avoid mistakes and missing significant findings.

Interpretation of chest X-ray examination

The following practical advice will help in interpreting the chest X-ray:

- **Patient data** Check for patient's name, date and time of the examination. Look out for any notations on the film written or labelled, for example supine, mobile, AP (anterior-posterior) or PA (posterior-anterior).
- **Technical adequacy** The chest X-ray must be technically acceptable. Ensure the exposure, symmetry and inspiratory/expiratory phases are taken into account. A well-centred film should have the thoracic spinous process centred equidistant from the medial aspect of the clavicles. Film rotation can cause significant confusion in the analysis of the mediastinal configuration and make one lung more translucent (darker) than the other. An adequate exposure is one where the thoracic disc spaces in the lower chest are visualized behind the heart.
- **Cardio-mediastinum** The cardio-mediastinal outlines should be observed. Changes in sequential films are more important in the CCU than a solitary film, as the anatomy in the cardio-mediastinum can be quite variable because of patient position and the AP projection. The great vessels and trachea should not be displaced. The area behind the heart and anterior to the thoracic vertebrae should not have a mass density. No air should outline the mediastinum or within the cardiac silhouette.[1] Sharply demarcated lucencies within the cardio-mediastinum should raise the suspicion of pneumopericardium or pneumomediastinum (see Fig. 15.1).
- **Lung fields** The lung fields should be systemically analysed, dividing the lung fields into the upper, mid and lower zones. The right and left upper zone should be compared together, then the middle and lower zones. The differences in translucencies

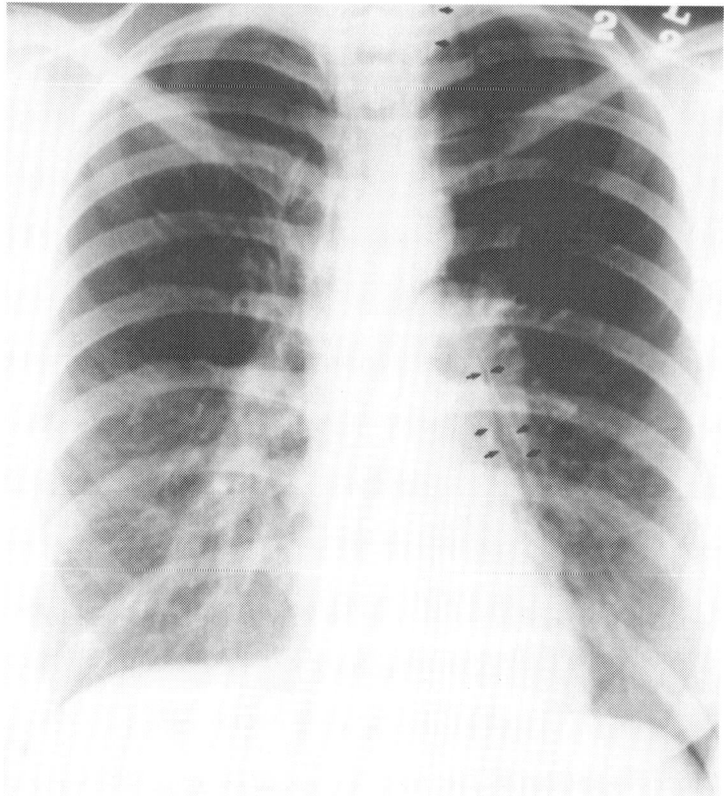

Fig. 15.1 Pneumomediastinum. Black arrows indicate air tracks.

may be due to film rotation and therefore the position of the thoracic spine should be checked in relation to the medial aspects of the clavicle. Lobar pneumonias and collapses are well demarcated by the fissures. Diffuse patchy shadowing is more commonly seen in pulmonary oedema. Pulmonary oedema is usually bilateral in the mid and lower zones but it can be unilateral or segmental.

- **Pleura** The pleura is not usually seen unless there is either a pneumothorax, pleural effusion or calcification. The costophrenic angles should remain sharp, unless there is an effusion. In the supine patient, pleural effusion and pneumothorax may be difficult to visualize. If either of these is suspected, a decubitus film can be performed on the patient's bed. A pleural effusion will then be easily visualized on the dependent side and the pneumothorax on the non-dependent side (see Fig. 15.2). In addition, this position would also highlight the lower lung base on the non-dependent side to advantage—for example, differentiating a pneumonic consolidation from an effusion.
- **Thoracic cage** Finally, a quick look at the thoracic cage may give some information regarding the density of the bones. Osteolytic or osteosclerotic lesions may indicate metastasis. New or healing fractures of the ribs or humerus may provide an unexpected clue in undiagnosed chest or shoulder pains.

Common abnormalities seen on chest X-rays[2]

Lobar collapse (atelectasis)

Lobar collapse may involve entire lobes, segments or only subsegments. When an entire lobe has collapsed the following abnormalities occur:

- loss of lung volume
- displacement of fissures and vascular markings
- mediastinal and tracheal shift to the involved side
- elevated diaphragm
- confluent density within lung substance
- rapid improvement following re-expansion.

The posterior segments of the upper and lower lobes are more frequently involved due to secretions in dependent zones. Distinction between collapse, pleural effusion and consolidation may be difficult. The common causes of lobar collapse are sputum retention and malpositioning of endotracheal tubes. Lobar atelectasis has been reported in 8.5% of chest X-rays reviewed; 66% involve the left lower lobe, 22% the right lower lobe and 11% the right upper lobe.[3]

Lobar consolidation

Lobar consolidation is rarely seen in critically ill patients. Lung infiltrates are often patchy and may be particularly hard to distinguish

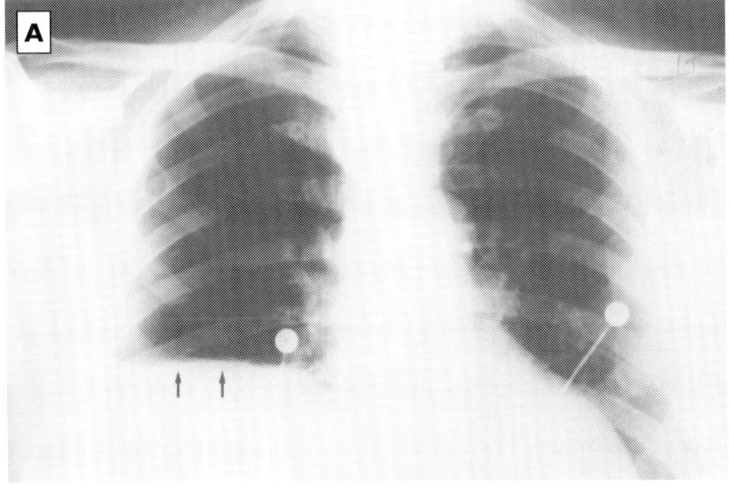

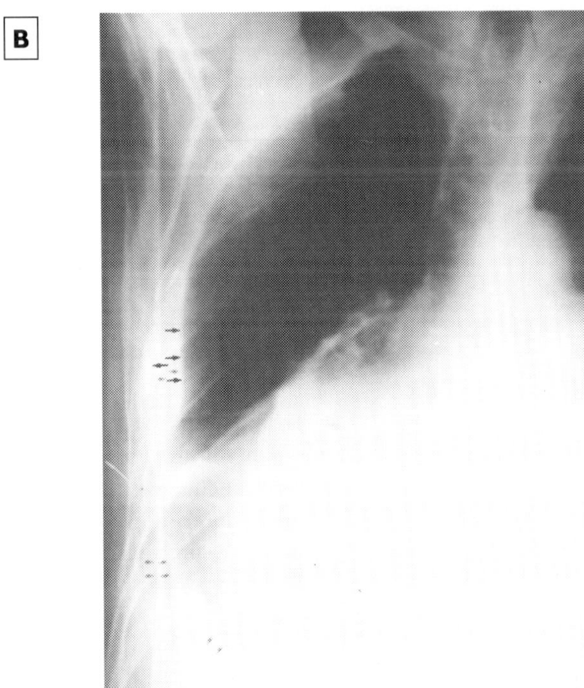

Fig. 15.2 [A] Elevated right diaphragm on supine film. On lateral decubitus view [B], black arrows indicate fluid tracking along lateral chest wall, confirming a subpulmonic pleural effusion.

aetiologically. The pattern of infiltration bears little relation to the likely pathogen. Coexistent collapse is common. Consolidation has the following features:

- homogenous shadowing confined to segments and bounded by fissures, diaphragm, pleura and chest
- no loss of lung volume
- air bronchograms
- relative consistency 'from day to day'.

Barotrauma

Pseudopneumothorax

The film cassette is usually made of heavy plastic and this adheres to moist skin and can produce a pseudopneumothorax (see Fig. 15.3). (This is the reason why cassettes are kept in a pillow cover when positioned behind a patient). The pseudopneumothorax is easily differentiated from a pneumothorax by the presence of lung markings traversing the area. It is usually seen bilaterally in the outer and upper aspects of the chest.

Pneumothorax

The commonest form of barotrauma is a pneumothorax. In the supine patient, a pneumothorax is rarely seen in the upper zones. Most pneumothorax in supine patients are situated in the anteromedial (38%) or subpulmonic (26%) recesses.[4] If a pneumothorax is suspected, a lateral decubitus film would help confirm it.

Important diagnostic features of a pneumothorax are:

- a white, visible air/lung interface
- mediastinal shift to the opposite side (tension pneumothorax)
- hypertranslucency of affected hemithorax (looks darker)
- lack of lung markings crossing the air/lung interface.

Pneumomediastinum (Fig. 15.1)

This is rare in CCU patients. Mediastinal gas may persist for up to 7 weeks after a cardiac surgical

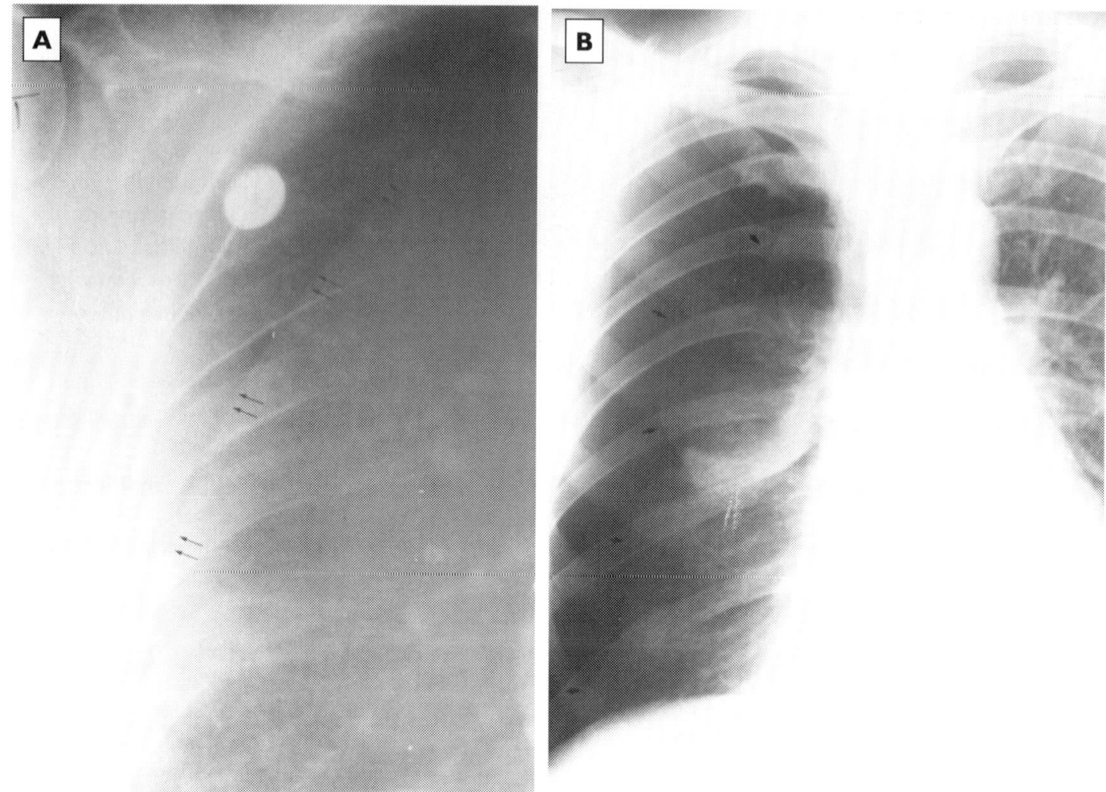

Fig. 15.3 [A] Pseudopneumothorax—note vascular markings beyond, compared to a true pneumothorax [B] where no vascular markings are seen beyond the lung.

procedure without clinical significance.

Pleural effusions

Important features identifying pleural effusions are:

- A fluid meniscus, usually seen in an erect film. As most films are supine, this feature is not evident. Instead, there is a homogenous increase in density from the bases to the mid zones. This can be confirmed by a decubitus film with the patient lying on the dependent side.
- diaphragmatic and cardiac obscurity
- no loss of any thoracic volume
- possible shift of the mediastinum away from a large effusion.

Pulmonary oedema

The commonest pulmonary abnormality in CCUs is pulmonary oedema. This is usually cardiac in origin; however, non-cardiac causes can produce similar appearances. The distinction is often difficult even with the aid of a Swan–Ganz catheter.[2] Several radiological features may help differentiate these entities. In cardiogenic pulmonary oedema:

- The distribution of blood flow is usually to the upper zones and this is increased;
- The distribution of the infiltrates is basal and perihilar;
- The pulmonary blood volume is either normal or increased;
- Peribronchial wall cuffing, subtle lines and pleural effusions are common in cardiogenic pulmonary oedema (whereas they are rare in non-cardiogenic pulmonary oedema);
- The heart is usually enlarged in the former, but is normal in the latter.

It must be remembered that radiographic evidence of left ventricular failure may precede clinical symptoms, especially in bed-ridden patients. Right heart failure and cor pulmonale may cause pleural effusions and enlargement of the azygos vein and superior vena cava. Pulmonary oedema and congestion are usually due to left

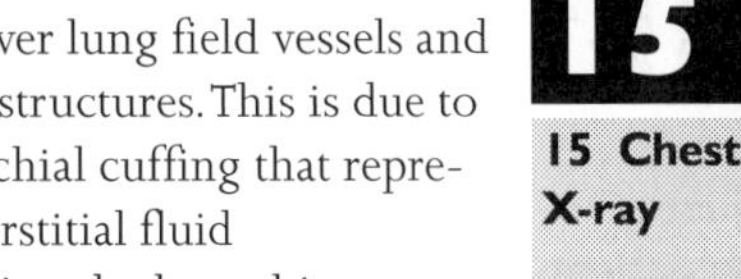

ventricular failure, but can sometimes be due to mitral stenosis or regurgitations.

For descriptive purposes, there are three distinct stages of left ventricular failure:

Stage 1, pulmonary venous congestion;
Stage 2, interstitial oedema;
Stage 3, alveolar pulmonary oedema.

Stage 1—pulmonary venous congestion

In a normal erect chest film, the upper lobe blood vessels are smaller than the lower lobe vessels due to hydrostatic pressure. However in the supine patient this relationship is lost and the sizes of the pulmonary vessels are equal both in the upper and lower zones. In congestive cardiac failure, in the supine chest X-ray, the upper lobe blood vessels have to enlarge to 1.5 times the size of lower lobe vessels before one considers it to be due to upper lobe blood diversion. The pulmonary vessels are usually the same diameter as the adjacent bronchus in normal people, and if the pulmonary vessels are larger than the adjacent bronchus then upper lobe blood diversion is confirmed. Pulmonary vascular markings clearly visible in the outer third of the lung fields in the upper zones indicate upper lobe blood diversion.

Stage 2—interstitial oedema

When the hydrostatic pressure within the vessels exceeds the ability of the vessels to retain the increased fluid load, fluid extravasates into the pulmonary interstitium. This causes thickening of the interstitial tissues and is manifested by a reticular pattern and septal lines. These are fine, branching lines that follow many directions. The commonest is the Kerley B line (see Fig. 15.4). These are dilated interlobular septa and they run horizontally over a length of 1–2 cm. They abut the pleura and extend medially. They are best appreciated along the periphery of the bases. Kerley A lines also represent dilated interlobular septa but they radiate from the periphery to the hilum and are usually 3–7 cm long. Kerley A lines do not occur without Kerley B lines. In stage 2 there is loss of definition of the lower lung field vessels and perihilar structures. This is due to peribronchial cuffing that represents interstitial fluid surrounding the bronchi.

Stage 3—alveolar pulmonary oedema

When the intravascular and interstitial fluid pressures exceed the intra-alveolar air pressure, fluid leaks into the alveoli (Fig. 15.5). In stage 3 there is an alveolar infiltrate in the perihilar regions (butterfly or batwing appearance) or in the lower zones with or

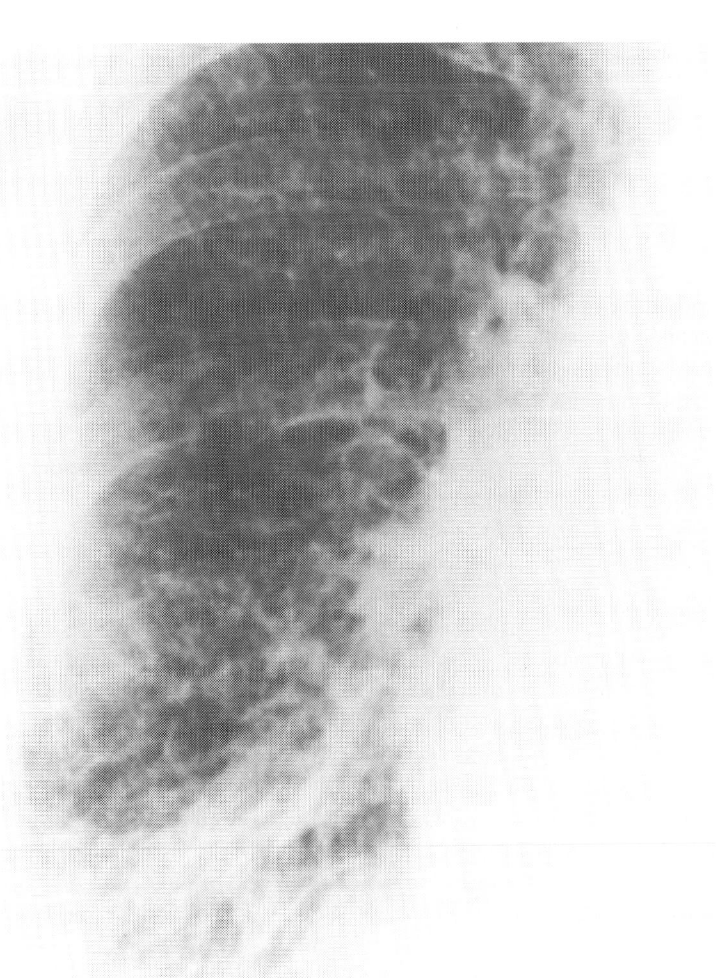

Fig. 15.4 Interstitial pulmonary oedema: note Kerley lines.

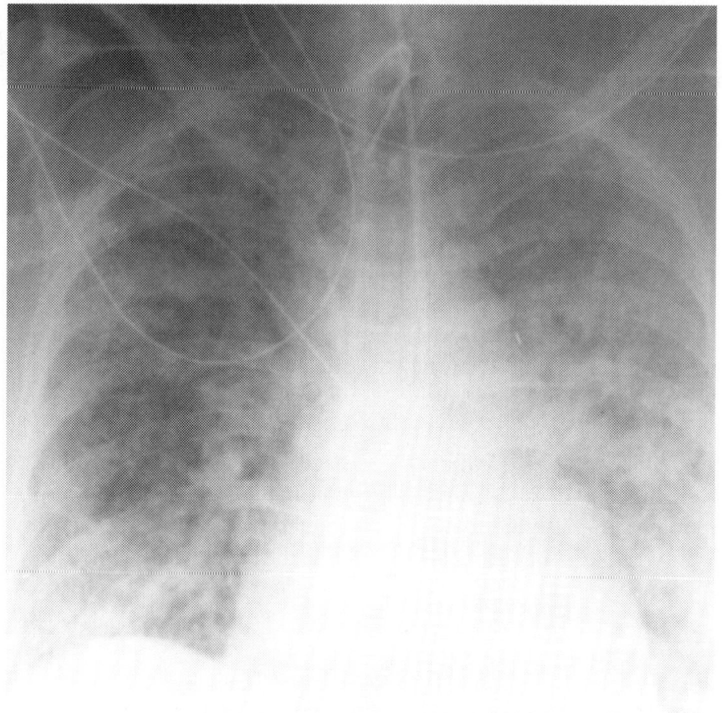

Fig. 15.5 Alveolar pulmonary oedema.

without air bronchograms. In addition to this, the Kerley B lines and loss of definition of vessels in all the lung fields may be present. The pleural fissures may be thickened and this is mainly due to fluid within them. The features in stage 3 can also occur in patients in renal failure and in overhydration. Left ventricular failure may infrequently produce pleural effusion in the absence of radiographic findings of alveolar pulmonary oedema. Cardiac enlargement may not be present in left ventricular failure of acute onset (for example, following AMI or ruptured papillary muscle). Patients lying on one side for prolonged periods may have unilateral pulmonary oedema. On occasions, localized pulmonary oedema may mimic pneumonitis (rapid clearing on sequential films after diuretic therapy favours pulmonary oedema).

Abnormal position of monitoring and life support devices

Transvenous catheters

Catheters used for infusion of fluids or drugs or used for monitoring right atrial, ventricular or pulmonary arterial pressures are often seen on CCU chest X-rays. The site of insertion, either through the antecubital vein in the arm, or through either subclavian vein or internal jugular veins, is usually evident. The infusion catheter tip should be placed in the superior vena cava, superior to the right atrium. The tips of these catheters should be in the midline of the superior vena cava. A satisfactory position is when the catheter tip is at the level of the azygos vein (approximately at the tracheo-right bronchial junction). Catheters inserted from the left subclavian vein or through the left jugular line may have their tips abutting against the lateral wall of the superior vena cava and this has a slightly increased incidence of perforation (see Fig. 15.6). Because of this theoretical possibility of perforation, catheters inserted from the left side should preferably be the pigtail variety rather than the straight catheters. The commonest complication following catheter insertion from the subclavian approach is a pneumothorax or extravasation of blood into the pleural or pericardial spaces. In the latter case, this can result in a haemopericardium.

The tip of the pressure monitoring catheter (Swan–Ganz catheter) should be in the main pulmonary arteries some 5–8 cm distal to the pulmonary bifurcation. Catheters lying more distally into the lobar branches of the pulmonary artery are prone to thrombosis and pulmonary infarction. These catheters are designed to 'float' when the balloon is distended into one of the lower lobe arteries for wedge pressure measurement. Following deflation of the balloon, these catheters should recoil back into the main pulmonary artery. If wedging is evident after balloon deflation, the catheters should be withdrawn 2–3 cm and the chest X-ray repeated.

Pacing wires

Pacing wires are usually placed through the subclavian approach

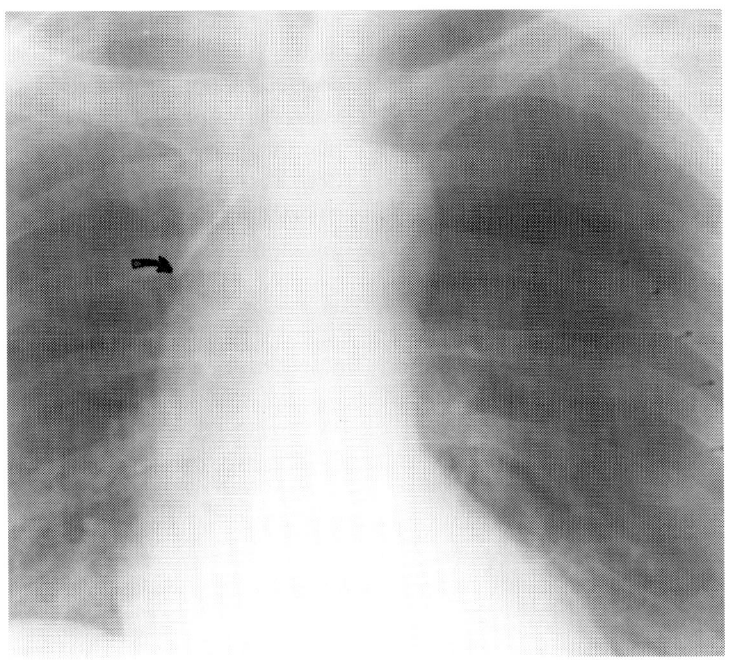

Fig. 15.6 Central venous line abutting against lateral wall of superior vena cava. Incidental left pneumothorax.

and hence common complications are malposition, pneumothorax, haemothorax or haemopericardium. An X-ray after placement of these wires is necessary to check for position and integrity of wire and to exclude complications. These wires should have smooth curves rather than sharp angulations as the latter are prone to fractures. Wire fractures are unusual, occurring in approximately 3% of cases.[5] The tips of the pacing wires are usually in the apex of the right ventricle and these are projected on the frontal view approximately 3–4 cm lateral to the thoracic vertebral body. On the lateral chest view, these pacing wire tips are situated anteriorly. Occasionally, pacing wires can perforate the myocardium and cause a haemopericardium. The tip of the catheter clearly outside the cardiac silhouette will confirm this. Sometimes catheters 'float' into the main pulmonary artery or may be placed in the coronary sinus. The coronary sinus runs in the posterior atrioventricular groove, and hence on the frontal view these malpositioned pacing wires point medially and upwards towards the left main pulmonary artery and on the lateral view they are positioned posteriorly.

Endotracheal and tracheostomy tubes

The carina is the junction between the right and left main bronchus. It is usually projected at the T6 vertebral body. Flexion and extension of the head and neck cause considerable forward and backward movement of an endotracheal tube. Since the tube is fixed at the nose or mouth, only the distal tube moves with head and neck movement. Flexion of the neck causes an inferior movement of the tube by 2 cm and extension causes superior movement of the tube by a similar distance.[6] This combined excursion of 4 cm is approximately one third the length of the trachea, which measures 12 cm in the average adult. Hence, a tube which is in a satisfactory position in the middle of the trachea during extension may extend into the right main bronchus during flexion. In the neutral neck position, the endotracheal tube is ideally in the mid-trachea some 5–7 cm from the carina. If the endotracheal tube lodges itself in the right main bronchus, this will cause atelectasis of the left lung, resulting in a smaller left hemithorax appearing a little more radio-opaque (white) (see Fig. 15.7).

Occasionally, an endotracheal tube is inadvertently placed in the oesophagus. This may not be apparent on a frontal chest X-ray. The stethoscope will come in handy.

Tracheostomy tubes do not suffer from malposition during flexion or extension of the neck. The tip of the tracheostomy tube should be approximately half to two-thirds the distance between the stoma and the carina. Long-term placement of endotracheal and tracheostomy tubes can result in mucosal ulceration of the trachea and perforation. Granuloma formation has been noted in some patients, resulting in stridor.[7]

Intercostal tubes

These are placed for the treatment of pneumothorax or for the drainage of pleural effusions. As most of these patients are supine, an intercostal catheter for the treatment of pneumothorax

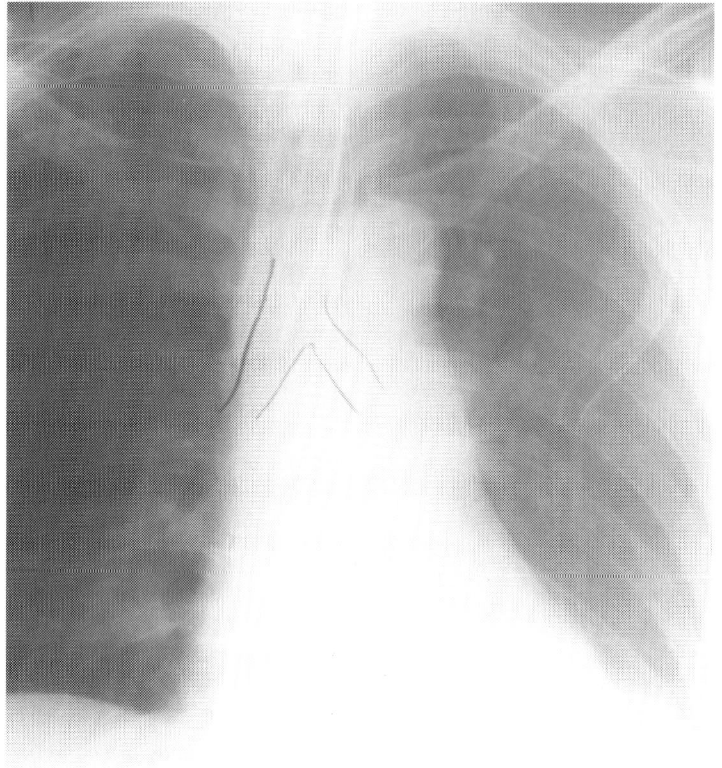

Fig. 15.7 Endotracheal tube in right main bronchus causing hyperventilation of right lung but partial collapse of left lung.

should be placed anteriorly and inferiorly where free air normally collects in the supine position. However, if intercostal catheters are placed for drainage of effusions they should be placed posteriorly and towards the apex, as in the recumbent position fluid collects posteriorly. Sometimes, following removal of intercostal catheters, a residual pleural tract is left which though not significant may be confusing. These pleural tracts are due to pleural thickening around the previous intercostal catheter. They disappear within a few days. However they should not be confused with pneumothorax.[7] Comparison with an earlier chest X-ray will confirm that these tracts relate to the position of a previously placed intercostal tube.

Intra-aortic balloon pumps

Intra aortic balloon pumps[8], sometimes known as intra-aortic counter pulsation balloon catheters, are used quite frequently to improve cardiac function in the setting of cardiogenic shock or high risk cardiac surgery. The device consists of an inflatable balloon, some 25 cm long. This balloon is inflated during diastole and deflated during systole and the timing is triggered by the ECG. Radiographically the device appears as a catheter with the distal end having a metallic marker. The position of this distal end should be below the left subclavian artery. Malposition can result in the catheter being placed in the left subclavian artery with subsequent thrombosis or rupture. During catheter placement, the possibility of aortic dissection has to be considered. Since these catheters have a large bore, they may occlude the femoral artery and cause vascular insufficiency to the lower limb.

Pulmonary embolism and infarction

The chest radiograph in pulmonary embolism is non-specific. A patient with pulmonary embolism can have a completely normal chest radiograph. However, in angiographically proven cases more than 50% of these patients would have some abnormality on a chest radiograph.[1] Though none of them are specific, a summation of findings, such as pleural effusion, elevation of a hemidiaphragm, subsegmental atelectasis and patchy consolidation may indicate a pulmonary embolism.

In pulmonary infarction a pleural based, wedge-shaped consolidation may be present. The apex of this consolidation points toward the heart and this represents the bronchovascular orientation of a segment of lung. This is sometimes called a Hampton's Hump. Rarely, a segmental pulmonary oligaemia is demonstrated on chest X-rays, especially in portable films.

If a pulmonary embolism is suspected, then a technetium 99m-labelled macro-aggregated albumin perfusion scan would be helpful. If the diagnosis is still in doubt, a pulmonary angiogram may need to be performed.

Mediastinal widening

This is one of the commonest findings on a supine chest radiograph. An easy and cheap way of excluding a suspicion of mediastinal widening would be to perform an erect chest film. Elderly patients, especially with hypertension and atherosclerotic disease, may have a widened mediastinum because of unfolding and tortuosity of the aortic arch (see Fig. 15.8). This is not pathological. However, this condition has to be differentiated from a dissecting aortic aneurysm especially with patients who present with chest pain. Comparison with an old chest film which may have calcification in the aortic knuckle is a simple and cost-effective way to help differentiate a recent aortic dissection. In this situation, the calcification in the sub-intimal layer of the aortic arch will be displaced medially in sequential films (Fig. 15.9).

Apart from the above simpler and economical methods of assessing mediastinal widening, there are other modalities which will help confirm the presence of an aortic dissection. Computed tomography scanning, which is now widely available, can rapidly demonstrate the dissected aorta and classify it into Type 1 or Type 2 (see Fig. 15.10).

Transoesophageal echocardiography (Ch 16) is another method to assess aortic dissections. However, it is limited to the descending portion of the aorta and hence only Type 2 dissections would be visible. The Type 1 dissections which involve the ascending aorta may not be well visualized.

Magnetic resonance imaging (Fig. 15.11) has laid claim to being the gold standard in aortic dissection (see Chs 20, 70). However, this modality is limited

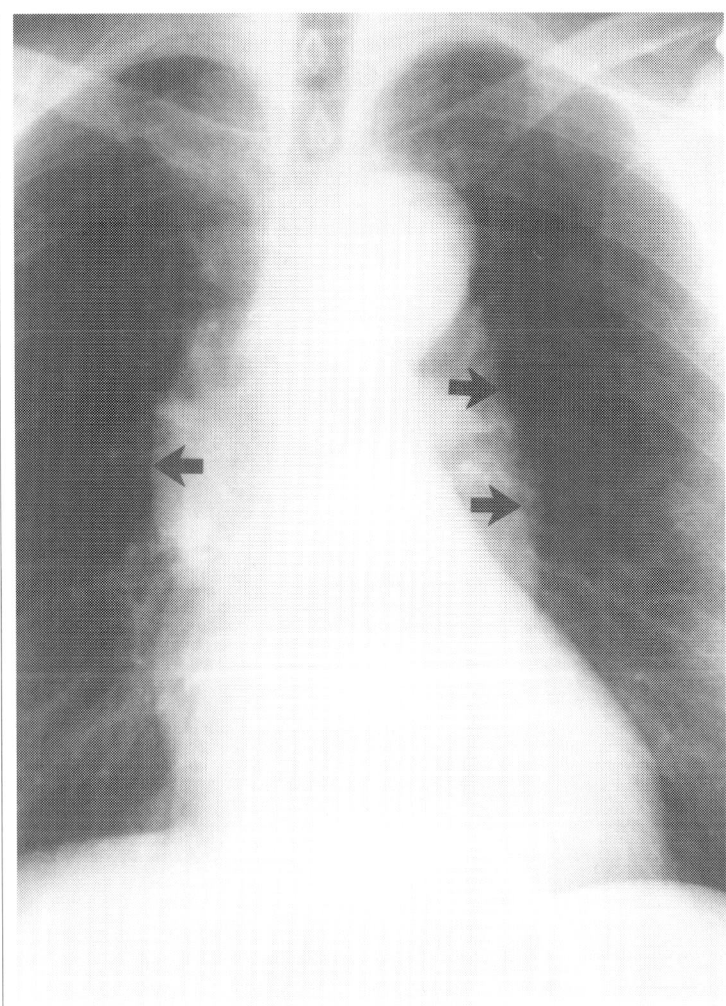

Fig. 15.8 Mediastinal widening due to tortuous aorta.

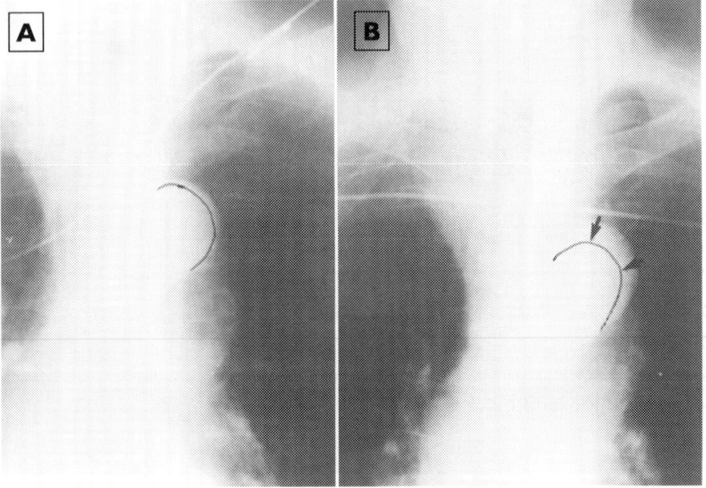

Fig. 15.9 Aortic dissection. The calcified aortic knuckle has been outlined in black [A], [B]. Note the displacement medially in aortic dissection [B].

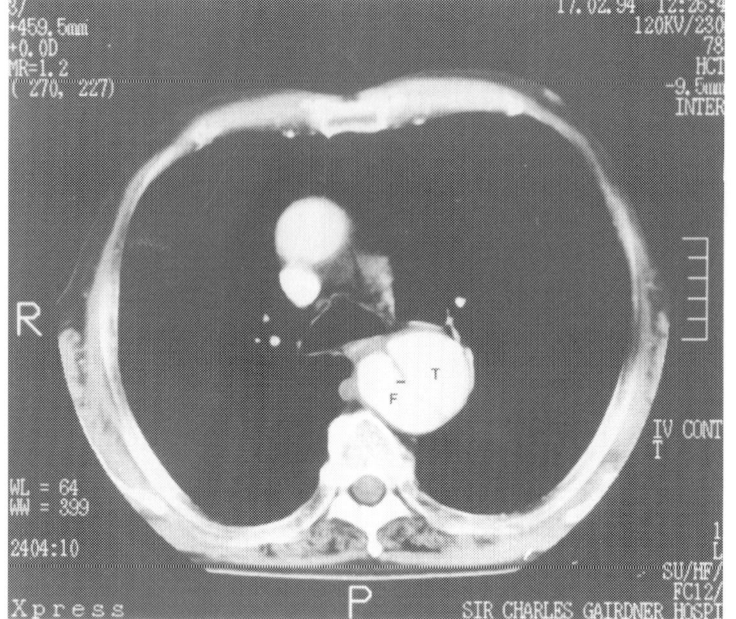

Fig. 15.10 Computed tomography of aortic dissection. F=false lumen; T=true lumen; –=intima.

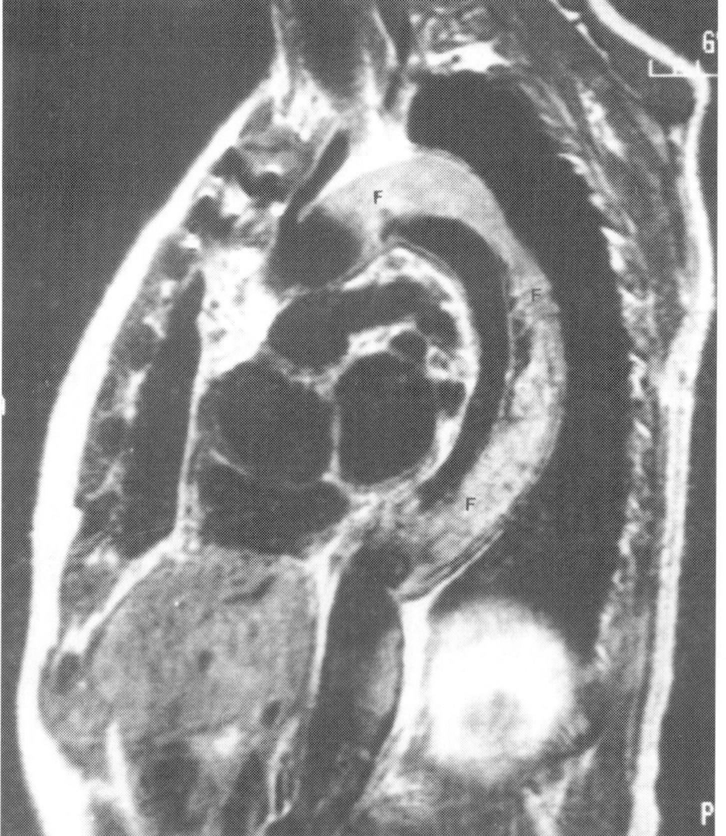

Fig. 15.11 Magnetic resonance imaging of aortic dissection false lumen (F). True lumen in black.

by virtue of its cost, availability and contraindications such as the presence of pacemakers.

Cardiac enlargement

Cardiac enlargement is usually a sign of long-standing left ventricular dilatation and dysfunction. As such, it indicates a poor prognosis in AMI. Assessing heart size on an anterior-posterior chest film is fraught with difficulty, but on a posterior-anterior film, a cardiothoracic ratio of greater than 0.5 is usually abnormal. Traps leading to inaccurate assessment of heart size include a poorly inflated film, epicardial fat pads and obscuring of the cardiac apex or right atrial border by pleural effusion, pulmonary oedema or consolidation. A globular heart shape may suggest pericardial effusion, but this can only be recognized reliably with echocardiography.

Conclusion

Chest radiography in CCUs is an essential component of clinical patient management. Various cardiopulmonary abnormalities and malposition of various life-saving devices are frequently detected. Technical factors may limit the resolution of the AP radiograph; however, close consultation between the cardiologist and radiologist will contribute to better patient care.

References

1. Rosen P, Doris PE, Barkin RM, Barkin SZ, Markovchick VJ. Diagnostic radiology in emer-

gency medicine. St Louis: Mosby, 1992
2. Oh TE. Intensive care manual. 3rd ed. London: Butterworths, 1990
3. Shevland JE, Hirleman MT, Hoang KA, Kealy GP. Lobar collapse in the surgical intensive care unit. Br J Radiol 1983;56:531–4
4. Tocino IM, Miller MH, Fairfax WR. Distribution of pneumothorax in the supine and semi-recumbent critically ill adult. Am J Roentgenol 1985;144:901–5
5. Swenson SJ, Peters SG, Le Roy AJ et al. Radiology in the intensive care unit. Mayo Clin Proc 1991;66:396–410
6. Courardy PA, Goodman LR, Lainge F, Singh MM. Alteration of endotracheal tube position: flexion and extension of the neck. Crit Care Med 1976; 4: 8–12
7. Goodman LR, Putman CE. Critical care imaging. 3rd ed. Philadelphia: Saunders, 1992
8. Sutton D. A textbook of radiology and imaging. 5th ed. London: Churchill Livingstone, 1993:491

16 Echocardiography

S Mark Nidorf

The role of echocardiography in the coronary care unit

Because two-dimensional echocardiography is non-invasive, has a rapid acquisition time and can be brought to the bedside, it is an ideal means of assessing the heart in the CCU, especially as there is often an urgent need for accurate diagnosis in order to plan appropriate patient care. Accordingly, echocardiography now has an established role in the assessment of patients with myocardial infarction (MI) as well as other clinical problems in the CCU.

The role of echocardiography after myocardial infarction

Although not routinely required, echocardiography may prove valuable in:

- the diagnosis and assessment of the site and extent of MI
- the diagnosis of the acute, clinically overt complications of MI
- the detection of clinically silent changes in ventricular structure after MI
- the assessment of ventricular function.

The diagnosis and assessment of the site and extent of myocardial infarction

The diagnosis of MI by echocardiography is suggested by the presence of abnormal regional wall motion.[1–3] Regional myocardial function is appreciated by assessment of the degree of endocardial motion and the degree of myocardial thickening, and is described qualitatively as being either normal, hypokinetic (moving in the proper direction but at a slower rate and to a smaller extent than normal), akinetic (not moving), or dyskinetic (moving outward in systole). Clinical studies have demonstrated a close relation between the site and extent of regional dysfunction and other markers of the site and extent of MI.[4–6] A clear relation has also been demonstrated between the site of abnormal wall motion and vascular territories.[7] Specifically, occlusion of the left anterior descending coronary artery invariably affects the apex, and when more proximal, also affects the anterior wall and septum. In contrast, occlusion of the circumflex or right coronary artery invariably affects the base of the ventricle, and if the vessel is large, the infarct will extend towards the papillary muscle and/or ventricular apex. Importantly, the extent of abnormal wall motion assessed by echo has also been correlated with clinical, haemodynamic and radionuclide indices of infarct severity.

Pitfalls in the echocardiographic diagnosis of myocardial infarction

Although echocardiography is a sensitive means of detecting abnormal wall motion, after small, usually non-Q, infarctions, the ventricle may appear normal despite other clear evidence of MI.[8] In part, this is because the sensitivity of echocardiography is very operator-dependent, being limited by: incomplete visualization of the ventricle and/or ventricular endocardium (especially the apex); misinterpretation of non-cardiac motion (rotation, translation) as endocardial motion; and misinterpretation of off-axis images.

Importantly, the presence of abnormal wall motion is not specific for MI.[9,10] For example, abnormal septal activation, which occurs following thoracotomy, in left bundle branch block (LBBB), or with cardiac pacing, may be misinterpreted as antero-septal infarction unless the apex is adequately visualized. In addition, abnormal regional wall motion can occur following focal myocarditis, or following transient myocardial ischaemia due to stunning rather than infarction. Indeed, this forms the basis for stress echocardiography.

Assessing the extent of myocardial dysfunction after myocardial infarction

Although many reputable echocardiographers and cardiology units report only subjective assessments of the extent of abnormal wall motion and overall ventricular function, echocardiography does allow for quantitative estimates of both indices of the extent of infarction to be made.[11] The usefulness and accuracy of estimates of ejection fraction after MI, however, may be of limited value for the following reasons:

- In the early post-infarct period there may be compensatory hyperkinesis in the non-infarct regions resulting in normalization of ejection fraction; hence the ejection fraction may be an insensitive marker of the extent of myocardial damage
- The formulae used in the two-dimensional echocardiographic assessment of ejection fraction rely heavily on assessment of function at the base of the heart, and are only valid in patients with a normally symmetrical or non-distorted ventricle; hence after anterior infarction, failure to account for dysfunction of the apex may lead to an over-estimate of global ventricular function, whereas after infero-basal infarction, estimates of ejection fraction may overestimate the extent of global ventricular dysfunction.

For these reasons, the extent of MI is best assessed by estimation of the extent of abnormal wall motion. Although highly sensitive methods for this purpose have been developed, they currently require the use of off-line computer analysis for accurate quantification. While useful for research purposes,[8] in the clinical setting more simple means of quantifying the overall extent of abnormal wall motion are sufficient for prognostication and decision-making purposes. The most simple of these methods is to divide the ventricle into segments of approximately equal size, and to assign a functional 'score' to each segment based upon qualitative (visual) assessment (normal=0, hypokinesis=1, akinesis=2 and dyskinesis=3). In this way, patients with extensive areas of infarction have higher scores. Overall scores derived by this approach have been shown to correlate with clinical, haemodynamic and radionuclide indices of infarct severity.[3,4,13] An alternative approach is to express the extent of abnormal wall motion as a percentage of the ventricle which appears abnormal.[8] This can be done by determining the proportion of the length of the ventricle that appears abnormal in the long axis, and multiplying this by the proportion of the circumference of the ventricle in the short axis which appears abnormal.

Diagnosis of the acute complications of myocardial infarction

The acute mechanical complications of MI, including papillary muscle and ventricular septal rupture, are most commonly seen after large infero-posterior and infero-septal infarctions.[14] Clinically both conditions present with a sudden deterioration in haemodynamic status and the development of a new pan-systolic murmur. Although clinical and haemodynamic variables may allow accurate differentiation of these complications, echocardiography provides a rapid and reliable means of distinguishing the two conditions, since the echocardiographic features of each are specific.[15] In patients with *papillary muscle rupture*, one or other mitral leaflet becomes flail and the head of the ruptured papillary muscle can be seen to prolapse in and out of the left atrium with each cardiac cycle[16] (see Fig. 16.1).

Further, as a consequence of the acute onset of regurgitation the non-infarcted myocardium is seen to be hyperdynamic, and colour Doppler confirms the presence of a large, usually eccentric, jet of mitral regurgitation into a slightly dilated atrium. In contrast, in patients with *acute septal rupture* the mitral apparatus is intact and colour Doppler can be used to accurately locate the septal defect.[17–19] Continuous wave Doppler can be used to determine the peak velocity of interventricular shunt flow, and thus predict the gradient between the left and right ventricles (by using the simplified Bernoulli equation), and from this information the pulmonary artery pressure can be estimated.

Urgent bedside echocardiography can be invaluable in assessing the cause of haemodynamic collapse, and differentiating cardiac rupture from other causes of electromechanical dissociation. *Rupture of*

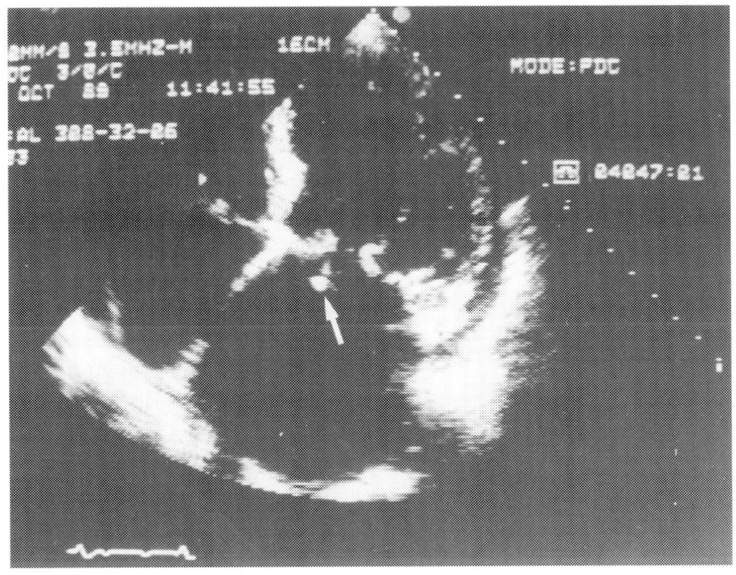

Fig. 16.1 An apical four chamber view in a patient who presented with a new murmur 24 hours after the onset of MI. The image shows a flail of the anterior mitral leaflet protruding into the left atrium in systole. The tip of the papillary muscle head is also seen (arrow).

the free wall of the ventricle may occur even after small infarctions, and is most often rapidly fatal due to acute pericardial tamponade. In some instances, however, the extent of pericardial bleeding may be limited by pericardial adhesions (either from past pericarditis or prior coronary surgery) and result in the formation of a localized *pseudoaneurysm*.[20] In contrast, true aneurysms usually form after large infarctions affecting either the anterior septal wall, or less commonly the inferior base of the heart.[21]

Detection of clinically silent changes after myocardial infarction

Patients surviving the acute phase of MI may develop clinically silent changes in both the infarcted and non-infarcted regions of the heart.[5,23–25] It is possible for the infarct zone to increase in size due to either *infarct expansion* (seen as thinning and bulging of the infarct segment) or *infarct extension* (seen as infarction of myocardium adjacent to the infarct zone). Further, *ventricular dilatation*, a global increase in ventricular size proportional to the extent of abnormal wall motion following MI, may occur due to an increase in the size of the non-infarcted myocardial segments. It has been demonstrated that these otherwise 'silent' changes in the infarct and non-infarcted regions of the heart bear independent prognostic information.[26–28] For example, patients with evidence of regional infarct expansion have been shown to be at high risk of early sudden death, while patients with a global increase in ventricular size are shown to be at high risk for late cardiac death after MI.

Left ventricular aneurysms are a clear expression of infarct expansion. They are characterized by areas of thinning and dyskinesia and may predispose to thrombus formation. *Apical thrombus* is usually evident as a collection of echogenic material in the region of abnormal wall motion, and may be detectable within days of MI.[29–31] Thrombus may either embolize acutely or organize to become laminated and calcified over time. In the acute phase, ventricular thrombi may be laminar, sessile or independently mobile. Although the degree of echogenicity is variable, it bears some relation to the age of the thrombus, with older thrombi tending to appear brighter as they become more organized. Ventricular thrombi should be differentiated from false tendons, apical scar and chest wall artefacts.[32,33] This is usually possible since thrombi are typically seen in at least two views, do not appear as distinct linear mid-ventricular structures, and tend to form in regions of abnormal wall motion. The risk of systemic embolism following MI has been demonstrated to be greater in patients with echocardiographic evidence of thrombus, and in these patients the risk has been demonstrated to be related to the size and mobility of the thrombus.[34,35]

The role of echocardiography in the approach to common diagnostic dilemmas in coronary care

Unexplained acute pulmonary oedema

The onset of pulmonary oedema is most often due to AMI. In some instances, however, especially in patients without overt clinical or electrocardiographic MI, echocardiography may prove invaluable in excluding other causes of this syndrome.

Specifically, echocardiography, in a patient with a small heart on chest X-ray, may lead to the diagnosis of previously *unsuspected mitral stenosis, atrial myxoma* or *acute partial flail* of the aortic or mitral valve due to infection or spontaneous chordal rupture. If these are excluded, the diagnosis must then be entertained of non-cardiac pulmonary oedema due to acute pneumonitis or aspiration. In contrast, acute breathlessness in a patient with an enlarged cardiac silhouette on chest X-ray would suggest the presence of a *dilated cardiomyopathy* or *pericardial effusion with pericardial tamponade*, a distinction which can be made readily by cardiac ultrasound. (For discussion on tamponade, see below.)

In patients with *prosthetic heart valves*, acute pulmonary oedema may mark the presence of acute prosthetic regurgitation or obstruction. Valvular *regurgitation* may occur as a consequence of valvular dehiscence or leaflet flail. Dehiscence of a prosthetic valve is usually due to perivalvular infection, and is suggested by independent motion or 'rocking' of the prosthesis. This occurs when at least 30% of the valve ring has become unstable.[36] Leaflet flail is seen most commonly with tissue valves and may not be appreciated by transthoracic imaging. Acute prosthetic *obstruction* is usually due to thrombosis and/or infection, and is more common on disc valves. The diagnosis is suspected by observing the pattern of disc motion. Although transthoracic imaging is useful in most cases of suspected acute prosthetic dysfunction transoesophageal imaging should be performed if any doubt exists as to the normality of valvular function.

Enlarged cardiac silhouette on chest X-ray

An enlarged cardiac silhouette on chest X-ray is a frequent diagnostic dilemma in the CCU. While the cause may relate to an underlying cardiomyopathy or unsuspected valvular heart disease, it is important to consider the possibility of right heart dilatation secondary to pulmonary hypertension, and pericardial effusion. In any instance, echocardiography can be used to rapidly resolve the issue.

Echocardiography is well established as a sensitive technique for the detection and localization of *pericardial effusions* (see Fig. 16.2). Serous pericardial fluid does not reflect ultrasound and therefore appears as an echolucent area within the boundaries of the pericardial sac. The size of the pericardial effusion is usually described semi-quantitatively as being small, moderate or large. When the effusion is large, the heart can be seen to swing freely in the pericardial space.[37] In some instances large fluid collections in the pleural space surround the heart and can be difficult to distinguish from fluid within the pericardial space. The distinction can usually be made by noting the relation between the fluid, the posterior surface of the heart and the descending thoracic aorta. Pericardial fluid extends between the descending aorta and left atrium. In contrast, the aorta remains closely apposed to the atrio-ventricular groove in the presence of pleural fluid.

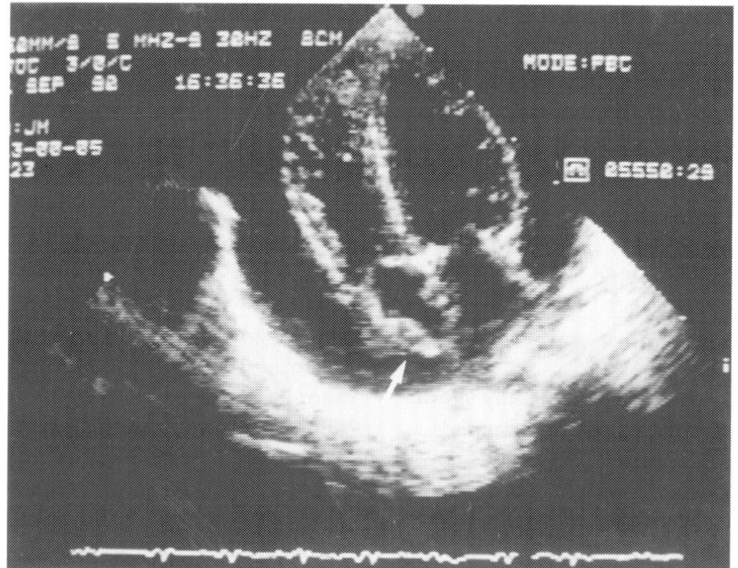

Fig. 16.2 Apical four chamber view in a patient presenting with dyspnoea, a raised jugular venous pressure and an enlarged cardiac silhouette on chest X-ray. The image shows a large circumferential pericardial effusion. Right atrial inversion is also evident (arrow).

Echocardiography has also proven useful in determining the haemodynamic significance of pericardial fluid collections. Specifically, *pericardial tamponade*, defined as an increase in intra-pericardial pressure relative to atrial and ventricular pressure, causes inversion of the right atrial free wall at the end of atrial systole (early ventricular diastole), and inversion of the right ventricular free wall in early diastole.[38] Right ventricular inversion has been shown to be both sensitive and specific for clinically apparent cardiac tamponade. In contrast, right atrial inversion has been demonstrated to be a more sensitive but less specific marker of tamponade. This is not surprising given the thin nature of the right atrial wall and the low pressure within this chamber, which together make the right atrium more sensitive than the right ventricle to subtle changes in pericardial pressure. Nonetheless, it has been demonstrated that when right atrial inversion persists more than one third of the cardiac cycle, correlation with haemodynamic evidence of tamponade is stronger than for detection of atrial inversion per se.[38]

Doppler ultrasound has also proven useful in the assessment of the haemodynamic significance of pericardial effusions.[39] In particular, it is possible to detect exaggerated respiro-phasic variation in right and left ventricular inflow and aortic and pulmonary outflow, consequent to the inability of the heart both to fill normally and to eject a normal stroke volume in the presence of a tense, fluid-filled pericardium. In effect therefore the exaggerated respiratory variation in the Doppler profiles is the equivalent to 'pulsus paradoxus'.

Atypical chest pain

In the patient with severe but atypical chest pain, the clinician must consider MI pericarditis, pulmonary embolism and aortic dissection. Although the role of echocardiography must be individualized in these patients, useful information can be obtained if there is a specific question in mind. Importantly, although abnormal wall motion might favour a diagnosis of myocardial ischaemia, a small pericardial effusion might favour the diagnosis of pericarditis, and a dilated right heart might suggest pulmonary embolism, a normal transthoracic echocardiographic study in these patients does NOT exclude these diagnoses. The most challenging diagnosis in such patients, especially when they have severe pain, is that of *aortic dissection*. Transthoracic echocardiography allows routine assessment of the ascending and abdominal portions of the aorta in adults, and variable imaging of the transverse arch and descending thoracic aorta. More complete examination of the aorta in adults is aided by the use of transoesophageal imaging.[40]

Proximal aortic root disease may be evidenced by an increase in aortic root dimension. In patients with Marfan's syndrome, dilatation typically occurs at the level of the aortic sinuses and the ascending aortic root appears relatively normal.[41] In contrast, in patients with either atherosclerotic or luetic-related aortic aneurysms, the aorta appears diffusely thickened and dilatation occurs beyond the level of the sino-tubular junction.[42] In these patients, discrete atheromatous plaques may be seen as irregular thickening of the vessel wall, or as areas of discrete calcification. On occasion, evidence of focal plaque rupture may also be seen, with linear mobile echodensities attached to the abnormal vessel wall.

The diagnosis of *aortic dissection* is suggested further by the presence of aortic root dilatation and a discrete dissection flap, which partitions the aortic lumen.[43,44] Typically the true lumen is smaller than the false lumen; however, the true lumen can also be recognized by an increase in its size during systole, and by the presence of high velocity flow within it (see Fig. 16.3). Once the diagnosis of aortic dissection is confirmed it is important to determine whether the dissection has involved the ostia of either the coronary or head and neck vessels, whether it has disrupted the aortic valve, or whether it has resulted in pericardial haemorrhage.

Although the diagnosis of dissection of the proximal aorta can occasionally be made with certainty by transthoracic imaging, the diagnosis can be made with much higher sensitivity, and almost complete specificity, by transoesophageal imaging.[45] The two examinations may be complementary, however, for while transoesophageal imaging is particularly valuable for assessing patency of the proximal left and right coronary ostia, transthoracic imaging is more sensitive for the detection of aortic regurgitation and assessing the presence and haemodynamic significance of

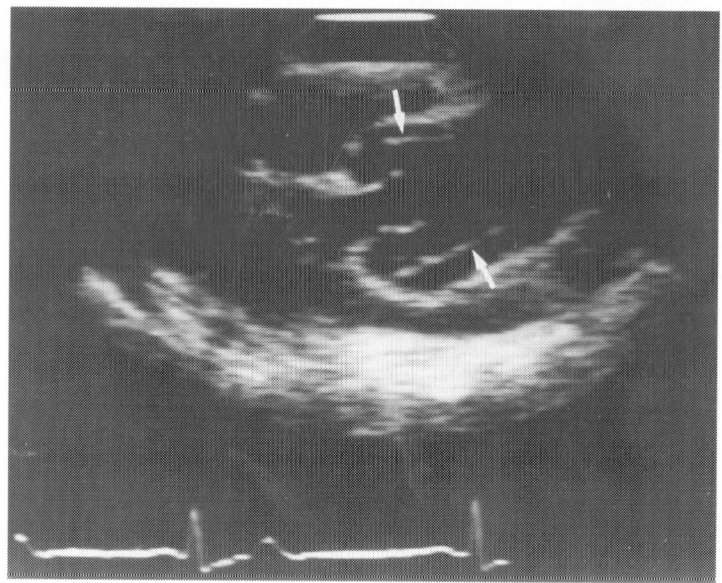

Fig. 16.3 Parasternal long axis view showing dissection of the proximal aortic root. Arrows point to the intimal lining dissected from the vessel wall.

any pericardial fluid collection. Unfortunately, both transthoracic and transoesophageal imaging cannot routinely exclude occlusion of the proximal aortic arch vessels in any given patient.

False positive and negative results are obtained by echocardiography. False positive diagnoses may be made when intra-aortic echoes from either the left atrium or subclavian lines are mistaken for an intimal flap. False negative studies are uncommon, but will occur if the aortic arch is not fully visualised. If doubt regarding the diagnosis exists, the patient should be sent for a computed tomography (CT) scan.

References

1. Mann DL, Gillam LD, Weyman AE. Cross-sectional echocardiographic assessment of regional left ventricular performance and myocardial perfusion. Prog Cardiovasc Dis 1986; 29(1): 1–52
2. Weyman AE, Peskoe SM, Williams ES, Dillon JC, Feigenbaum H. Detection of left ventricular aneurysms by cross-sectional echocardiography. Circulation 1976; 54(6): 936–44
3. Gibson RS, Bishop HL, Stamm RB, Crampton RS, Beller GA, Martin RP. Value of early two-dimensional echocardiography in patients with acute myocardial infarction. Am J Cardiol 1982; 49(5): 1110–9
4. Nishimura RA, Tajik AJ, Shub C et al. Role of two-dimensional echocardiography in the prediction of in-hospital complications after acute myocardial infarction. J Am Coll Cardiol 1984; 4(6): 1080–7
5. Picard MH, Wilkins GT, Ray PA, Weyman AE. Natural history of left ventricular size and function after acute myocardial infarction: assessment and prediction by echocardiographic endocardial surface mapping. Circulation 1990; 82: 484–94
6. Weiss JL, Bulkley BH, Hutchins GM, Mason SJ. Two-dimensional echocardiographic recognition of myocardial injury in man: comparison with post mortem studies. Circulation 1981; 63: 401–8
7. Heger JJ, Weyman AE, Wann LS, Dillon JC, Feigenbaum H. Cross-sectional echocardiography in acute myocardial infarction: detection and localization of regional left ventricular asynergy. Circulation 1979; 60: 531–8
8. Weyman AE. Left ventricle III: Coronary artery disease—clinical manifestations and complications. In: Principles and practice of echocardiography. 2nd ed. Philadelphia: Lea & Febiger, 1994: 657–86
9. Force T, Bloomfield P, O'Boyle JE et al. Quantitative two-dimensional echocardiographic analysis of motion and thickening of the interventricular septum after cardiac surgery. Circulation 1983; 68: 1013–20
10. Weyman AE. Cross sectional echocardiography. Philadelphia: Lea & Febiger, 1982
11. Starling MR, Crawford MH, Sorensen SG, Levi B, Richards K, O'Rourke RA. Comparative accuracy of apical biplane cross-sectional echocardiography and gated equilibrium radionuclide angiography for estimating left ventricular size and performance. Circulation 1981; 63: 1075–84
12. Weyman AE. Left ventricle II: quantification of segmental dysfunction. In: Principles and practice of echocardiography. 2nd ed. Philadelphia: Lea & Febiger, 1994: 625–55
13. Kisslo JA, Robertson D, Gilbert BW, von Ramm O, Behar VS. A comparison of real-time, two-dimensional echocardiography and cineangiography in detecting left ventricular asynergy. Circulation 1977; 55: 134–41
14. Barbour DJ, Roberts WC. Rupture of left ventricular papillary muscles during acute myocardial infarction: analysis of 22 necropsy patients. J Am Coll Cardiol 1986; 8: 558–65

15. Smyllie JH, Sutherland GR, Geuskens R, Dawkins K, Conway N, Roelandt JRTC. Doppler color flow mapping in the diagnosis of ventricular septal rupture and acute mitral regurgitation after myocardial infarction. J Am Coll Cardiol 1990; 15: 1449–55
16. Erbel R, Schweizer P, Bardos P, Meyer J. Two-dimensional echocardiographic diagnosis of papillary muscle rupture. Chest 1981; 79: 595–8
17. Farcot JC, Boisante L, Rigaud M, Bardet J, Bourdarias JP. Two-dimensional echocardiographic visualization of ventricular septal rupture after acute myocardial infarction. Am J Cardiol 1980; 45: 370–7
18. Scanlan JG, Seward JB, Tajik AJ. Visualization of ventricular septal rupture utilizing wide-angled two-dimensional echocardiography. Mayo Clin Proc 1979; 54: 381–4
19. Miyatake K, Okamoto M, Kinoshita N et al. Doppler echocardiographic features of ventricular septal rupture in myocardial infarction. J Am Coll Cardiol 1985; 5: 182–7
20. Roberts WC, Morrow AG. Pseudoaneurysm of the left ventricle. An unusual sequel of myocardial infarction and rupture of the heart. Am J Med 1967; 43: 639–44
21. Schiehter J, Hellerstein KH, Katz LN. Aneurysms of the heart: correlative study of 102 proven cases. Medicine 1954; 33: 43
22. Jeremy RW, Allman KC, Bautovitch G, Harris PJ. Patterns of left ventricular dilation during the six months after myocardial infarction. J Am Coll Cardiol 1989; 13: 304–10
23. Eaton L, Weiss JL, Bulkley BH, Garrison JB, Weisfeldt ML. Regional cardiac dilatation after acute myocardial infarction. N Engl J Med 1979; 300: 57–62
24. Schuster EH, Bulkley BH. Expansion of transmural myocardial infarction: a pathophysiologic factor in cardiac rupture. Circulation 1979; 60: 1532–8
25. Lamas GA, Pfeffer MA. Increased left ventricular volume following myocardial infarction in man. Am Heart J 1986; 111: 30–5
26. Hochman JS, Bulkley BH. The pathogenesis of left ventricular aneurysms: an experimental study in the rat model. Am J Cardiol 1982; 50: 83–8
27. Matsumoto M, Watanabe F, Goto A et al. Left ventricular aneurysm and the prediction of left ventricular enlargement studied by two-dimensional echocardiography: quantitative assessment of aneurysm size in relation to clinical course. Circulation 1985; 72: 280–6
28. Picard MH, Wilkins GT, Gillam LD, Thomas JD, Weyman AE. Immediate regional endocardial surface expansion following coronary occlusion in the canine left ventricle: disproportionate effects of anterior versus inferior ischaemia. Am Heart J 1991; 121: 753–62
29. Visser CA, Kan G, David GK, Lie KI, Durrer D. Two-dimensional echocardiography in the diagnosis of left ventricular thrombus. A prospective study of 67 patients with anatomic validation. Chest 1983; 83: 28–32
30. DeMaria AN, Bommer W, Neumann A et al. Left ventricular thrombi identified by cross-sectional echocardiography. Ann Intern Med 1979; 90: 14–8
31. Asinger RW, Mikell FL, Francis G, Elsperger KJ, Hodges M, Sharma B. Serial evaluation of left ventricular thrombus during acute transmural myocardial infarction using two-dimensional echocardiography. Am J Cardiol 1980; 45: 483
32. Asinger RW, Mikell FL, Sharma B, Hodges M. Observations on detecting left ventricular thrombus with two-dimensional echocardiography: emphasis on avoidance of false positive diagnoses. Am J Cardiol 1981; 47: 145–56
33. Straton JR, Lighty GW, Pearlman AS, Ritchie JL. Detection of left ventricular thrombus by two-dimensional echocardiography: sensitivity, specificity and causes of uncertainty. Circulation 1982; 66: 156–66
34. Visser CA, Kan G, Meltzer RS, Dunning AJ, Roelandt J. Embolic potential of left ventricular thrombus after acute myocardial infarction: a two-dimensional echocardiographic study of 119 patients. J Am Coll Cardiol 1985; 5: 1276–80
35. Kupper AJF, Verheugt FWA, Peels CH, Galema TW, Roos JP. Left ventricular thrombus incidence and behavior studied by serial two-dimensional echocardiography in acute myocardial infarction: left ventricular wall motion, systemic embolism and oral anticoagulation. J Am Coll Cardiol 1989; 13: 1514–20
36. Weyman AE. Echo-Doppler assessment of prosthetic heart valves. In: Principles and practice of echocardiography. 2nd ed. Philadelphia: Lea & Febiger, 1994: 1198–230
37. Weyman AE. Pericardial disease. In: Principles and practice of echocardiography. 2nd ed. Philadelphia: Lea & Febiger, 1994: 1102–34
38. Gillam LD, Guyer D, Stewart WJ, Clark MC, King ME, Weyman AE. A comparison of right atrial and right ventricular inversion as echocardiographic markers of cardiac tamponade. J Am Coll Cardiol 1983; 1: 738
39. Picard MH, Sanfilippo AJ, Newell JB, Rodriguez L, Guerrero JL, Weyman AE. Quantitative relation between increases in intrapericardial pressure and Doppler flow velocities during experimental cardiac tamponade. J Am Coll Cardiol 1991; 18: 234–42
40. Nanda NC et al. Transesophageal biplane echocardiographic imaging: technique, planes, and

clinical usefulness. Echocardiography 1990; 7: 771
41. Come PC, Fortuin NJ, White R, McKusick VA. Echocardiographic assessment of cardiovascular abnormalities in the Marfan syndrome. Am J Med 1983; 74: 465–74
42. DeMaria AN, Bommer W, Neumann A, Weinert L, Bogren H, Mason DT. Identification and localization of aneurysm of the ascending aorta by cross-sectional echocardiography. Circulation 1979; 59: 755–61
43. Erbel R, Engberding R, Daniel W, Roelandt J, Visser C, Rennollet H. Echocardiography in the diagnosis of aortic dissection. Lancet 1989; 1: 457–61
44. Engberding R, Bender F, Grosse-Heitmeyer W et al. Identification of dissection of aneurysm of the descending thoracic aorta by conventional and transesophageal two-dimensional echocardiography. Am J Cardiol 1987; 59: 717–20
45. Nienaber CA, Spielmann RP, von Kodolitsch Y et al. Diagnosis of thoracic aortic dissection. Magnetic resonance imaging versus transesophageal echocardiography. Circulation 1992; 85: 434–47

17 Exercise testing

Peter L Thompson

Introduction

Until the mid-1970s recent myocardial infarction (MI) was thought to be an absolute contraindication to exercise testing. Reasons for this included fear of cardiac rupture, ventricular arrhythmias and cardiac aneurysm formation during exercise in the presence of fresh myocardial necrosis.[1,2] Scandinavian investigators in the mid-1970s showed that early exercise testing after MI was safe[3] and in the late 1970s Jelinek in Australia demonstrated that exercise testing could be performed in selected low risk patients as early as 7–8 days post infarction.[4,5] Changing attitudes to post-infarction exercise testing were confirmed in a survey of physician practices in the United States by Wenger et al in 1982,[6] compared with a survey a decade later showing that the use of post-infarction exercise testing had increased from 24.4% of cardiologists in 1970 to 83.2% in 1979.[7] The safety of carefully selected pre-discharge limited or submaximal exercise testing is now widely accepted[2,8,9] and its use as the predictor of the low-risk patients suitable for early hospital discharge has been investigated.[10]

Technique

Exercise testing for the patient who has been in the coronary care unit is best performed adjacent to the CCU in an area fulfilling the usual quality and safety standards.[9] Either treadmill or bicycle ergometry protocols are suitable. Although there are selected reports demonstrating the safety of symptom-limited exercise testing as early as one week post infarction,[4] symptom-limited tests almost invariably produce higher peak heart rates and work loads than submaximal tests set to pre-specified limits.[11] A variety of indices have been used for specifying the level for submaximal testing but the near-routine use of beta blockers post infarction invalidates the usual formulas for tests based on a percentage of maximal heart rate. The widespread use of multiples of resting oxygen consumption (METS) has simplified the standardization of exercise testing and allowed comparison between bicycle and treadmill protocols.[9] The usual recommendation is that pre-discharge exercise testing should be limited to approximately 5 METS and the post discharge testing at 3 weeks to several months post infarction should use a symptom-limited protocol[8,9] There is some evidence that a post-discharge higher level test provides additional information to the predischarge submaximal test.[12]

Careful patient selection is needed to ensure the safety and maximize the value of post-infarction exercise testing. Patients who are too frail or immobilized by neurologic or musculo-skeletal problems are clearly unsuitable for exercise testing. Patients with continuing post-infarction symptoms of ischaemia or cardiac failure should be excluded, as should patients with persistent post-infarction arrhythmias. In usual clinical experience and most of the published studies, about one third of patients are unsuitable for pre-discharge exercise testing.

In addition to the usual safety and quality standards, the post-infarction patient requires particular emphasis on assessment of symptoms and meticulous monitoring of electrocardiograph (ECG) changes, cardiac arrhythmias and systolic blood pressure.[9] The usual indications for stopping prior to the pre-determined exercise level of approximately 5 METS are the development of angina, the development of ST segment depression greater than 2 mm, provocation of high grade arrhythmias and a drop in systolic blood pressure greater than 10 mmHg from the resting level. Each of these indicates significant inducible myocardial ischaemia which requires further evaluation.

Prediction of death and reinfarction

Most of the studies on the prognostic value of exercise testing were conducted prior to the widespread introduction of thrombolytic therapy for the treatment of MI. The most influential early report was that from Theroux et al in 1979.[13] In a study of 210 patients they showed that the finding of ST segment depression of greater than 1 mm in a pre-discharge exercise test was highly predictive of death in the subsequent year. 27% of patients with a positive test died, compared with only 2% of patients with a negative test.[13] Subsequent studies have failed to confirm this striking predictive value of ST segment depression. However, the use of other exercise indices such as greater degrees of ST segment depression and duration of exercise,[14] and the inclusion of other end points besides death, such as reinfarction or other coronary events, confirmed that the early exercise test after MI is of considerable value in predicting coronary events in the pre-thrombolysis era of management of MI. A review of 15 studies by Kulick and Rahimtoola[16] summarized the incidence of late events in patients with abnormal tests as ranging from 6 to 41%, whereas those with normal tests range from 0 to 8% in the published studies. The sensitivity of the exercise test to predict subsequent coronary events ranged from 19 to 100%, the specificity from 35 to 93% and the predictive accuracy from 92 to 100%. Debusk et al demonstrated that the predictive value of exercise testing is maximized when clinical features are included to stratify patients into high and low risk prior to their exercise test.[15]

A significant problem with exercise testing as a prognostic indicator is the inability of a significant proportion of post-infarction patients to perform the exercise test. The range of such patients in the published studies is 10–22% and this group of patients consistently has a high mortality in the subsequent year.[16]

Prediction of multi-vessel coronary artery disease

Exercise testing is frequently used to predict the presence of significant coronary artery disease after MI and is frequently recommended as a cost-effective strategy in selecting patients for cardiac catheterization.[8,17,19] Analysis of the reliability of exercise testing in predicting multi-vessel disease post infarction showed a range of sensitivities from 42 to 96% and specificities from 41 to 94% in the published studies reviewed by Kulick and Rahimtoola. In the majority of the series the sensitivity was less than 75%. Although this indicates that there may be 25% of patients with multi-vessel disease who fail to have it detected by exercise testing, it is not clear that the multi-vessel disease necessarily requires interaction in the absence of inducible myocardial ischaemia on exercise testing.

Studies of exercise testing in the 'Reperfusion era'

The data derived from patients not treated with thrombolytic therapy may not be applicable to patients who have been treated with thrombolysis or other forms of reperfusion. They may have a greater likelihood of patency of the infarct-related artery. The studies which have evaluated this question have failed to confirm the predictive value of pre-discharge exercise testing. Chaitman studied nearly 2000 patients who had been included in the TIMI II trial and found that an abnormal exercise test on pre-discharge exercise testing did not predict coronary events within the first 6 months following discharge.[18] These results were confirmed in an analysis of the 10,000 post-thrombolysis patients in the GISSI data base, which showed no predictive value when all tests were analyzed,[18a] or only weak predictive value of symptomatic ischaemia (RR 2.07) and low work capacity (RR 1.78) when submaximal tests were excluded.[18b]

The reasons for the disappointing results with thrombolysis treated patients compared with the earlier experience is not clear. A possible explanation is the low risk of death in post thrombolysis patients who are capable of performing an exercise test. The six month death rate in the exercise tested patients in the GISSI data base was only 1.3%. As in the pre thrombolysis studies, the death rate for those unable to exercise was far higher (7.1%).

Other uses of exercise testing in patients admitted to the coronary care unit

In addition to its role in prognostic stratification and selection of patients for further investigation, exercise testing has considerable value in the post-infarction patient in evaluating suitability for discharge, helping to establish the patient's confidence prior to discharge and setting guidelines for exercise levels and exercise training at home.[8] In addition to evaluation of the post-infarction patient, exercise testing is frequently used in evaluating the patient who has been admitted to the CCU with chest pain. In the patient with the intermediate likelihood of the chest pain being due to myocardial ischaemia, a limited exercise test is a relatively simple and cost-effective method of detecting inducible myocardial ischaemia, which may increase the likelihood that the chest pain was due to underlying coronary artery disease and warrant further investigation. In the patient with a negative exercise test early discharge is warranted.

In patients with medium to low likelihood of the chest pain being due to ischaemia, the stress test can be a valuable method of reassurance. Of course the use of exercise testing for this purpose must be done with appropriate regard to the sensitivity, specificity and the pre-test likelihood of disease. Two recent studies have evaluated the role of stress testing in patients with recent unstable angina. Moss et al[19] showed on post-discharge exercise tests that a combination of ST segment depression of greater than 1 mm and an exercise duration of less than 9 minutes identified patients with a 3.4-fold to 1.9-fold increase in risk of cardiac events. The RISC group[20] showed in pre-discharge exercise tests that a large number of leads with ST segment depression and a low maximal work load independently predicted 1 year infarct-free survival.

Conclusion

After 15 years' intensive evaluation and widespread use, the exercise test has a clear role in the evaluation of patients admitted to the CCU. The post-infarction patient can be evaluated with a pre-discharge submaximal exercise test of 5 METS. Analysis of ST segment depression alone will be of limited value. A composite analysis of the degree and location of ST segment shifts, associated symptoms, blood pressure response, arrhythmia response, and duration of exercise can provide valuable information on the degree of inducible myocardial ischaemia to assist in prognostic stratification and selection of patients for more detailed investigation.

Further studies are needed to clarify the role of exercise testing in patients who have received thrombolytic therapy. Stress testing has a wider role in evaluating exercise capacity and restoring patient confidence following a coronary event. It can be used as a simple cost-effective method of triaging patients admitted to hospital with unstable angina.

References

1. Hamm LF, Stull GA, Crow RS. Exercise testing early after myocardial infarction: historic perspectives and current uses. Prog Cardiovasc Dis 1986; 28: 463–76
2. Miller DH, Borer JS. Exercise testing early after myocardial infarction: risks and benefits. Am J Med 1982; 72: 427–38
3. Ibsen H, Kjoller S, Styperek J, Pedersen A. Routine exercise ECG three weeks after acute myocardial infarction. Acta Med Scand 1975; 198: 463–9
4. Jelinek VM, Ziffer RW, McDonald IG, Wasir H, Hale GS. Early exercise testing and mobilisation after myocardial infarction. Med J Aust 1977; 2: 589–93
5. Jelinek VM, McDonald IG, Ryan WF, Ziffer RW, Clemens A, Gerloff J. Assessment of cardiac risk 10 days after uncomplicated myocardial infarction. Br Med J 1982; 284: 227–30
6. Wenger NK, Hellerstein HK, Blackburn H, Castranova SJ. Physician practice in the management of patients with uncomplicated myocardial infarction: changes in the past decade. Circulation 1982; 65: 421–7
7. Wenger NK, Hellerstein HK, Blackburn H, Castranova SJ. Uncomplicated myocardial infarction: current physician practice in patient management. JAMA 1973; 224: 511–4
8. ACC/AHA Task Force Report. Guidelines for the early management of patients with acute myocardial infarction. J Am Coll Cardiol 1990; 16: 249–92
9. Guidelines for exercise testing. A report of the ACC/AHA Task Force on assessment of diagnostic and therapeutic cardiovascular procedures. (Subcommittee on exercise testing). J Am Coll Cardiol 1986; 8: 725–38
10. Topol E, Burek K, O'Neill W et al. A randomized controlled trial of early hospital discharge three days after myocardial infarction

in the era of reperfusion. N Engl J Med 1988; 318: 1083–8
11. Debusk RF, Haskell W. Symptom limited vs heart rate limited exercise testing soon after myocardial infarction. Circulation 1980; 61: 738–43
12. Stone PH, Turi ZG, Muller J and MILIS 5 Study Group. Prognostic significance of the treadmill exercise test performance six months after myocardial infarction. J Am Coll Cardiol 1986; 8: 1007–17
13. Theroux P, Waters DD, Halphen C, Debasieux JC, Mizgala HF. Prognostic value of exercise testing soon after myocardial infarction. N Engl J Med 1979; 301: 341–5
14. Weld FM, Chu KL, Bigger JT Jr, Rolnitzky LM. Risk stratification with low-level exercise testing two weeks after acute myocardial infarction. Circulation 1981; 64: 306–14
15. Debusk RF, Kraemer HC, Nash E. Stepwise risk stratification soon after myocardial infarction. Am J Cardiol 1983; 52: 1161–6
16. Kulick DL, Rahimtoola SH. Assessment of the survivors of acute myocardial infarction: the case for coronary angiography. In: Gersh BJ, Rahimtoola SH. Acute myocardial infarction. New York: Elsevier, 1991
17. Ross J, Gilpin EA, Madsen EB et al. A decision scheme for coronary angiography after acute myocardial infarction. Circulation 1989; 79: 292–303
18. Chaitman BR, McMahon RP, Terria M et al for the TIMI Investigators. Impact of treatment strategy on predischarge exercise test in the Thrombolysis in Myocardial Infarction (TIMI)-II trial. Am J Cardiol 1993; 71: 131–8
18a. Volpi A, De Vita C, Franzosi MG, et al. Determinants of 6-month mortality in survivors of myocardial infarction after thrombolysis. Results of the GISSI-2 data base. Circulation 1993; 88: 416–429
18b. Villella A, Maggioni AP, Villella M et al. Prognostic significance of maximal exercise testing after myocardial infarction treated with thrombolytic agents: the GISSI-2 data base. Lancet 1995; 346: 523–529
19. Moss AJ, Goldstein RE, Hall WJ et al. Detection and significance of myocardial ischaemia in stable patients after recovery from an acute coronary event. Myocardial Ischaemia Research Group. JAMA 1993; 269: 2379–85
20. Nyman I, Larsson H, Areskog M et al. The predictive value of silent ischaemia at an exercise test before discharge after an episode of unstable coronary artery disease. RISC Study Group. Am Heart J 1992; 123: 324–31

18 Nuclear imaging

Geoff Groom

Nuclear medicine provides a physiologic means of investigating coronary artery disease (CAD) and disorders of ventricular function. Radionuclide imaging can be employed to evaluate myocardial perfusion, to calculate global and regional left ventricular ejection fraction, and to diagnose and localize myocardial infarction (MI).

This chapter will describe the most commonly utilized radionuclide studies and then attempt to place their use in routine clinical practice in context. Before the various nuclear medicine studies that can be performed to evaluate the heart are outlined, the individual characteristics of the commonly used radiopharmaceuticals will be reviewed.

^{201}Tl thallous chloride

This is the oldest myocardial perfusion agent, and the utility of newer agents is measured against this isotope. Thallium is taken up within the myocardium via the sodium/potassium pump and is distributed intracellularly like potassium. It is not 'fixed' in the tissues but is 'washed in' and 'washed out', according to regional blood flow and the characteristics of the tissue being perfused.[1] For example, although an area of MI has reduced blood flow, thallium will 'wash out' from the infarct region at a similar rate as from normally perfused heart muscle, whereas ischaemic myocardium, with exactly the same blood flow as infarcted tissue, will 'wash out' thallium at a much slower rate, or may even accumulate thallium over a period of hours. Thus the distinction between ischaemic and infarcted muscle can be made on the basis of thallium redistribution. Significant uptake of thallium in the lungs, when injected during exercise or pharmacologic stress, is a sensitive indicator of left ventricular dysfunction.[2]

Unfortunately, the imaging characteristics of the photon emissions from thallium (predominantly low energy X-rays) are not ideal for imaging on the standard gamma camera, with the result that:

- overall image quality is only adequate
- relatively little thallium can be administered due to its long half-life
- image interpretation is hampered by attenuation artefacts due to soft tissues such as the diaphragm and the breasts.

Technetium-99m Sestamibi

^{99m}Tc Sestamibi is an isonitrile, and like ^{201}Tl, is distributed according to regional blood flow. Once delivered to the myocardial cell, it is bound in the mitochondria with very little redistribution.[3] As Sestamibi is labelled with ^{99m}Tc (which has a shorter half-life than thallium and an ideal gamma ray emission), larger amounts of activity can be administered for the same radiation dose to the patient and better image quality is achieved.

^{99m}Tc labelled red blood cells

Red blood cells can be easily labelled with ^{99m}Tc. This is usually performed in the laboratory after approximately 5 ml of blood has been taken from the patient. The labelled red cells are then reinjected into the circulation where they are rapidly mixed with the unlabelled red cells. The gamma camera is then used to quantitate the amount of radioactivity within the cardiac chambers during systole and diastole in order to calculate left (or right) ventricular ejection fraction.

^{99m}Tc pyrophosphate

Pyrophosphate binds to extracellular calcium. Hence, with release of calcium after breakdown of the myocardial cell membrane in MI, ^{99m}Tc pyrophosphate can be used to identify non-viable cardiac muscle cells, both for diagnostic purposes and to document the site and size of MI.

Types of nuclear medicine imaging studies

Myocardial perfusion imaging

The basic requirement for the evaluation of coronary artery blood flow is a pharmaceutical which is distributed within the myocardium according to blood flow at the time of its administration and can be labelled with radioactivity without changing its properties. This 'tracer' must either be fixed in the myocardium, or its rate of 'wash out' from the heart must be slow enough to allow imaging with a standard gamma camera. Suitable agents include ^{201}Tl thallous chloride, ^{99m}Tc Sestamibi and ^{99m}Tc Teboroxime (although Teboroxime washes out of the myocardium very quickly, limiting its utility). New technetium-based tracers continue to be developed.

If coronary artery blood flow is impaired, then less tracer is deposited in the heart muscle per unit time than in areas of normal blood flow. Consequently, when the heart is imaged in either two (planar) or three dimensions (single photon emission computed tomography or SPECT), the amount of radiotracer uptake in any region of the heart will be proportional to blood flow at the time of injection. (A complete account of the techniques employed in nuclear medicine is found elsewhere.)[4]

Under basal conditions of coronary artery blood flow, stenoses reducing the vessel diameter by greater than 90% can be detected. By increasing coronary artery blood flow by a factor of 2–4 (for instance, with maximal exertion or pharmacologic vasodilatation), lesions of greater than 50% can be demonstrated.

Various types of myocardial perfusion imaging studies can be performed. These include:

- **Resting study**. The injection of a radioisotope at rest evaluates coronary blood flow under basal conditions. Myocardial viability can be determined (with thallium) and the test can be used to assess rest pain of uncertain aetiology.
- **Exercise study**. In addition to information regarding the patient's functional capacity, the injection of a perfusion tracer at near peak exercise provides improved sensitivity and specificity for the diagnosis of CAD when compared with standard exercise electrocardiography.
- **Pharmacologic 'stress'**. By causing coronary artery vasodilatation, dipyridamole can be used to unmask coronary artery stenoses. Because a stenosed artery will be unable to dilate to the same extent as a normal vessel, relative blood flow to myocardium downstream from the stenosis will be significantly reduced, when compared to myocardium supplied by normally dilated arteries. Dipyridamole and adenosine act via the same mechanism (dipyridamole increases plasma levels of adenosine) to cause coronary artery vasodilatation; however, adenosine is shorter acting. Dobutamine, a synthetic sympathomimetic, can also be used to increase myocardial blood flow by increasing myocardial oxygen consumption.

Most nuclear medicine departments routinely collect myocardial perfusion studies using the SPECT technique, in which multiple views of the heart are acquired as the gamma camera moves around the patient in a circular or elliptical orbit. Images are presented in short axis, vertical and horizontal long axis slices. Stress (either exercise or pharmacologic) and resting images are presented side by side for visual analysis, with computer

Fig. 18.1 [A]: ^{201}Tl thallous chloride SPECT images performed after bicycle stress and at rest (after ^{201}Tl reinjection), in a patient with inferior myocardial ischaemia. Rows 1 and 2: the short axis image set. Apical slice is at the left, basal slice at the right. Rows 3 and 4: the vertical long axis, septal slice at left and lateral wall slice at right. Rows 5 and 6: the horizontal long axis views, the most inferior slice at left, the most anterior slice at right. For each image set, the stress images are presented above the rest (reinjection) images. The short axis and vertical long axis image sets best show the almost completely reversible inferior defect (arrows).
[B]: Polar or bull's-eye map of the same study as in [A]. Short axis slices are represented as a single image: the apical short axis slice at the centre of the bull's-eye; slices progressing towards the base of the heart by the concentric circles enlarging from the centre of the image; the outermost circle of the bull's-eye represents the basal short axis slice. Upper row: distribution of myocardial blood flow in the heart at stress and reinjection. Lower row compares the patient's data to a database of patients of the same sex with normal coronary arteries. Again, the inferior defect is identified on the stress images, with near complete normalization on the reinjection images. (Image collected on Siemens MULTISPECT 2 gamma camera. Quantitative analysis performed using Cedars-Sinai interpretive program—CTQ.)

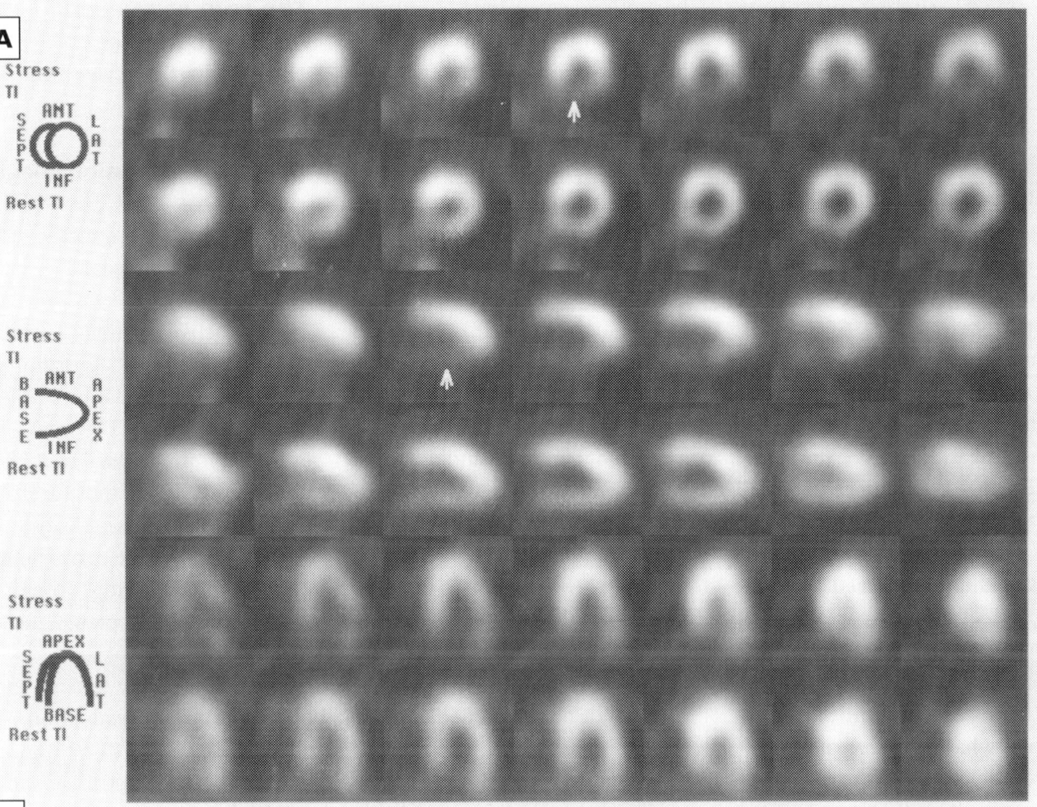
A
Stress Tl
ANT
SEPT
LAT
INF
Rest Tl
Stress Tl
ANT
BASE
APEX
INF
Rest Tl
Stress Tl
APEX
SEPT
LAT
BASE
Rest Tl

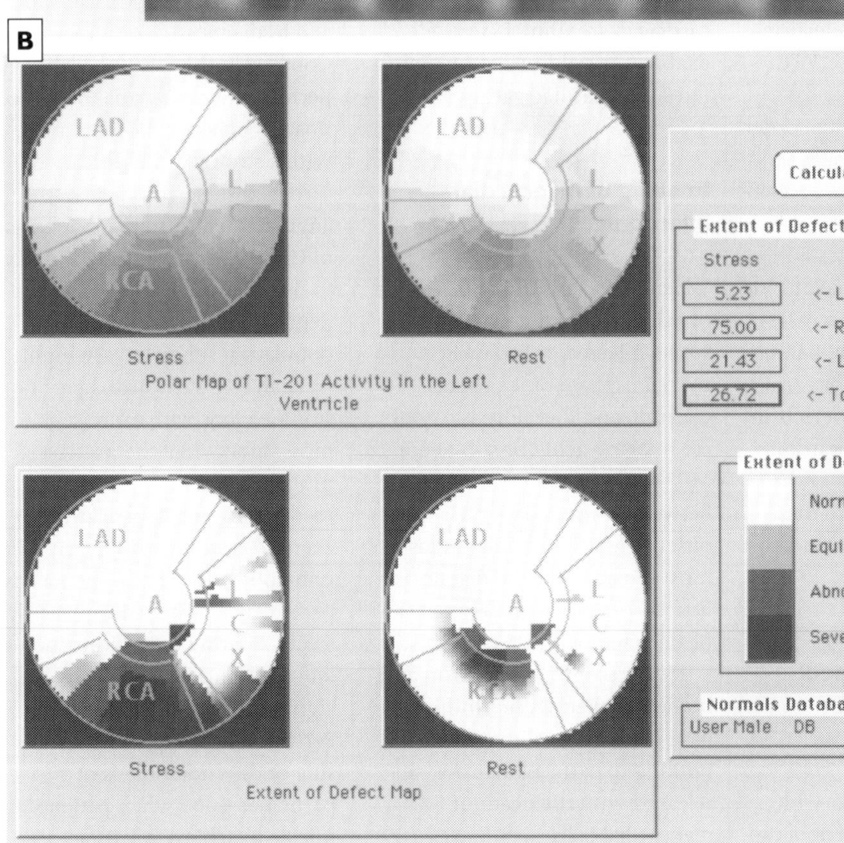
B
LAD
A
RCA
L
C
X
Stress
Rest
Polar Map of Tl-201 Activity in the Left Ventricle
Calculate Results
Extent of Defect Percentages
Stress
Rest
5.23 <- LAD % -> 2.61
75.00 <- RCA % -> 0.00
21.43 <- LCX % -> 0.00
26.72 <- Total % -> 8.65
Extent of Defect Color Key
Normal
Equivocal
Abnormal
Severely Abnormal
Normals Database used
User Male DB
Stress
Rest
Extent of Defect Map

generated 'bull's-eye' maps (two-dimensional representations of blood flow to the left ventricle) allowing confirmation of the visual findings and comparison to normal databases (see Fig. 18.1 A,B). Occasionally, three planar views of the heart, instead of SPECT imaging, are collected. Generally, planar imaging would be performed only if SPECT were not practicable, for instance, if a patient is extremely obese, or if arthritis of the left shoulder prevents full abduction of the arm.

The major advantage of SPECT imaging is to separate adjacent areas of abnormal and normal myocardium; if imaged using the planar technique, an area of abnormality may not be appreciated due to overlying normally perfused myocardium. SPECT imaging has been shown to be more sensitive and specific than planar imaging for the detection of coronary artery disease. With thallium SPECT, sensitivity for multi-vessel disease is in the order of 92%, with normalcy rates of 84% (specificity figures are somewhat lower due to post-test angiography referral patterns).[5]

Perfusion defects in the inferior wall of the left ventricle in males, and the anterior wall in females, have a lower specificity for coronary artery disease than defects in other regions of the myocardium. This is due to attenuation of the radioactivity emitted from these regions by the diaphragm and breast tissue respectively.

Gated cardiac blood pool imaging (radionuclide ventriculography)

By labelling red blood cells with ^{99m}Tc, images of the blood pool can be captured either in two or three dimensions. The patient's ECG is used to image the radioactivity in the left ventricle during different parts of systole and diastole (routinely the cardiac cycle is divided into 16–32 'gates'). Multiple cardiac cycles are averaged (an 'average cardiac cycle play-back' can be generated), and left ventricular ejection fraction can be determined by subtracting the radioactivity in the left ventricle during systole from the activity measured in diastole and dividing by the diastolic counts (see Fig. 18.2). Similar information can be gained about right ventricular function; however, due to the anatomy of the right ventricle, less accurate results are obtained.

Radionuclide ventriculography (RNV) can be performed at both rest and exercise, but becomes less accurate when significant cardiac dysrhythmia (for example, atrial fibrillation) interferes with cardiac gating.

Imaging of myocardial infarction

When MI occurs, there is leakage of calcium into the extracellular space. Injected ^{99m}Tc-labelled pyrophosphate binds to this calcium, and therefore is useful for imaging acute or sub-acute MI. Uptake of tracer is maximal between 2 and 5 days after the onset of MI. SPECT imaging is most sensitive for the diagnosis; infarcts of approximately 6 g can be detected by this technique.[6]

More recently, antimyosin antibodies labelled with ^{111}indium have been used to image MI, binding to extracellular myosin released with the death of myocardial cells.[7]

The role of nuclear medicine in the evaluation of cardiac disease

Myocardial perfusion imaging

The diagnosis of suspected coronary artery disease

The predictive accuracy of a diagnostic test will vary according to the prevalence of disease in the population (Bayes' Theorem). For example, if myocardial perfusion imaging has a sensitivity and specificity of 90% and 80% respectively, but the test is being performed in a young woman with atypical chest pain, a negative test adds little to the diagnostic accuracy that is gained by simple clinical evaluation, whereas a positive study is more likely to be falsely positive and add to diagnostic confusion. Conversely, there is little value in performing myocardial perfusion imaging in a middle-aged man, with a strong family history of cardiac disease and typical angina, to confirm the diagnosis of CAD; a negative study is likely to be falsely negative, as the incidence of disease in this population subset is very high.

Therefore myocardial perfusion imaging with exercise is of most value when the pre-test probability of CAD is intermediate, or when standard exercise electrocardiography is unhelpful either because of a suspected false positive result, or due to pre-existing conditions such as left ventricular hypertrophy or right bundle branch block. Perfusion imaging using adenosine or dipyridamole is of particular value when patients are unable to achieve a satisfactory

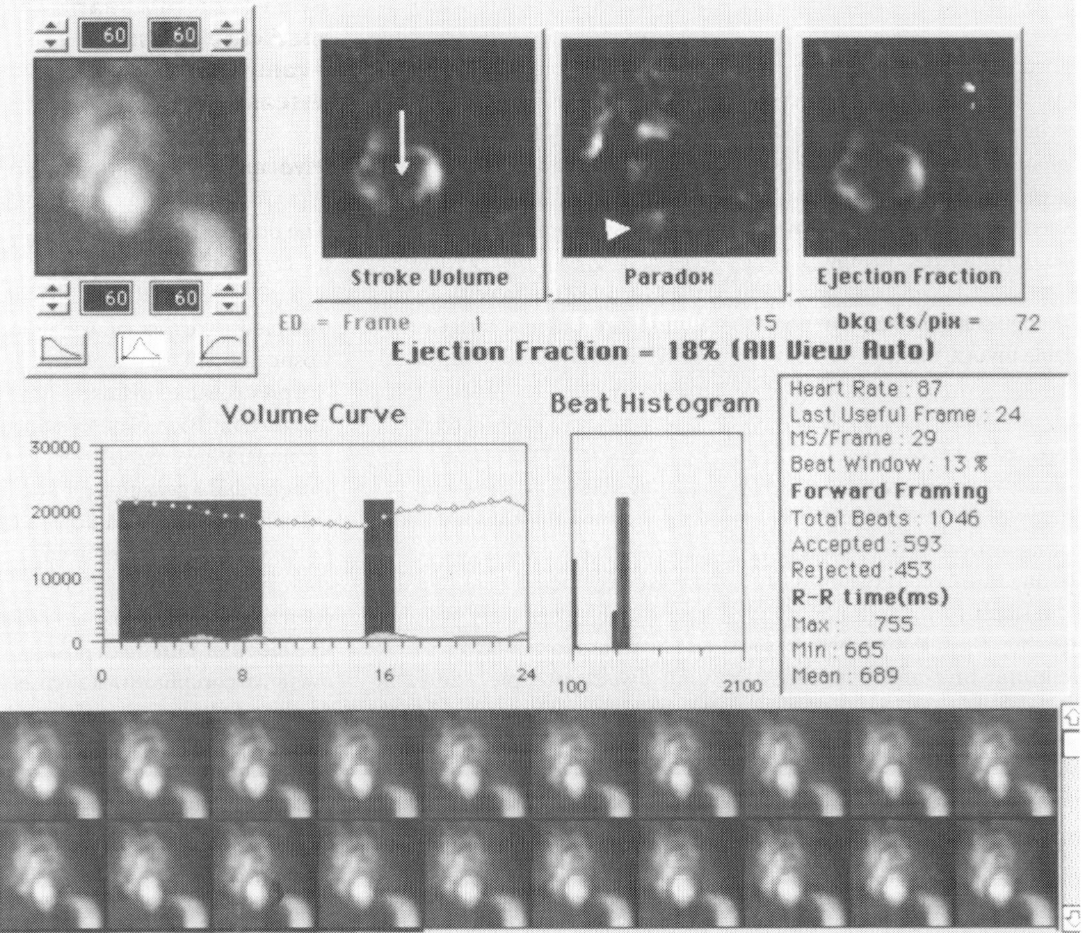

Fig. 18.2 Gated cardiac blood pool data from a patient with severe LV dysfunction and apical dyskinesis. LV ejection fraction is calculated at 18% (normal ≥ 55%). Arrow on the stroke volume image shows reduced contraction of the septum and apex; arrow head on the paradox image demonstrates dyskinetic motion of the apical wall. (Collected on Siemens MULTISPECT 2 gamma camera, analysis on ICON software.)

cardiovascular workload—this may be due to lack of fitness, physical handicap, obesity or even lack of motivation, to name some of the more common reasons. Because dipyridamole and adenosine cause broncho-constriction, the use of these agents is contraindicated in patients with asthma. Drugs such as theophylline and caffeine must be avoided prior to pharmacologic stress using dipyridamole or adenosine as they interfere with vasodilatation. Dobutamine can be used as the pharmacologic stress in patients with asthma when performing myocardial perfusion imaging.

Patients with left bundle branch block undergoing myocardial perfusion imaging should be evaluated using a vasodilator, rather than with exercise or dobutamine, as false positive results with the latter are common. The reasons for this are uncertain; one possible explanation is that delayed septal contraction leads to a reduced septal metabolism (and hence blood flow requirement), which is more marked with exercise.[8] By using a vasodilator, falsely positive 'reversible' defects are uncommon; however, it is not unusual to see fixed perfusion defects in the septum in the absence of CAD.

Assessing the functional significance of CAD

Myocardial perfusion imaging can be used to assess patients with known CAD. It is especially useful in establishing the culprit lesion in patients with angiographically documented multi-vessel disease,[9] when angioplasty is being considered. After a myocardial infarction, myocardial perfusion imaging can be used to demonstrate the presence or absence of residual ischaemia, especially in patients who have had thrombolytic therapy.[10]

Distinguishing viable from non-viable myocardium

It is now well established that impaired left ventricular function is not always irreversible.[11] Examples are stunned or hibernating myocardium (see Ch. 8). Resting injection of thallium, with late (usually 24-hour) re-imaging, is a sensitive method for evaluating myocardial viability. It has been shown that if thallium uptake is more than 50% of the normal value in the territory of MI, this indicates that revascularization of this territory will lead to improved regional contraction.[12]

Positron emission tomography (PET) using ^{18}F FDG or ^{11}C acetate is a more sensitive method for diagnosis of myocardial viability; its utility is limited however by the expense of PET technology, and the number of patients who would benefit from metabolic PET imaging after an equivocal SPECT thallium study is relatively small (see Ch. 20).

Evaluating the efficacy of revascularization procedures

Myocardial perfusion imaging can be used to demonstrate successful reperfusion following coronary artery bypass grafting (CABG) and angioplasty. Follow-up can be performed with exercise or pharmacologic stress and is especially useful when post-operative ECG abnormalities preclude interpretation of a standard exercise ECG. Myocardial perfusion imaging is superior to standard treadmill electrocardiography for assessing patients after multi-vessel angioplasty. The timing of myocardial perfusion imaging is critical in relation to angioplasty. Patients with early recurrence of typical symptomatology are often re-catheterized in preference to investigation with myocardial perfusion imaging.[9] Those patients who develop atypical symptomatology, or who are asymptomatic after a procedure which is considered to have a high risk of early restenosis, should not be tested until 4 weeks post procedure.[13] It has been shown that although an early negative test has a high negative predictive value,[9] the incidence of a positive myocardial perfusion imaging study in the presence of a widely patent angioplasty site is unacceptably high.[14] It is postulated that this is due to abnormal flow across the angioplasty site as endothelial remodelling occurs, or due to abnormalities in coronary vascular tone.[15] It is generally considered that exercise myocardial perfusion imaging is preferable to pharmacological stress in patients without physical limitations.

Assessing prognosis post myocardial infarction

Both submaximal pre-discharge exercise myocardial perfusion imaging[16] and early dipyridamole myocardial perfusion imaging[17] have been shown to be useful predictors of outcome and detection of triple vessel CAD in asymptomatic patients following uncomplicated MI. Positive submaximal exercise myocardial perfusion imaging identifies patients at higher risk for cardiac death and reinfarction. Dipyridamole thallium scintigraphy can be performed safely in the early post-MI period (3–5 days post uncomplicated MI) and provides similar prognostic information.

Dipyridamole thallium imaging has been used to evaluate peri-operative prognosis in patients undergoing major vascular surgery. Dipyridamole-induced myocardial perfusion abnormalities identified pre-operatively increase the likelihood of intra- and post-operative complications such as death and MI.[18] Cardiac catheterization may be indicated prior to the planned surgery, especially if the perfusion abnormalities are large or cover more than one vascular territory.

Radionuclide ventriculography

The advent of echocardiography has seen a decline in the number of RNV studies performed in Australia over the last 10 years. Echocardiography is clearly superior to (and slightly less expensive than) RNV for the overall assessment of myocardial structure and function, particularly with the advent of Doppler flow capability. Only occasionally when echocardiography is technically difficult is RNV superior. There is no doubt that the RNV is a sensitive test for evaluating overall and regional ventricular function, and that post-MI resting ejection fractions of less than 40% confer a higher risk of subsequent cardiac events.[19] One area where RNV remains the investigation of choice is the evaluation of cardiac function before and during treatment with cardiotoxic drugs such as adriamycin. In this setting, RNV's precision with repeated measurement of ejection fraction comes to the fore.[20]

Exercise RNV has been used both for the diagnosis of CAD and for prognostication. The development of regional wall motion abnormalities during exercise is a very sensitive indicator of CAD, as is a fall in ejection fraction (EF) (or failure to rise by greater than 5%) at peak workloads. It may be that the EF at peak exercise is the greatest prognostic indicator.[21] The use of exercise RNV has fallen in concert with the use of the resting RNV. This probably reflects the fact that stress myocardial perfusion imaging is easier to perform, and the perception that myocardial perfusion imaging has greater sensitivity and specificity for the detection of CAD, although recent studies have refuted this belief.

Myocardial infarction imaging

With the advent of rapid and accurate assays for MB-creatine kinase and other biochemical markers, and the improvement of echocardiographic techniques, nuclear medicine physicians are being asked to perform infarct avid imaging very infrequently. This study may be useful in documenting the site and size of MI in patients with uninterpretable ECGs and a previous history of MI.

Occasionally the diagnosis of MI can be made or excluded in situations such as late presentation, the perioperative period or post cardioversion, but generally echocardiography is the preferred alternative. Certainly, there has been some recent work combining perfusion imaging and infarct imaging to clearly define the ischaemic penumbra post MI.[22]

Summary

The role of nuclear medicine in the evaluation of coronary artery disease continues to evolve. Clearly, functional imaging of coronary artery perfusion and demonstration of myocardial viability complements the information that can be gained from other non-invasive and invasive investigative modalities. Future developments in the areas of improved tissue attenuation correction to reduce the numbers of falsely positive myocardial perfusion imaging studies and the development of new radiopharmaceuticals will ensure the continuing utility of nuclear medicine in the diagnosis, assessment and prognostic evaluation of cardiac disease.

References

1. Beller GA, Watson DD, Pohost GM. Kinetics of thallium distribution and redistribution: clinical applications in sequential myocardial imaging. In: Strauss HW, Pitt B (eds). Cardiovascular nuclear medicine. 2nd ed. St Louis: Mosby, 1979: 225–42
2. Gill JB, Ruddy TD, Newell JB, Finkelstein DM, Strauss HW, Boucher CA. Prognostic importance of thallium uptake by the lungs during exercise in coronary artery disease. N Engl J Med 1987; 317: 1486–9
3. Berman DS, Kiat H, Maddahi J. The new ^{99m}Tc myocardial perfusion imaging agents: ^{99m}Tc-sestamibi and ^{99m}Tc-teboroxime. Circulation 1991; 84: I-7–21
4. Zaret BL, Wackers FJT, Soufler R. Nuclear cardiology. In: Braunwald E (ed). Heart disease: a textbook of cardiovascular medicine. 4th ed. Vol. 1. Philadelphia: Saunders, 1992: 276–311
5. Beller GA. Myocardial perfusion imaging with thallium-201. J Nucl Med 1994; 35: 674–80
6. Jansen DE, Corbett JR, Wolfe CL et al. Quantification of myocardial infarction: a comparison of single photon-emission computed tomography with pyrophosphate to serial plasma MB-creatine kinase measurements. Circulation 1985; 72: 327–33
7. Lahiri A, Bhattacharya A, Carrio I. Antimyosin antibody imaging of myocardial necrosis. In: Zaret BL, Beller GA (eds). Nuclear cardiology: state of the art and future directions. Philadelphia: Mosby–Year Book, 1993: 331–8
8. Hirzel HO, Senn M, Nuesch K, Buettner C, Pfeiffer A, Hess OM, Kragenbuehl HP. Thallium-201 scintigraphy in complete left bundle branch block. Am J Cardiol 1984; 53: 764–9
9. Miller DD, Verani MS. Current status of myocardial perfusion imaging after percutaneous transluminal coronary angioplasty. J Am Coll Cardiol 1994; 24: 260–6
10. Zaret BL, Wackers FJ. Nuclear cardiology (Pt 1). N Engl J Med 1993; 329: 775–83
11. Dilsizian V, Bonow RO. Current diagnostic techniques of assessing myocardial viability in patients with hibernating and stunned myocardium. Circulation 1993; 87: 1–20

12. Gibson RS, Watson DD, Taylor GJ, Crosby IK, Wellons HL, Holt ND, Beller GA. Prospective assessment of regional myocardial perfusion before and after coronary revascularization surgery by quantitative thallium-201 scintigraphy. J Am Coll Cardiol 1983; 1: 804–15
13. Hirzel HO, Nuesch K, Gruentzig AR, Luetolf UM. Short- and long-term changes in myocardial perfusion after percutaneous transluminal coronary angioplasty assessed by thallium-201 exercise scintigraphy. Circulation 1981; 63: 1001–7
14. Powelson SW, DePeuy EG, Roubin GS, Berger HJ, King SB. Discordance of coronary angiography and 201-thallium tomography early after transluminal coronary angioplasty. Abst. J Nucl Med 1986; 27: 900
15. Bates ER, McGillem BMJ, Beals TF, DeBoe SF, Mikelson JK, Mancini GBJ, Vogel RA. Effect of angioplasty-induced endothelial denudation compared with medial injury on regional coronary blood flow. Circulation 1987; 76: 710–6
16. Gibson RS, Watson DD, Craddock GB, Crampton RS, Kaiser DL, Denny MJ, Beller GA. Prediction of cardiac events after uncomplicated myocardial infarction: a prospective study comparing predischarge exercise thallium-201 scintigraphy and coronary angiography. Circulation 1983; 68: 321–36
17. Moshiri M, Groom G, Hands M, Hung J, van der Schaaf A. Prediction of multivessel disease or clinical outcome by dipyridamole thallium early after myocardial infarction. Abst. Aust NZ J Med 1992; 22: 403
18. Eagle KA, Coley CM, Newell JB et al. Combining clinical and thallium data optimizes preoperative assessment of cardiac risk before major vascular surgery. Ann Intern Med 1989; 110: 859–66
19. Shah PK, Pichler M, Berman DS, Maddahi J, Peter T, Singh BH, Swan HJC. Non invasive identification of a high risk subset of patients with acute inferior myocardial infarction. Am J Cardiol 1980; 46: 915–21
20. Schwartz RG, McKenzie WB, Alexander J et al. Congestive heart failure and left ventricular dysfunction complicating doxorubicin therapy. Seven-year experience using serial radionuclide angiocardiography. Am J Med 1987; 82: 1109–18
21. Lee KL, Pryor DB, Pieper KS et al. Prognostic value of radionuclide angiography in medically treated patients with coronary artery disease. A comparison with clinical and catheterization variables. Circulation 1990; 82: 1705–17
22. Yoshida H, Mochizuki M, Kainouchi M et al. Clinical application of indium-111 antimyosin antibody and thallium-201 dual nuclide single photon emission computed tomography in acute myocardial infarction. Ann Nucl Med 1991; 5: 41–6

19 Positron emission tomography

Kevin C Allman and George Bautovich

Background

Left ventricular contractile dysfunction in patients with chronic coronary artery disease continues to confer a limited prognosis. This is despite advances in medical management of heart failure and the advent of cardiac transplantation.

Such cardiac dysfunction may be irreversible in the presence of widespread scarring from prior infarction. It may also be reversible when secondary to hibernating myocardium,[1,2] which shows reduced contraction related to low coronary blood flow and reduced nutrient supply. Such myocardium is viable (alive) but its function is jeopardized and its metabolism altered. Restoration of oxygen delivery and energy supply through successful coronary revascularization will normalize both processes, leading to improved regional and global function (and hopefully improved prognosis).

Since impaired systolic function increases the risks associated with revascularization procedures, diagnostic methods are required to accurately identify patients with hibernating myocardium, so they may be appropriately targeted for revascularization. Such methods should also allow those patients with irreversible dysfunction to be spared high risk revascularizations which are unlikely to result in functional improvement.

Technique and applications

Positron emission tomography (PET) imaging employs short-lived tracers of blood flow and metabolism to assess myocardial viability. The tracers most commonly used in clinical studies are shown in Table 19.1. These tracers emit high energy (511 KeV) gamma rays in opposing pairs.

These are detected in the PET tomograph (coincidence detection), resulting in high count, high resolution, attenuation-corrected images. A detailed discussion of PET imaging technology is provided by Bacharach.[3]

The most widely validated approach employed to assess viability combines resting blood flow imaging (using one of the tracers listed, such as N-13 ammonia), with metabolic imaging utilizing the glucose analogue F-18 fluorodeoxyglucose (FDG).[4] This traces the transport of glucose into the myocyte and its initial metabolism to FDG-6-phosphate. Thus FDG images in the heart reflect myocardial glucose uptake and utilization.

As part of its metabolic adaptation, hibernating tissue

Table 19.1 Positron emitting tracers in cardiac PET

Flow tracers	Half-life (minutes)	Production	Type
O-15 water	2.04	cyclotron	diffusible
N-13 ammonia	10.0	cyclotron	trapped
Rb-82 chloride	1.25	generator	cation
Cu-62 PTSM*	9.74	generator	trapped
Metabolic tracers			
F-18 fluorodeoxyglucose	110	cyclotron	glucose analogue
C-11 acetate	20	cyclotron	oxidative metabolism

* PTSM: pyruvaldehyde bis (N^4 thiosemicarbazone)

preferentially utilizes glucose, rather than free fatty acids (which are the usual myocardial energy substrate).[5] Thus, following tracer injection, hibernating myocytes accumulate FDG. Conversely, scar tissue, which is not metabolically active, does not accumulate tracer. This difference in behaviour forms the basis for the use of FDG to detect hibernating myocardium and differentiate it from scar.

Myocardial segments can be classified into three broad types according to the flow/metabolism patterns observed. These are shown in Table 19.2. In particular, hibernating myocardium will show reduced blood flow with preserved FDG uptake. This pattern is termed flow/metabolism mismatch. An example of a study demonstrating this pattern is shown in Figure 19.1.

Other potential clinical uses for PET imaging in the coronary care patient setting may come to include characterization of extent and severity of coronary artery

Table 19.2 PET flow/metabolism patterns

Segment	Flow	Metabolism (FDG)	Pattern
Normal	normal	normal	normal
Hibernating	decreased	preserved	mismatch
Scar	decreased	decreased	matched reduction

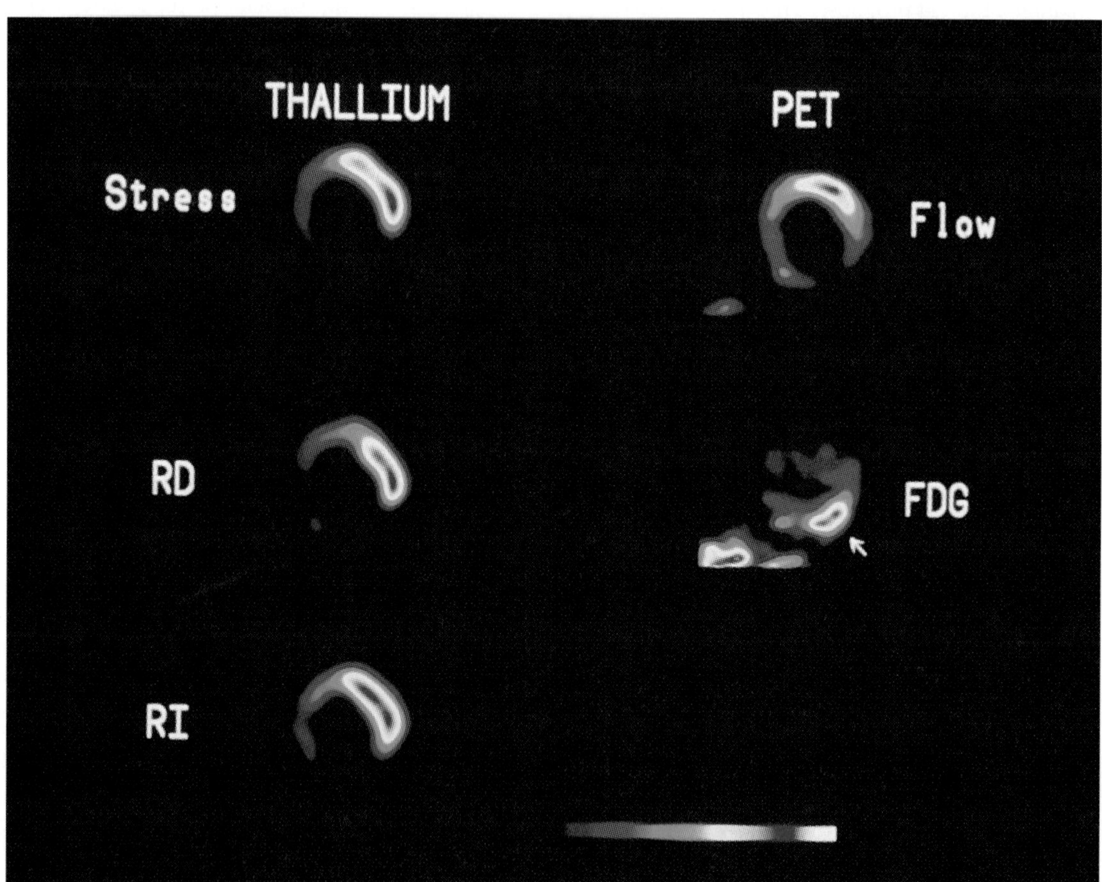

Fig. 19.1 Representative mid-ventricular short axis images from studies performed in a patient with prior MI to investigate myocardial viability. The left panel is from an initial thallium-201 study demonstrating severe reduction in tracer counts throughout anteroseptal, septal and inferior walls (3–12 o'clock) on the stress image (top left), which appears unchanged on a redistribution (RD) image performed 3 hours later (middle left) and on a subsequent rest-reinjection (RI) image (bottom left). Corresponding PET images on the right again demonstrate reduction in counts in the same regions on the N-13 ammonia resting flow image (top right). However, preserved FDG uptake is found in the inferolateral wall (arrow) on the metabolic study (lower right). This flow/metabolism mismatch indicates hibernating myocardium. (Images courtesy of Division of Nuclear Medicine, University of Michigan. Reproduced with permission.)

disease, differentiation of ischaemic from idiopathic cardiomyopathy and detection of resting ischaemia, as well as the assessment of efficacy of interventions such as thrombolysis and coronary angioplasty.

Patient studies

Patients being referred for clinical cardiac viability PET studies will have documented impairment of left ventricular global and/or regional function and be considered suitable candidates for intervention. Coronary angiography may be performed before or after the PET study depending on individual laboratory practice.

PET studies may be performed in the fasting state, with oral glucose loading, or in the case of diabetic patients, with insulin administration[6] to encourage FDG uptake into myocytes.

Quantitative research studies with flow/FDG PET may take several hours to complete. However, qualitative and semi-quantitative clinical studies, particularly in newer tomographs, can be accomplished with shorter imaging periods, which are better suited to patients with heart failure.

Diagnostic performance

Flow/FDG PET data for the prediction of reversibility of regional wall motion abnormalities have been reported from seven centres and the results have been summarized by Maddahi et al.[7] These studies demonstrate positive and negative predictive accuracies ranging from 72 to 95% and 75 to 100% respectively for changes in regional function.

Two studies have examined changes in global left ventricular function post revascularization (see Table 19.3) in patients with and without flow/metabolism mismatches.[8,9] These both demonstrated improved contractile function in patients with mismatch and unchanged function in those without mismatch.

Outcome data

Two retrospective clinical series examining one year outcome in selected patients have been reported from major centres.[10,11] These showed lower one year mortality in patients with PET mismatch who were revascularized versus those treated medically (see Table 19.4). In addition, in the study of Di Carli et al only those patients with PET mismatch who were revascularized had improvement in functional class. This study also demonstrated that the extent of mismatch in the left ventricle predicted the magnitude of improvement in left ventricular function.

Other PET approaches for viability

Several other methods for the evaluation of myocardial viability with PET have been proposed, including Rubidium-82 assessment of myocyte membrane integrity; perfusible tissue fraction of myocardium with O-15 water; and assessment of oxidative metabolism in myocardium with C-11 acetate. These approaches have not yet emerged as routine clinical studies in patients. The reader is referred to a recent review for further discussion of these methods.[12]

Conclusion

Flow/FDG PET has emerged as a clinically useful tool for the identification of hibernating

Table 19.3 PET and left ventricular function post revascularization

Author	Year	Patients	Mismatch		No mismatch	
			Pre-EF	Post-EF	Pre-EF	Post-EF
Tillisch[8]	1986	17	30±11	45±14	30±11	31±12
Besozzi[9]	1992	56	29±12	41±11	43±10	39±16

Pre = pre-revascularization; Post = post-revascularization; EF = ejection fraction

Table 19.4 Mortality in patients with PET mismatch

Author	Year	Patients	EF	Mortality	
				Intervention	No intervention
Eitzman[10]	1992	44	34	1/26	6/18
Di Carli[11]	1993	43	25	3/26	7/17

EF = ejection fraction pre-revascularization

myocardium and prediction of improvement in left ventricular function with revascularization. As such, it provides an effective tool in planning appropriate prognostic interventions in patients with advanced cardiac contractile dysfunction related to coronary artery disease.

While powerful diagnostic information is available from PET imaging, its clinical application remains limited by relative expense and reduced availability compared with other imaging modalities, such as echocardiography and single photon emission computed tomography (SPECT) nuclear imaging. However, there is little doubt that it will be more widely used for the evaluation of post-infarction and other coronary care patients in the future.

Update

Flow/FDG viability studies with SPECT imaging have recently been shown to be feasible using conventional gamma cameras with minor modifications. Early reports demonstrate diagnostic performance comparable to studies acquired in the less widely available PET tomographs.[13,14]

References

1. Braunwald E, Rutherford J. Reversible ischemic left ventricular dysfunction: evidence for the 'hibernating myocardium'. J Am Coll Cardiol 1986; 6: 1467–70
2. Rahimtoola S. The hibernating myocardium. Am Heart J 1989; 117: 211–21
3. Bacharach S. The physics of positron emission tomography. In: Bergmann S, Sobel B (eds). Positron emission tomography of the heart. Mount Kisco, New York: Futura Publishing, 1992: 13–44
4. Schelbert H. Metabolic imaging to assess myocardial viability. J Nucl Med 1994; 35: 8S–14S
5. Marshall R, Tillisch J, Phelps M et al. Identification and differentiation of resting myocardial ischemia and infarction in man with positron emission computed tomography, 18-F labelled fluorodeoxyglucose, and N-13 ammonia. Circulation 1983; 67: 766–78
6. Besozzi M, Smith G, Scott J. PET in clinical cardiology. In: Hubner K et al (eds). Clinical positron emission tomography. St Louis: Mosby-Year Book, 1992: 28–41
7. Maddahi J, Schelbert H, Brunken R, Di Carli M. Role of thallium-201 and PET imaging in evaluation of myocardial viability and management of patients with coronary artery disease and left ventricular dysfunction. J Nucl Med 1994; 35: 707–15
8. Tillisch J, Brunken R, Marshall R et al. Reversibility of cardiac wall motion abnormalities predicted by positron emission tomography. N Engl J Med 1986; 314: 884–8
9. Besozzi M, Brown M, Hubner K et al. Retrospective post-therapy evaluation of cardiac function in 208 coronary artery disease patients evaluated by positron emission tomography. Abst. J Nucl Med 1992; 33: I–199
10. Eitzman D, Al-Aouar Z, Kanter H et al. Clinical outcome of patients with advanced coronary artery disease after viability studies with positron emission tomography. J Am Coll Cardiol 1992; 20: 559–65
11. Di Carli M, Davidson M, Little R et al. Value of metabolic imaging with positron emission tomography for evaluating prognosis in patients with coronary artery disease and left ventricular dysfunction. Am J Cardiol 1994; 73: 527–33
12. Schelbert H. Merits and limitations of radionuclide approaches to viability and future developments. J Nucl Cardiol 1994; 1: S86–S96
13. Burt R, Perkins O, Oppenheim B et al. Direct comparison of fluorine-18-FDG SPECT, fluorine-18-FDG PET and rest thallium-201 SPECT for detection of myocardial viability. J Nucl Med 1995; 36(2), 176–9
14. Martin W, Delbeke D, Patton J, et al. FDG-SPECT: correlation with FDG-PET. J Nucl Med 1995; 36(6): 988–95.

20 Magnetic resonance imaging

Gregory B Cranney

Cardiovascular magnetic resonance imaging (MRI) is an evolving technology with the potential to provide comprehensive data on morphology, function, perfusion, flow and metabolism using a single imaging modality. Images are generated by laying the patient in a strong magnetic field and then applying radiofrequency pulses while at the same time modulating the localized strength of the magnetic field in three-dimensional space using rapidly changing gradient coils. The radiofrequency coil is then used to 'listen' to the radio signals being emitted by the perturbed nuclei in the body. These protocols are controlled by 'pulse sequences', which physicists can create to perform a myriad of different functions.[1,2]

By creating various pulse sequences, physicists can obtain morphology images (with different tissue characterization), create cine images to observe function, create 'tissue tags' to measure localized tissue function, measure flow vectors in three-dimensional space, measure tissue perfusion with and without the use of contrast agents, use spectroscopy to determine localized metabolic function and use blood pool sequences to obtain 3D angiograms of almost any circulation in the body.[3]

Compared to other organs, the heart presents special problems due to cardiac and in particular respiratory movement during the period of acquisition. These problems are gradually being overcome by strategies which shorten the imaging time, and will be overcome in the future by 'real time' imaging. Meanwhile, arrhythmias, such as atrial fibrillation, continue to degrade image quality on most systems.

Major absolute contraindications to MRI include ferromagnetic cerebral aneurysm clips, pacemaker or defibrillator implants and the uncommon pre-6000 series Starr–Edwards prosthetic valves, which have a metallic ball. A patient with a partially dehisced prosthetic valve should probably not be imaged. Other prosthetic valves, sternotomy wires, graft markers post coronary artery bypass surgery, and internal mammary artery staples have not presented problems. Metallic coronary care unit (CCU) chest electrodes should be replaced with non-ferromagnetic electrodes suitable for use in the MRI systems. Otherwise, MRI is a very safe imaging modality which does not use ionizing radiation and usually does not require any intravenous injections. The reader is referred to other publications for a full discussion of any potential biomedical implant hazards.[2,4]

The following is a brief summary of the major clinical issues in patients who present to a CCU, where MRI has the potential to provide useful data either in the acute or follow-up phase.

Ventricular function

MRI is an excellent technique for assessment of ventricular function. Early studies, comparing with contrast X-ray angiography, demonstrated a good correlation with global and regional left ventricular function using equivalent biplane long axis views.[5,6] End-systolic volume can be accurately obtained and this has been suggested to be a more important determinant of prognosis post MI than ejection fraction.[7] Recent 'breath-hold' techniques now permit rapid acquisition of stacked cine short axis slices from apex to base (each slice approximately 15–20 seconds). Using these data sets, three-dimensional reconstruction of regional left ventricular (LV) function is possible.

An exciting MRI approach tags myocardium in either a radial or 'cross hatched' fashion at the beginning of systole and then follows the tagged myocardium throughout the cardiac cycle. This can visualize radial and circumferential contraction of the myocardium and can distinguish subendocardial from epi-myocardial function.[8]

Acute infarct size

Infarct size is a major determinant of prognosis after MI. Ejection fraction correlates poorly with infarct size. Various MRI techniques have been used to calculate infarct size independent of regional function.[9,10] Early approaches in animals used time-consuming T2 weighted imaging techniques to visualize the infarct region. These correlated well with post mortem studies but overestimated the infarct size as the technique essentially measures oedema.[9]

Paramagnetic agents such as gadolinium diethylenetriamine penta-acetic acid (DTPA) or dysprosium DTPA magnetic susceptibility improve contrast between normal and infarcted myocardium and continue to be evaluated in both humans and animal models after MI.[11]

Detection of coronary artery disease and myocardium at risk

Post MI, the extent of myocardium at risk depends on:

- residual viable myocardium in the territory supplied by stenotic arteries
- the functional severity of the stenoses
- the function of collaterals supplied by other coronary arteries which may also be compromised.

'Stress' thallium imaging and echocardiography have been used previously and rely on creating differential flow or ischaemia in compromised zones.

As physical exercise is not practical within the confines of current MRI imaging systems, initial studies used cine MRI to detect reversible wall motion abnormalities induced by dipyridamole infusion. In 40 patients with angina and previously positive stress ECG, Pennell et al showed that the site of the wall motion abnormality was always the site of a reversible thallium defect.[12] However, the sensitivity for detection of reversible thallium defects was only 67%. More recent dipyridamole cine MRI studies[13] have found sensitivities of 73–88% for detection of angiographic 70% diameter stenoses.

Dobutamine infusions during cine MRI offer more promise. Using this approach in 25 patients, Pennell et al have improved the sensitivity for detection of angiographic significant coronary artery disease to 91% with a similar concordance with dobutamine thallium.[14]

Myocardial viability

Identification of regional myocardial viability is essential for determining the likely success of revascularization procedures post MI. Three MRI approaches have been described:

- Examining differences in signal intensity on spin echo images, with or without injection of contrast agents. This approach often overestimates infarct size during the first weeks due to surrounding oedema.[9,15]
- In chronic infarcts (greater than 16 weeks), lack of viability may be inferred but not proven by thinned asynergic myocardium.[16]
- Lastly, measurement of high energy phosphate metabolites is possible using MR spectroscopy; however, phosphorous nuclei imaging has poor spatial resolution compared to standard MR imaging with hydrogen nuclei and will probably require higher strength magnets.

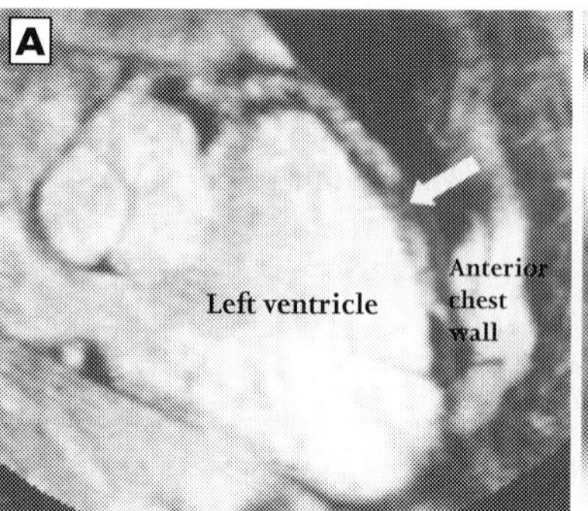

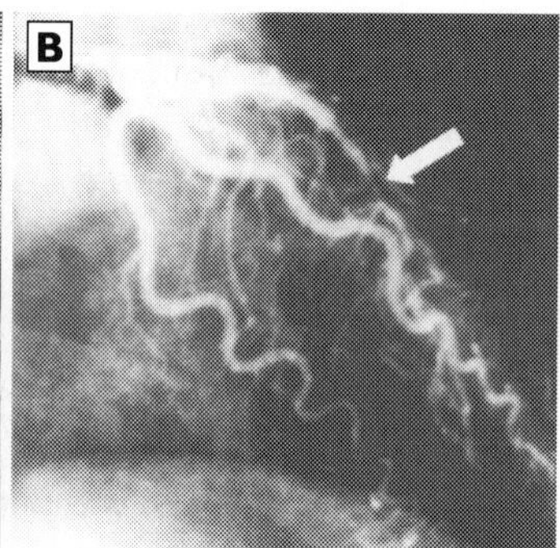

Fig. 20.1 Detection of critical coronary artery lesion in the left anterior descending coronary artery by magnetic resonance imaging (left). Confirmed on coronary angiography (right). Reproduced with permission of heart 1996; Pennell DJ, Assessment of Coronary Artery Stenosis by magnetic Resonance Imaging. Heart 1996; 75: 127–133.

Ventricular remodelling

Remodelling of the left ventricle after MI is highly variable and the mechanisms remain largely unknown. For measurement of ventricular volumes, regional wall thinning and overall shape of the left ventricle, MRI offers unsurpassed techniques for serial evaluation.

MRI 'tagging' of the myocardium uniquely permits assessment of regional wall motion, differentiation of epimyocardial and endomyocardial function, and circumferential and longitudinal myocardial shortening analysis. Kramer et al have used this approach in a post-MI animal model to detect different mechanisms of remodelling between adjacent and remote non-infarcted myocardium.[17]

Post-reperfusion myocardial haemorrhage has been postulated to play a role in remodelling after MI. Spin echo techniques have been used to detect this in an animal model.[18]

Coronary angiography

Non-invasive coronary angiography remains the 'Holy Grail' of MRI. Cardiac and respiratory motion and epicardial fat surrounding the epicardial coronary arteries have been stumbling blocks for development of a robust technique. ECG gated acquisition eliminates cardiac motion artefact in patients with regular rhythm. New techniques now permit images to be acquired during a breath-hold (approximately 18 seconds) to decrease respiratory motion artefact. Fat-suppression pulse sequences reduce the signal from epicardial fat.[19,20]

Using these methods Manning et al[19] evaluated 39 patients scheduled for elective cardiac catheterization with coronary angiography. For detecting 50% angiographic stenosis the sensitivity and specificity were: left main (100, 100%), left anterior descending (87, 92%), circumflex (71, 90%), right coronary (100, 78%) and overall (90, 92%). Total imaging times averaged less than 45 minutes. The same group has applied MRI velocity sequences to measure blood flow in the proximal left anterior descending and mid right coronary arteries and has demonstrated significant increases with adenosine infusion.[21]

Coronary artery bypass graft patency has been evaluated by cine MRI with sensitivities of 88%;[22] however, graft stenosis has not yet been properly evaluated.

Other CCU problems

Post-infarct ventricular septal defects

MRI can easily detect ventricular septal defects (VSD)[2] and may occasionally be useful either when echocardiography is not diagnostic or in detecting complications post-surgical repair.

Aortic dissection

MRI is an excellent modality for assessment of aortic dissection.[2,3] However, due to the instability of these patients, transoesophageal echocardiography currently is more practical in most units as it can be performed at the bedside and can usually resolve the main dilemma in acute dissections—determining whether the ascending aorta is involved (see Chs 8, 16, 70). In some units where logistic constraints are satisfied, short MR imaging protocols (less than 10 minutes) could be used for initial assessment. For less acute conditions and for subsequent follow-up, MRI permits better visualization of the distal ascending aorta and arch and is non-invasive. MRI may also be more useful for detecting and characterizing intramural haematomas.

Pulmonary embolism

Pulmonary MR angiography sequences are being developed which allow complete visualization of the main pulmonary arteries. Their potential role in detecting and assessing acute pulmonary embolism remains to be evaluated.

Summary

To date, MRI and in particular cardiovascular MRI has not been widely available for assessing patients in the CCU, and given the wealth of other cardiac imaging techniques there has not been a significant demand despite its apparent superiority in assessing regional ventricular function. It is of proven value in the follow-up of patients with aortic dissection and could be used for initial assessment in some units. Cardiovascular MRI techniques are rapidly evolving and coronary angiography, perfusion and tagging techniques are still in an embryonic stage. Further reductions in imaging times with 'echo-planar' approaches will make MRI cost-competitive with other imaging modalities and then MRI will start playing a more significant role in clinical practice as well as research.

References

1. Doyle M, Cranney GB, Pohost GM. Basic principles of magnetic resonance. In: Pohost GM, O'Rourke R (eds). Principles and practice of cardiovascular imaging. Boston: Little Brown, 1991
2. Blackwell GG, Cranney GB, Pohost GM (eds). MRI: cardiovascular system. New York: Gower Medical Publishing, 1992
3. Cranney GB, Lotan CS. Cardiovascular applications of magnetic resonance imaging. In: Pohost GM, O'Rourke R (eds). Principles and practice of cardiovascular imaging. Boston: Little Brown, 1991
4. Shellock FG, Morisoli S, Kanal E. MR procedures and biomedical implants, materials, and devices: 1993 update. Radiology 1993; 189: 587–99
5. Lotan CS, Cranney GB, Bouchard A, Bittner V, Pohost GM. The value of cine nuclear magnetic resonance imaging for assessment of regional ventricular function. J Am Coll Cardiol 1989; 14: 1721–9
6. Cranney GB, Lotan CS, Dean L, Baxley W, Bouchard A, Pohost GM. Left ventricular volume measurement using cardiac axis NMR imaging—validation by calibrated ventricular angiography. Circulation 1990; 82: 154–63
7. White HD, Norris RM, Brown MA, Brandt PW, Whitlock RM, Wild CJ. Left ventricular end-systolic volume as the major determinant of survival after recovery from myocardial infarction. Circulation 1987; 76: 44–51
8. Clark NR, Reichek N, Bergey P et al. Circumferential myocardial shortening in the normal human left ventricle. Assessment by magnetic resonance imaging using spatial modulation of magnetization. Circulation 1991; 84: 67–74
9. Bouchard A, Reeves RC, Cranney GB, Bishop S, Pohost GM. Assessment of myocardial infarct size using T2 weighted proton NMR imaging. Am Heart J 1989; 117: 281–9
10. Johns JA, Leavitt MB, Newell JB et al. Quantitation of acute myocardial infarct size by nuclear magnetic resonance imaging. J Am Coll Cardiol 1990; 15: 143–9
11. Yu KK, Saeed M, Wendland MF et al. Comparison of T1-enhancing and magnetic susceptibility magnetic resonance contrast agents for demarcation of the jeopardy area in experimental myocardial infarction. Invest Radiol 1993; 28: 1015–23
12. Pennell DJ, Underwood SR, Ell PJ, Swanton RH, Walker JM, Longmore DB. Dipyridamole magnetic resonance imaging: a comparison with thallium-201 emission tomography. Br Heart J 1990; 64: 362–9
13. Baer FM, Smolarz K, Jungehulsing M et al. Feasibility of high-dose dipyridamole magnetic resonance imaging for detection of coronary artery disease and comparison with coronary angiography. Am J Cardiol 1992; 69: 51–6
14. Pennell DJ, Underwood SR, Manzara CC et al. Magnetic resonance imaging during dobutamine stress in coronary artery disease. Am J Cardiol 1992; 70: 34–40
15. Baer FM, Theissen P, Schneider CA, Voth E, Schicha H, Sechtem U. Magnetic resonance tomography imaging techniques for diagnosing myocardial vitality. Herz 1994; 19: 51–64
16. Baer FM, Smolarz K, Jungehulsing M et al. Chronic myocardial infarction: assessment of morphology, function, and perfusion by gradient echo magnetic resonance imaging and ^{99m}Tc-methoxyisobutyl-isonitrile SPECT. Am Heart J 1992; 123: 636–45
17. Kramer CM, Lima JA, Reichek N et al. Regional differences in function within noninfarcted myocardium during left ventricular remodeling. Circulation 1993; 88: 1279–88
18. Lotan CS, Bouchard A, Cranney GB, Bishop SP, Pohost GM. Assessment of post-reperfusion myocardial hemorrhage using proton NMR imaging at 1.5 Tesla. Circulation 1992; 86: 1018–25
19. Manning WJ, Li W, Edelman RR. A preliminary report comparing magnetic resonance coronary angiography with conventional angiography. N Engl J Med 1993; 328: 828–32
20. Pennell DJ, Keegan J, Firmin DN, Gatehouse PD, Underwood SR, Longmore DB. Magnetic resonance imaging of coronary arteries: technique and preliminary results. Br Heart J 1993; 70: 315–26
21. Edelman RR, Manning WJ, Gervino E, Li W. Flow velocity quantification in human coronary arteries with fast, breath-hold MR angiography. J Magn Reson Imaging 1993; 3: 699–703
22. Aurigemma GP, Reichek N, Axel L, Schiebler M, Harris C, Kressel HY. Noninvasive determination of coronary artery bypass graft patency by cine magnetic resonance imaging. Circulation 1989; 80: 1595–1602

21 Coronary angiography

Phillip EG Aylward

Introduction

Coronary angiography defines the anatomy of the coronary arteries.[1,2] It enables visualization of the major coronary arteries and provides assessment of stenoses responsible for the clinical syndromes: stable angina, unstable angina and acute myocardial infarction (AMI) (see Fig. 21.1).

Coronary angiography is performed for two indications: a) uncontrolled symptoms; b) prognostic reasons when symptoms are absent or controlled. Although angiography does not give information about the physiological significance of a lesion,[3] it remains the gold standard for decisions about intervention with angioplasty or coronary bypass surgery.

Right anterior oblique

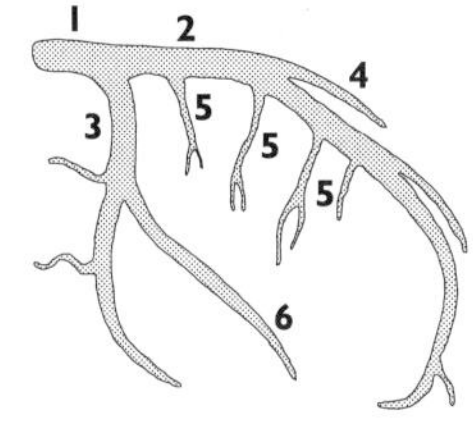

1. Left main
2. Lad
3. Circumflex
4. Diagonals
5. Septals
6. Obtuse marginals

Left anterior oblique

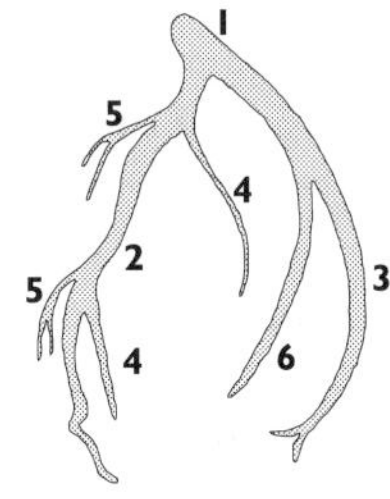

Right anterior oblique

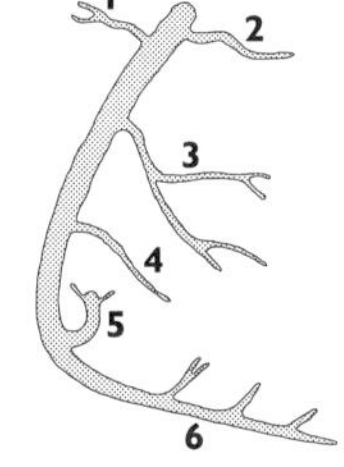

1. S.A. nodal
2. Conus
3. R.V. branch
4. Acute marginals
5. P.L.V. branch
6. P.D.A.

Left anterior oblique

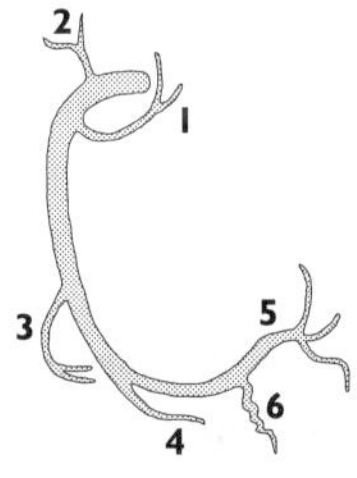

Fig. 21.1 Diagrammatic representation of coronary arteries. In the upper panel, left coronary artery and its main branches. In the lower panel, right coronary artery and its main branches.

Methodology and risks

Coronary angiography involves the passage of catheters under fluoroscopy from a peripheral arterial access point, usually the femoral or brachial artery, via the descending and ascending aorta to the coronary arteries. Contrast medium is injected into the coronary arteries, which are imaged on a cine film or by digital techniques.

The left main and right coronary arteries are selectively catheterized and several views of the left coronary and right coronary systems are obtained. The usual projections are the right anterior oblique (RAO) and left anterior oblique (LAO) (see Fig. 21.1) but often special positioning is required for optimal views of the coronary anatomy.

Since the introduction of coronary angiography there have been major improvements in all aspects of the procedures. In particular, better vascular protection by sheaths, improved catheters, new contrast media and high quality digital X-ray imaging have made the procedure easier for both patient and operator. The risks of routine angiography are now very small. Mortality is approximately 0.1%, and stroke 0.07%.[4] Of note Hildner et al[5] demonstrated that the incidence of these major complications in a 24-hour period just prior to angiography was exactly the same as on the day of angiography. This suggests that in patients with coronary vascular disease there is always a risk of these events and that the risk of the procedure itself is even lower than the above figures.

Procedure-related complications due to the catheterization do, however, occur. These relate to trauma at the vascular access site (0.5%) and minor (3%) and major (0.1%) reactions to the contrast media. In the setting of the CCU, vascular access site complications predominate.

Indications for coronary angiography in the coronary care unit

Acute myocardial infarction (AMI)

Angiography may be performed under a number of different circumstances in association with acute AMI.

Early angiography

Early angiography can be defined as angiography taking place immediate after or within a few hours of admission to hospital with AMI. It is performed as a prelude to acute percutaneous transluminal coronary angioplasty (PTCA) or to assess coronary artery patency after thrombolytic therapy.

Acute PTCA

Acute PTCA is an accepted treatment for AMI. It has been demonstrated to restore coronary patency, reduce mortality and have a low incidence of complications.[6,7,8]

Assessment of patency

The patency of the infarct-related coronary artery is an important determinant of subsequent outcome.[9] The only technique for assessing patency is coronary angiography. Non-invasive techniques are not adequate. Figure 21.2 shows serial angiograms in a patient who received thrombolysis therapy and failed to achieve early patency but late patency was documented.

Assessment of patency may be required for:

- **Clinical trials**. Early angiography to assess coronary patency is utilized in the assessment of drugs or techniques for the treatment of MI and in particular thrombolytic or adjuvant therapies. Improvement in 90-minute patency suggests the agent will improve overall outcome, although this will need to be tested in large trials to evaluate mortality and other complications such as stroke.
- **Rescue angioplasty**. If a coronary artery fails to reopen with thrombolytic therapy, particularly in patients with anterior infarction, there appears to be benefit from opening the artery late with angioplasty, so-called rescue angioplasty.[10] This is still an area of debate but may be the treatment of choice in patients with ongoing symptoms and ST elevation on their ECG 2 hours after the delivery of thrombolytic therapy (see Ch. 45).
- **Diagnostic reasons**. Early angiography may be used to make a diagnosis when the symptoms and signs of clinical investigations do not clearly delineate the problem.

Risks of early angiography

Angiography in a setting of early infarction carries small additional risks compared to routine elective angiography. The additional risk of major events including death and stroke have not been clearly delineated. They are small compared to the risk of the condition being treated. Mortality is reduced if the information gained from angiography is used to direct intervention with urgent surgery or angioplasty. Importantly, the risk of stroke with angiography is less than with thrombolytic therapy.[6]

The major problem of early angiography relates to the vascular access site and bleeding. Most of these patients are on anticoagulants and many will have received thrombolytic therapy (see below).

Late elective angiography

Late angiography is angiography performed during the hospital admission for AMI but is not part of the treatment of the initial event. Usually thrombolytic therapy and anticoagulants would have been stopped by this time.

Late angiography may be performed either in selected patients on the basis of ongoing symp-

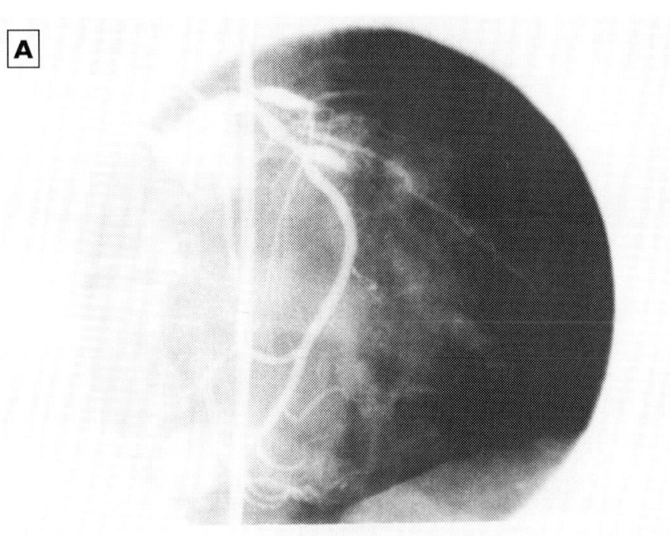

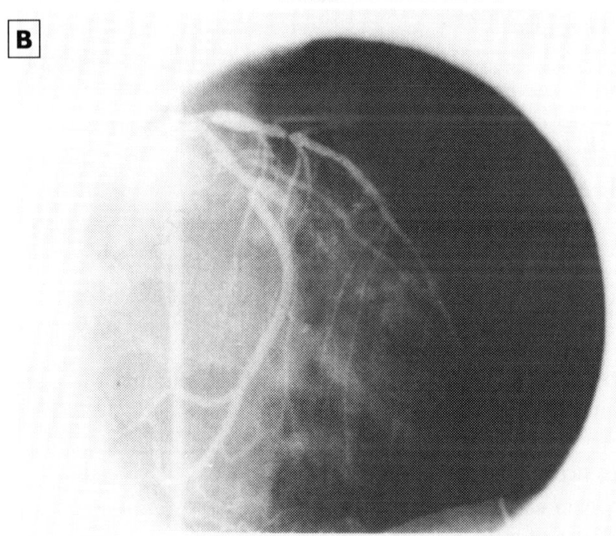

Fig. 21.2 A Coronary angiogram (right interior oblique) taken at 90 minutes after administration of a thrombolytic agent, showing total occlusion of the proximal left anterior descending (LAD) coronary artery in a patient with acute anterior myocardial infarction. B 48 hour coronary angiogram showing tight residual stenosis of the previously totally occluded LAD. In both angiograms the large obtuse marginal branch of the circumflex is totally occluded.

toms or positive exercise test, or in all patients as a routine to assess prognosis and allow risk stratification and intervention if necessary. This is a controversial area and available data would tend to support a more selective approach. Even utilizing the selective approach on the basis of symptoms, 25% of all AMI patients will undergo investigation within 6 months. However, as the presence of a patent coronary artery at discharge has now been shown to be an independent prognostic indicator,[11] there will be ongoing debate as to whether coronary patency should be routinely assessed in all patients with AMI.

Figure 21.3 shows typical angiographic findings in patients recovering from recent inferior AMI.

Urgent coronary angiography

Urgent coronary angiography is an unplanned procedure carried out at any point in the first few hours after thrombolytic therapy to the time of discharge, and is prompted by clinical events.

Haemodynamic compromise

Patients with haemodynamic compromise and in particular cardiogenic shock require rapid assessment of their coronary anatomy with a view to revascularization. Patients who develop mechanical defects such as mitral regurgitation or ventricular septal defect should, if possible, undergo angiography prior to surgical repair.

Ongoing ischaemic symptoms

Urgent angiography may also be performed in patients who show evidence of ongoing ischaemia, particularly if associated with new ECG changes.

Unstable angina

Urgent angiography

Patients admitted with rest angina who continue to have symptoms despite maximum medical therapy should undergo urgent angiography with a view to intervention.

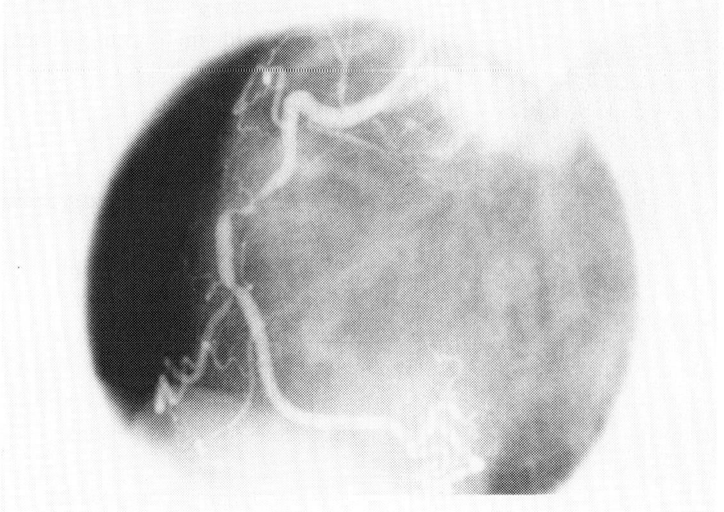

Fig. 21.3 A complex lesion strongly suggestive of thrombosis in an ulcerated atherosclerotic plaque in the right coronary artery of a patient with acute inferior MI.

Routine angiography

The role of routine angiography in patients with unstable angina is still debated. The TIMI-IIIB trial demonstrated that an early invasive policy (angiography 18–48 hours after admission) had a similar outcome to a conservative policy of angiography only for symptoms.[12] Of note, 64% of the patients treated by conservative strategy underwent angiography during the hospital admission. Either policy appears appropriate at the current time. The cost implications remain to be elucidated.

Other indications for angiography

Other indications for coronary angiography in patients in the CCU would include heart failure thought to be on an ischaemic basis or of unknown aetiology, intractable or difficult to manage arrhythmias, and other conditions which require cardiac surgery such as aortic dissection.

Special issues related to angiography in the coronary care unit

The major differences between routine elective angiography and those patients in the CCU undergoing the procedure relate to:

- the presence of full anticoagulation and/or thrombolytic therapy
- the presence of thrombus in the coronary artery
- the presence of impaired left ventricular function.

The presence of full anticoagulation and/or thrombolytic therapy results in problems with vascular access. The presence of thrombus in the coronary artery and impaired left ventricular function has implications for the choice of contrast medium.

Vascular access problems

Most of the patients undergoing angiography in the CCU will return with a sheath in situ in the femoral artery. This will include patients who have received thrombolytic therapy for AMI, patients on heparin for unstable angina and patients who have received high dose anticoagulants in the catheter laboratory for coronary procedures such as angioplasty and stent implantation.

Problems with groin bleeding and false aneurysm formation are significant in this group. The groin complications in patients who underwent angiography within 24 hours of thrombolytic therapy in the GUSTO angiography study are outlined in Table 21.1. Approximately 13% had minor bleeding, 6% had major bleeding requiring transfusion, and 1.4% required vascular repair. The incidence of bleeding and vascular repair following angioplasty and stent implantation are significantly greater than routine angiography[13] and are also shown in Table 21.1.

Sheath management

The sheath site and distal pulses must be closely observed by the nursing staff. This observation should be similar to those if the sheath is removed, viz: quarter-hourly for the first hour, half-hourly for the next 2 hours and hourly thereafter. The sheath should be sewn in, as death has been reported following a sheath falling out accidentally.

Patient comfort is a major issue, as lying flat for a prolonged period of time is often the major complaint of patients post procedures. Use of flexible sheaths may alleviate this problem but adequate analgesia and relaxants are essential.

Bleeding around the sheath is a common problem; manual pres-

Table 21.1 Number (and percentage) of patients with bleeding complications after reperfusion therapy*: results of two investigations

Severity of complication at catheterization puncture site	Streptokinase + SC Heparin (N = 442)	Streptokinase + IV heparin (N = 443)	Accelerated t-PA (N = 447)	Stent (N = 205)	Angioplasty (N = 202)
Major bleeding (transfusion)	24 (5.4)	33 (7.4)	19 (4.3)	10 (4.9)	5 (2.5)
Minor bleeding (no transfusion)	62 (14.0)	61 (13.8)	49 (11.0)		
Vascular repair	2 (0.5)	7 (1.6)	9 (2.0)	8 (3.9)	4 (2.0)

* Sources: (columns 2–4) The GUSTO Angiographic Investigators 1993;[9] (columns 5–6) Fischman DL, Leon MB, Baim DS et al, for the Stent Restenosis Study Investigators 1994.[13]

sure is required above the sheath site. If the bleeding is uncontrollable, the sheath should be removed. The clotting status may need to be returned to normal (see Ch. 34).

Sheath removal

The patient's coagulation status should be known prior to removal of the sheath. Activated clotting time (ACT) or activated partial thromboplastin time (APTT) should be measured. The ACT should have fallen to < 150 sec or the APTT to < 45 sec before removal of the sheath. Prolonged pressure will be required for at least half an hour and sometimes longer. Use of devices such as clamps and the 'Fem-Stop' (Radi Medical Systems) can be helpful.

Re-anticoagulation

In some patients there may be a need to re-anticoagulate as soon as possible, for example: stents and unstable angina with large thrombus in coronary artery. In each patient this would be an individual decision depending on the state of the groin and the clinical necessity for anticoagulation. In general, heparin can be restarted within 2 hours after sheath removal if the groin site is dry. The heparin may be restarted as an infusion alone or a small 2500 unit bolus and an infusion.

Contrast media

There have been significant developments in contrast media since coronary angiography commenced. Initially contrast medium had a high osmolality and was ionic (Diatrizoate [Urografin 76], Schering Pty Ltd) and this is still used in many centres. Non-ionic low osmolar contrast media (Iopromide [Ultravist], Schering Pty Ltd; Iohexol [Omnipaque], Sanofi–Winthrop) produce fewer allergic reactions, less nausea and depression of heart rate and contractility but have not been demonstrated to reduce major events such as stroke and death.[14] Non-ionic contrast medium costs significantly more than ionic, and debate continues as to the routine use for angiography. It is recommended that non-ionic contrast should be used in 'high risk' patients, those with ongoing ischaemic symptoms, or patients with haemodynamic compromise. It is particularly advantageous in patients with poor left ventricular function.

Recently it has been suggested that non-ionic contrast medium increases the thrombotic tendency[15] and should not be used in acute coronary syndromes in which thrombus is present in the coronary artery, for example AMI or unstable angina. Hexabrix (Ioxaglic Acid, Mallinckrodt Medical Pty Ltd), a low osmolar ionic contrast medium, is recommended as the best agent under these circumstances for coronary angiography.

The current recommendation for patients with acute coronary syndromes would therefore be to utilize Hexabrix for the coronary angiogram and a non-ionic low osmolar medium for contrast ventriculography if it is performed.

Summary

Coronary angiography is the gold standard in defining coronary anatomy as a prelude to intervention with angioplasty or cardiac surgery. It is mandatory in patients with ongoing symptoms as a guide to intervention, and is frequently used to define prognosis and allow risk stratification. It is a low risk procedure even in the setting of acute coronary syndromes, though bleeding from the vascular access site in relation to anticoagulation of thrombolytic therapy remains a major problem. The practical management of the patient undergoing coronary angiography and cardiac catheterization is discussed in Chapter 66.

References

1. Sones FM, Shirey EK. Cine coronary arteriography. Mod Concepts Cardiovasc Dis 1962; 31:735–8
2. Judkins MP. Selective coronary arteriography. I. A percutaneous transfemoral technique. Radiology 1967; 89:815–24
3. White CW, Wright CB, Doty DB et al. Does visual interpretation of the coronary arteriogram predict the physiologic importance of a coronary stenosis? N Engl J Med 1984; 310: 819–24
4. Kennedy JW. Complications associated with cardiac catheterization and angiography. Cathet Cardiovasc Diagn 1982; 8:5–11
5. Hildner FJ, Javier RP, Tolentino A, Samet P. Pseudo complications of cardiac catheterization: update. Cathet Cardiovasc Diagn 1982; 8:43–7
6. Grines CL, Brown KF, Marco J et al for the Primary Angioplasty in Myocardial Infarction study group. A comparison of immediate angioplasty with thrombolytic therapy for acute myocardial infarction. N Engl J Med 1993; 328:673–9
7. Gibbons RJ, Holmes DR, Reeder GS, Bailey KR, Hopfenspirger MR, Gersh BJ for the Mayo Coronary Care Unit and Catheterization Laboratory Groups. Immediate angioplasty compared with the administration of a thrombolytic agent followed by conservative treatment for myocardial infarction. N Engl J Med 1993; 328: 685–91
8. Zijlstra F, de Boere JM, Hoorntje JCA, Reiffers S, Reiber JHC, Suryapranata H. A comparison of immediate coronary angioplasty with intravenous streptokinase in acute myocardial infarction. N Engl J Med 1993; 328: 680–4
9. The GUSTO Angiographic Investigators. The effects of tissue plasminogen activator, streptokinase, or both on coronary artery patency, ventricular function and survival after acute myocardial infarction. N Engl J Med 1993; 329:1615–22
10. Ellis SG, Ribeiro da Silva E, Heyndrickx G et al for the RESCUE Investigators. Final results of the randomized RESCUE evaluating PTCA after failed thrombolysis for patients with anterior infarction. Abst. Circulation 1993; 88:2–106
11. White HD, Cross DB, Elliott JM, Norris RM, Yee TW. Long-term prognostic importance of patency of the infarct-related coronary artery after thrombolytic therapy for acute myocardial infarction. Circulation 1994; 89:61–7
12. The TIMI-IIIB Investigators. Effects of tissue-type plasminogen activator and a comparison of early invasive and conservative strategies in unstable angina and non-Q-Wave myocardial infarction: results of the TIMI-IIIB trial. Circulation 1994; 89:1545–56
13. Fischman DL, Leon MB, Baim DS et al for the Stent Restenosis Study Investigators. A randomized comparison of coronary-stent placement and balloon angioplasty in the treatment of coronary artery disease. N Engl J Med 1994; 331; 8: 496–501
14. Matthai WH, Kussmaul WG III, Krol J, Goin J, Schwartz JS, Hirshfeld JW. A comparison of low- with high-osmolality contrast agents in cardiac angiography. Identification of criteria for selective use. Circulation 1994; 89: 291–301
15. Esplugas E, Cequier A, Jara F et al. Risk of thrombosis during coronary angioplasty with low osmolality contrast media. Am J Cardiol 1991; 68:1020–4

22 Electrocardiographic monitoring

Wendy Bryson

History

Continuous electrocardiograph (ECG) monitoring is a key component of intensive coronary care. Technological advances, since the 1960s, have led to monitoring systems incorporating automated alarm systems, sophisticated analysis and trending of cardiac rhythm, haemodynamic monitoring parameters and a variety of accessories such as ST segment monitoring. Whilst the design, capabilities, reliability and cost of monitoring systems vary considerably, the optimal cost-benefit ratio will depend not only on the monitoring capabilities of the system but also on the type of patients to be monitored, staff-patient ratio and data storage requirements. However, the fundamental components of any cardiac monitoring system are simply to allow observation of the heart's electrical activity and identification of arrhythmic disturbances as they occur.

Detection of cardiac electrical activity

Monitoring electrodes placed on the skin surface of the chest will record atrial electrical activity, conduction system delay and ventricular electrical activity, corresponding to the P wave, PR interval and QRS complex respectively (see Figs 22.1 and 22.2).

Terminology

The standard terminology for the electrocardiographic waves and intervals is summarized in Figure 22.3. In the absence of normal atrial activity, P waves will be absent, and replaced by fibrillation or flutter waves.

Monitoring equipment

ECG paper

The waveforms produced during the cardiac cycle are recorded on standardized graph paper. Each of the lighter small squares (1 mm × 1 mm) represents 0.04 seconds in time and 0.1 mv in amplitude. The darker larger square (5 mm × 5 mm), composed of five smaller squares, represents 0.2 seconds in time and 0.5 mv in amplitude (see Fig. 22.4). Across the top of the paper various markings indicate measures of time at 1- and 3-second intervals.

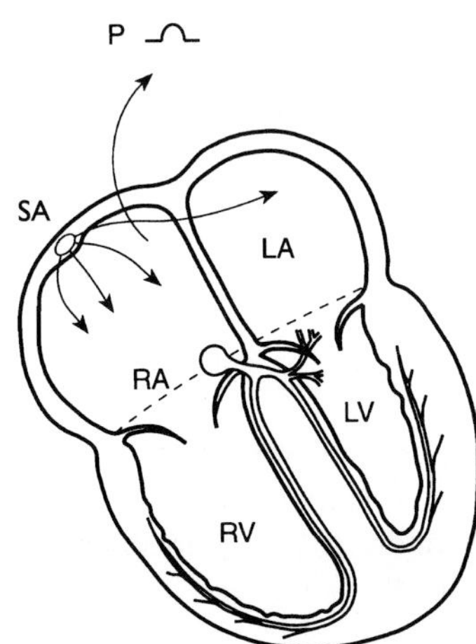

Fig. 22.1 Atrial depolarizations originating in the sino-atrial node (SA). Represented on the surface ECG by the P wave.

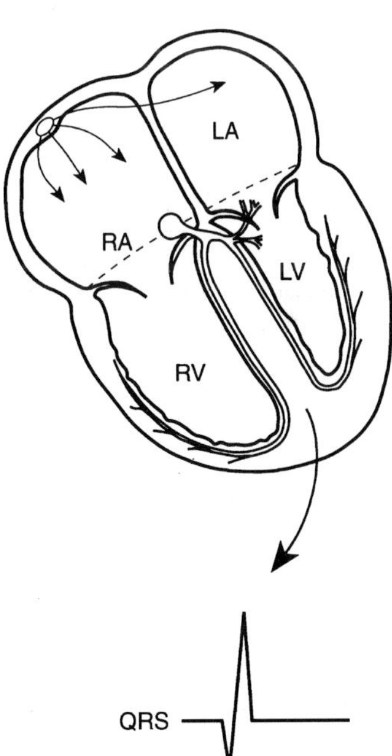

Fig. 22.2 Ventricular depolarization originating at the atrioventricular node, (AV), spreading through the specialized conduction tissue in the septum (His bundle, right, and bundle branches, left) and into the ventricular myocardium, via the Purkinje fibres. Represented on the surface ECG by the QRS complex.

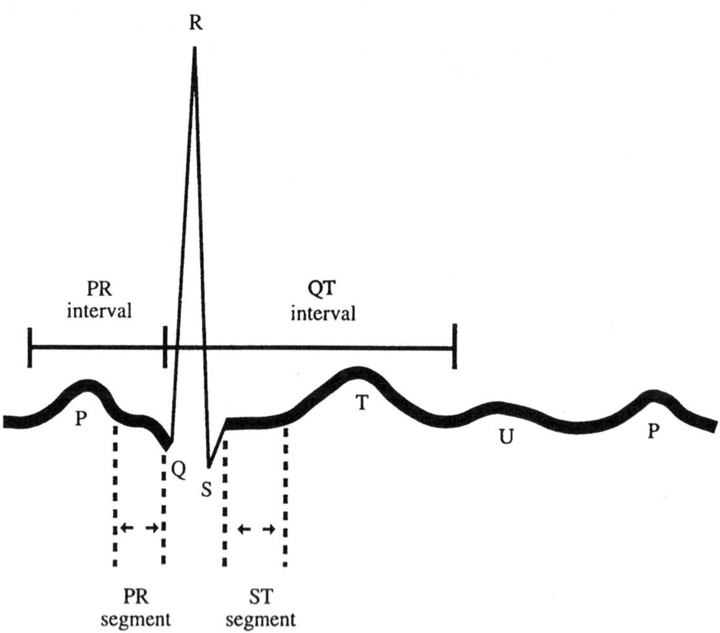

Fig. 22.3 A typical ECG representing a single cardiac cycle. Note the difference between the PR interval (from the beginning of the P wave to the beginning of the QRS) and the PR segment (from the end of the P wave to the beginning of the QRS). The QT interval is measured from the beginning of the QRS to the end of the T wave, and does not include the U wave.

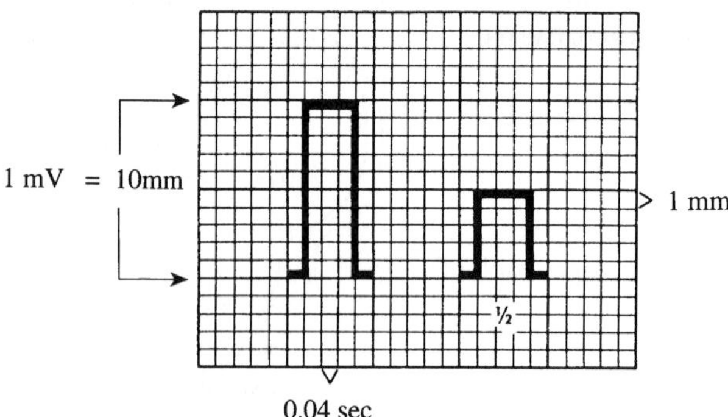

Fig. 22.4 Standardized ECG paper 10 mm = 1 mv amplitude and 25 mm/sec paper speed. These intervals will be inaccurate if the ECG recording is not standardized (e.g. double or half voltage) or the paper speed is slower (2.5 or 10 mm/sec) or faster (50 or 100 mm/sec) or if the machine is faulty.

The height or depth of a wave is measured from the isoelectric line (flat) representing a period of electrical quiet, usually just before the onset of the P wave.

12-lead ECGs usually display a standardized calibration of 1 mv being equal to 10 mm, or two large vertical squares. However it is important to realize that ECG monitoring systems are often not precisely standardized, and the complexes being recorded may be determined by the electrical positions which best display the cardiac rhythm.

Electrodes

Disposable electrodes generally consist of a disc area of conductive gel surrounded by adhesive material. The gel improves contact between the skin and the electrode and serves to reduce the electrical resistance from the skin surface, thereby improving conductivity and the quality of the cardiac electrical activity received via the electrode.

The clarity of the waveforms displayed on the monitor screen will be compromised and accurate arrhythmia analysis virtually impossible (despite sophisticated monitoring equipment) unless the signals are able to be detected clearly. For this reason the application of monitoring electrodes is of fundamental importance in obtaining clear and accurate waveforms when monitoring to detect cardiac arrhythmias.

Disposable adhesive type electrodes are manufactured in many sizes, shapes and colours. They are comfortable, easy to apply and relatively inexpensive. With more than 50 different disposable electrodes currently available, it is a worthwhile exercise to select and trial electrodes suitable for the monitoring situation in which they are to be used, i.e. short-term coronary care unit (CCU) monitoring or longer-term ambulatory telemetry monitoring. Whilst cost is a consideration, adherence, sensitivity and conductivity are of primary importance in selection. The convenience of a skin abrasive on the peel-off backing facilitates the prompt and effective application of electrodes. Specialized hypoallergenic electrodes provide an alternative for those patients who develop a skin irritation, usually to the adhesive component. Diaphoretic electrodes are available if adhesion to skin proves difficult.

Application of electrodes

Unless excellent contact is established between the skin and the monitoring electrode, the resulting waveforms will be distorted and interpretation difficult. When determining the location for electrode placement, avoid any skin abrasions, or areas of muscle mass. Ensure the chest lead positions are available for 12-lead ECG recordings and paddle positioning for emergency defibrillation.

Skin preparation

- If necessary hair is clipped from area approximately 7 cm around the proposed electrode location.
- Mild abrasion of the skin will decrease impedance between the skin and electrode, thereby reducing interference. Abrasion can be performed using the abrasive material on the backing of some electrodes or by using a dry gauze square.
- Moist skin should be dried to ensure adequate adhesion of the electrode. Application of tincture of benzoine to skin in contact with adhesive (tincture should be allowed to dry) prior to electrode application may promote adherence (or utilization of specialized diaphoretic electrode may be preferable).

Electrode preparation

- Use-by date should be checked on the electrode packet (the conductive gel can dry out).
- Snap-on leads are attached to the electrode, prior to attaching the electrode to the skin surface.
- Electrode backing is removed, exposing conductive gel disc.
- Electrode is attached to the prepared skin surface by applying firm pressure to the adhesive area surrounding the gel (pressure to the gel disc may result in a decrease in electrode conductivity and adherence).

Electrode care

- Staff should ensure monitoring leads are of adequate length and connections within the lead cable are supported, to prevent weight pulling on the electrodes.
- Clothing which rubs against or restricts access to the electrodes is removed, e.g. bra, singlet.
- It is recommended that electrodes are replaced 24 hours after initial application, to check for skin irritation and if necessary change to hypoallergenic electrodes.
- Electrodes are replaced as necessary to maintain optimal waveform (drying out of electrode gel will impair conductivity).

Leads

Technological advances now offer the opportunity to use either a 3- or 5-lead monitoring system. The 5-lead system provides the benefit of observing more than one lead simultaneously; this can be of significant value in arrhythmia analysis, providing an alternative view of the waveform.

Various colour coding exists to differentiate leads and facilitate rapid connection to the patient. The usual positions for the chest electrodes are shown in Fig 22.5 and are as follows:

- right arm – below right clavicle
- left arm – below left clavicle
- right leg – right rib margin
- left leg – left rib margin
- V1 or modified chest lead – right parasternal area in 4th interspace.

Each lead connects into a cable which transmits the electrical impulses to the monitor where they are displayed as waveforms.

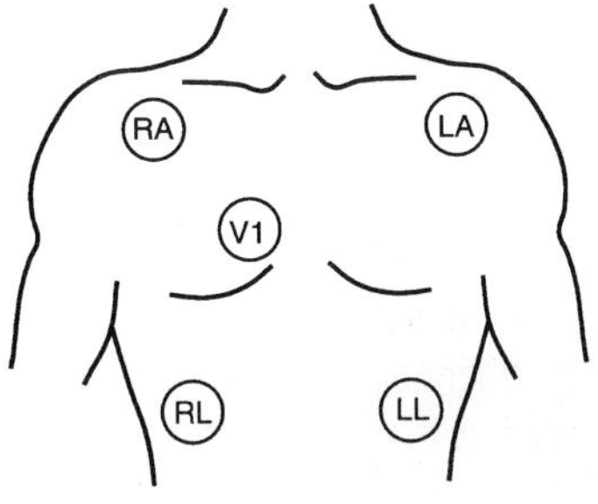

Fig. 22.5 5-lead system for continuous ECG monitoring. This system allows simultaneous dual channel recording or choice of leads approximately equivalent to leads I, II, III, AVR, AVL, AVF or V.

Monitoring lead positions

When monitoring for cardiac arrhythmias or changes in cardiac electrical axis, it is necessary to select a monitoring lead which will show clearly defined atrial activity and ventricular activity. The R wave configuration should be at least double the amplitude of the T wave, in order for the heart rate to be accurately displayed and computer rhythm analysis correct.

Standard ECG leads I, II, III, or MCLI (modified chest lead) similar to lead V, are commonly used for monitoring (see Fig. 22.6), with the availability of AVR, AVL, or AVF when using a 5-lead system. Once in place, switching between leads requires a simple monitor adjustment (or lead placement change, depending on the monitoring system).[2]

Monitoring in Lead II is often preferred, as it provides upright, positive waveforms with good P wave visualization. Lead II is used for analysis of atrial arrhythmias, differentiation of atrial and junctional arrhythmias, atrioventricular (AV) blocks, atrial pacing and inferior T wave changes.

Monitoring in lead MCLI is used for differentiation between ventricular and supraventricular arrhythmias, left from right ventricular ectopy, identification of bundle branch blocks,[2] atrial flutter waves and anterior T wave changes.

The ability to display two different leads simultaneously provides the benefit of two views of the rhythm for analysis.

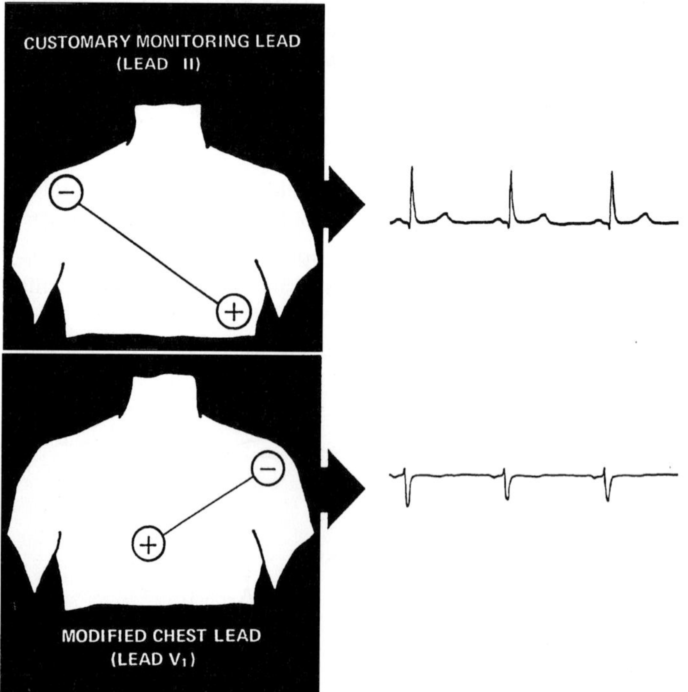

Fig. 22.6 Standard monitoring positions with wave forms. Adapted from Meltzer LE, Pinneo R, Kitchell JR (eds). Intensive coronary care: a manual for nurses. 4th ed. London: Prentice-Hall, 1983: 121.

Computerized arrhythmia analysis

Monitoring systems which detect, analyse, record and trend heart rate and rhythm are utilized to provide current information and accurate arrhythmia analysis. This information may provide a timely warning (e.g. ventricular tachycardia, missed beats), enabling preventive treatment to be initiated as appropriate.[3]

The computer programme is designed to recognize each R wave; analysis of waveforms then occurs by comparison with predetermined rhythm templates. Having analysed a rhythm the computer then classifies any waveform changes in accordance with pre-set arrythmia templates. This analysis, together with heart rate, may then be displayed as specific patient data on the monitor screen. Trending of this information occurs and it is stored to provide an accessible, ongoing record of monitoring data for each patient. The arrhythmia programme provides a visual and audible alarm system which can be adjusted to accommodate many rhythm disturbances. Programming of the system incorporates setting alarm parameters for each arrhythmia. When these limits are surpassed the respective alarm is activated and a rhythm strip recorded, with a record of the alarm stored as individual data.

Documentation

A direct print-out of the heart rhythm as seen on the monitor can be automatically generated as a result of an alarm state, or obtained manually, via the monitor printer. Rhythm strips generated automatically are usually of ten seconds' duration, whilst manually initiated strips can be of an individually determined length. The ability to generate rhythm strips from both the central station and the bedside provides immediate access to observed rhythm changes (in print). This documentation permits precise identification of arrhythmias and enables comparison with previously generated rhythm strips. Mounting of monitoring rhythm strips in chronological order provides a useful reference and ongoing arrhythmia record.[4–7]

Rhythm strips generated from a computerized system will usually be preceded by a 1 mv calibration indicator, seen as a deflection on the vertical axis at the commencement of the strip. This provides visual represention of the voltage scale, or height of waveforms; the height of the deflection indicator is automatically adjusted according to the waveform voltage. Other data, displayed on the top of the rhythm strip may include date, time of recording, patient or bed identification, heart rate, alarm activated (if appropriate) and monitored haemodynamic pressures (Fig. 22.7).

The monitoring lead should be documented on the rhythm strip and any change in lead accompanied by an appropriate rhythm strip.

Procedurally-induced arrhythmias, for example testing threshold of a temporary pacing wire, should be documented with appropriate rhythm strip. This avoids unexplained arrhythmias being found when reviewing a patient's alarm history.

Alarms

Staff should always check to ensure alarms are turned on.[5–7]

Pre-set default alarm limits are commonly programmed into modern monitoring systems, providing suggested alarm parameters, i.e. high rate set at 120 and low rate at 50, within which a particular patient's heart rate may, or may not, be confined. The continual sounding of alarms, despite reassurance that it is only a false alarm, may initiate unnecessary patient anxiety. Alarm parameters should therefore be adjusted according to the individual patient's prevailing heart rate, for example low rate alarm 30 and high rate alarm 80, if patient's prevailing heart rate is 40 beats per minute.

Audible and visual alarms should be validated as they occur, enabling the alarm to be reset and the ongoing analysis of lesser ranked alarms (programmed ranking) to continue. The computer programme has the provision to override an existing alarm, should any alarm condition of a higher ranking be detected. To ensure accurate arrhythmia detection, monitoring alarms should be reset as they occur, regardless of the alarm significance.

Pre-programmed rhythm analysis alarms may also need to be adjusted according to the patient's heart rhythm, for example by turning alarms off for ventricular premature beats > 5 per minute and for ventricular trigeminy, if this is not going to lead to any change in management. Other adjustments may include altering the size of the waveform, changing the monitoring lead, or reapplication of electrodes (see Fig. 22.8). Reviewing of individual monitor alarms should occur on a regular basis in order to ensure alarm parameters are changed to reflect changes in patient condition.

09 FEB 95 2035 MCL1 HR 55 VPB 0 ABP 124/58 (81) SPO2 98

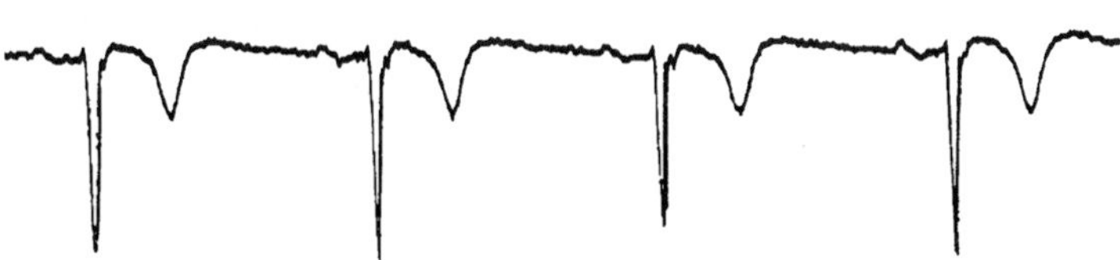

Fig. 22.7 Example of ECG recording from automated analysis systems, detailing date, time, lead, heart rate, arrhythmia, blood pressure, systolic and diastolic (and mean) blood pressure and oxygen saturation.

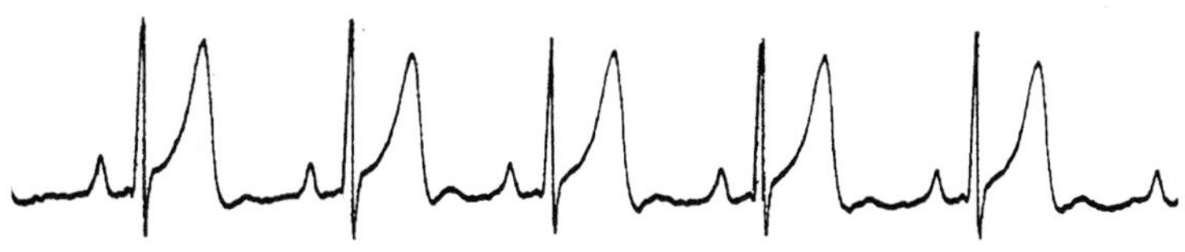

Fig. 22.8 ECG monitoring lead with tall T waves capable of generating an alarm for high heart rates by doubling the beats recorded.

Artefact/interference

Electrical artefact can produce extraneous waveform deflections. Inadequate electrode contact with the skin surface is the most frequent source of poor quality monitoring waveforms, resulting in artefact.[4–7] Causes of intermittent poor quality waveforms may include:

- muscle tremor
- patient movement
- damaged lead or cable
- equipment causing electrical interference.[1]

During muscle activity such as teeth cleaning, shivering, tremor or movement, electrical potentials are picked up by the electrodes and recorded as waveform irregularities and/or a grossly uneven base line (Fig. 22.9A). Direct contact with the monitoring electrode such as scratching may result in similiar waveform irregularities; however, continuation of the QRS complex throughout the bizarre pattern confirms that this is due to artefact and not ventricular tachycardia (VT) or ventricular fibrillation (VF) (see Fig. 22.9B).

Wandering of the waveforms up and down the monitor screen makes arrhythmia analysis difficult. This is usually transient as result of patient movement, or a cyclic pattern as a result of respiratory inspiration and expiration (see Fig. 22.9C). Electrodes should be moved away from the lower ribs to minimize the effect of chest wall movement on the waveform pattern.

Electrical currents from other electronic equipment, faulty grounding of equipment, loose connections or fractured monitoring leads may create interference with the monitor signal. Electrical interference from alternating current mains supply distorts the baseline and the baseline appears wide, making rhythm analysis difficult. This occurs as a result of regular deflections at the same amplitude as the alternating current (50–60 cycles per second) (see Fig. 22.9D).

Telemetry

Conventional monitoring systems connect the patient leads to the monitor via a cable. This significantly restricts the mobility, independence and environment of the patient. Telemetry monitoring eliminates the need for a monitor cable, by connection of

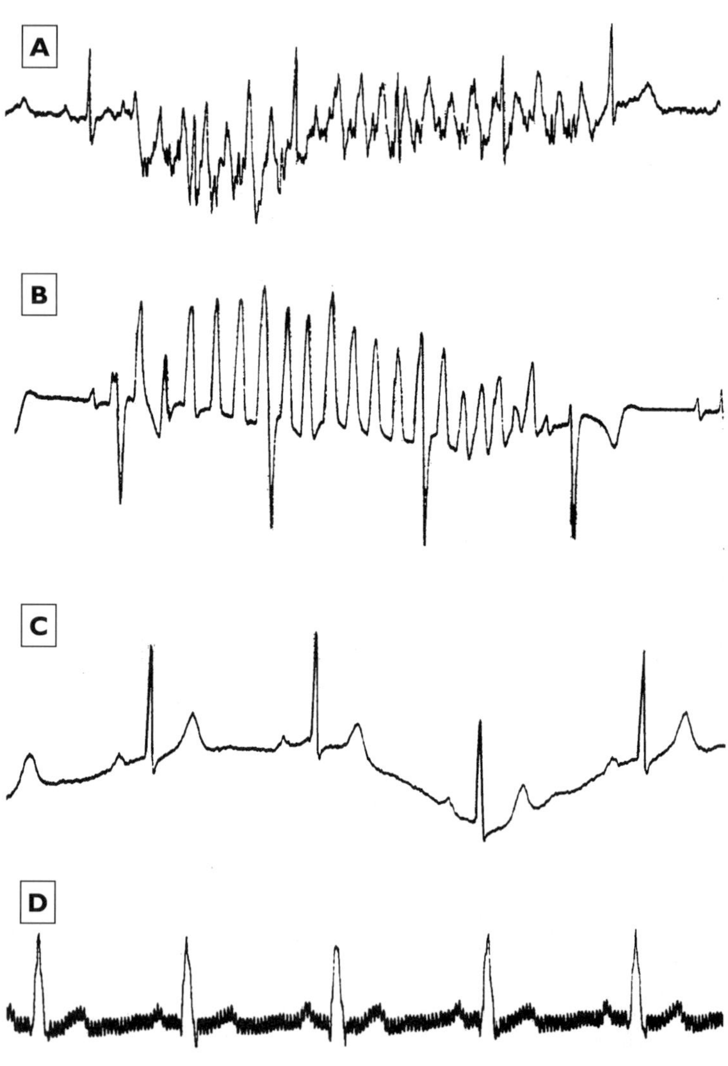

Fig. 22.9 Examples of ECG artefact recorded on monitoring: A Muscle tremor—the appearance of apparent ventricular tachycardia is due to the patient cleaning their teeth; B lead artefact—the patient was scratching near the electrode. In both A and B, the QRS complexes can be discerned at the same rate throughout the period of artefact C Wandering baseline due to poorly applied electrode. Note in the third complex the potential for misinterpretation of ST segment shift. D Alternating current (AC) interference at 60 cycles per second.

the leads to a small battery-operated radio transmitter.[7] The patient carries the transmitter (often waterproof) in a pocket or attached to them. The transmitter sends the electrical signals by radio frequency to a receiver, which then sends the signals into the monitoring system. Depending on the capabilities of the system and location of receivers, telemetry monitoring may occur on another floor or ward and while activities such as showering or exercising are being undertaken. This form of monitoring provides clear advantages for patients and allows greater accessibility to monitored beds within the CCU.

ST segment monitoring

Recent advances in technology have resulted in specialized monitoring equipment able to provide detailed analysis of ST segment waveforms in various monitoring leads. Deviations above and below the isoelectric line can be plotted providing an ST level for each lead using 12-lead monitoring systems.[8] The ST level for specific lead combinations is then averaged and trended. These ST segment trends can be valuable for monitoring a patient who is receiving thrombolytic therapy or has had mechanical reperfusion, and may allow early intervention in a patient at risk of re-occlusion (see Fig. 22.10).

References

1. Thaler M. The only EKG book you'll ever need. Philadelphia: Lippincott, 1988
2. Meltzer LE, Pinneo R, Kitchell JR (eds). Intensive coronary care: a manual for nurses. 4th edition. London: Prentice-Hall International, 1983: 121
3. Flynn J, Bruce N. Introduction to critical care skills. St Louis: Mosby Year Book, 1993
4. Dossey B, Guzzetta C, Kenner C. Essentials of critical care nursing: body—mind—spirit. Philadelphia: Lippincott, 1990
5. Casey P. Cardiac rhythms. In: Vazquez M, Lazear S, Larsen E. Critical care nursing. 2nd ed. Philadelphia: Saunders, 1992
6. Rainbow C. Monitoring the critically ill patient. Oxford: Heinemann Nursing, 1989
7. Nygaard T, Di Marco J. Cardiac monitoring. In: Shoemaker W, Abraham E (eds). Diagnostic methods in critical care: automated data collection and interpretation. New York: Marcel Dekker, 1987
8. Krucoff M, Croll M, Pope J et al. Continuously updated 12-lead ST segment recovery analysis for myocardial infarction artery patency and its correlation with multiple simultaneous early angiographic observations. Am J Cardiol 1993; 71: 145–51

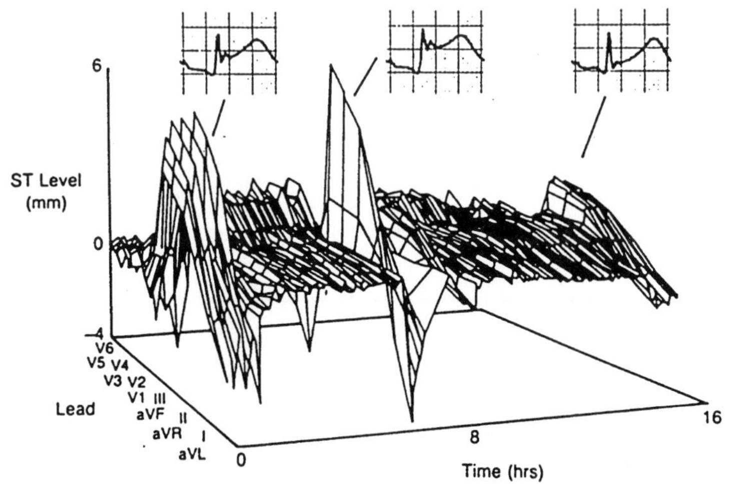

Fig. 22.10 Complete analysis of time-trends in ST segment deviation using continuous 12-lead ECG monitoring. Reproduced with permission Krucoff et al and the American Journal of Cardiology.[8]

23 Electrophysiology testing

David AB Richards, John B Uther and David Ross

Introduction

Philosophy of risk assessment

Following acute myocardial infarction (AMI), there is a significant risk of late mortality which cannot be adequately predicted by premonitory symptoms or clinical examination at follow-up. One approach to management after AMI is to institute prophylactic treatment in all patients, based on the results of large, well-conducted randomized controlled clinical trials. The other approach is to investigate individual patients in an attempt to define the risk of sudden death, and to institute some preventive therapy only in those at risk.

Implicit in the latter approach is the principle that the identified mortality risk relates to a particular complication for which there is effective treatment. Because of the reduced numbers of patients requiring such treatment, more costly therapies than those used for the whole population may be instituted in those at risk, within the same overall expenditure. A major advantage of the latter approach is that those at low risk for sudden unexpected death are greatly reassured and do not undergo unnecessary treatment, particularly when the treatments may be associated with troublesome or dangerous side-effects. Since the risk of sudden death may be multifactorial, the best overall result will be achieved by using whichever approach is most effective for each modifiable risk factor.

Pathogenesis of sudden death after myocardial infarction

Mortality following discharge from hospital after AMI is greatest in the first year. Most deaths are sudden, and most sudden deaths during the first year are due to spontaneous ventricular tachycardia or fibrillation. Asystole, bradycardia or electromechanical dissociation account for only about 15% of events.

Ventricular tachycardia and fibrillation may be due to ventricular electrical instability, where patchy scar at the border of the infarct forms a re-entrant circuit. Ventricular tachyarrhythmias may also occur secondary to further myocardial ischaemia or infarction, electrolyte disturbances, or acute heart failure with ventricular distension. Re-entrant ventricular tachycardia in patchy scar is probably the most common mechanism for sudden death after MI.

Evolution of electrocardiographic changes of AMI are seen in less than 15% of survivors of out-of-hospital cardiac arrest, even though coronary artery disease with prior MI is the commonest underlying heart disease in these patients. Cardiac arrest survivors with a history of prior AMI, but who do not have electrocardiographic changes of further acute infarction, usually have inducible monomorphic ventricular tachycardia at programmed electrical stimulation of the ventricles (electrophysiological study). Cardiac arrest and spontaneous episodes of ventricular tachycardia tend to recur in these patients.

Patients who have inducible ventricular tachycardia at electrophysiological study after MI[1–5] and/or delayed potentials due to slow conduction at the edge of the infarct[4–8] are much more likely to experience spontaneous ventricular tachycardia and sudden death than are those without inducible ventricular tachycardia and without delayed potentials.

Left ventricular (LV) hypertrophy is another important risk factor for sudden death. An increase in echocardiographic LV posterior wall thickness of 1 mm increases the risk of sudden death about sevenfold, independent of the degree of coronary disease present or whether or not coronary bypass grafting has been performed.[9] The pathogenetic mechanism is unclear.

Physiological regulatory systems in the peripheral circulation may exacerbate the effects of cardiac pathology and contribute to the suddenness of clinical events. Autoregulation in peripheral vascular beds (splanchnic, renal, skeletal muscle) normally allows local blood flow to be matched to local metabolic requirements. However, cardiac dysfunction which causes central arterial hypotension results in autoregulatory dilatation in all vascular beds simultaneously, thereby exacerbating hypotension. The hypotension may in turn worsen cardiac function if coronary blood flow is significantly reduced, creating a vicious cycle. Superimposed on this is the normal arterial baroreflex response to hypotension, which is generalized peripheral vasoconstriction, to elevate arterial pressure towards normal. Thus, factors such as initial ventricular function and baroreflex sensitivity become major determinants of the final outcome of the event.

Current therapeutic approaches to ventricular electrical instability

Routine empiric prophylactic use of Vaughan-Williams Class I antiarrhythmic drugs is no longer justifiable since the Cardiac Arrhythmia Suppression Trial (CAST) study,[10] and meta-analyses of other published trials, have shown that the incidence of sudden death is increased by these drugs.

Randomized clinical trials after AMI of beta blocking drugs without intrinsic sympathomimetic activity have shown a 20–30% reduction in overall mortality and risk of sudden death. In contrast to Vaughan-Williams Class I drugs, proarrhythmic effects of beta blocking drugs are rarely demonstrable in the laboratory at electrophysiological study. Antiarrhythmic effects at electrophysiological study of beta blocking drugs do not correlate well with, and cannot be used to predict, subsequent arrhythmia recurrence or sudden death.

Beta blocking drugs have long been widely recommended for prophylaxis after AMI. However, the prevalence of beta blocking drug therapy in patients with a history of prior infarction entering multicentre post-infarction clinical trials is only about 10%, suggesting that side-effects may limit their use in practice. Amiodarone reduces the recurrence rate and mortality following clinical episodes of spontaneous ventricular tachyarrhythmia. However, side-effects lead to withdrawal of therapy in up to 80% of patients within 2 years.

Electrical mapping of ventricular electrical activation and surgical, laser or cryoablation of re-entrant circuits in scarred myocardium in patients with clinical episodes of ventricular arrhythmia carries a 10–15% operative mortality, and has not been reliably curative. Radiofrequency catheter ablation of re-entrant circuits has a lower morbidity and mortality than surgery, but is presently not reliably curative.

Automatic implantable cardioverter defibrillators (AICDs) have gained increasing acceptance for patients surviving episodes of ventricular tachycardia or fibrillation. The size of AICDs has halved since their introduction. With transvenous electrode systems and better control logic, mortality at implantation has reduced to 0.4%[11,12] with approximately 90% overall survival to one year.[12] Randomized controlled clinical trials of these devices for managing recurrent ventricular tachyarrhythmias are in progress. Health economics estimates suggest that although AICDs are more costly, they are more effective than amiodarone therapy for such patients.[13]

In terms of dollar cost per Quality Adjusted Life-Year gained, AICD implantation for post-infarction ventricular tachyarrhythmias may be more cost-effective than primary prevention of heart attack with cholesterol lowering agents in hyperlipoproteinaemic patients.[14] The 1- and 2-year survival rates following successful implantation of AICDs for recurrent ventricular tachycardia are 89% and 84% respectively, whereas the 1- and 2-year survival rates for infarct survivors with ejection fraction <0.40 and inducible monomorphic ventricular tachycardia are only 70% and 54% respectively.[15]

There have so far been no randomized controlled clinical trials of surgery, catheter ablation, or AICDs in patients with inducible, but not spontaneous, ventricular tachycardia after AMI.

Assessment of risk of sudden death after myocardial infarction

Ideal investigations would test for the existence of potential intraventricular re-entrant circuits, determine whether sustained ventricular tachycardia could be induced, and would assess autonomic factors which might facilitate the late occurrence of ventricular tachycardia.

Since patients with low ejection fraction due to extensive AMI are more likely to die than are patients with normal or near normal left ventricular function,[16] testing for inducible ventricular tachycardia may be more cost-effective when restricted to those patients with extensive myocardial scar and low ejection fraction.[17,18] Tests which are surrogate markers for myocardial damage, such as ejection fraction, high grade ventricular ectopy and reduced heart rate variability, might not be expected to be as valuable for identifying patients prone to spontaneous ventricular tachycardia, as a test specifically designed to detect whether the heart can sustain ventricular tachycardia (electrophysiological study).

Prior to the widespread use of revascularization by angioplasty and surgery, the presence of significant ST segment displacement during exercise was a good predictor for subsequent myocardial ischaemia and death due to fresh ischaemia.[19] However, nowadays the majority of patients with ongoing ischaemia after AMI are detected and revascularized early, so that exercise testing is now a less effective predictor of late mortality.

Individual predictors of risk

Electrophysiological testing

Patients with inducible ventricular tachycardia at formal electrophysiological study have a relative risk of spontaneous ventricular tachycardia 15 times greater than that of patients without inducible ventricular tachycardia.[17] Electrophysiological study utilizing programmed stimulation is the single best test to stratify patients into high and low risk for subsequent spontaneous ventricular tachycardia and sudden death.[17] Those studies which have failed to reproduce these observations have generally employed inadequate stimulation protocols in insufficient patients and did not record enough end points to detect a difference in survival between those with and without inducible ventricular tachycardia.[20]

Patients with inducible ventricular tachycardia 1 week after MI, but hitherto no spontaneous ventricular tachycardia, have essentially the same chance of experiencing spontaneous ventricular tachycardia within the next year as have patients with a history of spontaneous ventricular tachycardia in the context of chronic MI.

Electrophysiological testing is relatively simple and quick to perform. A temporary pacing wire is passed to the right ventricular apex, and comprehensive assessment by programmed stimulation can be completed within about an hour. The major disadvantage is that ventricular fibrillation may sometimes be induced in patients who are not prone to spontaneous ventricular tachycardia.[17,21]

Signal averaging

Low amplitude delayed potentials due to slow conduction through patchy scar at the edge of infarction are often associated with circuits which may sustain spontaneous re-entrant ventricular tachycardia.[4–8,22] However, delayed potentials in some patients may represent slow conduction in dead ends which do not form parts of re-entrant circuits. In other patients, slow conduction may not be present in sinus rhythm, and may only become evident following right ventricular pacing. The orthogonal vector cardiographic lead systems commonly employed for signal averaging fail to detect some electrical information, particularly relating to the inferior wall of the left ventricle. Multilead systems should increase the sensitivity of signal averaging to detect delayed potentials.

Holter monitoring

The presence of high grade ventricular ectopy is associated with an increased risk for sudden death due to ventricular tachycardia.[23] Unfortunately, some drugs (for example, flecainide) which suppress ventricular ectopic beats, increase rather than decrease the risk of sudden death after infarction.[10] Suppression of ectopic beats does not therefore equate with an improved prognosis.

Heart rate variability

Although decreased heart rate[24] is associated with significant myocardial damage and indicates an increased subsequent risk for cardiac death, it is not useful for modulating therapy to reduce the risk of death after MI.

Exercise testing

Patients with ST segment displacement during exercise often have significant reversible myocardial ischaemia. Nowadays, exercise testing is utilized as part of post-AMI assessment, to direct early revascularization, which if effective reduces subsequent cardiac morbidity and mortality due to further ischaemia. Thus, although exercise testing is useful in directing revascularization, it is no longer a good indicator for subsequent cardiac death.

Left ventricular ejection fraction

Low ejection fraction not only is an indicator of poor ventricular systolic function, but also is a non-specific indicator for predisposition to ventricular tachycardia.[16] This is because patients with extensive AMI are more likely to have viable muscle fibres interspersed with patchy scar which form re-entrant circuits which can sustain ventricular tachycardia.[22]

Comparison of electrophysiological study and other investigations after myocardial infarction

Before routine thrombolysis

During the period from 1985 to 1987, a single cohort of survivors of AMI was studied[17] in order to compare the relative values of inducible ventricular tachycardia, delayed ventricular activation (late potentials), low left ventricular ejection fraction, high grade ventricular ectopy, and ST segment displacement on exercise as predictors of electrical events (witnessed instantaneous death and spontaneous ventricular tachycardia or ventricular fibrillation) and cardiac death (witnessed instantaneous death, death due to fresh myocardial ischaemia or death due to cardiac failure) (see Table 23.1).

Inducible ventricular tachycardia at electrophysiological study is the single best predictor for subsequent electrical events. No combination of tests excluding electrophysiological study is as effective as electrophysiological study alone, or electrophysiological study in combination with other tests, to identify patients at risk for ventricular tachycardia.

Low ejection fraction, delayed potentials and inducible ventricular tachycardia are all similarly valuable as predictors for cardiac death (see Table 23.2). Predictive models which incorporate any two of the above parameters are almost equally effective.[17] Inclusion of other parameters such as ambulatory monitoring and exercise testing do not improve the predictive value of models which incorporate ejection fraction, signal averaging and electrophysiological study.

At this time, no study incorporating heart rate variability and programmed stimulation as well as other predictors has been reported. It is possible that inclusion of heart rate variability into predictive models may improve the effectiveness of such models.

The thrombolytic era

Patients who receive early thrombolysis following infarction are less likely to have inducible ventricular tachycardia than those who do not receive early thrombolysis.[25] It is possible that early reperfusion prevents some of the patchy scarring at the edge of

Table 23.1 Relative risk of an electrical event after acute myocardial infarction. Relative risk in the absence of the risk factor is unity. An electrical event is defined as spontaneous ventricular fibrillation, ventricular tachycardia, or witnessed instantaneous death.

Univariate analysis	Risk	P
Inducible VT at EPS	15.2	<0.001
LVEF <0.40 at gated heart pool scan	4.8	0.002
Heart size	4.5	0.002
Late potentials on signal averaged ECG	4.4	0.003
Holter	3.1	0.08
Multivariate analysis	**Risk**	**P**
Inducible VT at EPS	10.4	<0.001
LVEF <0.40 at gated heart pool scan	3.2	0.05

Inducible VT=inducible ventricular tachycardia with a cycle length >230 ms; EPS=electrophysiological study; LVEF=low left ventricular ejection fraction (<0.40) at gated heart pool scan; heart size=cardiomegaly (cardiothoracic ratio >0.50) on chest X-ray; ECG=electrocardiogram; Holter=high-grade ectopy on 24 hour ambulatory electrocardiogram.

Table 23.2 Relative risk of cardiac death after myocardial infarction. Cardiac death is defined as witnessed instantaneous death, death due to fresh myocardial ischaemia, or death due to cardiac failure. For further details see legend to Table 23.1.

Univariate analysis	Risk	P
Late potentials on signal averaged ECG	7.0	<0.001
Inducible VT at EPS	5.6	<0.001
LVEF <0.40 at gated heart pool scan	5.2	<0.001
Heart size	2.8	0.01
Multivariate analysis groupings	**Risk**	**P**
Late potentials	5.6	0.001
Inducible VT	4.2	0.01
LVEF < 0.40	4.7	0.001
Inducible VT at EPS	3.5	0.01
Late potentials	4.5	0.003
LVEF <0.40	3.1	0.03

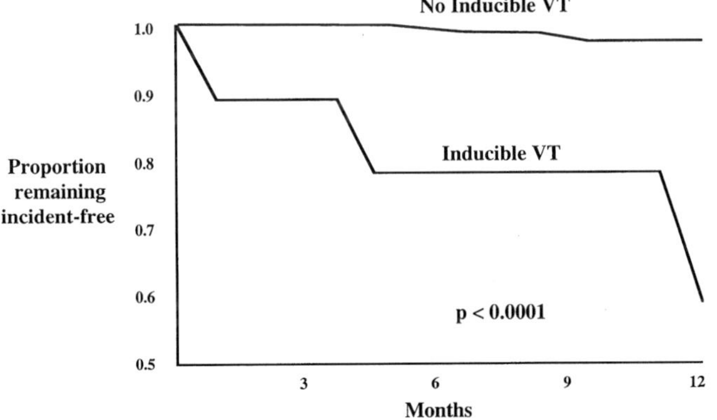

Fig. 23.1 Life table analysis of survival without sudden death or spontaneous ventricular tachycardia for 200 consecutive patients with (unstable) and without (stable) inducible ventricular tachycardia (cycle length ≥ 230 ms at programmed stimulation with up to five extra stimuli) after AMI. The difference in survival was highly statistically significant at 1 year. Reproduced with permission from Richards D, Taylor A, Fahey P et al. Identification of patients at risk of sudden death after myocardial infarction: the continued Australian experience. In: Brugada P, Wellens HJJ (eds). Cardiac Arrhythmia: where to go from here? New York: Futura, 1987: 329–41.

infarction, which otherwise would lead to slow conduction and the development of re-entrant ventricular tachycardia circuits.

Clinical significance of electrophysiological study and other tests

There is no doubt that electrophysiological study, alone or in combination with other tests, is a valuable technique to separate patients into high and low risk for subsequent ventricular tachycardia (see Fig. 23.1).

Although routine early thrombolysis has reduced the relative incidence of patients prone to ventricular tachycardia after AMI, there remains a significant small group of patients who are at risk of sudden death, and who can be identified. Prospective trials of therapeutic intervention are required to determine whether prognosis can be improved in these patients.

Summary

Death during the first year following AMI is most commonly due to spontaneous ventricular tachycardia, but may also be due to further myocardial ischaemia, cardiac failure and other causes. Inducible ventricular tachycardia at electrophysiological study is the single best predictor of spontaneous ventricular tachycardia after AMI. All-cause cardiac mortality after AMI is equally well predicted by electrophysiological study and by non-specific indicators of extensive AMI, including low left ventricular ejection fraction, high grade ventricular ectopy and impaired heart rate variability. Post-infarction management is facilitated by separating patients into high and low risk categories in order to focus therapeutic interventions on those patients who require them.

References

1. Hamer AR, Vohra J, Hunt D, Sloman G. Prediction of sudden death by electrophysiologic

studies in high risk patients surviving acute myocardial infarction. Am J Cardiol 1982; 50: 223–9
2. Richards DA, Cody DV, Denniss AR, Russell PA, Young AA, Uther JB. Ventricular electrical instability: a predictor of death after myocardial infarction. Am J Cardiol 1983; 51: 75–80
3. Waspe LE, Seinfeld D, Ferrick A, Kim SG, Matos JA, Fisher JD. Prediction of sudden death and spontaneous ventricular tachycardia in survivors of complicated myocardial infarction: value of the response to programmed extrastimuli. J Am Coll Cardiol 1985; 5: 1292–301
4. Denniss AR, Richards DA, Cody DV et al. Prognostic significance of ventricular tachycardia and fibrillation induced at programmed stimulation and delayed potentials detected on the signal averaged electrocardiogram of survivors of acute myocardial infarction. Circulation 1986; 74: 731–45
5. Breithardt G, Borggrefe M, Haerten K. Role of programmed ventricular stimulation and noninvasive recording of ventricular late potentials for the identification of patients at risk of ventricular tachyarrhythmias after acute myocardial infarction. In: Zipes D, Jalife J (eds). Cardiac electrophysiology and arrhythmias. Orlando: Grune & Stratton, 1983: 553–61
6. Simson MB. Use of signals in the terminal QRS complex to identify patients with ventricular tachycardia after myocardial infarction. Circulation 1981; 64: 235–42
7. Breithardt G, Becker G, Seipel L, Abendroth RR, Ostermeyer J. Noninvasive detection of late potentials in man: a new marker for ventricular tachycardia. Eur Heart J 1981; 2: 1–11
8. Kuchar DL, Thorburn CW, Sammel NL. Prediction of serious arrhythmic events after myocardial infarction: signal averaged electrocardiogram, Holter monitoring and radionuclide ventriculography. J Am Coll Cardiol 1987; 9: 531–8
9. Cooper RS, Simmons BE, Castaner A, Santhanam V, Ghali J, Mar M. Left ventricular hypertrophy is associated with worse survival independent of ventricular function and number of coronary arteries severely narrowed. Am J Cardiol 1990; 65: 441–5
10. Rogers WJ, Epstein AE, Arciniegas JG et al. The Cardiac Arrhythmia Suppression Trial (CAST) Investigators. Preliminary report: Effect of encainide and flecainide on mortality in a randomized trial of arrhythmia suppression after myocardial infarction. N Engl J Med 1989; 321: 406–12
11. EnGuard PFX clinical study update. Telectronics Pacing Systems Pty Ltd, Sydney, 1990
12. Saksena S, Mehta D. The PCD investigators and participating institutions. Long term results of implantable cardioverter-defibrillators using endocardial and epicardial defibrillation leads: a worldwide experience. Abst. PACE 1992; 15(II): 4
13. Cowley DE, Conway L, Hailey DM. Implantable cardiac defibrillators. Australian Institute of Health: Health Care Technology Series No. 5. Canberra: Australian Government Publishing Service, 1990
14. O'Brien BJ, Buxton MJ, Rushby JA. Cost effectiveness of the implantable cardioverter defibrillator: an analysis of the existing evidence. Hamilton, Ontario: McMaster University, 1991. CHEPA working paper No. 91-11
15. Uther JF. The automatic implantable defibrillator is the most realistic and cost-effective way of preventing sudden cardiac death. Aust NZ J Med 1992; 22(Suppl. V): 636–8
16. Schulze RA, Strauss HW, Pitt B. Sudden death in the year following myocardial infarction: relation to ventricular premature contractions in the late hospital phase and left ventricular ejection fraction. Am J Med 1977; 62: 192–9
17. Richards DAB, Byth K, Ross DL, Uther JB. What is the best predictor of spontaneous ventricular tachycardia and sudden death after myocardial infarction? Circulation 1991; 83: 756–63
18. Bourke JP, Richards DAB, Ross DL, Wallace EM, McGuire MA, Uther JB. Routine programmed electrical stimulation in survivors of acute myocardial infarction for prediction of spontaneous ventricular tachyarrhythmias during follow up: results, optimal stimulation protocol and cost-effective methods of screening. J Am Coll Cardiol 1991; 18: 780–8
19. Denniss AR, Baaijens H, Cody DV et al. Value of programmed stimulation and exercise testing in predicting one-year mortality after acute myocardial infarction. Am J Cardiol 1985; 56: 213–20
20. Uther JB, Richards DAB, Denniss AR, Ross DL. The prognostic significance of programmed ventricular stimulation after myocardial infarction: a review. Circulation 1987; 75 (Suppl. III): 161–5
21. Bourke JP, Richards DAB, Ross DL, McGuire MA, Uther JB. Does the induction of ventricular flutter or fibrillation at electrophysiology testing after myocardial infarction have any prognostic significance? Amer J Cardiol 1995; 75: 431–5
22. Denniss AR, Richards DA, Waywood JA, Yung T, Kam CA, Ross DL, Uther JB. Electrophysiological and anatomic differences between canine hearts with inducible ventricular tachycardia and fibrillation associated with chronic myocardial infarction. Circulation Research 1989; 64: 155–65

23. Mason JW. A comparison of electrophysiologic testing with Holter monitoring to predict antiarrhythmic-drug efficacy for ventricular tachyarrhythmias. N Engl J Med 1993; 329: 445–51
24. Kleiger RE, Miller JP, Bigger JT, Moss AJ. Decreased heart rate variability and its association with increased mortality after acute myocardial infarction. Am J Cardiol 1987; 59: 256–62
25. Bourke JP, Young AA, Richards DAB, Uther JB. Reduction in incidence of inducible ventricular tachycardia after myocardial infarction by treatment with Streptokinase during infarct evolution. Am Coll Cardiol 1990; 16: 1703–10

24 Haemodynamic monitoring

Philip A Cooke and Lillian J Barrie

Introduction

Haemodynamic monitoring in the coronary care unit (CCU) assists in the assessment and management of the patient with cardiac disease. The complexity of haemodynamic monitoring varies with the severity of the cardiac problem, ranging from non-invasive blood pressure monitoring to invasive pulmonary artery pressure monitoring and assessment of cardiac output. Invasive monitoring is rarely required in the patient with an uncomplicated myocardial infarction. The greatest danger of invasive haemodynamic monitoring is to neglect the acute management of the cardiac patient whilst being distracted by the intricacies of monitoring procedures. Resuscitation of the patient remains the priority.

Arterial pressure monitoring

Arterial blood pressure is an important indicator of clinical status in a patient with cardiac disease. Blood pressure can be measured by non-invasive and invasive methods.

Non-invasive blood pressure monitoring

Auscultation

The most common non-invasive technique of blood pressure measurement is by auscultation. Despite the increasing use of automated reference methods, auscultation remains the most frequently used method for blood pressure monitoring in the CCU; for this reason there must be adherence to accepted standards of measurement. The following points are recommended to ensure accurate and reliable readings:[1,2,3]

- bare arm positioned at heart level
- suitably sized cuff, bladder length 80% and width 40% of the arm circumference
- place bladder over the brachial artery, inflate to 30 mmHg above the pressure at which the radial pulse disappears
- deflate cuff at the rate of 2 mmHg per heart beat
- phase I Korotkoff sounds (onset of clear tapping sound that increases with intensity) recorded as the systolic pressure
- phase V (disappearance of sound) recorded as the diastolic pressure
- if the sound continues as pressure falls towards zero, phase IV (muffling of sound) is recorded as the diastolic pressure.

However, in low flow states resulting from hypotension, increased systemic vascular resistance, or a decrease in cardiac output, the accuracy of the auscultatory method may be unreliable as the vibrations produced may not be within the frequency range of the human ear. Obesity and peripheral oedema may also interfere with the transmission of sound.[4] Other causes of error include:

- inappropriate cuff size
- incorrect arm position
- poorly calibrated anaeroid manometer.

Automatic blood pressure monitors[3]

Virtually all automatic blood pressure monitors use a sphygmomanometer cuff operated by detection of Korotkoff sounds by oscillometry or ultrasound. This technique eliminates interobserver error, but otherwise the limitations are the same as for the auscultatory method of blood pressure measurement. The accuracy of the automatic blood pressure monitors is much the same as for the auscultatory method[4,5] and they all have the clear advantage that trends in blood pressure can be summarized graphically.

Invasive blood pressure monitoring

Intra-arterial cannulation provides continuous blood pressure monitoring and facilitates arterial blood sampling. Direct blood pressure monitoring can be achieved by cannulation of an artery and attachment of a fluid-filled transducer system which converts pressure to electrical impulses and displays this pressure on an oscilloscope.

The radial artery is the most common site for arterial cannulation. An Allen's test should be performed to ensure adequate collateral circulation. Other sites include the brachial, femoral and pedal arteries. The normal arterial waveform (see Fig. 24.1) is characterized by a rapid upstroke, followed by a dicrotic notch correlating with the closure of the aortic valve and signifying the onset of diastole which continues until the next systole. The arterial pressure differs in both contour and values in various locations. The systolic pressure is higher in the femoral artery than in the radial or brachial artery, with the diastolic value generally remaining the same. Additionally, the more distal the location of the arterial catheter, the sharper and later the upstroke and the less defined the dicrotic notch.[6]

Technique for direct bedside monitoring

Directly measured arterial pressure is generally more accurate than non-invasive measurement.[6] However, this method is subject to error in the set-up of the monitoring system, calibration and interpretation of the arterial waveform. The following steps should be followed when invasive monitoring is initiated:

- Prepare a closed continuous monitoring system to include a flow regulatory device, transducer, air port and non-compliant tubing.
- Prime monitoring set with normal or heparinized saline. Note: heparinized saline has been shown to increase catheter life.[7] Normal saline without heparin has the advantage of not interfering with coagulation profile.
- Inflate pressure bag to manufacturer's recommendation which enables the flow regulatory device to maintain catheter patency.
- Check the calibration of the monitoring system. Most monitors have a single command to institute the calibration process.
- Set appropriate scale on the monitor within physiological range of the pressure to be monitored.
- Secure primed monitoring system to the vascular access.
- Attach transducer cable from monitoring system to the external disposable transducer.
- Level the air reference port at the assumed level of the patient's right atrium at the fourth intercostal space and the mid axilla line.
- Adjust the stopcock on the transducer so that it is turned off to the patient and open to air. Zero the transducer. Zeroing ensures that the transducer reads zero relative to atmosphere. Most monitors have a single command to institute the zeroing process. Once completed, a message or signal will be displayed indicating successful zeroing of the transducer.
- Replace all vented caps with non vented caps.
- Commence monitoring.
- Set appropriate alarm limits and activate alarm.

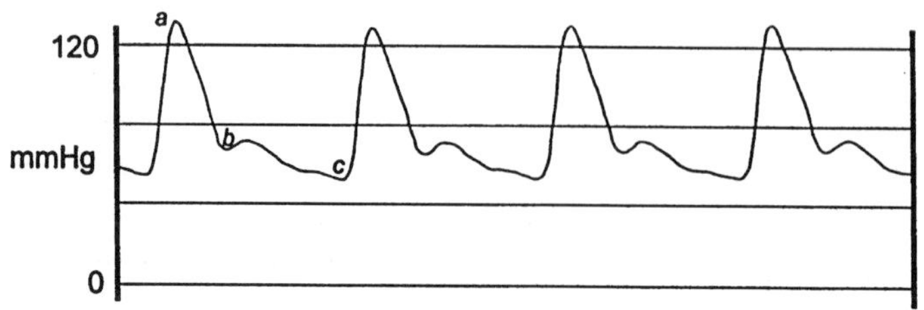

Fig. 24.1 Normal radial artery waveform, a) systole characterized by a rapid upstroke, followed by b) a dicrotic notch correlating with the closure of the aortic valve and signifying onset of diastole; c) diastole continues until the next systole.

Complications of invasive arterial pressure monitoring

Arterial thromboembolism

The incidence of arterial thromboembolism is less if a small (20 gauge) Teflon catheter is used. A higher incidence of thromboembolism occurs with brachial artery cannulation. Recanalization of the artery usually occurs following arterial thrombosis without major ischaemic complications.[8] Regular examination of the limb for ischaemic changes enables early detection of this complication.

Infection

Arterial cannulation can result in local or systemic infection. The incidence of infection can be reduced by utilizing an aseptic technique on insertion and adherence to infection control guidelines regarding frequency of line and cannula changes (see Chapter 83).

Haemorrhage

Haemorrhage usually results from disconnection of the monitoring set or dislodgement of the arterial cannula. Activation of the monitoring alarm and exposure of the insertion site enables expedient intervention.

Hyperextension of flexor tendons

Hyperextension should be avoided when positioning wrist with radial artery cannulation.

Non-invasive versus invasive arterial pressure monitoring

When a high degree of accuracy is required, such as in critically ill patients or with titration of cardioactive drugs, continuous direct arterial pressure monitoring is superior to indirect methods.[9]

Central venous pressure

Central venous pressure (CVP) measurement is an important monitoring parameter and has been widely used in the CCU for over 20 years.[10] CVP in conjunction with the clinical status is useful in the estimation of blood volume, adequacy of venous return and assessment of right ventricular function.

Normal CVP is 2–8 mmHg (3–10 cmH_2O) (see Fig. 24.2). The CVP waveform is characterized by three distinct waves, the *a*, *c* and *v* waves. The *a* wave correlates with atrial systole, the *c* wave correlates with closure of the tricuspid valve, and the *v* wave correlates with the upward movement of the tricuspid valve during ventricular systole.

CVP can be measured by a water manometer or displayed digitally on a pressure module and the waveform displayed on an oscilloscope. In the presence of left ventricular dysfunction, CVP may give a misleading impression of left ventricular filling pressures. Pulmonary artery pressure and pulmonary artery wedge pressure in this instance will provide a more accurate estimation (see pulmonary artery pressure monitoring, below).

Elevated CVP can be seen in:

- poor right ventricular function
- conditions causing restriction to cardiac filling—cardiac tamponade, constrictive pericarditis and restrictive cardiomyopathy
- pulmonary hypertension
- chronic left ventricular failure
- volume overload
- superior vena cava obstruction.

Waveform examination may be a useful adjunct for assessment and diagnosis of clinical problems in the CCU:

- Large *a* waves: right ventricular failure pulmonary hypertension
- Large *v* waves: tricuspid regurgitation
- Large *a* and *v* waves: cardiac tamponade constrictive pericarditis

Rise in right atrial pressure with inspiration (Kussmaul's sign) may be evident in constrictive pericarditis, cardiac tamponade and right ventricular infarction.

Pulmonary artery pressure monitoring

In the presence of right ventricular dysfunction the CVP may give a misleading impression of left heart filling pressures. Pulmonary artery pressure (PAP)

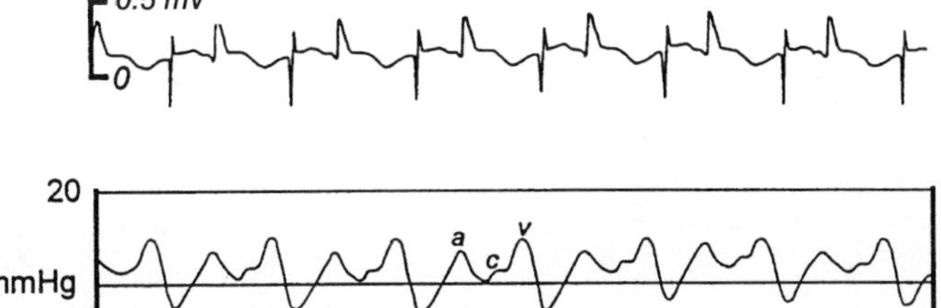

Fig. 24.2 Normal CVP waveform with *a*, *c* and *v* waves in atrial pacing.

and pulmonary artery wedge pressure (PAWP) monitoring provide a more accurate estimation of left atrial filling pressure. Additionally, pulmonary artery (PA) catheters facilitate measurement of cardiac output, from whence derived indices such as systemic vascular resistance (SVR) and pulmonary vascular resistance (PVR) can be calculated. These pressures and derived indices are, in turn, useful in assessing the patient's clinical status[10] and response to interventions affecting pre-load, afterload, ionotropic state of the myocardium, and heart rate. However, despite the advantages of having on-line monitoring of disordered haemodynamic states, the use of pulmonary artery catheters has not been shown to improve outcome,[11] and concerns have been expressed about their over-enthusiastic use.[12] In most CCUs the use of pulmonary artery pressure monitoring is now more selective than in the 1970s and 1980s.

Indications for pulmonary artery monitoring

The indications for pulmonary artery monitoring are as follows:

- hypovolaemia
- hypotension
- cardiogenic shock
- right ventricular infarction
- inotropic support and/or vasodilator therapy
- septal rupture
- papillary muscle rupture
- circulatory assist devices.

The most widely used pulmonary artery catheter is a 7.5 Fr, five lumen, balloon-tipped catheter with a thermistor at the tip (see Fig. 24.3). This is an updated version of the Swan–Ganz catheter introduced in the early 1970s.[15] The five lumens are labelled as follows:

- *distal lumen* is used for continuous PAP monitoring and mixed venous blood sampling
- *proximal lumen* terminates at 30 cm from the catheter tip and can be used for continuous right atrial pressure monitoring, infusion of fluid and drugs, and blood sampling
- *thermistor port* continuously monitors core temperature and is used for the measurement of cardiac output by the thermodilution technique
- *balloon inflation port* inflates balloon at catheter tip to obtain PAWP

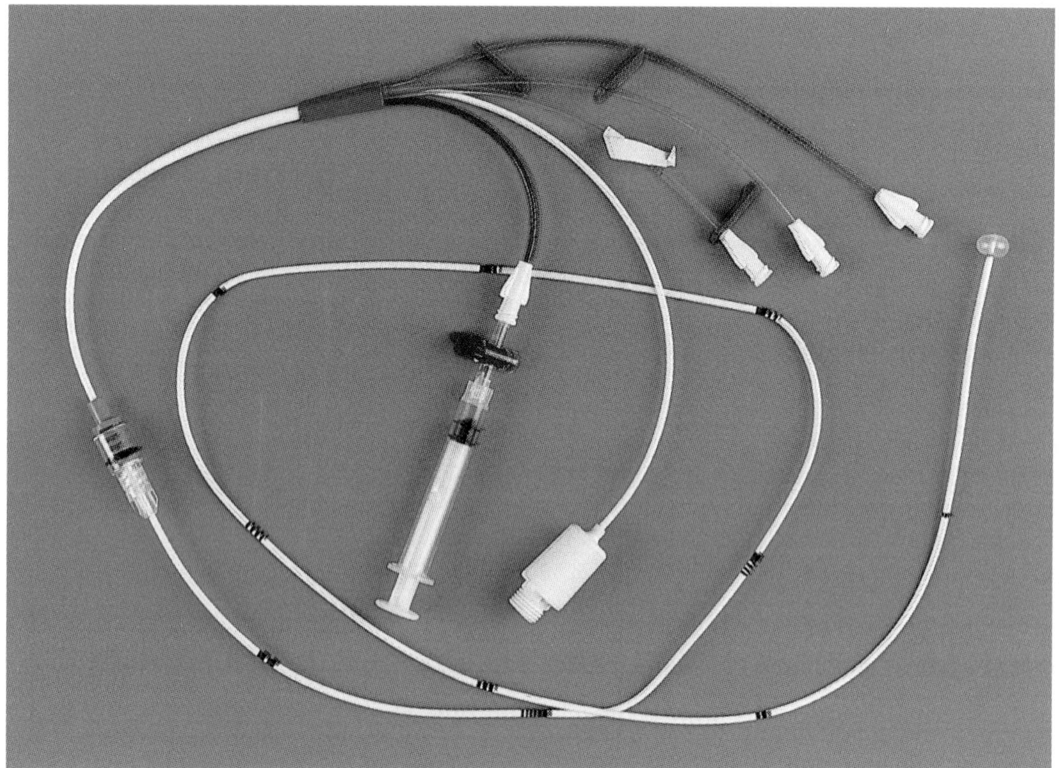

Fig. 24.3 The 7.5 Fr, 5 lumen, thermodilution PA catheter.

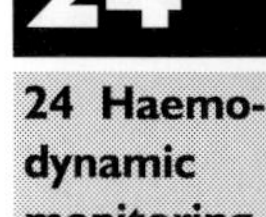

- *infusion port* provides an extra port for infusion of fluid or drugs.

The PA catheter is inserted through a venous sheath and guided sequentially into the right atrium (RA), right ventricle (RV), and pulmonary artery (PA) by following the characteristic pressures and waveform and/or with the aid of fluoroscopic imaging. When the PA catheter is properly positioned, the opening of the proximal port is located in the RA, allowing continuous monitoring of CVP. The distal port, located in the PA, allows monitoring of PAP and PAWP.

Insertion of PA catheter by visualization of pressure and waveforms

The insertion of the PA catheter by visualization of pressure and waveforms should be as follows:

- Set up transducer (see technique for bedside monitoring) and attach to the distal port of the PA catheter
- Level transducer to the level of the right atrium
- Zero transducer
- Set appropriate scale to enable visualization of the waveforms
- Check integrity of the balloon before insertion
- Pass PA catheter through sheath. As catheter is advanced into RA, the characteristic RA pressure and waveform is encountered (see Fig. 24.4)
- Inflate catheter balloon with 1.5 ml of air
- Advance catheter into the right ventricle. The RV waveform is characterized by a diastolic pressure of 0–6 mmHg and a systolic pressure of 20–30 mmHg (see Fig. 24.5).
- Elevated RV pressures may occur with pulmonary hypertension, pulmonary stenosis, chronic LVF, constrictive pericarditis and cardiac tamponade. Ectopy is frequently encountered as catheter is passed through RV, particularly the outflow tract. Continuous ECG monitoring is essential and emergency equipment should be readily available.
- Sudden elevation of diastolic pressure signifies position of catheter in the pulmonary artery (see Fig. 24.6). In the absence of pulmonary stenosis, RV systolic pressure should equal PA systolic pressure.
- With balloon remaining inflated, catheter should be further advanced until balloon wedges in a branch of pulmonary artery and the PAWP waveform is visualized. This can be recognized by the dampening of the PA waveform resulting in a contour

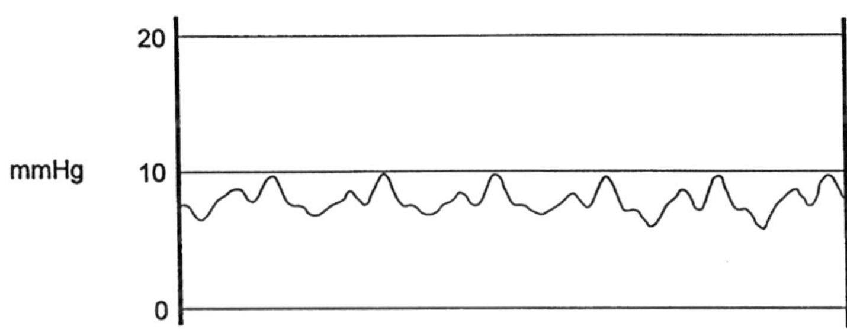

Fig. 24.4 The characteristic RA pressure and waveform.

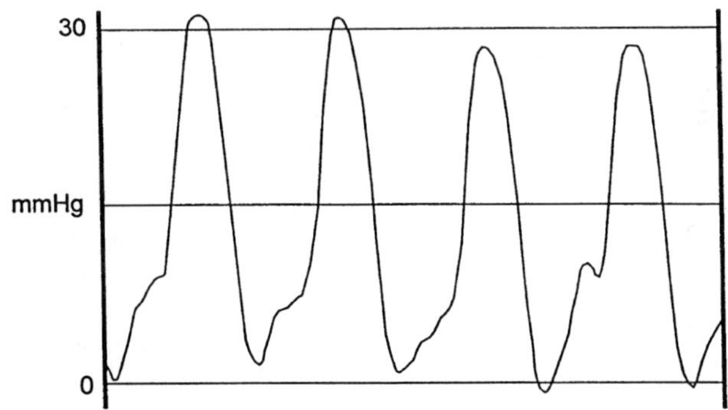

Fig. 24.5 The characteristic RV waveform, characterized by a low diastolic pressure.

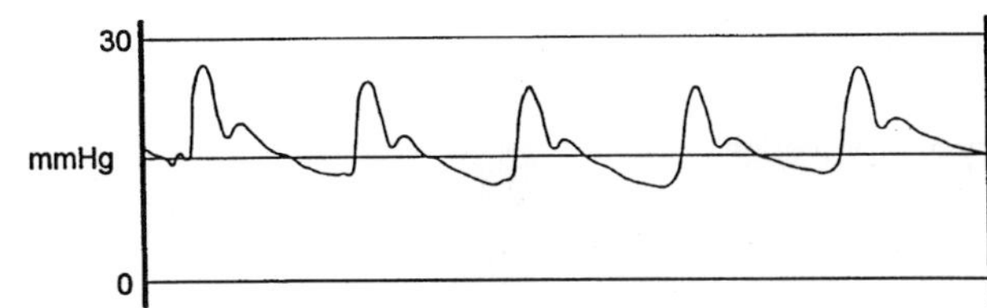

Fig. 24.6 The characteristic PA pressure and waveform.

resembling the RA pressure (see Fig. 24.7). The PAWP should be 2–3 mmHg less than the pulmonary artery end diastolic pressure (PAEDP).

- Once the PAWP waveform is visualized, balloon should be allowed to deflate passively and the PA pressure waveform will appear.
- To check position of catheter, reinflate balloon and observe for the PAWP waveform. The optimal volume for inflation of balloon is 1 ml of air. A PAWP waveform observed with balloon volume less than 1 ml suggests that catheter is placed too distally in the pulmonary artery.
- It is mandatory to check position of catheter with chest X-ray (see Fig. 24.8).
- Record length of catheter that has been inserted into the patient.

Pulmonary artery pressure

There is usually close correlation between the PAEDP and PAWP, and therefore PA monitoring facilitates safe continuous left ventricular end diastolic pressure (LVEDP) estimates without the need to wedge the catheter repeatedly. However PAEDP may not accurately reflect PAWP in conditions when the PA pressure is chronically elevated, acute pulmonary embolism or tachycardia. In these situations, PAWP should be performed to estimate LVEDP.

Pulmonary artery wedge pressure

The PAWP is obtained by inflating the balloon at the tip of the PA catheter and occluding a branch of the pulmonary artery. This effectively results in a 'closed' pressure system, and pressure changes in the next most distal chamber, the left atrium (LA), can be estimated via the distal catheter port.

Elevated PAWP occurs with LV failure, volume overload, mitral valve disease, constrictive pericarditis and cardiac tamponade. Low PAWP occurs with hypovolaemia.

PAWP, therefore, is an indirect estimation of LA pressure and this in turn estimates LVEDP. Where LA pressures are elevated significantly above LVEDP (in mitral stenosis or LA myxoma), PAWP does not approximate LVEDP. Other situations where PAWP does not accurately reflect LVEDP occur with elevated pleural pressures and when the PA catheter is placed in non-dependent lung zones.

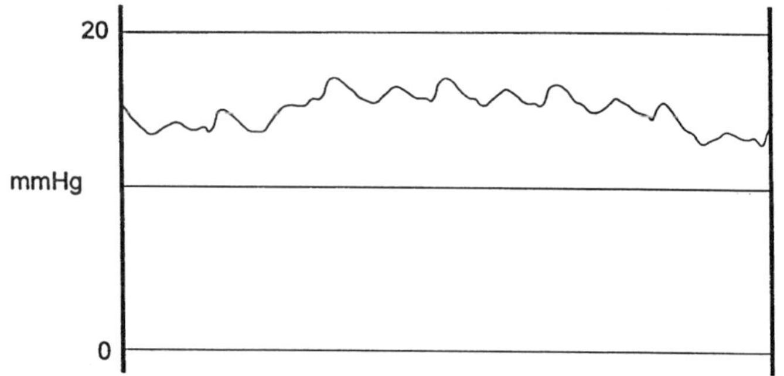

Fig. 24.7 The PAWP waveform.

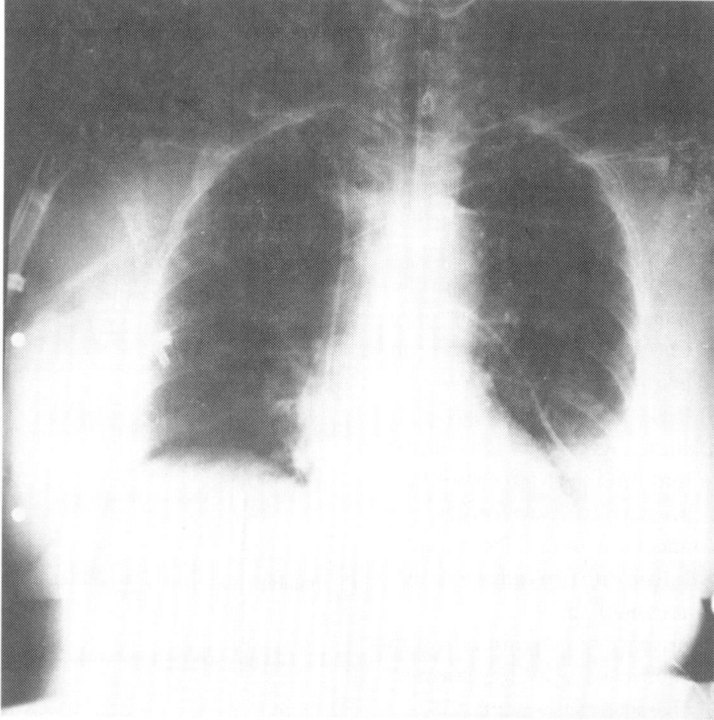

Fig. 24.8 Chest X-ray showing ideal position of the PA catheter.

Complications of pulmonary artery catheters

Major complications are reported to occur in 3–5% and minor complications in 20–25% of patients who have pulmonary artery catheters.[14]

Cardiac arrhythmia usually occurs during insertion of the catheter or migration of the catheter back into the RV. Right bundle branch block can occur as the catheter is advanced in the RV. This may result in complete heart block in patients with pre-existing left bundle branch block. Precautions taken during insertion should include continuous ECG monitoring, minimal manipulation of the catheter in the RV and preparation for the treatment of arrhythmias.

Thrombus formation is more likely to occur in patients with low cardiac output states. The risk is minimized by ensuring a continuous heparin flush is maintained by inflating the pressure bag to manufacturer's recommendations. Thrombus formation is reduced with heparin bonded catheters.

Pulmonary infarction can occur from thromboemboli, prolonged wedging and spontaneous wedging of a distally placed PA catheter (see Fig. 24.9).

Pulmonary artery rupture is usually fatal. It can be caused by over-inflation of the balloon, frequent wedging and use of excessive air in the balloon. The risk of pulmonary artery rupture is associated with pulmonary hypertension, the aged and abnormal coagulation profile. Pulmonary artery rupture should be suspected if haemoptysis occurs. Independent lung ventilation and surgical repair are indicated.

Infection from pulmonary artery catheterization can result in local or systemic infection. Infection can be minimized by aseptic insertion technique, minimal manipulation of the catheter once properly placed and removal of the catheter as soon as it is no longer required.

Knotting of the catheter prevents removal and in some instances surgery is indicated. Manipulation of the catheter under fluoroscopic imaging may be useful.

Balloon rupture may be caused by frequent inflations, over-inflation or active deflation. Lack of resistance on inflation, failure of passive deflation, blood in inflation syringe and inability to obtain PAWP are possible indications of balloon rupture. If balloon rupture is suspected, further attempts at inflation should be avoided.

Ventricular perforation and cardiac tamponade are rare complications of PA catheters.

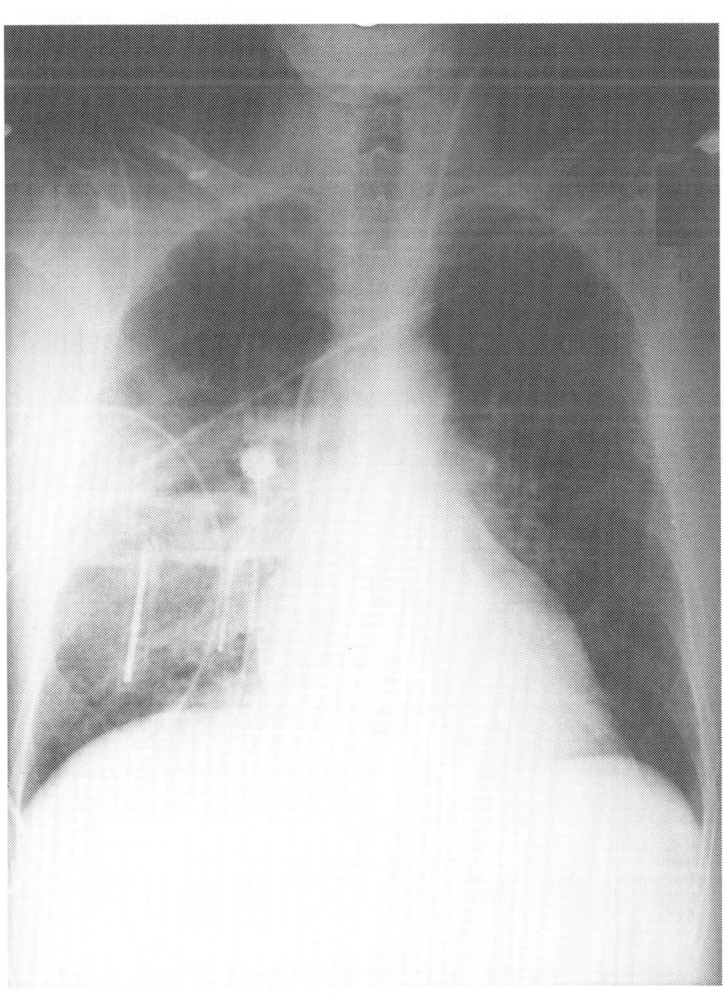

Fig. 24.9 Chest X-ray showing segmental lung infarction from a distally placed PA catheter.

Abnormalities and difficulties associated with invasive monitoring

Damping

Damping is characterized by poor systolic upstroke, rounding and flattening of the pressure waveform (see Fig. 24.10). In the arterial and pulmonary artery pressure waveforms, the dicrotic notch may be absent or difficult to discern. Damping of pressure waveform results in under-estimation of the pressure value.

The causes of damping are:

- fibrin clot on catheter tip
- catheter resting against vessel wall
- compliant tubing
- air bubbles in tubing
- kinking of tubing or catheter.

Pressure variation associated with respiration

The RAP, PAP and PAWP varies during respiration (see Fig. 24.11). In a patient breathing spontaneously, the pressure decreases with inspiration and increases with expiration. The pressure should be measured at end expiration where intra-thoracic pressure equals zero.

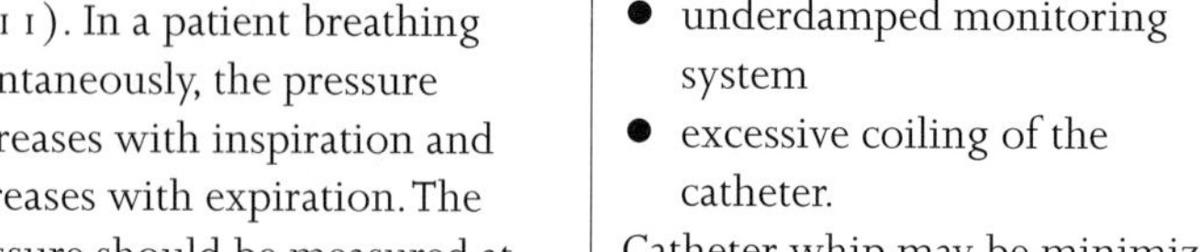

Catheter whip

Catheter whip is characterized by exaggerated oscillation of the pressure waveform causing incorrect estimation of the pressure value.

The causes of catheter whip are:

- catheter tip located near the pulmonary valve where the blood flow is turbulent
- underdamped monitoring system
- excessive coiling of the catheter.

Catheter whip may be minimized with manipulation and repositioning of the catheter.

Overwedging

Overwedging is characterized by flattening of the waveform with overshoot (see Fig. 24.12). Causes of overwedging include:

- overinflation of balloon
- eccentric balloon inflation
- catheter tip distally placed in the pulmonary artery.

Serious complications of overwedging include pulmonary artery rupture and pulmonary infarction. Overwedging results in incorrect estimation of PAWP. Except in mitral regurgitation, PAWP should be 2–3 mmHg less than PAEDP. In mitral regurgitation a large *v* wave is seen in the PAWP waveform (see Fig. 24.13). In instances other than mitral regurgitation where PAWP is greater than PAEDP, the technique of wedging should be reviewed.

Catheter migration

Post insertion, the position of the catheter should be checked by chest X-ray. Vigilant monitoring of waveform and pressure value will detect migration of the catheter.

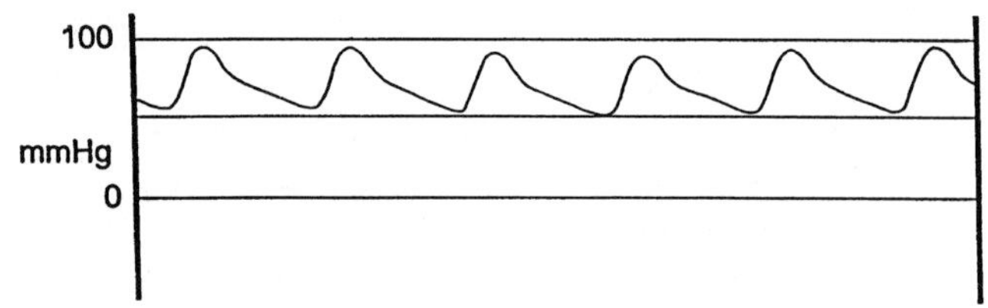

Fig. 24.10 Damping of arterial pressure waveform showing slow upstroke and poorly defined dicrotic notch.

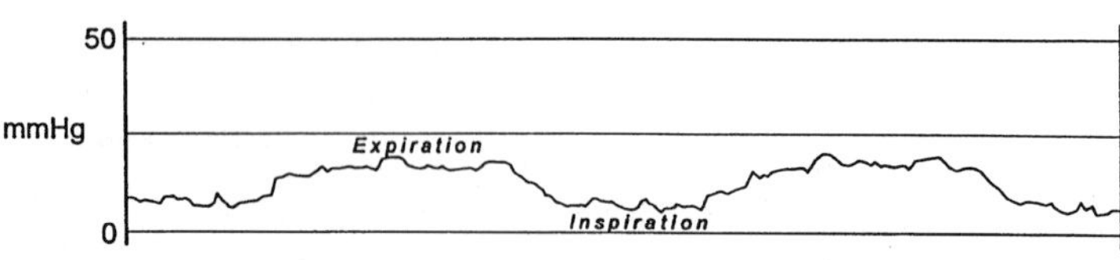

Fig. 24.11 PAWP waveform with respiratory variation in a spontaneously breathing patient. The pressure should be measured at end expiration.

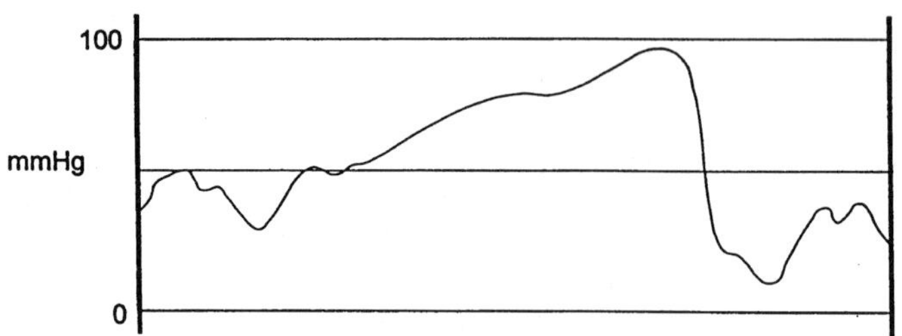

Fig. 24.12 PAWP waveform with overwedging.

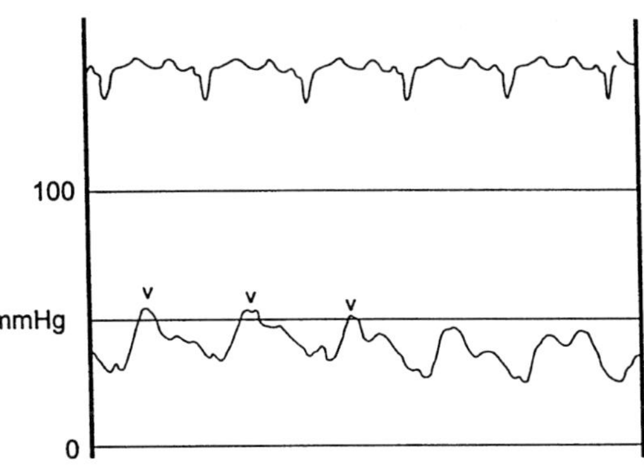

Fig. 24.13 PAWP waveform with large *v* wave indicating mitral regurgitation.

Spontaneous wedging

Spontaneous wedging occurs when the catheter is placed in a distal position and wedges without inflation of the balloon. Spontaneous wedging is recognized by visualization of the PAWP waveform. If unrecognized, spontaneous wedging can cause pulmonary infarction. Immediate withdrawal of the catheter should be carried out upon visualization of PAWP waveform in the absence of balloon inflation.

Intermittent wedging

Intermittent wedging is evidenced by a mixed PAP/PAWP pressure waveform which varies with respiration. Intermittent wedging can occur when the catheter is in a distal position without inflation of the balloon. In this case the catheter should be slightly withdrawn. Intermittent wedging can also occur during inflation of the balloon. Slight advancement of the catheter is required to obtain a PAWP waveform. The catheter should only be advanced if the sterility of the proximal end of the catheter is maintained.

Displacement of catheter into the right ventricle

Displacement of the catheter into the RV can be recognized by the visualization of the RV waveform and associated changes in the diastolic pressure. Upon recognition of catheter displacement into the RV, the balloon should be inflated immediately to reduce the incidence of ventricular arrhythmias. Attempts can be made to advance the catheter into the pulmonary artery. If this fails, the balloon should be deflated and the catheter pulled back.

Cardiac output measurement

Measurement of cardiac output (CO) via the pulmonary artery catheter can be achieved by the thermodilution method, which is in effect a modification of the Indicator Dilution Principle. The technique of thermodilution involves the injection of solution (usually normal saline) of known quantity and temperature into the right atrium. Dilution occurs in the right heart with the resulting change of temperature detected by the thermistor in the pulmonary artery. The flow (CO in L/min) is calculated from change in temperature versus time. Modern computerized monitoring systems automatically calculate CO from temperature variation, time and a computation constant dependent upon the catheter type, the volume and temperature of injectate. The thermodilution method for estimation of cardiac output is a simple, rapid, accurate and reproducible technique. However, there are many potential sources of error. To ensure consistency of technique, individual CCUs need to establish protocols to consider the following.

- *Temperature of injectate.* The reproducibility of CO estimation has been reported in using room temperature (23–28°C) and iced temperature injectate.[9–11] Iced temperature injectates are more likely to cause slowing of heart rate than room temperature injectates; hence underestimation of cardiac output. Iced temperature injectate is recommended for low and high cardiac output states.[12] Errors caused by rewarming of the injectate can be resolved with an in-line injectate temperature probe at the injection site.
- *Volume of injectate.* The volume of injectate is usually 10 ml, but this can be reduced to 5 ml in situations where volume is critical.
- *Injection technique.* It is recommended that the injectate be administered rapidly and evenly over 4 sec or less. Faulty injection techniques will be apparent from the thermodilution curves.

- *Respiratory variation*. The temperature of the PA blood varies during the ventilatory cycle. Hence injections timed to occur at one particular phase of the cycle may increase reproducibility, but may not reflect the mean flow rate per minute. Trends are often more clinically significant than true values; hence, some units opt to increase inter-observer reliability by timing injections at end expiration. Mean flow rate per minute can be achieved if CO determinations are made at various phases of the respiratory cycle.
- *Patient positioning*. Cardiac output may vary according to patient position. In order to minimize the effect of posture on CO and to improve reproducibility of results, measurements should be taken with the patient in the same position. The preferred position is supine with varying degrees of head elevation as tolerated by the patient.

Limitations

Cardiac output measurement will be inaccurate in the presence of intracardiac shunts (VSD and ASD). Significant tricuspid regurgitation will incorrectly estimate CO.

Derived cardiac indices

Derived cardiac indices are often automatically calculated by the modern computerized bedside monitoring system. Taken in isolation, derived cardiac indices are of limited use, but may be of considerable value when calculated serially to monitor response to

Common calculations of cardiac indices[13]

- Cardiac index = $\frac{\text{CO}}{\text{body surface area}}$ L/min/m^2
- Stroke index = $\frac{\text{cardiac index}}{\text{heart rate}}$ L/beat/m^2
- Systemic vascular resistance index = $\frac{\text{MAP} - \text{RAP}}{\text{CI}} \times 79.92$ $\text{dyne-sec/cm}^5\text{/m}^2$
- Pulmonary vascular resistance index = $\frac{\text{MPAP} - \text{PAWP}}{\text{CI}} \times 79.92$ $\text{dyne-sec/cm}^5\text{/m}^2$

CI = cordiac index.

therapeutic interventions. As derived indices the magnitude of errors may be compounded by inaccuracies in the basic haemodynamic measurements.

Continuous cardiac output measurement

A major advance in monitoring the critically ill is the capability to continuously measure cardiac output. This is achieved by modification of the PA catheter with a specialized filament that produces heat as the indicator. This enables continuous cardiac output monitoring by means of thermodilution principles. With correct positioning of the PA catheter the filament lies in the right ventricle. The monitor delivers random pulses of energy to the filament, raising the surface temperature of the catheter and surrounding blood to 44°C. The thermistor in the pulmonary artery detects the temperature change. The monitor continuously displays the CO and updates the CO estimation every 30–60 seconds.

Conclusion

As with any therapeutic manoeuvre, the potential risk to the patient from invasive monitoring needs to be weighed against the perceived benefits. The data obtained may assist in diagnosis and management but is no substitute for meticulous clinical assessment of the patient.

References

1. The management of hypertension: a consensus statement. Med J Aust 1994; March (Suppl. 21)
2. Hand HL. Direct or indirect blood pressure measurement for open heart surgery patients: an algorithm. Critical Care Nurse 1992; August: 52–60
3. Pickering TG. Ambulatory monitoring and blood pressure variability. London: Science Press, 1991
4. Henneman EA, Henneman PL. Intricacies of blood pressure measurement: re-examining the rituals. Heart & Lung 1989; 18(3): 263–71
5. Venus B, Mathru M, Smith RA, Pham CG. Direct versus indirect blood pressure measurements in critically ill patients. Heart & Lung 1985; 14(3): 228–31
6. Daily EK, Schroeder JK. Techniques in bedside haemody-

namic monitoring. St Louis: Mosby, 1994
7. Clifton GD, Kelly HJ, Record KE, Thompson JR. Comparison of normal saline and heparin solutions for maintenance of arterial catheter patency. Heart & Lung 1991; 20(2): 115–8
8. Bedford RF, Wallman H. Complications of percutaneous radial-artery cannulation. Anesthesiology 1973; 38: 228–36
9. Renner LE, Morton MJ, Sakuma GY. Indicator amount, temperature, and intrinsic cardiac output affect thermodilution cardiac output accuracy and reproducibility. Critical Care Medicine 1993; 21(4): 586–97
10. Forrester JS, Diamond G, Chatterjee K et al. Medical therapy of acute myocardial infarction by the application of haemodynamic subsets. N Engl J Med 1976; 295: 1356–62
11. Gore J, Goldberg R, Spodick D et al. A community-wide assessment of the use of pulmonary artery catheters in patients with acute myocardial infarction. Chest 1987; 92: 721–7
12. Robin E. Death by pulmonary artery flow-directed catheter. Chest 1987; 92: 727–31
13. Swan HJC, Ganz W, Forrester JS et al. Catheterisation of the heart in man with the use of a flow-directed balloon-tipped catheter. N Engl J Med 1970; 283: 447–51
14. Paglierello G. The pulmonary artery (Swan–Ganz) catheter. Int J Technology Assessment in Health Care 1993; 9: 202–9
15. Nishikawa T, Dohi S. Errors in the measurement of cardiac output by thermodilution. Canadian Journal of Anaesthesia 1993; 40(2): 142–53
16. Safcsak K, Nelson L. Thermodilution right ventricular ejection fraction measurements: room temperature versus cold temperature injectate. Critical Care Medicine 1994; 22: 1136–41
17. Wallace DC, Winslow EH. Effects of iced and room temperature injectate on cardiac output measurements in critically ill patients with low and high cardiac outputs. Heart & Lung 1993; 22(1): 55–61
18. Donovan KD. Invasive monitoring and support of the circulation. In: Dobb GJ (ed.) Clinics in Anaesthesia. London: WB Saunders, 1995: 909–54

Part 5
Drug therapies

25 Oxygen therapy

Paul E Langton

Oxygen therapy

A primary role of the circulation is the delivery of oxygen to tissues. Oxygen (O_2) delivery is dependent on:

- blood flow (cardiac output and regional perfusion)
- the O_2 content of blood (= [haemoglobin concentration × O_2 saturation (SaO_2) × 1.39] + [PaO_2 × 0.03])
- O_2 extraction by tissues.

In acute myocardial ischaemia there is impaired oxygen delivery to the myocardium itself, mainly due to severe local coronary stenosis or obstruction. More generally, impaired cardiac pump function reduces tissue oxygenation.

As myocardial function is largely aerobic, any compromise in O_2 delivery has the potential to cause (further) impairment in pump function and hence tissue blood flow and O_2 delivery. This leads into a potentially vicious cycle that contributes to the development of life-threatening pulmonary oedema and cardiogenic shock.

In optimizing myocardial function and/or minimizing the spreading wave of peri-infarction myocardial necrosis that is known to exist, one aims to ensure adequate oxygen saturation of haemoglobin (Hb).

Arterial oxygen saturation and the haemoglobin-oxygen dissociation curve

The nature of the haemoglobin-oxygen (Hb-O_2) dissociation curve (Fig. 25.1) is such that the incremental increase in O_2 carriage is relatively small once oxygen tension is over a critical level of approximately 93% (PaO_2 70 mmHg). A fall in PaO_2 below this however is associated with a rapid drop in O_2 content of blood, particularly once the saturation drops off the 'shoulder' of the curve at a tension of approximately 60 mmHg (SaO_2 ~90%).

Tissue oxygenation can also be altered by a shift of the Hb-O_2 curve secondary to changes in local milieu. Factors such as local tissue acidosis and stress-related increases in circulating cortisol

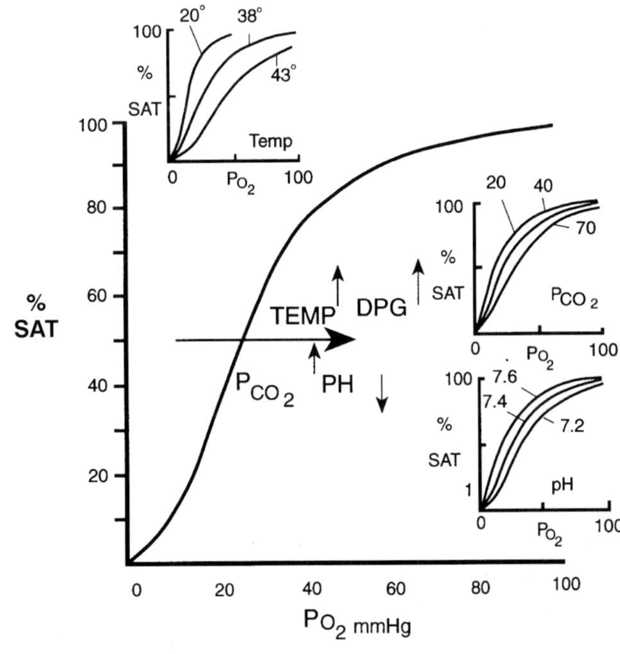

Fig. 25.1 Oxygen dissociation curve for haemoglobin. The incremental uptake of oxygen is relatively small once PaO_2 exceeds ~ 70 mmHg. The effect of acidosis, elevation of $PaCo_2$ and increasing DPG (diphosphoglycerate) enhance O_2 release to the tissues.

will shift the curve to the right. In doing so the affinity of Hb for O_2 is reduced and this allows for increased release of O_2 to tissues.

Hypoxaemia in myocardial infarction

Hypoxaemia has been a frequently recognized complication of acute myocardial infarction (AMI). The high pulmonary venous pressures associated with impaired pump function lead to degrees of pulmonary interstitial oedema with ventilation/perfusion mismatch and impaired gas diffusion, and hence hypoxaemia. Measured O_2 tensions correlate with indices of left ventricular pump function, most notably being inversely proportional to left ventricular end diastolic pressure (LVEDP).[1]

Data as to the frequency of significant hypoxaemia in a current coronary care population are relatively lacking. One series reported a frequency of significant O_2 desaturation (SaO_2<93%) in 19% of patients with MI who, at presentation, were otherwise uncomplicated (that is, without overt cardiac failure).[2] The incidence of hypoxaemia was also noted to be proportional to narcotic use. This suggests a role of narcotic-induced hypoventilation in contributing to hypoxia. Benefits, however, of preventing hypoxaemia are more presumed than proven.

Some clinical data have shown that supplemental O_2 in the setting of hypoxaemia post AMI is associated with reduction in the degree of ST segment elevation.[3] Information about more meaningful clinical endpoints (for example, infarct size, LV dysfunction, mortality) are lacking and in the current setting are unlikely to be generated.

Therefore, although reasonably based in theory, O_2 therapy is used empirically. A target level of 93% saturation (PaO_2 ~ 70) would seem to be appropriate.

Oxygen delivery

Hospital oxygen supply is generally derived indirectly from high pressure stores via a reducing valve to a wall outlet. Portable O_2 cylinders can be used in some situations, such as patient transport. Cylinders generally have an inbuilt regulating valve. From either source O_2 flow is controlled by the appropriate valve and the amount measured by a flow meter. This is then connected via tubing to the patient, using various delivery systems. The most common of these are:

- nasal cannulae or prongs
- semi-rigid (Hudson-type) mask
- controlled flow (Venturi-type) mask
- reservoir mask
- CPAP (continuous positive airway pressure) masks.

Normal peak inspiratory gas flows in patients breathing at rest are in the order of 35 L/min. This can easily be increased to over 50 L/min in the setting of severe breathlessness. The delivered concentration of inspired O_2 (F_IO_2) with a semi-rigid mask or with nasal prongs is highly dependent on peak inspiratory flow rates, and hence the pattern of the patient's respiration.

Intra-nasal oxygen

With nasal prongs at moderate flow (2–4 L/min), a degree of O_2 accumulates in the nasopharynx between respirations. It is this stored O_2, rather than the relatively low ongoing flow rate during inspiration, that provides most of the supplemental O_2 entrained. Marked differences in effective F_IO_2 occur between habitual mouth breathers and nose breathers with the former deriving little or no benefit from nasal oxygen. A tendency to mouth breathing may be exacerbated by narcotics or sedation, and this further reduces the efficacy of this route. Likewise patients with impaired conscious state requiring a Guedel type airway will receive no useful O_2 supplementation from nasal prongs. The advantage of nasal O_2 is the maintenance of patient's ability to eat and drink and the tendency to cause less claustrophobia than a mask. There is also no potential for carbon dioxide (CO_2) rebreathing. The disadvantages are those of drying of the nasal mucosa, with discomfort and/or ulceration and risk of infection. This is increased at higher nasal O_2 flows (> 3 L/min). Also, there is the aforementioned potential for inadequate O_2 supplementation.

Semi-rigid mask

With a mask for gas delivery some O_2 will accumulate in the dead space of the mask between breaths where it provides a small reservoir of supplemental O_2 for the next inspiration. The delivered F_IO_2 will again vary with flow rates and the patient's pattern of breathing, but is independent of mouth versus nose breathing. There is minimal potential for CO_2 rebreathing and this can be avoided by use of flow rates ≥ 4 L/min which adequately flushes expired air from the mask dead space between respirations.

Table 25.1 gives approximate F_IO_2 derived from nasal prongs or a semi-rigid mask for given flow rates for patients breathing at rest.

With both standard semi-rigid masks and nasal prongs the oxygen supply should incorporate a method of humidifying the otherwise very dry gas source, as this helps minimize patient discomfort.

Venturi-type high flow masks

This variant on a standard semi-rigid mask uses the oxygen flow to entrain a larger volume of room air via a special valve. The Venturi effect of the resultant mix delivers a fixed F_IO_2 across most inspiratory flow rates (≤ 50 L/min) with only low O_2 flows required (4–8 L/min). Valves are available to deliver F_IO_2 of 0.24, 0.28, 0.31, 0.35, 0.40 and 0.50, (±5%) (c.f. room air F_IO_2 = 0.21). The high delivered flow rate eliminates CO_2 rebreathing and the entrainment of room air avoids the necessity for a humidifier in the O_2 circuit.

Other

Some patients with severe pulmonary congestion will require O_2 supplementation beyond that provided by the aforementioned standard systems. Special supply valves can provide flows of up to 30 L/min, although this is a relatively inefficient method of delivery. An alternative is the incorporation of a soft reservoir between the O_2 supply and the mask, allowing patients to breathe directly from the O_2 reservoir with relatively little entrainment of room air and hence delivery of a high F_IO_2. With such circuits there is a significant potential for CO_2 rebreathing unless a one-way valve is used to prevent the return of expiratory gases to the reservoir.

In certain circumstances positive pressure can be added to the gas circuit to facilitate respiration and reduce/reverse the tendency for formation of pulmonary interstitial and alveolar oedema. This is most commonly done with a CPAP circuit, of which there are a number of variants.

Hyperbaric oxygen

An extension on the routine use of supplemental O_2 is seen with the application of pharmacological concentrations of O_2 in the form of hyperbaric O_2 (HBO). Although this would generally be considered an experimental therapy some data exists to support its use. Animal data show marked increases in PaO_2 with reduction in coronary sinus lactate consistent with improvement in myocardial ischaemia. However, increases in peripheral resistance and decreases in cardiac output have also been observed.[4]

In the pre-thrombolysis era several small trials demonstrated favourable outcomes with HBO therapy. One randomized study of HBO (at two atmospheres) in 208 patients with AMI showed rapid symptom improvement and earlier resolution of ECG changes, with lower mortality in the treated group (16% versus 22%).[5] More recently Thomas et al, using a dog model of AMI, found that HBO in conjunction with TPA thrombolysis was able to prevent irreversible damage of 97% of the myocardium at risk, compared with only 29% salvage with TPA alone.[6] Only preliminary human data are available and have yet to be published in a peer-reviewed format.

HBO has also been applied as a prognostic aid in the post-infarct setting in conjunction with biplane transoesophageal ECHO to demonstrate improved contraction in hibernating myocardium.[7]

Use of oxygen

Oxygen is a drug and its use should be along the lines of any other frequently administered therapeutic agent. That is, it

Table 25.1 Delivered concentration of inspired oxygen (F_IO_2) with nasal prongs and semi-rigid mask with varying flow rates of 100% oxygen

Nasal prongs					
Flow rate (L/min)	1	1.5	2	2.5	3
F_IO_2 (%)	27	31	34	38	42
Hudson mask					
Flow rate (L/min)	2	4	6	8	10
F_IO_2 (%)	28	35	43	50	~60

should have a specific indication, method of administration, and dose (flow rate), with monitoring of response (e.g. oximetry) and stated end point (e.g. relief of angina).

The principal indication for continuous O_2 should be the relief of known (or presumed) hypoxia. It is also used intermittently in certain circumstances for the relief of temporary symptoms (that is, short-lived angina in the absence of significant hypoxia). As O_2 is generally treating the consequence of some underlying problem the physician needs to give consideration to the differential diagnosis of hypoxaemia. As well as the aforementioned cardiac causes a number of other conditions can cause dyspnoea and/or hypoxia (see Table 25.2).

The degree of hypoxaemia is generally easily assessed by the use of oximetry (via finger stall or ear probes). This only gives O_2 saturation and not O_2 carriage, the latter being critically dependent on the haemoglobin level. Assessment of arterial blood gases (O_2, CO_2, pH, etc.) is indicated if there is any doubt as to the accuracy of oximetry (for example, under-recording in the setting of poor peripheral perfusion/low cardiac output states). It is also necessary in any case where the possibility of significant CO_2 retention occurs (e.g. chronic obstructive lung disease).

Hypoxaemia without CO_2 retention

For empirical use in demonstrated or presumed mild hypoxaemia, O_2 should be given at low flows by either nasal prongs (2 L/min) or simple mask (4 L/min).

In more severe cases (PaO_2 $\leq$60 mmHg or SaO_2 $\leq$90%) a mask with flows of 6–12 L/min will generally be necessary, and should be titrated to the patient's requirements as determined by regular SaO_2 monitoring. In patients with more extreme dyspnoea, systems with a reservoir circuit or high flow systems may be needed.

Moderate hypoxaemia with CO_2 retention

Some patients with chronic lung disease are dependent on a degree of hypoxaemia to provide ongoing respiratory drive. In these patients the administration of excessive O_2 therapy may be associated with severe respiratory depression, increasing CO_2 retention, acidosis, exacerbation of any cardiac dysfunction, arrhythmias, and in some instances, death. The aim of therapy is thus to provide only sufficient O_2 supplementation to partially relieve moderate to severe hypoxia, without removing ongoing respiratory drive. This is best achieved by controlled F_IO_2 with a Venturi-type mask with initially 24% or 28% O_2 delivery. As these patients are generally on the steep portion of the Hb-O_2 dissociation curve, even small increases in PaO_2 will be associated with significant improvement in O_2 content and tissue oxygenation. The endpoint of O_2 in these patients should generally be only a PaO_2 ~60 mmHg (SaO_2 ~90%).

Severe hypoxaemia or CO_2 retention

In extreme instances respiration is inadequate to continue to support life. Sometimes ventilation can be supported temporarily with CPAP masks while the underlying problem (such as severe pulmonary oedema) is brought under urgent control. If this is inadequate or if there is associated severe respiratory depression or impairment of conscious state then controlled ventilation is indicated.

Table 25.2 Causes of dyspnoea, and possibility of hypoxaemia

Cause	Hypoxaemia
Anxiety	Absent
Anaemia	Absent
Metabolic acidosis	Absent
Low cardiac output states	Variable
Left heart failure/high LVEDP	Usually present
Primary pulmonary disease	Present
Pulmonary embolism	Present

Oxygen measurement

Clinical assessment of blood oxygenation is relatively inaccurate. Indirect indices of the consequences of hypoxaemia, such as heart and respiratory rates, may be useful in certain circumstances. However, in the setting of the coronary care patient, the ischaemic process (particularly if anterior) itself, pain and anxiety may stimulate sympathetically mediated tachycardia. Conversely, inferior ischaemia or the negatively chronotropic effects of beta blockers and some calcium channel blockers can cause bradycardia and mask the effect of significant hypoxaemia. Narcotic analgesics and sedatives can suppress respiratory rate despite the presence of hypoxia, whereas anxiety and pain can drive respiration independently of adequate oxygenation. The detection of cyanosis is an unreliable and insensitive sign of hypoxaemia in clinical practice.

Oxygen is also a 'drug', and as such, the general principle of only using enough of the drug to correct the problem should apply. In excessive doses, oxygen is toxic. High inspired oxygen concentrations can cause local pulmonary damage, with non-cardiogenic pulmonary oedema, hyaline membrane formation and ultimately pulmonary fibrosis in severe cases. These changes can be first recognized within 48–72 hours of continuous exposure to inspired oxygen fractions (F_IO_2) of >60%. There is also potential systemic toxicity with increasing peripheral resistance and the increased propensity to the formation of oxygen free radicals. These free radicals are known to be involved in the genesis of reperfusion injury in the myocardium and other tissues. The exact role that supplemental oxygen may have in exacerbating reperfusion injury is however still conjectural.

Pulse oximetry

Non-invasive measurement of blood oxygenation is now routinely done via transcutaneous pulse oximetry.[8]

Pulse oximeters rely on differential spectrophotometric absorption of light wavelengths by different species of haemoglobin. Normal blood contains four species of haemoglobin, namely oxyhaemoglobin (HbO_2), deoxygenated haemoglobin (Hb), carboxyhaemoglobin (COHb) and methaemoglobin (MetHb). The latter two usually exist only in low concentration (i.e. <2%).

Current pulse oximeters usually derive functional oxygen saturation, as given by:

$$\text{Functional } SaO_2 = HbO_2 / HbO_2 + Hb,$$

and this represents the percentage of available haemoglobin loaded with O_2. The true fractional oxygen saturation is a more precise measure and corrects for haemoglobin unavailable for O_2 binding (i.e. COHb and MetHb). If significant proportions of these forms are present, then the functional SaO_2 will overestimate O_2 content.

Current generation pulse oximeters emit red (660 nm) and infrared (940 nm) wavelength lights. Absorption of the light occurs in tissue, capillarovenous blood and arterial/arteriolar blood. The oximeter measures absorbance with high frequency (30+times/sec) and can thus separate the absorption into non-pulsatile and pulsatile (AC) components (see Fig. 25.2).

The AC component is that attributable to arterial absorption. HbO_2 and Hb have different absorbances of light at the red and infrared wavelengths.

By determining the ratio of AC to BC absorption at each wavelength the relative proportion of HbO_2 to Hb is measured, and this is empirically related to functional SaO_2

Sources of error[9,10]

In situations of significant peripheral vasoconstriction there is a reduction in arterial flow and hence the relative amount of AC to BC absorption. The other source of 'pulsatile' variation in

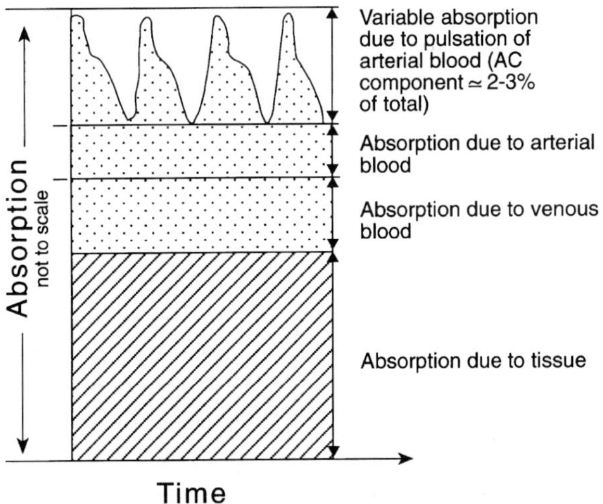

Fig. 25.2 Pulsatile or alternating component (AC) and non-pulsatile or background components (BC) of tissue light absorption.

absorption is that of the irregular effect of motion artefact. As the AC component is only a small percentage of the total, any distortion of this can markedly reduce the accuracy of the SaO_2. In circumstances where the pulse oximeter's oscillation (a bar graph display of the AC component) appears inadequate and/or the oximeter is not able to track heart rate accurately (compared to simultaneous ECG monitoring) one must doubt the reliability of SaO_2. Correlation with clinical indices and/or arterial blood gas estimation is recommended. New generation oximeters that incorporate an ECG-triggered gating mechanism are becoming available, and may help overcome the aforementioned problems.

Carboxyhaemoglobin is normally present in only low levels. Smokers however are reported to have up to 10–12% COHb, thus reducing their maximum blood O_2 content by a similar amount. Heavy exposures to car and certain types of smoke fumes can lead to significant elevation in COHb levels. COHb absorbs red wavelengths in a fashion similar to HbO_2; however, there is little absorption of infrared light. The effect of this is that standard oximeters will overestimate SaO_2. For a level of COHb ~10% this will be of ~2–3% saturation.

Methaemoglobin is formed by the oxidation of the ferrous (Fe^{++}) component of haem to ferric (Fe^{+++}). Background levels are usually <1–2%. Significant elevations can be seen in association with exposure to some drugs, particularly in patients who may have mild (and hence undiagnosed) congenital methaemoglobinaemia. The main drugs of concern in coronary care are the nitrates such as nitroglycerine. MetHb has a much greater absorbance at 660 nm than any of the other forms; hence as MetHb levels increase, the ratio of absorption will tend towards 1.0, which corresponds to an SaO_2 of 85%. In severe cases the patient will appear cyanosed, but has normal PaO_2 and is not improved by supplemental O_2 administration. Treatment is with the reducing agent methylene blue.

Occasionally external light sources can cause optical interference with the oximetry probe's photocells. Bright sunlight (uncommon in the CCU), surgical lamps, fluorescent lights and infrared heating lamps may lead to swamping of the photocell and inability to track pulsatile variation in light absorption. This situation can be easily remedied by covering over the oximetry probe.

Skin and nail pigmentation may reduce the accuracy of oximetry. This is presumed to be due to a reduction in the AC:BC ratio caused by the pigment. Dark nail varnishes (black, blue and green) can result in mild under-reading of SaO_2 by 3–6%. Use of the finger stall probe in a side-to-side manner (rather than front-to-back) overcomes this.

Arterial blood gas analysis

Direct measurement of blood gas content has necessitated arterial puncture, usually of the radial artery. Often in patients on intravenous heparin, and/or receiving thrombolytic therapy, there can be significant morbidity associated with arterial puncture(s), and hence this is now generally reserved for specific cases (see above).

Traditional analysis involves direct measure of pH, and the partial pressures of oxygen (PaO_2) and carbon dioxide ($PaCO_2$). Other parameters, including SaO_2, have been derived via inbuilt nomograms based on a number of assumptions, particularly to do with the shape of the Hb-O_2 dissociation curve.[8] The utility of PaO_2 is mainly in assessing changes on the plateau phase of the Hb-O_2 curve, as once SaO_2 is greater than 92% further increases are relatively small despite large changes in oxygenation. In this region PaO_2 is a more sensitive indicator, particularly of changes in gas exchange.

It must be remembered also that O_2 carriage may be severely compromised by anaemia with entirely normal PaO_2 and SaO_2, and functional Hb is necessary to determine arterial blood O_2 content.

New blood gas analysers are becoming available that directly measure SaO_2. Some also have the capacity to measure the concentrations of oxygenated and deoxygenated haemoglobin as well as abnormal isoforms (see above).

A further advantage of direct measurement of O_2 tension is in the estimation of efficiency of gas exchange at the alveolar level. Disturbance of alveolar function, either directly or due to alteration from optimal ventilation perfusion matching, will be reflected in an increased alveolar to arterial O_2 gradient ($P_{A\text{-}a}O_2$). This is calculated according to the formula

$$P_{A\text{-}a}O_2 = (149 - P_aCO_2/RQ) - PaO_2$$

where RQ = Respiratory Quotient and is assumed to be 0.8 in most circumstances, but can vary between 0.7 and 1.0 depending on metabolic substrate (carbohydrate or protein and fat respectively), and 149 is the partial pressure of oxygen in dry inspired air at sea level. Disturbances in ventilation-perfusion matching are the commonest cause of elevated $P_{A\text{-}a}O_2$. Less commonly one can see pure diffusion block or intrapulmonary shunt that increase the O_2 gradient.

Pulmonary thromboembolism is a common diagnostic possibility in patients presenting with chest pain, and can be a complicating factor in coronary care and surgical admissions (see Ch. 72). One characteristic feature is the presence of an elevated $P_{A\text{-}a}O_2$.

Functional indices of tissue perfusion

The measurement of oxygen tension or saturation is only indirectly relevant. The ideal parameter is one that reflects the tissue effect of O_2 or its lack. Tissue oxygenation may be adequate over a large range of delivered O_2 at rest, but conversely may be inadequate at normal O_2 deliveries in certain high demand states—for example, sepsis. Inadequate tissue oxygen delivery leads to anaerobic metabolism with lactate formation and hence acidosis. Arterial blood gases measure pH as an indirect measure of acidosis, but the more relevant figure is the base deficit, reflecting the metabolic component of acid balance (that is, removing any element of either concurrent respiratory acidosis or possibility of underestimating metabolic acidosis because of respiratory compensation). Occasionally metabolic acidosis can be driven by non-hypoxaemic means such as uraemia and certain toxins. In this circumstance measurement of arterial lactate may be feasible and will give more direct information about the adequacy of tissue oxygenation.

References

1. Fillmore SJ, Shapiro M, Killip T. Arterial oxygen tension in acute myocardial infarction. Am Heart J 1970;79:620–4
2. Evans SM, Richardson M, DeSomer EA, Barter C, Hockings BEF. Supplemental oxygen in uncomplicated myocardial infarction. Abst. Aust NZ J Med 1993;23:65
3. Madias JE, Hood WB. Reduction of precordial ST segment elevation in patients with anterior myocardial infarction by oxygen breathing. Circulation 1976;53:198–201
4. Cameron AJV, Hutton I, Kenmure ACF, Murdoch WR. Haemodynamic and metabolic effects of hyperbaric oxygen in myocardial infarction. Lancet 1966; I: 833–7
5. Thurston JGB, Greenwood TW, Bending MR, Connor H, Curmen MP. A controlled investigation into the effects of hyperbaric oxygen on mortality following acute myocardial infarction. Quart J Med 1973; 42: 751–70
6. Thomas MP, Brown LA, Sponseller DR, Williamson SE et al. Myocardial infarct size reduction by the synergistic effect of hyperbaric oxygen and tissue plasminogen activator. Am Heart J 1990; 120: 791–800
7. Swift PC, Turner JH, Oxer HF, O'Shea JP. Myocardial hibernation identified by hyperbaric oxygen treatment and echocardiography in post infarction patients. Am Heart J 1992;124:1151–8
8. Sykes MK, Vickers MD, Hull CJ. Acid-base, blood gas and other analysers used by clinicians. In: Principles of measurement and monitoring in anaesthesia and intensive care. Oxford: Blackwell Scientific, 1991:250–77
9. Clayton D, Webb RK, Ralston AC, Duthie D, Runciman WB. A comparison of the performance of twenty pulse oximeters under conditions of poor perfusion. Anaesthesia 1991;46:3–10
10. Ralston AC, Webb RK, Runciman WB. Potential errors in pulse oximetry. I: Effects of interference, dyes, dyshaemoglobins and other pigments. Anaesthesia 1991; 46: 291–5

26 Analgesic agents

P Vernon van Heerden

Introduction

'Pain is an unpleasant sensory and emotional experience associated with actual or potential tissue damage, or described in terms of such damage'.[1] Pain is a common problem in the coronary care unit (CCU), and its effective relief is an important responsibility of the CCU staff.

Besides the distress caused to the patient, there are other adverse aspects of pain which relate to extensive biochemical changes. These biochemical changes are due to the stress response evoked by the pain. Hawker[2] gives a full description of the stress response in the very ill patient.

The stress response induced by pain will result in activation of the sympathetic nervous system (SNS). In the patient in the CCU this may increase myocardial oxygen demand by increasing heart rate (reducing diastolic perfusion time of the left ventricle), blood pressure and myocardial contractility.[3] These changes will predispose to ongoing myocardial ischaemia and potentiate the pain associated with ischaemia. Histological evidence of myocardial damage has been shown in the animal model following an exaggerated stress response.[4]

Correct and effective treatment of pain will go some way to ameliorating the physiological responses which may impact on cardiac morbidity.

Assessment of pain

The experience of pain is entirely subjective, with a wide inter-patient variation in the perception of pain. Assessment and measurement of pain is therefore not an exact process, but relies on:

- *clinical assessment*, i.e. taking a history and examining the patient
- using simple measures, such as an *analogue score*, where a patient grades the pain experienced on a linear scale on which a score of zero indicates 'no pain' and a score of ten indicates the 'worst pain imaginable'. The analogue score has been shown to be highly reliable and reproducible[5]
- judging the *response to therapeutic measures*, for example, the patient reporting subjective relief after a dose of analgesic.

The patient's ranking of pain severity should be recorded during each episode of pain and again after attempts have been made to treat it.

Despite the subjectivity of the experience of pain, it is important to make a careful assessment of the patient in pain in order to be able to treat the pain effectively and avoid its pathological sequelae.

Methods of treatment of the patient in pain

The effective treatment of pain relies on non-pharmacological as well as pharmacological measures.

Non-pharmacological treatment

Adjunctive therapy

Empathic care by medical and nursing staff in a tranquil environment are very useful precursors to effective pain management. These will reduce the anxiety which is an almost invariable accompaniment of severe pain. This is all the more so when the emotive nature of cardiac disease is considered. Adjunctive measures such as bed-rest and effective oxygen therapy are also important. Once these measures are in place, the main thrust of management should be to treat the cause of the pain if possible.

While the cause of pain is sought and treated, pharmacological measures of pain control are employed (see below).

Treating the cause of pain

In the patient with coronary artery disease this process relies on correcting the imbalance between myocardial oxygen supply and demand. Supply may be improved by increasing circulating oxygen content (CaO_2) by optimizing plasma haemoglobin concentration and oxygen saturation (SaO_2). Ultimately myocardial oxygen supply may need to be assured by coronary artery dilatation (e.g. with calcium channel blockers or nitrates), thrombolysis, angioplasty or revascularization. Myocardial oxygen demand may also be reduced by non-specific measures (see 'Adjunctive therapy' above) and by specific treatment of tachycardia/tachyarrhythmias and hypertension with beta blockers.

Patients with pain of non-cardiac origin should similarly have the cause of the pain investigated and treated to avoid cardiac morbidity in the patient at risk. All potentially painful procedures in the patient with coronary artery disease should be undertaken with due regard for the risk/benefit ratio of the procedure and only after careful planning for adequate analgesia and anxiolysis during and after the procedure.

Pharmacological treatment of pain

The following relates mainly to the acute treatment of pain of cardiac origin and not to the treatment of other pain which may impact on the cardiovascular system. Considerations of chronic management of pain of cardiac origin, such as the indications for stellate ganglion blockade, are outside the ambit of this chapter. Management of pain in the post-cardiac surgical patient is discussed elsewhere.

Parenteral analgesics

The mainstay of analgesic therapy in the CCU patient is the opioid group of drugs, typified by morphine. These drugs all act at the opioid mu, kappa and delta receptors in the central nervous system (spinal and supraspinal).[6] The effects of morphine acting at the mu receptors are well known, and include:[7]

- spinal and supraspinal analgesia
- euphoria
- respiratory depression
- depression of gut motility
- meiosis
- dependence
- catalepsy
- bradycardia.

The safety of this group of drugs in the cardiac patient is borne out by the use of opioids in high dosage in the anaesthetic management of the cardiac surgical patient.[8] Side-effects include:[9]

- respiratory depression and loss of airway reflexes (if excessive sedation occurs)
- constipation and delayed gastric emptying
- nausea and vomiting
- dependence
- dysphoria
- hypotension (particularly in the elderly and in hypovolaemic patients) due to venous and arterial dilatation
- sedation
- tolerance to opioids
- urine retention.

Morphine and the semi-synthetic and synthetic opioids may all be used to good effect in the control of pain in the patient with coronary artery disease. Although there are many possible routes of administration of these drugs (for example: intrathecal, extradural, oral, transnasal, transcutaneous) the intravenous route of administration is the most useful in terms of titratability and safety in the CCU. The intramuscular route should be avoided because of delayed and unpredictable absorption, possible spurious rises in muscle enzyme levels in the plasma and increased risk of haematomata with thrombolytic therapy.

Intravenous (IV) administration may be further refined to:

- Intermittent IV administration. The simplest and most widely used method of administration: small, repeated doses (e.g. 1–2 mg of morphine) are titrated to analgesic effect, while avoiding unwanted side-effects, such as respiratory depression, which are possible after a large single dose.
- Continuous IV administration. A technique useful for prolonged or severe pain, continuous IV administration is safely performed using a dilute solution of drug (e.g. 1 mg/ml of morphine delivered via an infusion pump). An initial loading dose (Ld) (e.g. up to 0.1 mg/kg of morphine) is titrated intravenously

over 5 or 10 minutes. Once an adequate level of analgesia is obtained, as described under 'Assessment of pain' above, an infusion is commenced. The infusion rate is titrated upwards or downwards depending on the level of analgesia required, the upper limit being defined by the appearance of unwanted side-effects. In some circumstances, patient-controlled analgesia (PCA) may offer advantages over intermittent or continuous 'nurse-controlled' analgesia.

The side-effects posing the most danger to patients are respiratory depression and hypotension, particularly when associated with bradycardia. Careful monitoring of cardiovascular and respiratory parameters, as is usual in this group of patients in a CCU, is required to detect these side-effects before they pose a threat to patient safety. Monitoring should include an assessment of the level of analgesia (e.g. using an analogue score).

Morphine is the preferred opiate analgesic in the CCU. However, it has potential vagotonic properties which may accentuate a pre-existing tendency to bradycardia, as may occur with inferior myocardial infarction. In this situation pethidine (meperidine) may be used (see Table 26.1).

The specific antagonist, naloxone, which will rapidly reverse the respiratory depression and sedation associated with these drugs, should be readily available whenever opioids are administered. It should be noted that its duration of action is shorter than that of both morphine and pethidine and the patient should be carefully monitored for the possible return of potentially dangerous opioid side-effects. The usual dose of naloxone is 0.4 mg intravenously.

The nausea and vomiting associated with opioid administration can be very distressing, but can usually be controlled with antiemetics such as metoclopramide (10 mg IV).

Table 26.1 Comparison of morphine and pethidine (meperidine)

	Morphine	Pethidine
Respiratory depression	++	++
Vagal effect	vagotonic	vagolytic
Constipation	++	+
Nausea and vomiting	++	+++
Equipotent dose	0.1 mg/kg	1 mg/kg

Oral analgesics

For less severe pain, the oral route is effective. The most widely used agent is paracetamol, either alone in a dose of 500–1000 mg as necessary, or in combination with codeine. Paracetamol has no gastric or cardiac effects of note and does not interfere with warfarin therapy. In high doses it can cause hepatic necrosis and fulminant hepatic failure. The maximum daily dose should not exceed 5 g.

Inhalational analgesics

Short-acting analgesic agents administered via the inhalational route, such as nitrous oxide (N_2O) and methoxyflurane, are useful for the control of pain during short painful procedures. Side-effects such as euphoria and drowsiness may accompany the use of Entonox (N_2O 50% and O_2 50%), but these are rapidly reversed upon cessation of drug administration. These agents may be safely self-administered via facemask or mouthpiece. Careful patient monitoring during drug administration is required to avoid a depressed level of consciousness.

Adjunctive pharmacological therapy

Non-steroidal anti-inflammatory drugs (NSAIDS) are useful in certain conditions (e.g. pericarditis, fractured ribs post cardio pulmonary resuscitation, post-myocardial infarction syndrome, etc.).

The addition of *anxiolytics*, usually from the benzodiazepine group of minor tranquillizers, may reduce the requirement for opioid analgesics, but should never be used as a substitute for adequate analgesia.

The *major tranquillizers* should be used with caution in this group of patients because of the association with severe ventricular arrhythmias of some members of this group of drugs.[10]

Low doses of *cyclic anti-depressants* can often assist in the control of chronic pain.

Local or regional analgesia using local anaesthetic agents can sometimes be considered in the patient with intractable chest wall pain, where other causes of pain have been excluded and where the routine analgesic measures have not been effective.

Most pain is effectively managed by the attending team, but consultation with anaesthetic/pain management colleagues may be required when pain is difficult to control.

Conclusion

Comprehensive treatment of pain in the patient with cardiac disease involves more than choosing and administering an analgesic. Pathophysiological mechanisms in the genesis of the pain are considered, cardiovascular conditions optimized and appropriate treatment to counter the cardiovascular pathology embarked on prior to the considered introduction of appropriate analgesic agents. Familiarity with a small number of analgesic agents which are safe, simple to administer and of proven benefit is desirable. Addressing the anxiety component of pain is essential to good analgesic management.

References

1. Merskey H, Bonica JJ, Carmon A, Dubner R et al. Pain terms: a list with definitions and notes on usage. Pain 1979; 6: 249–52
2. Hawker F. Endocrine changes in the critically ill. British Journal of Hospital Medicine 1988; 39(4): 278–91
3. Drasner K, Katz JA, Schapera A. Control of pain and anxiety. In: Hall JB, Schmidt GA, Wood LDH (eds). Principles of critical care. New York: McGraw-Hill, 1992: 958–73
4. Novitzky D, Horak A, Cooper DK, Rose AG. Electrocardiographic and histopathologic changes developing during experimental brain death in the baboon. Transplant Proc 1989; 21(1): 2567–9
5. Chapman CR, Casey KL, Dubner R et al. Pain measurement: an overview. Pain 1985; 22: 1–31
6. Atcheson R, Lambert DG. Update on opioid receptors. British Journal of Anaesthesia 1994; 73: 132–4
7. Mather LE. Pharmacology of opioids. I. Basic aspects. Med J Aust 1986; 144: 474–541
8. Reiz S, Mangano DT. Anaesthesia and cardiac disease. In: Nimmo WS, Smith G (eds). Anaesthesia. Oxford: Blackwell Scientific, 1989: 875–7
9. Mather LE. Analgesic drugs. In: Nimmo WS, Smith G (eds). Anaesthesia. Oxford: Blackwell Scientific, 1989: 73–104
10. Zeifman CWE, Friedman B. Torsade de pointes: potential consequences of intravenous haloperidol in the intensive care unit. Intensive Careworld 1994; 11(3): 109–12

27 Antiarrhythmic drugs

Terence J Campbell

Antiarrhythmic drugs

Since the advent of coronary care units, antiarrhythmic drugs have formed the mainstay of the treatment of tachyarrhythmias, and a detailed understanding of the available agents is essential for those working in the field. Such an understanding must also include an awareness of the now well-demonstrated potential for these agents to aggravate or provoke arrhythmias, as well as their ability to treat them. These issues form the subject matter of the present chapter.

The cardiac action potential

Each heartbeat is triggered by a cardiac action potential, of which there are two fundamentally different types in the mammalian heart (see Ch. 9, Fig. 9.1). The first of these is seen with minor variations in working myocardium throughout the heart (atrium, ventricle and Purkinje fibre). The second is confined to the small but very important pacemaking cells of the sino-atrial node and the atrioventricular node. These nodes are truly automatic; they are modulated by nervous and hormonal inputs, but not dependent on them.

Antiarrhythmic drugs—classification

Any discussion of antiarrhythmic drugs, and particularly of the mechanisms by which they are thought to act, is complicated by our relatively sparse knowledge of the detailed causes of arrhythmias. This subject is dealt with in detail in Chapter 9, and some of the aspects of particular relevance to antiarrhythmic agents will also be covered later in this chapter. Let us consider first the way in which these agents are usually subclassified.

There have been many attempts in the last two decades to classify the growing number of antiarrhythmic agents, the most recent being an extremely complex schema, the so-called 'Sicilian Gambit'.[1] The classification proposed by Vaughan Williams[2,3] is the most widely used of these at present, and will provide the loose framework for our discussion (see Tables 27.1 and 27.2; Fig. 27.1).

It is important to note that this classification is based on the actions of the drugs and it is thus possible for one agent to exhibit more than one class of action. Indeed this is common, and the placing of drugs into particular classes for convenience is based on a judgment as to which is the most important action and sometimes on the historical sequence in which these actions were described.

Class I agents

The major effect of class I agents is to block the fast inward sodium

Table 27.1 Classification of antiarrhythmic drugs

	Drugs	Action
Class I	Quinidine, procainamide, disopyramide, lignocaine, mexiletine, flecainide	Block fast sodium current
Class II	Beta blockers	Block effects of catecholamines
Class III	Amiodarone, sotalol (D-sotalol, dofetilide, etc.)	Prolong action potential duration by blocking potassium current
Class IV	Verapamil, diltiazem	Block calcium current

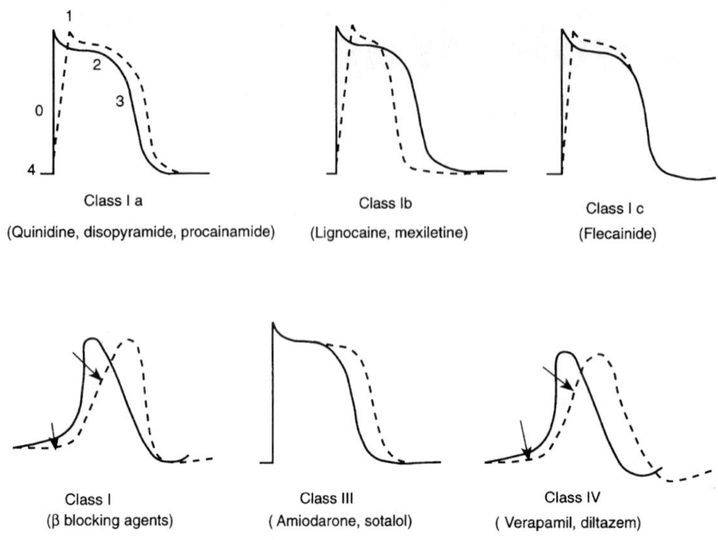

Fig. 27.1 The dominant effects of the three sub-classes of class I and of class III antiarrhythmic agents on typical ventricular action potentials and the effects of class II and class IV antiarrhythmic agents on typical sino-atrial or atrioventricular nodal action potentials. All class I agents block the fast inward sodium current which reduces the maximum rate of depolarization of phase 0. This in turn leads to a slowing of action potential conduction through the myocardium. For purposes of illustration the effect is grossly exaggerated in these diagrams. In addition to this the class Ia agents tend to prolong the action potential duration (APD), the class Ib agents tend to shorten APD and the class Ic agents have little or no effect on APD. Class II agents tend to reduce the slopes both of spontaneous diastolic depolarization and of phase 0 of pacemaker action potentials as illustrated. This is an indirect action due to blockade of the facilitating effect of catecholamines on the inward calcium current which is a component of both diastolic depolarization and phase 0 depolarization in these cells. Class III antiarrhythmic agents block the outward potassium current responsible for repolarization leading to a prolongation of APD. Class IV antiarrhythmic agents directly block inward calcium currents and thus have effects similar in nature but usually more marked than those seen with the class II agents.

Table 27.2 Subgroups of class I drugs

Class	Drugs	Effects on action potential	Summary of clinical effects
Ia	Quinidine, procainamide, disopyramide	Reduce rate of depolarization and prolong duration of action potential	Moderate slowing of cardiac conduction. Prolongation of refractory periods
Ib	Lignocaine, mexiletine	Reduce rate of depolarization selectively in ischaemic cells. Shorten action potential duration	Selective depression of ischaemic tissue. May shorten refractory periods
Ic	Flecainide, encainide	Marked depression of depolarization rate	Marked slowing of cardiac conduction. Small increase in refractory periods

current responsible for the fast upstroke and conduction of the action potential in atrial, ventricular and Purkinje cells[4] (see Fig. 27.1). This is also known as 'local anaesthetic' or 'membrane stabilizing' action. These drugs also tend to depress normal automaticity, particularly in Purkinje fibres. Class I comprises a large group of antiarrhythmic agents, many with different clinical electrophysiological properties. Table 27.2 is an attempt to subclassify some of these agents into homogeneous subgroups commonly referred to as class Ia, Ib and Ic.[3]

Class II agents

It is a common observation that arrhythmias are more frequently seen in the presence of enhanced sympathetic tone, which leads to both an increase in automaticity and a reduction in refractory periods and may facilitate potential re-entrant circuits. These conditions pertain particularly in the setting of acute myocardial infarction (AMI). The class II antiarrhythmic drugs, which are the beta-adrenergic blocking agents, are thought to exert their antiarrhythmic properties largely indirectly, by blocking these proarrhythmic effects of catecholamines.

In addition, because the slowly conducting calcium channel-dependent action potentials of the normal sino-atrial and atrioventricular nodes rely to some extent on sympathetic tone, class II drugs tend to depress conduction through these specialized tissues and to depress their automaticity. This can lead to bradycardia and heart block.

Class III agents

Drugs exhibiting this third class of action prolong the refractory period by increasing the duration of the cardiac action potential (especially phases 2 and 3; Fig. 27.1). This effect is produced largely by blockade of the major outward repolarizing current in these cells which is carried by potassium and commonly referred to as i_K. Repolarization is however a complex process involving a number of other poorly understood potassium channels, and the possibility that clinically important differences between class III antiarrhythmic agents may relate to differential effects on these various potassium channels is currently the subject of intense research.[5–7] Amiodarone and sotalol are the prototypes of class III and remain the only examples in widespread clinical use today, although a number of newer class III agents are currently at various stages of pre-clinical and clinical trials.

Class IV drugs

Class IV drugs ('calcium antagonists' or 'calcium channel blockers'), act by blocking the slow inward calcium current responsible for the slow upstroke and conduction of the action potentials of sino-atrial and atrioventricular nodal cells[4] (see Fig. 27.1). They therefore tend to suppress pacemaking activity in these cells, and can lead to bradycardia and heart block. As one would expect, re-entrant arrhythmias involving these calcium channel-dependent pathways are commonly aborted by these drugs.

Verapamil is the prototype for this class of drug. Diltiazem, which is currently used extensively for the management of hypertension and ischaemic heart disease, has similar antiarrhythmic properties, but is not widely used at present as an antiarrhythmic agent, although it is popular in some centres for slowing the ventricular response in atrial fibrillation. Nifedipine and related calcium antagonists have little or no clinically useful effects on myocardial calcium channels and no useful antiarrhythmic properties.

Miscellaneous antiarrhythmic agents (adenosine, digoxin)

A number of agents used for their antiarrhythmic properties do not fall within the Vaughan Williams classification. Two of these include adenosine and digoxin. Digoxin is reviewed in Chapter 31, and will not be further dealt with below. It has little or no direct antiarrhythmic properties of its own but is commonly a useful agent for slowing the ventricular rate in patients with atrial fibrillation or atrial tachycardia. It does this largely indirectly by enhancing the vagal tone on the atrioventricular node. This is a central nervous system effect primarily.

Adenosine is an endogenous nucleoside that is capable of causing atrioventricular nodal conduction block in humans. It also causes widespread vasodilatation. It seems to act via specific adenosine-sensitive receptors.[8,9]

Cellular electropharmacology of antiarrhythmic agents—antiarrhythmic and proarrhythmic actions

While a detailed coverage of the electrophysiological actions of antiarrhythmic agents is beyond the scope of this text, some understanding of the ways in which these drugs modify cardiac ion channels and action potentials is essential to their rational clinical use. In particular, such an understanding provides a rational basis for the paradoxical observation that many of these agents may be either antiarrhythmic as desired, or proarrhythmic in different patients. Indeed in some cases they may manifest both types of action in the same patient. As will be seen below, the majority of the direct cellular electropharmacological effects of antiarrhythmic agents can be considered under only three headings: suppression of automaticity, effects on conduction velocity and effects on refractory period. The reader wishing a deeper understanding of the ionic currents underlying the cardiac action potential is referred to recent reviews.[4,10,11]

Suppression of automaticity

Suppression of automaticity is a relatively simple concept (although the details of the mechanisms are still controversial), and will be dealt with only briefly. Automaticity due to spontaneous diastolic depolarization to a firing threshold is normally present in cells within the sinus and atrioventricular nodes (see Fig. 27.1). The currents involved in producing this phenomenon are both complex and controversial.[4,10,11] This type of automatic activity appears to be contributed to by several different inward and outward currents, and this fact probably explains the fortunate insensitivity of the sinus node to depression by antiarrhythmic drugs.

Automaticity can also arise in Purkinje fibres, particularly as an escape phenomenon, for example in the presence of atrioventricular block. It is then manifest as an action potential very similar to the typical fast upstroke potential seen normally in these cells (see Fig. 27.1), with the addition of spontaneous depolarization during diastole (phase 4). The mechanism in this case appears to be simpler and probably due almost entirely to a single inward current sometimes known as the 'pacemaker current' or I_f. I_f is suppressed by therapeutic concentrations of most class I antiarrhythmic agents. It is probably for this reason that Purkinje fibre automaticity is generally much more susceptible to depression by antiarrhythmic agents than is sinus node automaticity. Nonetheless clinical suppression of the sinus node leading to asystole, particularly in the presence of high vagal tone, commonly seen in the very early phases of AMI, is an uncommon but well-recognized complication of therapy with antiarrhythmic agents such as lignocaine and amiodarone.

Drug effects on conduction

A re-entrant circuit depends for its continuing existence on a fine balance between conduction time around the circuit and the refractory periods of the various components of the re-entrant pathway (see Fig. 27.2).[20] If the conduction time ever falls below the refractory period of part of the circuit then the 'excitable gap' will disappear, the advancing wavefront will meet only refractory tissue, and the arrhythmia will terminate. Theoretically, therefore, an ideal antiarrhythmic agent would tend to accelerate conduction and prolong refractoriness within the substrate for re-entry. Many of the drugs available to clinicians prolong refractory periods in myocardium, but none has been convincingly shown to accelerate conduction in therapeutic use. Almost invariably, in fact, conduction tends to be slowed. It can be seen from Figure 27.2 that this combination of conduction slowing and refractory period prolongation can be either proarrhythmic or antiarrhythmic. With currently available techniques, we really have no way of predicting which of these outcomes is likely for a given drug in a given patient. Of course, if the antiarrhythmic agent is able to reduce conduction velocity to zero at some point in the circuit, then this would always be an antiarrhythmic action. Some antiarrhythmic agents (e.g. lignocaine, amiodarone) show selectivity for depressing conduction in ischaemic or otherwise abnormal myocardium, so it is conceivable that a complete conduction block through an ischaemic segment of a re-entrant circuit is the mechanism of arrhythmia termination or prevention in many patients. This could occur without necessarily producing marked slowing of conduction elsewhere in the healthy myocardium.[12,13]

Drug effects on refractoriness

While most clinically useful agents prolong refractoriness, lignocaine, mexiletine and tocainide tend to shorten it, particularly in low concentrations. This latter mechanism may explain some cases of drug-associated arrhythmogenesis in patients with re-entrant tachycardias. Lengthening of refractoriness should in general be antiarrhythmic, but if conduction is slowed simultaneously, the net effect on the re-entrant circuit will determine the outcome (see Fig. 27.2).

Abnormal automaticity due to antiarrhythmic drugs—early afterdepolarizations and torsades de pointes

While the preceding section describes actions of antiarrhythmic agents which had the potential to be either therapeutic or harmful to the patient, the phenomenon to be described below is always an undesirable side-effect of certain antiarrhythmic agents. As noted above, most forms of automaticity known to cause tachyarrhythmia are suppressed by antiarrhythmic drugs. The major exception to this rule is the form of triggered automaticity due to so-called 'early afterdepolarizations' (see Fig. 27.3).

Early afterdepolarizations (EADs) can be defined as a marked slowing of repolarization which is easily visible on the action potential recording, and is due to reduction of the normal repolarizing outward potassium current. If the prolongation of depolarization is long enough, and the voltage conditions appro-

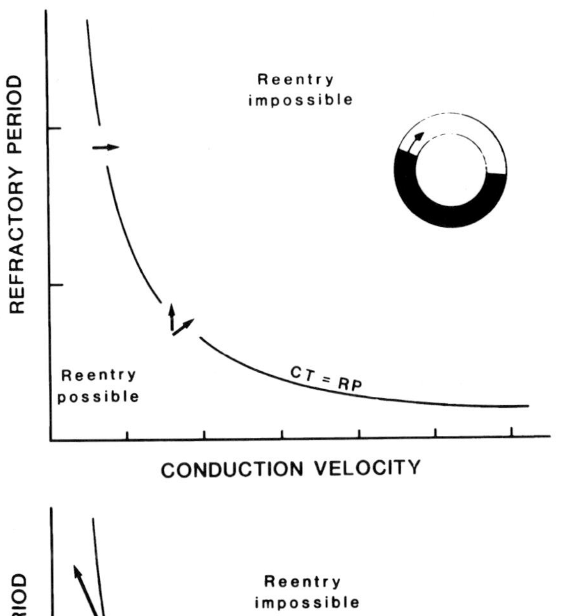

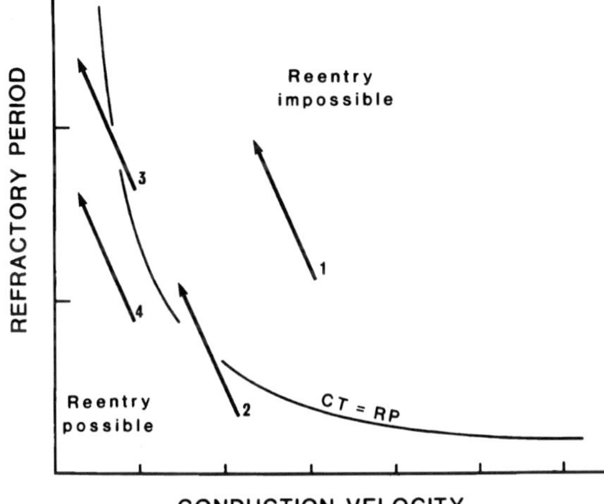

Fig. 27.2 This illustrates the close inter-relationship between the refractory period and the conduction velocity in a classical re-entrant arrhythmia. Refractory period is largely determined by action potential duration (APD) and conduction velocity is largely determined by maximum rate of depolarization of phase 0 and hence can be depressed by sodium channel blocking agents.
The re-entrant circuit depends for its existence on the maintenance of an 'excitable gap' of non-refractory tissue between the advancing wave front and its tail. This is illustrated by the half-shaded circle in the upper right of the figure. The curved arrow represents the direction of propagation of the action potential, and the dark area represents the refractory tissue behind it. This dark area is sometimes referred to as the 'wavelength' of the arrhythmia. The large curves (top and bottom) represent all possible combinations of conduction velocity and refractory period where the conduction time (CT) around the circuit is just equal to the refractory period (RP). For all points on and to the right of this curve, re-entry will be impossible (excitable gap < 0; or wavelength longer than circuit). For all points below and to the left, re-entry will be possible (excitable gap > 0). To have the best chance of moving a patient from the re-entry-possible to the re-entry-impossible side of the curves, an antiarrhythmic should theoretically increase either conduction velocity or refractory period, or both (horizontal, vertical, and diagonal arrows, respectively, in top section). Unfortunately most drugs in clinical use tend to reduce conduction velocity (or have no effect on it) and to increase refractory period (arrows 1 to 4 bottom section). It can be appreciated that whether this leads to an antiarrhythmic (arrow 2), a proarrhythmic (arrow 3), or a 'neutral' effect (arrows 1 and 4) will depend entirely on the initial conditions in the individual patient. In our present state of knowledge, this cannot usually be determined clinically. (Adapted from Aust NZ J Med 1990; 20: 275–82, with permission.)

priate, a series of automatic action potentials may be 'triggered'. The 'upstrokes' of these action potentials are thought to be due to inward current flow through the normal calcium channels which have inactivated, recovered from inactivation and found the membrane potential still in their activation range. They therefore reactivate and produce a secondary upstroke. This elevation of intracellular calcium concentration is then thought to trigger calcium-sensitive potassium channels to open, hence producing an acceleration of repolarization. This process can occur as a single event or as an oscillatory series of action potentials depending on the prevailing conditions of voltage, calcium levels, etc.[14,15]

The induction of early afterdepolarizations by cardioactive agents is currently the subject of intense research, and is thought to be the basis of the drug-induced long QT syndromes and their associated arrhythmias, including 'torsades de pointes'.[16–18] According to this theory, the slowing of repolarization (early afterdepolarization), leads directly to the QT prolongation, often with associated prominent, bizarre T-U waves, and if triggered activity occurs, ventricular tachyarrhythmias result. This idea has largely, though not entirely, replaced an alternative hypothesis which attributed torsades to increased dispersion of refractoriness.[19] The two concepts are not mutually exclusive and it may be that the two mechanisms coexist, or are complementary in some cases.

The class Ia antiarrhythmic agents quinidine, disopyramide and procainamide are all capable

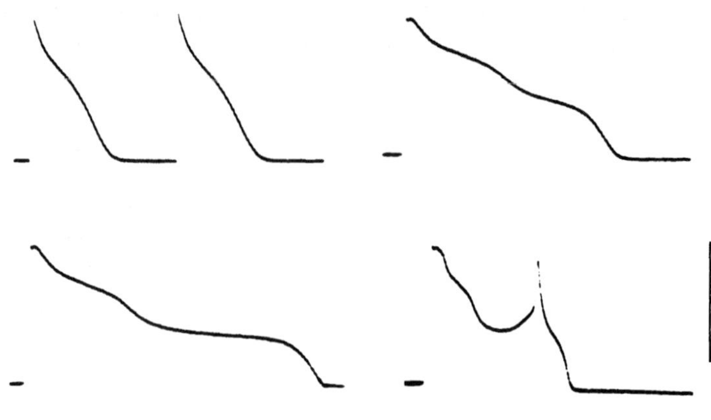

Fig. 27.3 Series of action potentials recorded in the author's laboratory from the same cell in a dog Purkinje fibre at varying times after exposure to quinidine 10μM. The upper left panel shows control action potentials. In this and all other cases the upstroke or phase 0 is not visible due to its high velocity. The remaining panels are potentials recorded from the same cell 10 minutes after exposure to quinidine. The potentials in the upper right and lower left show increasingly marked prolongation of repolarization (early afterdepolarizations, EAD). The potential in the lower right which is actually longer in duration than the others but recorded on a different time scale shows that the EAD is interrupted by a single triggered upstroke before repolarization finally occurs (triggered activity). Note differing baselines: horizontal callibration = 400 milliseconds for upper left, 800 milliseconds for upper right and lower left, and two seconds for lower right potentials. Vertical callibration = 100 mV for all panels.

of producing EADs and have all been reported to cause torsades de pointes.[16] This is also true of the class III drugs amiodarone and sotalol, although the incidence seems somewhat less. The class Ib agents lignocaine, mexiletine and tocainide do not produce EADs (indeed they tend to reverse them) and have not been convincingly reported to cause torsades de pointes. Arrhythmogenesis due to these agents probably relates to effects on conduction or refractoriness discussed above. This seems to be true also of the class Ic compounds which do not usually cause significant slowing of repolarization and have not been definitely shown to cause torsades de pointes. Proarrhythmia appears to be less of an issue with class II and IV drugs. Table 27.3 (p. 232) summarizes some of the information on proarrhythmia discussed above, and a brief clinical perspective of the problem is given below.

Proarrhythmia—clinical implications for antiarrhythmic therapy

The question of ventricular fibrillation and sudden death induced by the therapeutic use of antiarrhythmic agents, specifically quinidine, has been discussed in the literature since at least the 1920s,[20] but it is Selzer and Wray[21] who are usually given credit for making the link between 'quinidine syncope' and ventricular fibrillation, and Dessertenne,[22] who described what has become the classic form of quinidine-induced ventricular arrhythmia, torsades de pointes. Many cases of polymorphic ventricular tachycardia are probably also manifestations of this phenomenon. These early workers also realized what has sometimes been forgotten since, that most cases of quinidine-induced arrhythmia occur at therapeutic or subtherapeutic drug concentrations, and are not due to drug overdosage.

In 1982 the first of a series of papers appeared from Brigham and Womens' Hospital, Boston in which significant worsening of ventricular arrhythmias was documented on 80 of 722 (11.1%) antiarrhythmic drug tests in 155 patients.[23] The frequency of this complication for each of nine agents ranged from 5.9 to 15.8%. Further studies followed, documenting similar phenomena with large numbers of agents tested both non-invasively (ambulatory ECG monitoring) and by programmed ventricular stimulation studies.[24–26]

Quite recently, this message has been graphically reinforced by the results of the Cardiac Arrhythmia Suppression Trial (CAST), from the USA.[27] This large and expensive multicentre trial was funded by the National Heart Lung and Blood Institute. It was a placebo-controlled, randomized study designed to test the hypothesis implicit in the then widespread practice of treating asymptomatic ventricular arrhythmias in survivors of AMI, namely that suppression of the arrhythmias would improve survival. The class Ic drugs flecainide and encainide, and a novel class Ia compound, moricizine, were shown to produce adequate ectopic suppression in the target population, and were chosen as the active agents. In April 1989, the trial's Data and Safety Monitoring Board noted that there had been 56 deaths or non-fatal cardiac arrests among 730 patients assigned to encainide or flecainide and treated for a mean period of 10 months. This was significantly greater than the 22 such events seen in 725 patients on placebo. Accordingly recruitment to the flecainide and encainide limbs of the trial was ceased. Despite producing highly significant reductions in ventricular ectopic frequency (compared to patients on placebo), encainide and flecainide were associated with a relative risk of arrhythmic death or non-fatal cardiac arrest of 3.6 (95% confidence limits 1.7–8.5). The moricizine arm was initially modified, and later halted too. Moricizine significantly increased the risk of sudden death in the first two weeks, and was ineffective in the long term.[28]

Although possibly unfair to many who warned of the potential dangers of class I antiarrhythmic agents well before the publication of CAST, it is no exaggeration to say that from a practical point of view, the history of these agents can be divided into 'pre-CAST' and 'post-CAST' eras. Prior to CAST the concept that class I antiarrhythmic agents could cause death was widely acknowledged, but the main emphasis of clinical research in the field was on the efficacy of these drugs in suppressing arrhythmias. Since CAST and related studies, the emphasis has switched dramatically to the effects of antiarrhythmic agents on mortality. Until recently, papers on the issue of antiarrhythmic agents were generally confined to discussions of the relative merits of ambulatory ECG monitoring and invasive electrophysiology studies as measures of antiarrhythmic drug efficacy. Trials were generally not large enough to show clinically significant mortality differences, and trends in the direction of increased mortality on active agents were generally written off as being the play of chance.

The issue of the potentially lethal proarrhythmic effects of these agents can no longer be relegated to a small section in reports of drug efficacy trials under the heading 'Side-effects', but must form an integral part of any informed discussion of the pharmacotherapy of arrhythmias. Nor can the issue be swept under the carpet as being related solely to the class Ic agents such as flecainide and encainide. The IMPACT study from the early 1980s[29] was performed in a group of 630 patients similar to those entered in the CAST study, who were randomized to mexiletine or placebo. It was reported as showing no difference in mortality, but in fact the mortality in the mexiletine group was 7.6% (24 deaths), compared to 4.8% (15 deaths) in patients on placebo. If the relatively small numbers are taken into account it is possible that this may translate into a clinically significant proarrhythmic effect for mexiletine, although there remains a widespread clinical impression that class Ib agents such as mexiletine may be less likely to provoke arrhythmia than class Ic or class Ia drugs.[30] Data from recent meta-analyses of the use of quinidine in both supraventricular and ventricular arrhythmias[31,32] suggest that the risk of this agent in terms of proarrhythmia may well have been underestimated in the past, and in fairness to the class Ic agents, it should be pointed out that no class Ia drug has ever undergone such a rigorous investigation of its effects on mortality as was provided by CAST. The potential mechanisms of proarrhythmia with different subclasses of antiarrhythmic drugs are summarized in Table 27.3.

For some years now, Furberg, Yusuf and Teo have been reporting and updating what amounts to a cumulative meta-analysis of the randomized control trials of antiarrhythmic drug therapy in various subgroups of patients, particularly those with recent MI, congestive heart failure or serious clinical ventricular arrhythmias[33–35] (see Table 27.4). These data tend to suggest that class I (particularly 1c) and IV antiarrhythmic agents are of no benefit and may possibly be harmful in this setting. Meta-analysis of trials of class II and class III agents however indicates statistically significant improvements in overall mortality (see Table 27.4).

While it is difficult to be sure from data such as these that the class II and III drugs are acting as antiarrhythmic agents, these reports have led to a strong feeling that if antiarrhythmic therapy is indicated at all, post MI, then either beta blockers or class III drugs such as sotalol and amiodarone may well be safer and more effective alternatives to the traditional class I agents. Beta blockers have been known for many years to be cardio-protective following MI and there are some recent reports suggesting

Table 27.3 Mechanisms of proarrhythmia in different subclasses of antiarrhythmic drugs

Ionic mechanisms	Na channel blockade (class I)	K channel blockade (class III)
Cellular effects	Slowed conduction, increased refractoriness	Slowed repolarization =>EADs* ± triggered activity
ECG correlates	QRS prolongation when marked	QT prolongation ± bizarre TU waves ± torsades de pointes
Class Ia (quinidine, disopyramide, procainamide)	+	+++
Class Ib (lignocaine, mexiletine)	+	–
Class Ic (flecainide)	++	–
Class III (amiodarone, sotalol)	+ (amiodarone) – (sotalol)	++

* EAD: early afterdepolarization

Table 27.4 Meta-analysis of antiarrhythmic therapy after acute myocardial infarction[33–35]

Drug class	Placebo mortality (%)	Treated mortality (%)	Mortality reduction (%) (± SD)	P value
Ia	7.7	6.6	–20 ± 13	NS
Ib	4.3	4.0	– 6 ± 10	NS
Ic	7.4	6.0	–31 ± 24	NS
Class I—all	5.6	5.0	–14 ± 7	< 0.05
II	5.4	6.6	19 ± 13	< 0.00001
III (amiodarone)	9.9	13.0	29 ± 13	< 0.05
IV (verapamil and diltiazem)	10.0	10.6	5 ± 7	NS

that they may be quite effective in the management of ventricular arrhythmias per se.[36,37] The use of class III agents in this context is more controversial, but as will be discussed below, strong evidence is now emerging in support of such a practice.

Clinical pharmacology of antiarrhythmic drugs

Class Ia drugs

Quinidine, disopyramide, procainamide

In the clinical electrophysiology laboratory, these drugs produce very similar effects (see Table 27.2). Hence it is not surprising that all three compounds are useful in the treatment and prophylaxis of a variety of atrial and ventricular arrhythmias. All three have been used successfully for atrial flutter and fibrillation (both reversion and prophylaxis). If administered as the sole therapy for these arrhythmias, each of these drugs may produce an acceleration of the ventricular rate. This is due, in part, to a drug-induced reduction in atrial rate, and hence reduction in repetitive concealed conduction into the A-V node. As well as this, quinidine and disopyramide in particular exhibit vagolytic activity which can accelerate conduction through the A-V node.[38] For this reason, they are normally administered in conjunction with digitalis in the treatment of atrial flutter and fibrillation. Supraventricular tachycardia is most commonly and successfully treated with verapamil or adenosine, which block the calcium channel-dependent limb of the re-entrant circuit. The Ia drugs can however be used with moderate success for these arrhythmias. In these cases, the drugs probably act by blocking conduction in the sodium channel-dependent part of the circuit. Class Ia drugs are effective in approximately 50% of cases in suppressing ventricular ectopic beats.[39] Lignocaine and other antiarrhythmic drug agents have largely replaced these drugs for the treatment of ventricular tachycardia or fibrillation in association with AMI. All three agents have been used in the difficult clinical problem of chronic, recurrent ventricular tachycardia or fibrillation, although there are significant concerns about the safety of these agents in this setting.

Quinidine

Quinidine is usually administered orally as sulfate or gluconate, or in various long-acting forms. The usual dose of quinidine sulfate is 300–600 mg 6-hourly, and doses about 30% higher are used for the gluconate. Bioavailability is about 70% for both forms, but peak plasma levels are reached earlier for the sulfate (60–90 minutes) than for the gluconate. Protein binding is 70–80%, and the elimination half-life is 5–8 hours, with most of the drug (80%) being metabolized in the liver and the remainder excreted unchanged in the urine (see Table 27.5).

Sustained release formulations of both quinidine sulfate and gluconate are available, and produce adequate plasma concentrations for at least 8 hours.[40] A new steady-state is not achieved for at least 24–36 hours after a change in dosage or following the initiation of therapy with a sustained release formulation. As with all antiarrhythmic therapy, it is advisable where possible to adjust the dosage according to serum drug levels to ensure that these are in the therapeutic range (see Table 27.5).

The cardiovascular side-effects of quinidine include hypotension due to negative inotropic and alpha-adrenergic blocking actions, and proarrhythmic effects mediated both by conduction slowing and by action potential prolongation leading to a long QT on the ECG and sometimes to torsades de pointes. These phenomena are discussed in detail elsewhere in this chapter. Non-cardiac side effects include nausea, cinchonism (tinnitus, deafness, blurred vision, diplopia, headache, confusion), thrombocytopenia and drug-induced fever.

Quinidine has traditionally been used to treat virtually all types of arrhythmia, both

Table 27.5 Pharmacokinetics and therapeutic concentrations of some class I antiarrhythmic drugs

Drug	Approximate elimination half-life (hr)	Main routes of elimination	Approximate therapeutic range (μg/ml)
Quinidine	5–8	Hepatic	3–6
Procainamide	3–5	Hepatic	5–15
Disopyramide	4–6	Renal	2.8–7.5
Lignocaine	1.5–2.5	Hepatic	2–6
Mexiletine	6–12	Hepatic	0.6–1.7
Tocainide	12–20	Hepatic and renal	4–10
Flecainide	7–15	Hepatic and renal	0.2–1.2
Propafenone	2–12	Hepatic and renal	0.1–2.0
Moricizine	1.5–3.5	Hepatic and renal	0.1–3.5

supraventricular and ventricular. It has been particularly popular for most of this century for pharmacological conversion of atrial fibrillation, or for promoting maintenance of sinus rhythm following cardioversion from atrial fibrillation. A recent meta-analysis of reports of the use of quinidine for this latter purpose concluded that while it was significantly more effective than placebo at maintaining sinus rhythm in such patients there was also a significant increase in mortality in the treated group.[31] While quinidine is still in widespread use for atrial fibrillation, it seems reasonable to assume that its popularity is likely to continue to decline relative to the class III agents for this role. The safety of quinidine for the management of ventricular arrhythmias has also been seriously questioned by results from meta-analysis,[32,41] and it seems likely that its use for this indication will also decline in the future in favour of class III agents and implantable devices.

Procainamide

Procainamide also is usually given orally, to a total dose of 3–6 g per day. Bioavailability is high and peak plasma levels are achieved 1–2 hours after tablet ingestion. Protein binding is only 10–20% and the elimination half-life is quite short (3–5 hours).

Procainamide is eliminated by renal excretion and hepatic metabolism.[42] The major metabolite is N-acetylprocainamide (NAPA), which has potent class III and some class I antiarrhythmic activity.[43] In 'fast acetylators',[44] or in renal failure, as much as 40% of a dose of procainamide may be excreted as NAPA and blood concentrations of NAPA can exceed those of the parent drug.

Sustained release preparations are available and have been proved effective in ventricular arrhythmias.[45] Procainamide is sometimes given intravenously. The risk of significant hypotension is minimized by slow administration and regular monitoring of blood pressure. An acceptable intravenous regimen is 100 mg every 1–5 minutes, up to a maximum of 1–1.5 g.

The cardiovascular side-effects of procainamide are very similar to those of quinidine except that the drug has no alpha-adrenergic blocking activity. Non-cardiac side-effects include nausea, vomiting and diarrhoea, rashes, fevers, agranulocytosis and, rarely, mental disturbances. Approximately 40% of patients receiving long-term oral therapy with procainamide develop a syndrome resembling systemic lupus erythematosus.[46] This usually resolves after withdrawal of the drug.

The combination of a short half-life, necessitating frequent dosing or the use of slow-release preparations, and a high incidence of unwanted side-effects renders procainamide a less than ideal antiarrhythmic agent. It has in the past been used for both supraventricular and ventricular arrhythmias, and will no doubt continue to be used at least for some time to come in the minority of patients in whom it has been demonstrated effective.

Disopyramide

Disopyramide may be given orally or intravenously. Oral bioavailability is about 80%, and peak plasma levels occur at 1–2 hours.[47] The usual oral dose is 300–600 mg/day in three or four divided doses. Unlike most other antiarrhythmic drugs, protein binding of disopyramide shows non-linear, saturable characteristics. This is of clinical importance, since apparently small increases in total plasma level within the therapeutic range (see Table 27.5) may mask larger rises in free (active) drug concentration.[48] Furthermore, disopyramide binds significantly to alpha$_1$-acid glycoprotein, levels of which rise during many acute illnesses, including MI.[49] The elimination half-life in healthy volunteers is about 4.5 hours.[47] This rises markedly in renal failure, as 50–80% of the drug is normally excreted unchanged in the urine. There are several metabolites which probably do not contribute to the class I antiarrhythmic effect although they may promote action potential prolongation. Long-acting formulations of disopyramide are available and have been proved effective.[50] When administered intravenously, disopyramide is usually given as a bolus (1.5–2 mg/kg) followed by an infusion (0.4 mg/kg/hr). It produces hypotension less frequently than quinidine or procainamide. Disopyramide does produce a moderate negative inotropic effect, though this may to some extent be masked by a tendency to produce peripheral vasoconstriction.[51,52] Nevertheless this effect is capable of precipitating overt cardiac failure in patients with pre-existing depression of ventricular function.[53] More recently, this action has been harnessed in the treatment of hypertrophic cardiomyopathy.[54] Widening of the QRS complex, prolongation of the QT interval and drug-induced ventricular tachyarrhythmias have all been reported as occasional side-effects. The most common non-cardiac side-effects of disopyramide relate to its potent anticholinergic properties: dryness of the mouth, blurred vision, constipation, urinary hesitancy or retention, and impotence. Less frequently nausea, skin rashes and mental disturbances have been reported.[51]

Disopyramide, like quinidine, has been used both for supraventricular arrhythmias (including atrial fibrillation) and ventricular arrhythmias. Clinical trial data suggest that it is probably of comparable efficacy to quinidine.[55] There are fewer data available regarding its proarrhythmic properties, but there is no doubt that disopyramide is capable of causing arrhythmias, both on a re-entrant basis and due to the production of torsades de pointes along similar lines to quinidine.[16] There are no good data allowing a statement to be made regarding the relative arrhythmogenicity of the two agents. These concerns, coupled with only moderate efficacy, are likely to lead to a decline in the use of this agent in the future.

Class Ib drugs

Lignocaine

Because of extensive hepatic first pass metabolism to potentially toxic metabolites,[56] lignocaine must be administered parenterally. It has a volume of distribution at steady-state of about 1.3 L/kg, a distribution half-life of 8 minutes, and a plasma elimination half-life of approximately 2 hours. There are several effective dosage regimens in the literature aimed at rapidly producing therapeutic blood levels without causing toxicity. One such protocol is to inject a rapid bolus of 50 mg intravenously (which can be repeated after 1 or 2 minutes if ineffective), and to follow this with an infusion of 8 mg/min for 20 minutes and 2 mg/min thereafter. It is important to bear in mind that the maintenance infusion rate must be reduced for patients with cardiac failure or hepatic dysfunction, and for elderly patients because of their decreased capacity to metabolize lignocaine.[57] Plasma levels should be checked if the infusion is continued for more than 24 hours.

Lignocaine does have negative inotropic properties in vitro, but this is usually evident in clinical use only when the plasma drug level is well above the therapeutic range. Central nervous system effects may occur more commonly, including paraesthesia (often peri-oral), mental changes, tremor, convulsions and coma. There are usually no ECG changes.

Mexiletine

Mexiletine is structurally very similar to lignocaine, but is well absorbed after oral administration, with peak plasma levels occurring within 2–4 hours. Bioavailability is about 80%.[58] For oral doses of 100–600 mg/day there is a linear relationship between plasma concentration and dose. Mexiletine has a large volume of distribution (5–7 L/kg). Its plasma elimination half-life ranges from 6–12 hours in normals, and 11–17 hours in patients with arrhythmias.[58–60]

Mexiletine undergoes extensive metabolism in the liver to largely inactive compounds. About 15% of each dose of mexiletine is excreted unchanged in the urine. Mexiletine shares much of the side-effect profile of lignocaine, and in addition gastrointestinal symptoms, especially nausea, are relatively common, and tremor may be an unacceptable side-effect in some patients.

Class Ic drugs

Flecainide

Flecainide is very well absorbed orally with negligible hepatic first pass effect.[61] Elimination half-life ranges from 7–15 hours in healthy volunteers, and averages about 10 hours in patients with cardiac disease.[62] There is considerable variability, however, and plasma level monitoring is recommended. The drug is metabolized to compounds which are far less potent than the parent.[63] The usual starting dose is 100 mg 12-hourly in adults.

Intravenous flecainide is highly effective in terminating supraventricular tachycardia, intra-atrioventricular (AV) nodal tachycardia, atrioventricular re-entrant tachycardia and atrial fibrillation.[64] It is less successful in reverting atrial flutter. It has also proven to be particularly useful in supraventricular arrhythmias associated with the Wolff–Parkinson–White Syndrome.[65] Flecainide appears to be at least as good for atrial fibrillation as quinidine and disopyramide.[66,67] Its usefulness in this arrhythmia may well be related to the recent demonstration that even though flecainide is not generally regarded as having class III effects in traditional tests for this mechanism, it does appear to develop a class III effect in atrial myocardium (particularly human), at very fast stimulation rates such as those that would be seen during atrial fibrillation.[68,69] Enthusiasm for its use for this indication should be tempered, however, by reports of atrial proarrhythmic effects.[70]

Flecainide is extremely effective in eliminating ventricular ectopic beats and non-sustained ventricular tachycardia, and indeed it was its effectiveness for these indications in the Cardiac Arrhythmia Pilot Study[71] that led to its being chosen as one of the agents to be tested in the CAST study. Efficacy for treating these indications appears to come at the price of significant and serious proarrhythmic effects. These are more likely to occur in the presence of moderate or severely impaired left ventricular function (ejection from less than 35–40%), and patients in this category should probably not receive flecainide.

Flecainide should be reserved for patients in whom less potentially arrhythmogenic agents have failed or are contraindicated and in whom the left ventricular function is not significantly depressed. Serum concentrations should be monitored. While serious ventricular arrhythmias are the most feared complication of flecainide therapy, other side-effects may also occur. These include central nervous system toxicity (blurred vision, dizziness, headache, nausea, paraesthesias), which are generally dose-related. Flecainide is also well known to increase the ventricular pacing threshold, and this may from time to time present a clinical problem.[72]

Class II agents

Beta blockers

There are a large number of beta blocker agents available to the clinician. Table 27.6 gives some details on a few examples of this class. These agents have been selected because they are relatively more popular than many other available beta adrenergic blocking agents, though not necessarily clinically superior.

'Cardio-selective' (i.e. beta_1-selective) blockers, such as metoprolol and atenolol, have theoretical advantages over non-selective blockers such as propranolol in patients with peripheral vascular disease, diabetes or asthma. In practice no beta blocker is safe in asthmatics but if no alternative treatment is available, cardio-selective beta blockers can be used in low dose with careful monitoring of ventilatory function. The more lipophilic beta blockers such as propranolol are probably more prone to cause central nervous system disturbances (such as bad dreams) than the more hydrophilic drugs such as atenolol. Metoprolol exhibits intermediate behaviour in this regard.

Beta blockers are generally well absorbed from the gut (more than 90%), but some undergo

Table 27.6 Beta-adrenoceptor blocking drugs

Drug	Selectivity	Plasma solubility half-life (hours)	First pass metabolism	Site of metabolism elimination
Atenolol	Relatively selective for β_1-adrenoceptors	water soluble 6–7	–	Kidney
Metoprolol	Relatively selective for β_1-adrenoceptors	lipid soluble 3–7	++	Liver esterases
Propranolol	Non-selective	lipid soluble 3–6	+++	Liver
Timolol	Non-selective	moderately lipid soluble 4	–	Liver
Esmolol	Mainly selective for β_1-adrenoceptors	water soluble 0.15	–	Red cell esterases
Sotalol	Non-selective (also class III agent)	water soluble 10–15	–	Kidney

extensive first pass metabolism, for example metoprolol and propranolol. The half-lives of propranolol and metoprolol are only 2–3 hours with acute usage but this tends to rise to about 6 hours with chronic use due to decreased hepatic blood flow leading to decreased metabolism. The water-soluble compounds such as atenolol tend to be eliminated in the urine with minimal metabolism and hence have longer half-lives in renal disease.

Serious side-effects include bronchospasm and acute left ventricular failure, both of which may be life-threatening. 'Minor' side-effects may be quite troubling with these agents and are often underestimated in text books. A degree of weakness and lethargy may be present, and this may interfere with exercise tolerance particularly for vigorous sports. Depression and other mood disturbances may also be a problem. Impotence occurs in about 1–3% of males on long term beta blockers. Beta blockers may mask the adrenergic symptoms of hypoglycaemia. They also tend to have undesirable effects on plasma lipids with a tendency for high density lipoprotein (HDL) to fall and very low density lipoprotein (VLDL) cholesterol and triglycerides to rise. Total cholesterol may not change.

The toxic-to-therapeutic ratio for beta blockers tends to be much wider than for other antiarrhythmic agents and it is not usually necessary to monitor blood levels in using these agents. Usual oral doses of metoprolol are 25 mg 12-hourly up to 100 mg 12-hourly, and of atenolol 25 mg daily up to 50 mg 12-hourly. Intravenous metoprolol is typically given as a 5 mg bolus over 2–3 minutes which should be repeated once or twice at 5-minute intervals provided there are no untoward side-effects. In patients in whom there is particular concern about potential cardiac depression with intravenous beta blockade, esmolol may be of use because of its very short half-life. It may be administered as a bolus of 0.5 mg/kg over 1 minute and then an infusion titrated to the desired effect on ventricular rate, with a typical infusion rate ranging from 50 to 200 μg/kg/min.

It seems probable that the major mechanism of the acute antiarrhythmic effects of the beta blocking agents is their direct antagonism of the arrhythmogenic actions of endogenous catecholamines, but it is also possible that the class I activity exhibited by many of these drugs in high concentration may play some role.

Beta blocking agents are often effective both in reversion of, and in prophylaxis against, supraventricular tachycardia, where they probably act largely by prolonging refractoriness and slowing conduction in the AV node. Their role in this arrhythmia (particularly for 'acute' therapy) has, however, been largely overshadowed by the advent of verapamil. In atrial fibrillation and flutter (especially if due to thyrotoxicosis), beta blocking agents can be useful in slowing the ventricular response by their effect on the AV node, but they are generally of little use in restoring sinus rhythm. A possible exception to this is sotalol, which will be discussed with the class III drugs.

Beta blocking agents have some value in the therapy of ventricular tachyarrhythmias though they have not generally been regarded as first-line drugs. Exceptions to this include arrhythmias caused by increased circulating catecholamines (phaeochromocytoma, anxiety, exercise) and the arrhythmias of the congenital long QT syndrome.

Class III agents

Amiodarone

The best known drug of this class is amiodarone. It was first used in France, in 1962, as a vascular smooth-muscle relaxant, and has been widely used in Europe and South America as an antiarrhythmic agent for well over a decade. It did not, however, come into use in the United States and Australia until the 1980s. Apart from its marked ability to prolong the duration of the cardiac action potential (class III activity), amiodarone is also a smooth-muscle relaxant, a non-competitive anti-adrenergic agent (i.e. 'class II'), and demonstrates some degree of class I and IV activity, at least in vitro.

Whatever its basic mechanism (or mechanisms) of action, it is a very effective antiarrhythmic agent with demonstrated effectiveness in the therapy and prophylaxis of most types of arrhythmia.[39,73] It is particularly effective in the treatment of atrial fibrillation, supraventricular arrhythmias associated with the Wolff–Parkinson–White syndrome, ventricular arrhythmias complicating hypertrophic cardiomyopathy (which respond poorly to beta blocking agents or calcium antagonists),[74] and refractory, recurrent ventricular tachycardia and fibrillation.

Its clinical use is complicated by its very unusual pharmacokinetics and unwanted side-effects. These aspects are both well covered by recent reviews,[75–77] and will be only briefly outlined here.

The administration of amiodarone (normally by mouth) is complicated by a variable bioavailability (20–80%), and a terminal half-life of elimination which is usually 35–40 days, but may exceed 100 days. The major metabolite accumulates in high concentration in plasma and tissues, possessing very similar electrophysiological properties to amiodarone. Dosage regimens vary from clinician to clinician, but most recommend a loading dose of 600–2000 mg/day for 1–8 weeks, followed by reduction to a maintenance dose, usually of the order of 200–400 mg/day. Where rapid loading is desirable, amiodarone may be given intravenously (via a central vein). A suitable regimen would be 150–300 mg in 10–20 ml 5% dextrose given over 1–10 minutes, then a further 600–900 mg infused over 24 hours.

Many of the side-effects are dose-dependent and each patient should receive the minimum effective dose. Unfortunately with this agent, experience has generally been that blood level monitoring, other than to monitor compliance, is of limited benefit. The drug and its metabolite are found in tissues in enormously higher concentrations than in plasma.[78] There is some evidence that plasma levels above 0.5 μg/ml seem to be required for efficacy, but there are no convincing data showing a correlation between actual plasma level and antiarrhythmic effect.[79] Similarly while serious toxicity seems to be more likely at levels above 2.5 μg/ml,[80,81] its incidence is more reliably correlated with measures of total drug dosage, suggesting the importance of target tissue accumulation over time.

The cardiovascular side-effects can include hypotension and/or heart failure (especially with intravenous use but also seen with oral therapy at times),[82,83] bradycardia (which may be aggravated by concomitant therapy with beta blocking drugs or verapamil), and QT interval prolongation (normally therapeutic, but occasionally excessive and rarely associated with ventricular tachycardias).[84] Non-cardiac effects include photosensitivity, disturbances of sleep, resting tremor, thyrotoxicosis and hypothyroidism, and pulmonary alveolitis (sometimes fatal).[85,86] The interaction between amiodarone and the thyroid is complex and is well described elsewhere.[87] Suffice it to say that, while thyroid function should be assessed before the start of amiodarone therapy, overt thyroid disease develops in less than 2% of patients.

The most feared side-effect of amiodarone is pulmonary toxicity. This may develop within the first few weeks of therapy or may not appear for many months or years. Its onset is often quite insidious. Clinical symptoms include a troublesome cough or shortness of breath, and the chest X-ray may show evidence of patchy infiltration. In the early years of use of this agent the incidence was reported to be 5–15%. With the introduction of much lower long term dosage schedules the current incidence is probably between 1 and 5%. It has been reported at around 1% in many of the recent relatively short-term trials of amiodarone with follow-ups usually of the order of 1–2 years. There is no doubt, however, that this problem can present as a late complication, and the outcome of a missed diagnosis can be lethal.

One of the best known, but least important, side-effects of amiodarone therapy is the development of corneal microdeposits, which can be seen in 98% of patients receiving long-term treatment. These deposits rarely produce symptoms; blurred and halo vision occurs in 1–2% of cases and diminishes after reduction of the dose. Finally, it should be mentioned that amiodarone may interact with other drugs. Its additive effects with beta blocking agents and verapamil, and its ability to elevate serum digoxin levels, have already been noted. In addition, potentiation of the effects of warfarin may occur, which usually necessitates reduction of the anticoagulant dose by about half.[74]

Sotalol

Sotalol is a non-cardio-selective beta blocking agent with marked class III activity. Unlike other beta blocking agents the prolongation of the duration of the action potential is apparent at once (within minutes, if administered intravenously), and this drug is showing promise in clinical trials in the treatment of supraventricular and ventricular arrhythmias.[88–90] The oral bioavailability of sotalol is about 60%, and there is no significant hepatic first pass metabolism. More than half of the oral dose is recovered unchanged in the urine and there are no known active metabolites. The elimination half-life of sotalol is about 5–12 hours, but this is considerably lengthened in renal failure. The usual oral dose of sotalol is 80 mg 12-hourly to 160 mg 12-hourly. If urgent, the drug may be given intravenously (0.5–1.5 mg/kg over 10–20 minutes).

Sotalol can produce any of the characteristic side-effects associated with beta blockers, and in addition has been reported to cause polymorphic ventricular tachycardia (torsades de pointes) associated with lengthening of the QT interval. This side-effect, which may be fatal, is more common in the presence of high sotalol concentrations, potassium depletion or the co-administration of other drugs known to prolong the QT interval.

Other class III agents

As noted above, neither amiodarone nor sotalol is a 'pure' class III agent. This has naturally given rise to questions concerning the importance of the class III action in the therapeutic effects of these agents. A number of newer agents which possess the ability to prolong the action potential, but not the ancillary properties of amiodarone and sotalol, are currently under investigation. These include D-sotalol, dofetilide and E-4031. It will be very interesting to see whether agents whose only action is to prolong the refractory period by slowing cardiac repolarization can match their more complicated predecessors for efficacy.[90,91] It has also been widely postulated that the anti-sympathetic effects of sotalol and amiodarone, and in particular the calcium antagonist effects of amiodarone, may play an important role in minimizing the incidence of torsades de pointes. Very recently, a large scale trial of D-sotalol versus placebo in patients with ischaemic heart disease and depressed left ventricular function was aborted because of excess mortality in the treated group (SWORD study). Large trials of dofetilide both in patients with serious ventricular tachyarrhythmias and in patients with atrial fibrillation are currently in progress.

Class IV agents

Verapamil

Verapamil is the prototype for this class of drug.[92] It was introduced into clinical practice in 1966, and rapidly became the drug of first choice for the short-term therapy of supraventricular tachycardia, in which it acts by blocking the slow conducting (AV nodal) limb of the re-entrant circuit. Its role as drug of choice for this indication is currently being challenged by intravenous adenosine, which seems to be at least as effective and to offer the advantage of a very rapid onset and offset of effect (see below). This is particularly important in patients with ventricular impairment in whom the negative inotropic action of verapamil may be of significance and also patients undergoing electrophysiological studies in which repeated induction of arrhythmia may be necessary.

The usual dosage of verapamil is 5–10 mg administered intravenously over 5–10 minutes, with careful monitoring of the ECG and the blood pressure. In atrial fibrillation or flutter, verapamil will usually slow the ventricular response, but is unlikely to induce reversion to sinus rhythm. It is contraindicated in patients with Wolff–Parkinson–White syndrome because of the risk of accelerated preferential conduction down the bypass tract, leading to ventricular fibrillation.[93] Long-term oral therapy with verapamil can be useful in prophylaxis against recurrent supraventricular tachycardias, but can be complicated by the pharmacokinetics of the drug.

Verapamil is rarely of therapeutic value in treating ventricular tachyarrhythmias, with the exception of two small sub-groups of arrhythmias both of which occur in patients without otherwise identifiable cardiac disease. The first of these have ventricular tachycardia with a left bundle branch block and right axis deviation pattern which is triggered by exercise and isoprenaline but not reliably by programmed electrical stimulation.[94] The second group have ventricular tachycardia with a right bundle branch block and left axis deviation pattern and are usually inducible by both atrial and ventricular stimulation.[94]

Verapamil is well absorbed when taken by mouth, but undergoes very extensive first-pass metabolism in the liver so that its bioavailability in oral therapy is only 20–40%. Furthermore, its mildly active metabolite (norverapamil) has a longer half-life than the parent compound, and accumulates during long-term therapy. The usual oral dose of verapamil is 240–480 mg/day in three or four divided doses.

Cardiac depression is the most serious side-effect of verapamil. It is rarely a problem in patients with normal left ventricular function, but can be quite severe in already diseased or beta-blocked hearts, especially when administered intravenously.[95] Non-cardiac side-effects are occasionally a problem. These include tiredness, constipation, pruritus, headache and vertigo. Constipation in particular can be very troublesome, especially to elderly patients.

Because of their additive effects on the AV node and on myocardial contractility, the combination of verapamil and beta blocking agents is potentially dangerous. On occasions beta blocking eye drops used for glaucoma can cause clinically significant interactions with verapamil. Similarly, the combined administration of digoxin and verapamil may be useful, especially in atrial fibrillation, but caution must be exercised both because of their additive effects on AV conduction and because verapamil tends to elevate serum levels of digoxin.

Diltiazem

Diltiazem is the only example of the benzothiazepines in current clinical use.[96] It behaves rather more like verapamil than nifedipine and related compounds. It produces more vasodilatation than does verapamil, but less than nifedipine, and is somewhat less depressant than verapamil of atrioventricular conduction. Diltiazem is well absorbed orally (more than 90%), but its bioavailability is approximately 40% because of high first pass metabolism. Its elimination half-life is approximately 4–5 hours and it has no active metabolites. Renal dysfunction does not appear to influence its pharmacokinetics significantly, but severe liver dysfunction may do so.

Side-effects are mostly predictable, being due to either vasodilatation (resulting in headache or flushing and occasionally hypotension), or depression of the sino-atrial and AV nodes (resulting in bradyarrhythmias or heart block). Diltiazem has less propensity for negative inotropic effects than verapamil, but has certainly demonstrated an ability to provoke or worsen cardiac failure in patients with abnormal myocardium. Diltiazem like verapamil may elevate plasma digoxin concentrations 20–60% when these agents are co-administered orally. The usual starting dose of diltiazem is 30–60 mg 8-hourly or 6-hourly, increasing to a maximum of 120 mg 8-hourly or 6-hourly. Slow release forms of diltiazem (requiring dosing only 12-hourly), and so called 'controlled dose' forms (requiring only once daily administration), are available and appear to be effective, particularly for hypertension. Diltiazem is not commonly used to treat arrhythmias, although it is of some value in slowing the ventricular response in atrial fibrillation.

The co-administration of diltiazem with beta blockers has been strongly discouraged in the past, but has become a relatively common practice in cardiac referral units. Appropriate care should always be taken when using together two potentially powerful negative inotropic and chronotropic agents.

Adenosine

Adenosine is an endogenous nucleoside that causes atrioventricular nodal conduction block.[8,9,90] It is given only via the intravenous route, as a rapid injection through a large peripheral vein followed by a saline flush. Because its half-life is measured in seconds, intervals between doses can be as short as 1–2 minutes without cumulative effect. For normal sized adults, the dose is 6 mg initially, followed by 12 mg if the first dose is ineffective. Recent recommendations have suggested an initial dose of 3 mg because of symptoms of chest tightness and apprehension with the 6 mg dose. A further dose of 18 mg may be given if the 12 mg dose is ineffective but well tolerated by the patient. For smaller individuals (less than 55–65 kg), the dosing regimen is 0.05 mg/kg initially followed by 0.1 mg/kg if necessary.

Common side-effects include transient sinus bradycardia and ventricular ectopy particularly after termination of supraventricular tachycardia. Facial flushing, shortness of breath and chest pressure are also common and should be monitored.

Adenosine is contraindicated in patients with a history of asthma. Theophylline and caffeine antagonize the effects of adenosine, and alternative therapy such as verapamil should be considered in patients taking theophylline or who have consumed large quantities of coffee or tea in the preceding few hours. Dipyridamole (Persantin) is an adenosine agonist. It prolongs the elimination of adenosine, and may potentiate its effects. Adenosine should be avoided or given in decreased doses in patients currently taking dipyridamole.

References

1. Rosen MR, Schwartz PJ. The Sicilian gambit. A new approach to the classification of antiarrhythmic drugs based on their actions on arrhythmogenic mechanisms. Circulation 1991; 84(4): 1831–51
2. Vaughan Williams EM. A classification of antiarrhythmic actions reassessed after a decade of new drugs. J Cardiovasc Pharm 1984; 24: 129–47
3. Campbell TJ. Subclassification of class I antiarrhythmic drugs: enhanced relevance after CAST. Cardiovasc Drugs Ther 1992; 6: 519–28
4. Katz AM. Cardiac ion channels. N Eng J Med 1993; 328: 1244–51
5. Hondeghem LM, Snyders DJ. Class III antiarrhythmic agents have a lot of potential but a long way to go. Reduced effectiveness and dangers of reverse use dependence. Circulation 1990; 81: 686–90
6. Colatsky TJ, Follmer CH, Starmer CF. Channel specificity in antiarrhythmic drug action. Circulation 1990; 82: 2235–42
7. Hondeghem LM. Development of class III antiarrhythmic agents. J Cardiovasc Pharm 1992; 20(Suppl 2): S17–S22
8. Camm AJ, Garratt CJ. Drug therapy: adenosine and supraventricular tachycardia. N Engl J Med 1991; 325: 1621–9
9. Engelstein ED, Lippman N, Stein KM, Lerman BB. Mechanism-specific effects of adenosine on atrial tachycardia. Circulation 1994; 89: 2645–54
10. Noble D, Bett G. Reconstructing the heart: a challenge for integrative physiology. Cardiovasc Res 1993; 27: 1701–12
11. Noble D, Denyer JC, Brown HF, Difrancesco D. Reciprocal role of the inward currents i_b, Na and i_f in controlling and stabilizing pacemaker frequency of rabbit sino-atrial node cells. Proc R Soc Lond (Biol) 1992; 250: 199–207
12. Hondeghem LM. Antiarrhythmic agents: modulated receptor applications. Circulation 1987; 75: 514–20
13. Campbell TJ. Sodium channel blockers. In: Singh BN, Dzau VJ, Vanhoutte PM, Woosley RL (eds). Cardiovascular pharmacology and therapeutics. New York: Churchill Livingstone, 1994; 645–63
14. January CT, Riddle JM, Salata JJ. A model for early afterdepolarizations: induction with the Ca^{++} channel agonist Bay K8644. Circulation Res 1988; 62: 563–71
15. January CT, Moscucci A. Cellular mechanisms of early afterdepolarizations. Ann NY Acad Sci 1992; 644: 23–32
16. Jackman WM, Friday KJ, Anderson JL, Aliot EM, Clark M, Lazzara R. The long QT syndromes: a critical review, new clinical observations and a unifying hypothesis. Prog Cardiovasc Dis 1988; 31: 115–72
17. Bonatti V, Rolli A, Botti G. Recording of monophasic action potentials of the right ventricle in long QT syndromes complicated by severe ventricular arrhythmias. Eur Heart J 1983; 4: 168–79
18. Roden DM, Hoffman BF. Action potential prolongation and induction of a normal automaticity by low quinidine concentrations in canine Purkinje fibers. Circulation Res 1985; 56: 857–67
19. Surawicz B. Electrophysiologic substrate of torsade de pointes: dispersion of repolarization or early afterdepolarizations? J Am Coll Cardiol 1989; 14: 172–84
20. Askey JM. Quinidine in the treatment of auricular fibrillation in association with congestive failure. Ann Int Med 1946; 24: 317–84
21. Selzer A, Wray HW. Quinidine syncope. Paroxysmal ventricular fibrillation occurring during treatment of chronic atrial arrhythmias. Circulation 1964; 30: 17–26
22. Dessertenne F. La tachycardie ventriculaire à deux foyers opposés variables. Arch Mal Coeur 1966; 59: 263–72
23. Velebit V, Podrid PJ, Lown B, Cohen BH, Graboys TB. Aggravation and provocation of ventricular arrhythmias by antiarrhythmic drugs. Circulation 1982; 65: 886–94
24. Ruskin JN, McGovern B, Garan H, Dimarco JP, Kelly E. Antiarrhythmic drugs: a possible cause of out of hospital cardiac arrest. N Engl J Med 1983; 309: 1302–6
25. Hoffman BF, Dangman JH. The role of antiarrhythmic drugs in sudden cardiac death. J Am Coll Cardiol 1986; 8: 104A–109A
26. Rae AP, Kay HR, Horowitz LN, Spielman SR, Greenspan AM. Proarrhythmic effects of antiarrhythmic drugs with malignant ventricular arrhythmias evaluated by electrophysiologic testing. J Am Coll Cardiol 1988; 12(1): 131–9
27. The Cardiac Arrhythmia Suppression Trial Investigators. Preliminary report—effect of encainide and flecainide on mortality in a randomized trial of arrhythmia suppression after myocardial infarction. N Engl J Med 1989; 321: 406–12
28. Cardiac Arrhythmia Suppression II Investigators. Effect of the antiarrhythmic agent moricizine on survival after myocardial infarction. N Engl J Med 1992; 327: 227–33

29. IMPACT Research Group. International mexiletine and placebo antiarrhythmic coronary trial I. Report on arrhythmia and other findings. J Am Coll Cardiol 1984; 4: 1148–63
30. Morganroth J. Early and late proarrhythmia from antiarrhythmic drug therapy. Cardiovasc Drugs Ther 1992; 6: 11–14
31. Coplen SE, Antman EM, Berlin JA et al. Efficacy and safety of quinidine therapy for maintenance of sinus rhythm after cardioversion: a meta-analysis of randomized control trials. Circulation 1990; 82: 1106–16
32. Morganroth J, Goin JE. Quinidine-related mortality in the short- to medium-term treatment of ventricular arrhythmias: a meta-analysis. Circulation 1991; 84: 1977
33. Teo KK, Yusuf S, Furberg C. Effect on antiarrhythmic drug therapy on mortality following myocardial infarction. Circulation 1990; 82(suppl 4): III–197
34. Teo KK, Yusuf S, Furberg CD. Effects of prophylactic antiarrhythmic drug therapy in acute myocardial infarction. JAMA 1993; 270: 1589–95
35. Teo KK, Yusuf S. Overview of antiarrhythmic drug trials: implications for antiarrhythmic therapy. In: Singh BN, Dzau VJ, Vanhoutte PM, Woosley RL (eds). Cardiovascular pharmacology and therapeutics. New York: Churchill Livingstone, 1994; 631–45
36. Steinbeck G, Andersen D, Bach P et al. A comparison of electrophysiologically guided antiarrhythmic drug therapy with beta blocker therapy in patients with symptomatic, sustained ventricular tachyarrhythmias. N Engl J Med 1992; 327: 987–92
37. Antz M, Siebels J, Kuck KH. Metoprolol versus sotalol in ventricular tachycardia. Circulation 1992; 86(I): 720
38. Mirro MJ, Manalan AS, Bailey JC, Watanabe AM. Anticholinergic effects of disopyramide and quinidine on guinea pig myocardium. Circulation Res 1980; 47: 855–65
39. Salerno DM, Gillingham KJ, Berry DA, Hodges M. A comparison of antiarrhythmic drugs for the suppression of ventricular ectopic depolarizations: a meta-analysis. Am Heart J 1990; 120: 340–53
40. Taggart W, Holyoak W. Steady-state bioavailability of two sustained-release quinidine preparations. Clin Ther 1983; 5: 357–64
41. Morganroth J. Early and late proarrhythmia from antiarrhythmic drug therapy. Cardiovasc Drugs Ther 1992; 6: 11–14
42. Giardina EGV, Dreyfuss J, Bigger JT et al. Metabolism of procainamide in normal and cardiac subjects. Clin Pharm Ther 1976; 19: 339–51
43. Roden DM, Reele SB, Higgins SB et al. Antiarrhythmic efficacy, pharmacokinetics and safety of N-acetyl-procainamide in human subjects: comparison with procainamide. Am J Cardiol 1980; 46: 463–8
44. Reidenberg MM, Drayer DE, Levy M, Warner H. Polymorphic acetylation of procainamide in man. Clin Pharm Ther 1975; 17: 722–30
45. Giardina E, Fenster P, Bigger JT et al. Efficacy, plasma concentration and adverse effects of a new sustained-release procainamide preparation. Am J Cardiol 1980; 46: 855–62
46. Hoffman BF, Rosen MR, Wit AL. Electrophysiology and pharmacology of cardiac arrhythmias. (Pt VIII.) Cardiac effects of quinidine and procainamide. A Heart J 1975; 89: 804–8
47. Hinderling PH, Garrett ER. Pharmacokinetics of the antiarrhythmic disopyramide in healthy humans. J Pharmacokin BioPharmaceut 1976; 4: 199–230
48. Meffin PJ, Robert EW, Winkle RA et al. Role of concentration-dependent plasma protein binding in disopyramide disposition. J Pharmacokin Biopharmaceut 1979; 7: 29–46
49. Routledge PA, Stargel WW, Wagner GS, Shand DG. Increased alpha-1-acid glycoprotein and lidocaine disposition in myocardial infarction. Ann Int Med 1980; 93: 701–4
50. Fechter P, Ha H, Follath F, Nager F. The antiarrhythmic effects of controlled release disopyramide phosphate and long acting propranolol in patients with ventricular arrhythmias. Eur J Clin Pharm 1983; 25: 729–34
51. Heel RC, Brogden TM, Speight TM. Disopyramide: a review of its pharmacological properties and therapeutic use in treating cardiac arrhythmias. Drugs 1978; 15: 331–68
52. Kotter V, Linderer T, Schroder R. Effects of disopyramide on systemic and coronary hemodynamics and myocardial metabolism in patients with coronary artery disease: comparison with lidocaine. Am J Cardiol 1980; 46: 469–75
53. Podrid PJ, Schoenenberger A, Lown B. Congestive heart failure caused by oral disopyramide. N Engl J Med 1980; 302: 614–17
54. Sumimoto T, Hamada M, Ohtani T et al. Effect of disopyramide on systolic and early diastolic time intervals in patients with hypertrophic cardiomyopathy. J Clin Pharm 1991;31:440–3
55. Campbell TJ. Clinical use of class Ia antiarrhythmic drugs. In: Vaughan Williams EM, Campbell TJ (eds). Antiarrhythmic drugs. Berlin: Springer-Verlag, 1989:175–200
56. Blumer J, Strong JM, Atkinson AJ. The convulsant potency of lidocaine and its N-dealkylated metabolites. J Pharm Exp Ther 1978;180:31–6

57. Harron DWG, Shanks RG. Clinical use of class Ib antiarrhythmic drugs. In: Vaughan Williams EM, Campbell TJ (eds). Antiarrhythmic drugs. Berlin: Springer-Verlag, 1989:201–34
58. Haselbarth V, Doevendans J, Wolf M. Kinetics and bioavailability of mexiletine in healthy subjects. Clin Pharm and Ther 1981;29:729–36
59. Pringle T, Fox J, McNeill JA et al. Dose independent pharmacokinetics of mexiletine in healthy volunteers. Br J Clin Pharm 1986;21:319–21
60. Campbell NPS, Pantridge JF, Adgey AAJ. Long-term oral antiarrhythmic therapy with mexiletine. Br Heart J 1978;40:796–801
61. Conard GJ, Carlson GL, Frost JW, Ober RE. Human plasma pharmacokinetics of flecainide acetate (R-818), a new antiarrhythmic, following single oral and intravenous doses. Abst. Clin Pharm Ther 1979;25:218
62. Hodges M, Haugland JM, Granrud G et al. Suppression of ventricular ectopic depolarizations by flecainide acetate, a new antiarrhythmic drug. Circulation 1982;65:879–85
63. Guehler J, Gornick CC, Tobler HG et al. Electrophysiologic effects of flecainide acetate and its major metabolites in the canine heart. Am J Cardiol 1985;55:807–12
64. Camm AJ, Hellestrand KJ, Nathan AW, Bexton RS. Clinical usefulness of flecainide acetate in the treatment of paroxysmal supraventricular arrhythmias. Drugs 1985;29(Suppl. 4):7–13
65. Fauchiel J, Cosnay P, Rouesnal P et al. Effects of oral and injectable flecainide in patients with accessory atrial ventricular pathways. Arch Mal Coeur 1985;78:81–90
66. Borgeat A, Goy JJ, Maendly R et al. Flecainide versus quinidine for conversion of atrial fibrillation to sinus rhythm. Am J Cardiol 1986;58:496–8
67. Gavaghan TP, Feneley MP, Campbell TJ, Morgan JJ. Atrial tachyarrhythmias after cardiac surgery: results of disopyramide therapy. Aust NZ J Med 1985;15:27–32
68. Wang Z, Pelletier LC, Talajic M, Nattel S. Effects of flecainide and quinidine on human atrial action potentials. Circulation 1990;82:274–83
69. O'Hara G, Villemaire C, Talajic M, Natter S. Effects of flecainide on the rate-dependence of atrial refractoriness, atrial repolarization and atrioventricular node conduction in anesthetized dogs. J Am Coll Cardiol 1992;19:1335–42
70. Feld GK, Chen PS, Nicod P et al. Possible atrial proarrhythmic effects of encainide and flecainide. Am J Cardiol 1990;66:378–83
71. CAPS Investigators. The cardiac arrhythmia pilot study. Am J Cardiol 1986;57:91–5
72. Nigro P, Ganci B, Picone I et al. Variations in ventricular pacing threshold and in paced QRS width in patients treated with flecainide and propafenone. New Trends Arrhythmias 1990;6:405–8
73. Haffajee CI. Clinical effects of class III antiarrhythmic agents. In: Reiser HJ, Horowitz LN (eds). Mechanisms and treatment of cardiac arrhythmias: relevance of basic studies to clinical management. Baltimore: Urban & Schwarzenberg, 1985:283
74. McKenna WJ, Rowland E, Krikler DM. Amiodarone: the experience of the past decade. Br Med J (Clin Res ed.) 1983;287:1654–6
75. Myers M, Peter T, Weiss D, Nalos PL, Gang ES, Oseran DS, Mandel WJ. Benefits and risks of long-term amiodarone therapy for sustained ventricular tachycardial fibrillation: Minimum of three-year follow-up in 145 patients. Am Heart J 1990;119:8–14
76. Bauman JL, Berk SI, Hariman RJ et al. Amiodarone for sustained ventricular tachycardia: efficacy, safety and factors influencing long-term outcome. Am Heart J 1987;114:1436–44
77. Singh BN, Sarma JSM. Amiodarone and amiodarone derivatives. In: Singh BN, Dzau VJ, Vanhoutte PM, Woosley RL (eds). Cardiovascular pharmacology and therapeutics. New York: Churchill Livingstone, 1994:689–710
78. Holt DW, Tucker GT, Jackson PR, Storey GCA. Amiodarone pharmacokinetics. Am Heart J 1983;106:840–7
79. Mitchell LB, Wyse G, Gillis AM, Duff HJ. Electropharmacology of amiodarone therapy initiation. Time courses of onset of electrophysiologic and antiarrhythmic effects. Circulation 1989;80:34–42
80. Rotmensch HH, Belhassen B, Swanson BN et al. Steady-state serum amiodarone concentrations: relationships with antiarrhythmic efficacy and toxicity. Ann Int Med 1984;101:462–9
81. Counihan PJ, McKenna WJ. Low-dose amiodarone for the treatment of arrhythmias in hypertrophic cardiomyopathy. J Clin Pharm 1989;29:436–8
82. Kowey P, for the IV Amiodarone Investigators. Overall safety data from the intravenous amiodarone trials. Circulation 1994;90(I):545
83. De Paola A, Horowitz L, Spielman S et al. Development of congestive heart failure and alterations in left ventricular function in patients with sustained ventricular tachyarrhythmias treated with amiodarone. Am J Cardiol 1987;60:276–80
84. Hohnloser S, Klingenheben T, Singh B. Amiodarone-associated proarrhythmic effects. Ann Intern Med 194;121:529–35
85. Magro SA, Lawrence C, Wheeler SH, Krafchek J, Lin H, Wyndham CRC. Amiodarone pulmonary toxicity: prospective evaluation

of serial pulmonary function tests. J Am Coll Cardiol 1988;12:781–8
86. Horowitz LN. Detection of amiodarone pulmonary toxicity: to screen or not to screen, that is the question. J Am Coll Cardiol 1988;12:789–90
87. Nademanee K, Singh BN, Callahan B, Hendrickson JA, Hershman JM. Amiodarone, thyroid hormone indexes and altered thyroid function: long-term serial effects in patients with cardiac arrhythmias. Am J Cardiol 1986;58:981–6
88. Nademanee K, Feld G, Hendrickson J, Singh PN, Singh BN. Electrophysiologic and antiarrhythmic effects of sotalol in patients with life-threatening ventricular tachyarrhythmias. Circulation 1985;72:555–64
89. Cobbe SM. Sotalol. In: Vaughan Williams EM, Campbell TJ (eds). Antiarrhythmic drugs. Berlin: Springer-Verlag, 1989:365–87
90. Campbell TJ. Class III antiarrhythmic action: the way forward. Med J Aust 1993;158:732–3
91. Colatsky TJ, Singh BN. Potassium channel blockers as antiarrhythmic agents. In: Singh BN, Dzau VJ, Vanhoutte PM, Woosley RL (eds). Cardiovascular pharmacology and therapeutics. New York: Churchill Livingstone, 1994:675–88
92. McTavish D, Sorkin EM. Verapamil. An update review of its pharmacodynamic and pharmacokinetic properties, and therapeutic use in hypertension. Drugs 1989;38:19–76
93. McGovern B, Garan H, Ruskin J. Precipitation of cardiac arrest by verapamil in patients with Wolff–Parkinson–White Syndrome. Ann Int Med 1986;104:791–4
94. Singh BN. Calcium channel blockers and adenosine as antiarrhythmic drugs. In: Singh BN, Dzau VJ, Vanhoutte PM, Woosley RL (eds). Cardiovascular pharmacology and therapeutics. New York: Churchill Livingstone, 1994:747–64
95. Rankin AC, Rae AP, Cobbe SM. Misuse of intravenous verapamil in patients with ventricular tachycardia. Lancet 1987;ii:472–4
96. Henry PD. Comparative pharmacology of calcium antagonists: nifedipine, verapamil and diltiazem. Am J Cardiol 1980;46:1047–58

28 Beta blocking drugs

Robin M Norris

Beta adrenergic blocking drugs are among the most effective of all those used in the treatment of ischaemic heart disease. Because the major trials of beta blockers were carried out 10–15 years ago, nearly all the important literature was published in the 1970s and 1980s. There is thus a danger that their proven benefits will be submerged by the flood of information on new drugs, most of which are now much more vigorously promoted by the pharmaceutical industry than are beta blockers. This review will focus on the use of beta blockers during and after myocardial infarction (MI) although their use in the treatment of stable angina and hypertension is of course equally important.

Pharmacology of beta blocking drugs

This has been extensively reviewed previously.[1,2] In summary, beta adrenergic antagonists act by blocking the receptors which mediate the activation by adrenaline and noradrenaline of the membrane-bound enzymes adenylate cyclase and guanylate cyclase to produce the second chemical messengers cyclic adenosine monophosphate (cyclic AMP) and cyclic guanosine monophosphate (cyclic GMP). Competitive blockade of the effects of these messenger substances on cardiac myocytes results in four important effects: these are reduction in the automaticity of the sinus node; reduction in the automaticity of subsidiary pacemakers; reduction in conductivity through the atrioventricular node; and reduction in contractility of both the atrial and ventricular myocardium. The effects are to slow heart rate, to reduce myocardial contractility (and thus to increase ventricular filling and ventricular size) and to reduce the arrhythmogenic effects of catecholamines. It follows that the effects of beta blockade are greatest when the activity of the agonists adrenaline and noradrenaline is highest, that is under conditions of heightened sympathetic activity.

The major classification of beta blocking drugs is into those which selectively block the cardiac effects of beta adrenergic stimulation described above (the $beta_1$ or cardiac-specific drugs such as atenolol and metoprolol) and the non-cardiac-specific drugs such as propranolol and timolol which in addition to $beta_1$ blockade also block the $beta_2$ receptors subserving bronchodilatation, vasodilatation and ion transport across cell membranes. Thus drugs such as propranolol are more likely than those such as atenolol (although the effect is quantitative and not absolute) to exacerbate asthma by causing bronchoconstriction or to exacerbate claudication by causing arteriolar constriction in the legs. The effect of $beta_2$ receptors on potassium transport across cell membranes could also conceivably affect the antiarrhythmic potential of non-specific versus cardiac-specific drugs (see later).

Other important classifications are into drugs (atenolol, metoprolol, propranolol, sotalol, timolol) whose action is solely to block the beta receptors and those such as acebutolol, oxprenolol, and pindolol which have an additional stimulatory effect, termed partial agonist activity or intrinsic sympathomimetic activity (ISA). Clearly this distinction is important in that it may be desirable to maximize the inhibitory effects of beta blockers for the treatment of, say, MI but perhaps less desirable to do so for the treatment of hypertension. Another distinction is into those drugs (e.g. atenolol) which are not lipid soluble and most other beta blockers which are lipid soluble and therefore penetrate the brain. In practice, however, this distinction has not been shown to be important. Newer drugs such as celiprolol and carvedilol which have an additional vasodilating action have not been extensively studied in the context of MI and will not be considered further. Much more important on present knowledge, at least in the context of acute coronary care, is sotalol, which in addition to its effect as a non-cardiac-specific beta blocker has additional antiarrhythmic effects conferred by its class III activity (to prolong the duration of the action potential). Recent evidence suggests that sotalol is the drug of choice for the acute reversion[3] as well as for the prophylaxis[4] of ventricular tachycardia.

Use of beta blockers during the acute phase of myocardial infarction

Early fears that IV beta blockade could be dangerous when given during acute infarction were refuted by Mueller[5] who showed generally favourable haemodynamic effects. Following Mueller's work, Norris and co-workers showed that propranolol given intravenously within 4 hours of onset and continued orally for 24 hours limited infarct size assessed by serial measurements of creatine kinase enzyme activity[6] and, in selected cases, prevented progression from threatened to completed infarction.[7] Both of these effects were confirmed by subsequent trials and meta-analyses[8,9] although the beneficial effects are modest and have in any case been overshadowed in recent years by the greater benefits from thrombolytic therapy. The effect of intravenous beta blockade on mortality was studied in the Metoprolol in Acute Myocardial Infarction study (MIAMI)[10] and in the First International Study of Infarct Survival (ISIS-1)[11] which used atenolol. Both of the studies showed a reduction in early mortality rate of 14%; this was statistically significant (2p = 0.04) in ISIS-1 but was not significant in MIAMI, no doubt because of the smaller number of patients enrolled. A meta-analysis of all available trial data shows a mortality reduction by intravenous beta blockade of 13% (p=0.03).[9]

Results from all of these trials are, to a degree, irrelevant to present-day practice because they were conducted before the era of thrombolytic therapy and routine administration of aspirin. The only trial of intravenous beta blockade in conjunction with thrombolysis was the Thrombolysis in Myocardial Infarction (TIMI) IIb study[12] in which metoprolol given intravenously within on average 3.3 hours of onset and continued orally was compared with oral metoprolol started on day 6. All patients received thrombolytic therapy with tissue plasminogen activator starting within 4 hours of onset. No benefit was shown for immediate over deferred treatment with metoprolol in terms either of mortality reduction or improvement in ventricular function. There was a reduction in reinfarction for the immediately treated group at 6 days and at 6 weeks after entry to the trial, but this was no longer apparent after 1 year. It seemed at least possible that similar benefits in prevention of early reinfarction could have been obtained by starting metoprolol orally on days 1 or 2 in the immediate group rather than by intravenous administration of the drug within 4 hours of onset.

Should beta blockers be given intravenously to patients with AMI in the thrombolytic era? Although the TIMI-IIb results were discouraging, the study lacked statistical power (1434 patients enrolled versus 16 027 in ISIS-1), so that a modest beneficial effect could well have been missed because of a type 2 error. Despite the widespread involvement in ISIS-1 by coronary care units in the United Kingdom, Europe and Australia and the recommended use of IV beta blockers in subsequent large international trials, IV beta blockade has never become popular. However, there are several factors favouring its use. First, some 50% of patients admitted to UK hospitals are ineligible for thrombolytic therapy[13] and the mortality rate for these patients is considerably higher than for patients who do receive thrombolysis. Second, there is evidence from the ISIS-1 trial that intravenous atenolol prevented cardiac rupture.[14] There is also evidence that cardiac rupture may be one reason for the well documented early hazard from thrombolytic therapy and this early hazard appears to be greatest for the elderly and for those receiving thrombolysis relatively late after the onset of infarction.[15] Although there is no trial evidence to support the practice, it would seem logical to give intravenous beta blocker therapy to patients who are ineligible for thrombolysis and to those patients, particularly if they are elderly, who receive thrombolysis late. The limiting factor is that the patients at highest risk, who have pulmonary oedema and cardiogenic shock (in addition to those with asthma), cannot be treated. However there is no evidence from the pooled results of early intervention trials that cardiac failure is exacerbated in patients who do not have overt evidence of failure before intravenous administration of the beta blocker.[8]

Use of oral beta blockers after recovery from myocardial infarction

The efficacy of beta blockers in prolonging life after recovery from MI was proven in three trials which were reported during the early 1980s;[16–18] a meta-analysis of the results of these and other trials (together involving more than 18 000 patients treated from 8 days to 1–3 years after infarction) showed an odds ratio of 0.77 (95% confidence interval 0.70–0.85) for all-cause mortality for those receiving beta blockers.[8] The mortality reduction appeared to be due almost entirely to prevention of sudden death (Fig. 28.1),[9] but recurrent non-fatal reinfarction was also prevented (odds ratio for treatment with beta blockers (r = 0.74; 95% confidence intervals 0.66–0.83). Since many of the prevented sudden deaths must have been caused by MI, the patients surviving to develop non-fatal infarction, the effect of beta blockers to prevent non-fatal reinfarction must have been underestimated.

Mechanism of protective action of beta blockers: the oxygen-sparing effect

Intravenous followed by oral propranolol causes a modest (about 20%) reduction in the product of systolic blood pressure and heart rate in patients with acute MI (see Fig. 28.2).[19] Since the double product is a reliable clinical indicator of myocardial oxygen demand,[20] the oxygen-sparing effect may explain the limitation of infarct size[6] and alleviation of chest pain[21] which follow early intravenous administration of a beta blocker. Suggestive evidence that the beneficial long-term effect of beta blockers may be linked to their benefits on myocardial oxygen consumption is provided by a comparison of the effects of individual drugs on resting heart rate with the mortality reduction achieved during long-term trials (Fig. 28.3).[22] Drugs which reduced resting heart rate by more than about 10 beats per minute, i.e. drugs devoid of ISA, showed better mortality reduction than did drugs with ISA which reduced heart rate by less than 10 beats per minute. Although the relationship is not strong (r = 0.6; $p<0.05$), it does support the notion that the oxygen-sparing effects of beta blockers are important predictors of efficacy, and that drugs devoid of agonist action should be preferred to those which have intrinsic sympathomimetic activity.

Mechanism of protective action: the antiarrhythmic effect

Although suppression of ventricular ectopic activity by beta blockers is only partial,[23,24] the prevention of sudden cardiac death is undoubted[9] (see Fig. 28.1). This is in contrast to some class I antiarrhythmic drugs which suppress ventricular ectopics but increase sudden death.[25] Although it is assumed that prevention of sudden cardiac death equates with prevention of ventricular fibrillation (VF), prevention of infarction by beta blockers (see next section) could

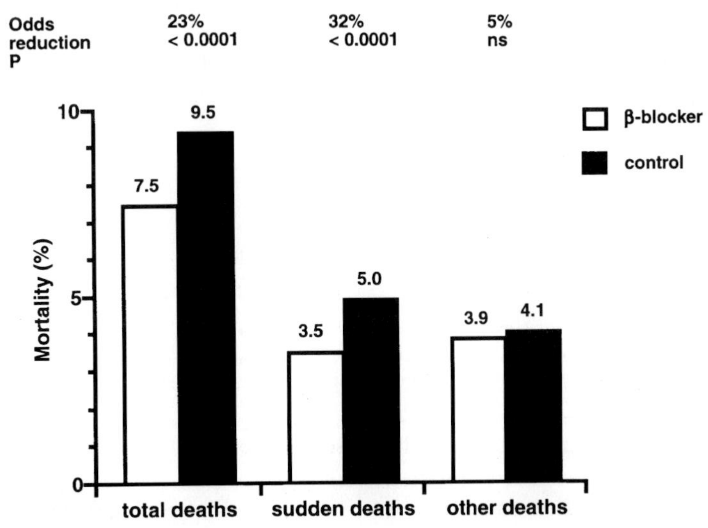

Fig. 28.1 Long-term beta blockade after MI. A meta-analysis of results from almost 20 000 patients[9] shows that the reduction in mortality is due to reduction in sudden death. (Redrawn with permission from the European Heart Journal 1988; 9: 8–16. The Beta Blocker Pooling Project)

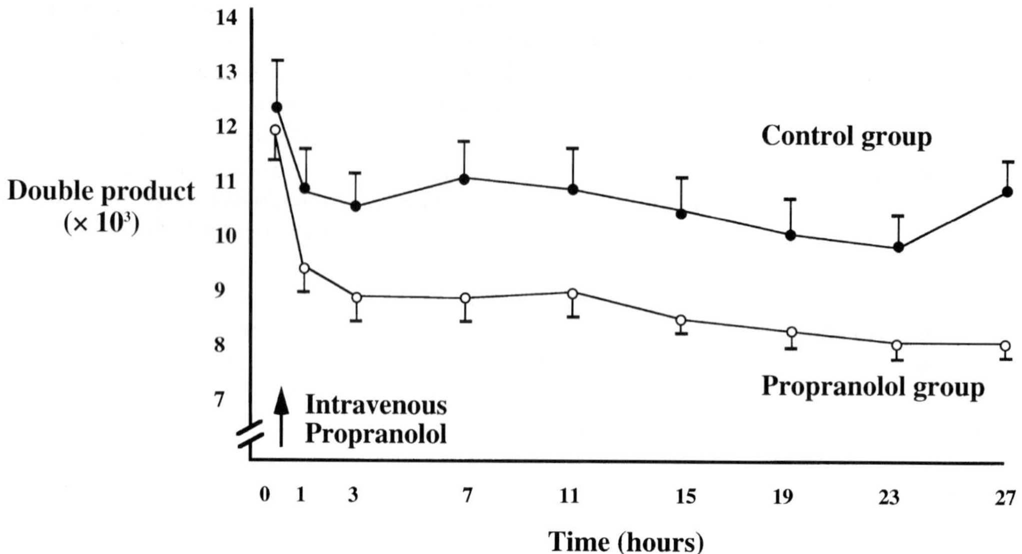

Fig. 28.2 The oxygen-sparing effect of beta blockers is shown by a reduction in double product (heart rate x systolic blood pressure) by about 20% after IV and oral propranolol.[19] (Reproduced with permission from the British Heart Journal 1985 54: 351–61.)

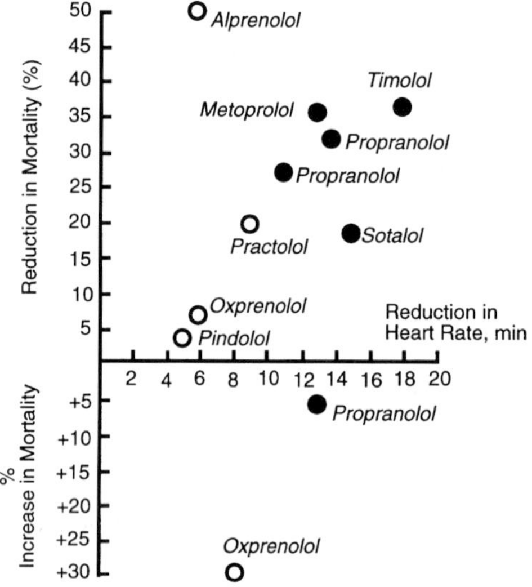

Fig. 28.3 Relation between the reduction in heart rate comparing treated groups with control groups and the percentage reduction in mortality in large post-infarction trials with beta blockers.[22] Open circles indicate beta blockers with ISA. Although the relationship is not strong ($r = 0.6$; $p<0.05$) it is suggestive that protection from beta blockers is due, in part at least, to their oxygen-sparing effect. (Reproduced with permission from the American Journal of Cardiology 1986 57: 3E–49E.)

account for some or conceivably even for all of the reduction in sudden death. Thus an antiarrhythmic basis for the efficacy of long-term beta blockade cannot be proven. Firmer evidence of antiarrhythmic activity must be sought from trials involving hospitalized patients during evolution of infarction, in whom, for all practical purposes, the arrhythmia which must be suppressed is VF.

Do beta blockers prevent VF during AMI? The evidence here is confusing for two reasons. First, VF occurs in two quite different clinical contexts: VF during the first 24–48 hours which is not necessarily associated with massive myocardial necrosis and is usually not recurrent if reverted (early VF), and VF occurring after a few days or longer which tends to be recurrent and to be associated with large myocardial scars (late VF). This fact has not been taken into account when the effect of beta blockers on the occurrence of VF is reported. Second, although there are good theoretical reasons for supposing that $beta_2$ blockade in addition to $beta_1$ blockade is desirable for prevention of early VF,[26–28] most evidence relates to the use of cardiac-specific beta blockers which are devoid of $beta_2$ blocking activity.[10,11,29,30]

If we consider early and late VF as separate entities, we find that the cardiac-specific blocker metoprolol prevented late VF in two trials,[29,30] the protective effect becoming apparent only after day 3 in one trial[29] and after day 6 in the other.[30] By contrast in the trial by Norris et al of intravenous followed by 24 hours of oral propranolol,[31] early VF appeared to be prevented (2/364 treated patients versus 14/371 controls; p=0.006) but late VF occurring after withdrawal of treatment was not prevented (5 vs 4 patients). Unfortunately no other trial using intravenous administration of a non-cardiac-selective beta blocker which was of sufficient size to confirm this experience has been reported. However, a small trial of intravenous timolol[32] did show directionally similar results, VF having occurred in 2/73 treated patients and 4/71 controls.

To summarize, the evidence strongly suggests that the salutary effects of beta blockade are due, at least in part, to an antiarrhythmic or, more specifically, to an antifibrillatory effect. There is some experimental and clinical evidence, by no means conclusive, that non-cardiac-specific beta blockers would be superior to cardiac-specific drugs in this regard, and in this reviewer's opinion a new clinical trial to prove or disprove this hypothesis is needed.

Mechanism of protective action: prevention of myocardial infarction

Prevention of non-fatal reinfarction is a powerful effect of long term beta blocker therapy started after recovery from an index infarct, having been shown in 13 of 15 trials.[33] Pooled data indicate that the odds of reinfarction are reduced by about one fourth (p<0.001)[8] and that prevention is a class effect and therefore presumably due to $beta_1$ blockade. Moreover, as mentioned earlier, some of the prevented sudden deaths in those trials must presumably have been associated with putative reinfarction, so the reduction in total reinfarction (fatal + non-fatal) by beta blockers must be greater than the reduction in non-fatal reinfarction.

The mechanism(s) by which beta blockers prevent MI are of great interest but are not at all clear. Some small infarcts, possibly those caused by a non-occlusive thrombus, may be prevented by the oxygen-sparing effect of beta blockers; this was the effect which we thought was operating in our trial of propranolol.[7] A further possible mechanism is prevention of platelet aggregation by beta blockers.[34,35] Perhaps the most attractive theory is that plaque rupture is in some way prevented by modification of sudden changes in coronary vasomotor tone,[33] since exercise-induced constriction of stenosed coronary arteries can be prevented by intracoronary injection of propranolol.[36] Whatever the mechanism, prevention of infarction by beta blockers is one of the most important effects favouring their use in patients with ischaemic heart disease.

Unwanted effects of beta blocker therapy

The only absolute contraindication to beta blocker therapy is bronchial asthma; other contraindications are relative and the importance of some has been overemphasized. In AMI hypotension (systolic blood pressure <100 mmHg) and clinically evident left ventricular failure are contraindications, but patients free from these complications before administration are no more likely to develop cardiac failure or shock if a beta blocker is given.[8] Similarly, there is no evidence that heart block is caused by beta blockers,[8] although established high grade atrioventricular block might be exacerbated and should still be regarded as a contraindication.

Unwanted effects would be expected to be more of a problem for patients on long-term beta blocker therapy than for those on short-term treatment in hospital. In fact, the number of patients who had to be withdrawn because of suspected side effects from the largest long-term study (BHAT) was quite small and the principal reason for withdrawal, cardiac failure, was no commoner in patients given propranolol (4.0%) than in controls (3.5%).[18] However, summation of all the complaints of side-effects made at any time did show an excess of complaints in the propranolol group of bronchospasm (31.3% versus 27%; p<0.005). Cold extremities (10.0% versus 7.7%; p<0.025), tiredness (66.8% vs 62.1%; p<0.005) and diarrhoea (5.5% versus 3.6%; p<0.01). The increased incidence of each individual side-effect was small, but taken together there was a price to be paid for the protective effect of the beta blocker. However if the benefits to quality of life by reduction in anginal attacks and improvement in exercise tolerance are taken into account, the picture is much more positive, a double-blind post-infarction trial having shown that patients taking metoprolol spent a significantly greater number of days in an optimum functional state than did those taking placebo.[37] For patients with angina beta blockers improve the quality as well as the quantity of life.

Which patients should receive a beta blocker and for how long?

As stated earlier, the benefits of beta blockade after MI are proven. But do all patients benefit or can subgroups be identified which benefit more than others? Retrospective analysis of results of the BHAT trial showed that the absolute reduction in mortality was greatest for those who had mechanical or electrical complications[38] and in particular for those with a history of congestive heart failure occurring either before or during their index infarction.[39] Indeed it appears from BHAT that propranolol given over a 25-month period to patients who had no previous cardiac failure saved about two lives per 100 patients compared with five lives per 100 for patients with previous failure. The proportionate reduction in mortality was similar, however, for both groups (25% reduction from 7.8% to 5.9% for patients without failure; 27% reduction from 18.4% to 13.3% for those with failure). These results were achieved without any important increase in mortality, even though more patients with a history of failure who took propranolol had a recurrence of failure within 30 days.[39] Provided cardiac failure is recognized and treated it is frequently unnecessary for beta blocker therapy to be withdrawn.[17,40]

These data clearly show that beta blockade is most effective for high-risk patients. However the goal posts have been moved in recent years by discovery of the protective effect of angiotensin-converting enzyme (ACE) inhibitors for high-risk patients with low ejection fraction,[41,42] the protective effect being, arguably, similar to that of beta blockers. Consequently, beta blockers are now less frequently used for patients with low ejection fraction. However it is of course not unlikely that the benefits from beta blockade and ACE inhibitors would be additive, and further clinical trials are badly needed to find this out.

Is there a group of post-infarction patients for whom the risk is so low that beta blocker therapy is unwarranted? The arguments here are more complex, but the question is so important both clinically and economically that it may be helpful to attempt to make them explicit.

For a patient under 60 years of age with completed infarction and normal left ventricular function who is followed up and managed appropriately in 1995, the annual mortality rate for the first 5 years after infarction should be no more than 1–2%. To show a 25% mortality reduction from this level due to beta blockers or any other form of treatment would require a trial many times larger than any which have been carried out. Thus it is hardly surprising that retrospective analyses of results from the largest trial[38,43] or even from a meta-analysis of all trials[44] have failed to find a protective effect in some low-risk subgroups. Nevertheless it would be surprising if the antiarrhythmic and infarct-preventing actions did not operate in all patients with ischaemic heart disease. It is a reasonable assumption that they do and consequently that one death and one non-fatal reinfarct would be prevented for every 200 to 400 patient years of treatment in low-risk patients. Assuming an annual cost of £100 (A$200) per annum for the medication, prevention of one death and one non-fatal infarct for this group of patients would cost between £20,000 and £40,000 (A$40,000 to A$80,000); this is not over-expensive compared with many treatments in other branches of medicine. It would seem reasonable to offer treatment to all low-risk patients so long as it is tolerated without side-effects, and the above argument could be put to individual patients when appropriate.

Thus this reviewer would advocate administration of a beta blocker to all post-infarct patients who do not have contraindications. It has been estimated however that about 30% of patients are unsuitable for treatment.[8,33] In actual practice, the rate of beta blocker use varies widely. In unpublished data from the United Kingdom Heart Attack study we have found that in three representative centres in the UK only about 50% of post-infarction patients are discharged from hospital taking beta blockers whereas in the Perth MONICA study,[45] the prescribing of beta blockers at the time of discharge from hospital rose from 50% to 75% from the mid 1980s to the 1990s. Only about 30% of patients with known ischaemic heart disease in the community who experience either a MI or sudden cardiac death are taking one of these drugs at the time of the event. Of course many patients with poor left ventricular function are now taking an ACE inhibitor in preference to a beta blocker. Nevertheless it seems to us that beta blockers are still under-used in long-term management after MI.

For how long after MI should the beta blocker be continued? Continued benefit was seen for up to 6 years after timolol,[46] and the same argument applies as for the treatment of low risk patients; it would seem reasonable to continue treatment indefinitely for a patient who is tolerating it well.

Which beta blocker should be used?

Strictly speaking, the recommendation should be that only those drugs proven by clinical trial should be used, and in the doses given in the trial. Results of meta-analyses[8,9] suggest, however, that both cardiac-specific and non-cardiac-specific drugs are equally effective for long-term treatment, but that drugs with partial agonist activity (as might be expected) may be less effective than those without. For intravenous use during evolution of infarction only the cardiac-specific drugs atenolol and metoprolol are commercially available although, as discussed earlier, there are reasons to believe that a non-cardiac-specific drug would be preferable for intravenous use and also, conceivably, for long-term use. Thus this reviewer's preference is for the non-cardiac-specific drugs propranolol or timolol over cardiac-specific atenolol or metoprolol.

Conclusions

Long term administration of beta blockers to patients after MI reduces sudden cardiac death and non-fatal reinfarction, both by about 25%. These drugs are still underused in clinical practice in post-infarction patients. The place of intravenous beta blockade during evolution of infarction is less well defined, mainly because comparatively little information is available on the combination of intravenous beta blockade with thrombolytic therapy. Again the drugs are probably underused, but more clinical trials are needed. Despite 30 years of use, uncertainties remain about the use of beta blockers in clinical practice. In particular, the possible antifibrillatory effect of $beta_2$ blockade over and above that of $beta_1$ blockade needs to be evaluated, as does the possibility of enhancement by beta blockade of the protective effect of ACE inhibition in patients with impaired left ventricular function.

References

1. Rutherford JD, Braunwald E, Sobel BE. In Braunwald E (ed). Heart disease, 3rd ed. Philadelphia: Saunders, 1988: 1330–2
2. Cruickshank JM, Prichard BNC (eds). Beta blockers in clinical practice. Edinburgh: Churchill Livingstone, 1988: 9–273
3. Ho DSW, Zecchin RP, Richards DAB, Uther JB, Ross DL. Double-blind trial of lignocaine versus sotalol for acute termination of spontaneous sustained ventricular tachycardia. Lancet 1994; 344: 18–23
4. Klein RC and the EVSEM investigators. Comparative efficacy of sotalol and class-1 antiarrhythmic agents in patients with ventricular tachycardia and fibrillation: results of the electrophysiology study versus electrocardiographic monitoring (EVSEM) trial. Eur Heart J 1993; (Suppl H): 78–84
5. Mueller H, Ayres SM, Religa A, Evans RG. Propranolol in the treatment of acute myocardial infarction. Effect on myocardial oxygenation and haemodynamics. Circulation 1974; 49: 1078–87
6. Peter T, Norris RM, Clarke ED et al. Reduction in enzyme levels by propranolol after acute myocardial infarction. Circulation 1978; 57: 1091–5
7. Norris RM, Clarke ED, Sammel NL, Smith WM, Williams B. Protective effects of propranolol in threatened myocardial infarction. Lancet 1978; ii: 907–9
8. Yusuf S, Peto R, Lewis J, Collins R, Sleight P. Beta blockade during and after myocardial infarction: an overview of the randomized trials. Progr Cardiovasc Dis 1985; 27: 335–71
9. Held PH, Yusuf S. Effect of beta blockers and calcium channel blockers in acute myocardial infarction. Eur Heart J 1993; 14(Suppl F): 18–25
10. The MIAMI trial research group. Metoprolol in acute myocardial infarction (MIAMI). A randomised placebo-controlled international trial. Eur Heart J 1985; 6: 199–226
11. ISIS-1 (First International Study of Infarct Survival) Collaborative group. Randomised trial of intravenous atenolol among 16 027 cases of suspected acute myocardial infarction: ISIS-1. Lancet 1986; ii: 57–66
12. Roberts R, Rogers WJ, Nueller HS et al. Immediate versus deferred beta blockade following thrombolytic therapy in patients with acute myocardial infarction.

Results of the thrombolysis in myocardial infarction (TIMI) IIb study. Circulation 1991; 83: 422–37
13. Norris RM, Roy S, Dixon GF. What proportion of patients with acute myocardial infarction should receive thrombolytic therapy? Abst. Br Heart J 1994; 71: 120
14. ISIS-1 (First International Study of Infarct Survival) Collaborative group. Mechanisms for the early mortality reduction produced by beta blockade started early in acute myocardial infarction: ISIS-1. Lancet 1988; i: 921–3
15. Fibrinolytic Therapy Trialists (FTT) Collaborative Group. Indications for fibrinolytic therapy in suspected acute myocardial infarction: collaborative overview of early mortality and major morbidity results from all randomised trials of more than 1000 patients. Lancet 1994; 343: 311–20
16. Hjalmarson A, Elmfeldt D, Herlitz J et al. Effect on mortality of metoprolol in acute myocardial infarction. A double-blind randomised trial. Lancet 1981; ii: 823–7
17. Norwegian multicenter study group. Timolol-induced reduction in mortality and reinfarction in patients surviving acute myocardial infarction. N Engl J Med 1981; 304: 801–7
18. Beta-blocker heart attack trial research group: A randomised trial of propranolol in patients with acute myocardial infarction. (Pt I.) Mortality results. JAMA 1982; 247: 1707–14
19. Brown MA, Norris RM, Barnaby PF, Geary GG, Brandt PWT. Effects of early treatment with propranolol on left ventricular function four weeks after myocardial infarction. Br Heart J 1985; 54: 351–6
20. Holmberg S, Varnauskas E. Coronary circulation during pacing-induced tachycardia. Acta Med Scand 1971; 190: 481–90
21. Ramsdale DR, Faragher EB, Bennett DH et al. Ischemic pain relief in patients with acute myocardial infarction by intravenous atenolol. Am Heart J 1982; 103: 459–67
22. Kjekshus J. Importance of heart rate in determining beta blocker efficacy in acute and long-term acute myocardial infarction intervention trials. Am J Cardiol 1986; 57: 3E–49E
23. Olsson G, Rehnquist N. Ventricular arrhythmias during the first year after myocardial infarction: influence of long-term treatment with metoprolol. Circulation 1984; 69: 1129–34
24. Bethge KP, Andersen D, Baisel JP et al. Effect of oxprenolol on ventricular arrhythmias: the European infarction study experience. J Am Coll Cardiol 1985; 6: 963–73
25. The Cardiac Arrhythmia Suppression Trial (CAST) Investigators preliminary report: effect of encainide and flecainide on mortality in a randomized trial of arrhythmia suppression after myocardial infarction. N Engl J Med 1989; 321: 406–12
26. Brown MJ, Brown DC, Murphy MB. Hypokalemia from $beta_2$ receptor stimulation by circulating epinephrine. N Engl J Med 1983; 309: 1414–9
27. Nordrehaug JE, von der Lippe G. Hypokalaemia and ventricular fibrillation in acute myocardial infarction. Br Heart J 1983; 50: 525–9
28. Hall JA, Ferro A, Dickerson JEC, Brown MJ. Beta adrenoceptor subtype cross regulation in the human heart. Br Heart J 1993; 69: 332–7
29. Herlitz J, Edvardsson N, Holmberg S et al. Goteborg Metoprolol Trial: effects on arrhythmias. Am J Cardiol 1984; 53: 27D–31D
30. The MIAMI trial research group. Arrhythmias. Am J Cardiol 1985; 56: 35g–38g
31. Norris RM, Barnaby PF, Brown MA, Geary GG, Clarke ED, Logan RL, Sharpe DN. Prevention of ventricular fibrillation during acute myocardial infarction by intravenous propranolol. Lancet 1984; ii: 883–6
32. The International Collaborative Study Group. Reduction of infarct size with the early use of timolol in acute myocardial infarction. N Engl J Med 1984; 310: 9–15
33. Chamberlain DA. Beta blockers and calcium antagonists. In: Julian D, Braunwald E (eds). Management of acute myocardial infarction. London: Saunders, 1994: 193–221
34. Callahan DS, Johnson AR, Campbell WB. Enhancement of the antiaggregatory activity of prostacyclin by propranolol in human platelets. Circulation 1985; 71: 1237–46
35. Winther K, Rein E. Exercise-induced platelet aggregation in angina and its possible prevention by $beta_1$ selective blockade. Eur Heart J 1990; 11: 819–23
36. Gaglione A, Hess OM, Corin WJ, Ritter M, Grimm J, Krayenbuehl HP. Is there coronary vasoconstriction after intracoronary beta adrenergic blockade in patients with coronary artery disease? J Am Coll Cardiol 1987; 10: 299–310
37. Olsson G, Larsen J, van Es GA, Rehnquist N. Quality of life after myocardial infarction: effect of long term metoprolol on mortality and morbidity. Br Med J 1986; 292: 1491–3
38. Furberg CD, Hawkins CM, Lichstein E for the Beta Blocker Heart Attack Study Group. Effect of propranolol in post infarction patients with mechanical or electrical complications. Circulation 1984; 69: 761–5
39. Chadda K, Goldstein S, Byington R, Curb JD. Effect of propranolol after acute myocardial infarction in patients with congestive heart

failure. Circulation 1986; 73: 503–10

40. Gunderson T. Influence of heart size in mortality and reinfarction in patients treated with timolol after myocardial infarction. Br Heart J 1983; 50: 135–9
41. Pfeffer MA, Braunwald E, Moye LA et al. The effect of captopril on mortality and morbidity in patients with left ventricular dysfunction after myocardial infarction. Results of the Survival and Ventricular Enlargement Trial. N Engl J Med 1992; 327: 669–77
42. The SOLVD Investigators. Effect of enalapril on mortality and the development of heart failure in asymptomatic patients with reduced left ventricular ejection fractions. N Engl J Med 1992; 327: 685–91
43. Gheorghiade M, Schultz L, Tilley B, Kao W, Goldstein S. Effects of propranolol in non-Q-wave acute myocardial infarction in the beta blocker heart attack trial. Am J Cardiol 1990; 66: 129–33
44. The Beta Blocker Pooling Project Research Group. The beta blocker pooling project (BBPP): subgroup findings from randomized trials in post-infarction patients. Eur Heart J 1988; 9: 8–16
45. Thompson PL, Parsons RW, Jamrozik KD, Hockey R, Hobbs MST, Broadhurst R. Changing patterns of medical treatment in acute myocardial infarction: observations from the Perth MONICA project. Med J Aust 1992; 157: 87–92
46. Pedersen TR for the Norwegian Multicenter Study Group. Six year follow-up of the Norwegian Multicenter Study on timolol after acute myocardial infarction. N Engl J Med 1985; 313: 1055–8

29 Calcium channel blockers

David T Kelly

Introduction

Calcium channel blockers are widely used in the coronary care unit (CCU), although a lack of support from clinical trials in myocardial infarction has seen a decline in their use in the 1990s.[1]

A large number of drugs are available. The reader is referred to one of the excellent monographs which describes these drugs in detail.[2,3]

The terminology for the drugs is confusing but the terms calcium antagonists, calcium channel antagonists, calcium entry antagonists, slow channel antagonists and calcium channel blockers are used interchangeably. The calcium channel blockers have heterogeneous chemical stuctures. The major groups are summarized in the information box.

The vascular and myocardial effects of the five major agents are summarized in Table 29.1.

The prototype dihydropyridine is nifedipine. Its potent vasodilating action and rapid onset of action are valuable properties in the relief of coronary spasm and in achieving rapid control of elevated blood pressure. However, it may produce a reflex tachycardia and neurohumoral activation which can have adverse effects in ischaemic heart disease and left ventricular dysfunction. This may explain the disappointing results post myocardial infarction (see below) and in unstable angina (see Ch. 60).

Modification of its delivery by retard preparations may modulate the reflex tachycardia and neuro-

Calcium channel blocker classification

Dihydropyridines

1st generation
- Nifedipine

2nd generation
- Amlodipine
- Felodipine
- Isradipine
- Nicardipine
- Nimodipine
- Nisoldipine
- Nitrandipine

Phenylalkylamines
- Verapamil

Benzothiazepines
- Diltiazem

Miscellaneous
- Lidoflazine
- Perhexiline
- Bedridil

Table 29.1 Characteristics of five commonly used calcium channel blockers

	Nifedipine	Amlodipine	Felodipine	Diltiazem	Verapamil
Heart rate	↑	0	0	↓	↓
A-V node conduction	0	0	0	↓	↓↓
Myocardial contractility	0	0	0	↓	↓↓
Coronary blood flow	↑↑	↑↑	↑↑	↑	↑
Peripheral vasodilatation	↑↑	↑↑	↑↑	↑	↑
Duration of action	+	++	+	+	+

↑ = increases; ↓ = reduces, 0 = no effect; + = 3–6 hours; ++ = 6–24 hours

humoral response but these preparations have not been tested in large post-infarction trials or unstable angina. The newer generation of dihydropyridines produce less neurohumoral activation and have a longer duration of action. They have found ready acceptance as anti-hypertensive agents. Amlodipine and felodipine have been shown to have anti-anginal properties but they have not been the subject of post-infarction or unstable angina survival studies. Because of their minimal chronotropic and negative inotropic properties the dihydropyridines can be used safely in conjuction with beta blocking drugs.

Diltiazem has peripheral and coronary vasodilating properties rendering it a highly effective anti-anginal and anti-hypertensive agent. Its effect on atrioventricular (AV) node conduction is less potent than that of verapamil but caution is required in its use in conjunction with beta blockers because of the sympathomimetic effect on myocardial contractility and AV node conduction.

Verapamil's actions are similar to diltiazem's apart from a more pronounced negative inotropic effect and its effect on delaying conduction through the AV node. The latter property underlies its efficacy as an effective agent for the treatment of re-entrant supraventricular tachycardia. Adverse interactions with beta blocking drugs are widely recognized, although with careful monitoring the combination has been used in the past. In practice the non-cardiac side-effects of verapamil, especially constipation in elderly patients, are often the limiting factor in verapamil therapy.

Less frequently used calcium channel blockers include lidoflazine, perhexilene and bepradil. The anti-anginal effect of lidoflazine has been limited by a reported pro-arrhythmic effect. Perhexilene has some use as an anti-anginal agent. Bepradil is an anti-arrhythmic agent also limited by pro-arrhythmic properties and marked prolongation of the QT interval.

Use in myocardial infarction

Calcium channel blockers in experimental myocardial infarction have been shown to reduce myocardial necrosis and preserve left ventricular function.[2,3] The mechanism of action may include reduced afterload, direct coronary vasodilatation and decreased intracellular calcium overload to minimize further myocardial damage.[4]

These encouraging experimental results have led to many trials in myocardial infarction. At least 24 randomized trials of calcium antagonists have been reported in the acute phase or early after acute infarction.[5] The end points have included infarct size, reinfarction and mortality. Experience has been mainly with nifedipine, verapamil and diltiazem. Most of the trials are small but there are several large trials available with mortality and reinfarction as the primary outcomes. Figure 29.1 shows the overall effect on mortality and reinfarction.

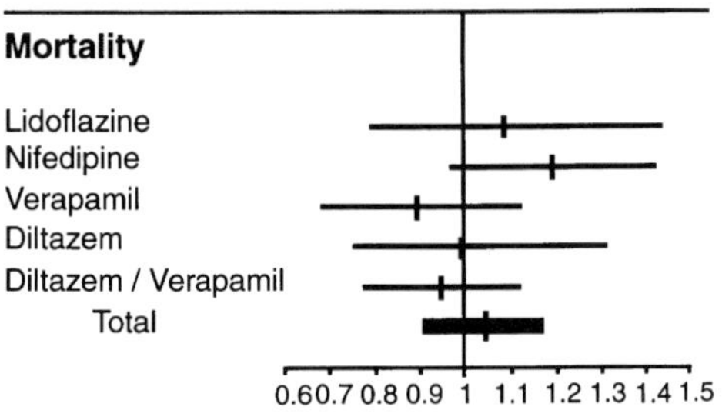

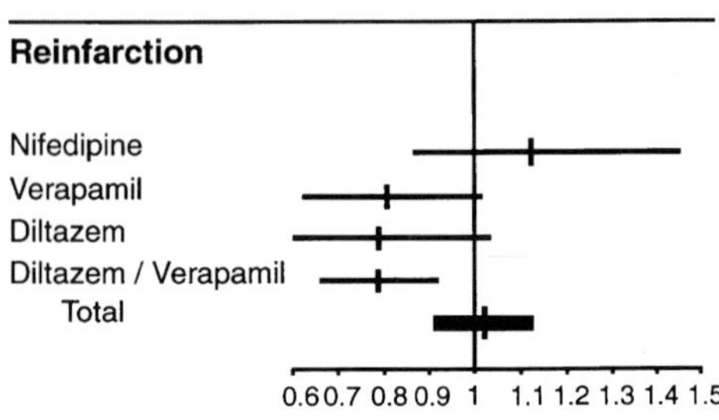

Fig. 29.1 Meta-analysis of trials of calcium channel blockers in myocardial infarction. (Adapted with permission from Held PH, Yusuf S. Coronary Artery Disease 1994; 5: 21–26.[5])

Nifedipine

Overall, nifedipine has been the most extensively studied with nearly 10 000 patients in thirteen trials.[5] Variations were seen in the dosage, duration and onset of treatment ranging from 2 days to 2 weeks and evaluation varying from 1 to 6 months. In nine trials designed to look at infarct size, no significant difference was noted between treatment and control. In the three trials specifically designed to study the effects on mortality, no difference was found. The commonly quoted trials are TRENT, SPRINT I and SPRINT II. The TRENT (Trial of Early Nifedipine in Acute Myocardial Infarction) compared administration of nifedipine and placebo for 1 month in 4491 patients.[6] No difference in one month's survival was seen. In SPRINT I, nifedipine was given 7–21 days post-infarction and no effects on mortality were seen in a mean 10 month follow-up of 2276 patients.[7] The trial was discontinued because no effect was found. In SPRINT II, which was confined to higher risk patients, those with anterior recurrent myocardial infarction, the study was discontinued because of a trend (non-significant) to a higher mortality in the nifedipine group.[8]

In summary, of the 13 trials no benefit was found therapeutically from the use of nifedipine either short or long term in patients who had suffered myocardial infarction.[5] There was a strong but not significant trend to higher mortality and reinfarction rates in the treatment group. Thus although these trials do not conclusively prove nifedipine is harmful, no benefit has been established and therefore its use is not recommended. By inference this would apply to other dihydropyridine calcium antagonists, although the smoother onset of action with less reflex tachycardia and neurohumoral activation seen in the second generation dihydropyridines, such as amlodipine or felodipine, could produce different results if they were subjected to large-scale post-infarction trials.

Verapamil

The major verapamil trials are the Danish DAVIT I and DAVIT II.[9,10] In DAVIT I, 3600 patients with suspected infarcts were randomized early and intravenous(IV) verapamil was given, followed by oral therapy for 6 months.[9] Patients taking beta blockers were excluded. No difference was noted in mortality rate but there was a high incidence of AV block and heart failure early, suggesting IV verapamil should have been avoided. In the later phase of follow-up, a decrease in reinfarction was noted. Because of this the DAVIT II trial was initiated, where therapy was begun between 1 and 3 weeks after acute infarction and patients with heart failure were excluded.[10] In 1800 patients randomly assigned, a positive benefit was suggested with a reduction in mortality of about 9% (non-significant). In addition there was a lower reinfarction rate.

Diltiazem

There are five published randomized trials with approximately 3100 patients. Only one large trial was conducted, the MDPIT study.[11] This involved 2500 patients followed for a mean of 25 months, with no difference in mortality between diltiazem and placebo. Patients with symptoms or signs of failure or low ejection rate had a significantly increased mortality rate. Non-fatal reinfarctions were less common. A further short-term trial showed that patients with non-Q wave infarction only, treated with Diltiazem for 14 days after admission, showed a 20% reduction of reinfarction (borderline statistical significance).[12] This trend is also found in the MDPIT trial at 1 year. These studies led to a Joint Taskforce of the American Heart Association and the American College of Cardiology to recommend that patients with non-Q wave infarction be given diltiazem orally in the first 24 hours and continued for 1 year. This is important, as beta blockers do not reduce death or reinfarction in these patients with non-Q wave infarction.[13]

Importance of heart rate reduction

The first generation dihydropyridines, mainly represented in published studies by nifedipine, with the attendant increase in heart rate, tend to increase the risk of death and reinfarction. This effect appears to be dose-related, with higher risks for patients taking moderate to high doses (>60mg) of rapidly acting nifedipine,[13a] although the magnitude of the adverse effect is debatable.[13b] In contrast the calcium antagonists that slow heart rate, namely verapamil and diltiazem, tend to decrease the rate of subsequent reinfarction and thus the long-term mortality.[5]

Current indications for the use of calcium antagonists in myocardial infarction

In the acute phase of infarction no calcium antagonist is recommended and may be deleterious. In patients with heart failure they are definitely contraindicated. In patients with non-Q wave infarction, who have normal left ventricular function and no failure, diltiazem has been shown to reduce the event rate and may be considered as appropriate therapy for these patients. Despite the promising experimental data, overall major clinical trials have shown no clinical benefit to suggest calcium antagonists are helpful in Q wave infarction. Although most patients have left the CCU by 11 days, the DAVIT II study suggests that there may be a beneficial effect of verapamil administered later in patients with normal ventricular function as this may decrease subsequent event rate and may be considered in patients where beta blockade is contraindicated following myocardial infarction.

Most of the calcium channel blocker trials were done prior to the advent of routine thrombolytic therapy in acute infarction. Boden has suggested that with recanalization of the coronary artery due to thrombolytic therapy, the therapeutic indications for calcium antagonists following infarction may be increased and important.[14] Proof of this however is awaited and because of the mainly negative effects of calcium antagonists, a cautious approach should be adopted.

Unstable angina pectoris

About 1000 patients have been included in clinical trials of calcium channel blockers in unstable angina. The largest and most influential was the HINT (Holland Interuniversity Trial) comparing nifedipine, metoprolol and placebo in a total of 515 patients.[15] Among the 338 patients not pre-treated with a beta blocker the incidence of infarction and recurrent ischaemia was 37% in the placebo-treated group, higher in the nifedipine-treated group (47%) and lower in the metoprolol-treated group (28%). Among the 177 patients pre-treated with a beta blocker the incidence of infarction and ischaemia was lower in the nifedipine-treated group (30%) than the placebo group (51%). The trial was terminated early because of the adverse trend with nifedipine. This has influenced practice against nifedipine monotherapy in unstable angina. However, nifedipine does appear to be safe in conjunction with a beta blocker in this situation. Trials of new generation dihydropyridines in unstable angina are awaited with interest.

Tachyarrhythmias

Verapamil has an established place in the management of re-entrant supraventricular tachycardia although it is no longer regarded as first line therapy because of wider availability of adenosine (see Ch. 27). Rarely verapamil is used in ventricular tachycardias due to triggered automaticity.

Other uses of calcium channel blockers

Calcium channel blockers are widely prescribed for hypertension.[13] A recent meta analysis concluded that short-acting nifedipine may have adverse effects in hypertension, but there is no evidence of harm for other preparations.[15a,15b] Sublingual nifedipine may be useful for hypertensive emergencies in the CCU (see Ch. 69). The use of calcium channel blockers in cardiac failure has been actively investigated because of their potent vasodilating and afterload reducing properties. The first generation agents have been unsuccessful and reports of adverse responses have resulted in cautions against their use.[16,17] However, encouraging results are now being reported with the second generation dihydropyridines.[18]

Anti-atherosclerotic effects of calcium channel blockers have been investigated following apparent benefits in experimental models of atherosclerosis.[19] The INTACT trial showed an apparent benefit in that fewer new lesions developed in patients treated with nifedipine compared with placebo[20] although this encouraging finding was somewhat overshadowed by a higher mortality in the nifedipine-treated patients. At present there is insufficient evidence to justify this application of calcium channel blockers.

In addition to many other therapies, calcium channel blockers have been used to treat restenosis after coronary angioplasty. Trials so far have shown no clear effect, although a preliminary report with diltiazem has been encouraging.[21] Calcium channel blockers are not routinely used to prevent re-stenosis, although they may have a role in the early stages post angioplasty when localized coronary artery spasm is suspected.

References

1. Thompson PL, Parsons RW, Jamrozik K et al. Changing patterns of medical treatment in acute myocardial infarction. Med J Aust 1992; 157: 87–92
2. Opie LH. Clinical use of calcium antagonist drugs. 2nd ed. Boston: Klinver, 1990
3. Nayler WG. Calcium antagonists. London: Academic Press, 1988
4. Kloner RA, Braunwald E. Effects of calcium antagonists on infarcting myocardium. Am J Cardiol 1987; 59: 84–94B
5. Held PH, Yusuf S. Calcium antagonists in the treatment of ischaemic heart disease: myocardial infarction. Coronary Artery Disease 1994; 5: 21–6
6. Willox RG, Hampton RF, Banks DC et al. Trial of early nifedipine in acute myocardial infarction. The TRENT study. Br Heart J 1986; 293: 1204–8
7. The Israeli SPRINT Study Group: Secondary Prevention Reinfarction Israeli Nifedipine Trial (SPRINT). A randomised intervention trial of nifedipine in patients with acute myocardial infarction. Eur Heart J 1988; 9: 354–64
8. Goldbourt U, Behar S, Reicher-Reiss H, Zion M, Mandelzweigh L, Kaplinsky E. Early administration of nifedipine in suspected acute myocardial infarction. The Secondary Prevention Reinfarction Israeli Nifedipine Trial 2 Study. Arch Intern Med 1993; 153: 345–53
9. Danish Study Group on Verapamil in Myocardial Infarction: verapamil in acute myocardial infarction. Eur Heart J 1984; 5: 516–28
10. The Danish Study Group on Verapamil in Myocardial Infarction: effect of verapamil on mortality and major events after acute myocardial infarction (The Danish Verapamil Infarction Trial II—DAVIT II). Am J Cardiol 1990; 66: 779–85
11. Multicenter Diltiazem Post-infarction Trial Research Group: the effect of diltiazem on mortality and reinfarction after myocardial infarction. N Engl J Med 1988; 319: 385–92
12. Gibson RS, Boden WE, Theroux P et al. Diltiazem and reinfarction in patients with non-Q wave myocardial infarction. N Engl J Med 1986; 315: 423–9
13. Ross J Jr, Brandenburg RO, Dinsmore RE et al. Report of American College of Cardiology, American Heart Association Taskforce on Assessment of Diagnostic and Therapeutic Cardiovascular Procedures. J Am Coll Cardiol 1987; 10: 935–50

13a. Furberg CD, Psaty BM, Meyer JV. Nifedipine: dose-related increase in mortality in patients with coronary heart disease. Circulation 1995; 92: 1326–31

13b. Opie LH, Messerli FH. Nifedipine and mortality: grave defects in the dossier. Circulation 1995; 92: 1068–73

14. Boden WE. Calcium channel blockers as adjuvant therapy post-thrombolysis. J Cardiovasc Pharmacol 1991; 18 (Suppl 10): S102–S106
15. The Holland Interuniversity Nifedipine/Metoprolol Trial (HINT) research group. Early treatment of unstable angina in the coronary care unit; a randomized, double blind, placebo controlled comparison of recurrent ischaemia in patients treated with nifedipine or metoprolol or both. Br Heart J 1986; 56: 400–413

15a. Psaty BM, Heckbert Sr, Koepsell TD, et al. The risk of myocardial infarction associated with antihypertensive therapies. JAMA 1995; 274: 620–25

15b. Buring JE, Glynn RJ, Hennekens CH. Calcium channel blockers and myocardial infarction: a hypothesis formulated but not yet tested. JAMA 1995; 274: 654–5

16. Packer M. Calcium channel blockers in chronic heart failure. Circulation 1990; 82: 2254–7
17. Editorial. Calcium antagonist caution. Lancet 1991; 337: 885–6
18. PRAISE trial. Preliminary results presented at American College of Cardiology 44th Annual Scientific Sessions in New Orleans, March 1995
19. Weinstein DB, Heider JG. Antiatherogenic properties of calcium antagonists. Am J Cardiol 1989; 86: 27–32
20. Lichtlen PR, Hugenholtz PG, Rafflenbeul W et al. Retardation of coronary disease in man by the calcium channel blocker nifedipine. Results of INTACT (International Nifedipine Trial on Antiatherosclerotic Therapy). Lancet 1990; 335: 1109–13
21. Unverdorben M, Kunkel B, Leucht M et al. Reduction of restenosis after PTCA by diltiazem. Abst. Circulation 1992; 86: 1–53

30 Nitrate therapy

John D Horowitz

Background

In the past ten years, extensive evidence has accumulated to engender the hypothesis that acute myocardial ischaemic syndromes can be regarded to a large extent as the consequence of a deficiency of endogenous homeostatic mechanisms ultimately involving the activation of soluble guanylate cyclase in vascular smooth muscle and platelets.[1–4] To a large extent, the relevant investigations suggest that in patients prone to the development of acute ischaemic syndromes there is a deficiency of production of nitric oxide (or of a chemically bound form of nitric oxide) by vascular endothelial cells.[1,2] This nitric oxide-like material (termed endothelium-derived relaxing factor) induces activation of soluble guanylate cyclase in vascular smooth muscle and platelets, leading to smooth muscle relaxation, and both inhibition and reversal of platelet aggregation.[3-5]

Recent studies have also demonstrated that there is a circulating 'pool' of S-nitrosoproteins in plasma, which probably induce background activation of soluble guanylate cyclase both directly and via transnitrosation to form smaller, more active, S-nitroso thiol molecules.[6,7] The relationship between the genesis of this circulating source of guanylate cyclase activation and variation of endothelial function is currently not well understood.

The potential pathophysiological impact of deficiency of endogenous guanylate cyclase activators in patients at risk of developing acute myocardial ischaemia is compounded by the intimate physiological relationship between endothelium-derived relaxing factor (EDRF) and a number of vasoconstrictor materials, particularly endothelin (Et). It appears probable that EDRF functions both as an inhibitor of Et release and as the most potent physiological antagonist of Et effect.[8,9] These various factors involving EDRF and other endogenous activators of soluble guanylate cyclase which may interface with the development of acute ischaemic syndromes are summarized in Figure 30.1.

In addition, it should be mentioned that experimental evidence is now accumulating implicating the release of nitric oxide or analogous materials from the endocardium and the coronary microvasculature in the process of left ventricular relaxation.[10] Hence it is possible that adequacy of such mechanisms may be critical to the maintenance of diastolic coronary perfusion in patients prone to myocardial ischaemia.

Organic nitrates

Exogenous activators of soluble guanylate cyclase

The finding that nitroglycerin (NTG; glyceryl trinitrate) acts as an activator of soluble guanylate cyclase (SGC) antedated the identification of EDRF.[11,12] It has also been apparent for many years that NTG and other organic nitrates are *indirect* donors of nitric oxide and hence activators of SGC; in vitro experiments indicate the presence of at least one enzymatic mechanism of bioconversion of NTG to yield less active dinitrates and nitric oxide. Isosorbide mononitrate and dinitrates also undergo enzymatic denitration to liberate nitric oxide. The process of activation of soluble guanylate cyclase by NTG in particular is critically dependent on the availability of certain sulphydryl (SH) compounds, with cysteine accelerating the bioconversion to nitric oxide approximately 100-fold.[13]

In contrast to the organic nitrates, a number of other agents are more direct donors of nitric

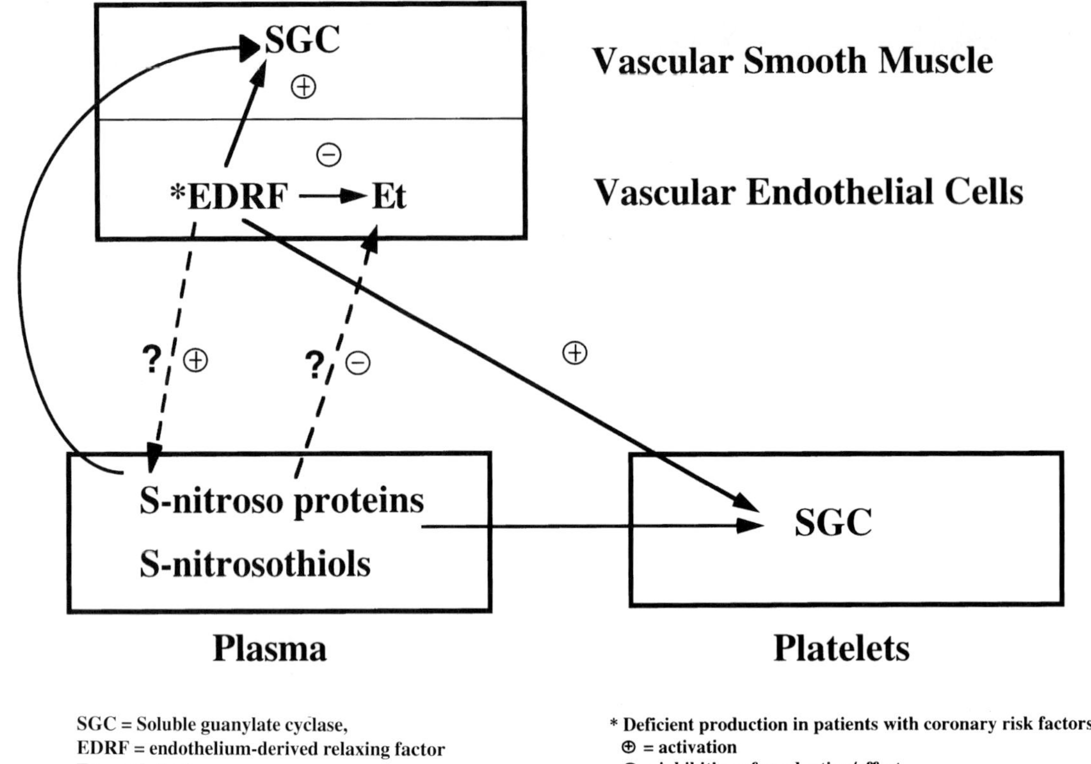

Fig. 30.1 Mechanisms of potential interaction between endogenous activators of soluble guanylate cyclase and the pathogenesis of acute myocardial ischaemia and infarction.

oxide. The actions of such agents (for example, sodium nitroprusside and molsidomine) are not critically modified by SH compounds.

Haemodynamic and anti-platelet effects of nitrates in acute ischaemic syndromes

It was once assumed on the basis of studies involving atrial pacing in patients with stable exertional angina that the anti-anginal actions of nitrates are independent of changes in either coronary haemodynamics or afterload, but are mediated entirely via changes in venous capacitance. More recent studies indicate that nitrates exert unique effects on coronary flow distribution, via a combination of dilatation of epicardial coronary arteries (including stenosed vessels), increases in collateral blood flow and redistribution of coronary flow from subepicardium towards the subendocardial area, which is more prone to ischaemic injury.[14,15] The effects of nitrates on afterload may also be relevant, with an improvement in arterial compliance detectable after administration of relatively small doses of NTG. Hence in patients without severe systolic heart failure, intravenous administration of NTG (5–10 μg/min) induces significant falls in both pulmonary capillary wedge pressure and systolic arterial pressure; changes in mean arterial pressure tend to be less pronounced.[16] Increases in coronary blood flow in similar patients occur after intracoronary injection of as little as 1 μg of NTG.[17]

The effects of nitrates on platelet aggregation, like those of nitric oxide, include both inhibition and reversal of aggregation.[3–5] Recent studies suggest that this effect may be a critical determinant of the efficacy of nitrates in the treatment of acute ischaemic syndromes. Indeed, in a canine model of coronary artery stenosis, NTG prevented the development of cyclic flow reductions due to intermittent platelet aggregation; this effect was potentiated by the SH donor N-acetylcysteine

(NAC).[18] Analogously, intracoronary injection of isosorbide dinitrate (ISDN) has been shown to stabilize coronary blood flow in patients prone to coronary reocclusion in the immediate peri-infarct period.[19]

Nitrate tolerance and pseudotolerance—mechanisms and clinical significance in acute ischaemia

The major factor limiting the therapeutic utility of nitrates for continuous administration is the potential loss of therapeutic effect. This attenuation of effect, which can be demonstrated in either intact animal models or isolated tissues after prolonged administration of any organic nitrate, appears to have two basic mechanisms:

- **Tolerance**. This is a loss of vascular responsiveness to nitrates, due to failure of the process of bioconversion which results in both progressive denitration and the release of nitric oxide. This process is relatively specific for nitrates, with intact responsiveness to direct nitric oxide donors and other vasodilators.
- **Pseudo-tolerance**. There is a progressive loss of *net* response to nitrates, due to increased activation of vasoconstrictor mechanisms (for example catecholamines and the renin-angiotensin system).[20]

The attenuation of response therefore reflects the simultaneous presence of vasodilator (nitrate) and vasoconstrictor tone within the vasculature. Sudden withdrawal of nitrate in this circumstance would lead to net vasoconstriction, the basis for a phenomenon of *rebound* aggravation of ischaemia.

At present there is no convenient way in vivo to differentiate the relative contribution of these two mechanisms to loss of nitrate effect in any individual patient. There is some evidence to suggest that pseudo-tolerance tends to be more marked when nitrates are administered to patients with systolic heart failure.[20] However, there is adequate clinical evidence in patients with stable angina to support the development of pseudo-tolerance in at least some individuals, with manifestations including both a clear-cut rebound phenomenon and the so-called 'zero-hour' phenomenon.[21] Furthermore there is currently inadequate evidence to support the contention that the extent of pseudo-tolerance can be minimized via co-administration of angiotensin-converting enzyme (ACE) inhibitors and/or calcium antagonists. Hence the potential development of this problem represents a major limiting factor to intermittent therapeutic administration of nitrates in patients with acute myocardial ischaemia.

Intravenous infusion of NTG—optimal methodology

Although some patients with unstable angina and/or AMI may experience symptomatic improvement when treated with oral or cutaneous nitrates, continuous intravenous infusion of NTG offers maximal control of nitrate delivery and minimal risk of adverse events.

As NTG and other nitrates are extensively adsorbed onto many plastics (notably PVC), it is important that NTG solutions be made up in glass bottles, with infusion via specialized non-adsorbent tubing. There is no practical alternative to this.

The optimal infusion rate of NTG has been the subject of controversy largely engendered by the use of suboptimal delivery systems and attempts to titrate infusion rates to a haemodynamic end-point (typically a 10% reduction in arterial pressure).[22] Studies in patients with angina show that in non-tolerant individuals systemic haemodynamic effects generally occur with infusion rates of approximately 5 μg/min. Higher infusion rates induce (initially) more extensive effects, but it is now clear that infusion rates greater than 20 μg/min are associated with development within 24 hours of extensive nitrate tolerance).[17]

For these reasons, it is to be recommended that NTG infusion rates for most individuals should not be increased to more than 10 μg/min for any length of time, irrespective of the extent of ischaemic symptoms. Occasional episodes of angina persisting despite intravenous NTG infusion are probably best managed by administering sublingual NTG on an intermittent basis. Indeed, occasional patients are very sensitive to NTG, and require lower infusion rates (1–2.5 μg/min) to prevent adverse effects such as headache and hypotension.[4]

A number of studies[23] have demonstrated that intravenous NTG may inhibit the anticoagulant effects of heparin, raising the possibility of significant fluctuations in partial thromboplastin time when NTG infusion is commenced or ceased in patients also receiving heparin. This interaction probably is only clinically relevant if NTG is infused at very high rates (greater than 50 μg/min).

The process of *withdrawal* from intravenous NTG therapy is important, especially in patients who have received relatively high infusion rates of NTG and in whom pseudo-tolerance may have developed. In general, a transition from intravenous to oral (or cutaneous) nitrate prophylaxis should be recommended, in order to minimize the risk of rebound aggravation of ischaemia.[24]

Therapy with oral or cutaneous nitrates in acute ischaemic syndromes

As indicated earlier, the potential development of nitrate tolerance generally limits the utility of nitrates to intermittent therapy. While this is adequate for most patients with predictable patterns of angina, it is not ideal for patients with acute ischaemic syndromes, in whom the occurrence of myocardial ischaemia is related primarily to changes in coronary blood flow, associated with intracoronary thrombosis and variable coronary vasomotor tone.

For this reason, therapy with transdermal NTG (which requires at least a 10-hour nitrate-free period to avoid tolerance) or sustained release isosorbide mononitrate (which provides a 'nitrate-poor' period of approximately 8 hours) is less than ideal for such patients, and cannot be recommended for very unstable ischaemic states. Intermittent isosorbide dinitrate is also suboptimal, with the necessity to limit therapy to a maximum of 8-hourly dosing in order to prevent development of tolerance.

Given the inadequacies of nitrates for 24-hour prophylaxis of ischaemia in such patients, there is a strong argument for simultaneous administration of other anti-ischaemic drugs in patients with acute ischaemic syndromes.

Co-administration of NTG and N-acetylcysteine (NAC)

It has been known for some time that NAC potentiates the haemodynamic[16,25] and anti-anginal[26] effects of nitrates. Furthermore NAC reduces the risk of occurrence of AMI in high risk patients with unstable angina.[27]

The mechanism of therapeutic interaction between NTG and NAC is incompletely understood. It is clear that NAC limits nitrate tolerance in some circumstances, but the extent of potentiation of NTG effects by NAC is largely independent of the development of tolerance. NAC also potentiates the effects of NTG in inhibiting platelet aggregation.[28]

In patients with myocardial ischaemia resistant to NTG infusion, co-infusion of NAC results in maintenance of anti-ischaemic effect. As intermittent administration of NAC may induce hypotension, NAC should be infused continuously at a rate of 10 g/24 h.[27] NTG infusion rates may need to be reduced simultaneously (for example to 2.5 μg/min), in order to reduce the risk of hypotension or development of headaches. Sublingual dosing with NTG should be limited to a maximum of 300 μg during NAC infusion, in order to minimize risk of hypotension.

Nitrate administration during evolving acute myocardial infarction: current status

Over the last 2 years, a number of studies have been undertaken to evaluate the potentially beneficial effects of nitrates and related nitric oxide donors in evolving AMI. These studies, GISSI-III,[29] ESPRIM[30] and ISIS-4,[31] are important in that they represent the only investigations reported to date which are large enough to examine effects on mortality. A previous meta-analysis of randomized trials involving NTG from the pre-thrombolytic era had suggested considerable reduction in mortality.[32] However, the more recent investigations cast some doubt upon this conclusion.

The GISSI-III[29] study evaluated the effects of lisinopril and/or NTG in 19 394 patients. NTG was infused at rates sufficient to reduce systolic blood pressure by at least 10%; such rates are likely to be associated with considerable extents of tolerance.[17] Subsequently, transdermal NTG was utilized in an intermittent manner. While evidence was obtained of an additive beneficial effect of lisinopril and NTG on 6-week mortality, NTG alone did not significantly reduce mortality.

The ISIS-4 study[31] involved 58 050 patients receiving as study drugs captopril, isosorbide mononitrate and/or magnesium sulphate. The major end-point was 5-week mortality, which was not significantly reduced by isosorbide mononitrate (although there was a trend in this direction). On the other hand, it was found that isosorbide dinitrate therapy was associated with a marked reduction in mortality on the first day of treatment. Furthermore, the frequency of utilization of intravenously infused NTG was high on the first day of treatment, irrespective of subgroup on randomization; apparent benefit of nitrate therapy.

These results suggest that there is little prognostic benefit associated with prolonged utilization of the nitrate treatment regimens from either GISSI-III or ISIS-4 after AMI. On the other hand, infusion of NTG at low rates, alone or together with NAC, may be beneficial in the short term. NTG/NAC reduces oxidative stress in streptokinase-treated patients with evolving MI[33].

References

1. Ludmer PL, Selwyn AP, Shook TL et al. Paradoxical vasoconstriction induced by acetylcholine in atherosclerotic coronary arteries. N Engl J Med 1986; 315: 1046–51
2. Chester AH, O'Neill GS, Moncada S, Tajkarimi S, Yakoub MH. Low basal and stimulated release of nitric oxide in atherosclerotic epicardial coronary arteries. Lancet 1990; 336: 897–900
3. Chirkov YY, Naujalis JI, Sage RE, Horowitz JD. Antiplatelet effect of nitroglycerin in healthy subjects and in patients with stable angina pectoris. J Cardiovasc Pharmacol 1993; 21: 384–9
4. Horowitz JD. Role of nitrates in unstable angina pectoris. Am J Cardiol 1992; 70: 64B–71B
5. Chirkov YY, Naujalis JI, Barber S et al. Reversal of human platelet aggregation by low concentrations of nitroglycerin in vitro in normal subjects. Am J Cardiol 1992; 70: 802–6
6. Stamler JS, Jaraki OA, Osborde DI et al. Nitric oxide circulates in mammalian plasma primarily as an S-nitroso adduct of serum albumin. Proc Natl Acad Sci USA 1992; 89: 7674–7
7. Scharfstein JS, Keaney JF, Slivka A et al. In vivo transfer of nitric oxide between a plasma protein-bound reservoir and low molecular weight thiols. J Clin Invest 1994; 94: 1432–9
8. Boulanger C, Luscher TF. Release of endothelin from the porcine aorta. Inhibition by endothelium-derived nitric oxide. J Clin Invest 1990; 85: 587–90
9. Yang Z, Buhler FR, Diederich D, Luscher TF. Different effects of endothelin-1 on cAMP and cGMP-mediated vascular relaxation in human arteries and veins: comparison with norepinephrine. J Cardiovasc Pharmacol 1989; 13: S129–131
10. Mohan P, Brutsaert DL, Sys SU. Myocardial performance is modulated by interaction of cardiac endothelium-derived nitric oxide and prostaglandins. Circulation 1994; 90(2): 648
11. Gruetter CA, Gruetter DY, Lyon JE et al. Relationship between cyclic guanosine 3′5′-monophosphate formation and relaxation of coronary arterial smooth muscle by glyceryl trinitrate, nitroprusside, nitrite and nitric oxide: effects of methylene blue and hemoglobin. J Pharmacol Exp Ther 1981; 219: 181–6
12. Katsuki S, Arnold WP, Murad F. Effects of sodium nitroprusside, nitroglycerin and sodium azide on levels of cyclic nucleotides and mechanical activity of various tissues. Adv Cycl Nucl Res 1977; 3: 239–47
13. Ignarro LJ, Gruetter CA. Requirements of thiols for activation of coronary arterial guanylate cyclase by glyceryl trinitrate and sodium nitrite. Possible involvement of S-nitrosothiols. Biochem Biophys Acta 1980; 631: 221–31
14. Cohn PF, Maddox D, Holman BL et al. Effect of sublingually administered nitroglycerin on regional myocardial blood flow in patients with coronary artery disease. Am J Cardiol 1977; 39: 672–8
15. Liu P, Houle S, Burns RJ et al. Effect of intracoronary nitroglycerin on myocardial blood flow and distribution in pacing induced angina pectoris. Quantitative assessment by single-photon emission tomography. Am J Cardiol 1985; 55: 1270–6
16. Horowitz JD, Antman EM, Lorell BH et al. Potentiation of the cardiovascular effects of nitroglycerin by N-acetylcysteine. Circulation 1983; 68: 1247–53
17. Meredith IT, Alison JF, Zhang F-M, Horowitz JD, Harper RW. Captopril potentiates the effects of nitroglycerin on the coronary vascular bed. J Am Coll Cardiol 1993; 22: 581–7
18. Folts JD, Stamler J, Loscalzo J. Intravenous nitroglycerin infusion inhibits cyclic blood flow responses caused by periodic platelet thrombus formation in stenosed canine coronary arteries. Circulation 1991; 83: 2122–7
19. Hackett D, Davies G, Chierchia S, Maseri A. Intermittent coronary occlusion in acute myocardial infarction. Value of combined thrombolytic and vasodilator therapy. N Engl J Med 1987; 317: 1055–9
20. Dupius J, Lalonde G, Lemieux R, Rouleau JL. Tolerance to intravenous nitroglycerin in patients with congestive heart failure: role of increased intravascular volume, neurohormonal activation and lack of prevention with N-acetylcysteine. J Am Coll Cardiol 1990; 19: 923–31

21. Demots H, Glasser SP. Intermittent transdermal nitroglycerin therapy in the treatment of chronic stable angina. J Am Coll Cardiol 1989; 13: 786–93
22. Jugdutt BI Sussex BA, Warnica JW, Rossall RE. Persistent reduction in left ventricular asynergy in patients with acute myocardial infarction by intravenous infusion of nitroglycerin. Circulation 1983; 68: 1264–73
23. Berk SI, Grunwald A, Pal S, Bodenheimer MM. Effect of intravenous nitroglycerin on heparin dosage requirements in coronary artery disease. Am J Cardiol 1993; 72: 393–6
24. Figueras J, Lidon R, Cortadellas J. Rebound myocardial ischaemia following abrupt interruption of intravenous nitroglycerin infusion in patients with unstable angina pectoris at rest. Eur Heart J 1991; 12: 405–11
25. Winniford MD, Kennedy PL, Wells PJ, Hillis LD. Potentiation of nitroglycerin-induced coronary dilation by N-acetylcysteine. Circulation 1986; 73: 138–42
26. Boesgaard S, Aldershvile J, Enghusen R, Poulsen H. Preventive administration of N-acetylcysteine and development of tolerance to isosorbide dinitrate in patients with angina pectoris. Circulation 1992; 85: 143–9
27. Horowitz JD, Henry CA, Syrjanen ML et al. Combined use of nitroglycerin and N-acetylcysteine in the management of unstable angina pectoris. Circulation 1988; 77: 787–94
28. Loscalzo J. N-acetylcysteine potentiates inhibition of platelet aggregation by nitroglycerin. J Clin Invest 1985; 76: 703–8
29. Gruppo Italiano per lo Studio della Sopravvivenza nel 'Infarto Miocardico: GISSI-III: effects of lisinopril and transdermal glyceryl trinitrate singly and together on 6-week mortality and ventricular function after acute myocardial infarction. Lancet 1994; 343: 1115–22
30. European Study of Prevention of Infarct with Molsidomine (ESPRIM) Group. The ESPRIM trial: short-term treatment of acute myocardial infarction with molsidomine. Lancet 1994; 344: 91–7
31. ISIS-4 Collaborative Group: ISIS-4. A randomised factorial trial assessing early oral captopril, oral mononitrate, and intravenous magnesium sulphate in 58 050 patients with suspected acute myocardial infarction. Lancet 1995; 345: 669–85
32. Yusuf S, Collins R, MacMahon S, Peto R. Effects of intravenous nitrates on mortality in acute myocardial infarction: an overview of the randomised trials. Lancet 1988; I: 1088–92
33. Arstall MA, Yang J, Stafford I, Betts WH, Horowitz JD. N-acetylcysteine in combination with nitroglycerin and streptokinase for the treatment of evolving acute myocardial infarction: safety and biochemical effects. Circulation 1995; 92: 2855–62

31 Diuretics, digoxin and electrolytes

Peter L Thompson

Diuretics

Intravenous diuretics

The most widely used intravenous diuretic is frusemide (furosemide). In patients with known sensitivity or refractoriness to frusemide, alternative loop diuretics such as bumetanide or ethacrynic acid can be used.

Frusemide

Intravenous frusemide is widely used for treatment of severe cardiac failure and pulmonary oedema. It has a rapid onset of action, is a powerful diuretic agent and also has venodilating properties.[1,2]

The diuretic action reaches a peak about 20 minutes after the IV injection but the venodilating effect will produce a lowering in pulmonary artery wedge pressure and sometimes clinical improvement before the diuretic effect is observed.

The initial dose of IV frusemide is 20–40 mg. The dose can be increased rapidly to 80, 160 or even 250 mg if there is no effect. In life-threatening pulmonary oedema, doses up to 80 mg can be given by slow intravenous injection. Higher doses of frusemide should be given by I.V. infusion at a rate not exceeding 4 mg/minute, ie 250 mg over 1 hour. To avoid accidental overdose, it is essential to distinguish the potent (250 mg in 25 ml) injection from the standard (20 mg in 2 ml) injection.

The major reason for refractoriness to frusemide is hypotension. It is sometimes necessary to use an inotropic agent to raise the systolic blood pressure and renal perfusion pressure to enable delivery of the frusemide to the nephron loop to allow its action to occur. Intravenous frusemide can be used in the presence of oliguria or renal failure.

The major side-effect of intravenous frusemide is hypokalaemia. Sudden shifts in potassium can cause severe hypokalaemia and provoke cardiac arrhythmias especially in the presence of digitalis intoxication. Hypomagnesaemia can also occur but this is usually a result of preceding diuretic therapy rather than a result of the acute diuresis. Hyperglycaemia may be accentuated in diabetic patients. Hypovolaemia is a serious complication of IV frusemide if a vigorous diuresis is initiated. On occasions careful haemodynamic monitoring is necessary to identify and treat hypovolaemia.

Ototoxicity with sudden hearing loss may be produced by high dose IV frusemide, but this is usually reversible. Skin sensitivity may occur, but usually only as a result of prolonged oral administration of frusemide.

Bumetanide, ethacrynic acid

Occasionally a history of hypersensitivity to frusemide or sulphonamides requires the use of alternative loop diuretics. Bumetanide is highly potent and it can be used as an alternative to frusemide in a dose of 1–3 mg. Ototoxicity is less but renal toxicity and elevation of creatinine may occur.

Ethacrynic acid may also be used as an alternative to frusemide. It must be used with caution in the presence of oliguria or anuria because ototoxicity can be permanent.

Oral diuretics

Loop diuretics

After initial IV therapy, diuretic therapy is usually continued with an oral once per day loop diuretic in the form of frusemide 40 mg or alternatively bumetanide 1 mg or ethacrynic acid 50 mg. Electrolyte disturbances can be corrected with intravenous administration of potassium or magnesium, or oral administration of potassium if there is persistent hypokalaemia. Short-term low dose administration of a loop diuretic has few metabolic side-effects. It is important to review daily the need for continuing diuretic therapy to ensure that treatment is not continued indefinitely. Inadvertent long-term administration is a common cause of hypotension and hypokalaemia and may cause inappropriate activation of the renin-angiotensin and adrenergic systems in the post-infarction patient.

If there is symptomatic evidence of continuing dyspnoea or clinical or radiographic evidence of persisting pulmonary congestion following MI, 12-hourly administration of 40 mg frusemide, or a higher daily dose, for example 80–120 mg per day of frusemide, may be necessary. In severe refractory cardiac failure even higher doses may be necessary, using a quarter or half a tablet of the high dose 500 mg frusemide tablet.

Thiazide diuretics

While once daily 12-hourly administration of loop diuretics is usually sufficient for control of acute left ventricular failure, the use of thiazide diuretics[3–5] is necessary for the occasional patient who needs combined thiazide and loop diuretic therapy, the patient who has been established on thiazide therapy prior to admission and patients who find the inconvenience of the acute diuresis induced by loop diuretics annoying.

In severe refractory cardiac failure the combination of a thiazide diuretic and a loop diuretic is occasionally effective in producing a diuresis when either agent alone is ineffective.[6] This strategy requires very careful attention to adverse effects that can result from the combination, such as hypovolaemia, hyponatraemia, hypokalaemia and hypomagnesaemia.

Patients who have been on thiazide diuretics prior to admission to the CCU are most likely to be suffering from the side-effects of the long-term administration. Unrecognized hypovolaemia from pre-existent diuretic therapy is an important cause of persisting hypotension and a differential diagnosis of cardiogenic shock. Hyponatraemia may be a cause of diuretic resistance in severe cardiac failure, and an important marker of adverse long-term diuretic effect. These patients are particularly prone to acute hypotensive response on administration of angiotensin-converting enzyme (ACE) inhibitors in the early stages after MI. Hypokalaemia in long-term diuretic administration can be a marker of significant potassium depletion requiring relatively large doses of oral or intravenous potassium for correction. Similarly, hypomagnesaemia may be an indication of long-term diuretic therapy and magnesium depletion which requires intravenous magnesium administration for correction. Hyperuricaemia may be a contributing factor to renal dysfunction or to the provocation of gout; the serum uric acid should be checked on admission in a patient on long-term diuretic therapy. Hyperglycaemia similarly may result from long-term diuretic therapy but rarely requires special attention unless the patient is diabetic. These metabolic side-effects tend to occur only with long-term administration and are not usually seen with the short-term de novo administration for treatment of recently developed cardiac failure.

On occasions oral administration of loop diuretics can cause a rapid diuresis which may cause inconvenience for elderly frail patients or for men with prostatic symptoms. In this situation administration of a longer acting thiazide diuretic is appropriate.

There is little to choose between the commonly available, well established thiazide diuretics such as chlorothiazide, hydrochlorothiazide, bendrofluazide and cyclopenthiazide.[5] They are mostly rapidly absorbed although there may be individual variations in bioavailability. The diuresis lasts for 6–12 hours. Metolazone is a very useful addition to the group. It is characterized by greater potency, longer duration of action and effectiveness even in the presence of renal dysfunction.[7] For this reason it is effective in combination with frusemide, particularly in patients with refractory cardiac failure and renal dysfunction.[8] Indapamide is a milder diuretic agent and more widely used for treatment of hypertension than cardiac failure.

Potassium-sparing diuretics[9]

Amiloride and triamterene are relatively weak diuretics but have potassium-sparing properties which are useful, and combination diuretics with these agents are widely used.

Spironolactone is a more potent diuretic than amiloride or triamterene and is occasionally used when there is evidence of hyperaldosteronism, especially in right heart failure with ascites.

Hyperkalaemia with the potassium-retaining diuretics can occur and this is of particular importance with ACE inhibitors, which themselves have potassium-retaining properties. Inadvertent co-administration of potassium-retaining diuretics with ACE inhibitors in the presence of mild renal failure can cause clinically significant hyperkalaemia.

Diuretic resistance

Resistance to diuretic therapy in the CCU can be due to:

- Hypotension with reduced renal blood flow. This can be corrected by infusion of fluids, inotropic therapy or stimulation of dopaminergic receptors with low dose dopamine.
- Incorrect diagnosis of cardiac failure—for example, elevated venous pressure in right ventricular infarction, basal crackles due to causes other than left ventricular failure such as obstructive airways disease, chest infection, pulmonary fibrosis, or peripheral oedema due to causes other than right heart failure such as venous thrombosis or hypoalbuminaemia.
- Hyponatraemia due to previous diuretic administration.
- Non-steroidal anti-inflammatory drug (NSAID) therapy.[10]

Effect on prognosis

There have been no randomized studies of the effect of diuretics on short- and long-term survival after MI or other coronary events. Depletion of potassium and magnesium have been implicated in the poor survival of patients with other causes of heart disease treated with long-term diuretics.[3,4]

Digoxin

Despite controversies surrounding its role in AMI and cardiac failure, and the availability of alternative drugs for supraventricular arrhythmias, digoxin remains a widely prescribed drug.

Role in myocardial infarction

The use of digoxin in MI has always been controversial. The adverse effects of increased contractility and transient increased systemic vascular resistance, and possible provocation of arrhythmias, may outweigh the benefits of possible increases in cardiac performance.[11] Despite widespread concerns about the adverse effects, the administration of digoxin in MI does appear to be reasonably safe if administered slowly in non-toxic doses in the absence of hypokalaemia. However, there is no clear-cut role for its use in early MI in the absence of rapid atrial fibrillation. In the early management of MI, symptomatic left ventricular failure is usually managed with diuretics and left ventricular dilatation with ACE inhibitors, and advanced pump failure is managed best with potent IV inotropic agents or circulatory support. For the long term administration after MI there is considerable controversy about the possible adverse effect of digoxin.[12] Retrospective non-randomized observations have highlighted a higher mortality in patients treated with digitalis therapy post MI.[13–18] In these studies it has been almost impossible to separate the likelihood that the LV dysfunction which is being treated is the major determinant of an adverse prognosis or whether there is a direct toxic effect of digitalis therapy.[19] Although sophisticated statistical techniques have been used to tackle this question the lack of truly comparative groups for treatment versus non-treatment cannot be overcome. Critical review of the evidence indicates that a randomized trial is the only way to clarify the issue[12] and this is currently under way.

Role in cardiac failure

The role of digitalis in cardiac failure remains controversial despite its having been used for over 200 years for this purpose.[20] The reason for the controversy is that digitalis is a relatively weak inotropic agent and its benefits on contractility have been difficult to establish.[21] Furthermore, several studies have shown that digoxin can often be stopped in patients on long-term therapy without adverse effect, although these studies fail to confirm whether the use was ineffective or inappropriate.[22] Studies showing clear-cut short-term effects on contractility have not been thought relevant to the question of whether digoxin confers a sustained benefit. The controversy is now clarified by the finding in three separate studies that digoxin does indeed confer a long-term benefit on systolic function. In the comparison of captopril and digoxin, ejection fraction improved and the number of hospitalizations due to cardiac failure was reduced.[23] In a comparison of xamoterol and digoxin, there was a reduction in the signs of cardiac failure in the digitalis treated group.[24] In a milrinone/digoxin trial there were improvements in ejection fraction and exercise tolerance attributable to the digoxin.[25]

Furthermore, studies on the randomized withdrawal versus continuation of digoxin therapy in cardiac failure have shown evidence of deterioration within a few weeks of withdrawal of digoxin,[26] despite the continued administration of ACE inhibitors.[27] There is considerable evidence that the benefits of digoxin therapy in cardiac failure may be due to modulation of the neuro-humoral response rather than a direct inotropic effect.[28,29]

Digoxin is now rarely prescribed for its inotropic effect in cardiac failure due to MI. It remains third line therapy after ACE inhibitors and diuretics for chronic cardiac failure. There is some evidence that digoxin is additive to ACE inhibitors and diuretics in preventing worsening heart failure.[29a] Digoxin seems to be helpful particularly when there is the persistence of signs of left ventricular dilatation, tachycardia and third heart sound.

There is some hope that the role of digoxin therapy in cardiac failure may be clarified by an ongoing randomized (DIG) trial.[30]

Use in supraventricular arrhythmias

Digoxin retains an important role in slowing the ventricular rate in supraventricular arrhythmias, particularly atrial fibrillation. The benefit is due to a dual direct and indirect vagal effect on the atrioventricular node.[31]

Therefore, in situations where there is rapid atrial fibrillation and LV dysfunction digoxin is of prime importance; however in the absence of LV dysfunction alternative methods of slowing the ventricular response such as beta blockers or verapamil may be equally effective (see Ch. 62). Furthermore, digoxin is no more effective than placebo than effecting reversion to sinus rhythm in recent onset atrial fibrillation.[32]

Contraindications to digoxin[33]

Digoxin should not be used in:

- Hypertrophic cardiomyopathy. The inotropic effect can worsen outflow tract obstruction.
- Rapid atrial fibrillation with known or suspected Wolff–Parkinson–White syndrome. Selective blocking of the atrioventricular (AV) node and acceleration of conduction through the accessory pathway can precipitate ventricular tachycardia or fatal ventricular fibrillation.
- Atrio-ventricular block. First or second degree AV block may be worsened to complete heart block with digoxin.

Administration of digoxin

Intravenous digoxin is not required for cardiac failure but may sometimes be used to treat rapid atrial fibrillation. An intravenous loading dose of 0.5–1.0 mg given slowly (over 15–30 minutes) should be accompanied by 0.25 mg orally, and subsequent doses adjusted according to clinical response and digoxin blood levels.

For less rapid administration of digoxin a loading dose regimen is less used than previously because, apart from in rapid atrial fibrillation, there is little to be gained from rapid administration. If an oral loading dose is used, the usual regimen is 0.75–1 mg over 24 hours with subsequent doses adjusted according to clinical response and digoxin blood levels.

The maintenance dose of digoxin can vary from 0.0625 mg per day in elderly patients or those with renal dysfunction, up to 0.25 mg per day in otherwise healthy patients. In the occasional large-framed patient with rapid atrial fibrillation a higher dose up to 0.25 mg twice daily may be necessary.

Digoxin interactions

Co-administration of verapamil, amiodarone, flecainide or quinidine will increase plasma digoxin levels, potentially provoking atrio-ventricular block with verapamil and amiodarone and ventricular arrhythmias with flecainide and quinidine.

Co-administration of diuretics may produce hypokalaemia with increased risk of ventricular arrhythmias.

Monitoring digoxin therapy[20]

Monitoring of plasma levels is of most value in chronic administration or when digoxin toxicity is suspected. There is little to be gained from monitoring of plasma levels during acute administration as plasma levels in this situation bear little relationship to the clinical response. Levels which would be regarded as 'toxic' during chronic administration are commonly seen after intravenous or oral loading doses.

During maintenance therapy the main value of digoxin plasma levels is to check for compliance and ensure that plasma levels are being achieved and to check that toxicity has not occurred. There is poor correlation between the clinical response and plasma levels within the therapeutic range of 0.5–2.0 ng/ml (nanograms/ml). Above 2.0 ng/ml the likelihood of toxicity increases with increasing levels, but levels >2 ng/ml do not automatically equate with digitalis toxicity. To ensure that samples are taken in a steady state, a delay of a minimum of 5–6 hours should be allowed after oral administration. The major factor affecting renal plasma levels is renal dysfunction, and particular care is needed to regularly monitor digoxin levels if there is known renal dysfunction.

Digitalis toxicity[34–36]

Toxicity can occur with continued administration in the presence of reduced renal clearance or with intentional overdose.

The first sign of toxicity in long-term administration is nausea and anorexia. At higher levels of toxicity there may be visual disturbance, vomiting and cardiac arrhythmias. Cardiac arrhythmias include ventricular irritability, the development of atrial tachycardia and high grades of atrio-ventricular block. The combination of atrial tachycardia with atrio-ventricular block (so-called PAT with block) is a classic digitalis toxicity arrhythmia. The degree of AV block and the rate of the atrial arrhythmia are determined by the degree of toxicity and the extent of the underlying heart disease. The rate of firing of the atrial tachycardia and the degree of AV block fluctuate according to the degree of toxicity.

With massive intentional overdosage the cardiac response will vary according to the extent of associated heart disease. In healthy young patients who have massive digoxin overdosage with suicidal intent, extremely high levels of plasma digoxin can be achieved with the only resultant cardiac arrhythmia being atrio-ventricular block. When there has been prior heart disease the response is more likely to be ventricular tachyarrhythmias.

Associated hypokalaemia may increase the likelihood of high grade ventricular arrhythmias in digitalis toxicity. With massive overdosage of digoxin there can be severe hyperkalaemia which can be of fulminant onset and may require urgent treatment.

Treatment of mild degrees of digitalis intoxication is usually achieved with the cessation of digoxin administration. If there is high grade atrio-ventricular block, temporary pacing may be necessary. The development of ventricular arrhythmias may require treatment with intravenous lignocaine. If there is associated hypokalaemia, administration of potassium may be necessary but this should be done cautiously because of the risk of acute hyperkalaemia with advanced digitalis toxicity. Purified digoxin-specific Fab fragments of digoxin antibody have been used to achieve rapid binding of digoxin and reversal of toxicity.[37] Digoxin immune Fab is used when there is severe toxicity as evidenced by toxic serum digoxin levels with ventricular tachycardia or complete atrioventricular block. Even in the absence of cardiac arrhythmia, digoxin toxicity with rising potassium levels >5 mE/L, ingestion of >10ng of digoxin or plasma levels of >10ng/L are indications for urgent treatment with digoxin immune Fab.

Dosage is determined by serum digoxin concentrations and body weight (approximately 1 vial of 40 ng per serum digoxin level in ng/ml per 10 kg of bodyweight). An 80 kg person with a serum digoxin level of 8 ng/ml will require 6 vials. Serum potassium levels must be monitored carefully during infusion.

There is increased sensitivity to electrical cardioversion in digoxin toxicity and this should be avoided wherever possible but may, on occasions, be necessary in life-threatening ventricular tachyarrhythmias.

Electrolyte disturbances

Hypokalaemia[38,39]

Hypokalaemia may occur as a result of increased renal loss, particularly with diuretic therapy and more rarely with gastrointestinal loss with vomiting and diarrhoea. Acute catecholamine release, as occurs in the early stages of MI, may cause sudden potassium shifts with acute hypokalaemia. There is a close correlation between the severity of hypokalaemia and the risk of ventricular fibrillation in AMI.[40,41]

Mild degrees of hypokalaemia are treated with oral administration of potassium-retaining diuretics or oral administration of slow release potassium, 10 mmol 8-hourly. Sometimes oral administration of potassium chloride is necessary.

Intravenous administration of potassium chloride must be performed with great care. It should never be given as a bolus as it can be potentially cardiotoxic but administration of 10 mmol per hour is usually safe. The solution should always be dilute (<30 mmol/L). Infusions of solution stronger than 30 mmol/L can cause pain at the infusion site.

Correction of hypokalaemia, even of a mild degree, is an important component of the management of ventricular arrhythmias particularly during MI. Whilst a mild degree of hypokalaemia is acceptable during chronic administration, every effort should be made to maintain serum potassium level above 4.0 milli equivalents per litre in the patient being treated for AMI in the CCU.

Hyperkalaemia

Hyperkalaemia may occur with the ACE inhibitors and inappropriate use of K^+ retaining diuretics or K^+ supplementation in the presence of renal dysfunction. The typical electrocardiographic signs are tall 'tented' T waves progressing to lengthening of the PR interval, widening of the QRS complex and eventual asystole. Urgent treatment is required if the serum K^+ exceeds 7.0 m Eg/L. Falsely high serum K^+ levels can result from haemolysis of the blood sample, and unexpected hyperkalaemia should be confirmed with an urgent repeat laboratory estimation. Management consists of cessation of the K^+ supplement, infusion of glucose, insulin (e.g. 10–20 units of insulin in 1 litre of 10% glucose infused at 300–500 ml/hour), and in the presence of life-threatening cardiac arrhythmias, 10 ml of 10% calcium gluconate over 1–5 minutes and oral or rectal administration of an ion-exchange resin.

Hypomagnesaemia

Hypomagnesaemia can result from long-term diuretic administration particularly in the chronic alcoholic patient.[42] Hypokalaemia frequently coexists with hypomagnesaemia.

Unfortunately, the serum magnesium level is not an accurate indicator of magnesium deficiency; however, a magnesium level consistently below 0.7 mmol/L (1.4 m Eg/L) is almost always an indication of significant magnesium depletion. Hypo- magnesaemia is an important cause of cardiac arrhythmias and its correction can be an effective antiarrhythmic therapy. It should be maintained above 1.0 mmol/L. Administration of IV magnesium has been studied in detail in AMI. A meta-analysis of seven small studies of IV magnesium suggested a benefit,[43] and the results of the LIMIT 2 study suggested an improvement in survival of 25%;[44,45] however, the larger ISIS-4 study recently completely failed to show any benefit of magnesium administration.[46] At present the administration of magnesium should be confined to patients with confirmed hypomagnesaemia or known risk factors for hypomagnesaemia such as long-term diuretic administration or chronic alcoholism but should not be used as a routine in AMI.[47,48]

Hyponatraemia

Hyponatraemia is commonly seen in aggressive diuretic therapy in cardiac failure. Mild hyponatraemia between 120 and 130 milli equivalents per litre usually responds to fluid restriction. Severe hyponatraemia, less than 120 milli equivalents per litre, may be associated with mental obtundation and may require administration of IV sodium chloride. This must be done with great care in the presence of cardiac failure or MI and administration should be with haemodynamic monitoring.

References

1. Dikshit K, Vyden JK, Forrester JS et al. Renal and extrarenal haemodynamic effects of furosemide in congestive heart failure after acute myocardial infarction. N Engl J Med 1973; 288: 1087–90
2. Biddle TL, Yu PN. Effect of furosemide on haemodynamic and lung water in acute pulmonary edema secondary to myocardial infarction. Am J Cardiol 1979; 43: 86–90
3. Lant A. Diuretics. Clinical pharmacology and therapeutic use. (Pt 1.) Drugs 1985; 29: 57–87
4. Lant A. Diuretics. Clinical pharmacology and therapeutic use. (Pt II.) Drugs 1985; 29: 162–88
5. Puschett JB. Clinical pharmacologic implications in diuretic selection. Am J Cardiol 1986; 57: 6A–13A

6. Oster JR, Epstein M, Smoller S. Combined therapy with thiazide type and loop diuretics for resistant sodium retention. Ann Int Med 1983; 99: 405–6
7. Kiyingi A, Field MJ, Pawsey CC et al. Metolazone in treatment of severe refractory congestive heart failure. Lancet 1990; 335: 29–31
8. Ghose RR, Gupta SK. Synergistic action of metolazone with 'loop' diuretics. Br Med J 1981; 282: 1432–5
9. Potassium sparing diuretics. Spironolactone v triamterene and amiloride. Drug and Therapeutics Bulletin 1972; 10: 30–2
10. Webster J. Interactions of NSAIDs with diuretics and beta blockers. Mechanisms and clinical implications. Drugs 1985; 30: 32–41
11. Marcus FI. Use of digitalis in myocardial infarction. Circulation 1980; 62: 17–19
12. Yusuf S, Wittes J, Bailey K, Furberg C. Digitalis—a new controversy regarding an old drug—the pitfalls of inappropriate methods. Circulation 1986; 73: 14–23
13. Moss AJ, Davis HT, Conard DL, De Camilla JJ, Ordroff CL. Digitalis-associated cardiac mortality after myocardial infarction. Circulation 1981; 64: 1150–6
14. Ryan TJ, Bailey KR, McCabe CH et al. The effects of digitalis on survival in high risk patients with coronary artery disease. The Coronary Artery Surgery Study (CASS). Circulation 1983; 67: 735–42
15. Madsen EB, Gilpin E, Henning H et al. Prognostic importance of digitalis after acute myocardial infarction. J Am Coll Cardiol 1984; 3: 681–9
16. Bigger JT Jr, Fleiss JL, Rolnitzky LM et al. Effect of digitalis treatment on survival after acute myocardial infarction. Am J Cardiol 1985; 55: 623–30
17. Muller JE, Turi ZG, Stone PH et al. Digoxin therapy and mortality after myocardial infarction. Experience in the MILIS Study. N Engl J Med 1986 314: 265–71
18. Byington R, Goldstein S. Association of digitalis therapy with mortality in survivors of acute myocardial infarction: observations in the Beta Blocker Heart Attack Trial. J Am Coll Cardiol 1985; 6: 976–82
19. Remme WJ. Inotropic agents for heart failure—what if digoxin increases mortality? Br Heart J 1994; 72(Suppl.): 92–9
20. Smith TW. Digitalis. Mechanisms of action and clinical use. N Engl J Med 1988; 318: 358–65
21. Smith TW. Digoxin in heart failure. N Engl J Med 1993; 329: 51–3
22. Jaeschke R, Oxman AD, Guyatt GH. To what extent do congestive heart failure patients in sinus rhythm benefit from digoxin therapy? A systematic overview and meta analysis. Am J Med 1990; 88: 279–86
23. The Captopril-Digoxin Multicenter Research Group. Comparative effects of therapy with captopril and digoxin in patients with mild to moderate heart failure. JAMA 1988; 259: 539–44
24. German and Austrian Xamoterol Study Group. Double blind controlled comparison of digoxin and xamoterol in chronic heart failure. Lancet 1988; 1: 488–92
25. Di Bianco R, Shabetai R, Kostuk W et al. A comparison of oral milrinone, digoxin and their combination in the treatment of patients with chronic heart failure. N Engl J Med 1989; 320: 677–83
26. Uretsky BF, Young JB, Shahidi FE, Yellen LG, Harrison MC, Jolly MK on behalf of the PROVED investigative group. Randomized study assessing the effect of digoxin withdrawal in patients with mild to moderate congestive heart failure: results of the PROVED trial. J Am Coll Cardiol 1993; 22: 955–62
27. Packer M, Gheorghiade M, Young JB et al for the RADIANCE study. Withdrawal of digoxin from patients with chronic heart failure treated with angiotensin converting enzyme inhibitors. N Engl J Med 1993; 329: 1–7
28. Covit AB, Schaer GL, Sealey JE, Laragh JH, Cody RJ. Suppression of the renin-angiotensin system by intravenous digoxin in chronic congestive heart failure. Am J Med 1983; 75: 445–7
29. Ferguson DW, Berg WJ, Sanders JS, Roach PJ, Kempf JS, Kienzle MR. Sympathoinhibitory responses to digitalis glycorides in heart failure patients: direct evidence from sympathomimetic neural recordings. Circulation 1989; 98: 65–77
29a. Gheorghiade M. Digoxin: resolved and unresolved issues. ACC Educational Highlights 1996; 11: 1–6
30. Yusuf S, Garg R, Held P, Gorlin R. Need for a large randomized trial to evaluate the effects of digitalis on morbidity and mortality in congestive heart failure. Am J Cardiol 1992; 69: 64G–70G
31. Simpson RJ, Foster JR, Woelfel AK, Gettes LS. Management of atrial fibrillation and flutter: a reappraisal of digitalis therapy. Postgraduate Med 1986; 8: 241–53
32. Falk RH, Knowlton AA, Bernard SA, Gottlieb NE, Battinelli NJ. Digoxin for converting recent-onset atrial fibrillation to sinus rhythm. Ann Int Med 1987; 106: 503–6
33. Dollery C. Therapeutic drugs. Vol. 1. Digoxin P D125. Edinburgh: Churchill Livingstone, 1991
34. Smith TW, Antman EM, Friedman PL, Blatt CM, Marsh JD. Digitalis glycosides: mechanism and manifestations of toxicity. Part I. Prog Cardiovasc Dis 1984; 26: 413–58
35. Smith TW, Antman EM, Friedman PL, Blatt CM, Marsh JD. Digitalis glycosides: mechanism and manifestations of toxicity. Part II.

Prog Cardiovasc Dis 1984: 26: 495–540
36. Smith TW, Antman EM, Friedman PL, Blatt CM, Marsh JD. Digitalis glycosides: mechanism and manifestations of toxicity. Part III. Prog Cardiovasc Dis 1984; 27: 21–56
37. Smith TW, Butler VP Jr, Haber E et al. Treatment of life-threatening digitalis intoxication with digoxin-specific Fab fragments: experience in 26 cases. N Engl J Med 1982; 307: 1357–62
38. Mudge GH, Weiner IM. Agents affecting volume and composition of body fluid. In: Gilman AG, Race TW, Nies AS, Taylor P (eds). The pharmacological basis of therapeutics. 8th ed. Oxford: Pergamon Press, 1990
39. Arieff AI, De Fronzo RA. Fluid, electrolyte and acid-base disorders. New York: Churchill Livingstone, 1985
40. Nordrehaug JE, Johannesen KA, Van Der Lippe G. Serum potassium concentrations as a risk factor of ventricular arrhythmias in acute myocardial infarction. Circulation 1985; 71: 645–9
41. Solomon R. Ventricular arrhythmias in patients with myocardial infarction: the role of serum potassium. Drugs 1986; 31: 112–20
42. Lauler DP (ed). A symposium: magnesium deficiency—pathogenesis, prevalence and strategies for repletion. Am J Cardiol 1989; 63(14): 1G–3G
43. Teo KK, Yusuf S, Collins R, Held PH, Peto R. Effects of intravenous magnesium in suspected acute myocardial infarction. Overview of randomized trials. Br Med J 1991; 303: 1499–1503
44. Woods KL, Fletcher S, Roffe C, Haider Y. Intravenous magnesium sulphate in suspected myocardial infarction: results of the second Leicester intravenous magnesium intervention trial (LIMIT-2). Lancet 1992; 339: 1553–8
45. Woods KL, Fletcher S. Long term outcome after intravenous magnesium sulphate in suspected acute myocardial infarction: the second Leicester intravenous magnesium intervention trial (LIMIT-2). Lancet 1994; 343: 816–19
46. ISIS-4 (Fourth International Study of Infarct Survival) Collaborative Group. ISIS-4, a randomized factorial trial assessing oral captopril, oral mononitrate and intravenous magnesium sulphate in 58 050 patients with suspected acute myocardial infarction. Lancet 1995; 345: 669–85
47. Yusuf S, Flather M. Magnesium in acute myocardial infarction. ISIS-4 provides no grounds for its routine use. Br Med J 1995; 310: 751–2
48. Egger M, Davey Smith G. Misleading meta analysis. Lessons from 'an effective, safe, simple' intervention that wasn't. Br Med J 1995; 310: 752–4

32 Inotropic agents

Peter L Thompson

Introduction

Despite the wider use of circulatory support devices and the use of revascularization procedures for cardiogenic shock, inotropic agents are still used frequently in the coronary care unit. However, their role has changed from being the sole mode of management in cardiogenic shock to a bridging role towards more definitive treatment.

Mechanisms of action of positive inotropes

The final common pathway of positive inotropic agents is an increase in the availability of calcium ions to the myofibrillar contractile proteins. This is achieved by increasing levels of cyclic adenosine monophosphates (AMP) which in turn activate c-AMP-dependent protein kinases to increase the phosphorylation of calcium channels and permit entry of calcium ions.[1–3]

Increased cyclic AMP levels can be achieved by:

- beta adrenoceptor agonists which by interaction with the beta adrenergic receptor activate adenylate cyclase, which encourages the conversion of adenosine triphosphates (ATP) to c-AMP
- phosphodiesterase-3 enzyme inhibitors which achieve a similar effect by inhibiting the breakdown of c-AMP (see Fig. 32.1).

The adrenoceptors relevant to clinically used inotropic agents are the alpha$_1$, beta$_1$, beta$_2$ and dopaminergic adrenoceptor subtypes. Their cardiovascular effects are summarized in Table 32.1.

Beta adrenoceptor agonists

The actions of the clinically available beta adrenoceptor agonists are summarized in Table 32.2.

Dobutamine

Dobutamine is a synthetic derivative of isoproterenol and is almost a pure beta$_1$ selective adrenergic stimulating agent.[4,5] It thus produces a stronger inotropic than chronotropic effect and produces less

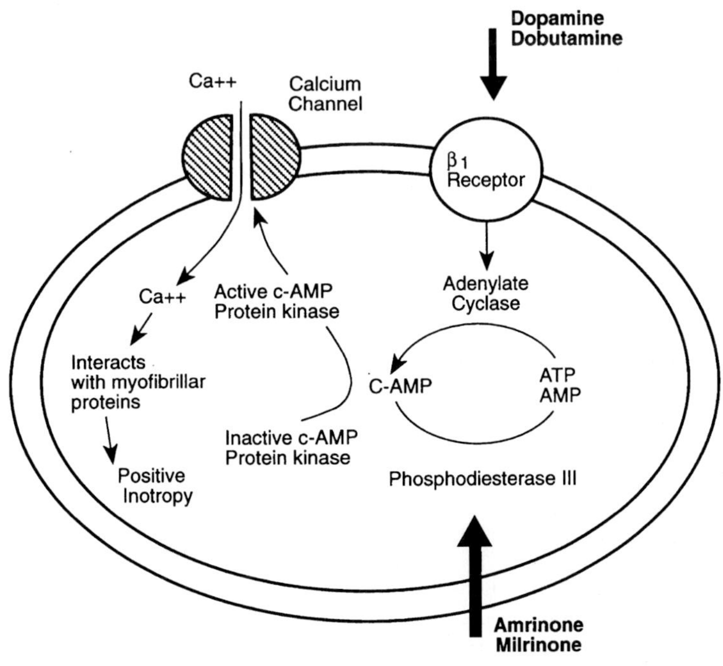

Fig. 32.1 Mechanism of action of intropic agents.

Table 32.1 Summary of cardiovascular adrenoceptor actions

Adrenoceptor type	Cardiovascular effects			
	Vasconstriction	Myocardial contractility	Tachycardia	Renal vasodilatation
$Alpha_1$	+	–	–	–
$Beta_1$	–	++	++	–
$Beta_2$	–	+	±	–
Dopaminergic	–	–	–	+

Table 32.2 Actions of clinically used sympathomimetic inotropic agents on adrenoceptors

	$Alpha_1$	$Beta_1$	$Beta_2$	Dopaminergic
Dopamine	±	++	+	+
Dobutamine	±	++	±	–
Adrenaline (Epinephrine)	+	+	+	–
Noradrenaline (Norepinephrine)	++	+	–	–
Isoprenaline (Isoproterenol)	–	+	+	–

peripheral vasoconstriction than dopamine at high dose. It does seem to have mild peripheral vasodilating effects but these are thought unlikely to be due to stimulation of vascular beta receptors but rather to relief of the sympathetic vasoconstriction with the increase in stroke volume. Concomitantly there is also a proportionate increase in coronary blood flow.[6] At high doses it may cause an increase in systemic vascular resistance.

These properties make it suitable as first line use in cardiogenic shock: in animal models it has not been shown to increase infarct size and in studies in patients it has not increased the plasma levels of cardiac enzymes.[7,8]

It does cause an increase in heart rate and can produce cardiac arrhythmias in higher dose, but because of the rapid clearance these are rarely troublesome.

The plasma half-life is 2.5 minutes. The standard dose is 2.5–10 mcg/kg per minute.

The usual indication is for cardiogenic shock with or without pulmonary congestion. It has been used for intermittent treatment of persistent pulmonary congestion in severe left ventricular dysfunction; however, a randomized trial of this approach had to be stopped because of an increase in mortality in the treatment group.[9]

Dopamine

Dopamine is a metabolic precursor of noradrenaline and adrenaline. It is a 'flexible molecule'. In addition to direct stimulation of $beta_1$ and $beta_2$ receptors and of $alpha_1$ receptors at high dose, it enhances the release of noradrenaline from cardiac nerve endings. It has the unique property at low concentrations of activating dopaminergic receptors producing renal and hepatosplenic vasodilatation resulting in increased renal blood flow.[10] It can induce a diuresis in patients with oliguria. These effects are produced at infusion rates of less than 5 mcg/kg per minute. At higher infusion rates dopamine can increase cardiac output by $beta_1$ stimulation as well as having $beta_2$ alpha stimulating properties. Although it will increase heart rate and contractility, cardiac arrhythmias are rarely seen in dosages under 10 mcg/kg per minute.

Combined dopamine/dobutamine

Combined treatment with dopamine and dobutamine combines the renal blood flow effects of dopamine at infusion rates less than 5 mcg/kg per minute whilst the rate of infusion of dobutamine is steadily increased from 2 to 10 mcg/kg per minute producing an increase in cardiac output but no increase in renal blood flow. The combination is especially beneficial in low output states with oliguria due to reduced renal blood flow.[11]

Other catecholamines

Noradrenaline (norepinephrine) as a sole infusion is rarely used but may be useful in situations where there is decreased cerebral perfusion and an increase in blood pressure is urgently required.

Adrenaline (epinephrine) and isoprenaline (isoproterenol) are rarely used in modern coronary care practice because of the marked increase in heart rate and propensity to increase myocardial oxygen consumption and extend infarct size. They are also associated with provocation of ventricular arrhythmias.

Dopexamine is a new dopamine analog with potent $beta_1$ and some dopaminergic properties said to have the properties of combined dobutamine and dopamine, particularly enhancement of renal blood flow and peripheral vasodilating properties at standard doses.[12]

Phosphodiesterase 3 inhibitors

Phosphodiesterase 3 inhibitors increase c-AMP levels by preventing its intracellular degradation. They produce potent inotropic stimulation and peripheral vasodilatation and for this reason have caused great interest as alternatives to catecholamine inotropes.[13]

Amrinone

Amrinone is a potent vasodilator with inotropic activity with minimal effects on heart rate and no effects on myocardial oxygen consumption, and can produce significant reduction in left ventricular filling pressure.[14] Prolonged infusion can produce thrombocytopenia.[15]

Milrinone

Milrinone, like amrinone, has potent vasodilating and inotropic properties and is 20 times more potent that amrinone.[16] It is available in oral form but the report of increased mortality in the orally treated group in a randomized placebo controlled trial has dampened enthusiasm for the use of oral phosphodiesterase inhibitors.[17] Intravenous infusion in patients with severe heart failure and cardiogenic shock has shown convincing early and substantial haemodynamic improvement with an infusion given at 0.5 mcg/kg/min after a loading dose of 50 mcg/kg.[18] The recommended dosage for IV infusion ranges from 0.375 mcg/kg/min to 0.75 mcg/kg/min. Frusemide should not be injected into intravenous lines containing milrinone as a precipitate may form.

Other phosphodiesterase inhibitors

Inoxemone and pimobendan are imidazole derivatives, both orally active.

Combined catecholamine and phosphodiesterase inhibitors

Combined amrinone or milrinone and dobutamine have been used to promote potent increase in contractility with peripheral vasodilatation.[19]

Combined sympathomimetic vasodilator therapy

On occasions increases in cardiac output are not sufficient to improve the patient's haemodynamic status and the combined use of catecholamines and vasodilators may produce benefits when the inotrope is associated with vasoconstriction or when the vasodilator is producing excessive hypotension.[20]

Cardiac glycosides

The role of digoxin as an inotropic agent is discussed in Chapter 31.

References

1. Marcus FI, Opie LH, Sonnenblick EH. Digitalis and other inotropes. In: Opie LH (ed.) Drugs for the heart. 3rd ed. Philadelphia: Saunders, 1991: Ch. 6
2. Cohn J. Inotropic therapy for heart failure. Paradise postponed. N Engl J Med 1989; 320: 729–31
3. Hoffman BB, Lefkowitz RJ. Catecholamines and sympathomimetic drugs. In: Goodman LS, Gilman AG (eds.) The pharmacological basis of therapeutics. New York: Pergamon Press, 1990: 187–220
4. Leier CV, Unverferth DV. Dobutamine. Ann Int Med 1983; 99: 490–6
5. Tuttle RR, Mills J. Development of a new catecholamine to selectively increase cardiac contractility. Circ Res 1975; 36: 185–96
6. Fowler MB, Alderman EL, Oesterle SN et al. Dobutamine and dopamine after cardiac surgery: greater augmentation of myocardial blood flow with dobutamine. Circulation 1984; 70: 1103–11
7. Maekawa K, Liang CS, Hood WB Jnr. Comparison of dobutamine and dopamine in acute myocardial infarction. Effect on systemic haemodynamics, plasma catecholamine blood flow and infarct

size. Circulation 1983; 67: 750–9

8. Francis GS, Sharma B, Hodges M. Comparative haemodynamic effects of dopamine and dobutamine in patients with acute cardiogenic circulatory collapse. Am Heart J 1982; 103: 995–1000
9. Dies F, Krell MJ, Whitlow P et al. Intermittent dobutamine in ambulatory outpatients with chronic cardiac failure. Circulation 1986; 74(Suppl II): 39
10. Beregovich J, Bianchi C, Robler S, Lomnitz E, Cagin N, Levitt B. Dose-related haemodynamic and renal effects of dopamine in congestive heart failure. Am Heart J 1974; 87: 550–7
11. Richard C, Ricome JC, Rimailho A, Bottineau G, Auzepy P. Combined haemodynamic effects of dopamine and dobutamine in cardiogenic shock. Circulation 1982; 67: 620–6
12. Leier CV, Binkley PF, Carpenter J, Randolph PH, Unverferth DV. Cardiovascular pharmacology of dopexamine in low output congestive heart failure. Am J Cardiol 1988; 62: 94–9
13. Colucci WS, Wright RF, Braunwald E. New positive inotropic agents in the treatment of congestive heart failure. Mechanisms of action and recent clinical developments. N Engl J Med 1986; 314: 349–58
14. Konstam MA, Cohen ST, Weiland DS et al. Relative contributions of inotropic and vasodilator effects to amrinone induced haemodynamic improvement in congestive heart failure. Am J Cardiol 1986; 57: 242–8
15. Wilmshurst PT, Webb-Peploe MM. Side effects of amrinone therapy. Br Heart J 1983; 49: 447–51
16. Baim DS, McDowell AV, Cherniles J et al. Evaluation of a new bipyridine inotropic agent—milrinone—in patients with severe congestive heart failure. N Engl J Med 1983; 309: 748–56
17. Packer M, Carver JR, Rodeheffer RJ et al and the PROMISE Study Investigators. Effect of oral milrinone in severe chronic heart failure. Results of the Prospective Randomized Milrinone Survival Evaluation (PROMISE). N Engl J Med 1991; 325: 1468–75
18. Klocke RK, Mager G, Kux A, Hopp H-W, Hilger HH. Effects of a twenty four hour milrinone infusion in patients with severe heart failure and cardiogenic shock as a function of the haemodynamic initial condition. Am Heart J 1991; 121: 1965–73
19. Gage J, Rutman H, Lucido D, Le Jemtel TH. Additive effects of dobutamine and amrinone on myocardial contractility and ventricular performance in patients with severe heart failure. Circulation 1986; 74: 367–73
20. Loeb HS, Ostrenga JP, Gaul W et al. Beneficial effects of dopamine combined with intravenous nitroglycerin on haemodynamics in patients with severe left ventricular failure. Circulation 1983; 68: 813–20

33 Angiotensin-converting enzyme (ACE) inhibitors

D Norman Sharpe

Introduction

Following their introduction in the late 1970s for the treatment of hypertension, angiotensin-converting enzyme (ACE) inhibitors were subsequently established in the treatment of heart failure. During the 1980s their application was extended further as they were proven beneficial in patients with left ventricular dysfunction following myocardial infarction (MI).

Clinical studies demonstrated prevention of progressive left ventricular (LV) dilatation and dysfunction in selected patients following Q wave MI.[1–3] Large scale studies then demonstrated reduced heart failure progression and hospitalization with survival benefit in similarly selected patients.[4,5] A neutral effect or small benefit has been shown with a non-selective early intervention approach in patients with MI generally.[6–8] More recently, improved outcomes with ACE inhibition in selected MI patients with clinical signs of heart failure,[9] extensive anterior infarction,[10] or echocardiographic evidence of LV dysfunction[11] have been confirmed.

The benefits from ACE inhibition in patients with LV dysfunction or heart failure following MI are thus clearly established. At issue is the optimal timing of intervention and whether an immediate non-selective or staged selective approach is more appropriate, particularly considering the need for other concomitant treatment such as thrombolysis and beta blockade. Review of all clinical trial data in the context of MI management generally allows the recommendation for a staged selective approach in patients with definite MI following consideration of ongoing ischaemia and the extent of LV dysfunction or evidence of heart failure. Importantly, treatment should be carefully individualized according to clinical characteristics and integrated with other management requirements.

The major clinical trials are summarized in Table 33.1 and a brief description of each follows.

SAVE

The SAVE (Survival and Ventricular Enlargement) study[4] selected patients who had suffered MI and with an ejection fraction of less then 40% detected on radionuclide ventriculography. Treatment was begun in hospital at a mean of 11 days after MI. The initial dose of captopril was 6.25 or 12.5 mg orally, titrated to 25–50 mg three times per day. A feature of the SAVE study was a delay in demonstrable benefit until 6 months after randomization, with benefit evident at 1 year and a significant 19% relative mortality reduction after a minimum 2-year follow-up. An additional feature was an apparent effect on fatal and non-fatal reinfarction, a feature also seen in the SOLVD (Studies of Left Ventricular Dysfunction) trial[5] and giving rise to speculation that ACE inhibitors may have a wider role in stabilizing myocardial ischaemia as well as left ventricular dysfunction.[13]

CONSENSUS II

The CONSENSUS II trial (Co-operative New Scandinavian Enalapril Survival Study II)[6] was planned to recruit 9000 patients for a study of the early administration of an ACE inhibitor within 24 hours of the onset of symptoms in acute MI. The study was terminated when 6090 patients had been entered and it was estimated that continuation of the study would not provide a definitive answer. ACE inhibitor therapy was initiated with an intravenous infusion of enalaprilat, followed by oral enalapril titrated up to 20 mg daily. The survival curves

Table 33.1 Post myocardial infarction ACE inhibitor mortality trials

Study	Drug	n	Selection	Entry post MI	Follow-up
SAVE[4]	Captopril	2231	LVEF <40%	3–16 days	2–4 yr
CONSENSUS II[6]	Enalaprilat IV Enalapril oral	6090	All	<24 h	6 mo
GISSI III[7]	Lisinopril	19 394	All	<24 h	6 wk
ISIS-4[8]	Captopril	58 050	All	<24 h	5 wk
AIRE[9]	Ramipril	2006	Heart failure	3–10 days	15 mo
SMILE[10]	Zofenopril	1556	Anterior MI	<24 h	6 wk
TRACE[11]	Trandolapril	1749	LV dysfunction (wall motion score)	3–7 days	2–4 yr
Chinese	Captopril	12 631	All	<36 h	4 wk

have been the only ones in the published series of major studies which have not demonstrated a benefit of ACE inhibitors at the termination of the study after 6 months' treatment. The possible adverse trend from this study has been widely quoted to suggest that too early administration of an ACE inhibitor may cause an excess of hypotensive response which outweighs any benefit and will produce an adverse effect on overall survival. However, the results are consistent with a neutral effect or even a benefit and the larger ISIS-4 and GISSI-III results indicated a modest benefit when treatment was begun similarly within the first 24 hours.

GISSI III

The GISSI III (Gruppo Italiano per lo Studio della Sopravvivenza nell'Infarto Miocardico) study[7] was a 2 × 2 factorial design comparing early treatment with oral lisinopril and IV/transdermal nitroglycerin versus placebo. A 12% relative mortality reduction was demonstrated at 6 weeks with lisinopril. The effect in high risk groups (patients over 70 years, and women) were of similar magnitude.

ISIS-4

The ISIS-4 (International Study of Infarct Survival) trial[8] randomized 58 050 patients in a 2 × 2 × 2 factorial design comparing oral captopril, oral slow release isosorbide mononitrate and IV magnesium versus placebo begun within 24 hours of the onset of infarction. All patients fulfilling the criteria for suspected acute myocardial infarction (AMI) according to the previous ISIS protocols were included. At the 5-week point there were no effects seen with magnesium and nitrates but a 7% relative mortality reduction with captopril.

AIRE

The AIRE (Acute Infarction Ramipril Efficacy) trial[9] selected patients with clinical evidence of heart failure following MI who were randomized to oral ramipril 2.5–5 mg twice daily or placebo at 3–10 days following MI. There was a substantial (27%) relative reduction in mortality after an average 15-month follow-up which emerged rapidly, approaching significance at 30 days after randomization.

SMILE

The SMILE (Survival of Myocardial Infarction Long Term Evaluation)[10] trial evaluated the effect of oral zofenopril commenced within 24 hours of onset of symptoms in patients with anterior MI not eligible for thrombolytic therapy. At 6 weeks there was a significant 34% relative reduction in the combined endpoint of death or severe congestive heart failure. Despite cessation of treatment at 6 weeks, there was a significant 29% mortality benefit after 1 year of observation.

TRACE

The Trace (Trandolapril Cardiac Evaluation) trial[11] selected patients on the basis of echocardiographic evidence of LV dysfunction within the first week after MI. Over a treatment period of 2–4 years a significant relative risk reduction of 22% was shown.

Chinese captopril

The Chinese Captopril study[12] compared captopril with placebo in the early stage of AMI. Patients were entered within 36 hours of suspected acute infarction and treated with captopril 12.5 mg three times daily or placebo for one month. 12 631 patients were randomized, approximately half with anterior infarction. Overall, a favourable trend in mortality reduction was seen and significant benefit for those with anterior infarction or those treated within 6 hours.

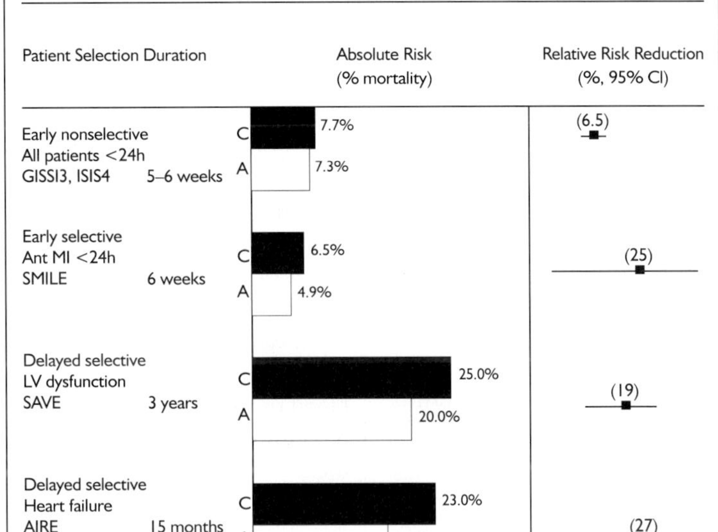

Fig. 33.1 Summary of clinical trial results of angiotension-converting enzyme inhibition after acute myocardial infarction.

Summary of clinical trial results

The results of these clinical trials, which have included over 100 000 post-infarction patients, are summarized in Figure 33.1. The trials can be categorized into early non-selective, early and delayed selective trials.

Immediate non-selective versus staged selective treatment

Major determinants of prognosis following MI are infarct artery patency and ventricular wall stress, which influence infarct size and subsequent LV remodelling. Thus thrombolysis and ACE inhibition are interventions which may be considered sequentially in eligible patients to improve outcome. Immediate treatment with ACE inhibition following definite MI offers the potential advantage of possible infarct size limitation and maximum prevention of early infarct expansion and LV dilatation, which can progress rapidly in the early hours following myocardial damage. These advantages may be offset by the difficulty of administering treatment early in unstable patients, the difficulty of co-administration of thrombolysis and the possibility of exacerbation of hypotension (particularly with streptokinase) and ongoing ischaemia. Many patients, particularly those with smaller infarcts without significant LV functional impairment, will be treated unnecessarily for no benefit.

In contrast, a staged approach with assessment and selection of relatively stable patients from 24–48 hours onwards should provide treatment for those most likely to benefit. With such an approach, however, further unnecessary delay should be avoided as most of the LV dilatation present at 6–12 months occurs during the first 1 week to 1 month. Clinical protocols should be designed to ensure that ACE inhibitor therapy in appropriate patients is commenced prior to discharge from the CCU. Patients with definite Q wave MI with evidence of LV dysfunction (LV ejection fraction less than 40–45%) or any evidence of clinical heart failure should be considered for treatment.

Patients with Q wave anterior infarcts in general will warrant treatment, although infarct size rather than location is the most important determinant of subsequent ventricular dilatation. Non-invasive assessment of LV volumes and function can guide management decisions, and echocardiography is useful in this respect. A test dose of captopril 6.25–12.5 mg, enalapril or ramipril 2.5 mg according to blood pressure is generally well tolerated, increasing gradually to captopril 25–50 mg tid or equivalent. Recent clinical reports indicate that initiation of therapy with a low dose once daily ACE inhibitor may be safe. A more cautious low dose titration approach will be required in patients with low blood pressure (<100 mmHg systolic), those who have received previous diuretic treatment and those on beta blocker treatment.

Patients with clinically evident ongoing ischaemia should, in the first instance, be treated with nitrates and beta blockers in preference to ACE inhibitors. Such patients may require further investigation and revascularization before later review and reconsideration of the need for ACE inhibition.

ACE inhibitors in combination with beta blockers

Definitive comparative studies of ACE inhibitors, beta blockers or a combination following MI have not been performed and appear impractical. The benefits of both treatments separately are clearly established and may be complementary working through different mechanisms.[13] ACE inhibitors have been tolerated and effective in patients receiving beta blocker treatment.[7–9] Choice of one or other agent or a combination will depend on consideration of infarct size, the degree of LV dysfunction, the presence of heart failure or ongoing ischaemia and arrhythmias. Low dose combination treatment may be optimal for many cases but may be limited by blood pressure, requiring careful monitoring and dosage adjustment.

Summary and recommendations

ACE inhibition should be considered for all patients following definite MI with significant LV dysfunction or clinical heart failure. Immediate treatment is an option but selection of stable patients with Q wave infarction from 24 to 48 hours appears more practical and is recommended. Echocardiographic evaluation of LV size and function can be useful in guiding management decisions. ACE inhibition can be combined with beta blockade in many cases to provide benefit through complementary mechanisms.

References

1. Sharpe N, Murphy J, Smith H, Hannan S. Treatment of patients with symptomless left ventricular dysfunction after myocardial infarction. Lancet 1988; 1: 255–9
2. Pfeffer MA, Lamas GA, Vaughan DE, Arisi AF, Braunwald E. Effect of captopril on progressive ventricular dilatation after anterior myocardial infarction. N Engl J Med 1988; 319: 80–6
3. Sharpe N, Smith H, Murphy J, Greaves S, Hart H, Gamble G. Early prevention of left ventricular dysfunction following myocardial infarction with angiotensin converting enzyme inhibition. Lancet 1991; 337: 872–6
4. Pfeffer MA, Braunwald E, Moye LA et al. Effect of captopril on mortality and morbidity in patients with left ventricular dysfunction after myocardial infarction—results of the Survival and Ventricular Enlargement Trial. N Engl J Med 1992; 327: 669–77
5. The SOLVD Investigators. Effect of enalapril on mortality and the development of heart failure in asymptomatic patients with reduced left ventricular ejection fractions. N Engl J Med 1992; 327: 685–91
6. Swedberg K, Held P, Kjekshus J, Rasmussen K, Ryden L, Wedel H. Effects of the early administration of enalapril on mortality in patients with acute myocardial infarction—results of the Cooperative New Scandinavian Enalapril Survival Study II (CONSENSUS II). N Engl J Med 1992; 327: 678–84
7. GISSI III: effects of lisinopril and transdermal glyceryl trinitrate singly and together on 6-week mortality and ventricular function after myocardial infarction. Lancet 1994; 343: 1115–22
8. ISIS Collaborative Group. ISIS-4: a randomised factorial trial assessing oral captopril, oral mononitrate and intravenous magnesium sulphate in 58 050 patients with suspected acute myocardial infarction. Lancet 1995; 345: 669–85

9. The Acute Infarction Ramipril Efficacy (AIRE) Study Investigators. Effect of ramipril on mortality and morbidity of survivors of acute myocardial infarction with clinical evidence of heart failure. Lancet 1993; 342: 821–8
10. Ambrosini E, Borghi C, Magnani B. The effect of the angiotensin converting enzyme inhibitor zofenopril on mortality and morbidity after anterior myocardial infarction. N Engl J Med 1995; 332: 80–5
11. Kober L, Torp-Pedersen C, Carlsen J et al. A clinical trial of the angiotensin-converting-enzyme inhibitor transdolapril in patients with left ventricular dysfunction after myocardial infarction. N Engl J Med 1995; 333: 1670–6
12. Tao Shou-chi. The use of captopril in the early stage of acute myocardial infarction: Chinese AMI Captopril Trial Proceedings 4th International—2nd Asian Pacific Symposium on ACE Inhibition, Beijing 1995; 2.4
13. Yusuf S, Pepine CJ, Garces C et al. Effect of enalapril on myocardial infarction and unstable angina in patients with low ejection fractions. Lancet 1992; 340: 1173–8

34 Thrombolytic therapy

Harvey D White

Acute myocardial infarction (AMI) is usually caused by thrombotic occlusion of a coronary artery[1] which results in myocardial ischaemia and necrosis. Reduction of infarct size,[2] preservation of ventricular function[3] and decreased mortality[4–7] can be achieved if thrombolytic therapy is administered early and reperfusion is established. The aim of thrombolytic therapy is to lyse intracoronary thrombi and to achieve sustained patency of the infarct-related artery as quickly as possible and in as many patients as possible. Patency of the infarct-related artery at 90 minutes after administration of a thrombolytic agent correlates with mortality reduction,[8] and long-term patency of the infarct-related artery is an independent favourable prognostic factor.[9]

Thrombolytic therapy reduces 35-day mortality by 18% for patients treated within 12 hours, with a saving of 18 lives per 1000 patients treated.[10] Increased survival is achieved with this therapy irrespective of age, sex, history of previous infarction, diabetes, heart rate or blood pressure on admission.

Despite compelling data from trials randomizing 7 100 100 patients, thrombolytic therapy continues to be under-utilized.[11,12] Approximately 75% of patients with acute infarction present within 12 hours with either ST elevation or bundle branch block.[13] Registry studies report that usage is only 35% in the United States[12] and 35–50% in the UK.[11] The elderly appear to be a group in which thrombolytic therapy continues to be under-utilized.[12] The elderly are at high absolute risk of dying and the number of lives saved by treating elderly patients may be greater than in younger patients. For example, in the Fibrinolytic Therapy Trialists' overview for patients aged 65 to 74 years, 26 lives were saved for each 1000 patients treated with thrombolytic therapy, whereas for patients aged <55 years, 12 lives were saved for each 1000 patients treated.[10] There should be no exclusion of patients on the basis of age alone.[14]

Who should receive thrombolytic therapy?

On the basis of clinical trials all patients presenting within 12 hours with prolonged ischaemic pain and ST segment elevation or a new bundle branch block pattern should receive thrombolytic therapy.[10] Its effectiveness is dependent on careful selection of eligible patients to maximize benefits and minimize risks.

Electrocardiographic criteria

Patients with anterior or inferior ST elevation should be treated. Although patients with inferior infarctions usually have smaller infarcts, the GISSI trial (Gruppo Italiano per lo Studio della Streptochinasi nell'Infarto Miocardico) showed that it was the amount of ST elevation and not the site of infarction that related to outcome and hence to likely benefit from thrombolytic therapy.[15] Patients with inferior infarction can develop complete heart block, and this is less frequent with thrombolytic therapy. Cardiogenic shock may develop from a large inferior infarction. Also, right ventricular infarction due to a proximal right coronary artery occlusion may result in a prolonged hospital stay. Furthermore patency of the infarct-related artery is likely to result in a better long-term outcome.[9]

At present patients with ST segment depression on the admission ECG should not be treated. Most patients with ST depression have non-occlusive thrombi in the ischaemia-producing coronary artery.[16] It is therefore unlikely that thrombolysis would improve perfusion. Also, thrombolytic therapy is procoagulant as it activates platelets[17] and exposes clot-bound thrombin which is a very powerful stimulus for platelet coagulation[18] and further thrombin generation.[19] These procoagulant effects could convert a non-occlusive thrombus to an occlusive one and result in infarction.[20]

In the Fibrinolytic Therapy Trialists' overview the mortality rate in the control patients with ST depression was 13.8% versus 15.2% in thrombolytic-treated patients. Patients with ST segment depression are a heterogeneous group. One group of patients with previous infarction and extensive coronary disease has a high mortality rate, while another group may have single-vessel disease with a posterior infarction and a low mortality rate. Mortality is related to the amount of ST depression.[21,22] There may be subgroups of patients who may benefit from thrombolytic therapy, but these have not been defined.

Patients with T wave inversion or a normal ECG have a low mortality rate and should not be treated with thrombolysis. However, the ECG should be repeated at 30 and 60 minutes as ST elevation could develop, making them eligible to receive thrombolytic therapy.

Contraindications

Thrombolytic therapy has been shown to be relatively safe, with a slight increase in total stroke (0.4%) depending on the thrombolytic regimen,[10] bleeding with a need for transfusion (0.9%) depending on the number of invasive procedures performed,[8,10] and a small risk of major allergy with streptokinase of about 0.3%.[13] Clinical situations such as aortic dissection, where there is a high risk of harm and no hope of benefit, are absolute contraindications for administering thrombolytic therapy.

The information boxes list contraindications for thrombolytic therapy and relative contraindications where the benefits and risks need to be assessed for the individual patient, taking into account other factors such as the size of the infarct, haemodynamic status, history of previous infarction, etc. In some patients the likelihood of clinical benefit may clearly outweigh the likelihood of causing harm, and these patients should be treated. Because of the urgency required to treat patients as early as possible, four questions can be asked that cover most contraindications:

- Have you ever had a stroke?
- Have you ever had any bleeding problems?
- Have you ever bled from the bowel, stomach or bladder?
- Have you had any recent surgery or trauma?

Stroke

The most important adverse event is intracranial haemorrhage. Risk factors for intracranial haemorrhage include hypertension on admission (systolic blood pressure ≥170 mmHg, diastolic blood pressure ≥110 mmHg), older age, low body weight, recent head trauma, previous stroke, and use of recombinant tissue plasminogen activator (r-TPA).[23]

The increased rate of intracerebral haemorrhage with r-TPA is also seen with a weight-adjusted infusion.[8] The reason for this

Contraindications for thrombolytic therapy

- Stroke within 6 months
- Head trauma or brain surgery within 6 months
- Internal bleeding within 2 weeks
- Known bleeding disorder
- Major surgery, trauma or bleeding within 2 weeks
- Traumatic cardiopulmonary resuscitation within 2 weeks
- Uncontrolled hypertension (systolic blood pressure > 200 mmHg, diastolic blood pressure > 110 mmHg)
- Acute pancreatitis
- Pregnancy or within 1 week postpartum

Relative contraindications for thrombolytic therapy

- Puncture of non-compressible blood vessel within 1 week
- Active peptic ulceration
- Infective endocarditis
- Active cavitating pulmonary tuberculosis
- Advanced liver disease
- Oral anticoagulant therapy
- Intracardiac thrombi

probably relates to its greater effectiveness in lysing old clots which may be protective in the brain. Also, the blood pressure-lowering effects of streptokinase may be beneficial.

Previous stroke is a major contraindication for thrombolytic therapy. A previous intracerebral bleed at any time should be an absolute contraindication.

Recent trauma, surgery or bleeding

Any recent head trauma, no matter how trivial, should be an absolute contraindication for thrombolytic therapy. Recent brain or spinal cord surgery is also an absolute contraindication.

With time, protective clots become relatively resistant to lysis. This takes about 10 days and therefore 2 weeks is taken as a reasonable time to withhold thrombolytic therapy. Clinically there are many circumstances where judgments have to be made about whether certain irreparable damage to the heart is outweighed by a bleeding risk which could be treated by transfusion.

Known bleeding disorders

The commonest bleeding disorder is von Willebrand's disease, which occurs in 0.1% of the population. Bleeding relates to abnormalities of platelet adhesion and aggregation and to the carrier for factor VIII procoagulant protein. Clinical manifestations are heterogeneous. If patients have had to receive transfusions then in general they should not be treated with thrombolytic therapy, whereas if there has only been mild bruising associated with trauma and the patient presents early with a large infarction, thrombolysis would be appropriate.

Cardiopulmonary resuscitation

Non-traumatic cardiopulmonary resuscitation should not be a contraindication, regardless of the length of resuscitation. Pooled data from small patient series have reported no significant complications if resuscitation was <10 minutes.[24–26] No bleeding has been reported with prolonged resuscitation up to 120 minutes or even when patients with rib fractures have been given thrombolysis.[27]

Hypertension

For patients with hypertension on admission the blood pressure should be lowered with IV nitroglycerin to <170 mmHg systolic and <105 mmHg diastolic before administering thrombolytic therapy. Although this approach has not been validated, it seems reasonable. It is not clear whether it is the driving head of systolic pressure which is the important factor predisposing to intracerebral bleeding, or the vascular disease relating to long-standing hypertension. It is likely that both factors are important. Although it is appreciated that 'time is of the essence', it would be appropriate to examine the fundi to assess the amount of vascular disease, and to not treat patients with advanced retinopathy.

Diabetes

Diabetic retinopathy should not be considered a contraindication as bleeding is very rare and not related to the coagulation system.[27a]

Acute pancreatitis

Thrombolytic therapy could potentially cause or aggravate haemorrhagic pancreatitis, and patients with acute pancreatitis should not be treated.

Pregnancy

Thrombolytic therapy should not be administered during pregnancy because of risks to the fetus. There is also a risk of bleeding in the first week postpartum.

Active peptic ulceration

Indigestion should not be a contraindication as there are many causes that may or may not be associated with an increased bleeding risk. Recent bleeding from peptic ulceration within 2 weeks can be considered a strong contraindication and between 2 and 6 weeks previously a relative contraindication.

Endocarditis

Because of the possibility of intracerebral haemorrhage from a mycotic aneurysm, endocarditis is a relative contraindication.

Active cavitating pulmonary tuberculosis

These patients are prone to haemoptysis which may be uncontrollable, and thrombolytic therapy is therefore contraindicated.

Liver disease

Because of the possibility of depletion of liver-produced clotting factors and the possible presence of oesophageal varices, severe liver disease is a contraindication.

Patients on oral anticoagulants

Patients on oral anticoagulants, which deplete the vitamin K-dependent clotting factors (II, VII, IX and X), are at increased risk of bleeding. If the international normalized ratio (INR) is <2.0, thrombolytic, antiplatelet and antithrombin therapy should be given as indicated. If the INR is in the therapeutic range, one approach is to administer simultaneously fresh frozen plasma to replenish the clotting factors or to give IV vitamin K and administer thrombolytic therapy 30 minutes later.

Risk of systemic embolism

Thrombolytic therapy should not be administered if there is a high risk of systemic embolism from dislodgement of a fresh left atrial or left ventricular thrombus.

Thrombolytic ineligibility

It is important to remember that ineligibility for thrombolytic therapy does not mean ineligibility for reperfusion. These patients should be considered for primary angioplasty if it is available.

Menstruation

Menstruation should not be a contraindication for thrombolytic therapy. Although menstrual blood does not clot due to small amounts of tissue plasminogen activator, bleeding is controlled mainly by uterine vessel contraction rather than haemostatic mechanisms. Although there is a small increment in vaginal bleeding, this is more than offset by the potentially life-saving effects of thrombolytic therapy.[28]

Thrombolytic agents

The different thrombolytic agents vary in their pharmacologic and safety profiles, as well as in their effectiveness and cost.

Streptokinase

Streptokinase is produced by Lancefield group C β-haemolytic streptococci. Streptokinase activates the fibrinolytic system by directly combining with circulating plasminogen and forms an activator complex which is able to convert both circulating plasminogen and thrombin-bound plasminogen to plasmin. Plasmin is then able to lyse fibrin with the thrombus to produce fibrin-degradation products. The amount of plasmin produced by the normal dose of streptokinase (1.5 million units) overwhelms the neutralizing capacity of α_2 antiplasmin. The circulating plasmin is able to degrade fibrinogen to produce a lytic state. There is no relation between the extent of the lytic state and the incidence of bleeding.[29] This is because most bleeding associated with thrombolytic therapy is a result of lysis of 'protective' haemostatic plugs rather than changes in the coagulation properties of the blood. The reduction in fibrinogen levels may reduce re-occlusion of reperfused infarct-related arteries.[29,30] Streptokinase has other effects which may be beneficial. A small decrease (5–10 mmHg) in systolic blood pressure may be related to the lower risk of cerebral haemorrhage with streptokinase compared to r-TPA.[5,8,31] Also, streptokinase has been shown to reduce infarct size even if the infarct-related artery remains occluded[32] and to reduce viscosity[33] which may improve the microcirculation to an ischaemic infarct-zone. The recommended dosage of IV streptokinase is 1.5 million units over 30–60 minutes.

The incidence of hypotension is greater with faster infusion (5–10%), but more rapid infusion may result in better reperfusion rates and clinical benefit. Prophylactic hydrocortisone is unnecessary.

Tissue plasminogen activator

Tissue plasminogen activator is a naturally occurring substance produced in small amounts by vascular endothelium and the uterus. r-TPA is produced by recombinant deoxyribonucleic acid (DNA) technology and is non-antigenic. The half-life is 2–5 minutes and r-TPA is metabolized in the liver. It requires fibrin in thrombus to act as a cofactor before converting plasminogen to plasmin. Because of its relative fibrin specificity, r-TPA degrades little circulating fibrinogen.

It should be given as a weight-adjusted accelerated regimen over 90 minutes, with a bolus dose of 15 mg, 0.75 mg/kg over 30 minutes (not exceeding 50 mg), and 0.5 mg/kg up to 35 mg over the next 60 minutes. This regimen has been shown to be as effective as alternative regimens such as 'double bolus' dosing.[33a]

Urokinase

Urokinase is produced from human urine and directly activates the conversion of plasminogen to plasmin. It is non-antigenic. Urokinase has been shown to reduce mortality[34] but is more expensive than streptokinase. A specific role may be for treatment of patients who have previously received streptokinase.[35] The usual mode of administration is 2 million units administered as an immediate bolus of 1 million units, repeated 60 minutes later.

Adverse events from thrombolytic therapy and recommended treatment

Bleeding: minor
- Slight oozing at puncture sites is common and should be treated with direct pressure

Bleeding: major
- Stop thrombolytic infusion, aspirin and heparin
- Reverse heparin with protamine sulphate
- Administer fresh frozen or freeze-dried plasma to replenish clotting factors and fibrinogen
- Consider administration of aminocaproic acid
- Consider fresh platelet transfusion
- Transfusion of whole blood should be avoided as far as possible unless the patient is symptomatic or haemoglobin falls ≥2 g/L

Hypotension
- Stop the infusion temporarily and restart at a slower rate when BP improves. Elevation of the patient's legs and infusion of volume is usually all that is necessary. Rarely inotropes may be required

Major allergy
- IV antihistamines and hydrocortisone may help. If the reaction is severe, adrenaline 0.5–1.0 mL (1/10 000) should be given as an IV bolus and repeated after 3 minutes if necessary

Adverse effects

Bleeding

The most important adverse effect of thrombolytic therapy is bleeding. Bleeding is related to lysis of 'protective' haemostatic plugs rather than to changes in coagulation factors. If bleeding occurs during infusion of a thrombolytic agent, the infusion should be stopped and general measures instituted (see the information box). The most devastating adverse event is the occurrence of haemorrhagic stroke. If this occurs the thrombolytic infusion and any antithrombin or antiplatelet therapy should be stopped. If heparin was being infused, IV protamine sulphate should be given immediately. Consideration should be given to the other treatments listed in the box. In most cases a computed tomography (CT) scan and a neurological opinion will be helpful in determining treatment and prognosis. Rarely surgical evaluation is indicated.

Allergy

As streptokinase is a foreign protein, allergic reactions can occur with fever, nausea or skin rash. Major reactions are rare. There were no episodes of anaphylactic shock in 8592 patients treated with streptokinase in the Second International Study of Infarct Survival (ISIS-2),[5] while in the GISSI trial the incidence was 0.1%[36] and in the Third International Study of Infarct Survival (ISIS-3), 0.3%.[13] Back pain may occur during infusion of streptokinase. Plasmacytosis with acute renal failure[37] and Guillain–Barré syndrome[38] have also been reported after administration of streptokinase.

Hypotension

Hypotension occurs with all thrombolytic agents but more commonly with streptokinase. In the blinded ISIS-3 trial hypotension occurred in 4.3% of patients treated with r-TPA and 6.8% of patients treated with streptokinase.[13] The development of hypotension is not an allergic reaction and is thought to relate to the effects of bradykinin produced after conversion of plasminogen to plasmin.

Adjunctive aspirin therapy

If there are no contraindications all patients with 20 minutes of ischaemic chest discomfort should immediately be given approximately 150 mg of aspirin (to be chewed if the preparation is enteric-coated). Acute administration of aspirin reduces mortality at 35 days by 20%.[5] Aspirin is cheap and effective with a low risk of either haemorrhagic or allergic reactions. The reduction in mortality is not time-dependent, but as patients die if this therapy is delayed, nurses should be instructed to give aspirin to most patients on admission to the CCU, and general practitioners and ambulances should carry aspirin for

Potential beneficial effects of heparin in acute myocardial infarction

- Improved early infarct artery patency
- Sustained infarct artery patency
- Decreased re-occlusion
- Decreased left ventricular thrombus
- Decreased deep vein thrombosis
- Improved collateral circulation

immediate administration. Long-term reinfarction, stroke and death are reduced by 25%.[39] Aspirin in a dose of 75–150 mg/day should be continued indefinitely.

Adjunctive heparin therapy

Both streptokinase and r-TPA produce procoagulant effects by activating platelets[17] and thrombin.[40,41] Streptokinase may have more prothrombotic effects than r-TPA.[42] Also with thrombolysis there is exposure of fibrin-bound thrombin which is very thrombogenic. Not only are platelets further activated[18] but thrombin is generated via a feedback mechanism 300 000 times.[19] The success of thrombolytic therapy therefore depends on the balance between the induced fibrinolytic activity and the induced procoagulant activity.

Heparin has a number of potential benefits (see the information box) and is effective at reducing increasing thrombin activity (as measured by fibrinopeptide-A levels) after administration of streptokinase or r-TPA.[40] Acute administration of heparin in the first 24 hours after the onset of AMI may promote the development of collateral circulation.[43]

The production of fibrin degradation products and lower fibrinogen levels may be expected to lessen the requirement for heparin with streptokinase, but as discussed above there are cogent reasons why heparin may also be beneficial.[44] In the GISSI-II trial (Gruppo Italiano per lo Studio Della Sopravvivenza Nell'Infarto Miocardico) with subcutaneous heparin at 12 hours hospital mortality was reduced 11% ($p<0.05$) when the patients not eligible to receive heparin were excluded—that is, those who died before 12 hours.[31] In ISIS-3 in a non-prespecified analysis administration of delayed subcutaneous heparin reduced mortality over the 7-day period that heparin was administered from 7.9% to 7.4% ($p=0.06$).[13] Reinfarction was also reduced from 2.8% to 2.4% ($p<0.01$). However, after the prespecified follow-up period of 35 days, there was no significant reduction in mortality (10.3% heparin versus 10.6% control) or reinfarction (3.5% heparin versus 3.2% control).

In neither trial were total stroke rates increased with heparin (see Table 34.1) and mortality was lowered by two lives per 1000 patients treated, non-fatal reinfarction by two per 1000 patients treated, with one extra non-fatal stroke and three extra transfusions per 1000 patients treated. On balance subcutaneous heparin could be considered modestly beneficial.

Several other trials also indicate that heparin may be beneficial with streptokinase. Intravenous heparin has been shown to reduce reperfusion time as measured by ST-segment monitoring, to result in lower creatine kinase MB peaks[45] and to increase early patency rates.[46] Also, when the effect of heparin without aspirin was evaluated, mortality was shown to be reduced from 8.8% to 4.6% ($p=0.05$) in the SCATI trial when a heparin bolus of 2000 units followed 9 hours later by 12 500 units 12-hourly was given subcutaneously.[47]

In the GUSTO trial (Global Utilization of Streptokinase and Tissue Plasminogen Activator for Occluded Coronary Arteries) an attempt was made to compare the effects of IV heparin to administration of subcutaneous heparin delayed for 4 hours after administration of streptokinase.[8] However, there was a large crossover (36%) of patients randomized to receive subcutaneous heparin, to the intravenous arm, considerably reducing the power of the study. There were no differences between these regimens. The mortality rate at 30 days was 7.2% in the intravenous heparin-treated patients and 7.4% in the group who received subcutaneous heparin with aggressive use of intravenous heparin if thought appropriate. Stroke and bleeding rates were also similar, while in the angiographic substudy there was an 11% absolute difference in infarct artery patency rates at 5–7 days in favour of IV heparin (83% versus 72%, $p<0.05$).[48]

Table 34.1 Overview of the addition of delayed subcutaneous heparin in the ISIS-3[13] and GISSI-II[73] trials for 1000 treated patients at 35 days

	ISIS-3	GISSI-II	Combined
Benefit			
Mortality reduction	−3	+1	−2
Reduced non-fatal reinfarction	−1	−2	−2
Risk			
Major bleeding	+2	+5	+3
Total non-fatal stroke	+1	+1	+1

Based on this evidence, either IV heparin (5000 unit bolus followed by 1000 units/h adjusted to an activated partial thromboplastin time (APTT) of 50–75 seconds) [48a] or subcutaneous heparin delayed 4 hours (12 500 units 12-hourly) could be administered, with administration of IV heparin for recurrent ischaemia in approximately one third of patients. In patients judged to be at higher risk of bleeding after streptokinase, for example those with hypertension, peptic ulceration or oral anticoagulant therapy, streptokinase may be administered without adjunctive heparin.

r-TPA has a short half-life and only a modest fibrinogen-lowering effect, with little production of fibrin degradation products. Several trials have reported high re-occlusion rates either in the absence of aspirin[49] or a small and possibly ineffective dose of 80 mg.[50] The European Trial gave 250–300 mg of aspirin intravenously and assessed patency at 3 days in patients randomized either to IV heparin or control. The absolute patency rate was 8% higher in the heparin-treated patients, 83% versus 75%.[51] It is therefore not known what effect adjunctive IV heparin has on patency rates in the first 24 hours following r-TPA when an adequate dose (≥150 mg) of aspirin is administered.

It is recommended that IV heparin be administered as a 5000 unit bolus followed by 1000 units/h, with the APTT adjusted to 50–75 seconds[48a] for 24–48 hours.[52] The possibility that mortality and re-occlusion after thrombolysis can be further reduced by specific antithrombin agents such as hirudin and hirulog (see Ch. 35) is currently under study. Recently reported results have shown that hirudin does not have a clear superiority over well controlled heparin therapy given after r-TPA.[52a] Hirulog administered after streptokinase achieves substantially higher early patency than heparin.[52b]

The importance of early treatment

Thrombolytic therapy is much more effective when given early. For each hour of delay 1.6 lives are lost per 1000 patients treated (see Fig. 34.1).[10] The early hours after the onset of infarction are when most deaths occur and early thrombolytic treatment has the most potential to achieve lysis of intracoronary thrombi and rapid early reperfusion with salvage of myocardium and preservation of left ventricular function.[2] Although pre-hospital administration of thrombolytic therapy is feasible, the most important practical approach is to reduce the 'door to needle' time in hospital. A recent registry report from the United States showed that the median delay from hospital arrival to administration of thrombolytic therapy was 99 minutes[12] whereas for the patients randomized in the GUSTO trial the delay was nearly one hour.[8] These unacceptable 'door to needle' times can be reduced by instituting review procedures.[55] The aims of treatment are listed in the information box.

Pre-hospital treatment

There have been a number of trials of pre-hospital thrombolysis. Pooled results from six trials in 6305 patients show an 18.4% reduction in short-term mortality from 10.7% to 9.1% ($p<0.05$).[56] In trials with less than an hour's difference between community and hospital treatment times there was little difference in mortality,[55,56] whereas in the GREAT trial[57] where there was a 139-

Aims of thrombolytic therapy

- To encourage patients to present for treatment as early as possible
- To obtain an ECG within 10 minutes of presentation
- To administer thrombolytic therapy within 30 minutes of arrival at hospital.*

* If there are no contraindication.

minute treatment difference, administration of pre-hospital thrombolysis halved mortality. These trials reported an increase in the incidence of pre-hospital ventricular fibrillation and it is therefore mandatory that if pre-hospital administration of thrombolysis is practised, well-trained staff and defibrillators are available. Pre-hospital management is discussed in more detail in Chapter 52.

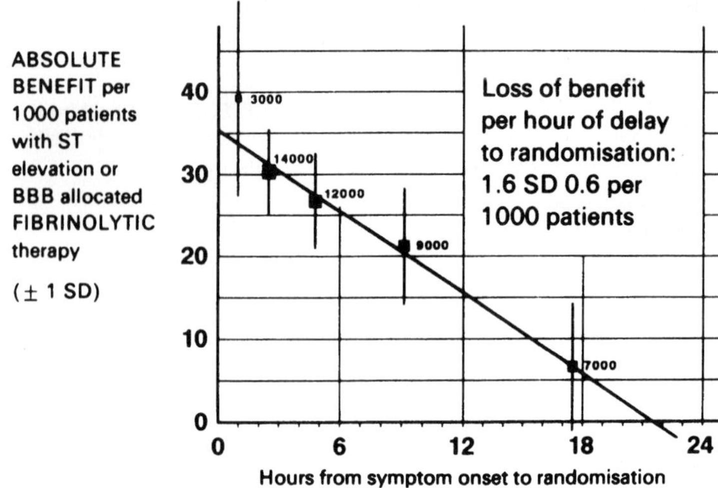

Fig. 34.1 Absolute reduction in 35-day mortality versus delay from symptom onset to randomization among 45 000 patients with ST elevation or bundle branch block. (All patients in ASSET[53] and LATE[54] are included because the tabular information available from these trials subdivided by delay was not subdivided by ECG.) For patients whose delays were recorded as 0–1, 2–3, 4–6, 7–12 and 13–24 hours, the absolute benefit (±SD) is plotted against the mean recorded delay time (0.98, 2.50, 4.79, 9.11 and 17.48 hours respectively). The area of each black square and the extent to which it influences the line drawn through five points is approximately proportional to the number of patients it is based on. Reproduced with permission from FTT Collaborative Group

Late thrombolytic therapy

For patients who present between 7 and 12 hours with ST elevation or bundle branch block pattern on their admission ECG, 35-day mortality is reduced by 13%.[10] This corresponds to about 16 lives saved per 1000 patients treated. For patients treated after 12 hours there is a non-significant 5% reduction in mortality corresponding to about five lives saved per 1000 patients treated (see Fig. 34.1). The confidence limits of this finding are wide but there may be some patients with continuing pain or heart failure who may benefit from treatment after 12 hours.

The mechanism of late treatment benefit may relate to a number of factors[58] including the difficulty of timing the onset of infarction. Infarction may be a stuttering process, with the infarct-related artery opening and closing, and presentation after 6 hours does not mean that the artery has been occluded for all of that time. Some patients will have collateral circulation supplying blood to the ischaemic zone, extending the time before myocardial necrosis occurs. As end-systolic volume is the most important modifiable prognostic factor after MI,[59] the most important mechanism may relate to patency of the infarct-related artery reducing infarct expansion and left ventricular remodelling and dilatation.[60] A patent artery is also associated with fewer late potentials[61] and propensity for ventricular arrhythmias.[62] A patent artery can also potentially provide a source of collaterals to a different infarct zone if occlusion of a different coronary artery subsequently occurs.[58] Patency of the infarct-related artery has also been shown to be a powerful long-term prognostic factor independent of left ventricular function.[9]

Thrombolytic therapy should be administered to all patients with ST elevation or bundle branch block presenting within 12 hours of the onset of ischaemic pain. Selected patients presenting after 12 hours may also benefit.

Readministration of thrombolytic therapy

Approximately 20% of patients admitted to CCUs with acute infarction have had a previous infarction.[10] An increasing proportion of these patients will have previously received thrombolytic therapy and be eligible for thrombolytic therapy again. Also, readministration of thrombolytic therapy may prevent reinfarction when there is threatened reocclusion of infarct-related arteries that may have been reperfused following thrombolytic therapy.[63,64] Rescue thrombolysis with re-administration of thrombolytic therapy when lack of reperfusion is identified[65] is likely to play an increasing role in the future.

Following the administration of streptokinase, antistreptokinase antibodies develop and streptokinase neutralizing titres rapidly increase so that by 3–4 days, the levels are sufficient to neutralize a standard dose of streptokinase. The levels remain elevated in 50% of patients 4 years after initial treatment.[66] The major concern with readministering streptokinase to patients with high antibody levels is that treatment may not be effective.[67] Also, allergic reactions may be more common with readministration. It is therefore recommended that streptokinase should not be re-administered except in the first 24 hours after the first treatment. Non-allergenic agents should be used for readministration, such as urokinase or r-TPA.[35]

Cardiogenic shock

Cardiogenic shock accounts for a large proportion of deaths after AMI and the mortality rate is in excess of 75%.[68] The most important treatment strategy is to open the occluded infarct-related artery. It is unclear which is the best approach to achieve this. Observational studies of angioplasty[69,70] or coronary artery bypass surgery[71,72] have reported lower mortality rates than historical controls, but there have been no randomized trials of angioplasty versus surgery or thrombolytic therapy. This evidence is presented in more detail in Chapter 57. Although the GISSI trial, comparing streptokinase to control treatment, showed no significant difference in survival of patients with cardiogenic shock, due to the small number of patients randomized, the results were consistent with a mortality reduction of 25–30%.[36] Furthermore in the Fibrinolytic Therapy Trialists' overview, for patients with a systolic blood pressure <100 mmHg and a heart rate >100/minute, the mortality rate was 61.1% among control patients and 53.8% among thrombolytic-treated patients.[10] Although this difference was not significant, it could result in a saving of 73 lives per 1000 patients treated.

Two trials have compared the effects of streptokinase versus r-TPA in patients with cardiogenic shock. In both trials the mortality rate was lower in streptokinase-treated patients. In the GISSI-II/International Study the hospital mortality rate was 64.9% in streptokinase-treated patients versus 78.1% in r-TPA-treated patients, a saving of 132 lives per 1000 patients treated ($p<0.05$).[73] In the GUSTO Trial the 30-day mortality rate was 55.6% in streptokinase-treated patients and 62% in r-TPA-treated patients ($p=0.06$).[8] Streptokinase can cause hypotension, but the incidence of this is not increased by a low pretreatment blood pressure.[5] Although these findings in two megatrials of a better outcome with streptokinase could have occurred by chance, it would seem reasonable to use streptokinase in these patients while being alert to the possibility of streptokinase-associated hypotension and the need for fluid loading. The mechanism of benefit may relate to reduction in viscosity and improved microvascular perfusion with streptokinase.[32]

Coronary artery bypass grafts

Patients with coronary artery bypass grafts make up a significant proportion of patients with MI.[8] The mortality rate for these patients is high. Often the vein graft supplying the infarct zone is full of thrombus, and the best treatment is unclear. In the GUSTO trial 30-day mortality was 8.3% in accelerated-r-TPA-treated patients with vein grafts, versus 11% in streptokinase-treated patients.[8] It would therefore seem reasonable to select r-TPA as the agent of choice for these patients.

Choice of agent

When administered in an accelerated regimen, r-TPA achieves higher rates of normal infarct artery blood flow (Thrombolysis in Myocardial Infarction (TIMI) grade 3 flow) at 90 minutes than streptokinase (54% versus 32%).[48] In the GUSTO trial this greater patency benefit translated into a 14% lower mortality rate (95% confidence interval 6–21%) with 10 additional lives saved per 1000 patients treated with r-TPA. As in previous comparative trials[13,73] the administration of r-TPA was associated with a higher stroke rate of 1.55% versus 1.22% for patients treated with streptokinase plus subcutaneous heparin and 1.4% for patients treated with streptokinase and IV heparin. For a combined end-point of mortality plus non-fatal disabling stroke, accelerated r-TPA resulted in a better outcome than streptokinase (6.9% versus 7.8%, $p<0.01$). The benefit of accelerated r-TPA in the GUSTO trial was seen across most groups and the benefit was in general greater in those patients at greater absolute risk of dying. This includes patients with large anterior infarcts and those with bypass grafts. There was no greater benefit in patients treated early, but there was a trend towards a smaller benefit in those treated late.[74]

Administration of r-TPA is associated with an increased risk of intracerebral haemorrhage. This needs to be considered when deciding treatment for an individual patient.[10] The greater expense of r-TPA over streptokinase also has to be taken into account when considering treatment for an individual patient: r-TPA costs approximately 4–7 times more than streptokinase. The appropriate selection of patients who are likely to benefit most is therefore very important. The overall cost-effectiveness ratio for accelerated r-TPA compared with streptokinase, based on data from the GUSTO trial, is US$32,678 per life year added.[77] It can be seen in Table 34.2 that for patients aged under 60 years with inferior infarctions or patients under 40 years with anterior infarctions the cost is nearly US$100 000 per life year added.

Table 34.3 lists clinical situations in which streptokinase or r-TPA may be recommended as the drug of choice. Streptokinase may be considered the treatment of choice for patients with small to moderate sized infarcts because of the risk of producing an iatrogenically-induced stroke in patients with a good prognosis, and also because of cost, particularly in patients under 60 years of age. Streptokinase is the drug of choice in patients who have an increased risk of stroke and may also be used in patients presenting after 6 hours. Streptokinase also has a role in the treatment of patients with cardiogenic shock.

There have been no comparative trials of thrombolytic agents in patients presenting after 6 hours. The aim of late treatment is to achieve sustained patency of the infarct-related artery for which the agents are the same at 3 hours after administration.[48] The drugs would therefore be expected to have the same benefits if achievement of infarct artery patency is the major mechanism of benefit, rather than salvage of myocardium. It would therefore be reasonable to choose either r-TPA or streptokinase for late treatment. However, the incidence of stroke is less with streptokinase.[54,75]

Accelerated r-TPA is the regimen of choice for patients at high risk, including patients with large anterior infarcts[76] and those with venous bypass grafts supplying the area of infarction. R-TPA is also an alternative to urokinase for readministration when streptokinase has been used previously.

Table 34.2 Incremental cost of accelerated r-TPA (tissue plasminogen activator) versus streptokinase per life year added in the GUSTO trial[77]

	Inferior infarction	Anterior infarction
≤40 years	US$99 510	US$76 417
41–60 years	US$46 639	US$35 123
61–75 years	US$24 956	US$21 885
>75 years	US$18 967	US$17 893

Table 34.3 Factors in choice of thrombolytic agent

	Streptokinase	r-TPA
Small infarction	✓	
Large infarction		✓
Young patients	✓	✓
Elderly patients		✓
Risk factors for stroke	✓	
Late treatment (>6 hours)	✓	
Previous streptokinase		✓
Previous CABG		✓
Cardiogenic shock	✓	✓
Cost constraints	✓	

CABG = coronary artery bypass grafing, r-TPA = tissue plasminogen activator

References

1. DeWood MA, Spores J, Notske R et al. Prevalence of total coronary occlusion during the early hours of transmural myocardial infarction. N Engl J Med 1980; 303: 897–902
2. Serruys PW, Simoons ML, Suryapranata H et al. Preservation of global and regional left ventricular function after early thrombolysis in acute myocardial infarction. J Am Coll Cardiol 1986; 7: 729–42

3. White HD, Norris RM, Brown MA et al. Effect of intravenous streptokinase on left ventricular function and early survival after acute myocardial infarction. N Engl J Med 1987; 317: 850–5
4. Gruppo Italiano per lo Studio della Streptochinasi nell'Infarto Miocardico (GISSI). Long-term effects of intravenous thrombolysis in acute myocardial infarction: final report of the GISSI Study. Lancet 1987; ii: 871–4
5. ISIS-2 (Second International Study of Infarct Survival) Collaborative Group. Randomized trial of intravenous streptokinase, oral aspirin, both, or neither among 17 187 cases of suspected acute myocardial infarction: ISIS-2. Lancet 1988; ii: 349–60
6. AIMS Trial Study Group. Long-term effects of intravenous anistreplase in acute myocardial infarction: final report of the AIMS Study. Lancet 1990; 335: 427–31
7. Wilcox RG, von der Lippe G, Olsson CG, Jensen G, Skene AM, Hampton JR. Effects of alteplase in acute myocardial infarction: 6-month results from the ASSET Study. Lancet 1990; 335: 1175–8
8. The GUSTO Investigators. An international randomized trial comparing four thrombolytic strategies for acute myocardial infarction. N Engl J Med 1993; 329: 673–82
9. White HD, Cross DB, Elliott JM, Norris RM, Yee TW. Long-term prognostic importance of patency of the infarct-related coronary artery after thrombolytic therapy for acute myocardial infarction. Circulation 1994; 89: 61–7
10. Fibrinolytic Therapy Trialists' (FTT) Collaborative Group. Indications for fibrinolytic therapy in suspected acute myocardial infarction: collaborative overview of early mortality and major morbidity results from all randomized trials of more than 1000 patients. Lancet 1994; 343: 311–22
11. Ketley D, Woods KL. Impact of clinical trials on clinical practice: example of thrombolysis for acute myocardial infarction. Lancet 1993; 342: 891–4
12. Rogers WJ, Bowlby LJ, Chandra NC et al. Treatment of myocardial infarction in the United States (1990 to 1993): observations from the National Registry of Myocardial Infarction. Circulation 1994; 90: 2103–14
13. ISIS-3 (Third International Study of Infarct Survival) Collaborative Group. ISIS-3: a randomized comparison of streptokinase vs tissue plasminogen activator vs anistreplase and of aspirin plus heparin vs aspirin alone among 41 299 cases of suspected acute myocardial infarction. Lancet 1992; 339: 753–70
14. White H, Cross D, Scott M, Norris R. Comparison of effects of thrombolytic therapy on left ventricular function in patients over with those under 60 years of age. Am J Cardiol 1991; 67: 913–8
15. Mauri F, Gasparini M, Barbonaglia L et al. Prognostic significance of the extent of myocardial injury in acute myocardial infarction treated by streptokinase (the GISSI trial). Am J Cardiol 1989; 63: 1291–5
16. DeWood MA, Stifter WF, Simpson CS et al. Coronary arteriographic findings soon after non-Q-wave myocardial infarction. N Engl J Med 1986; 315: 417–23
17. Fitzgerald DJ, Catella F, Roy L, Fitzgerald GA. Marked platelet activation *in vivo* after intravenous streptokinase in patients with acute myocardial infarction. Circulation 1988; 77: 142–50
18. Kroll MH, Schafer AI. Biochemical mechanisms of platelet activation. Blood 1989; 74: 1181–95
19. Mann KG, Tracy PB, Nesheim ME. Assembly and function of prothrombinase complex on synthetic and natural membranes. In: Oates JA, Harwiger J, Ross R (eds). Interaction of platelets with the vessel wall. Washington DC: American Physiologic Society, 1985: 47–57
20. Freeman MR, Langer A, Wilson RF, Morgan CD, Armstrong PW. Thrombolysis in unstable angina: randomized double-blind trial of t-PA and placebo. Circulation 1992; 85: 150–7
21. Lee HS, Cross SJ, Rawles JM, Jennings KP. Patients with suspected myocardial infarction who present with ST depression. Lancet 1993; 342: 1204–7
22. White HD, French JK, Norris RM, Williams BF, Hart HH, Cross DB. Effects of streptokinase in patients presenting within 6 hours of prolonged chest pain with ST segment depression. Br Heart J 1995; 73: 500–5
23. Simoons ML, Maggioni AP, Knatterud G et al. Individual risk assessment for intracranial haemorrhage during thrombolytic therapy. Lancet 1993; 342: 1523–8
24. Doorey AJ, Michelson EL, Topol EJ. Thrombolytic therapy of acute myocardial infarction: keeping the unfulfilled promises. JAMA 1992; 268: 3108–14
25. Neches RB, Goldfarb AM. Thrombolytic therapy after cardiopulmonary resuscitation in acute myocardial infarction. Am J Cardiol 1993; 71: 258
26. Scholz KH, Tebbe U, Herrmann C et al. Frequency of complications of cardiopulmonary resuscitation after thrombolysis during acute myocardial infarction. Am J Cardiol 1992; 69: 724–8
27. Weston CFM, Avery P. Thrombolysis following prehospital cardiopulmonary resuscitation. Int J Cardiol 1992; 37: 195–8

27a. Ward H, Yudkin JS. Thrombolysis in patients with diabetes: withholding treatment is probably mistaken: patients should be given a choice. Br Med J 1995; 310: 3–4
28. Karnash SL, Granger CB, White HD et al. Treating menstruating women with thrombolytic therapy: insights from the GUSTO-I trial. J Am Coll Cardiol 1995; 26: 1651–6
29. Sherry S, Marder VJ. Streptokinase and recombinant tissue plasminogen activator (rt-PA) are equally effective in treating acute myocardial infarction. Ann Intern Med 1991; 114: 417–23
30. Rapaport E. Thrombolysis, anticoagulation, and reocclusion. Am J Cardiol 1991; 68: 17E
31. Gruppo Italiano per lo Studio della Sopravvivenza nell'Infarto Miocardico. GISSI-II: a factorial randomized trial of alteplase versus streptokinase and heparin versus no heparin among 12 490 patients with acute myocardial infarction. Lancet 1990; 336: 65–71
32. Kopia GA, Kopaciewicz LJ, Ruffolo RR. Coronary thrombolysis with intravenous streptokinase in the anesthetized dog: a dose-response study. J Pharmacol Exp Ther 1988; 244: 956
33. Moriarty AJ, Hughes R, Nelson SD, Balnave K. Streptokinase and reduced plasma viscosity: a second benefit. Eur J Haemol 1988; 41: 25
33a. COBALT Investigators. Results of the Continuous Infusion Versus Double Bolus Administration of Alteplase (COBALT) study. Presented at European Society of Cardiology meeting, Birmingham, UK, 1996
34. Rossi P, Bolognese I, on behalf of Urochinasi per via Sistemica nell'Infarto Miocardico (USIM) Collaborative Group. Comparison of intravenous urokinase plus heparin versus heparin alone in acute myocardial infarction. Am J Cardiol 1991; 68: 585–92
35. White HD. Thrombolytic treatment for recurrent myocardial infarction: avoid repeating streptokinase or anistreplase. Br Med J 1991; 302: 429–30
36. Gruppo Italiano per lo Studio della Streptochinasi nell'Infarto Miocardico (GISSI). Effectiveness of intravenous thrombolytic treatment in acute myocardial infarction. Lancet 1986; i: 397–402
37. Chan NS, White H, Maslowski A, Cleland J. Plasmacytosis and renal failure after readministration of streptokinase for threatened myocardial reinfarction. Br Med J 1988; 297: 717–8
38. McDonagh AJG, Dawson J. Guillain–Barré syndrome after myocardial infarction. Br Med J 1987; 294: 613
39. Antiplatelet Trialists' Collaboration. Collaborative overview of randomised trials of antiplatelet therapy, Pt. I: prevention of death, myocardial infarction, and stroke by prolonged antiplatelet therapy in various categories of patients. Br Med J 1994; 308: 81–106
40. Eisenberg PR, Sherman LA, Jaffe AS. Paradoxic elevation of fibrin peptide A after streptokinase: evidence for intense thrombosis despite intense fibrinolysis. J Am Coll Cardiol 1987; 10: 527–9
41. Owen J, Friedman KD, Grossman BA, Wilkins C, Berke AD, Powers ER. Thrombolytic therapy with tissue plasminogen activator or streptokinase induces transient thrombin activity. Blood 1988; 76: 616–20
42. Eisenberg PR. Role of heparin in coronary thrombolysis. Chest 1992; 101(4) Suppl: 131S–9S
43. Ejiri M, Fujita M, Miwa K et al. Effects of heparin treatment on collateral development and regional myocardial function in acute myocardial infarction. Am Heart J 1990; 119: 248–53
44. White HD, Yusuf S. Issues regarding the use of heparin following streptokinase therapy. Journal of Thrombosis and Thrombolysis 1995; 2: 5–10
45. Melandri G, Branzi A, Semprini F, Cervi V, Galiè N, Magnani B. Enhanced thrombolytic efficacy and reduction of infarct size by simultaneous infusion of streptokinase and heparin. Br Heart J 1990; 64: 118–20
46. Col J, Decoster O, Hanique G et al. Infusion of heparin conjunct to streptokinase accelerates reperfusion of acute myocardial infarction: results of a double blind randomized study (OSIRIS) Abst. Circulation 1992; 86: I–259
47. The SCATI (Studio sulla Calciparina nell-Angina e nella Trombosi Ventricolare nell' Infarto) Group. Randomised controlled trial of subcutaneous calcium-heparin in acute myocardial infarction. Lancet 1989; ii: 182–6
48. The GUSTO angiographic investigators. The effects of tissue plasminogen activator, streptokinase, or both on coronary- artery patency, ventricular function, and survival after acute myocardial infarction. N Engl J Med 1993; 329: 1615–22
48a. Granger CB, Hirsh J, Califf RM et al. Activated partial thromboplastin time and outcome after thrombolytic therapy for acute myocardial infarction: results from the GUSTO-I trial. Circulation 1996; 93: 870–8
49. Bleich SD, Nichols TC, Schumacher RR, Cooke DH, Tate DA, Teichman SL. Effect of heparin on coronary arterial patency after thrombolysis with tissue plasminogen activator in acute myocardial infarction. Am J Cardiol 1990; 66: 1412–7
50. Hsia J, Hamilton WP, Kleiman N et al. A comparison between heparin and low-dose aspirin as adjunctive therapy with tissue plasminogen activator for acute

myocardial infarction. N Engl J Med 1990; 323: 1433–7
51. de Bono DP, Simoons ML, Tijssen J, for the European Cooperative Study Group (ECSG). The effect of early intravenous heparin on coronary patency, infarct size and bleeding complications after alteplase thrombolysis: results of a randomised double-blind European cooperative trial. Br Heart J 1992; 67: 122–8
52. Thompson PL, Aylward PE, Federman J et al. A randomized comparison of intravenous heparin with oral aspirin and dipyridamole 24 hours after recombinant tissue-type plasminogen activator for acute myocardial infarction. Circulation 1991; 83: 1534–42
53. Wilcox RG, von der Lippe G, Ollson CG, Jensen G, Skene AM, Hampton JR. Trial of tissue plasminogen activation for mortality reduction in acute myocardial infarction: Anglo-Scandinavian Study of Early Thrombolysis (ASSET). Lancet 1988; ii: 525–30
54. LATE Study Group. Late assessment of thrombolytic efficacy (LATE) study with alteplase 6–24 hours after onset of acute myocardial infarction. Lancet 1993; 342: 759–66
55. Weaver WD, Cerqueira M, Hallstrom AP et al. Pre-hospital-initiated vs hospital-initiated thrombolytic therapy. JAMA 1993; 270: 1211–6
55a. HERO Investigators. Preliminary results of the Hirulog Early Reperfusion/Occlusion (HERO) study. Presented at plenary session, American College of Cardiology, Orlando, Florida, March 1996
55b. GUSTO IIb Investigators. Results of the GUSTO IIb angioplasty substudy. Presented at plenary session, American College of Cardiology, Orlando, Florida, March 1996
56. The European Myocardial Infarction Project Group. Pre-hospital thrombolytic therapy in patients with suspected acute myocardial infarction. N Engl J Med 1993; 329: 385–9
57. Rawles JM, and the GREAT Group. Feasibility, safety, and efficacy of domiciliary thrombolysis by general practitioners: Grampian Region Early Anistreplase Trial. Br Med J 1992; 305: 548
58. White HD. Thrombolytic therapy for patients with myocardial infarction presenting after six hours. Lancet 1992; 340: 221–2
59. White HD, Norris RM, Brown MA, Brandt PWT, Whitlock RML, Wild CJ. Left ventricular end-systolic volume as the major determinant of survival after recovery from myocardial infarction. Circulation 1987; 76: 44–51
60. Hochman JS, Choo H. Limitation of myocardial infarct expansion by reperfusion independent of myocardial salvage. Circulation 1987; 75: 299–306
61. Gang ES, Lew AS, Hong M, Wang FZ, Siebert CA, Peter T. Decreased incidence of ventricular late potentials after successful thrombolytic therapy for acute myocardial infarction. N Engl J Med 1989; 321: 712
62. Sager PT, Perlmutter RA, Rosenfeld LE, McPherson CA, Wackers FJ, Batsford WP. Electrophysiologic effects of thrombolytic therapy in patients with a transmural anterior myocardial infarction complicated by left ventricular aneurysm formation. J Am Coll Cardiol 1988; 12: 19–24
63. White HD, Cross DB, Williams BF, Norris RM. Safety and efficacy of repeat thrombolytic treatment after acute myocardial infarction. Br Heart J 1990; 64: 177–81
64. Barbash GI, Hod H, Roth A et al. Repeat infusion of recombinant tissue-type plasminogen activator in patients with acute myocardial infarction and early recurrent myocardial ischemia. J Am Coll Cardiol 1990; 16: 779–83
65. White HD, Cross DB, Williams BF et al. 'Rescue' thrombolysis with intracoronary tissue plasminogen activator for failed intravenous thrombolysis with streptokinase for acute myocardial infarction. Am J Cardiol 1995; 75: 172–4
66. Elliott JM, Cross DB, Cederholm-Williams SA, White HD. Neutralizing antibodies to streptokinase four years after intravenous thrombolytic therapy. Am J Cardiol 1993; 71: 640–5
67. Cross DB, White HD. Allergic reactions to streptokinase: does antibody formation prevent reuse in a second myocardial infarction? Clin Immunother 1994; 2: 415–20
68. Goldberg RJ, Gore JM, Alpert JS et al. Cardiogenic shock after acute myocardial infarction: incidence and mortality from a community wide perspective 1975–1988. N Engl J Med 1991; 325: 1117–22
69. Lee L, Erbel R, Brown TM, Laufer N, Meyer J, O'Neill WW. Multicenter registry of angioplasty therapy of cardiogenic shock: initial and long-term survival. J Am Coll Cardiol 1991; 17: 599–603
70. O'Neill WW. Angioplasty therapy of cardiogenic shock: are randomized trials necessary? J Am Coll Cardiol 1992; 19: 915–7
71. DeWood MA, Notake RN, Hensley GR et al. Intraaortic balloon counterpulsation with and without reperfusion for myocardial infarction shock. Circulation 1980; 61: 1105–12
72. Moosvi AR, Khaja F, Villanueva L, Gheorghiade M, Douthat L, Goldstein S. Early revascularization improves survival in cardiogenic shock complicating acute myocardial infarction. J Am Coll Cardiol 1992; 19: 907–14

73. GISSI-II and International Study Group. Six-month survival in 20 891 patients with acute myocardial infarction randomized between alteplase and streptokinase with or without heparin. Eur Heart J 1992; 13: 1692–7
74. Topol EJ, Califf RM, Lee KL, on behalf of the GUSTO Investigators. More on the GUSTO Trial [letter]. N Engl J Med 1994; 331: 277–8
75. EMERAS (Estudio Multicéntrico Estreptoquinasa Republicas de América del Sul) Collaborative Group. Randomized trial of late thrombolysis in patients with suspected acute myocardial infarction. Lancet 1993; 342: 767–72
76. Thompson PL, Tonkin AM, Aylward P, White H. Thrombolysis '93—is there a consensus? Aust NZ J Med 1993; 23: 778
77. Mark DB, Hlatky MA, Califf RM et al. Cost effectiveness of thrombolytic therapy with tissue plasminogen activator as compared with streptokinase for acute myocardial infarction. N Engl J Med 1995; 332: 1418–24

35 Antithrombins

Joseph Hung

Role of antithrombin agents

Thrombin is a key regulator in thrombosis not only because it catalyyes the formation of the fibrin clot but it also amplifies its own generation through feedback activation of coagulation factors, notably factors V and VIII (see Fig. 35.1). Thrombin is also a potent platelet activator and stimulates platelet-rich thrombosis after vessel wall injury. Platelets in turn provide lipid surfaces for assembly of coagulation factors, notably the prothrombin activator (prothrombinase) complex, that greatly speeds thrombin generation. Heparin and direct antithrombin agents exert their antithrombotic action not only by inactivating thrombin but also by blocking thrombin generation through interruption of its autoamplification, and by preventing thrombin-enhanced platelet activation (see Fig. 35.1).

Heparins

Structure

Standard heparin is a mixture of sulfated glycosaminoglycans with an average molecular weight of 12 000–15 000 daltons.[1] McLean, a medical student, accidentally discovered heparin in 1916 but its first therapeutic use was not until 20 years later in 1937. Only about one third of the heparin binds to antithrombin III, and this portion is responsible for most of the anticoagulant action of heparin. Low-molecular weight heparins (LMWHs) are fragments of standard heparin, produced by chemical or enzymatic depolymerization, with mean molecular weights between 4000 and 6000, that still retain the antithrombin III binding site.[2]

Mode of action

The anticoagulant action of heparin is primarily through its binding to a plasma cofactor, antithrombin III, and the subsequent acceleration (1000-fold) of formation of complexes of antithrombin III with serine proteases of the coagulation system, notably thrombin (factor IIa) and factor Xa (see Fig. 35.1). For maximal heparin-enhanced inhibition of thrombin a ternary complex of heparin, antithrombin III and thrombin is required (see Fig. 35.2). The binding of thrombin to heparin is of an electrostatic nature and a larger heparin molecule increases the probability of interaction. In contrast, the inhibition of factor X is due to a binary complex between antithrombin III and factor Xa, in which heparin does not need to bind factor X (Fig. 35.2). Thus LMWHs like standard heparin can inactivate factor X but are less able to bind and inhibit thrombin. The theoretical rationale for LMWHs is that they can inhibit the coagulation cascade at an earlier stage (anti-Xa) and prevent its multiplying effect, while limited inhibition of thrombin may still allow normal haemostasis. Evidence suggests however that anti-Xa activity alone is not sufficient of itself for complete thrombosis prevention. Heparin may also have other useful roles apart from its anticoagulant action because it is lipolytic, suppresses smooth muscle cell proliferation, and is involved in angiogenesis.[1]

Pharmacokinetics

Heparin is not absorbed when given by mouth and needs to be administered by intravenous or subcutaneous injection. After IV injection, heparin is removed by both a saturable mechanism (rapid uptake by endothelium and macrophages) and by a slower linear mechanism (most probably renal excretion). The practical implication of these kinetics is that the dose-response

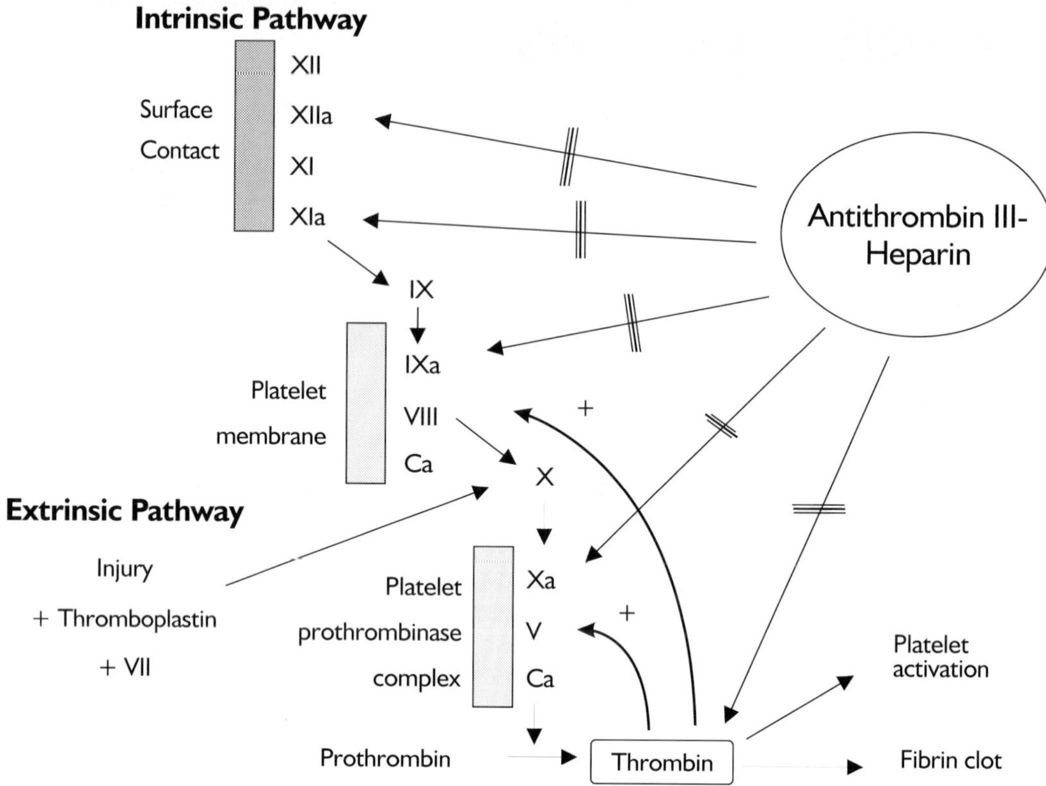

Fig. 35.1 The coagulation cascade with its sequence of amplifying proteolytic enzyme reactions resulting in thrombin generation. Thrombin-mediated positive feedback loops are shown. Lines with cross-hatching denote inhibitory activity of heparin-antithrombin III.

relation is not linear. With increasing dose of heparin there is a disproportionate increase in the duration and intensity of effect. For example, heparin has an approximate half-life of 30 minutes after 25 U/kg bolus but this increases to 60 minutes after 75 U/kg.[1] In circulation, heparin is bound to many plasma proteins and this contributes to individual variability in effect. Commercial LMWHs differ widely in their anti-Xa to anti-IIa activity but as a group they are readily absorbed from subcutaneous tissue, and are much less bound by endothelium and plasma proteins than standard heparin, resulting in good bioavailability at low doses and increased biologic half-life (see Table 35.1).

Limitations of heparin

Apart from its complex pharmacokinetics, other potential limitations of heparin are:

- Platelets release a heparin-neutralizing protein, called platelet factor 4.
- The prothrombinase complex on the platelet surface is protected from inhibition by heparin-antithrombin III.
- Thrombin bound within the fibrin clot is also resistant to inactivation by heparin-antithrombin III.
- Heparin increases the risk of microvascular bleeding through its effect on platelets and vascular permeability.

These limitations are less seen with the LMWHs.

Dosage

The clinical efficacy of heparin is usually optimized when heparin is monitored to maintain the patient's activated partial thromboplastin time (APTT) at a ratio of 1.5 to 2.5 of control value.[1] This corresponds to a heparin level of 0.2–0.4 U/ml by protamine titration. Unfortunately the thromboplastins used in APTT tests can vary greatly, making laboratory standardization difficult. Intravenous heparin therapy is usually started with a loading dose of 5000 U followed by 1000 U/h infusion. In well-

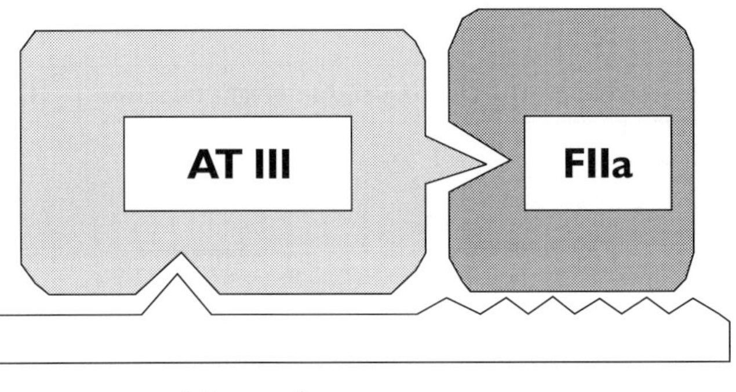

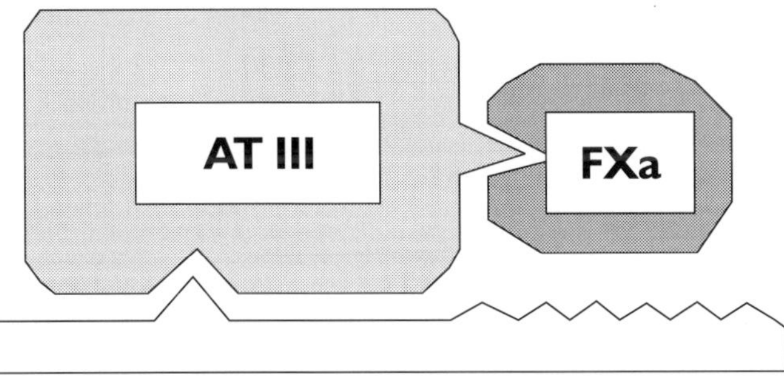

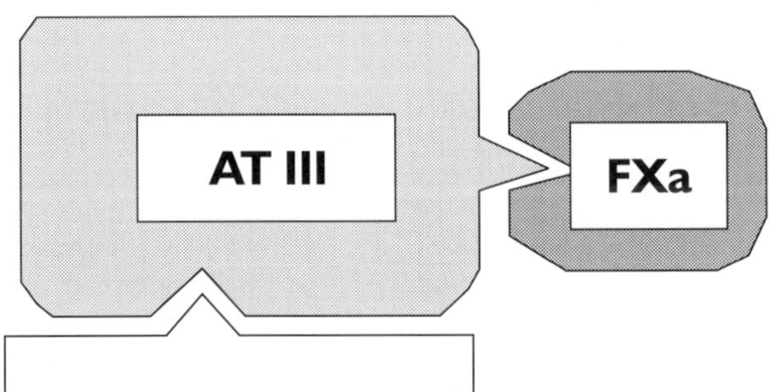

Fig. 35.2 Mechanisms of interaction between antithrombin III (AT III), thrombin (FIIa), factor Xa (Fxa) and heparin molecules of different molecular weight. LMWH denotes low-molecular weight derivative of standard heparin.

monitored studies the mean maintenance dose of heparin was approximately 30 000 U/24 h when given by continuous infusion and 35 000 U/24 h when given subcutaneously or by intermittent IV injection. LMWHs differ in their in vitro anti-Xa to anti-IIa activity and the latter may not correlate with their in vivo anticoagulant effect. Hence the recommended dosages for LMWHs have to be defined separately for each commercial preparation.[2] Because of their kinetics, LMWHs can usually be given once daily by subcutaneous injection without laboratory monitoring.

Clinical indications for heparin

Heparin has proven efficacy in the prevention and treatment of venous thromboembolism, in the prevention of mural thrombosis, for the treatment of evolving MI, in the prevention of coronary reocclusion after thrombolysis, for the treatment of unstable angina, and in the prevention of abrupt vessel occlusion after coronary angioplasty (see Table 35.2).

Prevention and treatment of venous thromboembolism

Low-dose subcutaneous heparin, 5000 U every 8–12 hours, is effective for the prophylaxis of venous thrombosis and pulmonary embolism in high risk surgical and medical patients.[3] In the treatment of established deep vein thrombosis or pulmonary embolism, high-dose heparin by continuous infusion, intermittent IV or subcutaneous administration, are effective provided heparin is maintained at therapeutic levels (on average 30 000–35 000 U/24 h). For venous thromboembolism, comparative studies suggest that LMWHs administered by subcutaneous once daily injection in a fixed or weight-adjusted dosage is as effective and safe as standard heparin given by continuous infusion.[2]

Left ventricular mural thrombus

Anticoagulation after acute myocardial infarction (AMI) is effective in reducing the incidence of mural thrombosis detected echocardiographically and the risk of systemic thromboembolism.[4] In randomized trials demonstrating

Table 35.1 Comparisons between standard unfractionated heparin, low-molecular weight heparins and hirudin

	Unfractionated heparin	Low-molecular weight heparins	Hirudin
Mean molecular weight, D	12 000–15 000	4000–6000	≅7000
Anti-Xa: Anti-IIa activity	1:1	2:1–4:1	Anti-IIa only
Subcutaneous absorption	+	+++	+++
Binding to endothelium	+++	+	No
Protein binding	++++	+	+
Half-life	Shorter	Longer	Shorter
Dose-dependent clearance	Yes	No	No
Bioavailability at low doses	Poor	Good	Good
Increases microvascular bleeding	++++	++	No

Table 35.2 Clinical uses of heparin

Condition	Recommended heparin regimen
Deep venous thrombosis and pulmonary embolism	
Prophylaxis	5000 U subcutaneously every 8–12 hours
Treatment	IV bolus of 5000 U, followed by 24 000 U/24 hours by IV infusion or subcutaneously, adjusted to maintain APTT at 1.5–2.5 times control value
Acute myocardial infarction	
Prevention of mural thrombosis, prevention of reinfarction and death	IV bolus of 5000 U, followed by 12 500 U subcutaneously 12-hourly (fixed dose)
Adjunctive therapy after thrombolysis	*Following r-TPA therapy*: IV bolus of 5000 U, followed by 24 000 U/24 hours, adjusted to maintain APTT at 1.5–2.5 times control value *Following streptokinase therapy*: Intravenous bolus of 2000 U, followed by 12 500 U subcutaneously 12-hourly (fixed dose)
Unstable angina	IV bolus of 5000 U, followed by 24 000 U/24 hours, adjusted to maintain APTT at 1.5–2.5 times control value

efficacy, heparin was given by infusion to maintain APTT above 1.5 times control or as a fixed dose of 12 500 U subcutaneously every 12 hours.[1]

Acute myocardial infarction

A meta-analysis of randomized trials of heparin therapy in evolving MI in the pre-thrombolytic era, totalling approximately 5700 subjects, found that heparin significantly reduced mortality by 16%, re-infarction by 22% and non-fatal stroke by 51%.[5] Similar results were obtained in the SCATI trial.[6] By comparison, aspirin was shown in the ISIS-2 trial comprising approximately 17 000 subjects to reduce vascular mortality by 23%, reinfarction by 49%, and non-fatal stroke by 46%—similar reductions to that seen with the combined heparin trials but with better statistical confidence.[7] Importantly aspirin is associated with a lower risk of bleeding than heparin therapy.

Hence the role of heparin in AMI is now largely adjunctive to aspirin and thrombolytic therapy except for the prevention of venous thromboembolism and mural thrombosis.

Adjunctive therapy after thrombolysis

The re-occlusion rate after thrombolysis is between 10% and 45% depending on the study being considered. Thrombolytic agents can paradoxically activate platelets and increase local thrombin generation from the dissolving clot, predisposing to re-thrombosis. Following tissue plasminogen activator (r-TPA) high-dose IV heparin has been shown to help sustain coronary patency.[8] Anticoagulation is less important following streptokinase, as the latter is associated with a temporary systemic fibrinolytic state. Current evidence, including the National Heart Foundation study of r-TPA in AMI[9] suggests that antiplatelet therapy, primarily aspirin, is as effective as anticoagulant therapy in maintaining long-term coronary patency after thrombolysis.[8] The conflicting evidence for the use of heparin after streptokinase (unfortunately not clearly resolved by the GUSTO trial[10]) and the persuasive evidence for the use of heparin after r-TPA are discussed in detail in Chapter 34.

In conclusion, all patients should receive aspirin as adjunctive therapy after thrombolysis. In those receiving r-TPA, heparin bolus should also be given with subsequent infusion for at least 48 hours monitored to an APTT 1.5–2.5 times control value. In those receiving streptokinase, heparin may have some advantage in reducing re-occlusion rate, but with an increased risk of bleeding complications; its use should be restricted in patients with an increased risk of bleeding.

Unstable angina

Aspirin has been shown in three large trials to reduce mortality in unstable angina.[11] High-dose IV heparin was more effective than aspirin in settling recurrent ischaemic symptoms in patients with unstable angina although not more effective in preventing subsequent non-fatal MI or death.[12] In randomized trials to date, the combination of heparin and aspirin has not been shown to provide a net benefit over aspirin alone in the rate of non-fatal MI or death.[13] However, in those patients not already on aspirin, the cessation of heparin therapy has been associated with an increased risk of rebound angina, MI and need for urgent revascularization.[14] Thus aspirin should be administered to all patients with unstable angina, and high-dose heparin infusion should also be strongly considered, particularly if ischaemic symptoms do not settle on admission.

Side-effects of heparin

The most common side-effect of heparin is bleeding. Factors associated with an increased incidence of bleeding include high-dose heparin, intermittent IV administration, patient factors such as increased age, female gender, renal failure, chronic alcohol abuse, serious concurrent illness, and concomitant aspirin use.[1] The experience of the recently aborted GUSTO IIa study showed that the risk of cerebral haemorrhage increased dramatically with ‘aggressive’ heparin regimens which aim to maintain APTT at over three times baseline values. An idiosyncratic heparin-induced thrombocytopenia, complicated or not by arterial thrombosis, occurs usually between days 7 and 11 of treatment and is related to immune platelet-heparin complexes. It occurs more commonly with bovine than porcine heparin and after previous exposure to heparin. LMWHs are probably as antigenic as unfractionated heparin. Other important side-effects of heparin include osteoporosis with long-term treatment, skin necrosis, hypersensitivity reactions, and suppression of aldosterone production, resulting in hyperkalaemia.[1]

Monitoring of anticoagulation

There is a large inter-individual variation in anticoagulant responses to heparin probably because of variations in plasma concentrations of heparin-binding proteins. Thus heparin treatment needs to be individually monitored. The most commonly used method of monitoring is by measurement of APTT with maintenance within a range of 1.5–2.5 times baseline APTT value. This ‘therapeutic’ range of anticoagulation appears to optimize the clinical efficacy of heparin treatment—that is, therapeutic benefit without excessive bleeding risk.[1] However, it should be emphasized that the thromboplastin reagents used in APTT tests can vary widely and the therapeutic range for any given APTT reagent should be established in each laboratory to correspond to a heparin level of 0.2–0.4 U/ml by protamine titration.[1] Heparin treatment in angioplasty laboratories is often monitored by measurement of activated clotting time (ACT) using portable coagulation instruments.[15] Although there is a general correlation of ACT with APTT values, the clotting time responds linearly to a wider range of heparin concentrations than APTT. For coronary angioplasty a much higher level of anticoagulation is required and only when ACT values approach or exceed 300 seconds is there a marked reduction in the incidence of abrupt re-closure.[15]

Direct thrombin inhibitors

Advantages of direct thrombin inhibitors

The limitations of heparin were previously discussed. It is further exemplified by the relative resistance of experimentally-induced arterial thrombi to heparin even in high doses.[16] In contrast, the direct thrombin inhibitors are antithrombin III-independent in action, are not significantly bound to plasma proteins, have a reliable dose-response effect, are not inactivated by platelet factors, are able to inactivate clot-bound thrombin, and are much more effective than heparin in experimental thrombosis.[16,17]

Structure and mode of action

Hirudin, the prototypic thrombin inhibitor, is a 65-residue polypeptide isolated from the saliva of the medicinal leech *Hirudo medicinalis*.[17] It is the most potent known inhibitor of thrombin and acts by simultaneous binding and inhibition of the anion-binding exosite (fibrinogen recognition site) and the active catalytic site of thrombin (see Fig. 35.3). Hirugen, a synthetic hirudin derivative, is a dodecapeptide that retains the portion of hirudin involved in blockade of the anion-binding exosite (Fig. 35.3). Because it leaves the catalytic site of thrombin free, it has much weaker antithrombotic activity than hirudin. Hirulogs are a group of peptides developed by linking the hirugen molecule to the N-terminal of hirudin. Like hirudin, hirulogs block both the anion-binding exosite and the catalytic sites of the thrombin molecule (see Fig. 35.3). PPACK is a synthetic tripeptide compound that has a structure very close to fibrinopeptide A. It acts as an affinity agent to thrombin, causing irreversible blockade of the active catalytic site (Fig. 35.3). Argatroban, an arginine derivative, binds adjacent to and blocks the active catalytic site of thrombin but unlike PPACK it is a competitive antagonist. DuP 714, a boroarginine tripeptide, combines the advantage of moderately high thrombin affinity with the potential for oral administration.

Pharmacokinetics

Hirudin is poorly absorbed orally and is administered by intravenous, intramuscular or subcutaneous route. The half-life is about 40 minutes after IV administration and almost 2 hours after subcutaneous injection (see Table 35.1). Most of the compound (over 90%) is renally excreted in its active form. Hirulog differs from hirudin in that its half-life is 15–20 minutes shorter after IV administration and it has more extensive metabolic clearance with only about 20% of the compound recovered in the urine. Hirudin and hirulog have demonstrated a good safety and anticoagulant profile in normal human subjects. They produce a linear dose-dependent

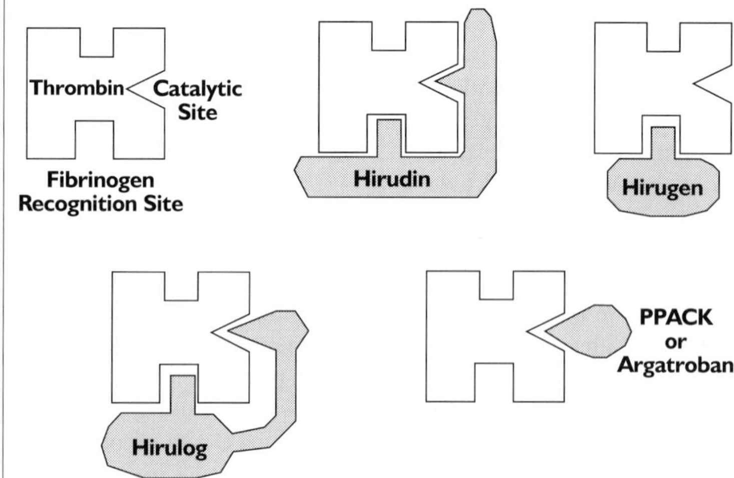

Fig. 35.3 Schematic of the thrombin molecule showing the key binding and catalytic sites. Sites of interaction of the thrombin molecule with the direct thrombin inhibitors, hirudin, hirugen, hirulog, PPACK, and argatroban are illustrated.

prolongation of coagulation parameters and a more predictable level of anticoagulation than heparin. Argatroban has also been shown to be well tolerated in humans with a dose-dependent prolongation of APTT which returns to baseline levels by 1 hour after IV administration.

Clinical uses of direct thrombin inhibitors

Experimental and clinical studies of direct thrombin inhibitors are largely focused on the prevention and treatment of arterial (platelet-rich) thrombosis which is relatively heparin resistant. Despite many efficacy and dose ranging studies, there are still relatively few randomized comparisons of direct thrombin inhibitors with heparin in patients with coronary artery disease.[17] Nevertheless experimental and clinical data do suggest that hirudin and other direct thrombin inhibitors may be more effective than heparin in facilitating and maintaining coronary patency after coronary thrombolysis, in preventing abrupt vessel closure after coronary angioplasty, and in the treatment of unstable angina.[17] Major bleeding risks associated with direct thrombin inhibitors have also been acceptably low and comparable with heparin when APTT on treatment is maintained at 1.5–2.5 times baseline value. The results of two randomized controlled trials comparing a direct thrombin inhibitor with heparin in acute coronary syndromes were recently reported.[18] In *GUSTO IIb*, which enrolled over 12 000 patients with AMI or unstable angina, hirudin was associated with a non-significant 10% reduction in deaths and non-fatal AMI at 30 days, although a significant reduction was seen at 24 hours.[18] Intracranial haemorrhage occurred more frequently with hirudin than heparin in unstable angina patients (0.2% vs 0.05% respectively). In the *HERO* trial, hirulog (2 doses) was compared with heparin in patients with suspected AMI treated with streptokinase and aspirin. 'High-dose' hirulog was associated with a significantly increased rate of TIMI-3 angiographic grade flow in the infarct-related artery, and did not increase the risk of severe bleeding.[18]

References

1. Hirsh J. Heparin. N Engl J Med 1991; 324: 1565–74
2. Hirsh J. Heparin and low-molecular weight heparins. Coronary artery disease 1992; 3: 990–1002
3. Collins R, Scrimgeour A, Yusuf S, Peto R. Reduction in fatal pulmonary embolism and venous thrombosis by perioperative administration of subcutaneous heparin; overview of results in randomized trials in general, orthopaedic, and urologic surgery. N Engl J Med 1988; 318: 1162–73
4. Thompson PL, Robinson JS. Stroke after acute myocardial infarction: relation to infarct size. Br Med J 1978; 2: 457–9
5. MacMahon S, Collins R, Knight C, Yusuf S, Peto R. Reduction of major morbidity and mortality by heparin in acute myocardial infarction. Abst. Circulation 1988; 78 (Suppl II): II–98
6. The SCATI Group. Randomised controlled trial of subcutaneous calcium-heparin in acute myocardial infarction. Lancet 1989; 2: 182–6
7. ISIS-2 (Second International Study of Infarct Survival) Collaborative Group. Randomized trial of intravenous streptokinase, oral aspirin, both or neither among 17 187 cases of suspected acute myocardial infarction: ISIS-2. Lancet 1988; 2: 349–60
8. Ridker PM, Hebert PR, Fuster V, Hennekens CH. Are both aspirin and heparin justified as adjuncts to thrombolytic therapy for acute myocardial infarction? Lancet 1993; 341: 1574–7
9. Thompson PL, Aylward PE, Federman J et al. A randomized comparison of intravenous heparin with oral aspirin and dipyridamole 24 hours after recombinant tissue-type plasminogen activator for acute myocardial infarction. Circulation 1991; 83: 1534–42
10. The GUSTO Investigators. An international randomized trial comparing four thrombolytic strategies for acute myocardial infarction. N Engl J Med 1993; 329: 673–82
11. Antiplatelet Triallists' Collaboration. Collaborative overview of randomised trials of antiplatelet therapy, Pt I. Prevention of death, myocardial infarction and stroke by prolonged antiplatelet therapy in various categories of patients. Br Med J 1994; 308: 81–106
12. Theroux P, Ouimet H, McCans J et al. Aspirin, heparin, or both to treat acute unstable angina. N Engl J Med 1988; 319: 1105–11
13. Holdright D, Patel D, Cunningham D et al. Comparison of the effect of heparin and aspirin versus aspirin alone on transient myocardial ischemia and in-hospital prognosis in patients with unstable angina. J Am Coll Cardiol 1994; 24: 39–45
14. Theroux P, Waters D, Lam J, Juneau M, McCans J. Reactivation of unstable angina after the dis-

continuation of heparin. N Engl J Med 1992; 327: 141–5
15. Ogilby JD, Kopelman HA, Klein LW, Agarwal JB. Adequate heparinization during PTCA: Assessment using activated clotting time. Cathet Cardiovasc Diagn 1989; 18: 206–9
16. Heras M, Chesebro JH, Webster MW et al. Hirudin, heparin, and placebo during deep arterial injury in the pig. The *in vivo* role of thrombin in platelet-mediated thrombosis. Circulation 1990; 82: 1476–84
17. Lefkovits J, Topol EJ. Direct thrombin inhibitors in cardiovascular medicine. Circulation 1994; 90: 1552–36
18. Reported at the 45th Annual Scientific Session, American College of Cardiology, Orlando, Florida, March 24–27, 1996

36 Antiplatelet agents

Joseph Hung

Role of platelets in thrombogenesis

Vascular endothelium is normally thromboresistant and produces platelet anti-aggregating substances, notably prostacyclin and endothelial relaxant factor (nitric oxide).[1] However after vascular injury, such as a plaque rupture, platelets adhere and their aggregation initiates occlusive thrombus formation along with activated coagulation. Initial activation of platelets occurs by exposure to collagen, thrombin, circulating adrenaline and high shear stress at the site of wall injury and underlying vessel stenosis (see Fig. 36.1). These extrinsic activators cause mobilization of intraplatelet calcium, platelet contraction, and release of adenosine diphosphate (ADP) and serotonin from dense granules. Released ADP and serotonin are further agonists for platelet aggregation. Arachidonic acid release from the platelet membrane represents a further major pathway for platelet activation. Enzyme cyclo-oxygenase converts arachidonic acid to labile prostaglandin endoperoxides (PGG_2/PGH_2) which are then converted to thromboxane A_2 (TXA_2) by thromboxane synthetase. TXA_2 is a potent platelet aggregating substance and vaso-

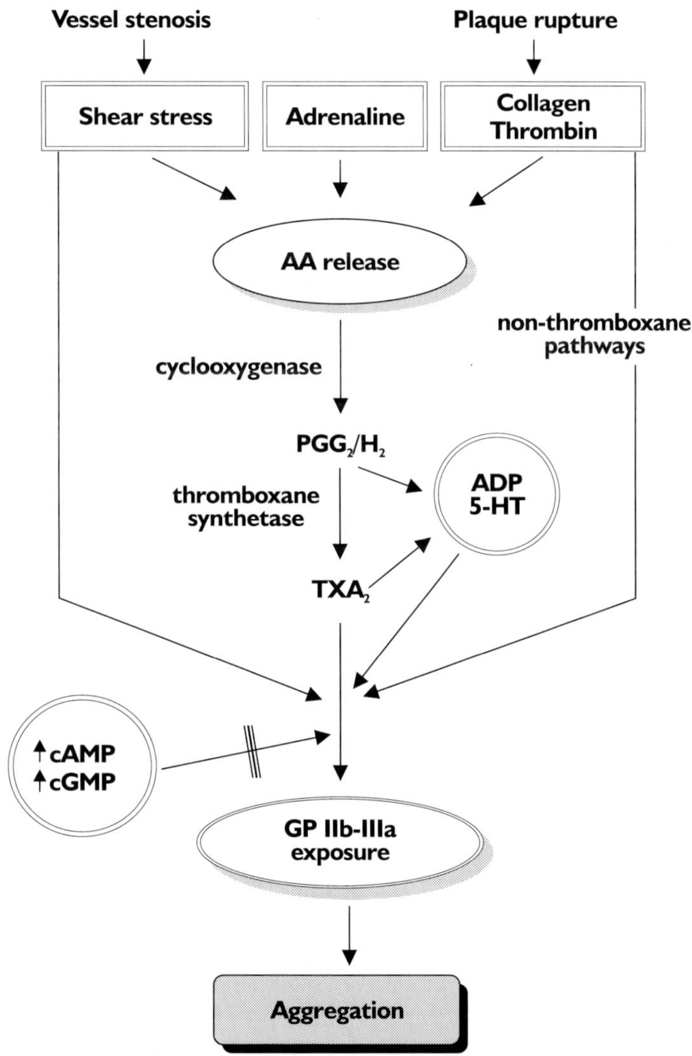

Fig. 36.1 Platelets are activated by agonists in vivo leading to exposure of the GP IIb-IIIa receptor via thromboxane- as well as non-thromboxane-dependent pathways. The Gp IIb-IIIa receptor causes platelet aggregation after binding to fibrinogen. Line with cross-hatching denotes inhibitory action.
AA=arachidonic acid; PGG_2/H_2=prostaglandin endoperoxides G_2 and H_2; ADP=adenosine diphosphate; 5-HT=5-hydroxytryptamine (serotonin); cAMP=cyclic adenosine monophosphate; cGMP=cyclic guanosine monophosphate.

constrictor. The final common pathway for platelet aggregation is the exposure of the platelet membrane receptor, GP IIb-IIIa (see Fig. 36.1). This receptor plays an essential role in platelet aggregation by binding to fibrinogen and other adhesive macromolecules, allowing platelet-platelet attachment and stabilization of the haemostatic plug.[1]

Antiplatelet agents

Agents that prevent platelet activation or interfere with platelet function have the potential to prevent thromboembolic disease. Aspirin is the most widely used antiplatelet agent but, despite its use, thromboembolic events still commonly occur. Other potentially more potent platelet inhibitors are currently under investigation. The pharmacology and mode of action of aspirin and other potential antiplatelet agents are reviewed in the following section (see the information box).[1–3]

Antiplatelet agents and mode of action

- Cycloxygenase inhibitors
  Aspirin
  Other non-steroidal anti-inflammatory drugs (NSAIDs)
- Thromboxane synthetase inhibitors
- Thromboxane/endoperoxide receptor antagonists
- Combined thromboxane synthetase inhibitor and thromboxane receptor antagonist
- Drugs that increase cAMP or cGMP
  Prostacyclin and its analogues
  Organic nitrates
  Dipyridamole
- Inhibitors of fibrinogen binding to GP IIb-IIIa
- Antagonists of pro-aggregating stimuli
  Thrombin inhibitors, e.g. heparin, hirudin
  Serotonin antagonists
  Inhibitors of ADP-induced platelet reaction, e.g. ticlopidine, clopidogrel

Aspirin

Mode of action

The major antithrombotic action of aspirin is associated with its ability to inhibit platelet TXA_2 synthesis via irreversible acetylation of the enzyme cyclo-oxygenase.[3] Because platelets cannot synthesize new enzyme, they are functionally impaired for their circulating life (7–10 days). Vessel wall cyclo-oxygenase is responsible for the conversion of arachidonic acid to prostacyclin, which has opposing actions to TXA_2. Because endothelial cells have the ability to synthesize new enzymes, it has been suggested that very low-dose aspirin (40 mg/day or less) may spare vessel wall prostanoid synthesis, although this remains uncertain.[3] Aspirin only partially inhibits platelet aggregation induced by ADP, collagen or thrombin. At higher agonist concentrations, as likely occurs in vivo, full platelet aggregation can still proceed via non-thromboxane-dependent pathways (see Fig. 36.1). The adherence of platelets to the subendothelium and the release of granule contents, such as platelet-derived growth factor, are also not prevented by aspirin.[1,3]

Clinical pharmacology

Aspirin (acetylsalicylic acid) is rapidly absorbed in the stomach and upper small intestine, with measurable plasma levels within 20 minutes of ingestion.[3] Oral aspirin has a poor systemic bioavailability and short half-life (15–20 minutes) because in the gut, liver and rest of the body it is rapidly hydrolysed by esterases to salicylic acid, which of itself has no significant antiplatelet effects. However the platelet inhibitory effect of aspirin occurs before its entry into the systemic circulation due to acetylation of platelet cyclo-oxygenase in the portal circulation, and its inhibitory effect lasts for the lifetime of the affected platelets.[3] Near complete inhibition of platelet TXA_2 synthesis can be shown within 1 hour of the ingestion of soluble aspirin (150–325 mg). Enteric-coated tablets may produce less gastrointestinal irritation but their absorption and antiplatelet effects may be delayed by 2–3 hours, a delay which is obviated by chewing the tablets before swallowing.

Other cyclo-oxygenase inhibitors

Non-steroidal anti-inflammatory drugs, such as ibuprofen and sulphinpyrazone, inhibit enzyme cyclo-oxygenase *in a reversible fashion* and are therefore less effective and have a shorter duration of action than aspirin. Their antithrombotic efficacy is uncertain and currently they are not recommended as antiplatelet agents.[1,2]

Inhibitors of thromboxane synthetase

Thromboxane synthetase inhibitors have been developed with the expectation of specific inhibition of thromboxane synthesis by platelets while sparing or even enhancing prostacyclin production by vascular endothelium. However, their clinical results have been disappointing.[1,2] This is probably due to incomplete suppression of TXA_2 by these inhibitors and the accumulation of precursor and pro-aggregatory prostaglandin endoperoxides.

Blockers of thromboxane receptors

The thromboxane receptor antagonists block the interaction of its receptor not only with TXA_2 but also the precursor prostaglandin endoperoxides, and so should inhibit platelet aggregation more effectively than thromboxane synthetase inhibitors. They are competitive antagonists, however, and high amounts of TXA_2 can displace the antagonist from its receptor. Drugs which combine the inhibition of thromboxane synthetase and blockade of the thromboxane/endoperoxide receptor have a theoretical advantage in that they offset each other's negative aspects. These agents have shown some promise in experimental and clinical studies.[1,2]

Drugs that increase platelet cAMP and cGMP

Exposure of the GP IIb-IIIa receptor can be inhibited by agents which increase cyclic adenosine monophosphate (cAMP) or cyclic guanosine monophosphate (cGMP). These agents have a much broader spectrum of activity as they affect the final common pathway of platelet aggregation and also inhibit platelet granule release (see Fig. 36.1).[1,2] Thus prostacyclin and nitric oxide, which stimulate platelet adenylate and guanylate cyclase respectively, are both potent endogenously-occurring anti-aggregating substances as well as vasodilators. A number of other substances, such as prostaglandin E_1, iloprost (a prostacyclin analogue), organic nitrates and adenosine exert their anti-aggregatory effects by a similar mechanism. Despite their antiplatelet effects, these agents have their main clinical use as vasodilators. Dipyridamole, which also increases platelet cAMP levels, has been widely used for its antiplatelet effects, but has been shown to be clinically ineffective by itself and of no additional benefit when combined with aspirin.[4]

Inhibitors of GP IIb-IIIa receptor binding to fibrinogen

Monoclonal antibodies or specific peptides that block the GP IIb-IIIa receptor binding of fibrinogen are very potent and broad in action because they block the final common pathway for platelet aggregation.[1,2] However it is likely that these agents will interfere with normal haemostasis because of their lack of selectivity. Their current human investigation is limited to acute thrombotic episodes (such as in acute myocardial infarction or unstable angina) because as they are peptides, oral administration is not feasible, their half-life is short and they are potentially immunogenic.

Antagonists of pro-aggregating stimuli

Thrombin is a powerful platelet activator and an important mediator of platelet-thrombus formation after vascular injury. Thus thrombin-induced platelet activation can be inhibited by heparin, an antithrombin III-dependent inhibitor, or by direct thrombin inhibitors such as hirudin (see Ch. 35). Ketanserin, a selective serotonin antagonist, prevents the proaggregating as well as vasoconstrictive effects of serotonin. It has been shown to exert some beneficial antithrombotic effects in animal models as well as humans.[1,2] Ticlopidine appears to inhibit ADP-induced platelet aggregation specifically, although its mode of action is not completely understood.[1,2] Platelet aggregation induced by thrombin, collagen, and TXA_2 are also inhibited by ticlopidine, but higher agonist concentrations may overcome these effects. Ticlopidine is a more potent antiplatelet agent than aspirin and it also does not impair prostacylin synthesis. Its onset of action is slow, and complete drug action is delayed for several days. After discontinuation the inhibition of platelet function may persist for 4–10 days.

Clinical indications for antiplatelet agents

The efficacy of antiplatelet agents, mainly aspirin, is now well established in patients at moderate to high risk of occlusive vascular disease. The following section summarizes the results of clinical trials of antiplatelet agents in different patient subsets (see Table 36.1). A more detailed overview including meta-analysis is provided by reports from the American Heart Association Special Working Group on Aspirin[5] and the Antiplatelet Trialists' Collaboration.[6]

Suspected or evolving myocardial infarction

The ISIS-2 trial, involving more than 17 000 patients, randomized patients to aspirin (162.5 mg/day), streptokinase, both or placebo within the first 24 hours (mean 5 hours) of suspected or evolving myocardial infarction (MI).[7] Compared to placebo, allocation to aspirin therapy for 1 month produced a highly significant 23% reduction in vascular death, 49% reduction in non-fatal reinfarction, and 46% reduction in non-fatal stroke. The reduction in deaths with aspirin was equivalent to that seen with streptokinase. Further, the benefit of aspirin was independent of streptokinase, and their combination was associated with a 49% reduction in vascular mortality. In absolute terms, aspirin treatment in acute myocardial infarction (AMI) could prevent 38 major vascular events (non-fatal infarction, stroke or death) per 1000 patients treated, with most benefit occurring in vascular deaths (24 prevented per 1000) (see Table 36.1).[6] It is important to note that the initiating dose of aspirin in ISIS-2 was 162.5 mg, chewed and swallowed for rapid absorption. There is no certainty that swallowing a low dose, for example a 75–100 mg tablet, especially if enteric-coated, will achieve the same benefit. Therefore treatment in AMI should be initiated with 150–325 mg aspirin, which if enteric-coated should be chewed before swallowing.

Patients with prior myocardial infarction

In 11 trials involving about 20 000 patients who survived a MI, aspirin treatment (300–1500 mg/day), with or without dipyridamole, produced an overall 25% reduction in the risk of a major vascular event after 2 years of treatment. In absolute terms, the treatment of 1000 patients with a history of MI will prevent 36 major vascular events, mainly non-fatal reinfarctions (18 prevented per 1000) and vascular deaths (13 prevented per 1000).[6]

Unstable angina or non-Q wave myocardial infarction

In seven trials involving about 4000 patients, aspirin treatment (75–1300 mg/day) given over 5 days to 1 year produced a 35% reduction in major vascular events.[6] The Swedish RISC trial in 796 men with unstable angina or non-Q wave MI was notable in showing that low-dose aspirin (75 mg/day) over 5 days reduced the risk of MI and death by 69% compared to placebo.[8] In absolute terms, aspirin treatment in 1000 patients could prevent 49 major vascular events, mostly non-fatal infarction.[6]

Medium risk patients with atherosclerotic vascular disease

Patients with stable angina, those who are post-coronary artery bypass grafting or coronary angioplasty, and those with peripheral vascular disease represent a medium risk group with an average annual mortality of 2–4%.[6] While sample size was not sufficiently large to test the efficacy of aspirin treatment in some of these clinical subsets, meta-analysis of 103 trials involving 22 000 patients (including patients with unstable angina) showed that antiplatelet therapy produced a highly significant 32% reduction in major vascular events (see Table 36.1).

In addition, aspirin treatment in patients undergoing vascular grafting or arterial angioplasty reduced the *early* risk of thrombotic graft or arterial occlusion by an average of 34%; a 6-month benefit of 93 occlusions prevented per 1000 treated.[9] Recent trials have also shown that lower aspirin doses (75–160 mg/day) are just as effective as higher doses in the prevention of vascular occlusion and cardiac events.[6,9] While aspirin has not been shown to reduce the incidence of coronary re-stenosis after angioplasty or late atherosclerotic graft occlusion, long-term aspirin therapy is still beneficial in preventing future vascular events in these patients.

Primary prevention

Table 36.1 Percent reductions in vascular events in trials of antiplatelet therapy among different patient risk groups: meta-analysis of 145 trials*

Category of trial	No. of trials	Percent odds reduction (SD)			Benefit per 1000 (SD) vascular events†
		Non-fatal MI	Non-fatal stroke	Vascular death	
Acute MI	9	54% (8) $2p<0.00001$	40% (17) $2p=0.02$	22% (4) $2p<0.00001$	38 (5)
Prior MI	11	31% (6) $2p<0.00001$	39% (11) $2p=0.0005$	15% (5) $2p<0.005$	36 (6)
Medium risk vascular disease‡	104	32% (7) $2p<0.0001$	46% (9) $2p<0.0001$	20% (7) $2p<0.001$	23 (4)
Prior stroke/TIA	18	36% (11) $2p=0.001$	23% (6) $2p<0.0005$	14% (7) $2p<0.05$	37 (8)
Low risk (primary prevention)	3	29% (8) $2p<0.0005$	–21% (13) NS	2% (10) NS	4 (3)

* From report of Antiplatelet Trialists' Collaboration. BMJ 1994; 308: 81–106.
Results are mean and standard deviation (SD). MI=myocardial infarction; TIA=transient ischaemic attack.
† Vascular events are non-fatal MI, stroke or vascular death.
‡ Medium risk vascular disease includes patients with unstable angina, post-coronary bypass grafting, post-angioplasty, stable angina, and peripheral vascular disease.

The case for aspirin in primary prevention is not yet proven. In the United States Physicians' Health Study of more than 22 000 male physicians, aged 40–84 years, those assigned to aspirin (325 mg every second day) had a significant 44% reduction in MI, a slight non-significant increase in haemorrhagic stroke (0.2% in the aspirin group versus 0.1% in the placebo group), and no difference in incidence of vascular deaths over 5 years compared to those on placebo.[5,6] In the British Doctors' trial of more than 5000 male physicians, aged 50–78 years, those assigned to aspirin (500 mg daily) compared to those instructed not to take aspirin (no placebo used) had no difference in the rate of MI and vascular death after 6 years, a slight non-significant increase in the rate of disabling stroke and a decrease in transient ischaemic attacks.[5,6]

When the trials are combined, there is a significant 29% reduction in non-fatal infarction but a non-significant 21% increase in non-fatal stroke. It should also be noted that the vascular mortality in these two primary prevention trials was only 2.0% over 5 years, and 1000 healthy subjects would need to be treated over 5 years to prevent four major cardiovascular events (see Table 36.1). Hence it is recommended that aspirin prophylaxis should only be considered in males over 40 years of age at high risk of MI.[5] The Thrombosis Prevention Trial is currently evaluating the effects of low-dose aspirin (75 mg daily) in asymptomatic men, aged 45–69 years, at high risk of coronary artery disease. Definitive recommendations for women will have to await the results of the Women's Health Study, a randomized trial of low-dose aspirin (100 mg second daily) in 40 000 nurses, aged 50 years or more, without a prior history of cardiovascular disease. Where aspirin is used to prevent MI, it should only be seen as adjunctive to the control of the patients' individual coronary risk factors.

Transient cerebral ischaemic attacks or ischaemic stroke

The efficacy of aspirin (50–1500 mg/day), alone and in combination with dipyridamole or sulphinpyrazone, has been studied in 18 trials including about 11 000 patients.[5,6] An overview of these trials suggests that antiplatelet therapy for about 3 years can significantly reduce the rate of major vascular events by an average of 22%. Thus treating 1000 patients with a history of cerebrovascular disease will prevent 37 vascular events, half of the events prevented being recurrent stroke and the other half being MI or vascular death.

Non-valvular atrial fibrillation

Warfarin is clearly effective for the prevention of strokes and thromboembolism in patients with non-valvular atrial fibrillation. Whether aspirin might also be useful was examined in two trials.[5] In the AFASAK trial, aspirin (75 mg daily) was associated with the same incidence of stroke as placebo treatment. In the SPAF study, aspirin (325 mg daily) significantly reduced the risk of stroke by 44% compared to placebo, but was not effective in patients more than 75 years old. Thus aspirin may have some stroke prevention benefit in younger patients with non-valvular atrial fibrillation unable to take warfarin.

Prevention of venous thrombosis and pulmonary embolism

A recent collaborative overview which pooled the results of antiplatelet therapy (mainly aspirin) involving over 8000 patients suggested that antiplatelet therapy could almost halve the risk of deep venous thrombosis and pulmonary embolism in high risk surgical and medical patients.[10] This is, in fact, similar to subcutaneous heparin, a proven form of thromboprophylaxis. However, aspirin should not be considered as standard therapy for this indication until the relative merits of antiplatelet, anticoagulant and combination therapy are tested in prospective randomized trials. One such Australasian trial (the Pulmonary Embolism Prevention Trial) is already in progress.

Dose of aspirin and side-effects

Gastrointestinal symptoms such as stomach pain, heartburn and nausea are the most common side-effects of aspirin and occur with increasing frequency with increasing doses. However, the reported incidence of these gastrointestinal symptoms in patients taking 75–300 mg/day of aspirin is often similar to those on placebo. A small but significant increase in gastrointestinal bleeding is observed with a dose of 75 mg/day; this risk is approximately doubled with a dose of 300 mg/day and increased fourfold with doses greater than 1200 mg/day.[3,5] Aspirin may also be associated with an increased incidence of haemorrhagic strokes. A positive trend was reported in the primary prevention trials and overall in the antiplatelet trials there was a non-significant 20% increase in haemorrhagic stroke. Importantly, though, its occurrence was very low (less than 0.3%), and in patients with atherosclerotic vascular disease, the potential benefits of aspirin against thromboembolic stroke far outweigh any possible increased risk of cerebral bleeding.[3,5]

Currently recommended doses of aspirin in cardiovascular disease are based on the knowledge that 75–100 mg daily is slightly in excess of the amount required to completely inhibit platelet thromboxane synthesis, and that higher doses (500–1500 mg/day) have not been shown to be more clinically effective than lower doses (75–325 mg/day) but are associated with more side-effects.[3,5,6] However, aspirin doses lower than 100 mg/day may take a few days to inhibit platelet thromboxane synthesis completely, and where immediate effect is desirable (such as in suspected heart attack), treatment should be initiated with a loading dose (150–325 mg), preferably of soluble aspirin dissolved in water before ingestion.[3,5]

Other antiplatelet agents

Despite demonstrated in vitro antiplatelet effects, neither sulphinpyrazone nor dipyridamole has been shown in clinical trials either to be an effective antithrombotic agent alone or to augment the effects of aspirin.[1,4] Ticlopidine has been found to be effective in patients with unstable angina and TIAs.[6] However ticlopidine is expensive and is associated with more major adverse reactions (diarrhoea, rash, neutropenia) than aspirin. A large randomized trial (CAPRIE) is ongoing which compares aspirin to clopidogrel, a related drug to ticlopidine, in patients with coronary, cerebrovascular and peripheral artery disease.

Abciximab, a c7E3, chimeric monoclonal antibody Fab fragment directed against GP IIb/IIIa receptor, was recently trialled (EPIC Investigators) as an adjunct to aspirin and heparin in patients undergoing high risk coronary angioplasty.[11] Patients randomized to abciximab had a statistically significant reduction in the primary composite endpoint (death, non-fatal AMI, or unplanned revascularization procedure) compared to placebo.[11] Subsequently, randomized trials of abciximab, in patients undergoing elective coronary angioplasty (EPILOG) and in patients scheduled for urgent angioplasty for refractory unstable angina (CAPTURE), were prematurely stopped because of a highly significant reduction in the primary composite endpoint of death, AMI, or need for urgent intervention in the group receiving abciximab.[12] While individual agents may differ in efficacy, these studies suggest that platelet GP IIb/IIIa receptor blockade is highly effective in reducing ischaemic and thrombotic complications in high-risk patients undergoing coronary interventions, although associated with an increased risk of major bleeding complications.[12]

Summary and recommendations

Aspirin is effective in a wide range of patients with occlusive vascular disease. It should be routinely recommended in nearly all patients with suspected, evolving or prior history of MI, those with stable or unstable angina, those undergoing coronary artery bypass surgery or coronary angioplasty, and those with stroke, TIA's or peripheral vascular disease. However, aspirin prophylaxis is *not* proven as yet for 'primary prevention' subjects at low risk of occlusive vascular events. In asymptomatic subjects with major coronary risk, aspirin may reduce the risk of MI, but the benefits of treatment must be carefully weighed against the potential side-effects. Low to medium dose aspirin (75–325 mg/day) is the most widely tested antiplatelet regimen, and no other regimen seems to be significantly more effective at preventing MI, stroke or death. However, thrombotic occlusions can still occur despite aspirin use and potentially more potent antiplatelet agents as well as combined antiplatelet and anticoagulant drug regimens need to be tested.

References

1. Stein B, Fuster V, Israel DH et al. Platelet inhibitor agents in cardiovascular disease: an update. J Am Coll Cardiol 1989; 14:813–36
2. Coller BS. Antiplatelet agents in the prevention and therapy of thrombosis. Annu Rev Med 1992; 43: 171–80
3. Patrono C. Aspirin as an antiplatelet drug. N Engl J Med 1994; 330: 1287–94
4. Fitzgerald GA. Dipyridamole. N Engl J Med 1987; 316: 1247–57
5. Fuster V, Dyken ML, Vokonas PS, Hennekens C. Aspirin as a therapeutic agent in cardiovascular disease. Circulation 1993; 87: 659–75
6. Antiplatelet Trialists' Collaboration. Collaborative overview of randomised trials of antiplatelet therapy (Pt I). Prevention of death, myocardial infarction, and stroke by prolonged antiplatelet therapy in various categories of patients. Br Med J 1994; 308: 81–106
7. ISIS-2. Second International Study of Infarct Survival Collaborative Group. Randomised trial of intravenous streptokinase, oral aspirin, both or neither among 17 187 cases of suspected acute myocardial infarction: ISIS-2. Lancet 1988; 2: 349–601
8. The RISC Group. Risk of myocardial infarction and death during treatment with low dose aspirin and intravenous heparin in men with unstable coronary artery disease. Lancet 1990; 336: 827–30
9. Antiplatelet Trialists' Collaboration. Collaborative overview of randomised trials of antiplatelet therapy (Pt II). Maintenance of vascular graft or arterial patency by antiplatelet therapy. BMJ 1994; 308: 159–68
10. Antiplatelet Trialists' Collaboration. Collaborative overview of randomised trials of antiplatelet therapy (Pt III). Reduction in venous thrombosis and pulmonary embolism by antiplatelet prophylaxis among surgical and medical patients. Br Med J 1994; 308: 235–46
11. The EPIC Investigators. Use of a monoclonal antibody directed against the platelet glycoprotein IIb/IIIa receptor in high-risk coronary angioplasty. N Engl J Med 1994; 330: 956–61.
12. Editorial. More evidence for the beneficial effect of platelet glycoprotein IIb/IIIa-blockade during coronary interventions. Latest results from the EPILOG and CAPTURE trials. Eur Heart J 1996; 17: 325–26
13. Ferguson JJ. EPILOG and CAPTURE trials halted because of positive interim results. Circulation 1996; 93: 637

37 Coumadins

Alexander S Gallus

The coumadins (typified by warfarin) are orally active anticoagulants with a venerable past: dicumarol entered clinical practice in 1941 and was in use by 1943 to treat myocardial infarction (MI). Warfarin was introduced soon after, in 1948, as the perfect rat poison.[1] Their long history is closely tied to the maturation of randomized clinical trials as a discipline and to better understanding of the blood clotting system. The study of their many and varied interactions with other drugs contributed greatly to the growth of clinical pharmacology.

There is a wide range of indications for oral anticoagulant therapy in cardiology, including its use to prevent systemic embolism after MI or in chronic heart failure, in atrial fibrillation, and in patients with prosthetic heart valves. The other major use for oral anticoagulant therapy is for the prevention and treatment of deep venous thrombosis and pulmonary embolism.

Using these drugs requires great care, since patients vary greatly in their dosage requirement and the penalties for incorrect treatment are severe: serious or fatal bleeding in the case of overdose and the underlying risk of thrombosis and embolism if the dose is too low.

Coronary care staff should therefore be very familiar with the indications for warfarin therapy, the practical aspects of treatment initiation and maintenance, and the management of overdose.

Oral anticoagulants in acute myocardial infarction

Thromboembolic complications relevant to MI include deep venous thrombosis (DVT), pulmonary embolism (PE), systemic embolism originating from intracardiac thrombosis triggered by transmural infarction, heart failure and/or atrial fibrillation (AF), coronary artery re-occlusion after initially successful thrombolytic therapy or angioplasty, and infarct extension or recurrence due to further coronary artery thrombosis.

Because these can all be prevented to some extent by antithrombotic treatment, as can the progression of unstable angina to MI, it is important for clinicians to decide, after reading the relevant clinical trials, about the likely relative benefits and hazards of heparin, warfarin and aspirin, given alone or in combination.

Preventing venous thrombosis and pulmonary embolism after MI

Risk factors for the onset of DVT or PE after MI include extensive MI, heart failure, prolonged bed-rest, and increasing age over the age of 50 years. In most people, the risk subsides with clinical recovery and is adequately dealt with by giving low doses of heparin (5000 i.u., subcutaneously, 8-hourly or 12-hourly) during the hospital stay.

Longer-term warfarin treatment targeting an INR (International Normalized Ratio) of 2.0–3.0 becomes appropriate in the presence of treatment-resistant heart failure, when it also serves to protect from mural thrombus formation and systemic embolism. All clinical trials of short- or long-term oral anticoagulant therapy after MI have consistently shown they can diminish the risk of developing DVT, PE and systemic embolism.[2]

Preventing systemic embolism after MI

70% of symptomatic systemic emboli cause stroke, often with significant residual disability, and 60% of strokes are embolic.[3] In population-based studies, almost 25% of people with a first ischaemic stroke have a potential cardiac source of embolism, and this is previous MI in nearly one quarter and atrial fibrillation in almost one half.[4]

In the absence of prophylaxis, 2–6% of people with anterior MI suffer a stroke within 28 days.[2,5] The cause is intracardiac thrombus formation, which is found at routine echocardiography in 20–40% of patients with anterior MI and especially when there is apical akinesis or dyskinesis, but only rarely after inferior MI. In one recent large but retrospective series, however, the risk of embolism was similar after anterior and after non-anterior MI.[6] Other risk factors are heart failure and atrial fibrillation.

Mural thrombosis within the first 10 days after MI can be prevented by high doses of subcutaneous heparin (12 500 i.u. 12-hourly, with indirect evidence that upward dose adjustment to prolong the activated partial thromboplastin time may increase efficacy).[7]

With regard to stroke after MI, an extensive overview shows that oral anticoagulants reduced this risk in seven of nine evaluations, mostly non-randomized, with a combined odds ratio of 0.46 for all studies (95% confidence interval = 0.30–0.64) and similar results in the two randomized trials.[8]

Most systemic embolism develops within 3 months of MI, although the greatest risk is in the first 10 days,[9] and the American Heart Association recommends routine warfarin therapy for 3 months after Q wave anterior MI.[2,5]

The combined risk of DVT, PE and arterial embolism in people with a large infarct, hypokinetic heart, and chronically resistant heart failure is sufficiently high to warrant long-term warfarin unless there is a strong contra-indication.[10]

Preventing a second systemic embolism after MI

Once MI has been complicated by systemic embolism, then initial heparin therapy should be followed by warfarin for a minimum of 3 months, or longer if there is continuing cardiac dysfunction.

Preventing coronary artery re-occlusion after successful thrombolytic therapy and/or angioplasty following MI

Aspirin and high dose IV heparin are both given to prevent early coronary artery re-occlusion after thrombolytic therapy and/or percutaneous transluminal coronary angioplasty (PTCA) following MI. Aspirin is then given after hospital discharge (as after any MI), but it remains uncertain how long-term warfarin therapy compares.

There is no good direct evidence, but extrapolation from trials of antithrombotic treatment after coronary artery bypass grafting (CABG) suggests the effects of warfarin and antiplatelet drugs may be similar. In one medium-sized trial, 2 months of warfarin improved graft patency from 85 to 90% ($p < 0.015$) but increased the bleeding risk when compared with aspirin plus dipyridamole; see review by Stein.[11] In a much larger trial, the patency rates for distal anastomoses were similar 1 year after CABG, regardless of treatment with warfarin, aspirin, or aspirin plus dipyridamole.[12] Five months of warfarin therapy in a small study failed to prevent late re-stenosis after PTCA.[11] Given this limited data, it is hard to support the use of warfarin for this purpose.

Preventing reinfarction with warfarin after MI

Opinion about the value of oral anticoagulants for preventing further coronary artery occlusion in people with MI has swung wildly over the years and is still greatly divided, although the balance of evidence now suggests a modest and clear-cut decrease in non-fatal reinfarction, but a much smaller effect on total mortality.

Oral anticoagulants were standard therapy after MI until the late 1950s, because the early, pioneering, large-scale evaluations found they prevented reinfarction and reduced mortality. But this indication was largely abandoned after later trials gave much less impressive results. Indeed, in a mordant overview (and one of the first for general readers to focus on clinical trial methodology) Gifford and Feinstein[13] found they performed well only when clinical trial design was poor.

And yet the issue would not die. It was pointed out that even 80% effectiveness in preventing thromboembolic deaths would have little impact on total post-infarct mortality, requiring much larger trials to demonstrate a benefit than any yet attempted.[14] By corollary, the sample size of existing trials was far too small to exclude even an important decrease of 20% in total mortality.[15]

Indeed, an early attempt at pooling the results in a total of 2500 patients, entered in nine controlled trials, had already suggested in 1970 that long-term oral anticoagulant therapy reduced mortality after MI in men by about 20%,[16] a deduction later supported by a more formal meta-analysis.[17] However, the radical changes in medical care and clinical outcomes during the decades between the first and last of these pooled studies, including the introduction of powerful diuretics, CCUs and the routine use of thrombolytics, aspirin and beta blockers after MI, make such meta-analyses largely irrelevant to modern clinical practice.[18,19]

For a long time, the field was also clouded by large variations in dosing regimens due to lack of any uniform measure of anticoagulant effect. This has now been largely overcome by widespread use of a standard method: the International Normalized Ratio (INR).

Early enthusiasm for coumadins after MI rapidly and almost completely dissipated in North America, the UK, Australia and New Zealand, but this indication was never abandoned in parts of Europe, and especially in Holland and Scandinavia,[20,23] where two large-scale double-blind, randomized and placebo-controlled clinical trials, the Dutch 'Sixty Plus' Reinfarction Study[24] and the Oslo based 'Warfarin Re-Infarction Study'[25] have reopened the case.

In the Dutch trial, 878 patients aged over 60 years, and previously treated with an oral anticoagulant for an average of 6 years after their index MI, were followed for another 2 years after random allocation to continued coumadin therapy or a change to placebo. The change to placebo treatment was followed by more recurrences of MI (15.9 versus 5.7%; p = 0.0001) and a higher cardiac mortality (13.4 versus 7.6%; p = 0.017). The targeted oral anticoagulant effect was a 'thrombotest' activity of 5–10% (corresponding to an INR of 2.7–4.5).[24]

A detailed response by Mitchell[26] highlighted the dilution of the measured effect on mortality when the 32% of patients with 'protocol deviation' who were excluded from the primary analysis were added back (placebo mortality now = 15.7%, anticoagulant mortality = 11.6%; p = 0.071; recurrent MI after placebo now = 14.6% and after anticoagulants = 6.6%, p = 0.005), and the fact that 'protocol deviants' were followed less carefully than those still taking trial drugs, making the diagnosis of recurrence after 'protocol deviation' suspect. The patients were highly selected, since they had already been taking an oral anticoagulant for some years after their MI, so that bleeding risk may have been atypically low; even so, coumadins caused a large excess of major bleeding events (27 patients versus three).

In the larger and prospective Oslo study of 1214 patients randomized an average of 27 days after MI and followed for an average of 37 months, warfarin therapy targeting an INR of 2.8–4.8 reduced total mortality from 20.3 to 15.5% (a risk reduction, or RR, of 24%; p = 0.027), non-fatal reinfarction from 20.4 to 13.5% (RR 34%; p = 0.0007), and cerebrovascular events from 7.3 to 3.3% (RR 55%; p = 0.0015).[25]

This was an 'intent to treat' analysis, where events were counted regardless of whether patients were still taking trial drugs or had discontinued them because of an end-point or side-effect. Major bleeding was rare (0.6% per annum) despite the high target INR. 182 of 1918 eligible patients (9.5%) were excluded because of bleeding risk.[25]

By contrast, there was a minimal effect on long-term mortality by oral anticoagulants in the recently published double-blind and randomized, multicentre 'ASPECT' study (again from Holland) where 3404 patients who entered the trial within 6 weeks of leaving hospital after MI were followed during an average 3 years of treatment with placebo or an oral anticoagulant.[27]

Active treatment aiming for an INR of 2.8–4.8 significantly reduced the incidence of non-fatal MI (hazard ratio = 0.47) and cerebrovascular events (hazard ratio = 0.60), but had a marginal impact on mortality (hazard ratio = 0.90; 95% confidence interval = 0.73–1.11). The penalty was an increase in the risk of major bleeding from 0.2 to 1.5 per hundred patient years.

A major hurdle to extrapolating from these results to standard clinical care is that aspirin was prohibited in all trials, there was no aspirin-treated comparison group, and the first two trials were done before thrombolytic therapy became routine. As a result it is best to wait for evidence from further studies before choosing warfarin over aspirin for routine secondary prevention after MI.

Atrial fibrillation

The importance of AF as a risk factor for stroke is well known, but in the past it was thought the risk of systemic embolism was too low, and the risk of bleeding too high, to justify long-term preventive warfarin therapy except when AF is combined with valvular heart disease or has already led to systemic embolism.

Five prospective, randomized, multicentre trials in people with AF, but without valvular heart disease and without a history of systemic embolism, have now generated entirely consistent results: in each case warfarin significantly prevented embolism without causing undue bleeding (see Table 37.1, from Laupacis[28] and Albers[29]).

Pooling of data from these trials by the investigators confirmed that warfarin reduced the risk of stroke across all trials by 68%, and this effect was consistent across all studies and subgroups of patient, including women. An equally valuable application of pooling was to identify risk factors for systemic embolism. These were increasing age, and a history of hypertension, diabetes, transient cerebral ischaemia, or stroke. In patients aged less than 65 years without risk factors (15% of all patients) the annual stroke rate was only 1%.[30]

Extrapolating these trial results to the population at large remains uncertain. Early stopping rules may have led to over-estimates of therapeutic benefit,[31] up to 93% of patients were excluded because of bleeding risk, the likelihood of poor compliance, and other reasons, and dose monitoring was more meticulous than might be expected in community practice.

A crucial question is the relative value of warfarin and aspirin. These were compared directly in two trials: AFASAK, where the risk reduction of 18% with aspirin was small and well short of that seen with warfarin; and SPAF I, where the risk reduction of 44% was more impressive (the pooled risk reduction derived from the two trials was 36% for aspirin, compared with 68% for warfarin).[28,20]

SPAF II, an extension of SPAF I, has brought some clarity: SPAF II compared warfarin (target INR of 2.0–4.5) with 325 mg/day aspirin in 715 patients aged 75 years or less and followed for 3 years, and in 385 patients aged over 75 years and followed for 2 years. Warfarin was slightly more effective than aspirin but caused more intracranial bleeding (especially in those aged over 75 years). In addition, aspirin-treated patients without hypertension, recent heart failure, or previous embolism had a very low rate of stroke and visceral embolism (0.5% per annum). It

Table 37.1 Primary endpoint events (% per annum) in oral anticoagulant trials in AF. Modified from Laupacis A et al 1992[28] and Albers GW 1994.[29]

Trial	Target INR	Patients	Mean follow-up	Warfarin (% p.a.)	Aspirin (% p.a.)	Placebo or control (% p.a.)
SPAF I	2.0–4.5	1330	1.3 yrs	2.3	3.6	7.4 6.3
SPAF II	2.0–4.5					
age ≤ 75		715	3.1 years	1.3	1.9	
age > 75		385	2.0 yrs	3.6	4.8	
AFASAK	2.8–4.2	1007	1.2 yrs	2.0	5.5	5.5
CAFA	2.0–3.0	383	1.3 yrs	3.5		5.3
BAATAF	1.5–2.7	420	2.2 yrs	0.4		3.0
SPINAF	1.4–2.8	525	1,8 yrs	0.9		4.3
EAFT	2.5–4.0	1007	2.3 yrs	8.0	15.0	17.0 19.0

All except EAFT enrolled patients without previous systemic embolism. To qualify for EAFT, patients with chronic or paroxysmal non-rheumatic AF were required to have had TIA or a minor ischaemic stroke within the past three months.

should be noted, however, that target INR in SPAF II was much higher than in two of the trials where warfarin was effective, that bleeding risk increases with increasing INR, and that many strokes in the warfarin group occurred in patients not taking warfarin at the time.[32]

Aspirin may be the drug of choice in people with AF and a low clinical risk of systemic embolism or a contraindication to warfarin, while warfarin is more appropriate for those at high risk.[32] What is quite definite, however, is that warfarin (INR = 2.5–4.0) is clearly superior to aspirin when people with AF have already suffered an embolic stroke or TIA. Not only is the risk of recurrence very high in this setting (see Table 37.1) but the risk of another stroke during warfarin therapy is about 60% below that seen with aspirin.[33]

The American College of Physicians recommends warfarin at a relatively low dose (target INR = 2.0–3.0) as the drug of choice in patients aged over 60 years with non-valvular atrial fibrillation, and recommends aspirin for people unwilling or unable to take warfarin.[34,35]

Warfarin and cardioversion

Cardioversion for AF can trigger systemic embolism, and retrospective studies suggest that warfarin should be used to prevent this. Preformed thrombi take some weeks to stabilize, and there is indirect evidence that the risk of embolism persists for some weeks after the intervention, so that prophylaxis should be started 3 weeks before and continued for 4 weeks after elective cardioversion.[28]

Unstable angina

Standard antithrombotic therapy for unstable angina consists of aspirin, heparin, or both.[5]

In a recent open, randomized, multicentre trial in 214 patients admitted to hospital with unstable angina or non-Q wave MI, the addition of heparin to aspirin in hospital followed by 3 months of warfarin plus aspirin gave better results than aspirin alone: combined therapy reduced ischaemic events at 14 days from 27 to 10.5% ($p = 0.004$) and at 12 weeks from 25 to 13% ($p = 0.06$), while major bleeding was increased from 0 to 2.9%.[36]

Warfarin

Warfarin interferes with blood coagulation by blocking the effect of vitamin K at a late step in the hepatic synthesis of the blood clotting factors II, VII, IX and X and of the 'natural anticoagulants', protein C and protein S: the γ-carboxylation of 10 or more glutamic acid residues. Without this modification, these proteins cannot bind calcium and cannot bind to phospholipid surfaces, and therefore take no part in blood coagulation.

The active hydroquinone form of vitamin K (vitamin KH_2) is an essential cofactor for γ-carboxylation, and is oxidized to form the inactive vitamin K_1 epoxide which must be cycled back through vitamin K to vitamin KH_2. Warfarin blocks the cycle by inhibiting vitamin K epoxide reductase.[2]

Warfarin is well absorbed after oral administration. Blood levels in healthy volunteers peak after about 90 minutes, the drug is bound to plasma proteins, and is cleared from the circulation with a half-life of 36–42 hours.

Both the pharmacokinetics and pharmacodynamics of oral anticoagulants vary widely and unpredictably between individuals, so that dosage is adjusted to maintain the anticoagulant effect within a recommended 'target range'. The most widely used measure is the prothrombin time (PT) ratio, which is derived by dividing the patient's PT by that of normal plasma. This is standardized by conversion to an International Normalized Ratio, or INR. Since the PT ratio reflects a balance between the synthesis and clearance of vitamin K-dependent clotting factors, the full effect of starting or changing warfarin therapy will always be delayed for several days.

Warfarin dose

Warfarin treatment is usually begun with 10 mg (5 mg/day when there is no urgency to reach a therapeutic effect, as in chronic atrial fibrillation without embolism, or when a reduced dose requirement is probable, as in the frail elderly and in severe heart failure) and further doses are titrated against each day's PT ratio. Dose-initiation algorithms take some of the guess-work from dose-adjustment and are no less successful than trainee clinicians in a teaching hospital.[37]

When treating an acute thromboembolic event, warfarin is given with heparin until the INR has exceeded its targeted minimum (usually 2.0) for 2–3 consecutive days. The INR is measured daily until heparin is stopped, and then 2–3 times per week for a further 1–2 weeks.

Once the daily maintenance dose is known (this normally averages about 4.5 mg/day but can be as little as 0.5 mg/day or as much as 15 mg/day) there are many people on long-term therapy whose PT ratio needs to be measured no more often than once in 4–5 weeks.

An absolute prerequisite for safe warfarin treatment is educating the patient to a full understanding of the process and its risks and benefits so that they become partners in management (see Ch. 76). A complete record of warfarin dose and INR effect kept by the patient is an important document that helps to prevent dangerous misunderstandings that can develop between managing doctors and between doctors and the patient.

Target INR

The recommended target range for warfarin therapy has changed over the years. At one stage, it was believed that a target INR of 2.0–3.0 was sufficient for preventing or treating venous thrombosis and pulmonary embolism, but that a higher target range was required to prevent systemic embolism and artery thrombosis.

The presently recommended target INR is 2.0–3.0 for all indications except for prosthetic heart valves, where the target range is 2.5–3.5 (or higher if there has been systemic embolism). Lack of evidence prohibits a solid recommendation about warfarin therapy to prevent coronary artery occlusion, although the target range in the relevant clinical trials was high (about 2.7–4.5).[38] A target range of 1.5–2.7 was effective in two of the atrial fibrillation studies. When aiming for these lower levels of target INR it is important to recognize the need for strict quality control of dose monitoring.

There is great variation between clinics in their ability to maintain patients within the target range of INR. In one comparison, 20% of results in one clinic, and 40% of results in another, were subtherapeutic.[39] Likely reasons include disparities in laboratory methods, the interval between clinic visits, patient education and communication, and compliance.

Warfarin dose adjustment

When adjusting warfarin dose up or down, it is important to remember that the INR response will be delayed for several days, and that small changes in warfarin dose can have a large effect on INR. It is therefore best to adjust in small increments and at intervals of several days. The alternative is wild swings in dose and effect. It also helps to use clinical judgment. If the dose and INR have been stable for some time, then it is often sensible to delay responding to small and unexplained variations from the target range until they have been confirmed by a repeat measurement some days later.

Duration of therapy

This is determined by clinical circumstance. If the intent is to prevent systemic embolism after MI, then 3 months is probably sufficient except when the risk factors for embolism remain. Other, ongoing indications (AF, resistant heart failure) require long-term therapy.

Interactions with other drugs

Oral anticoagulants are notorious for the number and variety of their interactions with other drugs.[40] A few drugs have been shown not to interact with warfarin. Others predictably increase or decrease the anticoagulant effect. Often information is incomplete, so that for most drugs it is best to assume an interaction is possible when they are introduced or withdrawn. This means weekly measurement of INR until it is seen to remain stable. Some commonly interacting drugs and their mechanism of action are shown in Table 37.2, modified from Hirsh and Fuster.[2]

Bleeding risk

Bleeding risk increases with INR, and especially once INR exceeds 4.0. An INR over 4.0 is the major risk factor for intracranial haemorrhage.[41] Other important risk factors include age over 70 years, female gender, and the presence of serious disease (cerebrovascular, kidney, heart and liver). Old age carries a lower warfarin requirement,[42] although, after allowing for co-morbidity, age in itself may not be a major risk factor for bleeding.[43] Investigation reveals an underlying lesion responsible for gastrointestinal or urinary bleeding in about one third of cases.[44–46] In one report, 83% of 52 patients having endoscopy for severe acute gastrointestinal bleeding while taking warfarin had a visible bleeding site.[47]

Table 37.2 Factors that alter the anticoagulant response to warfarin. Modified from Hirsh J, Fuster F 1994.[2]

Warfarin effect	Mechanism	Drugs or other source
Antagonize	Reduced warfarin absorption	cholestyramine
	Increased warfarin metabolism	barbiturates, rifampicin, carbamazepine
	Unknown	nafcillin
	Reduced anticoagulant effect	increased vitamin K intake (greens, nutritional supplements)
Potentiate	Inhibit warfarin metabolism	phenylbutazone, sulphinpyrazone, disulfiram, metronidazole, trimethoprim-sulphamethoxazole, cimetidine, amiodarone
	Pharmacodynamic effect (no effect on blood warfarin level)	clofibrate, heparin, second and third generation cephalosporins
	Unknown	erythromycin, anabolic steroids, ketoconazole, isoniazid, fluconazole, piroxicam, tamoxifen, quinidine, megadose vitamin E, phenytoin
	Increased anticoagulant effect	low vitamin K intake, reduced vitamin K absorption, liver disease, hypermetabolic states (e.g. fever)
Increased bleeding risk	Antiplatelet effect	aspirin and other NSAIDs, ticlopidine, carbenicillin and very high doses of other penicillins, moxalactam
	Gastric erosions	aspirin and other NSAIDs
No interaction		benzodiazepines, wine (small to moderate amounts)

NSAIDs = non-steroidal anti-inflammatory drugs

Non-bleeding side-effects

Warfarin, apart from the risk of bleeding, is remarkably safe. Occasional patients develop a fine, morbilliform skin rash, or complain of minor hair loss, but by far the most feared unusual complication is skin necrosis.[48] This extremely rare but potentially catastrophic event occurs in the first days of warfarin treatment and consists of the rapid spread of purple, painful, punched out, necrotic skin lesions affecting the fatty parts of the body (breasts, buttocks, abdomen, thighs). Skin biopsy shows thrombotic occlusion of small vessels. The cause is unknown, although it has been held to be at least partly triggered by the rapid fall in protein C level that follows the start of warfarin therapy. This comes with the fall in factor VII but precedes the decrease in clotting factors II, IX and X, perhaps causing a temporary 'hypercoagulable' state. This is one good reason to start treatment with a lower warfarin dose when there is no hurry and in the absence of heparin. In a poorly defined proportion of cases, there is an underlying deficiency of protein C or S.

Management is to stop warfarin, give heparin, and infuse fresh frozen plasma to replace protein C.

Reversing the anticoagulant effect

The warfarin effect can be reversed, depending on urgency, by stopping therapy, by giving vitamin K, and/or clotting factor infusion. When there is an excessive INR without bleeding, then the usual response is to stop warfarin with or without the addition of vitamin K. Stopping warfarin is followed by return of the INR towards normal over several days. 10–15 mg of vitamin K has an impact on the INR by 6 hours, but then makes people resistant to further warfarin therapy for several days. The INR will diminish in about 8 hours and may normalize within 24 hours after a smaller IV dose (0.5–2 mg) without interfering with continued warfarin therapy at a lower dose. Vitamin K is given when the INR is high enough to cause concern about spontaneous bleeding, but this level is a matter for individual judgment (one recommendation is to withhold warfarin if the INR is below 6, but add vitamin K if it reaches 6–10).[38] Clotting factor replacement is added if the patient is bleeding or the INR exceeds 8–10.

Vitamin K can be given orally, subcutaneously (sc) or intravenously (IV) but should not be given intramuscularly as the prolonged INR may result in local haematoma and poor absorption. Oral vitamin K is well absorbed in the absence of bowel disturbance or obstructive jaundice. Results are more predictable with IV than sc injection, but IV injection is, on rare occasions, followed by severe hypotension and cardiovascular collapse due to a massive and precipitous shift of fluid out of the circulation.

Response to bleeding

Bleeding during warfarin therapy may be spontaneous and induced by an excessive anticoagulant effect. When bleeding accompanies surgery or accidental injury, or complicates a pre-existing gastrointestinal or urogenital lesion, then it is aggravated by any level of anticoagulant effect, even one within the 'therapeutic range'.

Minor bleeding can often be managed with observation and a small decrease in INR. Major bleeding requires fresh frozen plasma and IV vitamin K. Prothrombin concentrate (containing factors II, IX and X) can be given with fresh frozen plasma but has, in the past, contained activated clotting factors capable of triggering thrombosis, especially in people with liver dysfunction, and should therefore still be used with caution.

Warfarin and pregnancy

Women of child-bearing age given warfarin must be strongly counselled against becoming pregnant while taking the drug. It is teratogenic during the sixth to twelfth weeks of gestation, and there have also been effects on development outside this timeframe.[49] Oral contraceptives are not contraindicated during warfarin therapy.

Future directions

Oral anticoagulants have been with us for 50 years, a very long time in modern therapeutics, and seem destined to remain with us for longer yet. They are cheap, well-absorbed, effective, and relatively safe when used with care. Despite their obvious disadvantages—the delayed onset of action, variable anticoagulant response, multiple drug interactions and bleeding risk—there is no obvious substitute. There are, however, two new lines of investigation: exploring the effects of very low doses of warfarin, and evaluating the combination of warfarin with aspirin.

'Mini-dose' warfarin, where 1–2 mg is given each day to marginally prolong the prothrombin time,[50] appears to prevent local thrombus formation after central venous catheter placement for cancer chemotherapy[51] and venous thromboembolism in patients given combination chemotherapy for metastatic breast cancer.[52] Raised factor VII activity is a strong risk factor for coronary artery disease (stronger, in some reports, than serum cholesterol level and on a par with fibrinogen concentration),[53] and is reduced by mini-dose warfarin, which is now undergoing clinical trial for the primary prevention of MI, both alone and combined with a small dose of aspirin.[54]

Warfarin has long been said to contraindicate aspirin treatment, but recent trials suggest that combined treatment may have advantages. In people with a prosthetic heart valve, the risk of systemic embolism is significantly reduced by the addition of enteric coated aspirin (100 mg/day) to standard dose warfarin (INR = 3.0–4.5). Minor bleeding is increased (as in other, similar trials) but the hazard from major bleeding is acceptable.[55] Aspirin alone is ineffective in this situation.

Whether there is any gain from the addition of 'mini-dose' warfarin to aspirin or another antiplatelet drug after MI or in atrial fibrillation is completely unknown and awaits the result of clinical trials.

New orally active anticoagulants, including orally active antithrombins, are under development but remain far from clinical use.

References

1. Mueller RL, Scheidt S. History of drugs for thrombotic disease. Discovery, development and directions for the future. Circulation 1994; 89: 432–491
2. Hirsh J, Fuster F. Guide to anticoagulant therapy (Pt 2). Oral anticoagulants. Circulation 1994; 89: 1469–80
3. Kistler JP. The risk of embolic stroke. Another piece of the

puzzle. N Engl J Med 1994; 331: 1517–9
4. Bogousslavsky J, Cachin C, Regli F, Despland P-A, Van Melle G, Kappenberger L. Cardiac sources of embolism and cerebral infarction—clinical consequences and vascular concomitants: the Lausanne Stroke registry. Neurology 1991; 41: 855–9
5. Cairns JA, Hirsh J, Lewis HDJ, Resnekov L, Theroux P. Antithrombotic agents in coronary artery disease. Chest 1992; 102: 456S–81S
6. Bodenheimer MM, Sauer D, Shareef B, Brown MW, Fleiss JL, Moss AJ. Relation between myocardial infarct location and stroke. J Am Coll Cardiol 1994; 24: 61–6
7. Turpie AGG, Robinson JG, Doyle DJ, Mulji AS, Mishkel GJ, Sealey BJ et al. Comparison of high-dose with low-dose subcutaneous heparin to prevent left ventricular mural thrombosis in patients with acute transmural anterior myocardial infarction. N Engl J Med 1989; 320: 352–7
8. Vaitkus PT, Berlin JA, Schwartz JS, Barbathan ES. Stroke complicating acute myocardial infarction. A meta-analysis of risk modification by anticoagulation and thrombolytic therapy. Arch Intern Med 1992; 152: 2020–4
9. Fuster V, Halperin JL. Left ventricular thrombi and cerebral embolism. N Engl J Med 1989; 320: 392–4
10. American College of Cardiology/American Heart Association Task Force. ACC/AHA guidelines for the early management of patients with acute myocardial infarction. Circulation 1990; 82: 664–707
11. Stein PD, Dalen JE, Goldman S, Schwartz L, Turpie AGG. Antithrombotic therapy in patients with saphenous vein and internal mammary artery bypass grafts following percutaneous transluminal coronary angioplasty. Chest 1992; 102: 508S–15S
12. CABADAS Research Group. Prevention of one-year vein-graft occlusion after aortocoronary-bypass surgery: a comparison of low-dose aspirin, low-dose aspirin plus dipyridamole, and oral anticoagulants. Lancet 1993; 342: 257–64
13. Gifford RH, Feinstein AR. A critique of methodology in studies of anticoagulant therapy for acute myocardial infarction. N Engl J Med 1969; 280: 351–7
14. Wessler S. Antithrombotic agents are indicated in the therapy of acute myocardial infarction. Cardiovascular Clinics 1977; 8: 131–8
15. Chalmers TC, Matta RJ, Smith HJ, Kunzler A-M. Evidence favoring the use of anticoagulants in the hospital phase of acute myocardial infarction. N Engl J Med 1977; 297: 1091–6
16. International Anticoagulant Review Group. Collaborative analysis of long-term anticoagulant administration after myocardial infarction. Lancet 1970; 1: 203–9
17. Leizorovicz A, Boissel JP. Oral anticoagulants in patients surviving myocardial infarction. A new approach to old data. European Journal of Clinical Pharmacology 1983; 24: 333–6
18. Goldman L, Feinstein AR. Anticoagulants and myocardial infarction. The problems of pooling, drowning, and floating. Ann Intern Med 1979; 90: 92–4
19. Selzer A. Use of anticoagulant agents in acute myocardial infarction: statistics or clinical judgment? Am J Cardiol 1978; 41: 1315–7
20. Rogel S, Bassan MM. Anticoagulants in ischemic heart disease. Arch Intern Med 1976; 136: 1229–30
21. Dalen JE, Goldberg RJ, Gore JM, Struckus J. Therapeutic interventions in acute myocardial infarction. Survey of the ACCP section on clinical cardiology. Chest 1984; 86: 257–62
22. Goldberg RJ, Gore JM, Dalen JE. The role of anticoagulant therapy in acute myocardial infarction. Am Heart J 1984; 108: 1387–93
23. Goldberg RJ, Gore JM, Dalen JE, Alpert JS. Long-term anticoagulant therapy after acute myocardial infarction. Am Heart J 1985; 109: 616–22
24. The Sixty Plus Reinfarction Study Research Group. A double-blind trial to assess long-term oral anticoagulant therapy in elderly patients after myocardial infarction. Lancet 1980; 2: 989–94
25. Smith P, Arnesen H, Holme I. The effect of warfarin on mortality and reinfarction after myocardial infarction. N Engl J Med 1990; 323: 147–52
26. Mitchell JRA. Anticoagulants in coronary heart disease—retrospect and prospect. Lancet 1981; 1: 257–62
27. ASPECT Research Group. Effect of long-term oral anticoagulant treatment on mortality and cardiovascular morbidity after myocardial infarction. Lancet 1994; 343: 499–503
28. Laupacis A, Albers G, Dunn MI, Feinberg WM. Antithrombotic therapy in atrial fibrillation. Chest 1992; 102: 426S–33S
29. Albers GW. Atrial fibrillation and stroke. Three new studies, three remaining questions. Arch Intern Med 1994; 154: 1443–8
30. Atrial Fibrillation Investigators. Risk factors for stroke and efficacy of antithrombotic therapy in atrial fibrillation. Analysis of pooled data from five randomized controlled trials. Arch Intern Med 1994; 154: 1449–57
31. Singer DE. Problems with stopping rules in trials of risky therapies: the case of warfarin to prevent stroke in atrial fibrillation. Clin Research 1993; 2: 482–6
32. Stroke Prevention in Atrial Fibrillation Investigators. Warfarin versus aspirin for pre-

vention of thromboembolism in atrial fibrillation: Stroke Prevention in Atrial Fibrillation II Study. Lancet 1994; 343: 687–91
33. EAFT (European Atrial Fibrillation Trial) Study Group. Secondary prevention in non-rheumatic atrial fibrillation after transient ischaemic attack or minor stroke. Lancet 1993; 342: 1255–62
34. Matchar DB, McCrory DC, Barnett HJM, Feussner JR. Medical treatment for stroke prevention. Ann Intern Med 1994; 121: 41–53
35. American College of Physicians. Guidelines for medical treatment for stroke prevention. Ann Intern Med 1994; 121: 54–5
36. Cohen M, Adams PC, Parry G, Xiong J, Chamberlain D, Wieczorek I et al. Combination antithrombotic therapy in unstable rest angina and non-Q-wave infarction in nonprior aspirin users. Primary end points analysis from the ATACS trial. Circulation 1994; 89: 81–8
37. Doecke CJ, Cosh DG, Gallus AS. Standardised initial warfarin treatment: evaluation of initial treatment response and maintenance dose prediction by randomised trial, and risk factors for an excessive warfarin response. Aust NZ J Med 1991; 21: 319–24
38. Hirsh J, Dalen JE, Deykin D, Poller L. Oral anticoagulants; mechanism of action, clinical effectiveness, and optimal therapeutic range. Chest 1992; 102: 312S–26S
39. Saour J, Gallus AS. Warfarin: is it time to reduce target ranges again? Aust NZ J Med 1993; 23: 692–6
40. Wells PS, Holbrook AM, Crowther NR, Hirsh J. Interactions of warfarin with drugs and food. Ann Intern Med 1994; 121: 676–83
41. Hylek EM, Singer DE. Risk factors for intracranial hemorrhage in outpatients taking warfarin. Ann Intern Med 1994; 120: 897–902
42. Isaacs C, Paltiel O, Blake G, Beaudet M, Conochie L, Leclerc J. Age-associated risks of prophylactic anticoagulation in the setting of hip fracture. Am J Med 1994; 96: 487–91
43. Fihn SD, McDonnell M, Martin D, Henikoff J, Vermes D, Kent D et al. Risk factors for complications of chronic anticoagulation. Ann Intern Med 1993; 118: 511–20
44. Levine MN, Hirsh J, Landefeld S, Raskob G. Hemorrhagic complications of anticoagulant therapy. Chest 1992; 102: 352S–63S
45. van der Meer FJM, Rosendaal FR, Vandenbroucke JP, Briet E. Bleeding complications in oral anticoagulant therapy. An analysis of risk factors. Arch Int Med 1993; 153: 1557–62
46. Landefeld CS, Beyth RC. Anticoagulant-related bleeding: clinical epidemiology, prediction, and prevention. Am J Med 1993; 95: 315–328
47. Choudari CP, Rajgopal C, Palmer CK. Acute gastrointestinal haemorrhage in anticoagulated patients: diagnosis and response to endoscopic treatment. Gut 1994; 35: 464–6
48. Colman RW, Rao AK, Rubin RN. Warfarin skin necrosis in a 33-year-old woman. Am J Hematology 1993; 43: 300–3
49. de Vries TW, van der Veer E, Heijmans HSA. Warfarin embryopathy: patient, possibility, pathogenesis and prognosis. Br J Ob Gyna 1993; 100: 869–71
50. Poller L, McKernan A, Thomson JM, Elstein M, Hirsch PJ, Jones JB. Fixed minidose warfarin: a new approach to prophylaxis against venous thrombosis after major surgery. Br Med J 1987; 295: 1309–12
51. Bern MM, Lokich JJ, Wallach SR, Bothe EJ, Benotti PN, Arkin CF et al. Very low doses of warfarin can prevent thrombosis in central vein catheters: a randomised prospective trial. Ann Intern Med 1990; 112: 423–8
52. Levine M, Hirsh J, Gent M, Arnold A, Warr D, Falanga A et al. Double-blind randomised trial of very low dose warfarin for prevention of thromboembolism in stage IV breast cancer. Lancet 1994; 343: 886–9
53. Meade TW, Mellows S, Brozovic M, Miller GJ, Chakrabarti RR, North WRS et al. Haemostatic function and ischaemic heart disease: principal results of the Northwick Park Heart Study. Lancet 1986; 2: 533–7
54. Meade TW, Roderick PJ, Brennan PJ, Wilkes HC, Kelleher CC. Extracranial bleeding and other symptoms due to low dose aspirin and low intensity oral anticoagulation. Thrombosis and Haemostasis 1992; 68: 1–6
55. Turpie AGG, Gent M, Laupacis A, Latour Y, Gunstensen J, Basile F et al. A comparison of aspirin with placebo in patients treated with warfarin after heart-valve replacement. N Engl J Med 1993; 329: 524–9

38 Lipid lowering after a coronary event

Brian L Lloyd

The presence of pre-existing coronary artery disease, and myocardial infarction (MI) in particular, indicates a major risk for future coronary events (see Ch. 5). Elevation of serum cholesterol, along with continued smoking and elevated blood pressure, also confers an unfavourable outcome in these patients. Recent evidence has demonstrated significant benefits of detection and treatment of elevated cholesterol in reducing the risk of future events following MI. Since most evidence has accumulated regarding changes in cholesterol and to a lesser extent low density lipoprotein (LDL), these will be principally discussed but triglyceride and high density lipoprotein (HDL) are reviewed where appropriate.

Elevated cholesterol and increased risk post myocardial infarction

Following MI, higher cholesterol levels are associated with increased, relative and absolute risk of future events including death.[1] Analysis of the absolute patient numbers post MI compared with results in a control population highlights the potential benefits of treatment in patients with established disease.

In the control group of the Coronary Drug Project, among men with prior MI the 5-year rate of death from ischaemic heart disease (IHD) was 129 per thousand for the lowest quintile of serum cholesterol and 196 per thousand for the highest quintile, representing an excess risk of 67 per thousand in the highest quintile.[2] The increased risk was graded across the quintiles. In contrast, in the absence of prior MI or disease, as in the Multiple Risk Factor Intervention Trial (MRFIT),[3] the corresponding lowest quintile risk was three per thousand and the highest quintile risk 11 per thousand, representing an excess risk of only eight deaths per thousand due to the increased level of cholesterol.

Benefits of reducing cholesterol levels post myocardial infarction

The benefits of reducing cholesterol following MI in the presence of coronary artery disease (diet and drug therapy) have been demonstrated in a number of ways:

- In serial angiographic studies disease progression of established coronary plaques is reduced and regression of plaques is more frequent.[4] New lesion formation appears reduced on treatment.
- Meta-analysis of previous studies by a number of groups has shown a significantly reduced event rate, reduced fatal MI rate and significant or near significant reduced total mortality.[1,5–7]
- Recent analyses of primary prevention and cohort studies suggest a significant benefit of lower cholesterol levels.[6]
- The large Scandinavian Simvastatin Survival Study showed significant benefits of treatment on mortality, fatal and non-fatal MI and need for intervention by angioplasty or coronary artery bypass graft (CABG)[8] a result supported by the results of the North American CARE Study.[8a]
- Reducing cholesterol following MI by ileal bypass surgery (rather than by drug therapy) resulted in a significant reduction in events (POSCH study) but not total mortality.[9]

Lipid lowering and disease regression

Considerable evidence indicates that lowering of cholesterol and LDL levels can modify progression of atheromatous plaques and cause regression in some patients, as demonstrated with repeat coronary angiograms. Four major studies on between 30 and 113 patients, three of which were randomized and used predominantly diet, but also modified other risk factors in two, showed less progression of disease and some regression. In two studies symptoms improved and in one, physical work capacity improved on diet.[10]

The results of randomized control studies employing repeated angiographic assessment were recently reviewed by Howes and Simons.[4] Their review included two studies without drug intervention and employing life-style change in one and ileal bypass surgery in the other. The remaining studies used drug therapy. They concluded there was a clear excess of regression or stable disease in those receiving active treatment. Further, the data provided suggestive evidence of a favourable clinical outcome in the active treatment groups, reaching statistical significance in three studies. Three further trials since the Howes and Simons review have shown broadly similar results.

Lipid lowering and reduced clinical events (including mortality)

While individual dietary trials in patients with coronary heart disease (CHD) have shown little conclusive benefit on clinical events, meta-analysis of these trials has shown an average reduction of 12–20% in clinical events. Holme demonstrated a reduced incidence of CHD (death from CHD and confirmed non-fatal MI) of 0.78 (confidence interval 0.63–0.96) but no change in total mortality.[9]

In his meta-analysis of dietary trials Truswell demonstrated reduced coronary events (13–30%) and total deaths (6–11%) on dietary therapy.[11]

Meta-analysis of drug treatment in 1990 by Rossouw et al[1] of eight secondary prevention trials showed a significant reduction in cardiovascular deaths, with odds ratio of 0.88 (confidence interval 0.77–0.99) but no significant change in total mortality (odds ratio 0.91, confidence interval 0.82–1.02). More recently in a further meta-analysis Davies-Smith analysed patient groups by risk of death in the control group and showed a reduced mortality in those whose randomized control group had the highest risk of death (greater than 5% annual mortality).[5]

Individual studies

A number of individual studies indicate a significant benefit on CHD events, CHD mortality and/or total mortality from cholesterol lowering, principally by drug treatment, following MI:

- In the Coronary Drug Project patients receiving niacin 3 g/day had a 9% fall in serum cholesterol and a significant reduction in non-fatal MI (26%). After MI fifteen-year follow-up, but not after five years, there was a significant reduction in CHD deaths (12%) and total mortality (12%).[12,13]
- In the Stockholm Ischaemic Heart Disease Secondary Prevention Study, combined treatment with clofibrate (2 g/day) and nicotinic acid (3 g/day) reduced CHD deaths by 36% and all-cause mortality by 25%.[14]
- In the Scandinavian Simvastatin Survival Study[8] 4444 patients, of whom 79% had prior MI with or without continuing angina, were studied on simvastatin or placebo. After median follow-up of 5.4 years mean changes in total cholesterol, LDL and HDL were 25% negative, 35% negative and plus 8% respectively. There were 189 coronary deaths in the placebo group and 111 in the simvastatin group (relative risk 0.58, 95% confidence interval 0.46–0.73). The results indicated that the addition of simvastatin 20–40 mg in every hundred patients can be expected over 6 years to succeed in preserving the 'lives of four of the nine patients who otherwise would die from CHD, prevention of non-fatal MI in seven of an expected 21 patients, and avoidance of myocardial revascularization procedures in six of the 19 anticipated patients'.[8]
- CARE trial[8a] – the results of a 5 year study in 4159 patients with documented MI 3–20 months prior to being randomly allocated to pravastatin 40 mg/day on placebo showed a statistically significant reduction of 24% in a composite endpoint of myocardial reinfarction or coronary heart disease death ($\beta = 0.002$). Patients in the CARE trial had plasma cholesterol levels <6.2 mmol and LDL cholesterol levels of 3.0–4.5 mmol on entry.
- POSCH Trial[10]—Between 1975 and 1983, 838 patients with hypercholesterolaemia having

survived MI were randomly assigned to diet therapy or diet plus partial ileal bypass surgery. Repeated coronary angiograms were compared in individual patients. Surgery resulted in sustained improvement in the blood lipid pattern and reduced subsequent morbidity due to coronary heart disease. A comparison of baseline coronary arteriograms with those obtained at 3, 5, 7 and 10 years consistently showed less disease progression in the surgery group.

Plaque modification and future events

Coronary plaques more likely to rupture and lead to unstable angina, MI and sudden death are those generally which are less stenotic, with most having less than 75% stenosis, and which have a higher cholesterol-rich lipid core with less thick fibrous cap.[15,16] It is these lesions which are best modified by cholesterol lowering therapy providing a basis for reduced events.[17]

Recent evidence also suggests that a beneficial effect on endothelial function is likely to be an important action of cholesterol lowering. The paradoxical vasoconstrictor effect of acetylcholine in arteries with atheroma is reversed after treatment.[18] Lipid lowering may also reduce platelet adhesion to plaques.[19]

Treatment criteria and goals of treatment

Levels of total cholesterol and LDL recommended for initiation of treatment in Australia, USA and Europe are shown in Table 38.1. Goals of therapy where recommended are shown. It should be noted that except for the guidelines of the National Heart Foundation of Australia, all other guidelines were established prior to publication of the 4S results, the inclusion criteria of which are also shown in this table.

Drug choice, dosages and side-effects

Recent evidence from meta-analyses has suggested that the degree of cholesterol lowering is the dominant influence on reduced CHD events and reduced total mortality for non-hormone and non-fibrate drugs.[7] Since HMG CoA reductase inhibitors give a consistently more marked reduction in cholesterol (25–35%) than bile acids sequestering agents (10–15%) and fibrates (10–15%), most would favour HMG CoA reductase inhibitors. This is particularly so in view of the very favourable outcome in the Scandinavian Simvastatin Survival Study and the low side-effect profile. Niacin, on the other hand, while producing substantial falls in cholesterol level with proven benefit, is not well tolerated and in many countries not a common drug of first choice. HMG CoA reductase inhibitors however are

Table 38.1 Levels of total cholesterol (TC) or low density lipoprotein (LDL) or triglyceride (TG) recommended for initiation of drug treatment after MI

Country/Study	Levels of TC, LDL, TG before drug treatment (mmol/L)	Target levels (mmol/L)
Australia, Pharmaceutical Benefits Advisory Committee (PBAC)	TC >6.5 or TC >5.5 if HDL <1.0	
Australia, National Heart Foundation, 1995	TC >5.5 or TC >5.0 and HDL <1.0 or TG >2.5 and HDL <1.0	TC <4.5 TG <2.0
USA	LDL ≥3.3	LDL ≤2.5
Europe	TC ≥6.5 or TC ≥5.2 with TG≥2.3†	TC 4.5–5.0 LDL 3.0–3.5
4S Study inclusion criteria	TC≥5.5 (with TG ≤2.5)	TC 3.0–5.2

† Uncommonly for patients who do not reach target levels after prolonged trial of conservative care.
4S = Scandinavian Simvastatin Survival Study

well tolerated, with low incidence of side-effects.[8]

Fibrates, and in particular gemfibrozil, are well tolerated but produce more modest reduction in cholesterol (10–15%). They are generally used for combined hyperlipidaemia where triglyceride elevation is substantial, generally greater than 4 mmol/L. Clofibrate, an early fibrate, was associated with increased mortality in primary prevention trials, and insufficient data exists for the new fibrates to exclude a similar effect. There is little data supporting their use as a secondary preventive agent although the Helsinki Heart Study (a primary prevention trial) demonstrated a benefit for reduced coronary events in certain subgroups, particularly those with elevated TG and lower HDL, but without reduced total mortality.[20]

The average changes expected in various lipid fractions with different treatments are shown in Table 38.2. Possible drug choices are shown in Table 38.3, and in Table 38.4 common dosages and possible adverse effects.

Measurement of lipids post myocardial infarction

Intercurrent illness, and MI in particular, results in marked changes in lipid levels with reduced plasma cholesterol and elevated triglyceride levels.[21,22] As the effect is manifested by 24 hours after the MI and lasts from 6–12 weeks, fasting lipids can only be assessed with reasonable accuracy if taken within 24 hours or after 3 months.

Timing of treatment initiation and repeat measurements

Little is known of the ideal time following MI to initiate treatment. In view of the significant delays in the benefits apparent in most studies, beginning around 1 year but potentially available

Table 38.2 Average changes in various lipid fractions on drug treatment

Drug	Cholesterol	TG	HDL	LDL
Simvastatin, Pravastatin, Fluvastatin	↓ 20–30%	↓ 12–18%	↑ 6–9%	↓ 30–40%
Cholestyramine, Colestipol	↓ 7–15%	↑ 10%	↑ 5%	↓ 20%
Gemfibrozil	↓ 11%	↓ 43%	↑ 10%	↓ 10%
Nicotinic acid	↓ 10–12%	↓ 28–34%	↑ 43%	↓ 9%

TG = triglyceride; HDL = high density lipoprotein; LDL = low density lipoprotein

Table 38.3 Treatment options. Modified from National Heart Foundation of Australia recommendations, 1995

Hyperlipidaemia	Initial	Alternative	Combination
Hypercholesterolaemia	Simvastatin Pravastatin Fluvastatin Cholestyramine Colestipol	Gemfibrozil Niacin	Resin + statin Resin + gemfibrozil Resin + niacin
Hypertriglyceridaemia	Gemfibrozil	Niacin Max EPA	Any of 2 of those nominated
Combined: Elevated TC and TG (mainly TC)	Simvastatin Pravastatin Fluvastatin	Gemfibrozil Niacin	Gemfibrozil + resin Niacin + resin Statin + Max EPA
Combined: Elevated TC and TG (mainly TG)	Gemfibrozil	Niacin Simvastatin Pravastatin Fluvastatin	Gemfibrozil and niacin Statin and n-3 fatty acids Gemfibrozil and statin

TC = total cholesterol; TG = triglycerides; Max EPA = concentrated fish oil capsules containing eicosapentaenoic acid

Table 38.4 Dosage, adverse effects and safety monitoring

Drug	Dose	Adverse effects	Safety monitoring	Contraindications
Simvastatin, Pravastatin, Fluvastatin	10–40 mg nightly	Muscle pains, muscle weakness, raised liver enzymes	Liver enzymes, creatine kinase	Caution with cyclosporine, fibrates
Cholestyramine	4–16 g daily	GI problems, drug interactions		High TG, peptic ulcer, haemorrhoids
Colestipol	5–20 g daily	As for cholestyramine		As for cholestyramine
Gemfibrozil	600 mg 12-hourly	GI discomfort, interact with statin or warfarin	Liver enzymes coagulation	? gallstones, caution with statins and warfarin
Nicotinic acid	100 mg 8-hourly titrating to 500 mg 8-hourly†	Flushing, raised glucose, urate and liver enzymes	Glucose, urate, liver enzymes	Liver disease, gout
MaxEPA (Eicosapentanoic acid)	6 g daily	Very few	Bleeding time	Hypercholesterolaemia

† Occasionally 1 g tds may be used.

earlier in individual patients, it may be argued that treatment be initiated within days or weeks following MI, assuming a reliable measurement of cholesterol is available and meets treatment criteria. Repeat measurements can be made after 3–6 weeks of initiating treatment and dosage adjusted if necessary. Appropriate diet ought to be maintained along with weight optimization.

While no lower limit of cholesterol level on treatment has been demonstrated to be adverse, most would favour that cholesterol should not be lowered below 3.0–3.5 mmol/L.

References

1. Rossouw JE, Lewis B, Rifkind BM. The value of lowering cholesterol after myocardial infarction. N Engl J Med 1990; 323: 1112–19
2. Coronary Drug Project Research Group. National history of myocardial infarction in the Coronary Drug Project: long term prognostic importance of serum lipid levels. Am J Cardiol 1978; 42: 489–98
3. Stamler J, Wentworth D, Neaton JD. Is relationship between serum cholesterol and risk of premature death from coronary heart disease continuous and graded? Findings in 356 222 primary screenees of the Multiple Risk Factor Intervention Trial (MRFIT). JAMA 1986; 256: 2823–8
4. Howes LG, Simons LA. Efficiency of drug intervention for lipids in the prevention of coronary artery disease. Aust NZ J Med 1994; 24: 107–12
5. Davies-Smith G, Song F, Sheldon TA. Cholesterol lowering and mortality: the importance of considering initial level of risk. Br Med J 1993; 306: 1367–73
6. Law MR, Wald NJ, Thompson BG. By how much and how quickly does reduction in serum cholesterol concentration lower risk of ischaemic heart disease? Br Med J 1994; 308: 373–9
7. Gould AL, Rossouw JE, Santanello NC, Heyse JF, Furberg CD. Cholesterol reduction yields clinical benefit. Circulation 1995; 91(8): 2274–82
8. The Scandinavian Simvastatin Survival Study Group. Randomised trial of cholesterol lowering in 4444 patients with coronary heart disease: the Scandinavian Simvastatin Survival Study (4S). Lancet 1994; 344: 1383–9

8a. Braunwald E, Pfeffer M, Sacks F. Cholesterol and recurrent events (CARE) Results preserved at American College of Cardiology. 45th Annual Scientific Sessions, March 1996

9. Holme I. Relation of coronary heart disease incidence and total mortality to plasma cholesterol reduction in randomised trials: use of meta-analysis. Br Heart J, 1993; 69: S42–S47
10. Buchwald H, Varco RC, Matts JP et al. Effect of partial ileal bypass surgery on mortality and morbidity from coronary heart disease in patients with hypercholesterolaemia. N Engl J Med 1990; 323: 946–55
11. Truswell AS. Review of dietary intervention studies: effect on coronary events and on total

mortality. Aust NZ J Med 1994; 24: 98–106
12. The Coronary Drug Project Research Group: clofibrate and niacin in coronary heart disease. JAMA 1975; 231: 360–81
13. Canner PL, Berge KG, Werge NK et al. Fifteen year mortality in Coronary Drug Project patients: long term benefits with niacin. J Am Coll Cardiol 1986; 8: 1245–55
14. Carlson LA, Rosenhamer G. Reduction of mortality in the Stockholm Ischaemic Heart Disease Secondary Prevention Study by combined treatment with clofibrate and nicotinic acid. Acta Med Scand 1988; 223: 405–18
15. Ambrose JA, Tannenbaum MA, Alexopoulos D et al. Angiographic progession of coronary artery disease and the development of myocardial infarction. J Am Coll Cardiol 1988; 12: 56–62
16. Taeymans Y, Theroux P, Lesperance J, Waters D. Quantative angiographic morphology of the coronary artery lesions at risk of thrombotic occlusion. Circulation 1992; 85(1): 78–85
17. Brown BG, Zhao X, Sacco DE, Albers JJ. Lipid lowering and plaque regression. New insights into prevention of plaque disruption and clinical events in coronary disease. Circulation 1993; 87: 1781–91
18. Leung WH, Lau CP, Wong CK. Beneficial effect of cholesterol lowering therapy on coronary endothelial dependent relaxation in hypercholesterolaemic patients. Lancet 1993; 341: 1496–500
19. Lacoste L, Lam JYT, Hung J et al. Hyperlipidemia and coronary disease: correction of the increased thrombogenic potential with cholesterol reduction. Circulation 1994; 92: 3172–3177
20. Mahnineu V, Elo MO, Frick MH et al. Lipid alterations and decline in the incidence of coronary heart disease in the Helsinki Heart Study. JAMA 1988; 260: 641–51
21. Avogaro P, Bon GB, Cazzo Lato G et al. Variations in apolipoproteins B and A_I during the course of myocardial infarction. Eur J Clin Invest 1978; 8: 121–9
22. Thompson GR. A handbook of hyperlipidaemia. 2nd ed. London: Current Science, 1994

Part 6
Non-drug therapies

39 Vascular access

Peter L Thompson, Bradley M Power and Philip A Cooke

Vascular access in the coronary care unit (CCU) can be literally a life-saving skill. Whilst correct technique is essential for a high success rate, there is no substitute for experience and constant practice. Junior medical staff should take every opportunity to perform vascular cannulation procedures, preferably under skilled supervision. The use of skilled nursing staff has been found in some units to improve success and reduce complication rates. The allocation of duties in vascular access, balancing training requirements with patient comfort and safety, is a matter for judgement in individual units.

This chapter will describe the techniques of cannulation of peripheral veins, access to central veins and right heart chambers and pulmonary artery as well as arterial cannulation. Access to the left heart is the province of the cardiac catheterization laboratory and will not be discussed.

Patient preparation

The patient should be comfortable and every attempt should be made to allay their apprehension about the procedure. A careful explanation should be given, but usually written informed consent is not required for vascular access procedures. However, if the operator considers that there is an element of risk, such as central venous catheterization in a patient with a bleeding tendency, formal informed consent is a wise precaution. For most procedures the patient can be in a comfortable semi-recumbent position but for some procedures such as femoral vein access, a supine position is necessary and for subclavian vein catheterization, a supine head down position may be optimum. On occasions, in a very apprehensive patient, a small intravenous (IV) injection of diazepam or midazolam may be necessary to avoid the patient's anxiety interfering with the procedure.

Aseptic technique

In emergency situations it is sometimes necessary to proceed with vascular access without aseptic precautions. In this situation the cannula or catheter should be replaced as soon as the life-threatening crisis has passed. Meticulous technique is necessary to minimize the risk of phlebitis[1] following the guidelines outlined in Ch. 86.

Local anaesthesia

Local anaesthesia (1% lignocaine) may cause venous spasm or haematoma but is suggested for all but emergency or small gauge peripheral intravenous cannula insertion. If a prolonged procedure is anticipated a longer acting agent such as bupivacaine (marcain) can be used. Reactions to local anaesthetics may include allergic reactions, which are managed with IV injection of antihistamine, or vasovagal bradycardia hypotensive response, treated with IV atropine, or neurotoxic effects due to inadvertent rapid IV injection. The latter are rare with 1% lignocaine as toxic plasma levels would require an injection of 100–150 mg (10–15 ml of 1%) or more.

Adequate local anaesthesia is usually obtained with local infiltration of 5–10 mg of lignocaine.

Initial skin puncture is achieved with a fine (25 gauge) needle raising a small weal on the skin and injecting gradually deeper layers with multiple injections. Each injection should be preceded by aspiration to reduce the risk of inadvertent intravascular injection. Local infiltration can usually be achieved through the single entry site. If deeper infiltration is required, the 25 gauge needle can be removed and replaced with a longer 23 gauge needle using the same entry site identified by a drop of blood on the skin or by leaving the finer needle in situ.

Lignocaine is usually effective in achieving local anaesthesia within 5 minutes, and lasts for approximately 1 hour.

Direct cannulation

Insertion of a cannula in a peripheral vein is usually a straightforward procedure. Shaving of hairy skin improves visualization of the vein and allows[3] application of an adhesive dressing. In difficult situations, tapping of the vein, dependency of the limb, application of warm compresses and local application of nitroglycerin cream or spray can all be attempted. With increasing use of anticoagulant and thrombolytic agents in the CCU, multiple venipuncture attempts should be avoided. If venous access has not been achieved after two or three attempts, more experienced assistance should be called for.

Seldinger technique

The Seldinger technique initially used for access to the arterial circulation[2] has become increasingly useful for access to the venous circulation for insertion of central venous catheters and pacing catheters via the subclavian, internal jugular and femoral veins.

- After infiltration of the area with local anaesthetic, a small nick in the skin 2–3 mm in length is made with sharp pointed No. 11 scalpel to prevent the skin tissues hindering access with the dilator and introducer.
- The vein or artery is located with a shallow bevelled needle containing a stylet or attached to a syringe containing heparinized saline.
- When a free flow of blood is obtained the needle is advanced slightly, ensuring that a free flow of blood continues.
- The floppy end of the guide wire is advanced through the needle into the vessel lumen and advanced approximately 15 cm past the tip of the needle.
- The needle is removed whilst maintaining the guide wire in the vessel. The guide wire is cleaned with moistened gauze.
- A firm dilator is passed over the guide wire until its tip rests at the skin entry site.
- The dilator is advanced over the guidewire using a rotating motion until the shoulder of the dilator has entered the vessel. It is then withdrawn leaving the guidewire in situ.
- A catheter (eg central venous catheter) may then be passed directly over the guidewire to a measured correct length after which the guidewire is withdrawn. Alternatively, an introducer (sheath) may be loaded onto the dilator which is then reinserted over the guidewire. Again a rotating motion is used as the sheath is advanced to its hub following which the guidewire and dilator are withdrawn. The introducer can now be used for infusion, or can be used for introduction of a pacing catheter or pulmonary artery catheter through its lumen.
- The introducer is passed over the dilator again in a firm rotating motion. The introducer is advanced to its hub and the dilator is removed. The introducer can now be used as an IV infusion site or can be used for introduction of a pacing catheter or pulmonary artery catheter.

Variations on the Seldinger technique include the use of a split sheath[3] which, following the introduction of a pacing catheter or pulmonary artery catheter, can be removed from the vein and separated into two halves.

Special precautions with the Seldinger technique[4,5]

- Never advance the guide wire if resistance is met.
- Always use the soft end, never use the firm end of the guide wire.
- Never withdraw the guidewire through the needle as this may cause guillotining and transection of the guidewire allowing embolization.
- Never force the dilator or introducer over the guide wire.
- If resistance to the guide wire is experienced, remove the needle and guide wire together, reinsert the needle through another entry site and ensure free flow of blood before reinserting the guide wire.
- To ensure vascular access, inject a small amount of contrast medium through the needle under fluoroscopy control.
- If vascular access is confirmed after injection of contrast medium and there is still resistance to passage of the guide wire, use a J-shaped guide wire instead of a straight guide wire.

- Prior to embarking on the Seldinger technique, ensure that the guide wire, dilator and introducer are all compatible.

Cut-down

Surgical cut-down is less frequently used now that the Seldinger technique is more widely used for venous access. However, it is still valuable if peripheral veins are not evident and the subclavian approach is thought to be too hazardous—for example, after thrombolytic therapy.

- Local anaesthesia is achieved by local infiltration and a horizontal intradermal bleb of local anaesthetic.
- A transverse incision is made over the vessel, deep enough to ensure that the dermal layer has been incised through to the subcutaneous tissues.
- Subcutaneous tissues are separated with blunt dissection using curved forceps.
- The vessel is identified and separated from adjacent tissues by longitudinal dissection.
- The point of the curved forceps is inserted behind the vessel, lifting it free from adjacent tissues.
- The vein is identified as a bluish vessel without pulsation. It is distinguished from the artery, which is white or pale cream with visible and palpable pulsations, and from nerve tissue which is non-pulsatile. If in doubt, a small gauge needle can be used to aspirate the vessel. Manipulation of a nerve may produce pain or discomfort in its area of distribution.
- Two catgut sutures are passed around the posterior aspect of the vessel by looping the catgut into the forceps and withdrawing behind the vessel then cutting to produce a distal and proximal ligature.
- The distal ligature is secured to close off the venous return. The proximal ligature is used for positioning the vessel for the incision into the vessel.
- A small incision, only slightly larger than the size of the cannula or pacing catheter, is made into the wall of the vein using a transverse incision with small sharp pointed scissors, or a longitudinal incision using a No. 11 scalpel blade with the sharp edge up.
- A small introducer is inserted into the proximal end of the incision, and the catheter or pacing wire is inserted into the lumen of the vessel and advanced proximally.
- When the catheter has been positioned, the incision in the vein is secured with the proximal ligature tight enough to prevent blood loss but not sufficiently tight to prevent withdrawal of the catheter at a later time.
- The incision is then closed in layers, using absorbable catgut in the deeper layers. Black silk sutures are used on the skin surface in case a haematoma develops and the incision needs to be reopened.
- The incision is dressed and sealed aseptically.

Special precautions with venous cut-down

- Venous spasm may occur. This can be reduced by avoiding excessive manipulation of the vein, by local warming, by IV injection of diazepam, by administration of sublingual nitroglycerin or direct application of papaverine.

Venous access sites

The various sites for access to the venous system are summarized in Table 39.1.

Peripheral venous access can be obtained by any peripheral vein. Veins in the dorsum of the hand are usually fragile and not suitable for long-term IV drip sites. Veins on the forearm are suitable but often not available because of previous attempts at intravenous cannulation. The antecubital veins are commonly used, but because of flexion of the elbow, are often not suitable for intravenous drip sites. Veins on the leg are available but cannulation of the saphenous vein may cause phlebitis which would render the use of the saphenous vein unsuitable for subsequent coronary artery bypass surgery. Similarly, veins in other locations should be used with circumspection because of the likelihood that patients with coronary heart disease will be needing coronary and intensive care on subsequent admissions for future episodes related to their coronary artery disease.

Of the sites used for central venous cannulation, the subclavian vein is the most widely used because of relative ease of access, low rate of complications and convenience for the patient.[4,5] The complication rates associated with the antecubital, internal jugular, subclavian, femoral and external jugular vein sites are summarized in Table 39.2.

Table 39.1 Indications and contraindications for venous access sites. Modified with permission from Daily EK, Tilkian AG 1986, reference 4

Site	Indications	Relative contraindications
Basilic or median cephalic vein	Administration of drugs and moderate volume of fluids Preferred route during CPR	Not ideal for long-term monitoring or pacing catheters Arm injury Local infection
Femoral vein	Administration of large volumes during emergency resuscitation	Severe obesity Local infection
Internal jugular vein	Placement of central catheter(s) Administration of large volumes of fluid Administration of irritating medications or hypertonic solutions	Neck injury Local infection Coagulopathies (thrombolytic treatment) CPR Severe agitation
Subclavian vein	Placement of central catheter(s) or temporary pacemaker Administration of large volumes of fluid Administration of irritating medications or hypertonic solutions	Severe scoliosis Chest trauma or deformity Severe agitation Coagulopathies Positive-pressure ventilation Emphysematous patient

CPR = cardiopulmonary resuscitation

As it is the most popular site for central venous cannulation, the infraclavicular approach to subclavian vein cannulation will be described in detail.

Subclavian vein—infraclavicular approach

Cannulation of the subclavian vein was first described in 1962.[6] Since then the infraclavicular approach has grown in popularity.[7] Comparison of the infraclavicular with the supraclavicular approach has shown that the infraclavicular approach is associated with a slightly higher proportion of subclavian artery cannulation and pneumothorax.[8] However, despite this the convenience for the patient and the suitability for long-term cannulation has ensured its wide application.

Anatomy

The anatomy of the subclavian vein in relation to the subclavian artery is summarized in Figure 39.1.

The subclavian vein drains the axillary vein and joins the internal jugular behind the sternoclavicular joint to form the innominate vein. It crosses the first rib and runs medial and inferior to the subclavian artery from which it is separated by the anterior scalenus muscle. The vein sits atop the apical pleura.

Surface markings

The vein is located at the junction of the medial and middle thirds of the clavicle immediately below the clavicular head of the sternomastoid.

Technique

The patient is supine, and in patients who are hypovolaemic, mild head down position is preferable. The breathless patient may be repositioned upright as soon as the guidewire is positioned in the vein. The skin is entered below the clavicle medial to the junction of the middle and medial third of the clavicle and just lateral to the clavicular head of the sternomastoid. A fine needle is used to palpate below the clavicle and above the medial aspect of the first rib. When the vein is entered a free flow of blood is obtained. The exploration needle is withdrawn from the vein and lignocaine is injected along the needle track and the line of the needle is memorized. The Seldinger technique is then used to enter the vein and insert a central venous catheter,

Table 39.2 Complications of different venous access sites. Reproduced with permission from Daily EK, Tilkian AG 1986, reference 4

Site	Insertion success rate (%)	Catheter malposition rate (%) (without fluoroscopy)	Complication rate (%)	Specific complications and rate (%)
Basilic	58–98	25–52	3–5	Thrombophlebitis (3–5) Thrombosis (< 1–5) Phlebitis/cellulitis (1–20)
Internal jugular	80–94	0–6 (right) 0–20 (left)	< 1–13	Carotid artery puncture (1–15) Myocardial perforation of pacing catheter (1–10) Pneumothorax (< 1) Haemothorax (< 1) Air embolism (< 1) Catheter embolism (< 1) Nerve damage (rare) Thrombosis (rare) Horner's syndrome (rare)
Subclavian vein	85–98	20–33	< 1–17	Pneumothorax (< 1–10) Subclavian artery puncture (1–20) Sepsis (< 1–2) Haemothorax (1) Hydrothorax (1) Air embolism (< 1) Thrombophlebitis (< 1) Thrombosis (rare) Catheter embolism (rare) Brachial plexus injury (rare) Phrenic nerve injury (rare) Sternoclavicular osteomyelitis (rare)
Femoral vein	89–95	None	4–20	Evidence of thrombus (15–20) Infection (3–20) Femoral artery puncture (4–10)
External jugular vein	61–99	6	0–4	Haematoma (< 5) Air embolism (rare) Thrombosis (rare)

pulmonary artery catheter or pacing catheter. The technique for right subclavian infraclavicular cannulation is demonstrated in Figure 39.2.

Complications[9]

Complications of the subclavian infraclavicular approach include:

- Air embolism.[10] Air can be aspirated into the venous system by a patient taking a deep breath in an upright position during cannulation. This can be prevented by asking the patient to maintain normal respiration with the patient in the supine position and with the head slightly down.
- Pneumothorax. Multiple attempts at cannulation should be avoided and preferably the vein should be identified with a narrow bore needle. Subclavian cannulation is best avoided in patients with hyper-expanded chests or emphysema.

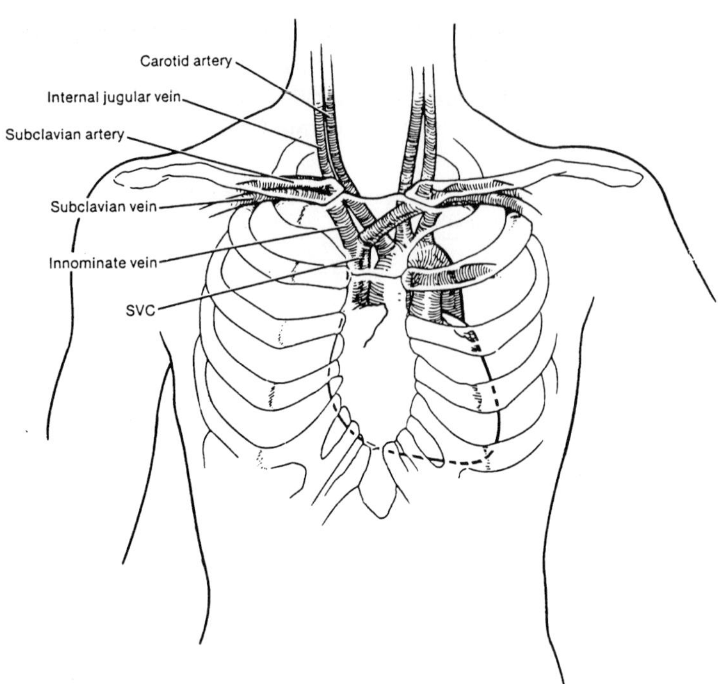

Fig. 39.1 Anatomy of the subclavian vein in relation to the clavicle, first rib and subclavian artery. Reproduced with permission from Daily EK, Tilkian AG 1986.[4]

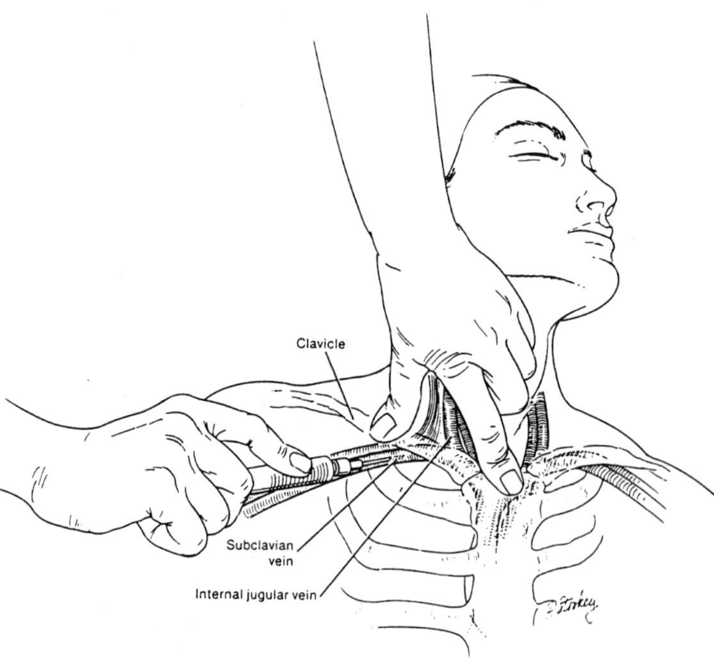

Fig. 39.2 Cannulation of the right subclavian vein by the infraclavicular approach. The technique for the left subclavian vein is identical; the left subclavian is preferable in the patient who may need a permanent pacemaker. Reproduced with permission from Daily EK, Tilkian AG 1986.[4]

- Subclavian artery cannulation.[10] This can be avoided by ensuring that the cannula is passed medially and not deeply. The vein is best located with a small bore needle. If subclavian artery perforation occurs, pressure over the clavicle on the first rib is usually sufficient to prevent major bleeding.
- Cannulation of the jugular vein.[10] The cannula or guide wire may enter the subclavian vein and redirect to the ipsilateral jugular vein. This can be detected by image intensifier control and can be corrected by having the patient bring their head or ear down to the shoulder on the site of insertion.

Subclavian vein—supraclavicular approach[7,8]

The supraclavicular approach to the subclavian vein has been reported as being safer with less chance of pneumothorax, and in skilled hands carries a greater rate of success, but the positioning of a cannula or pacing wire following insertion is less convenient and more uncomfortable for the patient than the infraclavicular approach because of the contour of the neck, clavicle and supraclavicular fossa.

Internal jugular vein

The internal jugular vein approach to venous cannulation[12–14] has gained in popularity in recent years because in contrast to the widely used infraclavicular approach to the subclavian vein, there is less risk of pneumothorax or arterial puncture and there is more direct access to the superior vena cava. Cannulation of the internal jugular vein can be life-saving during acute resuscitation when venous access is impossible via other routes. However, it is not an ideal site for elective cannulation for insertion of pulmonary artery catheters and temporary pacing catheters which may be in place for several days, because of difficulties in securing the catheter to the soft tissues of the neck, particularly in bearded males.

Patient preparation

The patient is prepared by lying in the supine position with extension of the neck, assisted by a small pillow under the neck, and the procedure is preferably performed in a slight head down position.

Entry sites

The right internal jugular is most commonly used because of ease of entry and ready access to the superior vena cava. Whilst a variety of entry sites have been described, including high entries lateral or medial to the sterno-clavicular muscle in the neck, the most commonly used entry site is the low central entry between the sternal and clavicular heads of the sternomastoid muscle.[14] The latter approach will be described here.

Technique

Following preparation of the patient, the surface landmarks are identified, preferably with a skin marker pen. The sternoclavicular heads are identified by asking the patient to turn their head laterally against resistance or lifting the head slightly off the pillow.

Routine preparation for the Seldinger technique is followed including check on compatibility of the guide wire, dilator, introducer and cannula and preparation for a small scalpel nick to allow the apparatus to be introduced.

The skin is entered in the centre of the triangle between the sternal and clavicular heads of the sternomastoid 3–4 cm above the medial aspect of the clavicle.

Local skin infiltration with 1% lignocaine is followed by locating the internal jugular with a fine needle. Leaving the needle in position, the Seldinger needle is used to enter the internal jugular vein at a 30 degree angle to the skin with the tip of the needle directed towards the ipsilateral nipple.

When the vein is entered and a free flow of blood is obtained the syringe is removed and the guide wire passed.

If the vein is not entered immediately the needle is passed more laterally. In a cooperative patient the Valsalva manoeuvre may help distend the vein, or in a less cooperative patient, an assistant applying abdominal compression may be helpful.

The guide wire is passed and the dilator and introducer are then passed in the usual Seldinger fashion with expiration and head down position being favoured to prevent air embolism. Following insertion of the cannula and removal of the dilator, the pacing catheter, central venous catheter or pulmonary artery catheter can then be passed.

In securing the catheter it is important to leave a loop on the skin sutured in position to the lateral aspect of the neck and medial aspect of the shoulder.

Complications of internal jugular cannulation

Complications include:

- Air embolism.[10] This can be avoided by performing the procedure in the head down position and ensuring that all manipulations are performed during expiration or with the Valsalva manoeuvre or manual abdominal compression.
- Carotid artery puncture.[15] Usually needle puncture of the carotid artery is not a major misadventure and local pressure for 5–10 minutes will prevent significant bleeding. In the elderly patient with known carotid atherosclerosis, manual compression may cause problems with central blood flow, and should be done with care; indeed a past history of transient cerebral ischaemia should be a contraindication to the jugular approach unless there are no alternative venous cannulation sites. If the Seldinger apparatus is inadvertently inserted into the carotid artery, skilled surgical removal or repair by a vascular surgeon will be necessary. Immediate notification to the vascular surgeons is imperative. This complication is unlikely to occur in the normotensive patient but in the shocked or hypotensive patient inadvertent carotid artery cannulation may occur. Pulsatile blood flow may be so compromised as to be unrecognizable and in this case urgent blood gas analysis may help to distinguish arterial from venous blood.

External jugular vein

Despite its obvious superficial location, the external jugular vein is not ideally suitable for venous cannulation because it is excessively mobile under the skin, making it difficult to enter on occasions and causing difficulties in passing the cannula into the great veins at the base of the neck.

However, on occasions venous cut-down to the external jugular can be a relatively simple procedure and passage of the guide wire can be facilitated by the use of a J-tip guide wire.[16] Nevertheless, if there is expertise in subclavian, internal jugular or femoral vein cannulation, the external jugular is best avoided.

Femoral vein

Although femoral vein cannulation is widely used in the cardiac catheterization laboratory for right heart catheterization, temporary pacing cover and electrophysiology study, it should not be used as a venous access site for the CCU if prolonged cannulation such as pulmonary artery catheter or temporary pacemaker is contemplated, because of the risk of deep vein thrombosis and pulmonary embolism.[17] Nevertheless, femoral vein cannulation can be a very useful route for venous access especially if emphysematous disease is likely to make subclavian cannulation hazardous or during resuscitation when cardiopulmonary resuscitation (CPR) and endotracheal intubation cause overcrowding at the upper half of the body and prevent clean access to the internal jugular. In the latter situation a long cannula to above the diaphragm should be used, as blood flow in the inferior vena cava may be minimal during CPR.[18]

The femoral vein lies medial to the artery and nerve in the femoral triangle.[4,5] The location of the vein can be identified by palpating along the length of the femoral artery. When the pulsations of the artery are recognized the vein should lie immediately medial to the pulsations. The artery can be moved laterally with the tips of three fingers and the skin entry site located approximately 1 cm medial to the pulsations. It is important to enter the vein below the inguinal ligament so that in the event of inadvertent femoral artery puncture or oozing from the femoral vein, bleeding can be controlled with local pressure rather than dealing with intrapelvic haematoma.

Following location of the vein and free flow of venous blood, the vein is entered with the usual Seldinger technique and the cannula is passed to the iliac vein, inferior vena cava and right heart under fluoroscopic control.[5]

Complications

Inadvertent puncture of the femoral artery can be dealt with by withdrawal of the needle and application of local pressure for 5 minutes (longer in the presence of anticoagulant or thrombolytic therapy).

Inadvertent needle puncture of the femoral nerve is recognized by the patient complaining immediately of searing pain down the medial aspect of the thigh. Immediate withdrawal of the needle usually avoids any femoral nerve damage.

Arterial access

Arterial access in the CCU is necessary for arterial puncture for blood gas analysis, for haemodynamic monitoring via the radial or femoral artery, or for percutaneous insertion of an intra-aortic balloon pump via the femoral artery.

Arterial puncture

Arterial puncture for blood gas analysis is performed with a heparin-loaded syringe using a small bore needle. Whilst a 26 gauge needle will reduce the risk of arterial damage or subsequent haematoma formation, it may not be of sufficient calibre to allow satisfactory aspiration of a blood sample; therefore a 23 gauge needle is usually used.

The radial artery is the preferred site. The hand is extended and the vessel palpated. In the most commonly used technique the vessel is transfixed by inserting the needle at a 45 degree angle and gradually withdrawing, allowing blood to well up into the barrel of the syringe under its own pressure. When a satisfactory sample has been withdrawn the needle is removed and bleeding from the arterial puncture site controlled by local pressure for about 2 minutes (longer in the anticoagulated or thrombolysed patient.)

Arterial blood sampling from the brachial artery or femoral arteries usually uses the direct cannulation technique rather than transfixion of the posterior wall. The brachial artery is located with the elbow extended and the site of maximal arterial pulsation identified. The femoral artery is entered approximately 2 cm below the inguinal ligament.

Arterial cannulation for pressure monitoring

The radial artery is the most widely used, although there is increasing use of the femoral artery.[19,20]

If the radial artery is to be used the adequacy of arterial blood supply to the hand must be assessed. If there is not adequate arterial collateral supply by the ulnar artery, radial artery spasm, thrombosis or compression can cause serious ischaemia of the hand. To ensure adequate collateral supply a modified Allen test is performed.[21] The patient's arm is elevated above the heart, and both radial and arterial pulses are occluded by thumb pressure for approximately 5 seconds. With the arterial compression maintained the hand is lowered and pressure from the ulnar site of the wrist is released. The hand should flush pink within fifteen seconds of lowering. If it does not do so this indicates that ulnar arterial blood supply is compromised and that problems with radial artery cannulation could have serious consequences. If the results of the manual Allen test are inconclusive, the use of Doppler flow probe over the ulnar artery may help to clarify the extent of arterial collateral blood supply.

Having confirmed adequate ulnar collateral supply, the radial artery is cannulated under local anaesthesia by direct cannulation or using a modified Seldinger technique. The artery is entered with a 20 gauge needle and a soft flexible guide wire is passed proximally. Having confirmed adequate ulnar collateral supply, the radial artery is cannulated under local anaesthesia **by direct cannulation** or using a modified Seldinger technique. The artery is entered with a 20 gauge needle and a soft flexible guidewire is passed proximally through the needle. A preloaded teflon catheter may then be passed over the needle and along the guidewire. The guidewire and needle are removed and connection follows to the arterial monitoring system (see CH. 24).

A similar technique is used for entry to the femoral artery or brachial artery. If the radial artery site is not suitable, femoral artery cannulation is preferred because this avoids the problems of elbow flexion with brachial artery cannulation.

Percutaneous femoral artery cannulation for intra-aortic balloon

Balloon catheters were initially inserted by a cut-down technique on the femoral artery, and while this is still often used by surgeons during cardiac surgery, percutaneous insertion has become the major method of insertion and is the preferred method in CCU.

Preparation

The patient's legs and vascular supply are examined, as are any angiographic studies which may suggest a favoured site of insertion. Previous vascular surgery is noted. An assistant (scrubbed) may help manoeuvre the long guide wire used during balloon insertion and can assist with control of blood loss from the femoral insertion site.

Procedure

Sheathed catheter insertion

- Standard preparation of the femoral artery for cannulation is made and local anaesthesia is introduced.
- Femoral artery puncture is made and a guide wire inserted by Seldinger technique.
- If fluoroscopy is available (recommended) and is to be used for insertion, the guide wire is advanced until it comes to lie at the level of the left subclavian artery.
- Serial dilators are then passed over the guide wire.
- A sheath (approximately 10 French) containing a dilator is then advanced over the guide wire until approximately 2–3 cm of sheath protrudes from the skin. Undue force should not be applied, to avoid femoral or iliac artery rupture.
- A haemostasis valve applied to the sheath prior to insertion helps minimize blood loss. The dilator is left in place until the balloon catheter is ready for insertion.
- Gentle suction is applied to the balloon inflation lumen through a one way valve which maintains the suction during insertion.
- The dilator is removed and the balloon catheter is advanced over the guide wire until the tip lies approximately 1–2 cm proximal to the left subclavian artery.
- The guide wire is removed and a heparinized pressure

monitoring line is connected to this lumen.

- The balloon inflation lumen is connected to the balloon console.
- The sheath is withdrawn until approximately 8–12 cm of sheath remains in the femoral artery. Care is taken not to retract the balloon catheter. A sheath locking device is used to lock the catheter in situ. The sheath is sutured in place.
- Where fluoroscopy is not available, the balloon catheter may be advanced directly through the sheath without the use of a guide wire. The length of balloon catheter should be measured prior to use. The length is measured from the manubrio-sternal joint to the umbilicus and from the umbilicus to the femoral insertion site.
- Post insertion, the limb is re-examined for presence of ischaemia. Sheath removal must be considered if ischaemic. Position of balloon catheter is reviewed on chest X-ray and this procedure is repeated daily.

Sheathless catheter insertion

This technique is similar to the above except that after dilation of the artery, the balloon catheter is inserted directly over the guide wire. Fluoroscopy is again recommended to assist balloon placement. A guide wire must always be used for this technique of insertion.

Balloon removal

- Check patient sedation and analgesia
- Check coagulation status and platelet count. Heparin ceased at least 4 hours
- Catheters implanted by surgical cut-down are best removed by surgical exploration and closure of the arteriotomy site.

Procedure

- Ballooning is ceased and the inflation lumen is disconnected allowing it to vent to atmosphere. All ties are removed and the sheath seal is loosened if a sheath has been used.
- The catheter is withdrawn until it just engages in the balloon sheath. Further attempts at retraction into the sheath may 'concertina' the sheath, increasing its diameter and causing increased vessel damage on withdrawal.
- The catheter and sheath are then withdrawn as a unit.
- The distal femoral artery is compressed to prevent clot passing down the leg. The proximal portion is then allowed to bleed for 1–2 seconds. The proximal artery is then compressed and back-bleeding from the distal artery is then briefly allowed.
- Pressure is then applied to the artery for a period of 30–60 minutes before checking for bleeding on release. Mechanical clamps are available for this compression. Pedal pulses are checked regularly and foot perfusion examined during this period.
- Where there is prolonged bleeding not attributable to coagulopathy, surgical exploration may be required.

Insertion of long-term central vein cannula

An indwelling cannula in the subclavian vein may be required where there is a requirement for long-term intravenous drug administration, such as with infective endocarditis.[24] These catheters are generally well accepted by patients, and allow out-patient treatment with a low incidence of major complications.[25]

Specialized sets are commercially available which provide all the equipment necessary for insertion of these long-term catheters (e.g. Hickman[24] Groshong[25] catheters*). An attractive more readily available alternative is the PICC (peripherally inserted central catheter) which can be inserted via the antecubital vein.

Procedure

A standard infra-clavicular subclavian vein puncture is performed under strict asepsis and local anaesthesia. A tearaway sheath is placed in the subclavian vein using the Seldinger technique. The dilator and J-wire are removed, and through the sheath a flexible silicon catheter is placed in the low superior vena cava (SVC). The tearaway sheath is then removed, as is the catheter's inner support wire.

After administration of more local anaesthetic, a 5–10 cm subcutaneous track is created (superficial to the pectoral muscles) with the metal spear provided. The catheter is attached to the end of this spear and then

*Groshong is a trademark of CR Bard Inc.

drawn through the track with constant, gentle traction. A small nylon tethering sleeve around the catheter should remain subcutaneous. Once the distal end of the catheter has been passed through the skin, the catheter should be cut just proximal to the spear attachment. A flushing port can then be attached, but blood should be aspirated before the catheter is flushed with heparinized saline.

Care should be taken to ensure the catheter does not kink, particularly at the site of the superior incision. The latter may need to be closed with a 3/0 silk suture. Maintenance of the catheter should follow manufacturer guidelines and strict infection control guidelines.

References

1. Schendorf WA, Brown RB, Sands M, Hosman D. Infections in a coronary care unit. Am J Cardiol 1985; 56: 757–9
2. Seldinger SI. Catheter replacement of the needle in percutaneous arteriography: a new technique. Acta Radiol Diagn 1953; 39: 368
3. Miller FA, Holmes DR, Gersh BJ, Maloney JD. Permanent transvenous pacemaker implantation via the subclavian vein. Mayo Clinic Proc 1980; 55: 309–14
4. Daily EK, Tilkian AG. Venous access. In: Cardiovascular procedures. Diagnostic techniques and therapeutic procedures. St Louis: Mosby, 1986: Ch. 2
5. Simon RR, Brenner BE. Procedures and techniques in emergency medicine. 2nd ed. Baltimore: Williams & Wilkins, 1987: Ch. 11
6. Wilson JN, Grow JB, Demong C. Central venous pressure in optimal blood volume maintenance. Arch Surg 1962; 85: 563
7. Linos DA, Mucha P, Van Heerden JA. Subclavian vein, a golden route. Mayo Clin Proc 1980; 55: 315–21
8. Dronen S, Thompson B, Nowak R, Tomlanovich M. Subclavian vein catheterization during cardiopulmonary resuscitation: a prospective comparison of supraclavicular and infraclavicular approaches. JAMA 1982; 247: 3227–30
9. Feliciano DR, Matlox KL, Graham JM, Beall AC Jr, Jordan GL Jr. Major complications of percutaneous subclavian vein catheters. Am J Surg 1979; 138: 869–74
10. Kashuk JL, Penn I. Air embolism after central venous catheterization. Surg Gynec Obstet 1984; 159: 249–52
11. Johnston AOB, Clark RG. Malpositioning of central venous catheter. Lancet 1972; 1: 1395
12. Brinkman AJ, Costley DO. Internal jugular venepuncture. JAMA 1973; 223: 182
13. Civetta JM, Gabel JC, Gemer M. Internal jugular vein puncture with a margin of safety. Anesthesiology 1977; 46: 362–4
14. Daily PO, Griepp RB, Shimway NE. Percutaneous internal jugular vein cannulation. Arch Surg 1970; 101: 534–6
15. Lipton JS, Trooskin SZ, Rosenberg N. Carotid artery injury during attempted jugular vein catheterization. Heart Lung 1984; 13: 416–8
16. Schwartz AJ, Jobes DR, Levy WJ, Palermo L, Ellison N. Intrathoracic vascular catheterization via the external jugular vein. Anesthesiology 1982; 56: 400–2
17. Swanson RS, Uhlig PN, Gross PL, McCabe CJ. Emergency intravenous access through the femoral vein. Ann Emerg Med 1983; 13: 244
18. Emerman CL, Bellon EM, Lukens TW, May TE, Effron D. A prospective study of femoral versus subclavian vein catheterization during cardiac arrest. Ann Emerg Med 1990; 19: 26–30
19. Soderstrom CA, Wasserman DH, Dunham CM, Caplan ES, Cowley RA. Superiority of the femoral artery for monitoring: a prospective study. Am J Surg 1982; 144: 309–12
20. Russell JA, Joel M, Hudson RJ, Mangano DT, Schlobohm RM. Prospective evaluation of radial and femoral artery catheterization sites in critically ill patients. Cor Care Med 1983; 11: 936–9
21. Kelly J, Braverman B, Land PC, Ivankovich AD. Comparison of Allen test, doppler and finger-pulse transducer to assess patency of ulnar artery. Anesthesiology 1983; 59: A178
22. Donovan KD. Invasive monitoring and support of the circulation. In: Dobb GJ (ed). Clinics in anesthesiology. London: Saunders, 1985; 3: 909–54
23. Lazar JM, Ziady GM, Dummer SJ, Thompson M, Ruffner RJ. Outcome and complications of prolonged intraaortic balloon counterpulsation in cardiac patients. Am J Cardiol 1992; 69: 955–8
24. Hickman RO, Buckner CD, Clift RA et al. A modified right atrial catheter for access to the venous system in marrow transplant recipients. Surg Gynecol Obstet 1979; 148: 871–5
25. Delmore JE, Horbelt DV, Jack BL, Roberts DK. Experience with the Groshong long-term central venous catheter. Gynecol Oncol 1989; 34(2): 216–8

40 Cardiopulmonary resuscitation

Peter L Thompson

Despite the many recent advances in management of acute coronary syndromes and cardiac arrhythmias, the coronary care unit (CCU) remains a high risk area for cardiac arrest. All staff working in the CCU or dealing with patients who are being admitted or discharged from the unit must have well developed skills in cardiopulmonary resuscitation (CPR). It is as important for allied health and technical staff as for medical and nursing staff to be familiar with the principles and techniques to buy time if immediate defibrillation is not available and to enhance the success of advanced cardiac life support techniques if necessary. To this end the CCU should be regarded as a centre of excellence in adherence to the latest standards in CPR, with a programme of re-certification of all staff in CPR skills, and should be a community resource to ensure that these skills are widely disseminated.

Standardization of techniques has been assisted in recent years by guidelines established by authoritative committees such as the Emergency Cardiac Care Committee of the American Heart Association,[1] the European Resuscitation Council,[2] the Australian Resuscitation Council[3] and the Heart Attack Committee of the Heart Foundation of Australia.[4]

Identification of cardiac arrest in the CCU

The patient who suffers cardiac arrest in the CCU is likely to be attached to the cardiac monitor, so the cause of the arrest can usually be identified immediately. Appropriate alarm systems should be in place to notify immediately of life-threatening arrhythmias as well as ready identification of artefacts due to electrode displacement and lead disconnection. Most cardiac arrests in the CCU environment are due to ventricular fibrillation (VF). The emphasis should be on rapid defibrillation rather than protracted CPR. It is important to distinguish true VF or ventricular tachycardia (VT) from electrode movement or muscle artefact as in seizure activity. Cardiac arrest due to asystole is less common and usually heralded by a protracted period of haemodynamic deterioration, usually with a poor outcome, or by the sudden failure of conduction in conduction system disease, in which there is usually a good outcome. Cardiac arrest with persistence of sinus rhythm on the ECG monitor indicates electromechanical dissociation and often indicates cardiac rupture or occasionally overwhelming ischaemic left ventricular dysfunction. The various types of cardiac arrest in ECG-monitored patients in the CCU are summarized in the information box.

Types of cardiac arrest in ECG-monitored patients in CCU

Good outcome
- VT with loss of consciousness
- Primary VF (i.e. VF without severe LV dysfunction)
- Asystole due to conduction system disease (sinus arrest, atrioventricular block)

Poor outcome
- Secondary VF (i.e. VF complicating severe LV dysfunction)
- Asystole with severe LV dysfunction
- Electromechanical dissociation (due to severe LV dysfunction or cardiac rupture)

VT = ventricular tachycardia; VF = ventricular fibrillation; LV = left ventricular

In the patient who is observed to collapse while not attached to the ECG monitor, it is usually safe to assume that the arrest is due to VF and arrange for immediate defibrillation, although of course confirmation of the cardiac arrhythmia is essential before defibrillation is initiated; this is possible with modern defibrillators with 'through the paddle' ECG monitoring capability. 'Blind' defibrillation without confirmation of the cardiac rhythm is no longer advocated.

If the patient not attached to an ECG monitor is found collapsed, and there is uncertainty about the cardiac rhythm or even the presence of any form of cardiac arrest, the usual 'shake and shout' algorithm should be followed (see Fig. 40.1).

COLLAPSE
CHECK RESPONSE TO SHAKE AND SHOUT
CONSCIOUS
MAKE COMFORTABLE
OBSERVE: AIRWAY
BREATHING
CIRCULATION
UNCONSCIOUS
TURN VICTIM ON SIDE
TURN FACE SLIGHTLY DOWNWARDS
CLEAR AIRWAY
APPLY HEAD TILT AND
JAW SUPPORT/JAW THRUST
CHECK FOR BREATHING
BREATHING
LEAVE ON SIDE
IN STABLE POSITION
OBSERVE: AIRWAY
BREATHING
CIRCULATION
NOT BREATHING
TURN VICTIM ON BACK
GIVE FIVE FULL INFLATIONS
WITHIN 10 SECONDS
CHECK FOR CAROTID PULSE
PULSE PRESENT
CONTINUE EAR
CHECK CAROTID
PULSE & BREATHING
AFTER ONE MINUTE
AND THEN AT LEAST
EVERY TWO MINUTES
PULSE ABSENT
BEGIN CPR (EAR & ECC)
CHECK CAROTID
PULSE & BREATHING
AFTER ONE MINUTE
AND THEN AT LEAST
EVERY TWO MINUTES
EAR = EXPIRED AIR RESUSCITATION
ECC = EXTERNAL CARDIAC COMPRESSION
CPR = CARDIOPULMONARY RESUSCITATION

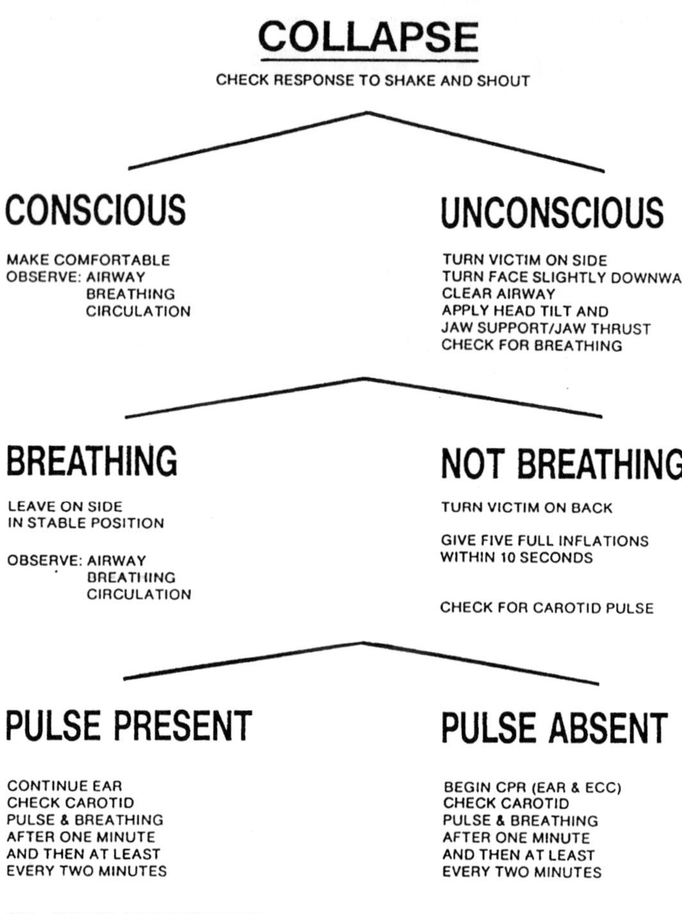

Fig. 40.1 Flow chart for assessment and action in suspected cardiac arrest. Reproduced with permission from Australian Resuscitation Council 1993.[3]

CPR procedure in the CCU

Each bed or room in the CCU should have an automatic alarm system which will alert staff that a cardiac arrest has taken place. This should activate a sequence which will bring immediately to the bedside the defibrillator, resuscitation drugs and appropriate staff. The CCU with adequate staffing levels will find it more convenient to deal with cardiac arrests 'in house' rather than activating the hospital cardiac arrest team which may be delayed and bring together a large number of personnel enthusiastic for the task but uninformed about the patient's medical background. In many cases a single defibrillating precordial shock will be adequate to resolve the crisis. If the cardiac arrest is due to other than primary VF or VT with loss of consciousness or transient asystole due to conduction system disease, full scale CPR needs to be immediately commenced.

Although there are some local variations it is usual to follow the ABC sequence of *airway, breathing and circulation*.

Airway

CPR can only be conducted with the patient supine—that is, flat on their back. In this position the tongue and epiglottis may obstruct the pharynx (see Fig. 40.2).

This can be overcome by the head-tilt, chin-lift manoeuvre, in which one hand is placed on the patient's forehead to tilt the head backwards and the other hand placed under the bony part of the lower jaw to lift the jaw forward. Alternatively the jaw can be thrust forward by bilateral forward lifting of the angle of the jaw. It is important before commencing any rescue breathing manoeuvres to ensure that the mouth is not blocked with dentures which can be readily removed, or food or vomitus which should be aspirated using a suction device. The latter manoeuvres should be performed with the patient lying on their side

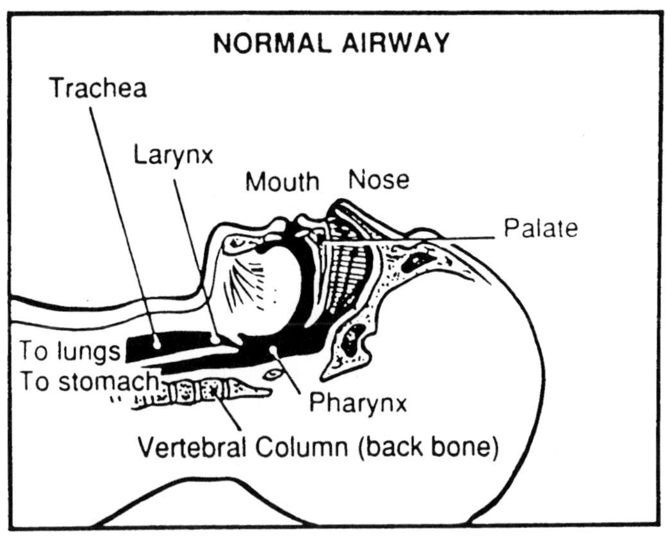

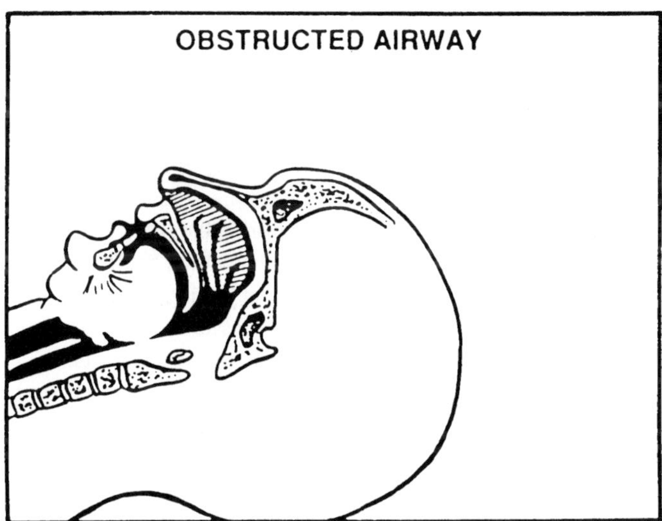

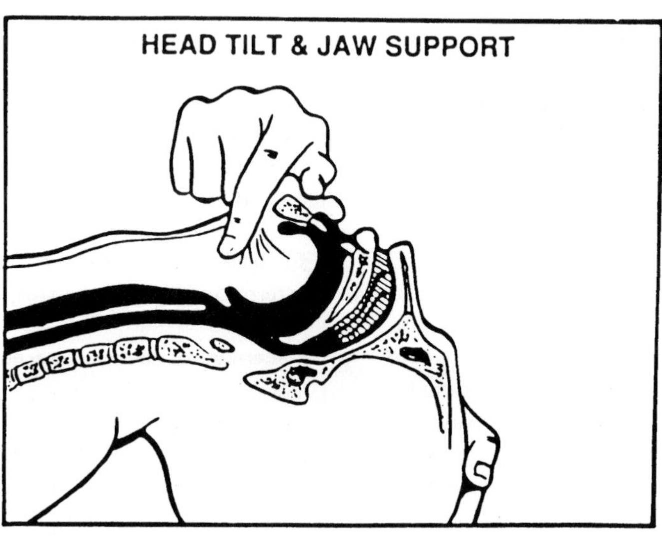

with the mouth facing downwards to allow the mouth and pharynx to drain naturally. Evidence of respiratory obstruction persisting despite these manoeuvres raises the possibility of foreign body obstruction of the pharynx. If the patient has been eating at the time of the arrest, food should be swept from the mouth by a gloved finger, or the possibility of impaction of a bolus of food in the pharynx should be considered and the Heimlich manoeuvre performed. This can be done with the patient supine by pressing firmly with the heel of one hand and the other hand placed over it applying quick upward thrust. This may be repeated up to five times.[1,5] The persistence of inspiratory efforts and gasping despite these manoeuvres may indicate laryngeal spasm or severe broncho-constriction and, if so, appropriate action should be taken.

Breathing

Expired air resuscitation

Expired air resuscitation is not usually necessary in the hospital or coronary care setting where face mask and intubation with respirator devices are usually available. In the setting where assisted ventilation devices are not immediately available, expired air resuscitation can be used. It has proven to be a highly effective method of resuscitation because of the relatively high level of oxygen in the expired air.[6] The mouth to mouth technique is the most widely used but the mouth to nose technique is

Fig. 40.2 Obstruction of airway in an unconscious patient and correction by head tilt. Reproduced with permission from Australian Resuscitation Council 1993.[3]

necessary when it is impossible to ventilate through the patient's mouth. For direct mouth to mouth or mouth to nose breathing, it is important that the rescuer opens the mouth widely over the victim's slightly open mouth sealing the nose with the cheek to blow effectively into the victim's lungs. The use of barrier devices to reduce the risk of cross infection has been attempted but only face masks with one way valves offer any protection. The flexible masks used for delivery of continuous oxygen therapy are not suitable for this purpose. An anaesthetic type face mask may be suitable as long as it is able to cover the mouth and nose of the patient and can provide an airtight seal, and does not provide any resistance to expired air flow. It is important that the narrow end of the mask is placed on the bridge of the nose and the mask is applied firmly to achieve an effective seal.[3]

Initial expired air resuscitation commences with two initial inflations over 1.5–2 seconds each (American Heart Association Recommendation[1]) or five full inflations within 10 seconds (Australian Resuscitation Council Recommendation[2]) and is then continued at the rate of 10–12 (AHA) or up to 15 (ARC) inflations per minute. Ventilation then continues in conjunction with external chest compression in a ratio of two breaths per 15 compressions for a single operator and one breath after five compressions for two operators.

Face mask and assisted ventilation

Despite the proven efficacy of rescue breathing with expired air resuscitation, there are understandable concerns about cross infection and aesthetics with this technique, particularly in the hospital setting when alternative methods are commonly available. In circumstances where ventilatory equipment is available the use of a face mask and assisted ventilation is the preferred method. Standards for bag-valve-mask units for assisted ventilation have been described and include easy cleaning and sterilization, low resistance to air or oxygen inflow, and standard fittings, and preferably should deliver oxygen rather than air.[7] Although these devices can be operated by a single operator, two operators are preferable to provide an adequate seal with the face mask and an adequate ventilatory volume. Oxygen-powered manual trigger devices and automatic devices are used in some centres but there are concerns about introduction of air into the stomach and difficulties in synchronizing with external cardiac compression.

Oropharyngeal or nasopharyngeal airways should be inserted where possible but care is required to ensure that the device is placed correctly to avoid impaction of the tongue against the pharynx.

Rescue breathing by any technique may be associated with the introduction of air into the stomach. This is avoided by ensuring an open airway with adequate head tilt, slow ventilation and limiting the inspiration to the point at which the chest wall rises adequately but not excessively. The temptation to relieve gastric insufflation by pressure over the epigastrium should be resisted as this frequently causes reflux of gastric contents into the airways.

Circulation

Before commencing external cardiac compression the absence of a carotid pulse should be confirmed by palpation of the carotid artery. Commencing at the larynx, two fingers are slid to the groove between the trachea and the sternomastoid as demonstrated in Figure 40.3. A decision on presence or absence of the carotid pulse should take no more than 2–3 seconds.

The technique of closed chest cardiac massage described by Kouwenhoven and co-workers in 1960[8] remains the basis of the technique used today. Properly performed external cardiac compression can produce arterial systolic blood pressures of 60–80 mmHg but with low diastolic blood pressures.[9] There has been considerable research on the mechanism of achieving cardiac output during external cardiac compression. Long-standing concepts that the technique depended on the direct compression of the cardiac chambers have been expanded to recognize a role for an overall increase in intrathoracic pressure.[10] However, to date this research has not resulted in significant changes to the technique of external cardiac compression.[11] The recent work on the role of intrathoracic pressure rise has not affected the recommendation that the patient should be supine on a firm surface to achieve effective external cardiac compression.

Placement of hands on sternum

There are two methods of identifying the correct position for the placement of the hands on the lower third of the sternum.

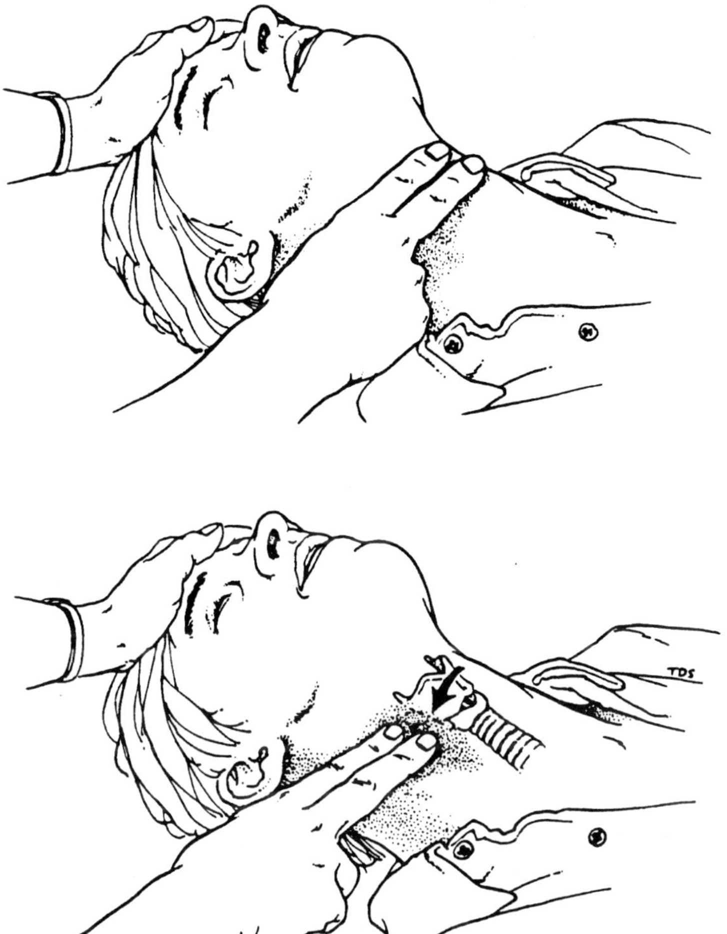

Fig. 40.3 Palpating for presence (or absence) of carotid pulsation in suspected cardiac arrest. From American Heart Association. JAMA 1992; 268: 2184–98. Copyright 1992, American Medical Association.

Caliper method

The resuscitator identifies the lower end of the sternum by running fingers on the lowest ribs on each side into the epigastrium until they meet in the middle. One index finger is left at the lower end of the sternum; the upper end of the sternum is detected with the other index finger in the notch between the clavicles. The thumbs of both hands are then used to identify the mid point of the sternum and the upper thumb is then left in position while the heel of the other thumb is placed immediately below it in the correct position to begin external cardiac compression.

Alternative method

The lower end of the sternum is detected in a similar manner as described above but the middle finger is used to mark the lower end of the sternum. The index finger of the same hand is placed adjacent to it and the heel of the other hand is placed immediately above the index finger in the correct position to begin external cardiac compression.

The heel of one hand is used for compression with the other hand either interlocking the fingers or grasping the wrist. The fingers should not press onto the thorax or the sternum during compression. The rescuer should kneel adjacent to the patient so that the arms are vertical above the thorax. The sternum should be compressed 1.5–2 inches (4–5 cm) with the heel of the hand. It is preferable to make a smooth prolonged compression rather than sharp thrusting jabs. Following compression the chest pressure must be released completely. Ventilation and chest compression should be combined in the following ratios, as described above: single operator—15 compressions and two breaths in 15 seconds; two operators—one compression per second and one breath after every five compressions.

On occasions the patient can initiate sufficient cardiac output by intrathoracic compression produced by a cough.[12] This technique is frequently used in the catheter laboratory to maintain cardiac output during bradycardias induced following coronary angiographic injection. On occasions it can be a suitable method to maintain the circulation pending the implantation of a pacemaker.

Monitoring the efficacy of resuscitation

The effectiveness of resuscitation is evaluated by checking the femoral or carotid pulse, the patient's overall colour and pupillary reactions. More reliable evaluation can be obtained from oxygen saturations or if necessary blood gas analysis.

Duration of CPR

CPR should be continued until the patient recovers or until it is clear that recovery is not going to occur despite the institution of all appropriate measures. The latter decision is frequently difficult and requires careful consideration by the most senior medical staff present.

Complications of CPR

Serious complications can occur during cardiac resuscitation including sternal fracture, rib fracture, flail chest, pneumothorax, haemothorax, contusion of the lung, laceration of the liver, rupture of the spleen and perforation of the stomach.[13] These complications are of greater concern in the current era of thrombolytic therapy and active antithrombotic therapy for acute coronary syndromes. However, normally conducted CPR without obvious bony injury is not a contraindication to subsequent thrombolytic therapy.[14]

Infection control

The major concerns during resuscitation are transmission of hepatitis B (HBV), human immunodeficiency virus (HIV), herpes simplex and tuberculosis. Adherence to standard infection control measures including the use of gloves during resuscitation and disposal of bodily fluids and sharps will reduce the risk of transmission (see Ch. 83). Transmission of HBV and HIV infection during mouth to mouth resuscitation is unlikely[15] and has not been documented to date,[1] but transmission of HIV from patients to health care workers by infected blood products through penetration of the skin has been documented in other circumstances[16] and instances of herpes transmission during CPR have been reported.[17] The risks are predominantly related to mouth to mouth resuscitation and can be substantially reduced by the preferential use of mechanical ventilation devices.

References

1. American Heart Association Emergency Cardiac Care Committee and Subcommittees. Guidelines for cardiopulmonary resuscitation and emergency cardiac care (Pt II). Adult basic life support. JAMA 1992; 268: 2184–98
2. European Resuscitation Council. Guidelines for basic and advanced life support. Resuscitation 1992; 24: 103–22
3. Australian Resuscitation Council. Cardiopulmonary resuscitation. Melbourne: Australian Resuscitation Council, 1993
4. National Heart Foundation. Cardiopulmonary resuscitation. Heart Lung Resuscitation. Canberra: National Heart Foundation, 1992
5. Heimlich HJ. A life-saving maneuver to prevent food choking. JAMA 1975; 234: 398–401
6. Safar P, Escarraga LA, Elam JO. A comparison of the mouth to mouth and mouth to airway methods of artificial respiration with the chest-pressure arm-lift methods. N Engl J Med 1958; 258: 671–7
7. Emergency Cardiac Care Committee and Subcommittees. Guidelines for cardiopulmonary resuscitation and emergency cardiac care (Pt III). Adult Advanced Cardiac Life Support. JAMA 1992; 268: 2199–241
8. Kouwenhoven WB, Jude JR, Knickerbocker GG. Closed chest cardiac massage. JAMA 1960; 173: 1064–7
9. Paradis NA, Martin GB, Goetting MG et al. Simultaneous aortic jugular bulb and right atrial pressures during cardiopulmonary resuscitation in humans: insights into mechanisms. Circulation 1989; 80: 361–8
10. Taylor GJ, Tucker WM, Greene HL, Rudikoff MT, Weisfeldt ML. Importance of prolonged compression during cardiopulmonary resuscitation in man. N Engl J Med 1977; 296: 1515–7
11. Sack JB, Kesselbrenner MB, Bregman D. Survival from in-hospital cardiac arrest with interposed abdominal counter-pulsation during cardiopulmonary resuscitation. JAMA 1992; 267: 379–85
12. Criley JM, Blaufuss AH, Kissel GL. Cough induced cardiac compression: self administered form of cardiopulmonary resuscitation. JAMA 1976; 236: 1246–50
13. Krischer JP, Fine EG, Davis JH, Nagel EL. Complications of cardiac resuscitation. Chest 1987; 92: 287–91
14. Neches RB, Goldfarb AM. Thrombolytic therapy after cardiopulmonary resuscitation in acute myocardial infarction. Am J Cardiol 1993; 71: 258
15. San De MA. Transmission of Aids: the case against casual contagion. N Engl J Med 1986; 314: 380–2
16. Marcus R. Surveillance of health care workers exposed to blood from patients infected with the

human immunodeficiency virus. N Engl J Med 1988; 319: 1118–23

17. Hendricks AA, Shapiro EP. Primary herpes simplex infection following mouth to mouth resuscitation. JAMA 1980; 243: 257–8

41 Advanced cardiac life support

Peter L Thompson

Introduction

The nature of cardiac arrest is such that randomized controlled data to guide best practice in advanced cardiac life support have been difficult to obtain. In the past, recommendations were based largely on individual experience and opinion, and as a result practice varied widely between hospitals. The situation is now changing rapidly and international sharing of data and experience at international symposia has allowed the development of some consensus. The recommendations of a large number of experts coordinated by the Emergency Cardiac Care Committee of the American Heart Association resulted in the publication of a consensus statement in 1992.[1] This detailed document is an authoritative and highly recommended statement, reprints of which should be available in every coronary care unit. A more succinct summary of recommendations has been developed to guide practice in Australia by the Advanced Life Support Committee of the Australian Resuscitation Council.[2] These two documents form the basis of the recommendations in this chapter.

Advanced cardiac life support in the CCU

Despite recent advances in acute cardiac care, cardiac arrest is still a frequent occurrence in most coronary care units (CCUs) and the CCU should be a centre of excellence in the management of this emergency. Basic life support with cardiac pulmonary resuscitation (CPR) (see Ch. 40) and more advanced cardiac life support frequently blend into each other in the CCU, because of ease of recognition of the cardiac rhythm, ready access to face mask and endotracheal intubation and the availability of venous access. Advanced cardiac life support is dealt with under the familiar CPR headings of ABC (*airway, breathing, circulation*) with the addition of DD (*defibrillation* and *drugs*). Frequently this sequence may need to be altered, and there are situations in the CCU where immediate defibrillation is more appropriate than standard CPR.

Airway

In CCU practice, resuscitation is usually commenced with a face mask and hand-operated bag of the Ambu or Oxyviva type. There are frequent difficulties in maintaining an adequate seal with the face mask, particularly in edentulous patients. The difficulties in face mask placement and operation of the ventilator bag frequently require two operators, and the pressures generated by the face mask may encourage gastric distension with the potential for aspiration of gastric contents. Therefore endotracheal intubation is the preferred method of maintaining the airway in any patient who does not stabilize immediately on initial resuscitation. However, endotracheal intubation requires a certain level of skill. Correct placement of the endotracheal tube can only be assumed when the entry of the tube through the vocal cords has been visualized through the laryngoscope. The tube is placed with the occlusive cuff just below the cords and the cuff is inflated with just enough air to occlude the airway. Correct placement of the tube is confirmed by auscultation over the epigastrium during the first inflation. If stomach gurgling occurs and no rise and fall of the thorax is observed, incorrect placement in the oesophagus must be assumed and the tube repositioned. When placement in the trachea is confirmed, auscultation over both lungs at the apex and base should be performed to ensure that the endotracheal tube has not preferentially intubated a main bronchus. When correct placement of the tube has been confirmed, the tube is secured. If feasible the correct position of the tube should be confirmed on a chest X-ray.

A variety of alternatives to the endotracheal tube have been described[1] but none is widely used.

Mechanical suction with a large bore non-kinking tube must be readily available to assist with suction of the oropharynx.

Breathing

Ventilation with a bag-valve-mask is the standard technique for initiating resuscitation. If endotracheal intubation is performed, resuscitation continues with the bag valve device. It is essential that all connectors in the CCU be compatible to ensure rapid transition of the bag valve device to the endotracheal tube. Oxygen-powered manually triggered ventilators are useful because they may free up staff for other tasks. However, high flow rates can be generated sufficient to cause gastric insufflation, and for this reason they should not be used with the face mask but their use restricted to the intubated patient.

Transportable automatic ventilators are available for out-of-hospital transport of intubated patients and may be used in hospital if prolonged transport is necessary and staff are not available for manual ventilation. Some studies have suggested an advantage of the automated ventilators over manual ventilation for prolonged resuscitation and transport of the intubated patient.[3,4]

Circulation

The technique of external cardiac compression for cardiopulmonary resuscitation has been described in Chapter 40. Transfer to clinical practice of the laboratory data on the role of abdominal compression in improving haemodynamics during cardiopulmonary resuscitation[5] has produced some encouraging preliminary reports[6] but not sufficient to modify the standard technique of external cardiac compression. A variety of mechanical chest compressors have been described to overcome fatigue in prolonged resuscitations and these can produce haemodynamics equivalent to manual compression.[7] Delays in setting up and the frequent need for repositioning of the head of the mechanical compressor over the sternum are irritations which can only be overcome with training and frequent use. A vest to encircle the trunk and produce a generalized increased in intrathoracic pressure, rather than sternal compression, has been studied and may produce improved haemodynamics but to date there is no data on improved survival.

Ventricular assist devices (see Ch. 47) have been used in some specialized units for intra-hospital transport of cardiac arrest patients.[9]

Defibrillation

In patients whose cardiac arrest is due to rapid ventricular tachycardia (VT) or ventricular fibrillation (VF), immediate defibrillation is the most effective element of the resuscitation. The delay between onset of arrest and defibrillation is the most important determinant of outcome.[10,11] In most situations when the patient is on continuous electrocardiogram (ECG) monitoring the cardiac rhythm will be clear. Occasionally low amplitude VF may be mistaken for asystole and it is important to check several ECG leads before excluding the possibility of VF.[12] Alternatively, patient movement or electrode interference may give the appearance of VF when the true cardiac rhythm is asystole. With modern 'through the paddle' defibrillation monitors there is little need for 'blind' defibrillation.

The initial pre-cordial shock should be 200 joules.[13] Following the first shock there is a drop in the transthoracic impedance, and a repeat shock of 200 joules will deliver a greater energy to the heart. If two shocks of 200 joules are ineffective, higher energy shocks up to the maximum output of the defibrillator (usually 360–400 joules) may be necessary. The usual defibrillator paddle positions are over the base of the heart slightly to the right of the sternum and the apex of the heart slightly lateral to the nipple. For refractory VF, antero-posterior paddle positions may be tried.[14] It is important to ensure that the paddle positions are not too close to each other to allow arcing between them or that there is too much gel on the chest to allow preferential passage of the shock around the chest wall rather than through the heart.

The defibrillator must be kept on immediate standby and in

excellent working condition in the CCU and any area where cardiac arrest is likely to occur. Development of staff skills in defibrillation is an essential component of staff development in the CCU and this is likely to be facilitated in the future with the introduction of 'intelligent' defibrillators which determine the need for defibrillation based on the electrocardiographic appearances.

Repeated shocks may sometimes be necessary in patients with protracted cardiac arrest. This may cause hyperaemia or even superficial burns which may require treatment with a soothing ointment or local application of a low dose steroid cream such as hydrocortisone 1%.

Precordial thump

A single precordial thump may sometimes revert ventricular tachycardia;[15] however it is ineffective for VF and may convert VT to asystole.[16] It may be considered as first line therapy if the rhythm is rapid VT while awaiting the arrival of the defibrillator, or as a single thump while clarifying the electrocardiographic diagnosis. It should never delay the institution of advanced cardiac life support and immediate defibrillation.

External cardiac pacing

The development of reliable transcutaneous cardiac pacing has been a significant advance in the management of patients with asystolic cardiac arrest.[17] It is effective only in patients with well preserved cardiac function whose cardiac arrest is due to bradycardia such as sinus arrest or complete atrioventricular block (see the information box). In such patients transcutaneous pacing can be effective for maintaining the cardiac rhythm while awaiting the implantation of a transvenous pacing wire. On occasions muscle twitching can be distressing but this can sometimes be overcome by repositioning the pacing electrodes or administration of a narcotic or benzodiazepine. Transcutaneous pacing is of no value in patients whose cardiac arrest is due to asystole following progressive cardiac dysfunction. The external pacemaker has been used for termination of ventricular tachycardia.[19]

Some modern defibrillators use adhesive conductive patches which can be used interchangeably for external pacing and defibrillation. In the patient at particularly high risk of cardiac arrest (see the box) such electrodes should be in position with the defibrillator/external pacemaker on standby.

Indications for emergent or standby pacing. Reproduced with permission from Journal of American Medical Association 1992.[1]

Emergent pacing

- Haemodynamically compromising bradycardias*
  (BP <80 mmHg systolic, change in mental status, myocardial ischaemia, pulmonary oedema)
- Bradycardia with malignant escape rhythms
  (unresponsive to pharmacologic therapy)
- Overdrive pacing of refractory tachycardia
  Supraventricular or ventricular (currently indicated only in special situations refractory to pharmacologic therapy or cardioversion)
- Bradyasystolic cardiac arrest
  Pacing not routinely recommended in such patients. If used at all, pacing should be used as early as possible after onset of arrest.

Standby pacing

- Stable bradycardias
  (BP >80 mmHg, no evidence of haemodynamic compromise, or haemodynamic compromise responsive to initial drug therapy)
- Prophylactic pacing in acute myocardial infarction
  Symptomatic sinus node dysfunction
  Mobitz II second-degree heart block
  Third-degree heart block
  Newly acquired: left bundle branch block, right bundle branch block, alternating bundle branch block or bifascicular block

*Include complete heart block, symptomatic second-degree heart block, symptomatic sick sinus syndrome, drug-induced bradycardias (i.e. digoxin, beta blockers, calcium channel blockers, or procainamide), permanent pacemaker failure, idioventricular bradycardias, symptomatic atrial fibrillation with slow ventricular response, refractory bradycardia during resuscitation of hypovolaemic shock, and bradyarrhythmias with malignant ventricular escape mechanisms.

Drugs

Venous access

Adequate venous access (Ch. 39) is essential for effective advanced cardiac life support. The patency of an indwelling intravenous (IV) line should be established and if such a line is not available it should be established immediately. If a peripheral vein cannot be accessed, central venous cannulation should be undertaken but it is important that this should not delay the performance of CPR, intubation or defibrillation. If a peripheral vein is used it is important to be aware that peripherally administered drugs may take 2–3 minutes to reach the central circulation and should be rapidly administered by bolus injection followed by a push of IV fluid and elevation of the extremity.[20] If the femoral vein is used, a long cannula should be positioned above the diaphragm as subdiaphragmatic blood flow may be minimal during resuscitation.[21]

The dosages for drugs used in advanced cardiac life support are summarised in Table 41.1, and the flow chart for administration is shown in Figure 41.1.

Endotracheal administration

On occasions if venous access is not achieved, drugs can be administered through the endotracheal tube. This can result in satisfactory absorption if the drug is administered in 10 ml of normal saline in a dose of 2–2.5 times the standard intravenous dose.[22]

Adrenaline (epinephrine)

Adrenaline (epinephrine) is now recommended as the initial drug therapy for cardiac arrest in view of its beneficial effects on cerebral and coronary blood flow and because of its alpha adrenergic properties.[23,24] (There have been concerns about the beta adrenergic effects causing increase in myocardial oxygen consumption, and there are still some reservations about its universal use for cardiac arrest in patients with MI.) These benefits are achieved with the standard dose of 1 mg. There has been careful examination of the role of higher doses such as 5 mg in cardiac arrest. Benefits were demonstrated in experimental models and in preliminary human application but there has been no improvement in outcome in randomized clinical trials of standard versus high dose adrenaline.[1] However, repeated doses of 1 mg can be used and are recommended.

Lignocaine (lidocaine)

Lignocaine is recommended as the first line antiarrhythmic drug when VF or VT persists after defibrillation and administration of adrenaline. The initial dose is 1–1.5 mg/kg (approximately 75–100 mg) given as a bolus. The dose can be repeated but there is a risk of lignocaine toxicity if the total dose exceeds 3 mg/kg (approximately 200 mg).[25]

Bretylium

Bretylium has anti-fibrillatory properties[26] but is no more effective than lignocaine in direct comparison.[27] It is used as a second line antiarrhythmic if defibrillation, adrenaline and lignocaine have failed to control VF. The dose is 5 mg/kg given intravenously as a bolus followed by defibrillation.

Atropine

Atropine is useful in cardiac arrest due to sinus bradycardia and sometimes in other bradyarrhythmias.[28] The dose is 0.5–1.0 mg intravenously. In the presence of MI the resultant increase in heart rate may cause extension of myocardial ischaemia[29] and there have been isolated reports of atropine-induced VF.[30]

Sodium bicarbonate

Tissue acidosis results from cardiac arrest due to low blood flow and inadequate ventilation. The routine reversal of this acidosis with sodium bicarbonate is no longer recommended in cardiac arrest because of potentially adverse effects and no demonstration of improved outcome.[31,32] However there may be a role for bicarbonate after protracted arrest, preferably guided by blood gas analysis. The initial dose is 1 mmol/kg intravenously.

Magnesium

Magnesium deficiency can be associated with cardiac arrhythmias, and supplementation can reduce the frequency of postinfarction arrhythmias;[33,34] however there has been no clear demonstration of the benefits of magnesium administration in MI. The dose of magnesium sulphate is 1–2 g (8–16 milli equivalents) in 50–100 ml of 5% dextrose administered over 5–60 minutes, followed by an infusion of 0.5–1 g (4–8 milli equivalents) per hour for 24 hours.

Potassium

In the patient with established hypokalaemia, the administration of potassium may be effective in refractory VF. A dose of 2–5 mmol is given intravenously.

Calcium

Calcium may be helpful in patients with hyperkalaemia, hypocalcaemia or overdose of calcium channel blocking drugs. The dose is 5–10 ml of 10% calcium chloride.

The dosages of drugs used in advanced cardiac life support are summarized in Table 41.1.

Algorithm/flow chart

The 1992 report from the Emergency Cardiac Care Committee of the American Heart Association contains a variety of detailed algorithms for the management of a variety of emergency situations requiring advanced cardiac life support. The algorithms are relatively complex and require careful study. The advanced life support flow chart recommended by the Advanced Life Support Committee of the Australian Resuscitation Council is reproduced in Figure 41.1 and provides a readily understandable flow chart for VF or pulseless VT, asystole or electromechanical dissociation.

For VF or pulseless VT it highlights the importance of several attempts at defibrillation before considering drug therapy. It recommends adrenaline as the initial drug therapy and only recommends antiarrhythmic drugs if VF persists despite initial measures.

In asystole and electromechanical dissociation, the first line of drug therapy is adrenaline, as electromechanical dissociation is frequently due to cardiac rupture. It is recommended that the cause be identified.

The use of sodium bicarbonate is no longer considered routine but may be considered if the arrest is protracted. Calcium chloride is also no longer routine but may be used in specialized circumstances.

Table 41.1 Summary of dosages of drugs used in advanced cardiac life support. Reproduced with permission from American Medical Association. JAMA 1992; 16: 268: 2199–2241. Copyright 1992.

Drug	Dose
Adrenaline (epinephrine)	1 mg repeated each 3–5 min
Lignocaine (lidocaine)	1.0–1.5 mg/kg
Bretylium	5 mg/kg
Atropine	0.5–1.0 mg
Sodium bicarbonate	1 mmol/kg
Magnesium (as $MgSO_4$)	1–2 g (8–16 m/Eq), then 0.5–1 g (4–8 m/Eq)/h for 24 hrs
Potassium	2–5 mmol
Calcium	5–10 ml of 10% calcium chloride

Breaking bad news

Breaking news of a cardiac arrest or death to family and friends should follow a set protocol. This is an important duty for coronary care staff, and performed in an inappropriate or apparently uncaring manner can have adverse emotional effects on survivors,[35,36] as well as potential medico-legal consequences. The following recommendations to improve communication in this area are partly derived from the 1992 publications of the Emergency Cardiac Care Committee of the American Heart Association.[1,37]

- Immediately notify the family (and others if appropriate) that the situation is serious. If they are not in the hospital, their immediate attendance should be advised. Sudden death should not be notified on the telephone.
- Relatives should be taken to a private room to await informed news or confirmation of death.
- A member of the staff familiar with details of the case should be responsible for communicating with the relatives. Progress reports during a prolonged resuscitation may be appropriate.
- In the event of death, briefly describe the circumstances. Avoid euphemisms such as 'he's passed on', 'she's no longer with us' or 'he's left us.' Instead use the words 'dying' or 'death'.
- Allow time. Share the human tragedy. 'You have my (our) sincere sympathy' is preferable to 'I am (we are) sorry.' Ensure the events leading to the death

are understood. Encourage grieving.

- Allow the immediate family the opportunity to see their relative; if monitoring and resuscitation equipment are connected, let them know, or preferably remove the equipment. The patient should be disconnected from the ECG monitor to avoid confusion from ECG artefacts.
- Know the sequence of death certificates, disposition of the body, to give clear instructions and support to the family.
- Ensure support from clergy, family friends, family physician where appropriate.
- Arrange follow-up and support during the bereavement.

Advanced life support flowchart

Arrest

- Witnessed/monitored → No pulse → Precordial thump → Basic life support
- Unwitnessed → No pulse → Basic life support

Basic life support →

VF or pulseless VT
→ Defibrillate 200 J
→ Defibrillate 200 J
→ Defibrillate 360 J
→ • Intravenous access • Adrenaline 1 mg bolus IV. Repeat every 3–5 min until return of spontaneous circulation • ETT + IPPV with 100% oxygen
→ Defibrillate 60 J if fails
→ Lignocaine 1 mg/kg IV CPR 60 s
→ Defibrillate 60 J if fails
→ Consider second line antiarrhythmic (bretylium 5 mg/kg IV)
→ Consider NaHCO3 1 mmol/kg IV +

Asystole
→ • Intravenous access • Adrenaline 1 mg bolus IV. Repeat every 3–5 min until return of spontaneous circulation • ETT + IPPV with 100% oxygen
→ Consider $NaHCO_3$ 1 mmol/kg IV + Atropine 1 mg IV

Electromechanical dissociation
→ Find and treat reversible causes
→ • Intravenous access • Adrenaline 1 mg bolus IV. Repeat every 3–5 min until return of spontaneous circulation • ETT + IPPV with 100% oxygen
→ Consider $NaHCO_3$ 1 mmol/kg IV

Note
- Minimise interruptions to CPR during manoeuvres
- Continued CPR between steps
- If no return of spontaneous circulation move to next step
- After initial steps seek cause (e.g., hypovolaemia, tension pneumothorax, acidosis, pulmonary embolus)
- If return of spontaneous circulation go to post-arrest management
- Consider calcium chloride 10% 5–10 mL in overdose of calcium channel blockers, hypocalcaemia and hyperkalaemia

Fig. 41.1 Advanced life support flow chart. Reproduced by permission of the Australian Resuscitation Council Advanced Life Support Committee from the Medical Journal of Australia 1993.[2]
Adrenaline = epinephrine; Lignocaine = lidocaine; ETT = endotracheal intubation; IPPV = intermittent positive pressure ventilation; J = joules.

References

1. American Heart Association. Emergency Cardiac Care Committee and Subcommittees. Guidelines for cardiopulmonary resuscitation and emergency cardiac care. Part III. Adult advanced cardiac life support. JAMA 1992; 16: 2199–241
2. The Advanced Life Support Committee of the Australian Resuscitation Council. Adult advanced cardiac life support. The Australian Resuscitation Council Guidelines. Med J Aust 1993; 159: 616–21
3. Weg JG, Haas CF. Safe intrahospital transport of critically ill ventilator-dependent patients. Chest 1989; 96: 631–5
4. Braman SS, Dunn SM, Amico CA, Millman RP. Complications of intrahospital transport in critically ill patients. Ann Intern Med 1987; 107: 469–73
5. Rudikoff MT, Maughan WL, Effron M, Freund P, Weisfeldt ML. Mechanisms of blood flow during cardiopulmonary resuscitation. Circulation 1980; 61: 345–52
6. Sack JB, Kesselbrenner MB, Bregman D. Survival from in-hospital cardiac arrest with interposed abdominal counter-pulsation during

cardiopulmonary resuscitation. JAMA 1992; 267: 379–85
7. Taylor CJ, Rubin R, Tucker M, Greene HL, Rudikoff MT, Weisfeldt ML. External cardiac compression: a randomized comparison of mechanical and manual techniques. JAMA 1978; 240: 644–6
8. Swenson RD, Weaver WD, Niskanen RA, Martin J, Dahlberg S. Hemodynamics in humans during conventional and experimental methods of cardiopulmonary resuscitation. Circulation 1988; 78: 630–9
9. Hartz R, LoCicero J III, Sanders JH Jr, Frederiksen JW, Joob AW, Michaelis LL. Clinical experience with portable cardiopulmonary bypass in cardiac arrest patients. Ann Thorac Surg 1990; 50: 437–41
10. Eisenberg MS, Copass MK, Hallstrom AP et al. Treatment of out-of-hospital cardiac arrests with rapid defibrillation by emergency medical technicians. N Engl J Med 1980; 302: 1379–83
11. Stults KR, Brown DD, Schug VL, Bean JA. Prehospital defibrillation performed by emergency medical technicians in rural communities. N Engl J Med 1984; 310: 219–23
12. Ewy GA, Dahl CF, Zimmerman M, Otto C. Ventricular fibrillation masquerading as ventricular standstill. Crit Care Med 1981; 9: 841–4
13. Weaver WD, Cobb LA, Copass MK, Hallstrom AP. Ventricular defibrillation; a comparative trial using 175-J and 320-J shocks. N Engl J Med 1982; 307: 1101–6
14. Kerber RE, Jensen SR, Grayzel J, Kennedy J, Hoyt R. Elective cardioversion: influence of paddle-electrode location and size on successful rates and energy requirements. N Engl J Med 1981; 305: 658–62
15. Pennington JE, Taylor J, Lown B. Chest thump for reverting ventricular tachycardia. N Engl J Med 1970; 283: 1192–5
16. Caldwell G, Millar G, Quinn E, Vincent R, Chamberlain DA. Simple mechanical methods for cardioversion: defence of the precordial thump and cough version. BMJ 1985; 291: 627–30
17. Zoll PM, Zoll RH, Falk RH, Clinton JE, Eitel DR, Antman EM. External noninvasive temporary cardiac pacing: clinical trials. Circulation 1985; 71: 937–44
18. Falk RH, Zoll PM, Zoll RH. Safety and efficacy of noninvasive cardiac pacing: a preliminary report. N Engl J Med 1983; 309: 1166–8
19. Rosenthal ME, Stamato NJ, Marchlinski FE, Josephson ME. Noninvasive cardiac pacing for termination of sustained, uniform ventricular tachycardia. Am J Cardiol 1986; 58: 561–2
20. Emerman CL, Pinchak AC, Hancock D, Hagen JF. The effect of bolus injection on circulation times during cardiac arrest. Am J Emerg Med 1990; 8: 190–3
21. Emerman CL, Bellon EM, Lukens TW, May TE, Effron D. A prospective study of femoral versus subclavian vein catheterization during cardiac arrest. Ann Emerg Med 1990; 19: 26–30
22. Aitkenhead AR. Drug administration during CPR: what route? Resuscitation 1991; 22: 191–5
23. Otto C, Yakaitis R. The role of epinephrine in CPR: a reappraisal. Ann Emerg Med 1987; 16: 743–8
24. Paradis NA, Koscove EM. Epinephrine in cardiac arrest: a critical review. Ann Emerg Med 1990; 19: 1288–301
25. De Silva RA, Hennekens CH, Lown B, Casscells W. Lignocaine prophylaxis in acute myocardial infarction: An evaluation of randomised trials. Lancet 1981; 2: 855–8
26. Koch-Weser J. Drug therapy: bretylium. N Engl J Med 1979; 300: 473–7
27. Haynes RE, Chinn TL, Copass MK, Cobb LA. Comparison of bretylium tosylate and lidocaine in management of out of hospital ventricular fibrillation: a randomized clinical trial. Am J Cardiol 1981; 48: 353–6
28. Stueven HA, Tonsfeldt DJ, Thompson BM, Whitcomb J, Kastenson E, Aprahamian C. Atropine in asystole: human studies. Ann Emerg Med 1984; 13(pt2): 815–7
29. Knoebel SB, McHeary PL, Phillips JF, Widlansky S. Atropine induced cardio-acceleration and myocardial blood flow in subjects with and without coronary artery disease. Am J Cardiol 1974; 33: 327–32
30. Cooper MJ, Abinader EG. Atropine induced ventricular fibrillation: case report and review of the literature. Am Heart J 1979; 97: 225–8
31. Bishop RL, Westfeldt ML. Sodium bicarbonate administration during cardiac arrest. JAMA 1976; 235: 506–9
32. Redding JS, Pearson JW. Resuscitation from ventricular fibrillation: drug therapy. JAMA 1968; 203: 255–260
33. Teo KK, Yusuf S, Collins R, Held PH, Peto R. Effects of intravenous magnesium in suspected acute myocardial infarction: overview of randomised trials. BMJ 1991; 303: 1499–503
34. Woods KL, Fletcher S, Roffe C, Haider Y. Intravenous magnesium sulphate in suspected acute myocardial infarction: results of the second Leicester Intravenous Magnesium Intervention Trial (LIMIT-2). Lancet 1992; 339: 1553–8
35. Parkes CM. Recent bereavement as a cause of mental illness. Br J Psych 1964; 110: 198–204
36. Dubin WR, Saunoff JR. Sudden unsuspected death; intervention with the survivors. Ann Emerg Med 1986; 15: 54–7
37. Burkle FM Jr, Rice MM. Code organization. Am J Emerg Med 1987; 5: 235–9

42 Cardioversion and defibrillation

Stephen PF Gordon

Definitions

Cardioversion refers to the delivery of a precisely timed electrical shock to the heart in order to revert certain susceptible arrhythmias (other than ventricular fibrillation).

Defibrillation refers to the delivery of a high energy non-synchronized shock to the heart for the emergency treatment of ventricular fibrillation (VF) or very rapid ventricular tachycardia (VT).

Theory

Modern defibrillators produce a direct current (DC) discharge which passes between two electrodes (hand-held paddles or adhesive patches) applied to the chest wall. The electrical current depolarizes the myocardium through which it passes, thus interrupting the continuous re-entry circuits which propagate many arrhythmias, and allowing restoration of normal rhythm.

Proper paddle position is important to ensure as much myocardium as possible is depolarized, as re-entry circuits may continue in non-depolarized tissue allowing continuation of the arrhythmia.

The amount of current passing through the heart is determined by both the energy level selected and the transthoracic impedance. The latter is determined by patient characteristics, such as chest wall shape and thickness, and physical factors such as paddle size and contact pressure.[1]

Arrhythmias which involve myocardial re-entry circuits (atrial fibrillation, atrial flutter, atrio-ventricular tachycardias, and ventricular tachycardia) tend to respond best to cardioversion, with a high success rate. Non-re-entry arrhythmias (accelerated idioventricular rhythm, parasystole, focal atrial tachycardias, triggered automaticity) tend to respond poorly, though cardioversion may occasionally be successful in some cases.

During cardioversion, precise timing of the electrical discharge is critical in order to avoid induction of ventricular fibrillation, the risk of which is greatest if the discharge falls in the 'vulnerable period' which is maximal in the 30 ms prior to the apex of the T wave (Fig. 42.1).

The defibrillator should therefore have a method of 'synchronizing' the shock with the patient's electrocardiograph (ECG) so that the discharge is delivered within the QRS complex, thus avoiding the vulnerable period.[2] Synchronization should be used in all arrhythmias except VF and very rapid ventricular tachycardia (ventricular flutter).

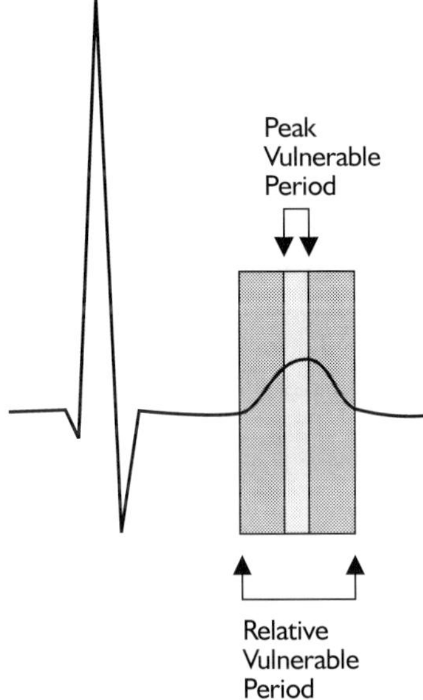

Fig. 42.1 The cardiac electrical cycle showing the 'relative vulnerable period' during which there exists a risk of inducing VF, and the 'peak vulnerable period' during which the risk of inducing VF is greatest.

Cardioversion

Indications

Urgent cardioversion is indicated in arrhythmias which are causing hypotension, acute cardiac failure, or acute ischaemia, or when drug therapy has failed to revert. Non-urgent cardioversion may be indicated in chronic arrhythmias which fail to revert after a period of drug therapy, or when drug therapy is contraindicated, or not tolerated.

Relative contraindications

- Digoxin toxicity may increase the risk of cardioversion, provoking high grade ventricular arrhythmias including ventricular fibrillation. Arrhythmias secondary to digoxin toxicity should not be cardioverted. If there is any doubt, an urgent digoxin assay should be sought.
- High risk of thromboembolism—for example, chronic atrial fibrillation without prior anticoagulation.
- Severe uncorrected electrolyte imbalance or metabolic disorder.
- Underlying sick sinus syndrome or severe conduction system disease.
- Where the chance of success is low, or the risk of arrhythmia recurrence is high (see below).

Equipment and facilities

The defibrillator should be capable of providing synchronized or non-synchronized DC shocks over a range of selected energies. The shock may be delivered through hand-held paddles or by self-adhesive pads applied to the chest wall.

The equipment should be checked regularly to ensure it meets accepted safety standards, including proper synchronization and programmed energy output.

Continuous ECG monitoring and full resuscitation facilities, with emergency drugs close at hand, are mandatory.

Preparation for cardioversion

Consent

It is important that the patient be adequately prepared for the cardioversion procedure (see checklist in the information box). If the patient's condition allows, a full explanation should be given and written informed consent obtained.

Fasting

The patient should be fasted for at least 6 hours prior to cardioversion to avoid aspiration during sedation and anaesthesia.

Optimize patient status

Except in emergency situations, the patient's metabolic and haemodynamic status should be optimized. This should include assessment and correction of any electrolyte or blood gas abnormalities, and exclusion of drug toxicity. Digoxin need not be withheld provided toxicity has been excluded.[3]

Anticoagulation

Where there is a risk of thromboembolism (e.g. chronic atrial fibrillation) warfarin anticoagulation at adequate level (consistent INR 2.5–3.5) for at least 2–3 weeks prior to, and following, cardioversion is indicated.[4]

Pre-cardioversion checklist

- Fast patient for 6 hours prior to procedure
- Review medications relevant to cardioversion,
  e.g. digoxin for possible digitalis excess,
  anticoagulants to ensure appropriate anticoagulation,
  diuretics for possible hypokalaemia
- Check blood test results.
  e.g. digoxin level INR/APTT, electrolytes
- Check that written informed consent has been obtained
- Ensure that patient has a patent IV line
- Ensure that lignocaine and atropine are at the bedside
- Ensure that drugs and equipment for advanced life support are readily accessible
- Apply ECG electrodes (ensure electrodes are away from proposed paddle positions, i.e. sternal and apex position)
- Select best lead positions to obtain mainly positive QRS complexes
- Remove nitroglycerin paste or patches from chest wall
- Apply oximeter and apply intranasal or facemask oxygen to achieve oxygen saturation > 95%
- Apply blood pressure monitor

Patient preparation

Patient preparation should include:

- ensuring good IV access throughout the procedure
- shaving of very hirsute patients
- continuous ECG monitoring throughout
- 100% oxygen administered for at least 5 minutes prior to cardioversion. Although there is no data on the relationship of hypoxia to success in synchronized cardioversion for supraventricular arrhythmias, it is well documented that hypoxia affects the success of ventricular defibrillation.[5] Ideally, oxygen saturation should be monitored through the procedure.
- It is important to ensure that the skin between the paddle positions is dry and free of any moisture or gel. Nitroglycerin patches must be removed from the skin, as there have been reports of localized explosions provoked by electrical sparking.[6]

Technique

Higher success rates and safer outcomes will be achieved with meticulous technique (see checklist in the information box below).

Anaesthesia

A short acting general anaesthetic agent should be used. Several agents have been evaluated and found useful including diazepam (5–20 mg intravenously), midazolam (2.5–10 mg), methohexitone (1 mg/kg), and propofol (1.5–2.5 mg/kg).[7,8]

Conductive gel

Conductive gel or gel-impregnated pads reduce transthoracic impedance[9] and should be placed on the chest wall or applied directly to the paddles.

Synchronization

Synchronized shocks should be used in all arrhythmias, except ventricular fibrillation and very rapid ventricular tachycardia associated with haemodynamic collapse. Modern defibrillators with rhythm displays allow visual confirmation of appropriate QRS complex sensing. Failure to sense appropriately the QRS, or inappropriate P or T wave sensing, may usually be overcome by adjusting the ECG gain, or using alternative monitoring lead configurations (see Fig. 42.2).

Paddle positions

Two positions are in common use. In the apex-anterior position one paddle is placed adjacent to the cardiac apex with the paddle centred in the mid-axillary line. The other paddle is placed to the right of the sternum just below the clavicle. In the apex-posterior position, the anterior paddle is placed over the cardiac apex, and the posterior paddle below the right scapula to the right of the spine.

In patients with permanent pacemakers, the paddle positions ought to be modified according to the position of the implanted pulse generator (see below).

Firm pressure is applied to both paddles to reduce transthoracic impedance.[1]

Delivery of the shock

Inspection is performed to ensure that no part of the patient is in contact with any metal object, and all attending personnel are warned to stand clear. If a synchronized shock is planned, a final check to ensure appropriate QRS sensing should be made before delivering the discharge.

Post cardioversion

The patient should be monitored for at least several hours post-reversion. Oxygen should be continued, and vital signs and airway monitored until full consciousness has returned (see checklist in the information box).

Cardioversion checklist

- Engage synchronization and check that it is synchronizing on 100% of QRS complexes. If not, change lead selection until 100% synchronization is achieved
- Apply defibrillator pads or electrode gel to chest wall; ensure clear separation of gel between the defibrillator paddle positions
- Administer sedation or light general anaesthesia
- Firmly apply defibrillator paddles ensuring no gaps between chest wall and paddles
- Re-check synchronization
- All staff stand clear from bed and contact with patient
- Deliver synchronized DC shock (see Table 42.1 for recommended energy levels)
- Check return to sinus rhythm and decide if additional DC shock necessary before sedation wears off
- Obtain ECG rhythm strip before, during and after procedure

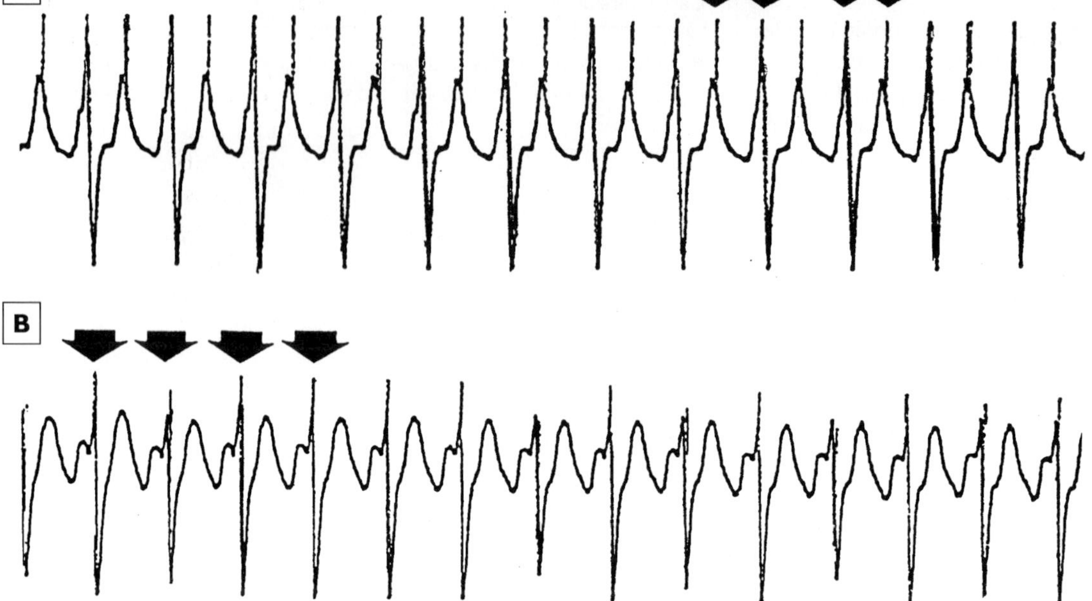

Fig. 42.2 A Defibrillator ECG strip showing inappropriate T wave sensing with sensing markers (spikes) on both QRS complexes and T waves (arrowed). B After adjustment of ECG gain and monitoring electrodes, proper sensing of only QRS complexes is obtained (arrows).

Post-cardioversion checklist

- Record vital signs and O_2 saturation immediately post procedure and each 5–10 minutes until stable
- Position patient to afford maximum airway protection
- Medical or nursing staff to remain with patient until vital signs, O_2 saturation and ECG are stable and patient can safely maintain their own airway
- Repeat 12 lead ECG post procedure
- Document drugs administered, cardioversion settings and the outcome of the procedure

Energy levels

In general the lowest possible initial energy ought be utilized, to minimize the risk of cardiac damage. It is often possible to revert ventricular tachycardia with very low energies of 10–20 joules.[10] If there is any possibility of digitalis excess a 'test dose' of 10 joules to expose ventricular arrhythmias may be considered.[3,10] Suggested initial energy levels for various arrhythmias are listed in Table 42.1. If the initial shock is unsuccessful, higher energy levels should be utilized incrementally. In resistant cases, an antiarrhythmic drug can be administered intravenously and cardioversion repeated.

Complications

- Arrhythmia: This usually occurs with improper synchronization, though occasionally a properly timed shock may induce ventricular fibrillation. This risk is greater with digitalis excess or hypokalaemia.[3] Bradycardia and asystole may occur but in most cases are transient.
- Thromboembolism: this may occur in up to 3% of patients with atrial fibrillation who have not had prior anticoagulation. Anticoagulation for a minimum of 2–3 weeks prior to cardioversion has become standard practice.[4]
- Cutaneous burns: the risk may be reduced by firm paddle pressure and correct use of conductive gel or pads. Slight reddening of the skin is common following the procedure and if necessary may be treated with topical steroid creams.
- Myocardial injury: significant myocardial necrosis is unusual.

Table 42.1 Suggested initial energy level for cardioversion/defibrillation (J = joules)

Initial energy	Arrhythmia
200 J	Ventricular fibrillation
100 J	Ventricular tachycardia
25 J	Supraventricular tachycardia
100 J	Atrial fibrillation
25 J	Atrial flutter

Total creatine kinase is often elevated following cardioversion but MB fractions are usually normal.[11] Transient ST segment elevation may occur but does not necessarily imply significant myocardial injury[12] See example on Fig. 42.3.

- Anaesthetic complications: aspiration and drug reactions may occur.
- Hypotension: hypotension is often transient and may be related to the anaesthetic agent.
- Pulmonary oedema: acute congestive cardiac failure occurs in a small number of patients.

Defibrillation

Once a diagnosis of ventricular fibrillation (or pulseless VT) is confirmed, defibrillation should be performed as quickly as possible as any delay reduces the chance of successful reversion. The shock should be unsynchronized with an initial energy setting of 200 J, and repeated immediately if unsuccessful on the first attempt. Paddle positions are the same as those described for cardioversion (see Ch. 41).

Special considerations

Atrial fibrillation

Certain parameters have been identified as predictors of a low chance of successful cardioversion, or a high risk of early recurrence. These include atrial fibrillation of greater than 12 months' duration, markedly enlarged left atrium (greater than 5 cm by echocardiogram), and atrial fibrillation associated with thyrotoxicosis, sick sinus syndrome, myocarditis/pericarditis, cardiomyopathy, and uncompensated lung disease.

Anticoagulation should be given for at least 2–3 weeks prior to cardioversion to reduce the risk of thromboembolism,[4] when the atrial fibrillation is of long-standing or unknown duration. Acute onset atrial fibrillation is generally cardioverted early provided conditions predisposing to atrial thrombus can be excluded clinically or echocardiographically and heparin has been administered. Transoesophageal echocardiography has been proposed as a method of excluding atrial thrombus prior to cardioversion.[13] As atrial mechanical function may take several weeks to return to normal following cardioversion, anticoagulation should be maintained for at least 4 weeks after successful reversion.

Pacemakers

Damage to the pulse generator is unusual, but current can be conducted through the pacing electrode causing endocardial injury, a rise in pacing threshold, and possible loss of capture. Reprogramming of selected pacing parameters may also occur. The lowest possible energies should be used, and the paddle positions modified according to the site of the implanted pulse generator to minimize current flow between the paddles and the generator. For generators in the right or left pectoral position, one paddle should be placed over the central sternum and the other below and lateral to the cardiac apex. For generators implanted in the abdomen, the apex-anterior position, described above, should be used. Facilities for re-programming pacing parameters, and if

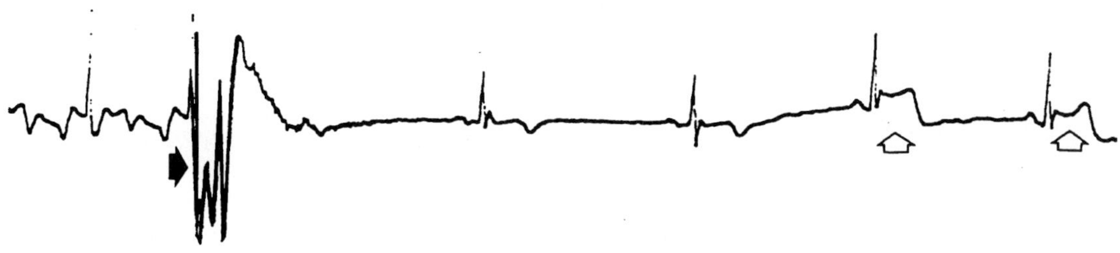

Fig. 42.3 Transient ST segment elevation (open arrows) occurring 2 beats after successful cardioversion (closed arrow).

necessary increasing pacing output, should be available immediately after cardioversion.[14,15] Back-up temporary pacing should be considered in pacemaker-dependent patients.

Pregnancy

Cardioversion during pregnancy has been reported to be safe, with the shock synchronized to the maternal ECG.[16,17] If possible, fetal ECG should also be monitored.

Care of the defibrillator/cardioverter

Immediately following the procedure, the defibrillator paddles should be washed to remove electrode paste in order to avoid pitting of the surface, which will interfere with current delivery in the future. The equipment should be stored according to the manufacturer's recommendations and there should be regular checks on the performance of the delivered dose and synchronizer mechanism. There should be a charge/discharge test of a low energy shock (e.g. 0.25 J) load on each CCU shift. It is particularly important with defibrillator/cardioverters which rely on battery power for portable use that battery levels are checked regularly.

References

1. Kerber RE, Grayzel J, Hoyt R et al. Transthoracic resistance of human defibrillation: influence of body weight, chest size, serial shocks, paddle size and paddle contact pressure. Circulation 1981; 63: 676–82
2. Wiggers CJ, Wegria R. Ventricular fibrillation due to single, localised induction and condensor shocks applied during the vulnerable phase of ventricular systole. Am J Physiol 1940; 128: 500
3. Lown B. Cardioversion and the digitalized patient. J Am Coll Cardiol 1985; 5: 889–90
4. Mancini GBJ, Goldberger AL. Cardioversion of atrial fibrillation: consideration of embolization, anticoagulation, prophylactic pacemakers and long-term success. Am Heart J 1982; 104: 617–21
5. Kerber RE, Sarnat W. Factors influencing the success of ventricular defibrillation in man. Circulation 1979; 60: 226–30
6. Babka JC. Does nitroglycerin explode? N Engl J Med 1983; 309: 379
7. Khan AH, Malhotra R. Midazolam as intravenous sedative for electrocardioversion. Chest 1989; 9: 1068–71
8. Bechleitner P, Genser N, Mitterschiffthaler G, Dienstl F. Propofol for direct current cardioversion in cardiac risk patients. Eur Heart J 1991; 12: 813–7
9. Aylward PE, Kieso R, Hite P, Charbonnier F, Kerber RE. Defibrillator electrode chest wall coupling agents: influence on transthoracic impedance and shock success. J Am Coll Cardiol 1985; 6: 682–6
10. De Silva RA, Graboys TB, Podrid PJ, Lown B. Cardioversion and defibrillations. Am Heart J 1980; 100: 881–95
11. Reiffel JA, Gambino SR, McCarthy DM, Leahey EB Jr. Direct current cardioversion: effect on creatine kinase, lactic dehydrogenase, and myocardial isoenzymes. JAMA 1978; 239: 122–4
12. Zelinger AB, Falk RH, Hood WB. Electrical-induced sustained myocardial depolarization as a possible cause for transient ST elevation post-DC elective cardioversion. Am Heart J 1982; 103: 1073–4
13. Manning WJ, Silverman DI, Gordon SPF, Krumholz HM, Douglas PS. Cardioversion from atrial fibrillation without prolonged anticoagulation with use of transesophageal echocardiography to exclude the presence of atrial thrombi. N Engl J Med 1993; 328: 750–5
14. Levine PA, Barold SS, Fletcher RD et al. Adverse acute and chronic effects of electrical defibrillation and cardioversion on implanted unipolar cardiac pacing systems. J Am Coll Cardiol 1983; 1: 1413–22
15. Gould L, Patel S, Gomes GI, Choksi AB. Pacemaker failure following external defibrillation. PACE 1981; 4: 575–7
16. Cullhed I. Cardioversion during pregnancy. Acta Med Scand 1983; 214: 169–72
17. Finlay AY, Edmunds V. DC cardioversion in pregnancy. Br J Clin Prac 1979; 33: 88–94

43 Cardiac pacemakers

Harry G Mond

The success and value of cardiac pacing in the treatment of a variety of bradyarrhythmias and tachyarrhythmias cannot be challenged. In recent years, marked advances in pacemaker battery technology, leads materials, microprocessor circuitry, programmability and telemetry together with improved implantation techniques has resulted in safe, reliable, long-life, physiologic pacing systems with remarkably few complications.

Pacemaker design

The artificial cardiac pacemaker is an integrated electrical system comprising a pulse generator and a lead. The remainder of the circuit is composed of living tissue (endocardium, myocardium and thoracic structures). The pulse generator has three major components: the encapsulating material, the power source and the electronic circuitry. The original encapsulating material was epoxy resin which, being permeable to water, allowed ingress of body fluids which destroyed the internal contents of the pulse generator. Consequently, hermetic sealing with a metal casing became essential. The major metals used today are titanium and stainless steel.

A number of power sources have been used for implantable pulse generators. The original was the alkaline zinc mercury battery which had a predicted life of 5 years but because of design limitations usually lasted less than 3 years. During the early 1970s, both a nuclear power source and a rechargeable nickel cadmium battery were used, but found wanting. At the same time the extremely reliable, hermetically sealed lithium iodine power source was introduced and this battery has completely revolutionized the pacemaker industry.

Marked developments have also occurred with pacemaker electronic circuitry. The original discrete components have now given way to sophisticated microprocessor-based circuits which allow complex physiologic pacemaker functions as well as memory, logic, programmability and telemetry. Programming is a non-invasive function which involves changing a pacing parameter by a radio-frequency link with a programmer. Telemetry involves a similar radio-frequency link in order to obtain the pacemaker status or internal measurements (real time telemetry).

The other major component of a pacemaker is the lead connecting the pulse generator to the heart. A pacemaker lead is composed of an insulated metal conductor with a connector at the proximal end which joins the lead to the pulse generator. At the distal end is the electrode; a small area of bare metal or carbon connected to the conductor responsible for transmission of the stimulus to the heart. Most pacemaker leads are implanted via the transvenous route and make contact with the endocardial surface. On occasion, the lead is attached directly to the epicardial surface or screwed into the epimyocardium.

With transvenous pacing, there must be a lead fixation device to prevent dislodgement. A simple passive fixation device such as tines behind the electrode which become anchored beneath or between trabeculae are very effective. Another fixation device is a retractable endocardial screw (see Fig. 43.1).

How pacemakers work

In order to create an electrical circuit there must be two poles. Current in the form of ions flows from the negative pole or cathode to the positive pole or anode.

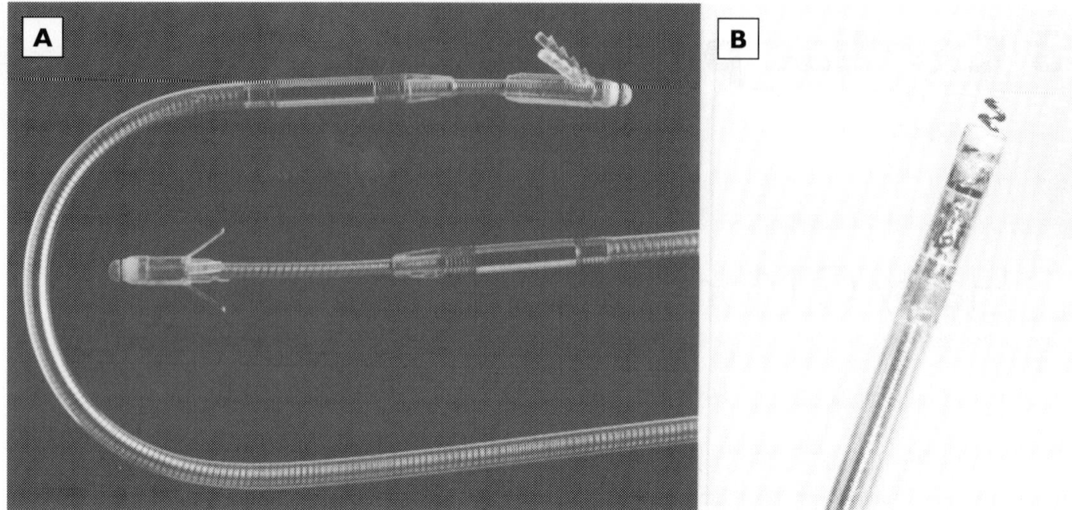

Fig. 43.1 A Tined leads. The J-shaped bipolar lead is designed for right atrial use and has two tines behind the electrode. The white collar between the tines and electrode is a silicone rubber steroid-eluting device. Following implantation, the steroid (< 1 mg dexamethasone sodium phosphate), elutes into the electrode-tissue interface and is responsible for keeping the stimulation threshold low. The straight ventricular lead is similar but has four tines.
B Retractable screw-in lead. The exposed screw for attachment to the endomyocardium is retracted at the time of implantation. When the desired position is obtained, the screw is extended using an implement at the proximal end.

Pacing leads may be unipolar or bipolar. With a unipolar system, only one electrode, the cathode, lies on the lead. The anode or metal indifferent plate lies on the surface of the implanted pulse generator. Bipolar leads have both poles on a single lead. The distal tip is the cathode and lying a short distance behind is the ring anode. A pacemaker system must pace the heart and be able to sense spontaneous intracardiac electrical potentials. Via the lead, the pacemaker will deliver, in a pulsed fashion, a small voltage to the heart. Following implantation, the electrode irritates or inflames the endocardium resulting in a rise of the stimulation threshold or amount of energy required to pace the heart. Although the initial stimulation threshold is usually less than one volt, the pulse generator must be able to cope with this rise and deliver at least 5 volts. New electrode designs, and in particular the use of steroid elution from behind the electrode or from a collar around it, will lower or even abolish this rise allowing more widespread use of programmed low voltages (see Fig. 43.1).

Types of pacing systems

A pacemaker that delivers an electrical impulse at a set repetition rate irrespective of the underlying rhythm is a fixed rate or asynchronous system. With the vast majority of pacing systems, spontaneous intracardiac potentials such as sinus beats or ectopics are recognized and the pacemaker responds appropriately, usually by inhibiting the next impulse. With modern pacing systems, all four cardiac chambers can be used for pacing or sensing. The simplest system uses only the right ventricle and is the ventricular inhibited system (see Fig. 43.2). For atrial inhibited pacing, the right atrium is used and the leads are usually inserted transvenously to the appendage as a J-tined lead or placed anywhere in the atrium using the screw-in design (Fig. 43.1). Because of atrioventricular dissociation, simple ventricular pacing is unphysiologic. The other disadvantage to ventricular pacing is the lack of rate-responsiveness which is the ability to change the rate of pacing with exercise or stress. Although atrial pacing reconstitutes atrioventricular synchrony, it nevertheless is not rate-responsive. Atrial pacing cannot be used in cases of suspected atrioventricular nodal or distal conduction tissue disease. Physiologic dual chamber pacing systems, using both atrial and ventricular leads, re-establish or maintain atrioventricular synchrony. The P wave can be sensed and after a set atrioventricular delay, the ventricle is paced. With this system, both atrioventricular synchrony and rate responsiveness are present (Fig. 43.2).

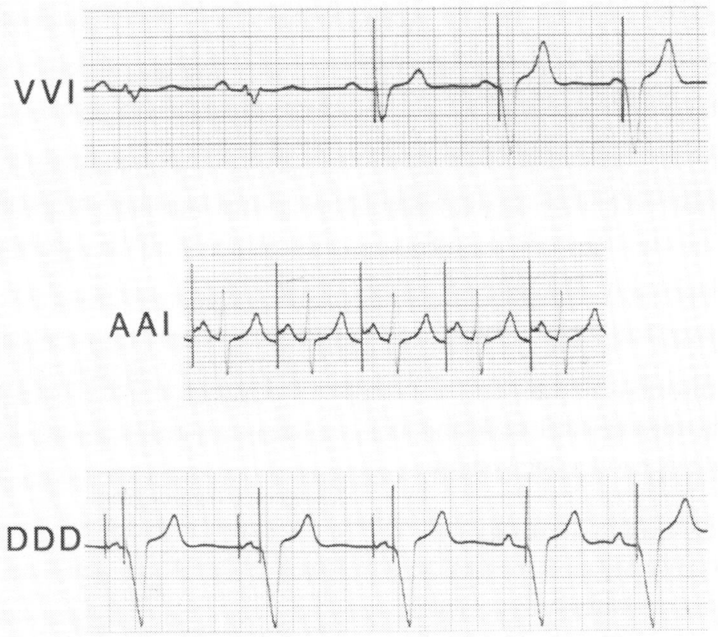

Fig. 43.2 ECGs, Lead II, demonstrating the common modes of cardiac pacing.
Above: VVI—ventricular inhibited pacing. The first two complexes are sinus and the last two unipolar ventricular pacing. With pacing, there is a prominent spike or stimulus artefact followed by a broad QRS and T wave. The middle complex is a fusion beat. Normally a sinus QRS would inhibit the pulse generator. With a fusion beat the sinus and pacing rates are similar. The atrium has depolarized and the wave of depolarization is being conducted through the ventricle but has not yet reached the pacemaker electrode. Hence this spontaneous QRS remains unsensed and the pulse generator delivers its energy into the ventricular myocardium. The resultant QRS is a hybrid of the two complexes. Fusion beats represent normal pacemaker function.
Middle: AAI—atrial inhibited pacing. There is a unipolar stimulus artefact followed by atrial depolarization and normal atrioventricular conduction. In the presence of normal sinus beats, the atrial output would be inhibited.
Below: DDD—dual chamber pacing. There is unipolar sequential atrioventricular pacing with a programmable atrioventricular delay. In the last two complexes, the sinus rate is faster than atrial pacing, resulting in atrial pacing inhibition. After a set atrioventricular delay, there is ventricular pacing.

An exciting new concept with physiologic pacemakers is rate-adaptive pacing. Instead of using the sinus mechanism to drive the ventricle, another physiologic sensor is utilized. The most popular system uses a standard lead and a vibration sensing piezo-electric crystal bonded to the inside of the pacemaker can or to the electronics. The other popular and highly physiologic sensor-based pacing system assesses changes in minute ventilation to determine the pacing rate. The system measures transthoracic impedance between a standard bipolar lead and the pulse generator casing. Both of these sensors have been incorporated into dual chamber pacemakers.

Because of the variety of pacing systems available, a three letter identification code has been developed with a fourth letter, 'R', to identify the presence of a rate-adaptive function (see the information box). Patients with electrically intact atria benefit more from single chamber atrial (AAI or AAIR) or dual chamber (DDD or DDDR) pacing compared with single chamber ventricular (VVI or VVIR) pacing. Atrial pacing and sensing results in fewer supraventricular tachyarrhythmias, fewer emboli, less stroke and cardiac failure, together with improved mortality. Most pacemaker implanters prefer dual chamber to pure atrial pacing. Because of inappropriate atrial sensing, patients with paroxysmal supraventricular tachyarrhythmias and high degree atrioventricular block have in the past been limited to ventricular pacing. Today, a variety of methods for ventricular rate protection have allowed dual chamber physiologic pacing to be more widely used in this group.[1]

Pacemaker testing

Testing of an implanted pacemaker system involves confirmation of pacing on the electrocardiogram (ECG) and measurement of battery status. When the pacemaker discharges its energy into the myocardium, a voltage deflection occurs on the ECG which is the stimulus artefact (see Fig. 43.2 above). Depending on the chamber being paced, P or QRS waves immediately follow. Not infrequently, when the ECG of a patient with a pacemaker is examined, no pacing complexes are noted. This will occur if the spontaneous rhythm is faster than the pacemaker rate and consequently inhibition of the pulse generator results (see Fig. 43.2). To confirm an intact pacing system, the pulse generator can be converted to asynchronous pacing by posi-

Three letter pacemaker code

First letter (chamber being paced); second letter (chamber being sensed)
- A—atrium
- V—ventricle
- D—atrium and ventricle

Third letter (mode or response to sensing)
- I—inhibited
- T—triggered
- D—inhibited and triggered

tioning a magnet over it. Determination of the pacemaker battery status can be assessed by measurement of the asynchronous pacing rate. Usually this falls as the power source is depleted. After a specified rate change, the pulse generator should be electively replaced. Battery status can also be determined by the use of telemetry.

Indications for pacing

The two major indications for cardiac pacing are *failure of cardiac impulse formation* and *failure of atrioventricular conduction*. These usually result from degenerative or atherosclerotic processes, which damage biological pacemaker and conductive cells as well as surrounding tissues. Indications can be divided into three classes:[2]

- Class I: there is general agreement regarding pacemaker implantation
- Class II: permanent pacemakers are frequently used, but there is a divergence of opinion with respect to the necessity of their insertion
- Class III: there is general agreement that pacemakers are unnecessary.

Disorders of the atrioventricular node and distal conducting system

Complete heart block

Permanent pacing for acquired complete heart block is usually indicated irrespective of symptoms. Asymptomatic patients are rare, and usually attribute their 'slowing down' to other age-related problems. Digitalis toxicity should be excluded. DDD pacing is indicated in patients with normal sinus activity and VVIR pacing for patients with established atrial fibrillation.

Second-degree atrioventricular block

Asymptomatic Mobitz type I block with Wenckebach phenomenon (narrow QRS) is stable and a class III indication unless the block is intra- or infra-His and hence clinically unpredictable (class II).

Mobitz type II block (wide QRS), whether permanent or intermittent, is unpredictable and progressive. Asymptomatic patients are class II and DDD pacing is preferred.

Bundle branch blocks

The presence of a bundle branch block may not be a predictor of complete heart block. Asymptomatic patients with isolated blocks, including bifascicular block and first degree atrioventricular block, are class III, but symptomatic patients (syncope) are generally regarded as class II. Alternating right and left bundle branch blocks usually require permanent pacing.

Congenital high-degree atrioventricular block

This condition is often well tolerated, especially if the ventricular escape rhythm is satisfactory. Symptomatic patients require DDD pacing. Pacing for asymptomatic patients depends on the prognosis and stability of the spontaneous ventricular pacing focus. Class II indications include competing ventricular foci, ventricular arrhythmias and ventricular rates < 45 bpm when awake.

High-degree atrioventricular block, post myocardial infarction

Indications for temporary and permanent pacing differ.

Inferior infarct—proximal block
- Temporary—for haemodynamic deterioration
- Permanent—for persistent high-degree block at the atrioventricular node (class II).

Anterior infarct—distal block with extensive septal infarction. The long term prognosis is primarily related to the extent of myocardial injury and the character of the intraventricular conduction disturbances rather than to the block itself.

- Temporary—for developing and progressive block
- Permanent—for persistent chronic high-degree atrioventricular block. Transient blocks are controversial but generally class III.

His bundle ablation

Radiofrequency His bundle ablation is very useful for intractable supraventricular tachyarrhythmias. VVIR pacing should be used for established tachyarrhythmias and DDD or DDDR pacing with ventricular rate protection if paroxysmal.

Disorders of impulse formation

The sick sinus syndrome constitutes a spectrum of episodic or persistent sinus bradycardia with periods of sinus arrest or sino-atrial block, with or without an escape junctional rhythm, and with varying degrees of atrioventricular block. Paroxysmal supraventricular tachyarrhythmias, and in particular, atrial fibrillation may also occur. Patients are usually elderly and permanent pacing is successful in eliminating or alleviating symptoms which include syncope, tiredness, congestive cardiac failure and angina. Permanent pacing is important where essential long-term drug therapy produces symptomatic bradycardia. The ultimate prognosis usually depends on the underlying cardiovascular disease. Asymptomatic patients are generally class III.

There are three levels of severity:

- Sinus bradycardia or slow junctional rhythm (chronotropic incompetence) is often benign as a result of increased vagal tone and may be physiologic in trained athletes. Symptomatic patients require permanent pacing and in particular DDDR pacing. Because of retrograde conduction, patients with single chamber ventricular pacing may become more symptomatic.
- Sinus arrest or sino-atrial block—patients may present with syncope. VVI pacing may be indicated for infrequent bradyarrhythmias, and DDDR pacing if sinus bradycardia is also present.
- Tachycardia/bradycardia syndrome—patients are usually symptomatic. DDDR pacing with ventricular rate protection is important.

Other symptomatic bradyarrhythmias

- **Combined high-degree atrioventricular block and sick sinus syndrome**. The *pan conduction defect*. DDDR pacing is usually indicated.
- **Atrial fibrillation with marked pauses**. VVI pacing is indicated in symptomatic patients and VVIR pacing if associated with slow atrial fibrillation. Digitalis toxicity must be excluded.
- **Prolonged QT interval and torsade de pointes**. AAIR, VVIR or DDDR pacing have been used together with beta blockade to prevent ventricular ectopic beats and syncope (class II).
- **Carotid sinus hypersensitivity and neuro-cardiogenic syncope**. In both groups, syncope is unpredictable and may be life-threatening. With carotid sinus hypersensitivity, a class I indication requires a > 3 second pause with minimal carotid sinus pressure. With neuro-cardiogenic (vasovagal) syncope tilt table testing helps identify a cardio-inhibitory group where rapid DDD pacing may be successful. AAI pacing is not recommended because of associated proximal atrioventricular block. Permanent pacing in the group with mixed cardio-inhibitory and vasodepressor responses is controversial and may result in an incomplete alleviation of symptoms.
- **Atrial inexcitability**. No mechanical, electrical or pacing activity in the atrium. Symptomatic patients require VVIR pacing.

Cardiomyopathy

DDD pacing with a short atrioventricular delay for committed ventricular pacing may result in a marked gradient reduction in patients with hypertrophic obstructive cardiomyopathy.

Tachyarrhythmias

With the introduction of radiofrequency ablative techniques, the need for special tachycardia reverting pacemakers has become rare. Such pacemakers are still available as part of an implantable cardioverter defibrillator for treatment of ventricular tachycardia.

Empirical indication

On occasion, life-threatening syncope presumed cardiac, but with no cause documented after extensive investigation including tilt table testing, may require implantation of a dual chamber pacemaker.

Pacemaker insertion and implantation

The techniques of pacemaker insertion and implantation are described in Chapter 44.

References

1. Mond HG, Barold SS. Dual chamber, rate adaptive pacing in patients with supraventricular tachyarrhythmias: protective measures for rate control. PACE 1993;16:2168–85
2. American College of Cardiology/American Heart Association. Guidelines for implantation of cardiac pacemakers and antiarrhythmia devices. A report of the American College of Cardiology/American Heart Association task force on assessment of diagnostic and therapeutic cardiovascular procedures (Committee on pacemaker implantation). JACC 1991;18:1–13

44 Pacemaker insertion

James S Robinson

Introduction

Transvenous endocardial pacing is the method of choice and for this, local anaesthesia is adequate. Insertion of a permanent pacing system should take place in an operating theatre under strict aseptic technique. In some clinical situations temporary pacing can be done at the bedside, but aseptic technique must be followed.

Temporary transvenous pacing

Venous access

Conventional temporary pacing is by infraclavicular percutaneous puncture of the subclavian vein. This is particularly so if temporary pacing will be required for a period of time, for example in profound bradycardia due to drug overdose, symptomatic drug resistant heart block in myocardial infarction, or the need to stabilize a patient's condition prior to permanent pacing, etc.

Either the right or left subclavian vein may be used, the right being favoured because of the familiar anatomical variant of left superior vena cava, which makes passing a ventricular electrode difficult.

The femoral vein may be used if pacing is required for only a short time, for example overdrive atrial pacing of atrial flutter, or pacing support during permanent pacemaker replacement in totally pacer-dependent patients. The patient's mobility is seriously impaired by femoral vein cannulation and it is an option for only brief periods of pacing.

The femoral vein is located just medial to the femoral artery just below the inguinal ligament. In femoral vein puncture the operator protects the femoral artery by placing an index finger on it, the other hand holding a 2–5 ml syringe containing 1–2 ml of normal saline, connected to a percutaneous entry needle, and passes the needle just medial to the protecting index finger at an angle of 45° to the patient's thigh. Suction is applied to the syringe and the needle advanced until venous flow is obtained. The syringe is removed and a guide wire inserted.

Passage of the electrode

Once the wire is positioned within the subclavian or femoral vein, a dilator and sheath are passed over the guide wire, then the wire and dilator are removed and the temporary electrode inserted via the sheath. Using X-ray control the electrode is passed to the right atrium. In ventricular pacing the electrode is passed across the tricuspid valve to the apex of the right ventricle (see Fig. 44.1), while in atrial pacing the J-lead is placed medially in the atrial appendage (see Figs 44.1, 44.2). Further details on placement of the electrode are given in the section dealing with the placement and electrical characteristics of permanent pacing electrodes.

Fixation

The electrode should be fastened by several firm silk ligatures passed in a purse string fashion at the point of exit from the skin. The electrode is fastened to the skin in two small tension-relieving loops and is then covered with a transparent adhesive dressing.

Permanent transvenous pacing

Skin preparation

The operative field should be prepared by shaving and cleaning the skin. The side of the neck and infraclavicular region is prepared

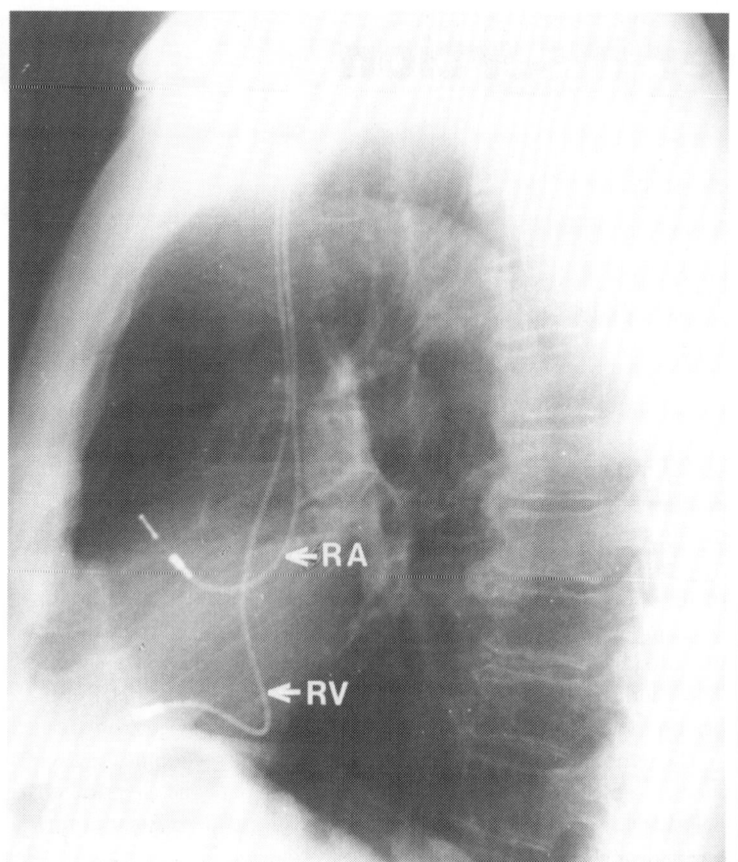

Fig. 44.1 Lateral view of dual chamber system with J-tip lead (RA) in the right atrium and the ventricular lead (RV) sitting anteriorly in the apex of the right ventricle.

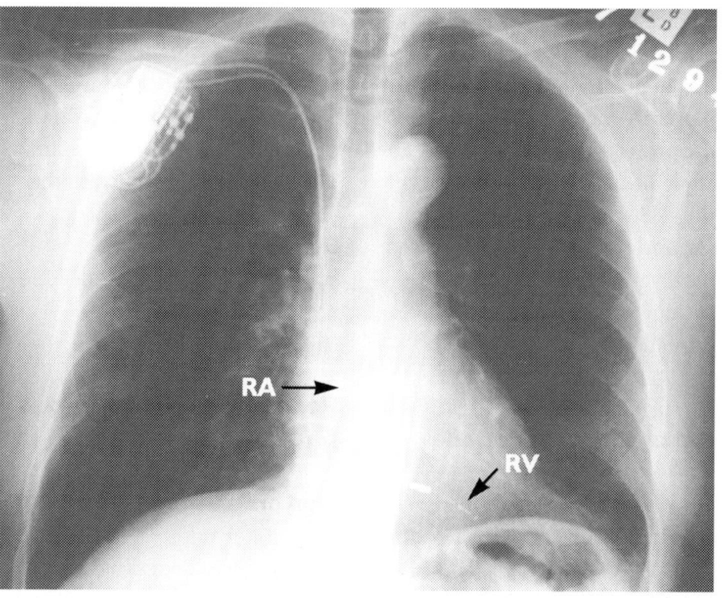

Fig. 44.2 PA view of ventricular pacing lead fixation in the apex of the right ventricle, and an atrial lead pointing medially in the atrial appendage.

with alcoholic providone-iodine 10% which is allowed to dry. Surgical drapes are applied so that the infraclavicular region is exposed as well as access to the homolateral internal jugular vein. The drapes can be held in place by adhesive 'Steri Drape'* applied over the skin and surrounding drapes. The skin is anaesthetized by infiltration of 10 ml of 1% lignocaine, the subcutaneous area by 20 ml of bupivacaine 0.5%. Prophylactic cephamandole nafate 1 g is given by IV injection soon after the procedure begins and is followed by cephalexin, 500 mg orally 6-hourly for several days.

Venous access—permanent pacing

The favoured vein is the cephalic vein, thus an incision is made over the delto-pectoral groove. The cephalic vein (if present) should be found beneath the fat pad and fascia in the delto-pectoral groove. The vein should be dissected free and raised by ligatures placed at the most proximal and distal parts. The distal ligature is tied, and the cephalic vein is opened by incision with small scissors, preferably at a point above its crossing by the thoraco-acromial artery. The vein lumen is opened with a small lifter and the electrode is introduced into the vein and passed proximally down its lumen.

If the cephalic vein is not available (anatomical variant), or has been used for a previous pacing system, then the subclavian vein is usually accessed by the stan-

* 'Steri Drape' incise drape 1040 3M

dard infraclavicular introducer technique.

If it is known that subclavian vein puncture is to be used, then the incision should be made parallel to the lower border of the clavicle with its medial extremity near the junction of the clavicle and first rib.

The introducer needle is passed across the first rib into the thoracic inlet, there entering the subclavian vein. This latter, and widely used, method has been associated with damage to the pacing electrode due to compression by the clavicle and first rib or to entrapment by the costo-clavicular ligament or subclavius muscle. This combination of bone and soft tissue compression stress is known as the 'clavicle first rib complex'. Hence extrathoracic approaches to subclavian vein puncture have been developed and should be considered.[1,2]

Here the subclavian vein is cannulated as it passes over the body of the first rib, and thus the pacing lead traverses the first rib in the subclavian vein groove (as it does in cephalic vein cut-down) and this protects the lead from damage by the clavicle first rib complex.

If the subclavian vein cannot be entered, then a supraclavicular approach to the subclavian vein or internal jugular vein may be used. This method will require a second incision, that is, above the clavicle, and a subcutaneous passage is prepared for the electrode to the infraclavicular site.

Venous access—dual chamber pacing

When instituting dual chamber pacing, it is often possible to pass both atrial and ventricular leads via the cutdown in the cephalic vein. If the second electrode cannot be manipulated into the cephalic vein then it is passed by the introducer technique as described above.

If the cephalic vein is not available and installation of both electrodes is required, it is possible to do this by a single venepuncture of the subclavian vein. An introducer one size larger than that required by the first electrode (for example, 11 Fr instead of 10 Fr), is passed and the first electrode introduced, but before tearing away the sheath, a guide wire is inserted down the sheath along with the first electrode; then, holding the wire and electrode in place, the sheath is removed. A second introducer can then be passed over the wire.

Passage of the electrodes

When introducing the permanent pacing electrode into the vein it is usual to have the stiffening stylet fully advanced. The electrode is advanced continuously, stopping only if resistance is encountered. Difficulty negotiating the cephalic-subclavian vein junction can usually be resolved by partially withdrawing the electrode; staff must ensure that the patient's head is turned to the opposite side and move the head temporarily off any pillow, then re-advance the electrode. If difficulty continues, then fluoroscopy should be used to determine if the electrode is turning toward the shoulder or down the chest wall; if it is, then it is in a branch of the cephalic and the site of entry into the cephalic was too distal, i.e. before the thoraco-acromial artery crossing. If despite repeated attempts the electrode continues to pass into the branch, it should be withdrawn and a more proximal entry made into the cephalic vein. This will usually be successful.

Once the electrode is within the subclavian system it can usually be advanced with ease, but if any resistance is encountered then the site should be screened while the electrode is slightly withdrawn. The electrode can in part be guided by withdrawing the stylet to make the end of the electrode floppy.

During the passage of dual pacing leads in the subclavian superior vena caval system it is common for the electrodes to become twisted together. To ease their subsequent manipulation and placement they should be untwisted, usually by partially withdrawing one electrode up into the superior vena cava or subclavian vein, then untwisting and readvancing under X-ray vision.

Ventricular lead passage in the ventricle

Tined leads are almost invariably used for pacing the ventricle and the passage of these across the tricuspid valve may be difficult, due to the tines being entrapped in the chordae of the tricuspid valve. To prevent damage to the tip of the electrode, the stylet should be fully advanced when crossing the tricuspid apparatus.

If the tines become entrapped (a tug can be felt on the electrode) and the electrode will not easily advance, it should be withdrawn using gentle traction and then re-manipulated. Sometimes the tricuspid valve can be negotiated by withdrawing the stylet, forming the electrode in the right atrium into a reversed C, advancing the back of the C through the tricuspid into the ventricle, then advancing the stylet into the electrode, straightening the curve while withdrawing the electrode. This often carries the tip of the electrode into the right ventricle.

Once in the right ventricle, the stylet is slightly withdrawn so that the tip of the electrode is not rigid. The tip of the electrode should be passed to the apex of the right ventricle with the remainder making a gentle C in the right atrium. On screening, the electrode tip will usually be seen to lie below the level of the left hemidiaphragm and if a lateral view is obtained the electrode should pass anteriorly. The stability of the lead should be checked by withdrawing the stylet; staff should then screen and have the patient cough and deep breathe.

Electrical characteristics—ventricular leads

Once the lead is considered to be in a suitable position the stylet is removed and the electrode is connected by sterile leads to an external pacemaker analyser. Pacing is initiated with the cathode connected to the distal electrode and the anode to the proximal ring electrode in bipolar pacing. In a unipolar system the cathode is applied to the pacing electrode while a pair of forceps applied to the subcutaneous tissues in the wound will suffice as the anode.

Measurements—ventricular lead

- Pacing threshold should be low, preferably below 0.5 volts at 0.5 milliseconds.
- Intrinsic sensed R wave is measured and ideally should be greater than 5 millivolts.
- Electrode resistance should be greater than 300 ohm and generally not greater than 1000 ohm.

Other features—ventricular leads

The paced QRS complex should have a left bundle branch block (LBBB) configuration. If it shows a right bundle branch block (RBBB) pattern, the electrode should be withdrawn until LBBB is seen, as the electrode has penetrated the ventricle or septum. In the RBBB situation the threshold will usually be unacceptably high.

With the analysers pacing output at 5 volts, the patient's lower left chest should be screened briefly to ensure that the left hemidiaphragm is not being paced. If it is, the lead is repositioned.

Fixation

Once satisfactory electrical characteristics are obtained and the electrode is considered to be in a stable position, it is fixed to pectoralis major by non-absorbable ligatures tied firmly around the movable protective plastic sleeve which has been moved close to the point of venous entry. Atrial leads are secured in a similar fashion.

Once no further electrode manipulations are required, haemostasis about the vein electrode interface is achieved by one or two gently tied purse string sutures through the close surrounding tissues.

Atrial leads—passage in the atrium

In dual chamber pacing the ventricular lead is placed first and secured in position. The atrial lead is then passed into the right atrium using a straight stylet. Once in the atrium the stylet is withdrawn and preformed electrodes will then assume a J shape. If the electrode is not preformed then a J-shaped stylet should be advanced to the tip of the electrode.

The J is moved to the mid-atrium with its tip medially directed, and under fluoroscopic control the electrode assembly is drawn upwards until the tip of the electrode engages in the right atrial appendage. Here in the PA view the electrode will sway from side to side 'like a dog's tail wagging'. In the lateral view the tip should pass anteriorly and the electrode has a J shape in expiration and an L shape in deep inspiration.

In some patients (particularly those who have had previous open heart surgery) it is often difficult to secure in place a tined atrial lead, and it may be necessary to use a screw-in atrial electrode, i.e. one that can be actively fixed in place to the atrial wall.

The lateral wall of the right atrium must be avoided because of the proximity of the right phrenic nerve and the resultant pacing of the right hemidiaphragm.

Measurements—atrial lead

- Pacing threshold should preferably be below 1 volt.
- Intrinsic sensed P wave should be greater than 0.75 millivolts.
- Electrode resistance should be greater than 300 ohm but generally not greater than 1000 ohm.

Pacemaker implantation

The electrodes have been secured in place; the pacemaker is now connected. Then by using a combination of sharp and blunt dissection, a space is made between the subcutaneous tissue and pectoralis major. Any redundant electrode is coiled into this space, followed by the pacemaker which sits on the surplus electrode. Using a non-absorbable suture, the pacemaker is fixed to the pectoralis major.

If a unipolar pacing system is used, the anodal surface of the pacemaker must be directed towards the subcutaneous tissue; otherwise, if directed toward the pectoralis major, an uncomfortable muscular twitch will occur with each pacing impulse.

Using interrupted sutures the subcutaneous tissues are closed over the pacing system. The skin is closed with a continuous subcutaneous stitch.

References

1. Byrd CL. Clinical experience with the extra-thoracic introducer insertion technique. PACE 1993; 16: 1781–4
2. Magney JE, Staplin DH, Flynn DM, Hunter DW. A new approach to percutaneous subclavian venipuncture to avoid lead fracture of central venous catheter occlusion. PACE 1993; 16: 2133–42

45 Percutaneous transluminal coronary angioplasty (PTCA)

I Nigel Sinclair and Peter L Thompson

Introduction

Shortly after introduction of the technique of percutaneous transluminal coronary angioplasty (PTCA) by Gruentzig and colleagues in the late 1970s,[1] the technique was used to treat acute coronary occlusion in patients with myocardial infarction (MI), both with and without thrombolytic therapy.[2,3] Since this early experience the use of PTCA in acute coronary syndromes has grown rapidly.[4,5]

A series of clinical trials has helped to clarify the role of angioplasty in acute myocardial infarction (AMI) and its relationship to coronary thrombolysis as a technique for achieving re-perfusion. These have recently been summarized[5,2a] and presented in a meta-analysis.[6]

Immediate PTCA after successful coronary thrombolysis

The apparent logic of attempting to restore normal coronary patency after thrombolytic therapy had achieved partial patency was subject to clinical trial in three separate studies.[7–9] The results are summarized in Table 45.1.

Although the design of the three trials was not identical, the results were strikingly similar. In the TAMI-I Study[7] a subset of patients was randomized to immediate angioplasty versus angioplasty deferred for a week. In the European Co-operative Study Group,[8] half the patients were randomized to immediate angioplasty and the other half to no angioplasty. In the TIMI-IIA Study[9] half the patients were randomized to immediate angioplasty versus angioplasty delayed for 18–48 hours. There were no statistically significant differences in mortality although there was a trend towards increased mortality in the angioplasty treated patients. There was an increased risk of bleeding requiring transfusion and emergency coronary artery bypass surgery. There were no differences in ejection fraction.

Each of the above trials was with tissue plasminogen activator. A randomized trial of similar design with streptokinase as the thrombolytic agent[10] showed no

Table 45.1 Trials of immediate PTCA after thrombolysis with r-TPA

Immediate post-thrombolysis PTCA

	TAMI-I*		ECSG**		TIMI-IIA***	
Drug	r-TPA		r-TPA		r-TPA	
Patients	386		367		389	
	PTCA	No PTCA	PTCA	No PTCA	PTCA	No PTCA
Mortality	4%	1%	7%	3%	7%	5%
Ejection fraction	53%	56%	51%	51%	50%	49%

* Thrombolysis and Angioplasty in Myocardial Infarction[7]
** European Cooperative Study Group[8]
*** Thrombolysis in Myocardial Infarction[9]

differences in angioplasty success, time to re-perfusion, 6-monthly re-stenosis, patency or left ventricular function with the less clot-specific agent. However, there was an increased need for urgent bypass surgery, transfusion requirement and an increased length of hospital stay in the patients who had received streptokinase prior to their angioplasty.

This series of trials clearly showed that angioplasty was unhelpful and potentially deleterious when partial lysis had been achieved with thrombolytic therapy in acute coronary occlusion. The reasons for this are not clear but may relate to a paradoxic increased activation of platelets and thrombin binding sites in the coronary thrombus resulting from thrombolytic therapy.[11] There is a possibility that more effective adjunctive anti-thrombotic therapy such as selective thrombin or platelet receptor antagonists could improve the results of both thrombolysis and PTCA.

Immediate PTCA after unsuccessful thrombolysis

In this approach, angioplasty is used when thrombolytic therapy has failed to achieve re-perfusion—so-called 'rescue angioplasty'. To date only about 500 patients have been subjected to clinical trials,[12] and less than 200 in randomized controlled trials comparing post-thrombolytic PTCA with no PTCA.[6,13] The approach has not found wide acceptance because it is an expensive approach to the management of MI, the rate of successful re-perfusion is disappointingly low (averaging 80% compared with the 95% success rates in direct angioplasty unassociated with thrombolysis) and there are concerns about haemorrhage and vascular complications from catheterization in a recently thrombolysed patient.

The early re-occlusion rates are relatively high, averaging 14% in the streptokinase/urokinase trials and 24% in the r-TPA trials. There was no demonstrable benefit in ventricular function. An additional significant problem is the difficulty in reliably recognizing the patient who has failed to achieve re-perfusion with thrombolysis.[14]

Despite the lack of support from clinical trials, rescue angioplasty may have a role in the patient with evidence of continuing ischaemia, particularly when there is associated haemodynamic deterioration.

Pre-discharge PTCA after thrombolysis

Two large trials[15,16] and a number of smaller trials[6] have evaluated a policy of routine angioplasty 24 hours or more after thrombolytic therapy (Table 45.2).

The TIMI-IIB Study[15] randomized 3262 patients to an invasive strategy compared with a conservative strategy. In the invasive strategy cardiac catheterization was performed routinely at 18–48 hours following administration of r-TPA and if the coronary anatomy was suitable PTCA was performed. In the conservative strategy cardiac catheterization was not performed unless there was continuing ischaemia.

In patients in the invasive strategy the rates of intervention within 6 weeks were 93% catheterization, 57% angioplasty and 12% bypass surgery. In the conservative strategy the 6-week rates of intervention were 33% catheterization, 16% angioplasty and 11% bypass surgery. At 6 weeks there were no differences in the rates of death or reinfarction between the two groups. Major criticisms of the TIMI-IIB study are the lack of adequate aspirin therapy, potentially increasing the risk of early re-stenosis after angioplasty, and the decision not to attempt angioplasty of totally occluded vessels.

Table 45.2 Trials of delayed PTCA after thrombolysis

	TIMI-IIB*		SWIFT**	
Drug	r-TPA		APSAC	
Patients	3262		800	
	PTCA	No PTCA	PTCA	No PTCA
Mortality	5.2%	4.6%	2.7%	3.3%
Reinfarction	5.9%	5.4%	12.1%	8.2%
Ejection fraction	50%	50%	52%	51%

* Thrombolysis in Myocardial Infarction[15]
** Should We Intervene Following Thrombolysis?[16]

Furthermore, the high rate of intervention in the 'conservative' group would be considered as a relatively aggressive strategy in most countries other than the USA and this high rate of intervention may have obscured differences between the groups.

In the SWIFT (Should We Intervene Following Thrombolysis?) trial[16] 800 patients were randomized to routine coronary angiography and angioplasty if the anatomy was suitable, versus conservative management. After thrombolytic therapy with anistreplase (APSAC), similar results to TIMI-IIB were obtained with no differences in ejection fraction, re-infarction or mortality between the angioplasty and the conservatively treated patients.

Meta-analysis of these and four smaller trials[6] demonstrated no differences at 6 weeks (odds ratio 1.06) or 1 year (odds ratio 0.99) in mortality or reinfarction in patients treated with an aggressive approach after thrombolysis. On the basis of these trials a policy of routine early pre-discharge angioplasty after thrombolysis cannot be justified.

It is important to note that both TIMI-IIB and SWIFT cannot answer the question of the benefits of late angioplasty of a persistent totally occluded infarct-related vessel as angioplasty of these was not attempted in either of these trials. There is considerable evidence that the restoration of patency even when delayed for some time after coronary occlusion may have benefits in preventing deterioration of LV function, improving long-term survival and improving chances of survival at a subsequent coronary occlusion.[17] The 'delayed' open artery hypothesis has been tested in only a small clinical trial (TAMI-6) which failed to demonstrate a benefit on left ventricular function at 6 months with angioplasty of a totally occluded vessel at 48 hours post thrombolysis.[18]

The role of selective PTCA in patients with continuing symptoms of ischaemia or a demonstrable area of ischaemic but viable myocardium post-infarction is discussed in Chapter 81.

Primary PTCA as an alternative to coronary thrombolysis

Clinical trial results

The feasibility of PTCA as primary treatment for coronary occlusion was demonstrated over a decade ago, but its use has tended to be restricted to specialized centres, highly skilled in coronary angioplasty.[2,3] Two small randomized trials did not show convincing benefits on early mortality or reinfarction.[19,20] Wider acceptance of this approach to the treatment of AMI did not occur until the simultaneous publication of three well designed randomized trials in 1993,[21–23] although none of these trials individually showed a benefit on mortality or reinfarction at 6 weeks. The cumulative experience in the published trials now totals over 1000 patients, with 21 deaths among the 571 patients treated with angioplasty and 37 deaths among the 574 patients treated with thrombolytic therapy.[21–26, and 5a, 6] A meta-analysis of these trial results by Michels and Yusuf has calculated an odds ratio of 0.56 (95% confidence intervals .33–.94).[6] There was a similar reduction in the rate of non-fatal reinfarction at 6 weeks totalling 14 out of 571 (2.5%) in the angioplasty treated patients and 26 of 574 (4.5%) in the thrombolysis treated patients (see Table 45.3). In contrast with these encouraging results, the GUSTO IIB results in 1138 patients showed no clear advantage of primary PTCA over thrombolysis (odds radio 0.80, 95% CI 0.49–1.30).[6a]

Rationale

These clinical trial results are consistent with the concept that early establishment of coronary patency is the key to improving survival in MI from acute coronary occlusion. The angiographic sub-study of the GUSTO trial has shown that improved survival in patients being treated with thrombolytic therapy is confined to those patients in whom there is restoration of normal coronary blood flow (TIMI grade III flow) (Fig. 45.1).

Extrapolation of the benefits anticipated from the angiographic sub-study to the observed benefits in the total study in the analysis by Simes et al[27] has demonstrated convincingly the need for establishing early and complete reperfusion of the infarct-related artery. The pooled angiographic patency rates which have been achieved with currently available thrombolytic regimens have achieved TIMI grade III rates below 50%,[28] but it is possible that this could be significantly improved with newer thrombolytic regimens such as double bolus r-TPA and newer thrombolytic agents. The most effective

Table 45.3 Randomized comparisons of primary angioplasty with thrombolysis for acute myocardial infarction. Based on Michels and Yusuf 1995[6]

	Thrombolytic agent	N	Deaths at 6 weeks PTCA	Deaths at 6 weeks thrombolysis
O'Neill et al.[9]	IC SK	56	2/29 6.9%	1/27 3.7%
DeWood et al.[20]	IV r-TPA	90	3/46 6.5%	2/44 4.5%
Grines et al.[23] (PAMI)	IV r-TPA	395	5/195 2.6%	13/200 6.5%
Zijlstra et al.[22] (Zwolle)	IV SK	301	3/152 2.0%	11/149 7.4%
Gibbons et al.[21] (Mayo)	IV r-TPA	103	2/47 4.3%	2/56 3.6%
Ribeiro et al.[25]	IV SK	100	3/50 6%	1/50 2%
Elizaga et al.[26]	Thrombolysis	100	3/52 5.8%	7/48 14.6%
Total		1145	21/571 3.7%	37/574 6.4%
ODDS RATIO (95% CI)	PTCA/thrombolysis		0.56 (0.33, 0.94)	

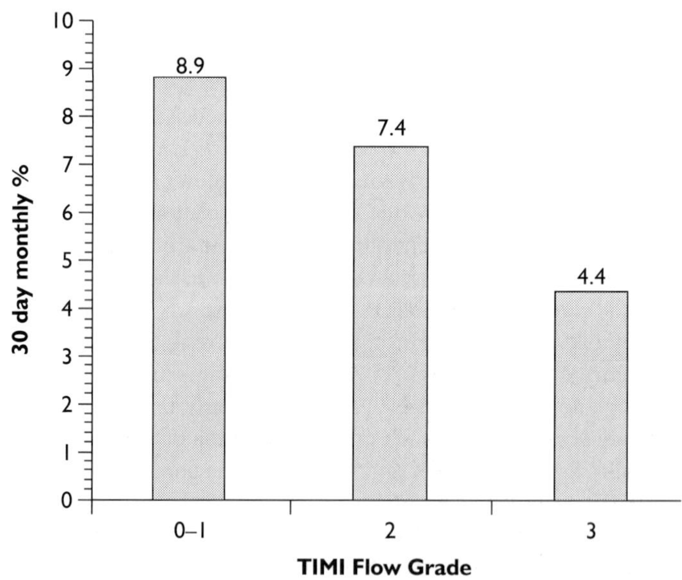

Fig. 45.1 30 day mortality and TIMI flow at 90 minutes in the GUSTO angiographic sub-study. Adapted from The GUSTO-1 Angiographic Investigators. All rights reserved.

thrombolytic regimen which has been demonstrated to date in a large clinical trial has been accelerated r-TPA, and this achieved grade III flow at 90 minutes in only 54% of patients, dropping to 46% at 24 hours.[29] In contrast the rates of TIMI grade III patency achieved in the angioplasty arms of the randomized trials[20–22] and in a primary angioplasty registry has approached 97%, demonstrating a clear superiority of primary angioplasty over the best currently available thrombolytic regimen (Fig. 45.2). It should be noted that the figure of 97% is an inflated estimate of the efficacy of angioplasty in acute MI as it is based only on those in whom angioplasty was attempted. When patients who are unsuitable for angiography or angioplasty are excluded, the figure is somewhat lower, but still well in excess of 90%.

Other benefits

Other benefits which have been claimed for primary angioplasty

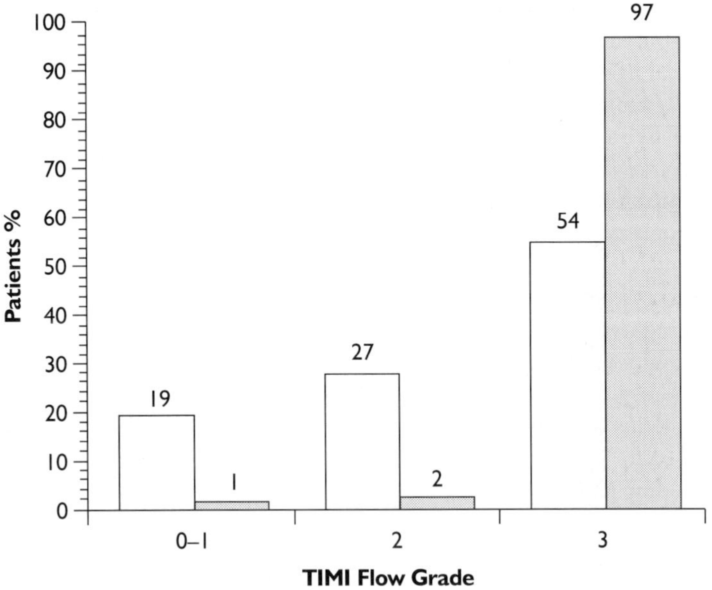

Fig. 45.2 Comparison of TIMI flow grades achieved with accelerated r-TPA in the GUSTO angiographic substudy[28] compared with those achieved by primary PTCA in the Primary Angioplasty Registry.[30] Adapted from The GUSTO-I Angiographic Investigators. All rights reserved.

compared with thrombolytic therapy have been reduced risk of stroke, shorter and more economical hospital stays and reduced risk of re-occlusion.

The logic of attempting to avoid the risk of haemorrhagic *stroke* with angioplasty rather than thrombolytic therapy is persuasive, but to date the data are inconclusive because the total number of patients in the randomized trials is only just over 2000. The rate of stroke in the angioplasty group in the PAMI trial was 0% and in the thrombolytic group was surprisingly high at 3.5% and quite out of line with the usual rate of 0.5% seen in most of the thrombolytic trials. A more realistic estimate of the risk of stroke with primary angioplasty comes from registry data showing that primary angioplasty is not totally protective against stroke. The data on comparison of *costs* is also unclear. The Mayo study[21] compared hospital charges and found a somewhat lower total for the angioplasty group, but there was considerable overlap of the confidence interval of these estimates, and furthermore, the estimates were for charges rather than true hospital costs. Comparisons of angioplasty with r-TPA regimens may not be representative of the costs if less expensive regimens such as streptokinase were compared. The Zwolle trial[22,24] estimated that the total 1-year costs of the angioplasty group were similar to those of the streptokinase group. It is conceivable that the savings resulting from shortened hospital stays with primary angioplasty treatment of MI could balance the costs of the procedure, but more detailed analysis of this proposition is required before it can be accepted. The available data suggest that the *re-occlusion* rate after angioplasty is low; patency rates remain high at 87–91% through to 6 months after MI treated with primary angioplasty.[24,30]

Reservations

The clear superiority of angioplasty in establishing early patency, and the available data on mortality and reinfarction from the clinical trials, lead to the conclusion that primary angioplasty is capable of achieving better early and late outcomes than thrombolytic therapy treatment of MI. However, many reservations and controversies remain.

The first reservation is that the weight of clinical trial evidence at present strongly favours thrombolytic therapy with over 150 000 patients treated in clinical trials with clear definition of the benefits, side-effects and limitations of the therapy (see Ch. 34). In contrast, the randomized clinical trial data to support primary angioplasty totals just over 2000 patients, at this stage without any individual trial showing a clear-cut benefit.

Secondly, the trials of primary angioplasty which have been reported have all been conducted in high-volume institutions where skills in coronary angioplasty have been well developed over many years, and there is considerable doubt that the same high patency rates and low complication rates could be achieved in institutions with less skilled operators and lower volumes of angioplasty cases.[31] This could explain the apparent lack of superiority of primary PTCA over thrombolysis in the GUSTO IIB study.[6a]

Thirdly, the analysis of the costs of this approach to the treatment of MI have to date been very superficial. The estimates quoted above indicating an apparent equivalence of costs by balancing the shorter hospital stays against the catheter laboratory costs are all based on high-volume institutions which have absorbed the costs of the primary angioplasty programme into previously established angioplasty programmes. There has been no published analysis of the costs of introducing primary angioplasty as a new service into a hospital as an adjunct to coronary care management. Furthermore, each of the major trials has reported high rates (nearly 50%) of in-hospital revascularization for the thrombolysis treated patients, thus increasing the costs of their care to approximately the cost of care of those who had immediate angioplasty.

Views about the role of primary angioplasty and AMI differ significantly among different countries.[31]

Recommendations

The eventual place of primary angioplasty in the treatment of AMI will depend on further clinical trial results, more sophisticated cost comparisons with thrombolytic agents, including the cheaper agents such as streptokinase rather than r-TPA, and the application of the technique in community hospitals with lower volumes of angioplasty procedures. At present, a sensible recommendation is that primary angioplasty should be considered as the preferred procedure in hospitals which are skilled in the technique with ready availability of a catheter laboratory, a skilled team and an operator with high-volume, recent experience in coronary angioplasty. To maximize the benefits and prevent a blowout in costs from the procedure, it needs to be balanced with a programme of early hospital discharge and follow-up. The current evidence would support the establishment of primary angioplasty programmes in those hospitals with well-established cardiac catheterization facilities and high-volume coronary angioplasty programmes. Within such hospitals certain sub-groups of patients could be selectively chosen for primary angioplasty, including patients who develop evidence of acute coronary occlusion within the CCU, or patients with haemorrhagic or other contraindications to thrombolytic therapy. Patients with cardiogenic shock are a particular sub-group in whom thrombolytic therapy has been less than effective, and stand to benefit most from revascularization[32] (see Ch. 57), but randomized trials are lacking.

New interventional devices

Coronary angioplasty is now used to treat up to 50% of patients who need revascularization for obstructive coronary artery disease. The major drawbacks to its even more widespread use are:

- the inability of the wire and the balloon to cross total obstructions (particularly those older than 3 months)
- acute re-closure within 24 hours which occurs in 2–9% of cases[33]
- re-stenosis post angioplasty occurring up to 6 months after the procedure in 20–50% of cases, depending on which definition is used.[34]

To help overcome these drawbacks a number of new devices have been trialed over the years and include stents, atherectomy devices, drills and lasers.

Stents

Stents are metallic mesh or coil splints which are placed inside arteries to brace them open and prevent collapse through dissections or elastic recoil. They were first applied by Dottor and co-workers in 1969 in the femoro-popliteal arteries and in the coronary arteries in 1986 by Sigwart et al. When first used in coronaries, the rate of sub-acute stent thrombosis was exceedingly high and a regimen of extensive anticoagulation using IV heparin and dextran, oral aspirin, dipyridamole and warfarin was required in the first few hours and weeks after stent placement.

This anticoagulation regimen was associated with a significant rate of major bleeding, particularly at the puncture site. Despite this, it has now been well demonstrated in both the BENESTENT[35] and STRESS trials[36] that there is improved procedural success with reduced long-term re-stenosis and a reduced need for coronary revascularization (see Table 45.4).

Colombo and co-workers from Milan, Italy, have recently challenged the need for such an extensive anticoagulation regimen.[37,38] They have found that as long as the stent is adequately dilated there is no difference in subacute thrombosis rates between patients orally anticoagulated and those who have an anticoagulation consisting of aspirin and ticlopidine only.

Table 45.4 Comparison of BENESTENT and STRESS Trials (combined results) with conventional angioplasty.

	Balloon angioplasty (mean)	Stents
Predilation diameter (mm)	0.93	0.92
Luminal diameter immed. post procedure (mm)	1.99	2.49
Gain immed. (mm)	1.06	1.57
Luminal diameter 6 mo (mm)	1.64	1.78
Net gain (mm)	0.71	0.86
Re-stenosis %	37.5	26.8
No coronary events %	73.3	80.2
Revascularization required %	21.4	14.9

Adequate stent dilatation is defined as a full round stent, closely applied to the underlying vessel wall, which is checked using intravascular ultrasound (IVUS). This device, which can be passed into the coronary artery, enables a view of the vessel lumen and wall to be obtained. Further studies will be needed to confirm these findings from other centres.

Current indications for stents include severe dissection or recoil of the vessel post angioplasty, and stenosis in the body of saphenous vein grafts, and may in the future be used more for initial angioplasties if the reduced rate of re-stenosis shown in the above trials is proven and as the anti-coagulation and post-operative bleeding is sorted out. However, concerns have been expressed about the need for this in every case, and the cost implications of choosing stent implantation as a primary procedure in coronary angioplasty.[39]

Directional atherectomy

Directional coronary atherectomy (DCA) is a means by which a cutting device is introduced into the coronary artery and obstructing atheroma is shaved off and removed. It was first developed by Simpson and co-workers and appears particularly indicated for eccentric obstruction, lesions in the proximal segment of the left anterior descending coronary artery and those at branch points. However, two recent trials (CAVEAT and CCAT)[40,41] failed to confirm that the early improvement in vessel diameter associated with use of this device continues long term. In fact the rate of cardiovascular events such as angina and MI was increased following their use. There has however been a vigorous debate concerning how well the device was used in these trials and suggestions that not enough atheroma was removed, and further trials are pending to test the hypothesis that 'bigger is better'. Again the use of the IVUS device will in the future enable increased atheroma removal with safety.

Rotational atherectomy

A percutaneous transluminal coronary rotational ablation device (Rotablator) consists of a high-speed rotating burr coated with diamond chips which is particularly useful for grinding hard calcific stenosis. Often these do not dilate satisfactorily with angioplasty balloons. The rotating action produces small particles which are cleared from the circulation by the reticulo-endothelial system. It is useful with hard calcific lesions and has also been used with some effect in extensively diseased vessels. Most patients require adjunctive balloon angioplasty to obtain a satisfactory result.[42] In the ERBAC Trial (Excimer Laser, Rotablator, Balloon Angioplasty for Complex Lesions),[43] 884 patients with complex lesions were randomized to undergo one of these procedures. Rotational atherectomy resulted in a significantly higher procedural success rate than the two other methods. Only 1.5% of patients undergoing rotational ablation suffered death, MI or emergency coronary artery bypass grafting compared with 7% of those who underwent balloon angioplasty.

Lasers

Lasers are devices which allow the transfer of large amounts of energy in the form of light to the tip of a catheter via fine glass fibres. This energy can be used to heat or vaporize tissue. Devices such as the laser balloon angioplasty system developed by Spears have however proved disappointing and currently the only laser devices used in cardiology are the Excimer laser systems. These use very short wavelength light to ablate tissue. Theoretically they can be used most effectively for the treatment of diffuse disease but in fact trial results do not demonstrate any superiority over using conventional angioplasty.[44,45] A laser wire which is under investigation for treatment of totally occluded arteries may prove useful in the future. In general terms lasers are investigational devices which currently display no clear superiority, although this may change in the future.

Transluminal extraction catheter

The transluminal extraction catheter (TEC) device with forward-facing cutting blades associated with aspiration capability could be useful in the treatment of old saphenous vein grafts which contain much friable material. This device has been under investigation for the last 5 years, but trial results are disappointing, and as yet no clear indication has been found for this device.[46]

Future interventional devices

Ultrasound angioplasty, whereby ultrasonic energy is transmitted to the end of the catheter via a thin wire embedded in the catheter and used to shatter atherosclerotic and particularly calcific material into small fragments, is undergoing early patient trials.[47] This is a promising new technology which employs different principles to get rid of the excessive material in the coronary arteries. However it will be some time before sufficient information is available about its capabilities and drawbacks, and its possible promise realized.

Drug delivery catheters are in their early stage of development. These generally allow seepage through small pores in the balloon of a drug material to reduce re-stenosis, with the medication effectively injected directly into the vascular tissue at the site of angioplasty. Other devices allow a pool of highly concentrated medication to be kept at one particular site in the vascular system for minutes or hours at a time. Medication such as heparin and other anticoagulants, or even cytotoxic drugs or modulators of gene expression materials, could be injected in this way. These theoretically could have an effect on the acute and long-term re-stenotic process.

In the future, stents which are increasingly resistant to local thrombosis will be employed. These may incorporate antithrombotic or cytotoxic drugs and could even be seeded with endothelial cells, perhaps altered by cellular genetic processes to reduce the chance of re-stenosis.[48] It is likely that revascularization will be increasingly performed using devices which are less invasive than coronary artery bypass grafting.

To date, few of these devices have been applied to deal with acute coronary thrombotic occlusion. The excellent early and late patency achieved with balloon angioplasty in acute coronary thrombosis makes it unlikely that the new devices will find a major role in this area.

References

1. Gruentzig AR, Senning A, Siegenthaler WE. Non operative dilation of coronary artery stenosis: percutaneous transluminal coronary angioplasty. N Engl J Med 1979; 301: 61–8
2. Hartzler GO, Rutherford BD, McConahay DR et al. Percutaneous transluminal coronary angioplasty with and without thrombolytic therapy. Am Heart J 1983; 106: 965–73
3. Meyer J, Merx W, Schmitz H et al. Percutaneous transluminal coronary angioplasty immediately after intracoronary streptolysis of transmural myocardial infarction. Circulation 1982; 66: 905–13
4. Detre K, Holubkov R, Kelsey S et al. Percutaneous coronary angioplasty in 1985–86 and 1977–81: the National Heart Lung and Blood Institute Registry. N Engl J Med 1988; 318: 265–70
5. Coronary Angioplasty 1993. A report of the National Heart Foundation of Australia. Report No. 9. Canberra: National Heart Foundation, 1993
5a. Lieu TA, Gurley RJ, Lundstrom RT, Parmley WW. Primary angioplasty and thrombolysis for acute myocardial infarction. J Am Coll Cardiol 1996; 27: 737–50
6. Michels KB, Yusuf S. Does PTCA in acute myocardial infarction affect mortality and reinfarction rates? A quantitative overview (meta-analysis) of the randomized clinical trials. Circulation 1995; 91: 476–85
6a. GUSTO IIB Angioplasty substudy. Preliminary report at American College of Cardiology 45th Annual Scientific Sessions, March 1996.
7. Topol EJ, Califf RM, George BS et al, and the Thrombolysis and Angioplasty in Myocardial Infarction Study Group: a randomized trial of immediate versus delayed elective angioplasty after intravenous tissue plasminogen activator in acute myocardial infarction. N Engl J Med 1987; 317: 581–8

8. Simoons ML, Arnold AER, Betriu A et al. Thrombolysis with tissue plasminogen activator in acute myocardial infarction: no additional benefit from immediate percutaneous coronary angioplasty. Lancet 1988; I: 197–202
9. Rogers WJ, Baim DS, Gore JM et al for the TIMI II-A Investigators. Comparison of immediate invasive, delayed invasive and conservative strategies after tissue-type plasminogen activator. Circulation 1990; 81: 1457–76
10. O'Neill WW, Weintraub R, Grines CL et al. A prospective, placebo-controlled, randomized trial of intravenous streptokinase and angioplasty versus lone angioplasty therapy of acute myocardial infarction. Circulation 1992; 86: 1710–7
11. Kerins DM, Roy L, FitzGerald GA et al. Platelet and vascular function during coronary thrombolysis with tissue-type plasminogen activator. Circulation 1989; 80: 1718–25
12. Ellis SG, Van de Werf F, Ribeiro da Silva E et al. Present status of rescue coronary angioplasty: current polarization of opinion and randomized trials. J Am Coll Cardiol 1992; 19: 681–6
13. Ellis SG, Ribeiro da Silva E, Heyndrickx GR et al for the Rescue Investigators. Final results of the randomized Rescue study evaluating PTCA after failed thrombolysis for patients with anterior infarction. Abst. Circulation 1993; 88(Suppl. 1): I–106
14. Califf RM, O'Neill W, Stack RS et al. Failure of simple clinical measurements to predict reperfusion status after intravenous thrombolysis. Ann Int Med 1988; 108: 658–62
15. The TIMI Study Group. Comparison of invasive and conservative strategies after treatment with intravenous tissue plasminogen activator in acute myocardial infarction: results of the Thrombolysis in Myocardial Infarction (TIMI) phase II trial. N Engl J Med 1989; 320: 618–27
16. SWIFT (Should We Intervene Following Thrombolysis?) Trial Study Group: SWIFT trial of delayed elective intervention vs conservative treatment after thrombolysis with anistreplase in acute myocardial infarction. Br Med J 1991; 302: 555–60
17. Califf RM, Topol EJ, Gersh BJ. From myocardial salvage to patient salvage in acute myocardial infarction: the role of reperfusion therapy. J Am Coll Cardiol 1989; 14: 1382–8
18. Topol EJ, Califf RM, Vandormael M et al and the Thrombolysis and Angioplasty in Myocardial Infarction (TAMI-6) Study Group. A randomized trial of late reperfusion therapy for acute myocardial infarction. Circulation 1992; 85: 2090–9
19. O'Neill W, Timmis GC, Bourdillon PD et al. A prospective randomized clinical trial of intra coronary streptokinase versus coronary angioplasty for acute myocardial infarction. N Engl J Med 1986; 314: 812–8
20. DeWood MA, Fisher MJ for the Spokane Heart Research Group. Direct PTCA versus intravenous r-TPA in acute myocardial infarction: preliminary results from a prospective randomized trial. Abst. Circulation 1989; 80(Suppl. II): I–418
21. Gibbons RJ, Holmes DR, Reeder GS et al. Immediate angioplasty compared with the administration of a thrombolytic agent followed by conservative treatment for myocardial infarction. N Engl J Med 1993; 328: 685–91
22. Zijlstra F, De Boer MJ, Hoorntje JCA et al. A comparison of immediate coronary angioplasty with intravenous streptokinase in acute myocardial infarction. N Engl J Med 1993; 328: 680–4
23. Grines CL, Browne KR, Marco J et al. A comparison of primary angioplasty with thrombolytic therapy for acute myocardial infarction. N Engl J Med 1993; 328: 673–9
24. DeBoer MJ, Hoorntje JCA, Ottervanger JP, Reiffers S, Suryapranata H, Zijlstra F. Immediate coronary angioplasty versus intravenous streptokinase in acute myocardial infarction—left ventricular ejection fraction, hospital mortality and reinfarction. J Am Coll Cardiol 1994; 23: 1004–8
25. Ribeiro EE, Silva LA, Carneiro R et al. Randomized trial of direct coronary angioplasty versus intravenous streptokinase in acute myocardial infarction. J Am Coll Cardiol 1993; 22: 376–80
26. Elizaga J, Garcia EJ, Delcan JL et al. Primary coronary angioplasty versus systemic thrombolysis in acute anterior myocardial infarction: in hospital results from a prospective randomized trial. Abst. Circulation 1993; 88: (Suppl. I) I–411
27. Simes RJ, Topol EJ, Holmes DR et al for the GUSTO-1 Investigators. Link between the angiographic sub-study and mortality outcomes in a large randomized trial of myocardial reperfusions; importance of early and complete infarct artery reperfusion. Circulation 1995; 91: 1923–8
28. Granger CB, Ohman EM, Bates E. Pooled analysis of angiographic patency rates from thrombolytic therapy trials. Abst. Circulation 1992; 86: I–269
29. The GUSTO-1 Angiographic Investigators. The effects of tissue plasminogen activator, streptokinase or both on coronary artery patency, ventricular function and survival after acute myocardial infarction. N Engl J Med 1993; 329: 1615–22
30. O'Neill WW, Brodie BR, Ivanhoe R, Knopf W, Taylor G, O'Keefe J et al. Primary coronary angioplasty for acute myocardial infarction.

The Primary Angioplasty Registry. Am J Cardiol 1994; 73: 627–34
31. International roundup. Primary angioplasty in myocardial infarction. Brit Heart J 1995; 73: 403–16
32. O'Neill WW. Angioplasty therapy of cardiogenic shock: are randomized trials necessary? J Am Coll Cardiol 1992; 19: 915–7
33. de Feyter PJ, de Jaegere PPT, Murphy ES, Serruys PW. Abrupt coronary artery occlusion during percutaneous transluminal coronary angioplasty. Am Heart J 1992; 123: 1633–42
34. Serruys PW, Luijten HE, Beatt KJ et al. Incidence of restenosis after successful coronary angioplasty: a time-related phenomenon. Circulation 1988; 77: 361–71
35. Serruys PW, de Jaegere P, Kiemeneij F et al. A comparison of balloon expandable stent implantation with balloon angioplasty in patients with coronary artery disease. N Engl J Med 1994; 331: 489–95
36. Fischman DL, Leon MB, Baim DS et al. A randomized comparison of coronary-stent placement and balloon angioplasty in the treatment of coronary artery disease. N Engl J Med 1994; 331: 496–501
37. Colombo A, Hall P, Almagor Y, Malello L et al. Results of intravascular guided coronary stenting without subsequent anticoagulation. J Am Coll Cardiol 1994; 335A
38. Hall P, Colombo A, Almagor Y et al. Preliminary experience with intravascular ultrasound guided Palmaz–Schatz coronary stenting: the acute and short-term results on a consecutive series of patients. J Interven Cardiol 1994; 7: 141–59
39. Topol EJ. The stentor and the sea change. Am J Cardiol 1995; 76: 307–8
40. Topol EJ, Leya F, Pinkerton CA et al. A comparison of directional atherectomy with coronary angioplasty in patients with coronary artery disease. N Engl J Med 1993; 329: 221–7
41. Adelman AG, Cohen EA, Kimball RP et al. A comparison of directional atherectomy with balloon angioplasty for lesions of the left anterior descending coronary artery. N Engl J Med 1993; 329: 228–33
42. Bertrand ME, Lablanche JM, Leroy F et al. Percutaneous transluminal coronary rotary ablation with the Rotablator (European experience). Am J Cardiol 1992; 69: 470–4
43. Vandormael M, Reifart N, Preusler WE et al. Comparison of excimer laser angioplasty and rotational atherectomy with balloon angioplasty for complex lesions: ERBAC study results. J Am Coll Cardiol 1994; 57A
44. Forrester JS, Litvack F, Grundfest WS. Laser angioplasty in cardiovascular disease. Am J Cardiol 1986; 57: 990–2
45. Bittl JA, Sanborn TA. Excimer laser-facilitated coronary angioplasty: relative risk analysis of acute and follow-up results in 200 consecutive patients. Circulation 1992; 86: 71–81
46. Mehta S, Kramer B, Margolis JR et al. Transluminal extraction. Cor Art Dis 1992; 3: 887–96
47. Siegel RJ, Gaines P, Crew J et al. Clinical results of percutaneous ultrasound angioplasty. J Am Coll Cardiol 1993; 22: 480–8
48. Clowes AW. Improving the interface between biomaterials and the blood: the gene therapy approach. Circulation 1996; 93: 1319–20

46 Coronary artery bypass graft surgery (CABG)

Mark AJ Newman

Introduction

Coronary artery bypass grafting (CABG) is a common method of myocardial revascularization[1–3] and coronary care staff will frequently be involved in the management of these patients. The technique usually involves the use of extra corporal cardiopulmonary bypass to allow cardiac arrest with cardioplegia.

The bypass conduits are anastomosed to the coronary arteries distal to the angiographically determined coronary lesions. Autogenous saphenous veins are commonly used conduits.[4] They have high (> 90%) early patency rates but due to progressive intinal hyperplasia and accelerated atherosclerosis in the veins, patency rates rapidly fall after about 10 years to about 25% at 15 years.

The internal mammary artery (IMA)[5] has much better long-term patency rates, especially when anastomosed to the left anterior descending (LAD) coronary artery. It is well established that survival and angina-free intervals are better with the IMA rather than saphenous vein anastomosed to the LAD.[6] There is less convincing evidence of improved results with multiple IMA grafts or IMA grafts to vessels other than the LAD. The IMA is also a smaller diameter vessel and may not supply adequate perfusion acutely in some situations. Also it may not be appropriate to use it for bypassing vessels with less than 60–70% obstructions due to competitive flow resulting in early closure of the IMA.

Alternative conduits such as arm veins, gastro-epiploic artery, inferior epigastric arteries, radial arteries and synthetic grafts have been used in special situations but with generally less favourable results than IMA or saphenous vein grafts.[7]

Effect of CABG on survival

The role of coronary artery bypass graft surgery in improving survival, compared with medical therapy, has been studied in a number of randomized trials.[8] These trials have been subjected recently to a helpful meta-analysis which clarifies the overall benefit and the subgroups most likely to benefit.[9] A total of 1324 surgically treated and 1325 medically treated patients were compared. At 5 years post randomization, the relative risk reduction in the surgically treated patients was 36% (10.2 versus 15.8% mortality). These benefits were maintained at 7 years (27% relative risk reduction) and 10 years (13% relative risk reduction). The 5-year relative risk reduction was greater in those with left main coronary disease (68%) than in those with three vessel disease (42%) and one or two vessel disease (23%). The benefit was five times greater in those with left ventricular (LV) dysfunction compared with normal left ventricular function.

A high crossover rate for medical to surgical therapy during the course of these trials (37% on average) may have diluted the impact of surgery on survival; furthermore, the trials were conducted at a time when surgical bypass techniques were less developed than at present and were associated with a higher operative mortality. On the other hand, the improvements in medical therapy in recent years and the overall decline in mortality would undoubtedly narrow the gap between medical and surgical treatment in the unlikely event of a modern day randomized comparison.

Nevertheless there is clear evidence from the clinical trials that in more advanced coronary artery disease, i.e. left main or three vessel with reduced LV function or severe myocardial ischaemia, CABG is the preferred therapy. The trials also show that for mild one or two vessel disease, surgical therapy has no advantage over medical therapy. Patients in the middle ground, whose coronary anatomy would be treatable with either CABG or percutaneous transluminal coronary angioplasty (PTCA), are currently the subject of a new series of trials, several of which have reported their results.[10–12] These trials show similar results: that is, in a carefully selected group (about 10% of those screened) whose coronary anatomy is suitable for either procedure, the mortality and myocardial infarction rates are similar with either CABG or PTCA. The PTCA group had a higher likelihood of recurrent angina requiring further revascularization procedures, but the CABG group had a higher rate of complications and longer hospital stays at the time of the procedure.

CABG surgery in the coronary care patient

The results of CABG surgery have improved markedly over the past twenty years[3] (see Fig. 46.1). However, emergency surgery, to treat acute ischaemic syndromes, still is a major risk factor for morbidity and mortality for CABG.

Mortality rates of less than 1% are now achieved for elective CABG, but urgent and emergency surgery can increase these risks fivefold. It has been shown experimentally that the recently infarcted heart is more sensitive to global ischaemia, induced during CABG, than the normal heart or heart with a healed infarct.[12a]

There are four major indications for CABG in the patient in the CCU. These are:

- CABG for unstable angina
- emergency CABG for evolving myocardial infarction (MI)
- urgent CABG for ongoing ischaemia post-infarction
- early elective CABG for post-infarction angina or for severe coronary disease.

Unstable angina

Patients with unstable angina can usually be settled with bed-rest, heparinization and nitrates (see Ch. 60).

However, there are a number of patients with severe coronary lesions who continue to have unstable angina despite maximal medical treatment. In these patients, urgent coronary angiography is indicated. Many patients will be suitable for balloon angioplasty (PTCA), but there will be some patients who have either severe triple vessel disease or coronary lesions unsuitable for PTCA. These patients are candidates for urgent CABG.

Before the use of intravenous nitrates, heparin and PTCA, many patients who came to early CABG for unstable angina were included in randomized comparisons of medical and surgical therapy in unstable angina. There were no clear benefits of surgery on survival,[13–14] except in patients with

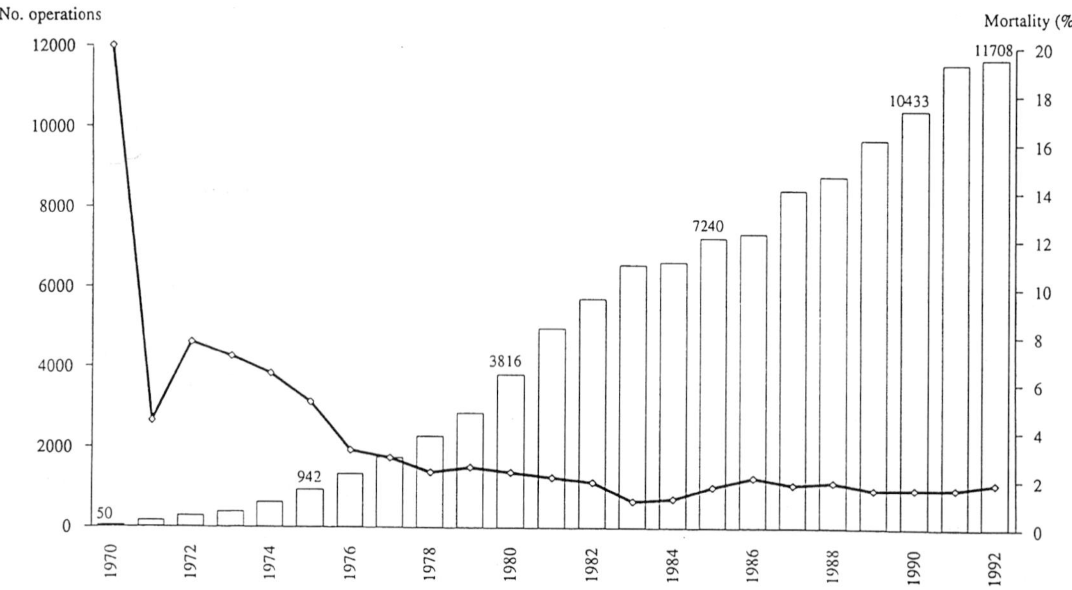

Fig. 46.1 Number of cases and operative mortality for coronary artery bypass surgery in Australia from 1970 to mid-1990s. Reprinted with permission from the National Heart Foundation of Australia.

depressed LV function,[15] but there were clear-cut benefits on symptoms and functional capacity in a majority of patients. It was shown that mortality with CABG was about twice as high for unstable patients as for stable patients.[16] The reason for this is not clear, but may relate to coronary spasm. Therefore if possible, unstable angina should be settled medically and CABG performed as an early elective procedure. There have been no randomized comparisons of treatment with PTCA versus CABG, in patients with similar anatomy, although the previously cited RITA,[10] GABI[11] and EAST[12] trials included many patients with unstable angina. A non-randomized comparison of over 9000 patients with unstable angina in the Duke database[17] attempted to draw conclusions on the efficacy of CABG or PTCA versus medical therapy after matching for baseline characteristics. They concluded that CABG produced better 5 year survival than PTCA or medical therapy in severe proximal LAD stenosis, but better outcomes with PTCA for less severe disease. There were no differences in survival in patients with single vessel disease.

The TIMI III-B Study[18] compared outcomes with a conservative strategy versus an aggressive strategy of early (less than 48 hours post admission) cardiac catheterization followed by revascularization if appropriate. Their choice of PTCA or CABG depended upon the coronary anatomy and LV function. No difference in 6 week survival was seen; however, revascularization within six weeks was deemed necessary in 61% of the conservatively treated group.

Aspirin is a very useful drug for unstable angina, but unfortunately causes a significant coagulopathy in many patients subjected to cardiopulmonary bypass.[19] Generally cardiac surgeons would like to cease the patients' aspirin at least 7 days prior to surgery.

Intravenous heparin is usually adequate in unstable angina without aspirin; however, some patients with critical coronary anatomy should remain on aspirin until the time of surgery. In patients on aspirin, aprotinin has been shown to reduce blood loss after CABG. Platelet transfusions may also be necessary post-operatively to control bleeding.

CABG for evolving myocardial infarction

Early reperfusion following acute coronary occlusion has been shown to significantly reduce infarct size and reduce mortality. Although the most expedient way to do this is with IV thrombolytic agents or if necessary with PTCA, there is a considerable volume of experimental evidence to show that controlled surgical reperfusion results in better preservation of myocardium in early infarction.[20] A solution which maintains cardioplegia and is alkalotic, hypocalcaemic, hyperosmolar and contains amino acid substrates has been shown to be very effective experimentally and clinically.

Although there have been encouraging reports of the use of CABG for emergency treatment of myocardial infarction,[21] surgical reperfusion must be performed within 6 hours of infarction. The logistics and cost of this form of treatment, at present, preclude its widespread use. Acute CABG may be indicated in acute infarction in the setting of failure or unsuitability for thrombolysis and PTCA.

The risk of CABG in this setting is a mortality of about 5–8%. The risk markedly increases, to a mortality of 30–50%, in the setting of cardiogenic shock.[22]

Urgent surgery for ongoing ischaemia post infarction

This group of patients is at a high risk of further infarction and death,[23] and urgent CABG is indicated for uncontrolled angina post myocardial infarction in patients unsuitable for PTCA.[24,25]

Risks for operation are about twice that for elective surgery and further increase when there is significant associated LV dysfunction. Risks are particularly high in women, in older patients and those with prior CABG surgery.[24,25] Surprisingly the timing of surgery after infarction has not been shown to be a risk factor except when surgery is performed within the first 2–3 days post infarction. The timing of surgery does not seem to be an important risk factor in patients with normal LV function but delayed surgery is safer than early surgery, when the LV function is significantly depressed.[26] Prior thrombolysis did not increase post-operative bleeding or mortality unless the operation was performed within 12 hours of streptokinase therapy.[27]

Early CABG for post infarction angina or severe coronary disease

Early investigation after AMI currently practised is based on observations that there is little to be gained by delaying surgery. The logistics of performing surgery during the same hospital stay often favour early intervention, but a delay of several weeks to allow healing of the infarct and haemodynamic stabilization is usually preferred. The TIMI-IIB study was not able to demonstrate a better survival for an aggressive early revascularization policy using either PTCA or CABG compared with a conservative policy of revascularization as determined by symptoms.[28]

Risk factors for mortality and morbidity from CABG

Many studies have looked at these factors and they have changed over the years as techniques of pre-operative management, anaesthesia, myocardial protection and post-operative management have improved.

Risks for mortality

At present the major risk factors for mortality are:

- risk doubles approximately for each decade after 60
- sex—risk factor is double for females
- emergency operation—risk is about five times elective risk
- very poor ventricular function—about two times risk
- re-operation—risk is doubled.

Risks for morbidity

Risks for morbidity include:

- Cerebro-vascular accident (CVA)—risk overall is about 1% and is increased with age, peripheral vascular disease, previous stroke, known carotid disease, left main disease and diabetes. Post-operative CVA is usually due to atheromatous emboli from the ascending aorta.
- Renal failure—risk is usually low but is increased in pre-operative renal impairment, poor ventricular function and diabetes.
- Infection—major sternal infection rates are about 1% overall. There is increased risk in diabetes, with use of bilateral internal mammary artery and in obesity.
- Bleeding—excess bleeding requiring return to theatre occurs in about 2% of patients. The risk of bleeding is increased in those on aspirin within 5–7 days of surgery, in the elderly (> 70 years), those with coagulopathy and in re-operation.

Pre-operative workup

In the history, specific enquiry should be made for evidence of past transient ischaemic attacks (TIAs) or CVAs or history of blood-borne viral diseases or transfusion reactions. A detailed cigarette smoking history is relevant. An accurate drug history is recorded. Presence of diabetes and its treatment are also important, as is use of systemic steroids.

Specific attention should be paid to certain areas of physical examination. This includes examination of:

- the peripheral pulses and listening for carotid bruits
- the state of the saphenous veins and amount of subcutaneous fat
- the sternal area for evidence of skin infection
- the state of the dentition
- the lungs for evidence of chronic airway disease etc.

Investigations should include:

- routine full blood count, renal and liver function tests and cardiac enzymes
- arterial blood gases for chronic lung disease
- electrocardiograms and chest X-rays
- carotid ultrasound and doppler are necessary if there is suspicion of carotid disease
- a coagulation screen in those with suspected coagulopathy
- cross matching of blood. For first time surgery, three units are usually sufficient and for re-do surgery, five units are ordered.

Drugs

The following should cease:

- aspirin at least 7 days pre-operatively if possible
- warfarin 7 days pre-operatively if possible.

If INR is high immediately pre-operatively, then Vitamin K should be given intravenously slowly (1 mg if there is need for re-warfarinization).

Patients will probably require fresh frozen plasma post-operatively as well.

The following should continue:

- beta blockers
- digoxin
- calcium antagonists
- nitrates

- ACE inhibitors for cardiac failure.

Staff should consider reducing ACE inhibitors or changing to another agent if used for hypertension, as the prolonged effect post-operatively can cause hypotension.

References

1. State of the art symposium on coronary arterial surgery. Circulation 1989; 79 (Suppl. I): I-1–I-192
2. Feinleib M, Havlik RJ, Gillum RF, Pokras R, McCarthy E, Moien M. Coronary heart disease and related procedures. National Hospital Discharge Survey Data. Circulation 1989; 79 (Suppl. I): I-1–I-18
3. Cardiac Surgery 1992. A report by the National Heart Foundation of Australia. Canberra: National Heart Foundation, 1993
4. Favaloro R. Saphenous vein autograft replacement of severe segmental coronary occlusion. Ann Thorac Surg 1968; 5: 335–9
5. Green GE. Internal mammary artery—coronary anastomosis: three year experience with 165 patients. Ann Thorac Surg 1972; 14: 260–71
6. Loop FD, Lytle BW, Cosgrove DM et al. Influence of the internal mammary artery graft on 10-year survival and other cardiac events. N Engl J Med 1986; 314: 1–6
7. Foster ED, Krane MAK. Alternative conduits for aorto-coronary bypass grafting. Circulation 1989; (Suppl. I): I-34–I-39
8. Frye RL, Fisher L, Schaff HV, Gersh BJ, Vliestra RE, Mock MB. Randomized trials of coronary artery bypass surgery. Prog Cardiovasc Dis 1987; 30: 1–22
9. Yusuf S, Zucker D, Peduzzi R et al. Effect of coronary artery bypass graft surgery on survival: overview of 10 year results from randomized trials by the Coronary Artery Bypass Graft Trialists Collaboration. Lancet 1994; 344: 563–70
10. RITA trial participants. Coronary angioplasty versus coronary artery bypass surgery: the Intervention Treatment of Angina (RITA) trial. Lancet 1994; 341: 573–80
11. Hamm CW, Reimers J, Ischinger T et al. A randomised study of coronary angioplasty compared with bypass surgery in patients with symptomatic multi-vessel coronary disease. N Engl J Med 1994; 331: 1037–43
12. King SB III, Lembo NJ, Weintraub WS et al. A randomised trial comparing coronary angioplasty with coronary bypass surgery. N Engl J Med 1994; 331: 1044–50

12a. Newman MA, Chen XZ, Rabinov M, Williams J and Rosenfeldt FL. Sensitivity of the recently infarcted heart to hypothermic cardioplegia: beneficial effect of orotic acid. J Thorac Cardiovasc Surg 1989; 97: 593–604

13. Luchi RJ, Scott SM, Dupree RH. Comparison of medical and surgical treatment for unstable angina pectoris. Results of a Veterans Administration Cooperative Study. N Engl J Med 1987; 316: 977–84
14. Russell RO, Moraski RE, Kouchoukos N et al. Unstable angina pectoris: national cooperative study group to compare surgical and medical therapy. Am J Cardiol 1978; 42: 839–48
15. Scott SM, Luchi RJ, Dupree RH. Veterans Administration Cooperative Study for treatment of patients with unstable angina. Results in patients with abnormal left ventricular function. Circulation 1988; 78 (Suppl. I): I-113–I-121
16. Kaiser GC, Schaff HV, Killip T. Myocardial revascularization for unstable angina. Circulation 1989; 79: I-60–I-67
17. Mark DB, Nelson CL, Califf RM et al. Continuing evolution of therapy for coronary artery disease. Initial results from the era of coronary angioplasty. Circulation 1994; 89: 2015–25
18. The TIMI-IIIB Investigators. Effects of tissue plasminogen activator and a comparison of early invasive and conservative strategies in unstable angina and non-Q-wave myocardial infarction. Results of the TIMI-IIIB Trial. Circulation 1994; 89: 1545–56
19. Ferraris VA, Ferraris SP, Lough WR et al. Perioperative aspirin ingestion increases operative blood loss after aortocoronary bypass grafting. Ann Thorac Surg 1988; 45: 71–4
20. Buckberg GD. When is cardiac muscle damaged irreversibly? J Thorac Cardiovasc Surg 1986; 92: 483–7
21. De Wood MA, Spores J, Berg R Jr et al. Acute myocardial infarction: a decade of experience with surgical reperfusion in 701 patients. Circulation 1983; 68: II-8–II-16
22. Laks H, Rosenkranz E, Buckberg GD. Surgical treatment of cardiogenic shock after myocardial infarction. Circulation 1986; 74: 11–16
23. Shuster EH, Bulkley BH. Early post infarction angina: ischaemia at a distance and ischaemia in the infarct zone. N Engl J Med 1981; 305: 1101–5
24. Kouchoukos NT, Murphy S, Philpott T, Pelate C, Marshall WG Jr. Coronary artery bypass grafting for post-infarction angina pectoris. Circulation 1989; 79(Suppl. I): I-68–I-72
25. Kennedy JW, Ivey TD, Misbach G et al. Coronary artery bypass grafting surgery early after acute myocardial infarction. Circulation 1989; 79: I-78
26. Hochberg MS, Parsonnet V, Gielinschky I et al. Timing of

coronary revascularization after acute myocardial infarction. Early and late results in patients revascularized within seven weeks. J Thorac Cardiovasc Surg 1984; 88: 914–21

27. Lee KF, Mandell J, Rankin JS et al. Immediate versus delayed coronary grafting after streptokinase treatment. Pre-operative blood loss and clinical results. J Thorac Cardiovasc Surg 1988; 95: 216–22
28. TIMI Study Group. Comparison of invasive and conservative strategies after treatment with intravenous tissue plasminogen activator in acute myocardial infarctions. Results of the Thrombolysis In Myocardial Infarction (TIMI) Phase II trial. N Engl J Med 1989; 320: 618–27

47 Circulatory assist devices including IABP

Bradley M Power

Introduction

Pharmacological agents such as inotropes and vasodilators remain the mainstay of treatment for acute myocardial dysfunction and cardiogenic shock. The use of such agents may be associated with significant problems. Inotropic therapy (see Ch. 32) improves cardiac output but at the cost of increased myocardial oxygen consumption (MVO_2). Vasodilators reduce left ventricular afterload but can worsen existing hypotension, aggravating myocardial ischaemia. Vasopressor therapy may increase coronary artery perfusing pressure, but at the expense of increased afterload resulting in possible increased MVO_2 or decreased stroke volume.

As a result of problems with pharmacological support, mechanical devices have been developed to allow the short-term support of the failing myocardium. Table 47.1 displays the mechanical devices which have been used to manage cardiovascular dysfunction.

Balloon counterpulsation

History

Kantrowitz (1968)[1] described the first clinical use of balloon counterpulsation in man, utilizing a technique outlined by Moulopoulos (1962)[2] in which a balloon catheter was positioned in the descending aorta and was inflated and collapsed in synchrony with cardiac relaxation and contraction respectively (that is, counterpulsation).

Recent developments in balloon pump technology have hinged upon the development of rapidly responsive aortic balloons which can be inserted at the bedside, of pumps capable of shuttling gas rapidly in and out of these balloons, and of improved timing against markers of ventricular contraction and relaxation.

Theory

The intra-aortic balloon pump (IABP) is a volume displacement device designed to provide partial assistance to the left ventricle by inflation and deflation of an intra-aortic balloon catheter synchronized with the cardiac cycle (see Fig. 47.1).

By deflating the balloon just prior to ventricular systole, inertial resistance to blood flow is reduced and left ventricular (LV) afterload falls. Balloon deflation thus results in reduced MVO_2 and/or increased stroke volume. Clinically effective ballooning results in increased stroke volume, slowing of the pulse rate, a fall in pulmonary artery wedge pressure (PAWP) and an increase in cardiac output of 10–40%[3] (see Table 47.2).

Inflation of the balloon at the commencement of diastole results in increased aortic diastolic pressure, and since diastolic blood flow is responsible for 70% of cardiac perfusion, coronary artery and collateral vessel flow should theoretically increase (see Fig. 47.2).

Detailed studies of coronary and myocardial blood flow during IABP counterpulsation of non-shocked patients with critical coronary artery stenosis have failed to show significant increase in coronary artery blood flow[4,5] suggesting benefits in this group to be mostly due to reduced myocardial work and oxygen demand. In the patient with severe hypotension or cardiogenic shock, augmentation of diastolic pressures is still a likely significant effect of counterpulsation.[6,7]

Standard 40 cc balloons are usually used, as these provide adequate volume displacement and incomplete aortic occlusion required for optimal ballooning; however, a smaller balloon may be required in small adults.

Laboratory and mathematical models have been used to

Table 47.1 Mechanical cardiac support devices

	Advantages	Disadvantages	Use
Short-term cardiac support			
Intra-aortic balloon pump (right ventricle support available)	Bedside insertion Common use Good safety profile Reduce MVO_2	Require stable rhythm Modest augmentation of Cardiac output (10–40%)	Post surgery Pre-op support High risk angio.
Percutaneous cardiopulmonary bypass	Decreased MVO_2 Independent of LV function & rhythm	No improvement coronary perfusion Perfusionist to control	Circulatory collapse Short-term post-op
External centrifugal & roller pumps (non-pulsatile)	LV or RV support Independent of LV function & rhythm Mod clinical experience Improves coronary perfusion	Require surgical insertion Require extensive supervision Non-pulsatile Expensive	Severe post-op dysfunction Circulatory collapse
External pulsatile ventricular assist device	RV or LV support Pulsatile flow	Difficult to insert Expensive	Investigation only
Intermediate/long-term devices			
Implantable LVAD (pulsatile)	Allow mobility	Extensive surgery needed LV support only	Investigation only Transplant bridge
Orthotopic ventricles (total artificial heart)	Long-term use (80% alive > 30 days)	High incidence of bleeding and infection	Transplant bridge

Table 47.2 The haemodynamic effects of intra-aortic balloon pumping. Reproduced with permission from Goldberg IF 1992, reference 3

Effects	% change
Peak systolic arterial pressure	5–15 decrease
Presystolic (end-diastolic) aortic pressure	20–30 decrease
Diastolic aortic pressure	70 increase
Mean aortic pressure	No significant change
Left ventricular end-diastolic pressure	10–20 decrease
Pulmonary artery wedge pressure	10–20 decrease
Peak dp/dt	10–20 decrease
Heart rate	5–10 decrease
V_{max}	25 decrease
Cardiac output	10–40 increase

quantify the relative effects of deflation and inflation upon cardiac metabolic parameters.[6] Optimal timing intervals for maximal afterload reduction and diastolic augmentation may overlap and vary with heart rate, baseline stroke volume and baseline mean aortic pressure. Clinical experience is essential to 'tailor' timing to the clinical situation.

Role of IABP counterpulsation in the coronary care unit

Early reports of the use of IABP counterpulsation in acute myocardial infarction (AMI) concentrated on its role in haemodynamic stabilization in patients with

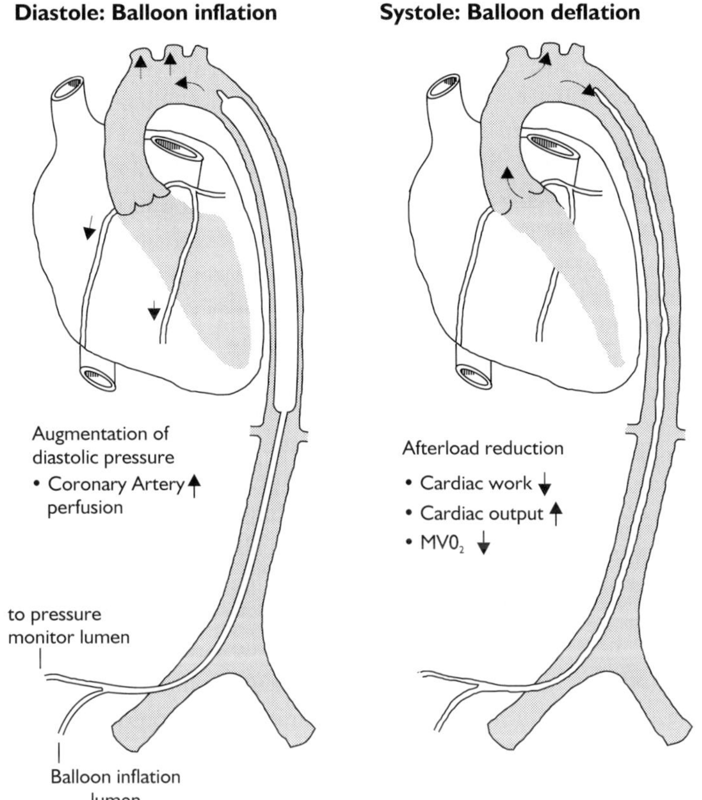

Fig. 47.1 Intra-aortic balloon catheter in the aorta.

cardiogenic shock and severe heart failure. This experience demonstrated that the patient's clinical state could be improved in about 70% of patients.[8–10] However, direct benefits in infarct size and survival could not be demonstrated in randomized trials.[11,12] As a result, IABP counterpulsation is now rarely used as the sole adjunct to pharmacologic therapy of cardiogenic shock and severe cardiac failure (see Chs. 56, 57). However, the capacity of IABP counterpulsation to achieve haemodynamic stabilization in most patients has necessitated a widening role in the management of patients with cardiogenic shock prior to angioplasty,[13] or bypass surgery[14] or for circulatory support after successful revascularization.[15]

IABP has been successfully used to support the circulation as an adjunct to the early surgical management of patients suffering mechanical complications of

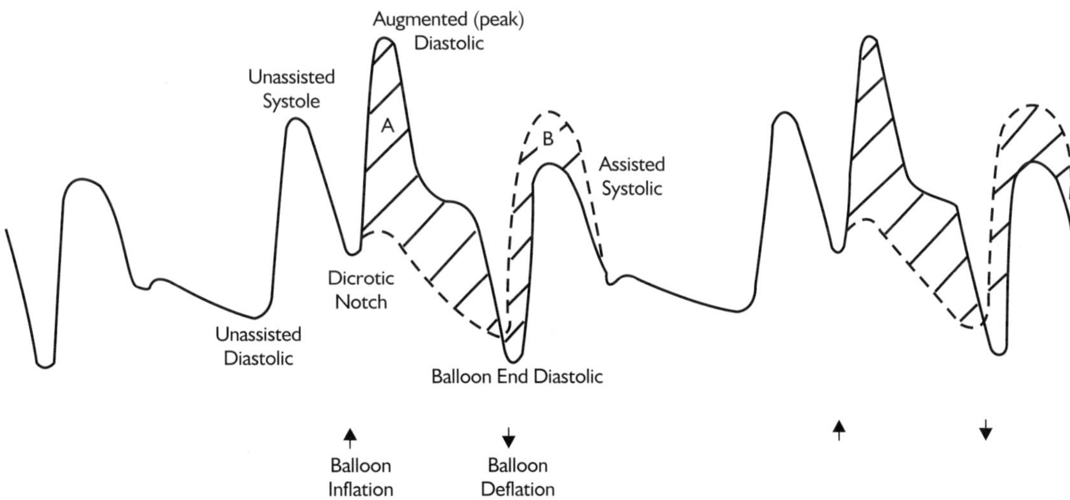

Fig. 47.2 Solid line displays arterial pressure trace with counterpulsation ratio set at 1:2. Dotted line shows theoretical non ballooned beats. Balloon inflation ↑ begins at the the dicrotic notch and deflation ↓ commences with the next systole. Balloon timing is determined with the balloon ratio on 1:2. Diastolic augmented pressure is usually greater than systolic pressures. Area A is related to the degree of diastolic augmentation. With effective balloon deflation, afterload is reduced. It is important to note that assisted diastolic (balloon end diastolic) is < unassisted diastolic, and assisted systolic < unassisted systolic. The size of these differences, or area B, is related to the degree of afterload reduction.

myocardial infarction such as septal rupture and papillary muscle rupture[16] or 'subacute' left free wall rupture.[17] The use of IABP for control of refractory arrhythmias after infarction[18] or for control of myocardial ischaemia[19] has been largely surpassed by the wider use of antiarrhythmia devices (see Chs. 49, 50) and revascularization techniques (see Chs 45, 46).

Indications

The balloon pump is suitable for support of the failing myocardium provided the condition is potentially reversible. Such conditions are summarized in the information box.[3,20,21]

While counterpulsation is generally used to assist the left ventricle, pulmonary artery counterpulsation to assist the impaired right ventricle is possible but rarely used. Again the existence of a reversible condition is the major imperative.

Contraindications

Contraindications to IABP counterpulsation include aortic regurgitation and thoracic aortic dissection.

Counterpulsation is not usually introduced in the presence of severe irreversible cardiac disease unless as a bridge to transplantation, nor when there is severe irreversible chronic disease. Severe aorto-iliac disease or previous arterial surgery may preclude femoral insertion and necessitate direct thoracic or axillary insertion. The increased risk of these insertions is judged against likely clinical benefit.

Complications

The possible complications[20,22] of IABP counterpulsation are summarized in the box.

Method

An intra-aortic balloon is usually inserted via the femoral artery and occupies the descending aorta distal to the left subclavian artery (Fig. 47.1). Balloon inflation and deflation is performed by the rapid shuttling of gas in and out of the balloon. Helium is the preferred agent because of favourable flow characteristics.

The trigger for balloon counterpulsation in routine use is best provided by the surface ECG. R waves are identified by the console and define the RR interval. Regular cardiac rhythms provide stable RR intervals used by algorithms within balloon consoles to then reference balloon deflation and inflation triggers to ventricular systole and diastole. Manual timing adjustment markers allow variations to the timing of inflation and deflation, necessary because of mechanical limits to balloon inflation and deflation, and because of dynamic, variable relationships between the R wave and ventricular contraction.

Because of mechanical limits to gas shuttling, early balloon pumps were required to 'predict' ventricular contraction by algorithms based on previous RR intervals.[23] This led to inefficient counterpulsation during ectopy and atrial fibrillation. Recently, improved computing and more efficient shuttling of gas has allowed 'real time' pumping such that balloon deflation is triggered by the actual R wave being sensed.[6,23] This has improved the ability of balloon pumps to supply afterload reduction and to remain inflated throughout diastole (improving diastolic augmentation).[6] Atrial fibrillation, however, still represents a challenge to effective ballooning.

Where the surface ECG does not provide sufficient signal, or where there is electrical interference (for example, diathermy) balloon timing may be performed using the arterial pressure trace or alternatively from pacemaker signals. Internal timing mode may be needed during cardiac arrest.

Indications for intra-aortic balloon pump (IABP) counterpulsation

- **Cardiogenic shock or pump failure**
  Post cardiopulmonary bypass
  AMI
- **Mechanical complications of AMI**
  VSD
  Acute mitral regurgitation
  Subacute free wall rupture
- **Prophylaxis during high risk angiography or angioplasty**
- **Prophylaxis during general surgery of patients with poor left ventricular function**
- **Bridge to transplantation**

Complications of IABP counterpulsation

- **Complications related to arterial insertion**
  Limb ischaemia—compartment syndrome and limb loss may occur if not recognized early
  Arterial wall damage and dissection
  Haemorrhage post-removal
- **Problems related to intravascular catheter**
  Infection
  Thrombosis and embolus including stroke
  Balloon entrapment (rare)
  Balloon rupture (rare)
  Renal artery obstruction
- **Errors of inappropriate timing**
  Increased afterload
  Coronary artery steal

Practical use

Intra-aortic counterpulsation is used as an adjunct to the management of severe cardiac dysfunction and is often performed in conjunction with inotropic therapy and afterload reduction, 'physiological pacing' and, if necessary, controlled ventilation. Invasive arterial pressure monitoring and cardiac output measurement (by flow directed Swan–Ganz catheter) are usually performed so that response to therapy can be assessed.

Balloon position

Insertion can be performed percutaneously or via cut-down of a femoral artery. The method of arterial access is described in detail in Chapter 39. The balloon is then positioned using image intensification or with a 'blind' technique following measurement of the desired catheter length and with analysis of balloon catheter inflation waveform if available. The tip is positioned 2–3 cm below the origin of the left subclavian artery, and the proximal end of the balloon will usually then lie above the renal arteries.

Timing

Optimal balloon timing is usually assessed by visual examination of the pressure trace printout while ballooning at a ratio of 2:1 which allows augmented and non-augmented pressure waves to be viewed simultaneously. The inflation marker is adjusted to allow inflation to occur after the dicrotic notch (aortic valve closure) thus causing maximal increase in diastolic pressures. The deflation marker is adjusted to cause maximal fall in end-diastolic pressure or maximal fall in systolic pressure between ballooned and non-ballooned beats (see Fig. 47.2) without intruding into the diastolic period. Caution is taken to avoid premature or delayed inflation and deflation. Regular checks should be performed to exclude poor timing of inflation and deflation and adjustments may be necessary where cardiac rate changes by more than 10 beats per minute from the baseline setting.

Regular cardiac rhythm

Regular cardiac rhythm provides the best substrate for balloon pumping. Ectopy sufficient to interfere with counterpulsation may require antiarrhythmic therapy, regularization of cardiac rate with overdrive pacing, or both.

Atrial fibrillation

AF is particularly difficult for all IABP consoles to track. Cardioversion should be considered. If this is not possible, slowing of ventricular rate and regularization with overdrive pacing should be considered where a ventricular pacemaker is present. If the ventricular response cannot be adequately controlled, some consoles require that the deflation timer be set to maximize chances of deflation upon detection of an R wave. This minimizes the risk of inadvertent increases in left ventricular afterload.

Rapid cardiac rates

This situation may not allow the balloon console to track and if they cannot be controlled (e.g. heart rate > 150 per minute), 2:1 counterpulsation may be necessary.

Console alarms

Console alarms readily alert the clinician to difficulties with balloon obstruction, gas leak and loss of trigger. Examination of balloon pressure traces if available, of chest X-rays, of arterial pressure traces and of clinical data at regular intervals are needed to ensure optimal balloon pump function.

Balloon weaning

Balloon weaning is generally undertaken when sufficient improvement in left ventricular function has occurred to allow removal. The technique of removal is described in Chapter 39. Inotropic support should usually be low, such that an increase in this therapy will cover the reduction in assistance consequent upon balloon removal. Weaning can be accomplished by reduction of balloon ratio to 2:1 and then 3:1, or alternatively by reducing balloon volume. Weaning by progressive reduction in balloon volume may be preferred to weaning by decreasing ballooning ratio in the patient with angina.[7]

Systemic anticoagulation

Systemic anticoagulation with intravenous heparin is usually commenced at the time of balloon insertion in the non-surgical patient and as soon as feasible in the post-operative patient. Continuous heparin infusion (low dose) is also connected to the pressure monitoring lumen at the time of insertion.

Pharmacological cardiac support

If optimal balloon pump augmentation is to be obtained, pharmacological cardiac support is usually necessary.

Monitoring

While examination of a balloon pump pressure trace gives the best indication of the adequacy of balloon inflation and deflation, it does not give any direct indication of the effects on myocardial oxygen supply and demand.[6]

Clinical effect must be judged by examination of clinical parameters such as cardiac output and PAWP, by review of markers of systemic perfusion and by assessment of ST segments where cardiac ischaemia is suspected. Traditionally charted variables such as systolic and diastolic blood pressure have less meaning (Fig. 47.2) and the best indicators of balloon function are probably the augmented diastolic pressure (as a marker of coronary perfusion), balloon aortic end-diastolic pressure (as an indication of afterload reduction) and mean aortic pressure (as an indication of systemic perfusion). The CCU should have policies regarding which parameters are recorded and which parameters to use when calculating derived cardiac indices.

Ventricular assist devices

Mechanical assist devices are used for temporary support of the failing ventricle where the ventricle has been or is unlikely to be responsive to a combination of pharmacological therapy and IABP and where there is reversible cardiac dysfunction. The invasive nature of these devices and the need for reversible cardiac dysfunction has seen their use largely confined to the post-cardiothoracic surgical population where sustained separation from bypass by conventional means has been impossible. Ventricular assist devices, unlike counterpulsation devices, can replace up to 100% of ventricular output on a temporary basis.

The Medtronic Biomedicus (Biomedica Comp) centrifugal pump is a commonly used ventricular assist device. Blood is taken from the left atrium and is replaced in the aortic root. Non-pulsatile blood flow at a rate of 2–5 litres per minute is generated by a rotor pump head, flow being adjusted to allow 'resting' of the ventricle but maintenance of systemic perfusion. The devices are usually used in combination with pharmacological therapy and often in association with a balloon pump, the latter assisting pulsatile flow. While they are most commonly used for support of the left ventricle (LVAD), they can be used to support the right ventricle (RVAD), and biventricular support (BIVAD) can also be provided.

Major complications of LVAD use are bleeding, thrombus formation, air embolism, infection and thrombocytopenia.[3] Heparin-bonded tubing reduces the risk of thrombus, but systemic heparinization is usually needed. Surgical assistance is needed for replacement of worn pump heads, for ultimate removal of cannulae and for final closure of the chest where this has not been possible.

Weaning is usually judged clinically by reducing blood flow through the pump and assessing the ability of the heart to cope. The benefit from continued ventricular assistance is balanced against the risk of thromboembolism and infection.

Other ventricular assist devices

A variety of mechanical assist devices are under investigation for circulatory support, although their use is not widespread. The devices available are summarized in Table 47.1.

References

1. Kantrowitz A, Tjonneland F, Freed PS, Phillips SJ, Butner AN, Sherman JL Jnr. Initial clinical experience with intra-aortic balloon pumping in cardiogenic shock. JAMA 1968; 203: 135–40
2. Moulopolis SD, Topaz S, Kolff WF. Diastolic balloon pumping (with carbon dioxide) in the aorta; a mechanical assistance to the failing circulation. Am Heart J 1962; 63: 669–75
3. Goldberg IF. Nonpharmacologic management of cardiac arrest and cardiogenic shock. Chest 1992; 102(Suppl. 5 No. 2) 596S–616S
4. Port SC, Patel S, Schmidt DH. Effects of intra-aortic balloon counterpulsation on myocardial blood flow in patients with severe coronary artery disease. J Am Coll Cardiol 1984; 3: 1367–74
5. MacDonald RG, Hill JA, Feldman RL. Failure of intra-aortic balloon counterpulsation to augment distal coronary perfusion during percutaneous translumenal coronary angioplasty. Am J Cardiol 1987; 59: 359–61
6. Barnea O, Moore TW, Dubin SE, Jaron D. Cardiac energy considerations during intraaortic balloon pumping. IEEE Transactions of Biomedical Engineering 1990; 37(ii): 170–81
7. Fuchs RM, Brin KP, Brinker JA et al. Augmentation of regional coronary blood flow by intra-aortic balloon counterpulsation in patients with unstable angina. Circulation 1983; 68: 117–23
8. McEnany MT, Kay HR, Buckley MJ et al. Clinical experience with intra-aortic balloon pump support in 728 patients. Circulation 1978; 58: I-124–32
9. Willerson JT, Curry GC, Watson JT et al. Intra-aortic balloon counterpulsation in patients with cardiogenic shock, medically refractory left ventricular failure and/or recurrent ventricular tachycardia. Am J Med 1975; 58: 183–91
10. Hagemeijer F, Laird JD, Haalebos MM, Hogenholtz PG. Effectiveness of intra-aortic balloon pumping without cardiac surgery for patients with severe heart failure secondary to recent myocardial infarction. Am J Cardiol 1977; 40: 951–6
11. O'Rourke MF, Norris RM, Campbell TJ, Chang VP, Sammel NL. Randomized controlled trial of intra-aortic balloon counterpulsation in early myocardial infarction with acute heart failure. Am J Cardiol 1981; 47: 815–20
12. Flaherty JT, Becker LC, Weiss JL et al. Results of a randomized prospective trial of intra-aortic balloon counterpulsation and intravenous nitroglycerine in patients with acute myocardial infarction. J Am Coll Cardiol 1985; 6: 434–46
13. Bengtson JR, Kaplan AJ, Pieper JS et al. Prognosis in cardiogenic shock after acute myocardial infarction in the interventional era. JACC 1992: 20: 1482–9
14. DeWood MA, Notske RN, Hensley GR et al. Intra-aortic balloon counterpulsation with and without reperfusion for myocardial infarction shock. Circulation 1980; 61: 1105–12
15. Ohman EM, George BS, White CJ et al. Use aortic counterpulsation to improve sustained coronary artery patency during acute myocardial infarction. Results of a randomised trial. Circulation 1994; 90: 792–9
16. Nishimura RA, Schaff HV, Gersh BJ, Holmes DP Jnr, Tajik AJ. Early repair of mechanical complications after acute myocardial infarction. JAMA 1986;256:47–50
17. Hochreiter C, Goldstein J, Borer JS et al. Myocardial free-wall rupture after acute infarction: survival aided by percutaneous intra-aortic balloon counterpulsation. Circulation 1982;65(6):1279–82
18. Hanson EC, Levine FH, Kay HR et al. Control of post infarction ventricular irritability with the intra-aortic balloon pump. Circulation 1980;62(2 Pt2): I 130–7
19. Levine FH, Gold HK, Leinbach RC, Daggett W, Austen WG, Buckley MJ. Management of acute myocardial ischaemia with intra-aortic balloon pumping and coronary bypass surgery. Circulation 1977; 58: (Part 2): I 69–72
20. Donovan KD. Invasive monitoring and support of the circulation. In Dobb, GJ (ed). Clinics in anaesthesiology. London: Saunders, 1985; 3: 909–54
21. Swanton RH. Who requires balloon pumping? Intensive Care Med 1984;10:271–3
22. Lazar JM, Ziady GM, Dummer SJ, Thompson M, Ruffner RJ. Outcome and complications of prolonged intraaortic balloon counterpulsation in cardiac patients. Am J Cardiol 1992; 69: 955–8
23. Gould KA. Perspectives on intra-aortic balloon-pump timing. Critical Care Nursing Clinics of North America 1989;1: 469–73

48 Cardiac transplantation

Anne M Keogh

Introduction

When the first human cardiac transplant was performed in 1967,[1] it initiated an early wave of interest which waned rapidly when graft rejection and poor survival became evident. Since then further developments of the surgical technique,[2] more effective management of graft rejection and associated problems during the 1970s[3] and the introduction of cyclosporin for effective immunosuppression in the 1980s,[4] allowed improved results establishing a clear-cut role for cardiac transplantation in the treatment of advanced cardiac disease in the mid 1990s.[5,6] As a consequence, coronary care unit (CCU) staff are likely to be involved in the pre-operative assessment or post-operative management of cardiac transplant patients.

Effect on survival

The expected survival after cardiac transplantation in Australia and New Zealand is 85% at 1 year and 78% at 5 years.[5–7] These estimates compare favourably with the survival of the typical transplant candidate with NYHA class 4 cardiac failure of less than 50% at one year.[8]

Who should be considered?

Cardiac transplantation may need to be considered in coronary care patients with:

- NYHA class 3 or 4 heart failure (despite optimal medications) and due to ischaemic heart disease, idiopathic dilated cardiomyopathy, valvular or congenital heart disease, peripartum or familial cardiomyopathy; expected survival should be less than 2 years and the quality of life poor due to symptoms.
- Angina (regardless of left ventricular [LV] function) resistant to maximal tolerated medications and where revascularization is not feasible or too risky.
- Recurrent life-threatening arrhythmias with implantable defibrillator where frequency of shocks causes an unacceptable lifestyle.

In the majority of cases with advanced cardiac failure, aggressive tailored therapy can achieve stabilization and discharge home[9] prior to transplantation. In some cases, however, haemodynamic stabilization cannot be achieved with maximal medical therapy and haemodynamic support with a mechanical device as a 'bridge' to transplant is necessary (see Ch. 47).

Assessing prognosis

Poor prognostic markers in potential transplant recipients include persistent class 3 or 4 symptoms, LV ejection fraction on radionuclide ventriculography less than 0.25, presence of four or more beat ventricular tachycardia on Holter monitoring, hyponatraemia,[10] and in ambulant patients MVO_2 less than 14 ml/kg/min (if not limited by inability to exercise or poor physical conditioning).[11] Inability to normalize haemodynamic measurements despite aggressive use of nitrates, hydralazine and ACEI is an important adverse prognostic sign.[12] Patients with LV ejection fraction < 0.25 treated with tailored therapy who are able to achieve a pulmonary capillary wedge pressure (PCWP) below 16 mmHg have an 83% 1-year survival compared with 38% 1-year survival where the wedge pressure is not able to be controlled. Not one but many factors are considered when estimating prognosis.

Criteria for acceptance for heart transplant

1. Less than 63 years of age (long-term results above 60 are suboptimal).
2. No significant renal or other organ dysfunction (except where related to hypoperfusion and showing signs of reversibility with congestive cardiac failure management). Renal impairment (creatinine ≥ 0.18 mmol/L) may warrant a trial of 3–4.5 mcg/kg/min dopamine. The other organ may be able to be transplanted (e.g. combined heart-kidney transplant).
3. No disease likely to interfere with longevity (e.g. malignancy).
4. No disease interfering with quality of life (e.g. inoperable peripheral vascular disease, diabetic retinopathy with visual loss, cerebral vascular accident with substantial deficit).
5. TPG ≤ 12 (TPG = MPAP minus PCWP) after vasodilator challenge.
6. No psychosocial instability likely to interfere with compliance (adolescents most at risk).
7. No current drug abuse (alcohol, cigarettes, illicit drugs).
8. No major active infection (treat infection first).
9. Not HIV positive or methicillin-resistant staphylococcus aureus (MRSA) carrier.

TPG = transpulmonary gradient; MPAP = mean pulmonary artery pressure; PCWP = pulmonary capillary wedge pressure

Factors affecting success of cardiac transplant

Criteria for acceptance which affect the success of a transplant are shown in the information box.

Effect of age

The upper age limit for recipients in most cardiac transplant centres is between 55 and 65. Although there have been reports of success in older patients, the likely presence of associated diseases increases long term morbidity.[13] Conversely, when hearts from older donors are used, there is a greater likelihood of implantation of coronary artery disease with the donor organ.

Renal and hepatic dysfunction

Cyclosporin nephrotoxicity is more problematic in patients with pre-transplant renal dysfunction or hepatic cirrhosis. It will be the individual choice of the unit whether hepatitis BsAg positive or hepatitis C carriers (on PCR) are acceptable. Long term results in hepatitis C positive patients may be limited by liver disease.[14] Additionally there is risk to staff and laboratory personnel.

Elevated pulmonary vascular resistance

An elevated transpulmonary gradient increases the risk of right heart failure after the transplant by exposing a normal donor right ventricle to a sudden pressure load.[15] It is important to determine the responsiveness of the transpulmonary gradient to vasodilators. Over 50% of patients with elevated pulmonary resistance will respond to an infusion of nitroglycerin or nitroprusside. If resistant to nitrates, reversibility may be demonstrated with prostacyclin infusion or nitric oxide inhalation. Continuous oxygen therapy or continuous positive airway pressure (CPAP) used for several months where there is substantial sleep apnoea may help. If the transpulmonary gradient does not fall to 12 units or less with these manoeuvres then heterotopic or heart-lung transplantation may be considered.

Diabetes

Diabetic patients may have an increased risk of infections and vascular complications but overall have acceptable survival after transplantation. The limitations are in diabetics with inoperable peripheral vascular disease, retinopathy with neovascularization and diabetic nephropathy.[16]

Donor availability and cost issues

Donor availability remains the limiting factor. The number of persons receiving cardiac transplants in Australia has stabilized at approximately 130 per year, although double the number of hearts could be utilized.
The cost of a heart transplant and the first 5 years follow-up is approximately half the cost of 5 years of renal dialysis, not taking into account that 75% of patients return to work after a transplant.[6]

Summary and conclusions

Cardiac transplantation is available for patients with advanced cardiac failure, intractable angina unsuitable for revascularization, and selected patients with refractory life-threatening cardiac arrhythmias. Coronary care staff need to be aware of the potential benefits and indications for transplantation to assist the transplant team in the selection of patients, preparation for the procedure and management of the patient before and after the transplant. The practical aspects of management of the transplant patient are described in Chapter 68.

References

1. Barnard CN. A human cardiac transplant: an interim report of a successful operation performed at Groote Schuur Hospital, Capetown. S Afr Med J 1967; 41: 1271
2. Stinson EB, Dong E Jr, Iben AR, Shumway NE. Cardiac transplantation in man. III: surgical aspects. Am J Surg 1969; 118: 182
3. Baumgartner WA, Reitz BA, Oyer PE et al. Cardiac homotransplantations. Curr Prob Surg 1979; 16: 24
4. Oyer PE, Stinson EB, Jamieson SW et al. Cyclosporin in cardiac transplantation. A two and a half year follow up. Transplant Proc 1983; 15: 246
5. O'Connell JB, Bourke RC, Costanzo-Nordin MR et al. Cardiac transplantation: recipient selection, donor procurement and medical follow up. A statement for health professionals from the Committee on Cardiac Transplantation of the Council on Clinical Cardiology, American Heart Association. Circulation 1992; 86: 1061–78
6. Keogh A, Kaan A. The Australian and New Zealand Cardiothoracic Organ Transplant Registry. First report 1984–1992. Aust NZ J Med 1992; 22: 712–7
7. The Registry of the International Society for Heart and Lung Transplantation. Ninth official report. J Heart and Lung Transplant 1992; 11: 599–606
8. The CONSENSUS Trial Study Group. Effects of enalapril on mortality in severe congestive heart failure. Results of the Co-operative North Scandinavian Enalapril Survival Study (CONSENSUS). N Engl J Med 1987; 316: 1429–35
9. Stevenson LW. Tailored therapy before transplantation for treatment of advanced heart failure: effective use of vasodilators and diuretics. J Heart and Lung Transplant 1991; 10: 468–76
10. Keogh A, Baron D, Hickie J. Prognostic guides in patients with idiopathic or ischaemic dilated cardiomyopathy assessed for cardiac transplantation. Amer J Cardiol 1990; 65: 903–8
11. Mancini M, Elsen H, Kussmaul W, Mull R, Edmunds L, Wilson J. Value of peak exercise oxygen consumption for optimal timing of cardiac transplantation in ambulatory patients with heart failure. Circulation 1991; 83: 778–86
12. Stevenson LW, Tillisch J, Hamilton M et al. Importance of haemodynamic response to therapy in predicting survival with ejection fraction less than or equal to 20% secondary to ischaemic or non ischaemic dilated cardiomyopathy. Am J Cardiol 1990; 66: 1348–54
13. Olivari MT, Antolick A, Kaye MP, Jamieson SW, Ring WS. Heart transplantation in elderly patients. J Heart Transplant 1988; 7: 258–64
14. Lake K, Milfred S, Reutzel T, Smith C, Allen J, Pritzker M, Emery R. Hepatitis C in cardiothoracic transplantation: Outcomes of seropositive candidates and seronegative recipients of seropositive organs. Abst. J Heart Lung Transplantation 1995; 14: 1: Pt 2; S69
15. Kirklin JK, Naftel DC, Kirklin JW, Blackstone EH, White-Williams C, Bourke RC. Pulmonary vascular resistance and the risk of heart transplantation. J Heart Transplant 1988; 7: 331–6
16. Ladowski J, Kormos RL, Uretsky BF, Griffith BP, Armitage JM, Hardesty RL. Heart transplantation in diabetic recipients. Transplant 1990; 49: 303–5

49 Catheter ablation therapy of arrhythmias

Michael JE Davis

Introduction

Catheter ablation has revolutionized the management of cardiac arrhythmias. Ablation using direct current shocks was first employed for the treatment of human cardiac arrhythmias in 1982.[1,2] After it had been demonstrated that atrioventricular conduction could be permanently interrupted, the technique was applied to a variety of re-entrant and ectopic arrhythmias. Introduced in 1987, radiofrequency (RF) has replaced direct current shock energy because of its relative ease of use (including administration without general anaesthesia), the smaller, homogeneous lesions it produces, and its greater safety (gradation in energy delivery without barotrauma or adverse effect on left ventricular function).[3] This chapter focuses on the use of RF since it is the energy source almost always now employed.

Although catheter ablation techniques have a very limited role in the situation of the coronary care of patients with acute myocardial infarction (AMI) or unstable myocardial ischaemia, ablation is now a first line therapy for a number of arrhythmias which might result in admission to a CCU. Furthermore, in some hospitals post-ablation monitoring is undertaken in the CCU, although increasingly ablation is an outpatient technique.[4]

Catheter ablation using RF can be used to produce a discrete scar virtually anywhere in the heart. A single carefully placed lesion can destroy a normal or abnormal connection or focus. Larger lesions, produced by delivering a sequence of RF pulses in linear fashion, have eliminated atrial flutter circuits and have even been used to prevent atrial fibrillation. Table 49.1 summarizes the current role of RF catheter ablation.

Radiofrequency energy

This form of electrical energy is the same as that employed for electrocautery or diathermy. Lower energies of 'pure' alternating current in a radiofrequency range of 300–1000 kHz allow heating of the distal tip of an electrode catheter without electrical arcing and thus burning of tissues. With catheter tip temperatures above 100°C, boiling occurs at the interface between electrode and tissue. Coagulum formation causes a rise in impedance, preventing current flow, and thus heating and charred tissue may weld the catheter to the point of contact. This was frequently seen when RF energy was delivered through standard electrode catheters.[5] Using larger tip catheters (typically 4 mm^2), application of around 500 mA current will allow resistive tissue heating to 50–80°C and result in a circumscribed area of homogeneous coagulation necrosis 0.5–1.0 cm^2 in diameter.[6] Catheters which incorporate a thermistor at the tip permit close monitoring of the tissue temperatures being achieved. Purpose-built RF generators without temperature monitoring incorporate an automatic cutoff if an impedance rise (due to coagulum forming over the electrode at temperatures in excess of 100°C) is detected. This may render the technique as safe as without temperature monitoring, but another advantage of the thermistor catheters is the detection of inadequate tip heating due to poor catheter tissue contact.

Technique

For many arrhythmias, catheter ablation is undertaken immediately following diagnostic electrophysiologic study. Once the arrhythmia substrate has been identified or confirmed, a 4 mm^2 tip steerable catheter is deployed

Table 49.1 The current role of catheter ablation for treatment of cardiac arrhythmias. IVC = inferior vena cava, CS – coronary sinus, WPW – Wolf Parkinson White Syndrome, CHB – complete heart block, RVOT – right ventricular outflow tract, BB = bundle branch

Arrhythmia	Target sites	Success	Role
Sinus tachycardia	Sinus node	50–70%	Where drugs have failed to control rate
Atrial tachycardia	Ectopic foci or re-entrant circuits left or right atrium	50–90%	First-line treatment
Atrial flutter	Between tricuspid annulus, IVC and CS	50–90%	Typical atrial flutter refractory to drug therapy
Atrial fibrillation	Accessory pathway (WPW)	95–98%	First-line treatment
	AV junction (induction of CHB—permanent pacemaker required)	95–98%	Where drugs have failed to prevent recurrences or to control rate
	AV junction (modification of conduction)	?70%	Where drugs have failed to prevent recurrences or to control rate
	Atria	?	Experimental
AV junctional tachycardia	Slow AV pathway	95–98%	First-line treatment in patients with incapacitating or life-threatening symptoms
	Fast AV pathway	95–98%	Largely superseded by slow pathway ablation
AV re-entrant tachycardia	Accessory pathway	95–98%	First-line treatment in patients with incapacitating or life-threatening symptoms
Ventricular tachycardia	Ectopic foci or re-entrant circuits left or right ventricle	70–100%	First-line treatment in structurally normal hearts esp. RVOT & BB tachycardia. Limited role in IHD

to map the precise location for RF delivery. This is introduced into the venous system for right-sided arrhythmia foci or pathways and for left-sided targets where a transeptal approach is considered appropriate. A stable catheter position for some right-sided targets is more easily achieved by a superior approach via the subclavian or jugular veins. For left-sided targets, retrograde positioning of the catheter via the femoral artery retrogradely across the aortic valve is most commonly used.

The catheter is advanced to the approximate target site for RF delivery under radiographic guidance, assisted by the location of the diagnostic electrode catheters. The precise location of the target site is determined either anatomically (once again using diagnostic catheter positions as landmarks) or electrically. Electrical mapping includes the use of electrogram activation sequences, local electrocardiographic characteristics and particular electrical signals (such as accessory pathway potentials). The response to brief RF application can also be helpful. RF current is delivered between the distal electrode of the ablation catheter and a large skin electrode placed between the scapulae (Fig. 49.1).

Catheter stability during energy delivery is ensured by fluoroscopic observation, with energy delivery terminated if excessive catheter movement is observed or if the impedance rises during energy delivery. A minimum of 2500 i.u. heparin is given to prevent thrombosis at the vascular entry site, with full coagulation being employed for long procedures and for left-sided ablation, particularly if many RF applications have been made.

For many arrhythmia substrates, success is immediately apparent (Fig. 49.2). For others, further electrophysiologic testing is necessary to ensure that the patient's arrhythmia cannot be reinitiated. This may require

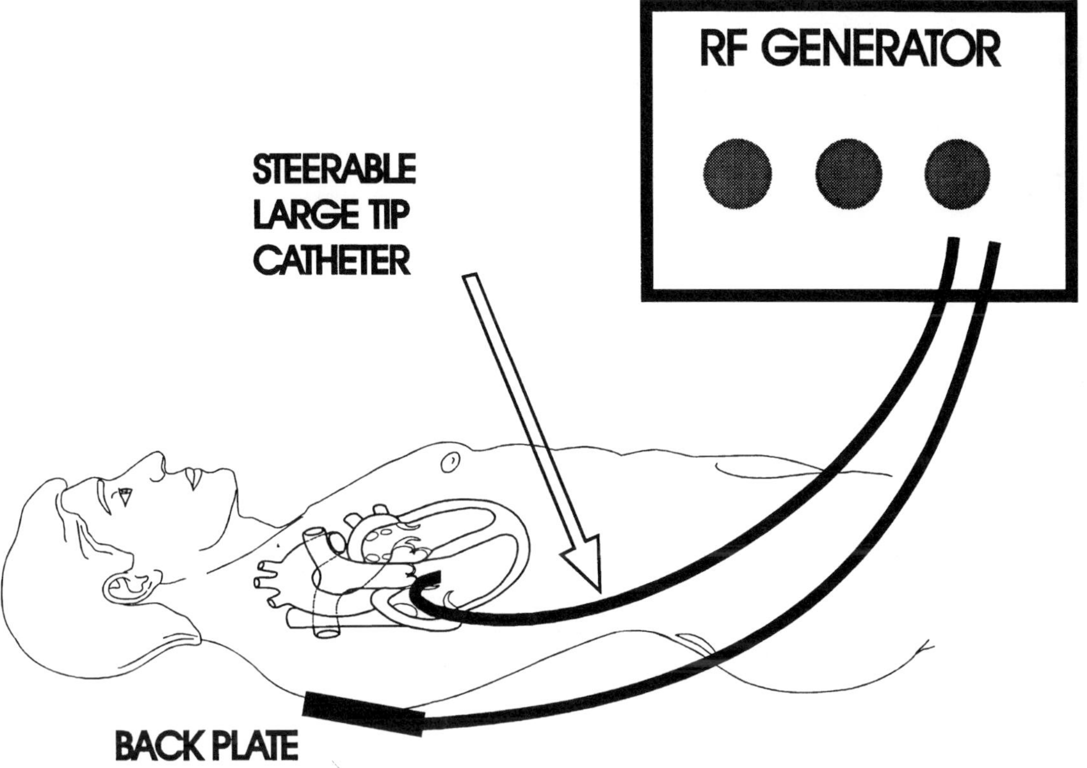

Fig. 49.1 Radiofrequency energy is delivered from a purpose-built electrosurgical generator in unipolar fashion to a large tip (usually 4 mm^2) electrode catheter. A common electrode plate is positioned between the scapulae.

cardiac stimulation both before and after infusion of isoprenaline. A catheter ablation procedure can take less than 30 minutes in straightforward cases, although procedure times of over 18 hours have been reported in difficult cases involving operators with extraordinary perseverance. Most cases take 1–2 hours. After a period of monitoring in the electrophysiology laboratory the patient may be admitted for overnight observation and ECG monitoring.

Risks

Coronary care staff should be aware of the risks of the technique, but detailed discussion of these is the responsibility of the cardiologist undertaking the procedure. Catheter ablation has been associated with an overall complication rate of around 5% in both adults and children.[7] This is similar to the early rates for diagnostic cardiac catheterization. As catheter ablation is a new procedure, learning curves for each institution are reflected in the published figures. There is no doubt that at tertiary referral centres the current risk is considerably lower than the published rates, reflecting both experience and improved equipment and techniques.[8] For the individual patient, the risk of the procedure needs to be considered in the context of the patient's underlying condition and the risks of long term antiarrhythmic medication or other treatment, bearing in mind that catheter ablation is usually curative rather than palliative.

The general risks of cardiac catheterization include death, cardiac perforation/tamponade, deep venous thrombosis and pulmonary embolism, sepsis, pneumothorax and ventricular fibrillation.

Specific risks of RF delivery include inadvertent heart block (with the need for permanent pacing) where RF delivery is close to the AV node, transient cerebral ischaemic attacks or stroke with left-sided ablation, and late sudden cardiac death, reported in only one patient without structural heart disease.[7]

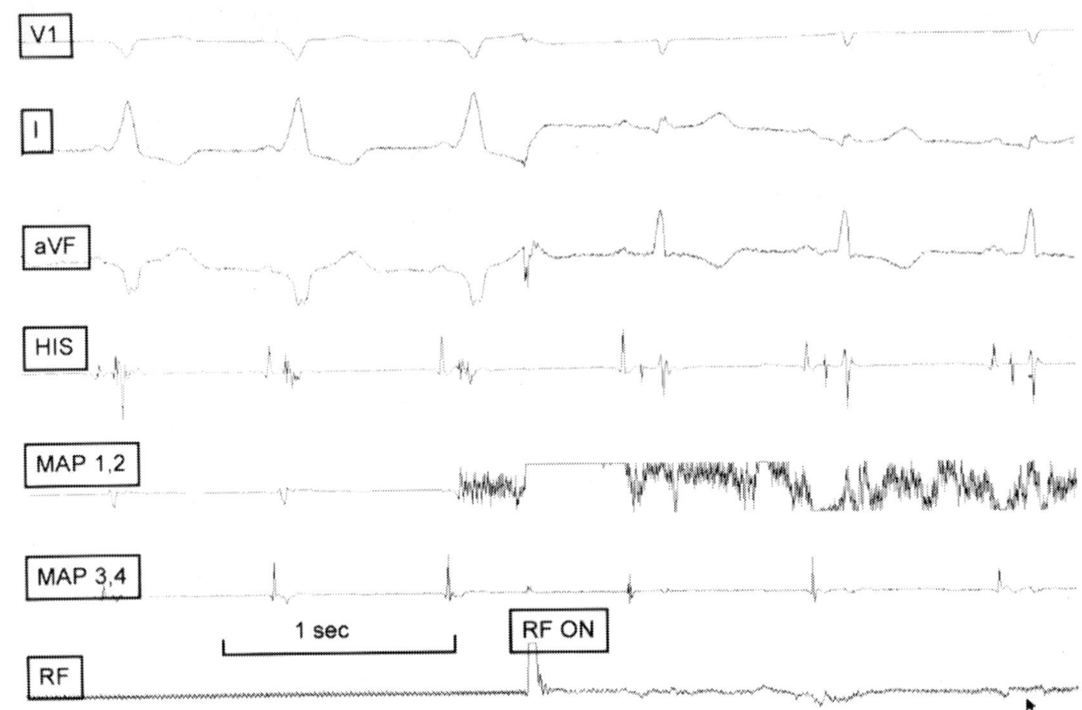

Fig. 49.2 Ablation of accessory pathway conduction within one second of the onset of radiofrequency current delivery in a patient with Wolff–Parkinson–White syndrome. V1, I, aVF = surface electrocardiographic leads V1, I and aVF. HIS, Map 1,2; Map 3,4 = intracardiac electrograms from a His bundle catheter and electrode pairs 1,2 and 3,4 of the mapping catheter. RF = Marker channel for RF (radiofrequency) current onset. Sec = second.

Specific techniques and results

The atrioventricular junction

Catheter ablation techniques were first employed in humans in 1982 with the use of direct current (DC) electric shocks to destroy the atrioventricular (AV) junction and produce complete heart block.[1,2] Initially AV junction ablation was reserved for highly symptomatic patients refractory to multiple pharmacological agents. Permanent pacemaker implantation before or immediately after the procedure was essential. The arrhythmias treated with this technique included atrial fibrillation and flutter, intra-atrial tachycardias, and AV junctional re-entrant and atrioventricular re-entrant tachycardias.

Using DC shocks, complete AV block was achieved in approximately 85% of patients, but with recurrence of AV conduction in around 20%. Approximately a quarter of patients required multiple procedures. There was early and late mortality of around 2% and a risk of early life-threatening complications of 4.8%.[7] For RF ablation the success rate for a single procedure has been around 95% with an early life-threatening complication rate of 1.6% and no reported mortality.[7]

In contrast with the lesions resulting from trans-catheter DC shock delivery, RF produces small well-circumscribed lesions which can be targeted to the proximal region of the AV junction. As a result, RF ablation of the AV junction is associated with development of a junctional escape rhythm, usually between 30 and 50 bpm, which has been shown to be stable in the long term.[9] While patients require permanent pacing, they are rarely rendered pacemaker-dependent.

With the development of more specific curative ablation techniques, the use of RF ablation of AV conduction has virtually been confined to the management of atrial fibrillation. It has been shown recently that it is possible to modify rather than to destroy AV conduction in patients with rapidly-conducted atrial fibrillation in order to slow the ventricular response while avoiding the need for permanent pacing.[10,11] RF energy is delivered to the posterior or mid septal right atrium, near the ostium of the coronary sinus. This is the region of the 'slow' AV nodal pathway (see below), and destruction of this pathway has been postulated as the mechanism of modification of AV conduction. Medium-term follow-up has shown clinically beneficial slowing in around 70% of patients.

It thus seems likely that the indication for catheter ablation (induction of complete heart block) which 'started it all' may be relegated to use only where more specific techniques have failed.

Atrioventricular nodal pathways

Atrioventricular junctional tachycardia (AVJRT, sometimes known as atrioventricular nodal re-entrant tachycardia or AVNRT) is the most common form of supraventricular tachycardia. RF catheter ablation for this arrhythmia has a reported success rate of 85–99%.[5,12,13] Ablation has greatly assisted in our understanding of its pathophysiology. The AVJRT circuit is composed of two pathways with distinct electrophysiologic properties classifying them as 'fast' or 'slow'. The perinodal atrial myocardium is usually also involved.

Either the slow or fast pathway can be ablated, but the reported incidence of complete antegrade AV block has been 8–21% and reversed re-entrant tachycardia (slow-slow tachycardia) has been seen occasionally following fast pathway RF ablation.[14,15] Slow pathway ablation eliminates AVJRT with little effect on resting antegrade AV node conduction[16,17,18] and is now generally preferred.

The target ablation site of slow pathway is situated within an area located in the region between the ostium of the coronary sinus and the His bundle. The recognized electrogram patterns predictive of success are small atrial and large ventricular electrograms without a His bundle potential. Recording a presumed 'slow pathway potential' has also been cited as a good predictor of successful ablation. McGuire et al have shown in a pig model that such potentials are most likely indicative of the anatomic location of slow pathways rather than arising from pathways themselves.[19] Accelerated AV junctional rhythm is often seen during energy delivery at successful sites.

Elimination of dual AV nodal physiology is not essential. Even with persistence of single AV nodal re-entrant beats, provided AVJRT cannot be initiated by atrial or ventricular stimulation (including during infusion of isoprenaline 1–4 mcg/min) the incidence of recurrent AVJRT is low (0–11%).[14,15,20,21]

Accessory atrioventricular pathways

Accessory AV pathways or connections are microscopic bundles of normal or fibrotic myocardium bypassing the AV annulus in the coronary sulcus.[22] They are usually epicardial, may be multiple, and sometimes traverse the AV groove obliquely. With the notable exception of 'Mahaim fibres', accessory pathways do not possess typical AV nodal decremental conduction properties: conduction is 'all or nothing', limited by the refractory period which can be as short as the normal myocardium. In the Wolff–Parkinson–White (WPW) syndrome the presence of an accessory pathway is apparent from the surface 12-lead ECG because of 'ventricular pre-excitation' (depolarization of ventricular myocardium before this occurs over the normal conducting system). Ventricular pre-excitation produces the typical 'delta wave' seen in sinus rhythm.

In the WPW syndrome there is a small risk of atrial fibrillation with the potential for extremely rapid ventricular rates and degeneration to ventricular fibrillation.[23] Differing degrees of ventricular depolarization via the normal conducting system or the accessory pathway result in the bizarre QRS complexes of differing width and axis seen in atrial fibrillation in patients with WPW. Patients with WPW who are symptomatic with palpitations or syncope should undergo electrophysiologic study: accessory pathway ablation would usually be undertaken at the same time, if warranted by the patient's symptoms or the finding of a short accessory pathway refractory period.

Accessory pathways may also be 'concealed' (not apparent on the surface ECG). Concealed pathways are the substrate for paroxysmal supraventricular tachycardia in approximately 40% of patients. Their presence is suggested by a very rapid heart rate or obvious retrograde P waves during tachycardia.

Accessory pathways can be located anywhere around the AV annulus except anteriorly on the left near the pulmonary artery. The most common site is the left free wall, followed by postero-septal and then anteroseptal locations. The pathways are occasionally multiple or associated with abnormal AV nodal pathways.

Accessory pathways can be ablated from either the atrial or ventricular side of the AV groove or occasionally from within the coronary sinus or its branches. The pathways can be mapped in sinus rhythm (in WPW), with the identification of the earliest site of ventricular activation, or by mapping earliest atrial activation during initiated AV re-entrant tachycardia or ventricular pacing. Particularly helpful in localizing a pathway is the recording of an accessory pathway 'potential'.

The overall success rate for accessory pathway ablation now exceeds 95% in experienced centres and is close to 100% for left sided pathways.[24–27]

Atrial foci and re-entrant circuits

Atrial tachycardias arise above the AV junction and are distinguished from atrial fibrillation or flutter and multifocal atrial tachycardia. Most are 'ectopic' rather than re-entrant and are notoriously resistant to pharmacological therapy.[28] Patients, many of whom are children or adolescents, often have incessant arrhythmia. This may result in secondary cardiac failure and make pharmacological or surgical treatment more hazardous.

There have been a number of reports of early experience with RF catheter ablation of atrial tachycardia.[29–33] The success rate has varied from 69 to 98% but there has been recurrent tachycardia in around 10% of patients. Even in the technique's infancy, these results compare more than favourably with surgery and with a considerably lower morbidity.[34]

Recent human studies have demonstrated that in most cases atrial flutter is due to re-entry in the right atrium.[35] The critical area in the re-entrant circuit, which is probably the exit site from the area of slow conduction, is the isthmus of tissue between the inferior vena cava and the tricuspid ring. Electrical mapping using the activation sequence, identification of abnormal electrical activity and/or entainment pacing, has been used to identify this area, with RF delivery abolishing flutter in most cases.[36] Delivery of RF pulses to this anatomic area without electrical mapping, less time-consuming, has also been shown to abolish atrial flutter successfully.[37] During short-term follow-up a few patients have developed atrial fibrillation, but these early results are certainly encouraging for an arrhythmia which can be very difficult to treat medically and where AV junction ablation with pacemaker implantation is not ideal.

Ventricular foci and re-entrant circuits

The role of catheter ablation in ventricular tachycardia (VT) is limited. The ideal candidate has no structural heart disease and a single morphology of haemodynamically well-tolerated tachycardia. Undertaken in experienced centres, the technique is a first line treatment modality in such patients. Right ventricular outflow tract or idiopathic LV tachycardias have been ablated with a success rate approaching 100%.[38–41]

With structural heart disease catheter ablation has a role which is adjunctive to other therapies, being useful for frequent or incessant tachycardia primarily with a single origin.[42–44] Unfortunately ventricular tachycardia usually occurs in hearts with diffuse disease and multiple sites or potential sites for re-entry. Recurrences in patients where catheter ablation has initially seemed curative have been shown to be due to VT arising from a different site.[45] When VT arises in a structurally abnormal heart, progression of ventricular damage may create new re-entry sites at any time. For this reason, few patients with structural heart disease are discharged off antiarrhythmic therapy after catheter ablation.[8,9]

Thus of the patients with VT who require definitive treatment, the majority—those with damaged hearts and poorly tolerated ventricular arrhythmias—are the least suitable candidates for catheter ablation. Recent reports from tertiary referral centres suggest that less than 10% of referred patients with VT related to coronary artery disease will be suitable candidates.[46]

Cost-efficacy

The cost-effectiveness of RF catheter ablation compared with traditional treatments for supraventricular tachycardia is well established.[47,48] The mean cost of undertaking catheter ablation as a day case procedure in an Australian teaching hospital has been estimated to be less than $A2000 (1994).[49] This contrasts with a cost of over $10 000 for surgical therapy and around $4000 (for 10 years' ongoing care) in patients treated with drugs.[48] Analysis of quality of life clearly favours catheter ablation.

References

1. Gallagher JJ, Svenson H, Kasell JH et al. Catheter technique for closed chest ablation of the atrioventricular conduction system: a therapeutic alternative for the treatment of refractory supraventricular tachycardia. N Engl J Med 1982; 306: 194–200
2. Scheinman MM, Morady F, Hess DS et al. Catheter-induced ablation of the atrioventricular junction to control refractory supraventricular arrhythmias. J Am Med Assoc 1982; 248: 851–5
3. Huang SK, Bharati S, Graham AR et al. Closed chest catheter desiccation of the atrioventricular junction using RF energy—a new method of catheter ablation. J Am Coll Cardiol 1987; 9: 349–58
4. Weerasooriya HR, Wang L, Davis MJE. Day stay transcatheter radiofrequency ablation for supraventricular tachyarrhythmias. Med J Aust 1995; 162: 204–5
5. Weerasooriya HR, Murdock CJ, Davis MJE. Early experience with radiofrequency ablation for supraventricular tachyarrhythmias related to accessory pathways and dual atrioventricular nodal pathways. Med J Aust 1993; 159: 97–102
6. Haines DE, Watson DD. Tissue heating during radiofrequency catheter ablation: a thermodynamic model and observations in isolated perfused and superfused canine right ventricular free wall. PACE 1989; 12: 962–76
7. Scheinman M, Olgin J. Catheter ablation of cardiac arrhythmias of atrial origin. In: Zipes D (ed). Catheter ablation of arrhythmias. Armonk: Futura, 1994: 129–49
8. Davis MJE, Murdock CJ, Weerasooriya R. Early experience with transcatheter radiofrequency ablation for the treatment of supraventricular tachycardia: the effect of equipment and experience. Abst. Aust NZ J Med 1993; 23: 612
9. Alison JF, Yeung-Lai-Wah JA, Schulzer M et al. Characterization of junctional rhythm after atrioventricular node ablation. Circulation 1995; 91: 84–90
10. Williamson BD, Ching Man K, Daoud E et al. Radiofrequency catheter modification of atrioventricular conduction to control the ventricular rate during atrial fibrillation. N Engl J Med 1994; 331: 910–7
11. Feld GK, Fleck P, Fujimara O et al. Control of rapid ventricular response by radiofrequency catheter modification of the atrioventricular node in patients with medically refractory atrial fibrillation. Circulation 1994; 90: 2299–307
12. Jazeyeri MR, Hempe SL, Sra JS et al. Selective transcatheter ablation of the fast and slow pathways using radiofrequency energy in patients with atrioventricular nodal reentrant tachycardia. Circulation 1991; 85: 1318–28
13. Lee MA, Morady F, Kadish A. Catheter modification of the atrioventricular junction with radiofrequency energy for control of atrioventricular nodal reentry tachycardia. Circulation 1991; 83: 827–35
14. Lee MA, Morady F, Kadish A et al. Catheter modification of the atrioventricular junction with radiofrequency energy for control of atrioventricular nodal reentrant tachycardia. Circulation 1991; 83: 827–35
15. Jazayeri MR, Hempe SL, Sra JS et al. Selective transcatheter ablation of the fast and slow pathways using radiofrequency energy in patients with atrioventricular nodal reentrant tachycardia. Circulation 1992; 85: 1318–28
16. Kay GN, Epstein AE, Dailey SM et al. Selective radiofrequency ablation of the slow pathway for the treatment of atrioventricular nodal reentrant tachycardia: evidence for involvement of perinodal myocardium within the reentrant circuit. Circulation 1992; 85: 1675–88
17. Haissaguerre M, Gaita F, Fischer B et al. Elimination of atrioventricular nodal reentrant tachycardia using discrete slow potentials to guide application of radiofrequency energy. Circulation 1992; 85: 2162–75
18. Chen SA, Chiang CE, Tsang WP et al. Selective radiofrequency catheter ablation of fast and slow pathways in 100 patients with atrioventricular nodal reentrant tachycardia. Am Heart J 1993; 125:1–10
19. McGuire MA, de-Bakker JM, Vermeulen A et al. Origin and significance of double potentials near the atrioventricular node. Correlation of extracellular potentials, intracellular potentials and histology. Circulation 1994; 89: 2351–60
20. Wang L, Weerasooriya HR, Davis MJE et al. Comparison of the early and late results of radiofrequency catheter ablation of fast and slow atrioventricular nodal pathways. Med J Aust 1995. In press
21. Lindsay BD, Chung MK, Gamache C et al. Therapeutic end points for the treatment of atrioventricular node reentrant tachycardia by catheter-guided radiofre-

quency current. J Am Coll Cardiol 1993; 22: 733–40
22. Hackel DB. Anatomic basis for preexcitation syndromes. In: Benditt DG, Benson DW (eds). Cardiac preexcitation syndromes: origins, evaluation and treatment. Boston: Martinus Nijhoff Publishing, 1986: 31
23. Klein GJ, Badshore TM, Sellers TD et al. Ventricular fibrillation in the Wolff–Parkinson–White syndrome. N Engl J Med 1979; 301: 1080–5
24. Jackman WM, Wang X, Friday KJ et al. Catheter ablation of accessory atrioventricular pathways (Wolff–Parkinson–White syndrome) by radiofrequency current. N Engl J Med 1991; 324: 1605–11
25. Kuck KH, Schluter M, Geiger M et al. Radiofrequency current catheter ablation of accessory atrioventricular pathways. Lancet 1991; 337: 1557–61
26. Calkins H, Langberg J, Sousa J et al. Radiofrequency catheter ablation of accessory atrioventricular connections in 250 patients: abbreviated therapeutic approach to Wolff–Parkinson–White syndrome. Circulation 1992; 85: 1337–46
27. Lesh MD, Van Hare GF, Schamp DJ et al. Curative percutaneous catheter ablation using radiofrequency energy for accessory pathways in all locations: results in 100 consecutive patients. J Am Coll Cardiol 1992; 19: 1303–9
28. Swerdlow CD, Liem LB. Atrial and junctional tachycardias: clinical presentation, course and therapy. In: Zipes DP, Jalife J (eds). Cardiac electrophysiology; from cell to bedside. Philadelphia: Saunders, 1990: 742–55
29. Walsh EP, Saul JP, Hulse JE et al. Transcatheter ablation of ectopic atrial tachycardia in young patients using radiofrequency current. Circulation 1992; 86: 1138–46
30. Sperry RE, Ellenbogen KA, Wood MA et al. Radiofrequency catheter ablation of sinus node reentrant tachycardia. PACE 1993; 16: 2202–9
31. Chen SA, Chiang CE, Yang CJ et al. Sustained atrial tachycardia in adult patients: electrophysiological characteristics, pharmacological response, possible mechanisms, and effects of radiofrequency ablation. Circulation 1994; 90: 1262–78
32. Wang L, Weerasooriya HR, Davis MJE. Radiofrequency catheter ablation of atrial tachycardia. Aust NZ J Med, 1995. In press
33. Lesh MD, Van Hare GF, Epstein LM et al. Radiofrequency catheter ablation of atrial tachyarrhythmias. Results and mechanisms. Circulation 1994; 89: 1074–89
34. Prager NA, Cox JL, Lindsay BD et al. Long-term effectiveness of surgical treatment of ectopic atrial tachycardia. J Am Coll Cardiol 1993; 22: 85–92
35. Puech P, Gallay P, Grolleau R. Mechanisms of atrial flutter in humans. In: Touboul P, Waldo AL (eds). Atrial arrhythmias: current concepts and management. St Louis: Mosby-Year Book 1990: 190–209
36. Feld GK, Fleck P, Chen P et al. Radiofrequency catheter ablation for treatment of human type I atrial flutter. Circulation 1992; 86: 1233–40
37. Kirkorian G, Moncada E, Chevalier P et al. Radiofrequency ablation of atrial flutter: efficacy of an anatomically guided approach. Circulation 1994; 90: 2804–14
38. Wilber DJ, Baerman J, Olshansky B et al. Adenosine-sensitive ventricular tachycardia. Clinical characteristics and response to catheter ablation. Circulation 1993; 87: 126–34
39. Klein LS, Shih H-T, Hackett K. Radiofrequency catheter ablation of ventricular tachycardia in patients without structural heart disease. Circulation 1992; 85: 1666–74
40. Nakagawa H, Beckman K, McClelland J et al. Radiofrequency ablation of idiopathic left ventricular tachycardia guided by a Purkinje potential. Abst. PACE 1993; 16: 890
41. Tanno K, Kobayashi Y, Yoshiro J et al. Radiofrequency catheter ablation for idiopathic left ventricular tachycardia. Abst. PACE 1993; 16: 860
42. Davis MJE, Murdock CM. Radiofrequency catheter ablation of refractory ventricular tachycardia. PACE, 1988; 11:725–9
43. Stevenson WG, Sager PT, Khan HH et al. Identification of reentry circuit sites during catheter mapping and ablation of ventricular tachycardia late after myocardial infarction. Abst. PACE 1993; 16: 859
44. Borgreffe M. Radiofrequency catheter ablation in patients with incessant ventricular tachycardia. Abst. PACE 1993; 16: 859
45. Cohen TJ, Chien WW, Lurie KG et al. Radiofrequency catheter ablation for treatment of bundle branch reentrant ventricular tachycardia: results and long-term follow-up. J Am Coll Cardiol 1991; 18: 1767–73
46. Morady F, Harvey M, Kalbfleisch SJ et al. Radiofrequency catheter ablation of ventricular tachycardia in patients with coronary artery disease. Circulation 1993; 87: 363–72
47. Weerasooriya HR, Harris AH, Murdock CJ et al. The cost-effectiveness of treatment of supraventricular arrhythmias related to an accessory atrioventricular pathway: comparison of catheter ablation, surgical division and medical treatment. Aust NZ J Med 1994; 24: 161–7
48. Kalbfleisch SJ, Calkins H, Langberg JJ et al. Comparison of the cost of radiofrequency catheter modification of the atrioventricular node and medical therapy for drug-refractory atrioventricular node reentrant

tachycardia. J Am Coll Cardiol 1992; 19: 1583–7
49. Weerasooriya HR, Harris AH, Davis MJE. Cost-effectiveness of day stay versus inpatient radiofrequency catheter ablation for the treatment of supraventricular tachyarrhythmias. Aust NZ J Med, 1995. In press

50 Implantable cardioverter defibrillator

Jitu Vohra

Background

Despite all the recent advances in the management of heart diseases, sudden arrhythmic death remains a major problem. Implantable cardioverter defibrillator (ICD) was conceived and developed by Dr Michel Mirowski in the 1970s as an answer to this problem. More than 50 000 devices have been implanted worldwide since the first human implant in 1980 and this number is increasing rapidly.

Recent models of ICD are referred to as third generation ICD and are capable of detecting ventricular tachycardia (VT) and ventricular fibrillation (VF) by detecting rate. They have the functions[1] shown in the information box.

Figure 50.1 illustrates various functions of a recent Telectronics ICD model 4211.

Functions of currently available implantable cardioverter defibrillators

- Tachycardia detection
- Anti-tachycardia pacing (ATP)
- Bradycardia support pacing
- Low energy cardioversion (LEC 0.4–4 joules)
- High energy cardioversion up to 34 joules
- Ability to programme all the above functions and provide a tiered therapy
- Telemetry of tachycardia events and therapy, provision of snapshots of ECG during and after reversion
- Non-invasive programme stimulation (NIPS) for VT/VF induction

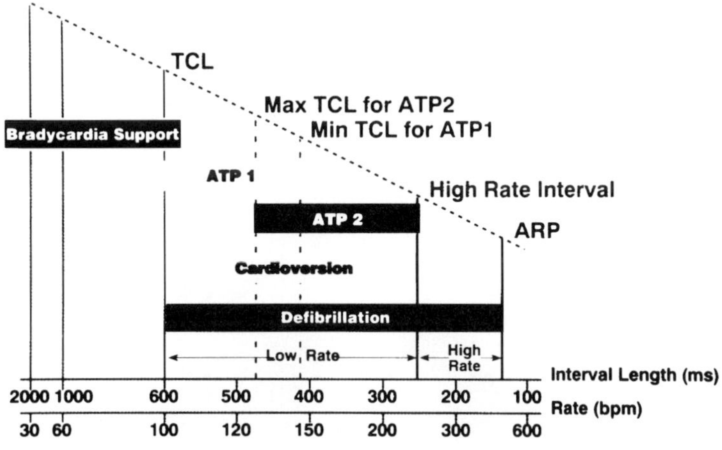

Fig. 50.1 Sequencing of therapy for implantable cardioverter defibrillator. ATP = anti-tachycardia pacing. TCL = tachycardia cycle length.

Thoracotomy and non-thoracotomy ICD implantation

Earlier ICD models used monophasic truncated exponential shock for defibrillation. Recent alternatives have included sequential monophasic shocks or a single biphasic shock. It is now generally accepted that biphasic shocks give lowest defibrillation thresholds (DFT) and all recent models of ICD use biphasic shock or provide it as a programmable function.

Advance in lead technology has allowed the use of transvenous defibrillating coil electrodes with the tip of the right ventricular (RV) electrode providing sensing and pacing.

It is now possible to use a transvenous system with or without a subcutaneous (SC) patch and thus avoid thoracotomy in patients requiring ICD without concomitant cardiac surgery. ICD implantation is now further simplified with the availability of a single lead unipolar transvenous defibrillator with an active can or 'hot can' where the generator with a titanium shell acts as a cathode (Medtronic 7219C). Thoracotomy ICD implantation with epicardial patches is now necessary only in occasional patients where adequate DFT is not achieved with the transvenous system. Even in patients requiring thoracotomy for other cardiac surgery, transvenous implantation as a separate procedure is preferable. Further reduction in the size of the generators will make ICD implantation similar to pacemaker implantation. Figure 50.2 shows pectoral ICD implantation of Medtronic 7219C with a single lead and an active can.

Implantation procedure

Implantation of an ICD whether thoracotomy or non-thoracotomy should be performed under strictly sterile conditions as infection of the ICD system is a serious complication.

Patients requiring epicardiol patches have an RV sense pace lead through the left cephalic or subclavian vein and epicardial defibrillator patches. All leads are tunnelled through to the left hypochondriac or pectoral region where the device is implanted.

Patients having a non-thoracotomy ICD have leads positioned through the left cephalic and/or subclavian vein and the generator is implanted in the pectoral region or the left hypochondrial region depending on the size of the device and the size of the patient.

Before implantation of the device, sensing and pacing thresholds are measured. Ventricular fibrillation is induced and DFT is checked to ensure that the DFT allows adequate safety margin for any possible rise in the DFT post-implant.

Following the ICD implantation the patient undergoes a detailed ICD check under general anaesthesia where all measurements mentioned earlier, including the DFT, are checked again and where appropriate antitachycardia pacing (ATP) function is checked and programmed by inducing VT.

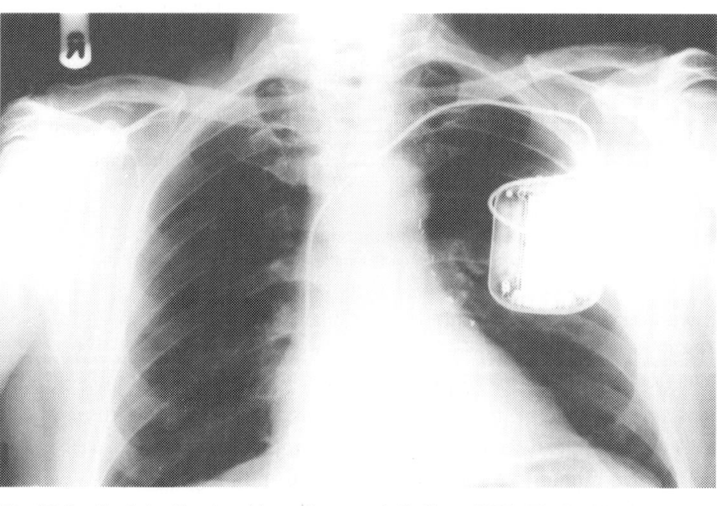

Fig. 50.2 Single lead implantable cardioverter-defibrillator (ICD). The lead in the right ventricle is the anode and the titanium shell of the ICD is the cathode ('hot can' system).

Clinical indications for ICD implantation

Guidelines for ICD implantation were drawn up by the North American Society of Pacing and Electrophysiology, American College of Cardiology and American Heart Association in 1991. Indications were divided in three categories.[2] With increasing ease of insertion and reduced size of ICD units there is likely to be a trend to earlier implantation in high risk cases.

Assessment of patients being considered for ICD

Potential candidates for ICD implantation require precise structural, functional and aetiological diagnosis. All patients should have assessment of left ventricular ejection fraction (LVEF), electrophysiological (EP) study and coronary angiography. The patient's age, quality of life, general condition, life expectancy and psychological profile are also important considerations.

Indications for ICD in coronary artery disease

Patients with coronary artery disease (CAD) who have survived one or more episodes of cardiac arrest form the largest group of patients who are considered for ICD implantation. The 'usual' patient has been very well described by Klein and Trappe and is a male between 55 and 70 years, who has survived one episode of cardiac arrest, has an ejection fraction of about 25%, has probably had previous myocardial infarctions, has two or three vessel coronary artery disease and inducible VT > 200/min that is non-pace-terminable.[3]

The next group are CAD patients with frequent episodes of monomorphic ventricular tachycardia at a rate of less than 200/min that are pace-terminable.

ICD in dilated cardiomyopathy

While coronary artery disease patients account for more than 70% of patients who are considered for ICD implantation, the next major group are patients with dilated cardiomyopathy who have survived cardiac arrest or have drug-resistant recurrent monomorphic VT.[4]

Other indications for ICD

Other indications for ICD implantation include primary electrical arrhythmia where no structural abnormality has been found, and this condition accounts for some 7% of survivors of cardiac arrest.[5]

Mitral valve prolapse, prolonged QT interval, arrhythmogenic RV dysplasia and hypertrophic cardiomyopathy are some of the other conditions for which ICDs have been used.

ICD as a bridge to cardiac transplant

Patients who are in NYHA class 3 and 4 with LVEF < 20% are probably best served by cardiac transplant as these patients have a high incidence of death due to progressive heart failure. Once a decision to refer a patient for cardiac transplant is made, there is a waiting period during which there is significant sudden death mortality. As the results of cardiac transplants are very good, the use of ICD as a bridge to transplant is considered economically worthwhile. ICD may be necessary in some of these patients who have had VT/VF.

Follow up of ICD patients

Patients with ICD are given a letter detailing the ICD programme. They also carry a card supplied by the manufacturer with specifications of the ICD model. Patients need to be seen at regular intervals for ICD checks and they also need follow-up by their cardiologists for general cardiological management.

Patients are advised to phone medical or paramedical personnel if they experience a shock. Unless the patient has experienced multiple shocks they are not admitted in hospital but have their device interrogated and treatment reviewed. Patients who have experienced multiple shocks frequently require admission and monitoring. They may require reprogramming of their device or alteration of antiarrhythmic drug regimen. Inappropriate ICD discharges due to supraventricular arrhythmias, atrial fibrillation, lead malfunctions or electrical 'noise' may require the ICD to be turned off while the patient is being monitored and corrective measures are taken. Improvement in telemetry has demonstrated that even modern ICDs do not always deliver appropriate treatment at times and careful examination of telemetered data and signals are frequently required.

In ICD patients undergoing other forms of surgery requiring diathermy, the ICD should be programmed off during surgery.

Quality of life after ICD implantation

Most patients enjoy a full, active and good quality life after ICD implantation. Psychological problems have declined with the reduction in inappropriate discharges and the use of ATP therapy to prevent shocks for termination of recurrent VT. A proportion of patients, particularly those who have received a large number of shocks in quick succession, become apprehensive and require psychological support in addition to measures to prevent frequent discharges.

Patient education, education of relatives in cardiopulmonary resuscitation (CPR), proper patient selection, pre-implant discussion, regular follow-up visits and good rapport with the medical and paramedical staff are all helpful in this regard.

Driving after ICD implant is an important quality of life issue. Driving after ICD is not forbidden unless the patient is considered to be at high risk of syncopal ventricular arrhythmias. Commercial driving is not recommended after ICD implantation.

Revascularization without ICD

Amongst survivors of cardiac arrest there are clearly patients who require only revascularization. These patients generally have a history of ischaemic chest pain prior to cardiac arrest, left main coronary stenosis or significant obstructive coronary artery disease. The ejection fraction is frequently higher than 30% and EP study is either negative or produces VF. These patients should have coronary bypass grafts without an ICD.

The use of antiarrhythmic drugs post ICD implant

While ICD implantation allows considerable reduction, or even omission, of antiarrhythmic drugs in many patients after ICD implant, at least 50% require some antiarrhythmic therapy.

Beta adrenergic blockers are often employed to reduce sinus tachycardia or frequency of supraventricular or ventricular arrhythmias.

Many patients require sotalol or amiodarone to suppress uncontrolled atrial fibrillation or non-sustained ventricular arrhythmias or to reduce ICD activations or discharges.

Some of the antiarrhythmic drugs, particularly class Ic drugs, may affect pacing and defibrillation threshold and this aspect should be kept in mind. Bradyarrhythmia and atrioventricular block, either due to the natural progression of the disease or due to side-effects from antiarrhythmic drugs, may require a dual chamber pacemaker implant, as at this stage ICDs incorporate only VVI pacing—which is not the ideal form of pacing for most of these patients who generally have poor LV function. Interactions between the implanted pacemaker and ICD may cause problems in VT/VF detection and careful planning and consultations with the manufacturers are required to avoid these problems.

Controversies

While there is general agreement that ICDs lower the incidence of sudden cardiac death to 1–2% per year, whether they reduce total mortality or just change the mode of death from sudden arrhythmic to non-sudden has been a topic of controversy, and a large number of ongoing trials are expected to provide an answer.[6,7]

Some of the major randomized trials prospectively assessing survival benefit from ICDs include AVID (Antiarrhythmics Versus Implantable Defibrillators), CIDS (Canadian Implantable Defibrillator Study) and CASH (Cardiac Arrest Study Homburg). Other multicentre prospective trials include Coronary Artery Bypass Graft Patch (CABG Patch), Multicenter Unsustained Tachycardia Trial (MUSTT) and Multicenter Implantable Defibrillator Trial (MADIT).

Economic aspects of ICD

The cost of ICD based on 5-year device life has been estimated at US$7430 per additional patient life year. Saksena and Camm suggest highest cost efficacy for patients with EF < 30% who are EP inducible and have drug resistant arrhythmias. Patients with EF < 30% regardless of EP results are considered to be the next cost efficient group for ICD, while ICD as a bridge to cardiac transplant is also very cost-efficient according to these authors.[8] Implantation of an ICD costs approximately $A40 000.[9]

Conclusion

Therapeutic alternatives in the management of malignant ventricular arrhythmias include various strategies that include coronary revascularization, antiarrhythmic treatment, mapping guided arrhythmia surgery, ICD implantation and combination of these different strategies. Recent advances in ICD technology have increased reliability and safety of these devices and have reduced cost. If the ongoing trials show a significant reduction in total mortality then prophylactic implantation for high risk groups may become a reality. Until such time, rational decisions regarding ICD indications need to be made using existing guides that need continuous scrutiny and updating as more definitive information becomes available.

References

1. Furman S, Gimoss JN, Kim SG, Ben-Zur U, Andrews C, Fisher J. The implantable cardioverter defibrillator. ACC Current Journal Review 1994; 3: 41–3
2. Lehman MH, Saksena S, for NASPE Policy Conference Committee. NASPE Policy Statement: Implantable cardioverter defibrillators in cardiovascular practice: Report of the Policy Conference of the North American Society of Pacing and Electrophysiology. PACE 1991; 14: 969–79
3. Klein H, Trappe H. Implantable cardioverter defibrillator therapy:

indications and decision making in patients with coronary artery disease. PACE 1992; 15: 610–15
4. Borggrefe M, Chen X, Block M et al. The role of the ICD in patients with dilated and hypertrophied cardiomyopathy. PACE 1992; 15: 627–30
5. Almendral J, Ormaetxe J, Delcan JL. Idiopathic ventricular tachycardia and fibrillation: Incidence, prognosis and therapy. PACE 1992; 15: 627–30
6. Sweeney MO, Ruskin JN. Mortality benefits and the implantable cardioverter defibrillator. Circulation 1994; 89: 1851–8
7. Zipes DP. Implantable cardioverter defibrillator. Life saver or a device looking for a disease? Circulation 1994; 89: 2934–6
8. Saksena S, Camm AJ. Implantable defibrillator for prevention of sudden death; technology at a medical and economic crossroad. Circulation 1992; 85: 2316–21
9. Uther JFB. The automatic implantable defibrillator is the most realistic and cost effective way of preventing sudden cardiac death. Aust NZ J Med 1992; 22: 636–8

51 Exercise

Tom G Briffa

Benefits of exercise in cardiac rehabilitation

Exercise is considered an essential part of the rehabilitation process for all cardiac patients. The goal of exercise cardiac rehabilitation is to decrease activity-induced symptoms and improve functional work capacity.

The benefits of exercise conditioning for patients recovering from myocardial infarction (MI), cardiac surgery or percutaneous transmural coronary angioplasty (PTCA) are summarized in the information box and discussed below.

Increased functional work capacity

Typically, cardiac patients show a considerable improvement in functional work capacity after engaging in exercise rehabilitation programmes, ranging from 10 to 60%, for up to 6 months of conditioning.[1–4] Considerable improvement occurs at intensities and amounts below traditional high intensity exercise.[1–2] The greatest improvement is seen in those patients with the lowest initial functional work capacity. However, a major part of this improvement occurs naturally and with the resumption of activities of daily living. The improvement in functional work capacity for most cardiac patients appears to be predominantly due to peripheral adaptations resulting in an increase in oxygen extraction and utilization by active skeletal muscles and an associated increase in arterial oxygen extraction.[3–7]

Improvement in cardiovascular efficiency

Regular exercise is accompanied by a lower heart rate, systolic blood pressure, and rate pressure product (RPP) that decreases the myocardial oxygen demand at any given submaximal workload in most patients with coronary heart disease. The threshold for exertional ischaemia is also increased.[3–7] These adaptations provide patients with greater tolerance for activities of daily living. Everyday activities are performed at a lower percentage of maximum, resulting in greater endurance and less exertional fatigue and dyspnoea. Patients with angina pectoris frequently perform more physical activity before the onset of symptoms. Patients with angina can increase symptom-limited maximal work capacity by 32–56% after exercise conditioning.[3]

Potential for improved coronary blood flow

Froelicher et al[8] and Hung et al[9] provided indirect evidence of improved coronary blood flow, as shown by increased thallium perfusion following exercise training. Diminished exercise-induced ST segment abnormalities,[10] increased ejection fraction and stroke volume, and increased ischaemic threshold have also been demonstrated with exercise conditioning.[5]

Benefits of exercise training for the cardiac patient

- Improves functional work capacity
- Improves cardiovascular efficiency
- Potential for improved coronary blood flow
- Reduces coronary risk profile for heart disease
- Reduces recurrent cardiac events
- Improves psychosocial function

Other associated changes with endurance exercise conditioning are a lower rest and submaximal exercise heart rate. This is accompanied by reduced myocardial oxygen demands and coronary blood flow requirements. Also, the slowing of heart rate provides increased time for coronary blood flow by lengthening diastole.

Reduction in coronary risk profile

Endurance exercise in healthy persons and those with coronary heart disease increases high-density lipoprotein cholesterol levels, reduces mild hypertension, lowers body weight, and improves carbohydrate metabolism.[11] Ornish et al reported a reduction in the severity of angiographically demonstrated coronary atherosclerosis at one year, in post-MI patients randomized to comprehensive exercise rehabilitation, compared to controls.[12]

Reduction in recurrent cardiac events

Controlled secondary prevention trials after MI demonstrate a reduction in mortality for those participating in exercise conditioning,[13–16] with only one trial attaining statistical significance.[15] These studies are limited by the low patient numbers, treatment crossover and poor compliance.

However, meta-analyses[17–19] of these controlled trials revealed that patients assigned to exercise rehabilitation following MI had about 20–25% lower rate of fatal cardiovascular events and total mortality than did control subjects; no differences were observed in the rate of non-fatal recurrent MI. However, most trials included comprehensive lifestyle intervention, therefore making it impossible to assess the independent contribution of exercise to the prevention of future cardiac events.

Improvement in psychosocial function

The benefits of exercise conditioning for psychological well-being are unclear. Exercise studies involving healthy volunteers suggest reduced muscular tension, mental depression, and anxiety.[20–21] Several studies in post-MI patients have failed to document sustained psychosocial benefits with exercise conditioning.[13,24] However, in highly selected patients with heart disease, a significant improvement in psychological parameters occurred after a comprehensive 12-week exercise rehabilitation programme that included stress management and counselling.[22] Worcester et al[23] reported favourable changes in psychological social adjustment scores in post-MI patients following comprehensive rehabilitation. Therefore, currently scientific evidence is inadequate to attribute to exercise an independent role in improving the psychosocial function of most cardiac patients.[5]

Exercise in heart failure

Increasingly, exercise rehabilitation is reportedly safe among patients with heart failure with increases in functional work capacity of 18–34% after 2–6 months' conditioning.[25–26] Patients with heart failure experience fewer symptoms, increase anaerobic threshold, lower minute ventilation and improve oxygen delivery to the working muscles following exercise conditioning.[25–29]

Safety

The international trend to earlier mobilization after MI has been achieved without any adverse effect on mortality or reinfarction.[30] However, there has been a recent re-examination of the role of exercise in precipitating MI.[31] Although there have been no reports of adverse effects of early mobilization on ventricular remodelling after infarction, over-enthusiastic mobilization or exercise early after a large infarction may conceivably worsen left ventricular dilatation or infarction expansion.

Cardiac arrest is the most common complication during exercise cardiac rehabilitation, occurring seven times more frequently than recurrent non-fatal MI.[32] The survey was based on data obtained from 167 randomly selected programmes from throughout the United States involving 51 303 patients, who exercised a total exceeding 2 million hours during the period 1980–1984. 21 cardiac arrests (18 successfully resuscitated and three fatal) and eight non-fatal AMI were reported. The rate of complications was one cardiac arrest per 111 996 hours, one AMI per 293 900 hours and one fatality per 783 976 hours of prescribed exercise. These data suggest an improvement in the cardiac complication rates as compared to a survey performed a decade earlier by Haskell[33] which reported one cardiac arrest for every 33 000 hours of patient activity and one death for every 120 000 patient hours.

References

1. Goble AJ, Hare DL, MacDonald PS et al. Effect of early programmes of high and low intensity exercise on physical performance after transmural myocardial infarction. Br Heart J 1991;65:126–31
2. Blumenthal JA, Rejeski WJ, Walsh-Riddle M et al. Comparison of high- and low-intensity exercise training early after acute myocardial infarction. Am J Cardiol 1988;61:26–30
3. Clausen JP. Circulatory adjustments to dynamic exercise and physical training in normal subjects and in patients with coronary artery disease. In: Sonnenblick EH, Lesch M (eds). Exercise and the heart. New York: Grune & Stratton, 1977:39–75
4. Thompson PD. The benefits and risks of exercise training in patients with chronic artery disease. JAMA 1988;259:1537–40
5. Leon AS. Position paper of the American Association of Cardiovascular and Pulmonary Rehabilitation. Scientific evidence of the value of cardiac rehabilitation services with emphasis on patients following myocardial infarction. I. Exercise conditioning component. J Cardiopulmonary Rehabil 1990:1079–87
6. DeBusk RF, Blomqvist CG, Kouchoukos NT et al. Identification and treatment of low-risk patients after acute myocardial infarction and coronary artery bypass graft surgery. N Engl J Med 1986;314:161–6
7. Detry JM, Rousseau M, Vandenbrouche G et al. Increased arteriovenous oxygen difference after physical training in coronary heart disease. Circulation 1986;74:350–8
8. Froelicher V, Jensen D, Genter F et al. A randomised trial of exercise training in patients with coronary artery disease. JAMA 1984; 252: 1291–7
9. Hung J, Gordon EP, Houston N et al. Change in rest and exercise myocardial perfusion and left ventricular function 3 to 26 weeks after clinically uncomplicated acute myocardial infarction: effects of exercise training. Am J Cardiol 1984; 54: 943–50
10. Rogers MA, Yamamoto C, Hagberg JM et al. The effect of 7 years of intense exercise training on patients with coronary artery disease. J Am Coll Cardiol 1987; 10(2): 321–6
11. Leon AS. Effects of exercise conditioning on physiological precursors of coronary heart disease. J Cardiopulmonary Rehabil 1991; 11: 46–57
12. Ornish D, Brown SE, Scherwitz LW et al. Can lifestyle changes reverse coronary heart disease? The Lifestyle Heart Trial. Lancet 1990; 336: 129–33
13. Shaw LW. Effects of a prescribed supervised exercise programme on mortality and cardiovascular morbidity in patients after myocardial infarction. Am J Cardiol 1981; 48: 39–46
14. Vermuelen A, Lie KI, Durrer D. Effects of cardiac rehabilitation after myocardial infarction: changes in coronary risk factors and long term prognosis. Am Heart J 1983; 105: 798–801
15. Hamalainen H, Luurila OJ, Kallio V. Long-term reduction in sudden deaths after multifactorial intervention programme in patients with myocardial infarction: 10-year results of a controlled investigation. European Heart Journal 1989; 10: 55–62
16. Rechnitzer PA, Cunningham DA, Andrew GM et al. Relation of exercise to recurrence rate of myocardial infarction in men. Ontario Exercise-Heart Collaborative Study. Am J Cardiol 1983; 51: 65–9
17. May GS, Eberlein KA, Furberg CD et al. Secondary prevention after myocardial infarction: A review of the long-term trials. Prog Cardiovasc Dis 1982; 24: 331–62
18. Olderidge NB, Guyatt GH, Me F et al. Coronary rehabilitation after myocardial infarction. Combined experience of randomised clinical trails. JAMA 1988; 260: 945–50
19. O'Connor GT, Burning JE, Yusuf S et al. An overview of randomised trials of rehabilitation with exercise after myocardial infarction. Circulation 1989; 80: 234–44
20. Dishman RK. Medical psychology in exercise and sports. Med Clin North Am 1985; 69: 123–43
21. Hughes JR. Psychological effects of habitual aerobic exercise. A critical review. Prev Med 1984; 13: 66–78
22. Dracup K, Moser DK, Marsden C et al. The effect of a multidimensional cardiopulmonary rehabilitation program on psychological functioning. Am J Cardiol 1991; 68(1): 31–4
23. Worcester MC, Hare DL, Oliver RG et al. Early programmes of high and low intensity exercise and quality of life after acute myocardial infarction. Br Med J 1993; 307: 1244–7
24. Blumenthal J, Emery CF, Rejeski WJ. The effects of exercise and psychosocial functioning after myocardial infarction. J Cardiopulmonary Rehabil 1988; 8(5): 183–93
25. Coats AJ, Adamopoulos S, Radaelli A et al. Controlled trial of physical training in chronic heart failure: exercise perfor-

mance, hemodynamics, ventilation and autonomic function. Circulation 1992; 85: 2119–31

26. Koch M, Douard H, Broustet JP. The benefit of graded physical exercise in chronic heart failure. Chest 1992; 101 (Suppl. 5): 231–5S
27. Sullivan MJ, Higginbotham MB, Cobb FR. Exercise training in patients with severe left ventricular dysfunction: hemodynamic and metabolic effects. Circulation 1988; 78: 506–15
28. Sullivan MJ, Higginbotham MB, Cobb FR. Exercise training in patients with chronic heart failure further delays ventilatory anaerobic threshold and improves submaximal exercise performance. Circulation 1989; 79: 324–9
29. Coats AJ, Adamopoulos S, Meyer TE et al. Effects of physical training in chronic heart failure. Lancet 1990; 335: 63–6
30. Topol EJ, Burek K, O'Neill WW et al. A randomized controlled trial of hospital discharge after myocardial infarction in the era of reperfusion. N Engl J Med 1988; 318: 1083–8
31. Willich SN, Lewis M, Lowel H et al. Physical exertion as a trigger of acute myocardial infarction. N Engl J Med 1993; 329: 1684–90
32. Van Camp SP, Peterson RA. Cardiovascular complications of outpatient cardiac rehabilitation programmes. JAMA 1986; 256: 1160–3
33. Haskell WL. Cardiovascular complications during exercise training of cardiac patients. Circulation 1978; 57: 920–4

Part 7

Acute myocardial infarction

52 AMI: Pre-hospital coronary care

Michael F O'Rourke

Introduction

While a book such as this is directed at hospital practice in coronary care, readers must recognize that the greatest challenges yet to be faced lie outside hospital, where afflicted persons first suffer the symptoms of heart attack (see Ch. 3). Despite public education campaigns, and despite individual education of patients during previous admission for myocardial infarction (MI), delays after symptom onset average 2.5–3 hours before presentation to hospital.[1–3] It is during this time that most deaths occur from heart attack—twice as many as occur in hospital, and most from potentially reversible ventricular fibrillation (Fig. 52.1).[4]

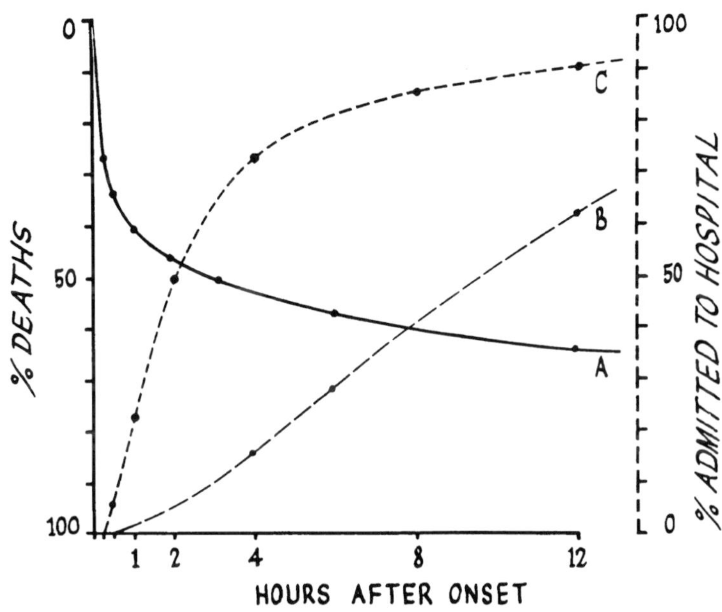

Fig. 52.1 Time course of death (curve A; left axis) and of time to come under intensive care (curves B, C; right axis) after onset of symptoms of acute coronary occlusion. Curve B refers to patients seeking hospitalization in the usual way. Curve C refers to those attended by the coronary ambulance service in Belfast. From Pantridge 1994.[31]

It is during this time too that MI commences. After onset of coronary occlusion by thrombus, some 30 minutes elapse before infarction commences in the region furthest from collateral vessels, and infarction proceeds to involve 50–70% of the region by 3 hours after occlusion and symptom onset (Fig. 52.2).[5]

By the time most patients present, potential benefits of thrombolysis are thus limited to well under 50% of the myocardium afflicted, and unfortunately to well under this again by the time that thrombolytic therapy is administered, and less still by the time that this has been effective and has re-opened the thrombosed artery.

A number of initiatives have been taken to improve pre-hospital coronary care. The most obvious is to shorten the time taken for persons to seek medical attention. In Australia, in the USA, and in many other countries, public education campaigns have been conducted to explain the major symptoms of heart attack, and to outline the need for, and mechanisms for, getting promptly to hospital.[3,6] In the pre-thrombolytic era, the only reason for such action was to provide facilities for treatment of ventricular fibrillation. This need was difficult to communicate without inducing alarm. Nowadays, another reason can be truthfully given. Irreversible heart muscle damage can be limited or even prevented by expeditious diagnosis and use of thrombolytic agents. Such a reason is muted by

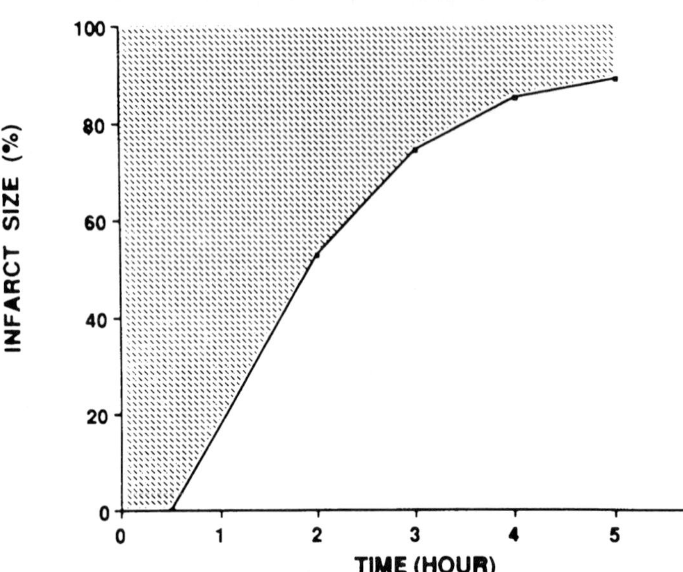

Fig. 52.2 Time course of infarction after onset of symptoms of acute coronary occlusion. From Carroll et al.[30] after data presented by Hugenholtz.[5]

the term 'myocardial infarction'. 'Coronary occlusion' or 'coronary thrombosis' are more realistic terms.[7] Professional communicators prefer the lay term of 'heart attack'. Those involved with community education programmes are often disappointed that they are not more successful.[1,3] Such disappointment should not induce inertia. Professional communicators and advertisers know only too well that the population as a whole does respond, but only when a message is repeated, reinforced, and repeated again.

Such public education campaigns stress the major problem of having a person with symptoms of coronary occlusion recognize the symptoms as of sufficient concern to call for assistance. The next delay, getting to an appropriate medical facility, is usually relatively short. In Australia as in most Western countries, ambulance services recognize chest pain or discomfort as a possible manifestation of coronary occlusion, and assign a top priority for fast response.

Pre-hospital ambulance services

The concept of pre-hospital coronary care was popularized by Pantridge and Geddes in Belfast during 1965.[8,9] Recognizing that most deaths had occurred before presentation to hospital, Pantridge arranged for ambulance vehicles located next to the Royal Victoria Hospital in Belfast to collect nurse and doctor with defibrillator and ancillary equipment from the hospital before proceeding to the call. The aim was to take coronary care to the patient. This proved very effective, not only in preventing death from ventricular fibrillation, but also for treating other complications and for expediting passage through the emergency department to the coronary care ward. This system was taken up in many other countries, including Australia—notably in Perth and Sydney.[10] A different approach was adopted in the USA, with emergency ambulance officers (usually fire-fighting personnel) trained in defibrillation and other procedures.[11] This 'paramedic' system had ambulance and other specially trained personnel provide emergency services outside hospital according to set protocols, and without direct medical supervision. In Sydney and Melbourne, this system was adopted, continued, and expanded from the early 1970s.[12,13] The paramedic system proved very effective, particularly for management of ventricular fibrillation and heart attack. However, such a system is only practicable in major cities where population density enables prompt response, and also sufficient exposure to emergencies for skills at electrocardiogram (ECG) interpretation and in various procedures to be maintained. Something different was required for country towns, for rural areas, and for the outskirts of the major cities.

The provision of pre-hospital cardiac care has been improved in such areas by the introduction of semi-automatic defibrillators, instruments that can identify ventricular fibrillation as well as providing counter shock.[14] Such instruments have now been installed in regular ambulance vehicles, and with staff appropriately trained in their use in many communities, including the whole of Scotland[15] and the Australian state of New South Wales (NSW).[16] Results of treatment for ventricular fibrillation outside hospital approximate those obtained by trained paramedics who have other drugs (for example, adrenaline, lignocaine) and procedures (endotracheal intubation) available.[17] It appears that the benefits of shortening the time for defibrillation by use of a regular ambulance vehicle make up for extra benefits of such ancillary treatment as paramedics can provide. In NSW, during 1992, 1047 cases of cardiac arrest with ventricular fibrillation (VF) or ventricular tachycardia (VT) were treated by the ambulance service. Survival to hospital discharge for out-of-hospital defibrillation in patients with VF was 13% overall, and 32% in those (210) defibrillated less than 5 minutes after witnessed cardiac arrest.

Pre-hospital medical care

In major cities and most country towns, medical practitioners have little role in treatment of acute heart attack, except for providing solace and explanation, and for expediting transfer to hospital. Most physicians do not carry oxygen, let alone a defibrillator or an ECG machine. They can, however, liaise effectively with ambulance officers. In Sydney, ambulance officers are taught to accept the pre-eminence of the medical practitioner, and to defer to him/her when present. Sensible medical practitioners recognize the skills of ambulance officers and liaise effectively with them. Administration of aspirin (300 mg) to chew should be routine, and a small dose of nitroglycerin (300–600 mg) sublingual or by buccal spray, may be used for pain relief. If narcotic analgesics are necessary, morphine 1–2 mg IV, repeated as necessary, can be given.[18,19]

In some situations, medical practitioners have to do much more. The Australian resort region of Ayers Rock (Uluru) is an example. There is no hospital, just an air service with the Alice Springs Hospital some 300 miles distant. Medical officers in the medical centre are often called on to treat patients with heart attack as though they were in hospital; even fibrinolytic therapy can be initiated under these circumstances. Naturally, such patients need to be transported by air or surface with full ambulance paramedic facilities, including defibrillator deployed.

Public access defibrillation

Ventricular fibrillation outside hospital is the most common cause of death following coronary occlusion. This may be the first symptom, or may occur before the afflicted person recognizes the significance of their symptoms or has sought emergency care. But ventricular fibrillation can also occur under other circumstances such as an 'electrical accident' of cardiac rhythm in a patient with longstanding ventricular scarring or disease.[20,21] Hence, VF cannot always be foreseen. It can occur at any time, and is most likely to be seen when large numbers of people congregate, especially when there is a good deal of bustle or excitement. The father of pre-hospital coronary care, Professor Frank Pantridge of Belfast, was the first to champion public access defibrillation, by providing a small inexpensive non-advisory defibrillator, which he urged to be used as is a fire extinguisher in the case of fire, but by any member of the public who is faced with a person in cardiac arrest.[9] Pantridge rightly pointed out that if a person was in asystole, no harm would be done, whereas if he was in ventricular fibrillation, his life might be saved. As with his initial concept of pre-hospital coronary care, Pantridge was well ahead of his time. The concern with unappropriate use, as in persons with a simple faint, discouraged development of this device.

The situation has now changed with development of algorithms capable of recognizing VF, and their installation into implantable automatic and external semi-automatic defibrillators.[14] With further miniaturization and decreasing cost of these devices, the American Heart Foundation has set up a task force for implementing a programme of public access defibrillation with the expectation that this may save up to 100 000 lives per year in the United States. This task force held its first open meeting with cardiologists, engineers, industry and government agencies in Washington in December 1994.[21a]

Programmes for use of defibrillators in aircraft and in airport terminals have been approached in the past, notably by British Caledonian Airlines, prior to the merger of this company with British Airways. The Australian carrier Qantas installed defibrillators in all its international fleet of 53 Boeing 747 and 767 aircraft in 1991 and trained staff in their use and in handling of cardiac arrest.[21,21b] To date, there have been two survivors of ventricular fibrillation in flight, and at least one more survivor was possible had terminal facilities been adequate on arrival (at a minor port).[21b] Survival rate for ventricular fibrillation in the air terminal approaches that of treatment by paramedics. Death in aircraft (87 per million sectors, 0.72 per million passengers)[21b] are greater than reported from the (incomplete) data previously published.[22] The Qantas experience provides support for availability of defibrillators on aircraft, though pointing out that the utilization is infrequent, and that their present provision forms part of a safety network whose value is hard to estimate on economic grounds.

Pre-hospital thrombolysis

Pre-hospital fibrinolysis has been used and evaluated in a number of different settings—in the ambulance vehicles staffed by medical practitioners in Israel,[23] in Northern Ireland and France,[24] and in the paramedic-staffed ambulances in Seattle, Rotterdam and Sydney.[25–27] All have been successful, with early initiation of therapy and minimal inappropriate use, and with complication rates no different from that in hospital. Overview of the clinical trials has shown that pre-hospital initiated thrombolysis is associated with a 17% reduction in 30-day mortality.[28] Benefits however arise from early treatment; identical benefit might be expected if patients could be evaluated expeditiously and treated promptly on arrival in hospital. The downside of this is practicability. In Seattle, Rotterdam and Sydney, some 20 persons were attended by ambulance officers and subjected to full evaluation, including 12-lead ECG, for every patient fulfilling criteria for, and receiving, thrombolytic therapy. In the major cities, it should be more practicable to expedite evaluation of patients with suspected coronary thrombosis on arrival in a hospital emergency department.

Pre-hospital fibrinolysis has proved of greatest value in sparsely populated communities.[29] When transportation delays are considerable and when medical practitioners are willing and able to initiate thrombolytic therapy in the home, definite benefits have been shown.[30,31] Pre-hospital fibrinolysis is also practicable, desirable, and effective in ambulance vehicles staffed by medical officers, as in the major cities of Israel[23] and some European cities.[24]

Summary

Pre-hospital coronary care is the first step in the 'chain of survival' and commences with a person (after previously being healthy) recognizing the need to call for emergency assistance. The next step is an efficient emergency service which can provide resuscitation and defibrillation if required while transporting the patient expeditiously to hospital. Both steps are enhanced by a community education process, which also ensures that members of the public are trained in cardiac pulmonary resuscitation so that resuscitative measures can be initiated and maintained prior to arrival of an emergency vehicle if this should be required.

References

1. Bett JHN, Aroney G, Thompson PL. Delays preceding admission to hospital and treatment with thrombolytic agents of patients with possible heart attack. Aust NZ J Med 1993; 23: 312–3
2. Kereiakes DJ, Weaver WD, Anderson JL et al. Time delays in the diagnosis and treatment of acute myocardial infarction: a tale of eight cities. Am Heart J 1990; 120: 773–80
3. Bett JHN, Aroney G, Thompson PL. Impact of a national education campaign to reduce patient delay in possible heart attack. Aust NZ J Med 1993; 23: 157–61
4. Martin CA, Hobbs MST, Armstrong BK. Estimation of myocardial infarction mortality from routinely collected data in Western Australia. J Chron Dis 1987; 661–9
5. Hugenholtz PG. Acute coronary artery obstruction in myocardial infarction: overview of thrombolytic therapy. J Am Coll Cardiol 1987; 6: 1375–84
6. O'Rourke MF, Ballantyne K, Thompson PL. Community aspects of thrombolysis: public education and cost effectiveness. In: Julian DG et al (eds). Thrombolysis in cardiovascular disease. New York: Dekker: 1989: 309–24
7. O'Rourke MF. Early thrombolytic treatment in acute coronary thrombosis. Aust NZ J Med 1993; 23: 742–4
8. Pantridge F, Geddes JS. A mobile intensive care unit in the management of myocardial infarction. Lancet 1967; 2(510): 271–3
9. Geddes JS. The management of the acute coronary attack. London: Academic Press, 1986
10. Staff of the Cardiovascular Unit at St Vincent's and Prince of Wales Hospitals, Sydney. Modified coronary ambulances. Med J Aust 1972; 1: 875–8
11. Cobb LA, Baum RS, Alvarez H, Schaffer WA. Resuscitation from out of hospital ventricular fibril-

lation: four years follow-up. Circulation 1975; 52: 223–8
12. Luxton M, Peter T, Harper R, Hunt D, Sloman G. Establishment of the Melbourne Mobile Intensive Care Service. Med J Aust 1975; 1: 612–5
13. O'Rourke MF, Ladd-Hudson K, Sloman G. Establishment of pre-hospital emergency services in Australia. Canberra: National Heart Foundation of Australia Technical Paper, 1985
14. Weaver WD, Hill DD, Fahrenbruch CE et al. Use of the automatic external defibrillator in the management of out-of-hospital cardiac arrest. New Engl J Med 1988; 319: 661–6
15. Cobbe SM, Redmond MJ, Watson JM, Hollingworth J, Carrington DJ. 'Heartstart Scotland'—initial experience of a national scheme for out-of-hospital defibrillation. Br Med J 1991; 302: 1517–20
16. O'Rourke MF, Hall J. Pre-hospital cardiac arrest in New South Wales 1992. Aust NZ J Med 1994; 24: 619
17. Sammel NL, Taylor K, Selig M, O'Rourke MF. New South Wales intensive care ambulance system: outcome of patients with ventricular fibrillation. Med J Aust 1980; 2: 546–50
18. Weston CFM, Penny WJ, Julian DG, on behalf of the British Heart Foundation Working Group. Guidelines for the early management of patients with myocardial infarction. BMJ 1994; 308: 767–71
19. National Heart Foundation of Australia, Heart Attack Committee. Emergency coronary care. Guidelines for the treatment of patients with suspected coronary occlusion. Canberra: National Heart Foundation, 1995
20. Weaver WD, Cobb LA, Hallstrom AP, Fahrenbruch CE, Copass MK, Ray R. Factors influencing survival after out-of-hospital cardiac arrest. J Amer Coll Cardiol 1986; 7: 752
21. O'Rourke MF, Donaldson E. An airline cardiac arrest programme. Circulation 1994. 90: Suppl I: 287
21a. Weisfeldt ML, Kerber RE, McGoldrick RP, Moss AJ, Nichol G, Ornato JP, Palmer DG, Riegel B, Smith Sc. American Heart Association Report on the Public Access Defibrillation Conference December 8–10, 1994. Circulation 1995; 92: 2740–7
21b. O'Rourke MF, Donaldson E. Successful Management of Ventricular Fibrillation in Commercial Airliners. Lancet 1995; 345: 515–6
22. Cummins RO, Chapman PT, Chamberlain DA, Schubach JA, Litwin PE. In-flight deaths during commercial air travel. J Amer Med Assoc 1988; 259: 1983–8
23. Weiss AT, Fine DG, Applebaum D et al. Pre-hospital coronary thrombolysis: a new strategy in acute myocardial infarction. Chest 1987; 92: 124–8
24. European Myocardial Infarction Project Group. Pre-hospital thrombolytic therapy in patients with suspected acute myocardial infarction. N Engl J Med 1993; 329: 383–9
25. Weaver WD, Cerqueira M, Hallstrom AP et al. Pre-hospital-initiated vs thrombolytic therapy. JAMA 1993; 270; 1211–6
26. Simoons ML. Cardiology in the community. The Thoraxcenter Journal 1991; 3(3): 50–2
27. Gallagher DE, O'Rourke MF, Healey J et al. Paramedic-initiated pre-hospital thrombolysis using urokinase in acute coronary occlusion (TICO 2). Coronary Artery Disease 1992; 3: 605–9
28. Weaver WD. Time to thrombolytic treatment: factors affecting delay and their influence on outcome. J Am Coll Cardiol 1995; 25(Suppl. 7) 35–95
29. GREAT Group. Feasibility, safety and efficacy of domiciliary thrombolysis by general practitioners. Grampian Region early Anistreplase trial. Br Med J 1992; 305: 548–53
30. Carroll G, O'Rourke MF, Feneley M. Preventive strategies in management of myocardial infarction. Aust NZ J Med 1990; 20: 615–20
31. Pantridge TF. Mobile intensive care in the management of myocardial infarction. Coronary Artery Disease 1994; 1: 294–302

53 AMI: Emergency department care

Peter L Thompson and John E Morgan

Introduction

The emergency department (ED) has a key role in the management of the patient with suspected acute myocardial infarction (AMI).[1–3] In the pressured working conditions of the emergency room, the patient with acute coronary thrombosis who is conscious and without visible signs of trauma may be competing with patients with other medical emergency conditions which may have a greater visual or emotional impact in setting priorities for medical or nursing attention. It is absolutely essential that emergency medicine staff approach the patient with acute coronary thrombosis as a patient who is at imminent risk of death from ventricular fibrillation (VF) and from permanent cardiac damage and disability if restoration of blood flow to the ischaemic myocardium is not achieved immediately. A variety of strategies have been suggested to highlight the emergency needs of the patient with suspected acute coronary thrombosis.[4] The most persuasive strategy may simply be to abandon the diagnostic term 'acute myocardial infarction' and to define the clinical problem as a threatening and rapidly deteriorating process of 'acute coronary thrombosis with myocardium infarcting.'[5] In this way the patient's needs can be recognized and the process can be modified if not totally aborted.

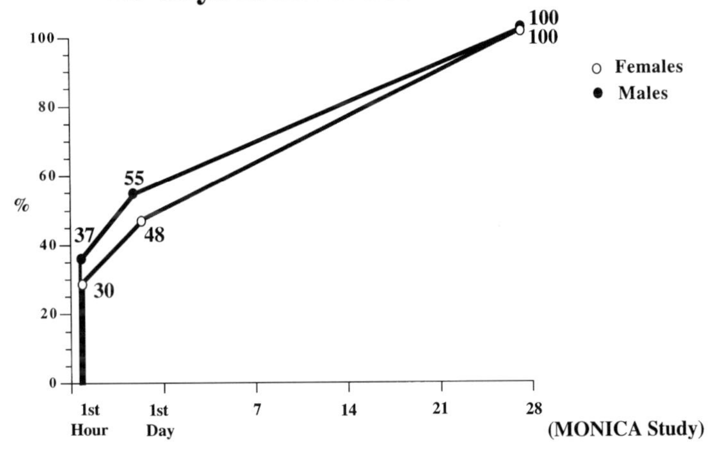

Fig. 53.1 Cumulative pattern of coronary deaths from onset to 28 days after the event. Of the deaths which occur in the first month, one third occur in the first hour. Data from 48 communities in the MONICA study.[6] NB Time axis not to scale.

Need for urgent action

The key pathophysiologic and clinical trial data pertaining to the emergency department management of acute coronary thrombosis are displayed in Figures 53.1 and 53.2.

Figure 53.1 shows the pattern of coronary heart disease deaths following the onset of an event. Of the patients who are destined to die in the month after onset of AMI, one third of the deaths will occur in the first hour.[6] Many of these occur outside of hospital and are not amenable to any form of treatment, but a considerable proportion are due to VF which can be treated by an emergency medical service or hospital emergency department. The importance of encouraging patients to call an ambulance or to present to hospital to have the benefit of a defibrillator needs constant repetition in community education campaigns.[7]

The large GISSI-I[8] and ISIS-2[9] trials established the importance of early treatment with thrombolysis, with approximate halving of early mortality in patients treated

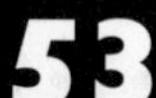

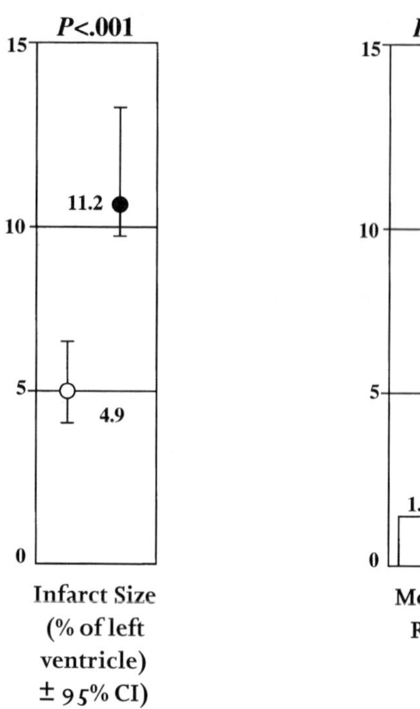

Fig. 53.2 Impact of initiating thrombolytic therapy early (either out of hospital or in the emergency department). Data from the MITI (Myocardial Infarction and Triage Intervention) trial.[17] Reproduced with permission from the American College of Cardiology (Journal of the American College of Cardiology 1990; 15: 925–31)

in the first hour. Figure 53.2 demonstrates even more clearly the critical time-dependency of reperfusion therapy. Patients in the MITI (Myocardial Infarction Triage and Intervention) trial who were treated in the first hour had dramatically better left ventricular function and survival than patients treated later. These benefits were achieved with thrombolytic regimens which we now know achieve early patency in less than half of patients treated.[10] The benefits of aggressive early therapy with modern reperfusion strategies, which include more effective thrombolytic therapy regimens and (possibly) primary coronary angioplasty in selected patients, highlights the key role of the emergency department in improving outcome in acute coronary occlusion.[11]

Management plan

The key components and outcome indicators in the emergency department plan for management of acute coronary occlusion are shown in Table 53.1.

The overall plan of management needs to be developed in consultation between the community emergency medical services, the hospital emergency department and the CCU to ensure that the responsibilities of each area are quite clear, that there is an approved plan of triage, an agreement on early management procedures, agreement on outcome indicators and agreement on the principles of monitoring and review of the outcomes. Having established these principles of management it is important that they be reviewed from time to time. A member of the emergency medicine staff should be responsible at each shift for chest pain and 'myocardium infarcting' patients to be dealt with expeditiously.

Management of chest pain and the 'myocardium infarcting' patient

Relief of pain and anxiety

Reassurance, application of oxygen and narcotic analgesics as required will help to allay the patient's pain and anxiety, reduce the likelihood of VF and speed the process of haemodynamic stabilization. Oxygen therapy should be instituted immediately on arrival in the ED. Sublingual or buccal spray administration of nitroglycerin 0.3 mg should be routine.

Prevention of death from ventricular fibrillation

The incidence of VF is highest in the first few hours after the onset of AMI.[12] Rapid application of a cardiac monitor is essential to monitor the cardiac rhythm, and venous access is essential to administer antiarrhythmic or beta blocking drugs as necessary. Application of the ECG monitor and the insertion of the IV line should be achieved within minutes of arrival in the emergency department. All staff in the emergency department should be familiar with the principles of cardiopulmonary resuscitation (CPR—see Ch. 40) and the techniques of advanced cardiac life support and defibrillation (see Chs 41, 42). It should be possible to achieve defibrillation within 15 seconds of the onset of VF. If this

Table 53.1 Monitoring emergency department management of acute coronary occlusion

Key principles of management	Outcome indicator	Target
Relief of pain and anxiety	Time to application of oxygen	Immediately on arrival
Prevention of death from VF	Time to insertion of IV Delay in defibrillation	Minutes from arrival 15 seconds from onset of VF
Early coronary reperfusion	Door to needle time	30 minutes from arrival

can be achieved, protracted CPR may not be necessary. To achieve this, the defibrillator must be readily accessible and functioning satisfactorily. It should be assumed that the patient presenting to the emergency department with symptoms suggestive of acute coronary occlusion may develop VF.

The use of prophylactic antiarrhythmic drugs has been only partly effective in preventing fibrillation and has not affected mortality[12] but the use of intravenous beta blockers, particularly in patients with obvious anxiety, resting tachycardia and hypertension, is helpful.[14] The patient who is showing frequent salvos of ventricular premature beats with ventricular tachycardia (VT) may benefit from treatment with intravenous antiarrhythmic therapy. Although there will be occasions when a patient with overwhelming myocardial necrosis will die as a result of VF, the death of a patient from primary VF should normally be regarded as unacceptable and a reason for review of protocols and procedures for dealing with this emergency. Deaths from VF should be so rare as to render it unhelpful as an outcome indicator.

Early coronary reperfusion

The overwhelming data that thrombolytic therapy[15] and more recently coronary angioplasty[16] can dramatically improve survival from acute coronary occlusion by restoration of coronary patency has revolutionized the management of this condition in the past decade. The critical time dependency of the benefits to be achieved from coronary reperfusion are demonstrated in Figure 53.2. The maximum benefits are obtained in the first hour after the onset and this has been referred to as the 'golden hour' of treatment opportunities for acute coronary occlusion. Whilst the extension of this pre-hospital thrombolysis is logical (see Ch. 52 for detailed discussion), the rather limited benefits demonstrated in clinical trials,[17,18] the complex logistics and the medico-legal concerns about responsibility for complications, have limited the application of this approach except in specialized circumstances.[19] Therefore it is even more important for the emergency departments of major hospitals to ensure that the procedures for rapid decision making and administration of reperfusion therapy where appropriate are in place and functioning effectively. The simplest outcome indicator of the effectiveness in dealing with acute coronary occlusion is the *door to needle time*, that is the delay between the arrival of the patient at the front door of the hospital and the administration of thrombolytic therapy.[1,3] Despite the overwhelming clinical trial benefits demonstrated and the increased awareness of the need to act decisively, it has been universal experience that hospitals which measure their door to needle time are shocked at the delays which still exist in emergency management.[3,20] The National Heart Attack Alert Program co-ordinating committee,[1,3] the American Heart Association's emergency cardiac care committee[5] and most other committees which have evaluated this problem have recommended that eligible patients be identified and treated with thrombolytic therapy within 30–60 minutes of their arrival in the emergency department and that staff should strive to treat all patients within 30 minutes of arrival. Further breakdown of the door to needle time delays have been suggested by dividing the delay into three components from the time of arrival (*Door*), obtaining an ECG (*Data*), deciding to treat with thrombolytic therapy (*Decision*) and initiating thrombolytic therapy (*Drug*). The pharmaceutical industry has collaborated actively with this approach and has produced timing devices with clipboards to monitor the *Door-Data-Decision-Drug* times and provide software for monitoring and analysis of trends. The template for obtaining this data is reproduced in Table 53.2.

The early delivery of reperfusion therapy requires the cooperation not only of medical and nursing staff but also the emergency clerical staff and triage nurse. Guidelines for ensuring early recognition and rapid triage of possible coronary occlusion have been suggested by the US National Heart Attack Alert Program.[3] These are reproduced in Table 53.3.

The "fast-track" flow chart used by the Australian National Heart Foundation and College of Emergency Medicines is reproduced in Figure 53.3.

In recent years primary angioplasty has been considered as an alternative to thrombolytic therapy because of encouraging preliminary evidence from clinical trials[16] and persuasive evidence that this is able to achieve a higher rate of TIMI Grade 3 coronary patency than even the most effective thrombolytic drug regimens. While this procedure is available in only a few centres with high volume angioplasty programmes, it is essential that the CCU, catheter laboratory and emergency department have clear-cut protocols to identify patients who may be considered for angioplasty rather than thrombolytic therapy.[21] It is important that the expectations of patient and family should not be raised unnecessarily as this procedure is critically dependent on the availability of a catheter laboratory and high volume angioplasty programme and operator. In the absence of these, thrombolytic therapy remains the most effective reperfusion treatment for suspected coronary occlusion.

Table 53.2 The Four Ds for assessing components of door to needle time

- *Door* Time of arrival in the emergency department
- *Data* Time of obtaining 12 lead ECG
- *Decision* Time thrombolytic drug ordered
- *Drug* Time thrombolytic drug infusion started

Table 53.3 Triage guidelines for suspected acute myocardial infarction ('myocardium infarcting') in the emergency department. A detailed medical history is not an essential requirement for reperfusion therapy. Source: National Heart Attack Alert Program Coodinating Committee, 60 Minutes to Treatment Working Group. Ann Emerg Med 1994; 23: 311–29

NHAAP TRIAGE GUIDELINES

Guidelines for ED registration clerk's and/or triage nurse's identification of AMI patients.

Registration/clerical staff

Patients more than 30 years old with the following chief complaints require immediate assessment by the triage nurse and *should be referred for further evaluation:*

Chief complaint

- Chest pain, pressure, tightness, or heaviness; radiating pain in neck, jaw, shoulders, back, or one or both arms
- Indigestion or 'heartburn'/nausea and/or vomiting
- Persistent shortness of breath
- Weakness/dizziness/light headedness/loss of consciousness

TRIAGE NURSE

Patients with the following symptoms and signs require immediate assessment by the triage nurse *for initiating the AMI protocol:*

Chief complaint

- Chest pain. Patients more than 30 years old with chest pain or severe epigastric pain, non traumatic in origin, having components typical of myocardial ischaemia or infarction:
  - central/substernal compression or crushing chest pain
  - pressure, tightness, heaviness, cramping, burning, aching sensation
  - unexplained indigestion/belching
  - radiating pain in neck, jaw, shoulders, back or one or both arms
- Associated dyspnoea
- Associated nausea/vomiting
- Associated diaphoresis

If these symptoms are present, obtain stat ECG

Medical history

The triage nurse should do a brief, targeted, initial history assessing for current or past history of:

- coronary artery bypass graft (CABG), angioplasty, coronary artery disease, or AMI
- Nitroglycerin use to relieve pain
- Risk factors, including smoking, hyperlipidaemia, hypertension, diabetes mellitus, family history and cocaine use

This brief history *must not* delay entry into the AMI protocol.

Special considerations

- Questions have been raised as to whether women may present more frequently with atypical chest pain and symptoms.
- Diabetic patients may have atypical presentations due to autonomic dysfunction.
- Elderly patients may have stroke, syncope, or change in mental status.

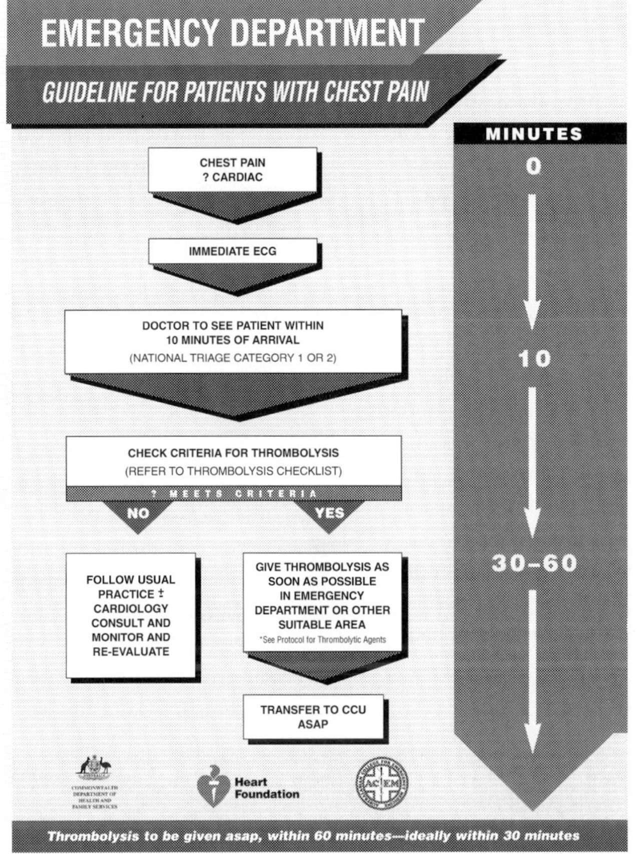

Fig. 53.3 Fastrack guideline for triage of chest pain in the Emergency Department (National Heart Foundation of Australia and Australian College of Emergency Medicine).

Specific management recommendations

Analgesia

Often administration of oxygen and sublingual nitroglycerine is sufficient. If it is not, the most effective analgesic remains small repeated boluses (1–2 mg) of intravenous (IV) morphine sulphate as required up to 8–10 mg. Higher doses may induce unnecessary mental obtundation, prolonged nausea and respiratory depression increasing the risk of pulmonary complications with MI.

Venous access

Venous access and infection control guidelines should be agreed between the emergency department and CCU. Thrombolytic therapy can be administered via a peripheral vein. The most suitable access sites are the antecubital veins or the veins on the dorsum of the forearm. Access via central veins may cause later complications with thrombolytic and anticoagulant therapy.

Oxygen

Commence oxygen therapy on arrival at 6–8 litres per minute via face mask. Monitor with an oxygen saturation monitor, aiming to achieve a saturation over 97%.

High flows of oxygen can cause respiratory depression in patients with severe obstructive airways disease, but the frequency of this problem is overrated. Oxygen delivery should not be compromised for fear of this relatively infrequent problem.

Nitroglycerin

Sublingual nitroglycerin (see Ch. 30) may have beneficial systemic venodilating effects and coronary vasodilating effects in acute coronary occlusion. Acute hypotensive reactions may occur including an hypotensive bradycardiac response thought to be due to a vagal response to coronary reperfusion (the Bezold–Jarisch reflex).[22] Treatment can be initiated with half a nitroglycerin tablet (300 micrograms) or a single rather than double puff of nitroglycerin spray. Intravenous infusion of nitroglycerine may be indicated in some patients.

Beta blockers

Intravenous beta blockers (see Ch. 28) have demonstrated benefits in controlled clinical trials[14] but problems with inducing hypotension and bradycardia have limited the widespread uptake of this procedure. There are clear-cut indications for the patient with persistent tachycardia, particularly associated with hypotension (systolic BP greater than 160 mmHg) or the patient with frequent ventricular ectopic beats associated with a sinus tachycardia. Administration of IV beta blockers is as follows: atenolol 5 mg followed by a further 5 mg after 10 minutes or IV metoprolol 5 mg injections at 5-minute intervals to a maximum of 15 mg, monitoring the heart rate to ensure that it does not drop below 50 beats per minute and the blood pressure to ensure that it does not drop below 100 mmHg systolic.

Antiarrhythmic drugs

Prophylactic antiarrhythmic drugs are no longer used. For sustained VT or repeated short salvos of VT, lignocaine remains widely used in a dose of 50–100 mg intravenously. There is increasing use of IV sotalol (75–100 mg over 10–20 minutes) and IV amiodarone 300 mg for control of high grade ventricular arrhythmias. See chapter 27 for a more detailed review of antiarrhythmic drugs.

Aspirin

All patients with suspected acute coronary thrombosis should receive aspirin 300 mg as soon as possible, but the time dependency is not as critical as with thrombolytic therapy. See chapter 36 for further details.

Thrombolytic therapy

The guidelines for thrombolytic therapy in the emergency department are identical to those in the CCU. See also Chapters 34 and 54. The guidelines for reperfusion therapy recommended by the National Heart Foundation of Australia and the Australian College of Emergency Medicine are reproduced in Fig. 53.4.

Management of complications

Atrial fibrillation

Rapid atrial fibrillation (see Ch. 62) may occur during the early stages of AMI. It can be treated with IV digoxin 0.25 mg administered over 10 minutes or with IV beta blockers (see above) or IV amiodarone.

Pulmonary oedema

Pulmonary oedema (see Ch. 56) is common in the early stages of AMI. It is treated with IV frusemide 40 mg repeated and increased as necessary, morphine 5 mg, sublingual nitroglycerin, intravenous nitroglycerine and if necessary continuous positive airways pressure via occlusive

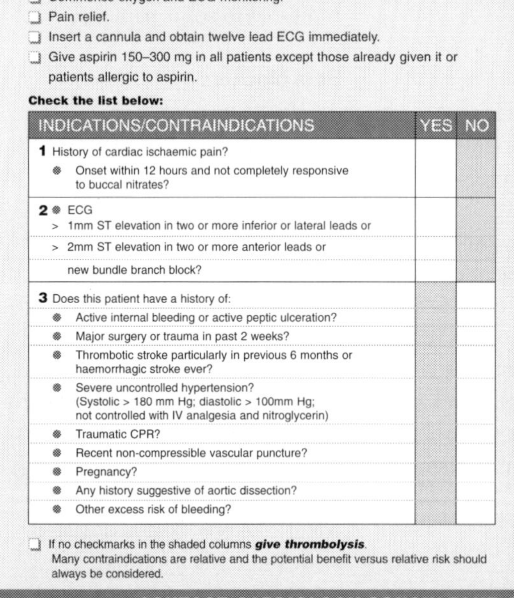

INDICATIONS FOR THROMBOLYTIC THERAPY

EARLY THROMBOLYSIS SAVES MYOCARDIUM AND LIVES

THROMBOLYSIS CHECK LIST

- ❑ Commence oxygen and ECG monitoring.
- ❑ Pain relief.
- ❑ Insert a cannula and obtain twelve lead ECG immediately.
- ❑ Give aspirin 150–300 mg in all patients except those already given it or patients allergic to aspirin.

Check the list below:

INDICATIONS/CONTRAINDICATIONS	YES	NO
1 History of cardiac ischaemic pain?		
• Onset within 12 hours and not completely responsive to buccal nitrates?		
2 • ECG		
> 1mm ST elevation in two or more inferior or lateral leads or		
> 2mm ST elevation in two or more anterior leads or		
new bundle branch block?		
3 Does this patient have a history of:		
• Active internal bleeding or active peptic ulceration?		
• Major surgery or trauma in past 2 weeks?		
• Thrombotic stroke particularly in previous 6 months or haemorrhagic stroke ever?		
• Severe uncontrolled hypertension? (Systolic > 180 mm Hg; diastolic > 100mm Hg; not controlled with IV analgesia and nitroglycerin)		
• Traumatic CPR?		
• Recent non-compressible vascular puncture?		
• Pregnancy?		
• Any history suggestive of aortic dissection?		
• Other excess risk of bleeding?		

❑ If no checkmarks in the shaded columns ***give thrombolysis***. Many contraindications are relative and the potential benefit versus relative risk should always be considered.

THROMBOLYTIC AGENT

rt-PA

- ❑ Previous use of streptokinase

Consider rt-PA especially if:

- ❑ Age < 75 years
- ❑ Evolving anterior infarct
- ❑ Thrombolytic can be administered within 4 hours of onset of symptoms

Streptokinase

- ❑ All others eligible for thrombolysis

- ❑ PTCA: In a small number of tertiary centres with an experienced angioplasty team, primary PTCA for acute coronary occlusion is being used.

PROTOCOL FOR THROMBOLYTIC AGENTS

rt-PA Administration

- ❑ IV heparin 5,000 units bolus
- ❑ IV bolus rt-PA 15mg *then*
- ❑ 50 mg over 30 minutes *(or 0.75 mg/kg in patients < 70kg) then*
- ❑ 30–35 mg over 60 minutes *(0.5 mg/kg in patients < 70kg)* Maximum total dose = 100mg
- ❑ Maintain heparin infusion at 1,000 units/hour

SK Administration

- ❑ 1.5 million units SK in 100 ml normal saline over 60 minutes using infusion pump and peripheral line

COMMONWEALTH DEPARTMENT OF HEALTH AND FAMILY SERVICES

ACEM

Heart Foundation

CONTACT CARDIOLOGY CONSULTANT OR CORONARY CARE REGISTRAR URGENTLY

Fig. 53.4 Summary protocols for assessment and decision-making for reperfusion therapy in emergency department as recommended by the National Heart Foundation of Australia and the Australian College of Emergency Medicine.

face mask or intubation with intermittent positive pressure ventilation.

Cardiogenic shock

Patients with cardiogenic shock (see Ch. 57) should have treatment initiated with IV dobutamine and be transferred immediately to the CCU for consideration of intra-aortic balloon pumping, urgent cardiac catheterization and angioplasty if available. Patients with cardiogenic shock do not respond well to thrombolytic therapy.

References

1. National Heart Attack Alert Program (NHAAP). Staffing and equipping emergency medical services systems: rapid identification and treatment of acute myocardial infarction. US Department of Health and Human Services NIH, 1993: Publication No. 93–3304
2. American Heart Association Emergency Cardiac Care Committee and Subcommittees. Guidelines for cardiopulmonary resuscitation and emergency cardiac care. III. Adult advanced cardiac life support. JAMA 1992; 268: 2199–241
3. National Heart Attack Alert Program (NHAAP) Coordinating Committee, 60 minutes to treatment working group. Emergency department: rapid identification and treatment of patients with acute myocardial infarction. Ann Emerg Med 1994; 23: 311–29
4. National Heart Foundation of Australia Heart Attack Committee. Emergency coronary care. Guidelines for treatment of the patient with suspected coronary occlusion. Canberra: National Heart Foundation of Australia, 1995
5. RO Cummins (ed.) Textbook of advanced cardiac life support. American Heart Association, 1994
6. World Health Organization. Myocardial infarction and coronary deaths in the World Health Organization MONICA project. Registration procedures, event rates and case fatality rates in 38 populations from 21 countries in four continents. Circulation 1994; 90: 583–612
7. Bett JHN, Aroney G, Thompson PL. Impact of a national education campaign to reduce patient delay in possible heart attack. Aust NZ J Med 1993; 23: 157–161
8. Gruppo Italiano Per Lo Studio Della Streptochinasi Nell'Infarto Miocardico (GISSI). Effectiveness of intravenous thrombolysis treatment in acute myocardial infarction. Lancet 1986; 1: 397–401
9. ISIS-2 Collaborative Group. Randomised trial of intravenous Streptokinase, oral aspirin, both or neither during 17 187 cases of suspected acute myocardial infarction (ISIS-2). Lancet 1988; 2: 349–60
10. The GUSTO-I Angiographic Investigators. The effects of tissue plasminogen activator, streptokinase, or both on coronary patency, ventricular function and survival in acute myocardial infarction. N Engl J Med 1993; 329: 1615–22
11. Ornato JP. Role of the emergency department in decreasing time to thrombolysis therapy in acute myocardial infarction. Clin Cardiol 1990; 13(Suppl. V): V48–52
12. McNeilly RH, Pemberton J. Duration of last attack of 998 fatal cases of coronary artery disease and its relation to possible cardiac resuscitation. Br Med J 1968; 3: 139–42
13. MacMahon S, Collins R, Peto R, Kotter RW, Yusuf S. Effects of prophylactic lidocaine in suspected acute myocardial infarction: an overview of results from the randomized controlled trials. JAMA 1988; 260: 1910–6
14. Yusuf S, Wittes J, Friedman L. Overview of results of randomized clinical trials in heart disease. Treatments following myocardial infarction. JAMA 1988; 260: 2088–93
15. Fibrinolytic Therapy Triallists (FTT) Collaborative Group: indications for fibrinolytic therapy in suspected acute myocardial infarction: collaborative overview of mortality and major morbidity results from all randomised trials of more than 1000 patients. Lancet 1994; 343: 311–22
16. Grines CL, Browne KF, Marco J et al for the PAMI Study Group. A comparison of immediate angioplasty with thrombolytic therapy for acute myocardial infarction. N Engl J Med 1993; 328: 673–9
17. Weaver WD, Eisenberg MS, Martin JS et al. Myocardial Infarction Triage and Intervention Project—Phase I: patient characteristics and feasibility of prehospital indication of thrombolytic therapy. J Am Coll Cardiol 1990; 15: 925–31
18. GREAT Group. Feasibility, safety and efficacy of domiciliary thrombolysis by general practitioners: Grampian Region Early Anistreplase Trial. Br Med J 1992; 305: 548–53
19. Weston CFM, Penny WJ, Julian DG. Guidelines for the early management of patients with myocardial infarction. Brit Med J 1994; 308: 767–71
20. MacCallum A, Stafford P, Jones C et al. Reduction in hospital time to thrombolytic therapy by audit of policy guidelines. Eur Heart J 1990; II: 48–52
21. International Roundup. Primary angioplasty in myocardial infarction. Br Heart J 1995; 73(5): 403–16

22. Mark AL. The Bezold–Jarisch reflex revisited; clinical implications of inhibitory reflexes originating in the heart. J Am Coll Cardiol 1983; 1: 90–102

54 AMI: CCU admission and care

Peter L Thompson

Introduction

Despite the widening role of the coronary care unit (CCU), the management of the patient with suspected acute myocardial infarction (AMI) remains its 'core business.' The principles of management of the CCU have been discussed in Chapter 2. This chapter will discuss the management of the individual patient who presents with symptoms suggestive of AMI.[1–3] Following initial assessment and pain relief, aims are to prevent death from ventricular fibrillation, preserve cardiac function and improve prognosis with coronary reperfusion, and prevent and manage complications.

AMI: Initial management and pain relief

Initial management
- reassurance and explanation
- intranasal oxygen 2–4 L/min
- insertion of IV with 5% dextrose
- attachment to cardiac monitor
- 12-lead ECG

Initial blood sampling
- electrolytes, urea, creatinine, full blood examination, cardiac enzymes and other biochemical markers, hepatic function, coagulation screening

Additional evaluation as necessary
- chest X-ray, echocardiography, O_2 saturation monitoring

Pain relief
- morphine 1–2 mg IV (bolus as required)

Nausea relief
- metoclopramide 5 mg IV

Routine orders (see text)

Feedback to patient, family and referring medical practitioner

Initial assessment and pain relief

Initial management and pain relief are summarized in the information box.

The patient who has experienced chest pain suggestive of AMI will invariably be apprehensive, fearful of the unfamiliar events taking place around them and very likely concerned for their survival. An essential part of the early management is reassurance of the patient and family that pain and other symptoms can be relieved and that most MIs have an uncomplicated course with an excellent prognosis. Part of the reassurance process is to ensure that the admission to the CCU is uncomplicated by delays and that the patient is greeted immediately with an air of quiet efficiency and concern for their welfare. Each step during the application of oxygen, insertion of intravenous drip, application of electrocardiogram (ECG) monitoring electrodes and performance of the 12-lead ECG and chest X-ray, will need a brief explanation of the purpose of the procedure.

Initial management

Initial management consists of:
- patient sitting in a comfortable semi-recumbent position
- intranasal or face mask oxygen at 2–4 litres per minute
- insertion of an intravenous cannula with blood sampling for tests (see below) and infusion of 5% dextrose
- application of chest electrodes and commencement of continuous ECG monitoring
- vital signs including blood pressure, pulse, respiratory

rate and application of automated blood pressure (BP) monitor if available
- 12-lead ECG
- application of finger stall for O_2 saturation monitoring if available
- detailed nursing assessment
- detailed medical assessment.

Initial blood sampling

Included in initial blood sampling will be:

- urea, electrolytes and creatinine
- cardiac enzymes or other biochemical markers
- full blood examination including platelet count
- screening tests of hepatic function including transaminase, alkaline phosphatase and bilirubin
- screening tests for coagulation including activated partial thromboplastin time (APTT).

Additional evaluation

Additional evaluation may require the following when appropriate:

- portable chest X-ray
- echocardiography
- arterial blood gas analysis
- O_2 saturation monitoring

Pain relief

Pain relief is not only essential for humane management of the distressing event, but there is evidence that it can speed haemodynamic stabilization and reduction in the frequency of arrhythmias. The use of a simple 0–10 grading system for the severity of chest pain and its response to the administration of analgesics is a very useful system for charting the response to therapy as well as providing a baseline for evaluating recurrences of chest pain.[5] Initial analgesia is usually with small doses of IV narcotics such as morphine 1–2 mg repeated as required.[6] If the chest pain is clearly due to persisting myocardial ischaemia, intravenous nitroglycerin should be used but with the caution that adjustments in the rate of delivery of nitroglycerin may have a delayed effect because of the slow rate of infusion and absorption from the tubing.[7] If more immediate pain relief is required, the use of sublingual nitroglycerin or nitroglycerin spray may be necessary[8] (see Ch. 30).

Nausea

Nausea may result from the MI or the narcotic analgesic and should be treated with IV metoclopramide (Maxolon) 5 mg repeated as necessary to a maximum of four doses in 24 hours.

Routine orders

Following the initial assessment, orders are written to ensure that the following are performed:

- fasting serum lipids (on the morning after admission)
- fasting blood glucose (on the morning after admission)
- cardiac enzymes or biochemical markers (12-hourly for 36 hours and then daily)
- urea, electrolytes and creatinine daily
- full blood examination daily
- 12-lead ECG daily and immediately on the development of chest pain, cardiac arrhythmia or major change in status.

Feedback to patient and family

Following the initial assessment it is essential that the patient and family be given some preliminary feedback on the presumed diagnosis and whether the diagnosis of MI is confirmed or still in doubt, the extent of likely damage to the heart, a brief review of the expected duration of coronary care and hospital stay and anticipated procedures. It is helpful if this information can be supplemented with a culturally appropriate information leaflet or booklet. Preliminary experience with the use of critical pathways in the CCU[4] has suggested that patients and family gain some reassurance from seeing the pathway for a typical case charted against the pathway which they are likely to follow as determined by the initial assessment.

As soon as the patient is able to comprehend what has happened to them, the process of discharge planning, rehabilitation and education should begin and it is essential that this should not be delayed until late in the hospital course. Having the necessary information is reassuring for the patient and family; having the wrong information or allowing misconceptions to remain uncorrected can have serious long term consequences. All members of the coronary care team must be involved in this process, which is overseen by a rehabilitation coordinator (see Ch. 76). Feedback to the patient's own or referring practitioner is a courtesy which is appreciated and will enhance future management.

Prevention of death from ventricular fibrillation (VF)

It is usual to make a distinction between *primary* VF which occurs in the patient with normal or only mildly impaired haemodynamic status and *secondary* VF which occurs as one of the agonal rhythms in a patient dying from progressive pump failure.[9] Although on occasions there will be difficulties in categorizing an individual case of VF as primary or secondary, as in the patient who develops VF during progressive but potentially retrievable cardiogenic shock, in most cases the distinction between primary and secondary VF is clear.

In the modern CCU, VF will be relatively infrequent. In the coronary care reports from the 1960s, VF occurred in up to 10% of patients.[9,10] In recent reports from databases and clinical trials, the incidence of primary VF complicating MI in the CCU has been below 5%.[11,12] Death from primary VF should occur rarely in a well run CCU; occasionally it may be the mechanism of death in patients with overwhelming myocardial ischaemia and infarction from recent acute coronary thrombosis.

The factors in preventing the onset of primary VF are shown in the information box discussed in more detail below.

Relief of anxiety

Although it is difficult to obtain controlled clinical trial data on this point, there does seem to be an association between uncontrolled anxiety and the onset of VF.[13] The process of anxiety relief involves a strategy of pain relief, reassurance and explanation as outlined above.

Maintenance of serum potassium above 4.0 mmol/L

There is a clear-cut relationship between hypokalaemia and the onset of ventricular fibrillation.[14,15] Hypokalaemia appears to be associated with increased levels of circulating catecholamines.[16] Although clinical trial data have been lacking to confirm the benefits of restoration of the serum potassium, a routine of maintaining the potassium level above 4.0 mmol/L appears to be a sensible policy.

Early administration of beta blockers

Administration of beta blockers improves the prognosis in AMI and is of most benefit in patients at high risk (see Ch. 28). The mechanism is of benefit partly due to a reduced incidence of ventricular fibrillation.[16,17] Despite the benefits demonstrated in clinical trials, IV beta blockers in AMI remain under-utilized.[18,19] They should preferentially be given in patients with persistent heart rates above 100 per minute, particularly if there is associated hypertension with systolic blood pressure above 160 mmHg.

Avoidance of unnecessary intracardiac cannulation

Ventricular fibrillation on occasions can be precipitated by manipulation of haemodynamic monitoring catheters or pacing catheters within the right ventricle.[20] Unnecessary manipulation of catheters within the ventricles should be avoided and haemodynamic monitoring and right ventricular pacing limited to those cases where there are clear-cut indications (see Chs 24, 43).

Treatment of high grade ventricular arrhythmias

Clinical trials of prophylactic lignocaine showed a slight reduction in ventricular fibrillation but no improvement in outcome and therefore this policy has now been abolished.[21] In the past decade there has been a declining use of antiarrhythmic drugs.[22] Antiarrhythmic therapy should be limited to patients with frequent salvos of ventricular ectopic beats or ventricular tachycardia with haemodynamic effects (see Chs 55, 63). While lignocaine remains widely used for this purpose there is an

AMI: Prevention of death from ventricular fibrillation

Prevention of VF
- relief of anxiety
- maintenance of serum K^+ above 4.0 mmol/L
- early administration of beta blockers
- avoidance of unnecessary intracardiac cannulation
- treat sustained ventricular tachycardia

Treatment of VF
- electrical defibrillation 200 joules within 20–30 seconds
- recheck serum K^+ to maintain above 4.0 mmol/L

increasing use of Class 3 agents such as IV sotalol[23] or amiodarone.[24] There are not sufficient clinical trials to guide the choice of agent.

Immediate treatment of VF

VF should be recognized immediately and treated within a few seconds with electrical defibrillation. Time should not be wasted with external cardiac compression and assisted ventilation. Upon reversion to sinus rhythm, the serum potassium should be rechecked.

Preservation of cardiac function by coronary reperfusion

Re-establishing coronary patency as early as possible has now become a major focus in the management of AMI. The data from the coronary thrombolytic trials (see Ch. 34) has demonstrated a clear-cut survival benefit for patients treated with thrombolytic therapy, with an advantage of accelerated r-TPA over streptokinase (SK) particularly in selected subgroups of high risk patients. A smaller series of trials with coronary angioplasty has demonstrated a possible advantage of angioplasty over thrombolytic regimens (see Ch. 45). These clinical trial data are consistent with angiographic observations which show clearly that restoration of TIMI Grade 3 flow is necessary to achieve the benefits of reperfusion therapy. All trials have shown a benefit in achieving patency early rather than later. The ISIS-II Trial has shown the importance of a supporting role for aspirin. The r-TPA-heparin studies have highlighted the importance of heparin accompanying r-TPA but its importance is less clear for streptokinase.

AMI: Coronary reperfusion therapy to preserve LV function

- **Earliest possible reperfusion strategy** to achieve normal patency in the infarct related artery
- Patients **suitable for thrombolytic therapy** (ST elevation or BBB, within 12 hours of onset, no contraindications):
  - **accelerated r-TPA** is preferable in patients with previous SK therapy, extensive infarction, and treatment within 4 hours of onset
  - **streptokinase** is a satisfactory and less expensive alternative in other patients
  - **aspirin** for all patients
  - **heparin IV** for r-TPA patients, not necessarily for streptokinase patients
  - **primary PTCA** if high-volume lab, team and operator available and a structured primary PTCA programme in place
- Patients **not suitable for thrombolytic therapy**:
  - **PTCA** if early treatment can be achieved by a high volume lab team and operator
  - **routine management** if PTCA not available
  - **cardiac catheterization** for impending cardiogenic shock, then PTCA or (high risk) CABG depending on coronary anatomy

PTCA = percutaneous transluminal coronary angioplasty; CABG = coronary artery bypass graft

From this wealth of clinical trial information, strategies for reperfusion in the CCU are clear-cut.[2,3,25] These are summarized in the information box and discussed in more detail below.

Early reperfusion

The CCU must be an integral part of community emergency services for chest pain, which include public education, rapid response ambulance service and emergency departments to ensure the earliest possible treatment of patients with suspected MI.

Appropriate reperfusion strategy

The reperfusion strategy most appropriate to each patient should be implemented as early as possible (see Ch. 34). For the patient thought suitable for thrombolytic therapy, the choice of agent will depend on availability, cost and the clinical setting. Both r-TPA and streptokinase should be available in the CCU. Staff should be aware of the price differential for streptokinase and r-TPA therapy, as well as the results of comparative clinical trials. In most countries the cost of streptokinase is approximately one tenth of the cost of r-TPA. Though r-TPA achieved better survival in direct comparison with streptokinase in the GUSTO trial, this was achieved at a slightly higher risk of intracerebral haemorrhage. The benefits were most obvious in patients with more extensive infarction who were able to have treatment early. Patients with prior streptokinase therapy may develop antibodies which inactivate future doses of streptokinase. Therefore, patients with prior streptokinase or who have extensive infarction and who can be treated within 4 hours are clear candidates for r-TPA in preference to streptokinase.

Aspirin

All patients receiving thrombolytic therapy should receive aspirin 300 mg initially followed by 100–150 mg per day (see Ch. 56).

Heparin

Patients who receive intravenous r-TPA should have accompanying IV heparin 5000 units bolus followed by 1000 units per hour continued for 24–48 hours to maintain the APTT level at 60–85. IV heparin need not accompany streptokinase especially if there is a risk of bleeding, but may be used if there is another indication for anticoagulation or concern about recurrent occlusion, when heparin can be given intravenously or subcutaneously (see Chs 34 and 35).

PTCA

Patients who are ineligible for thrombolytic therapy may be considered for primary angioplasty if a skilled, high-volume angioplasty laboratory and operator are readily available (see Ch. 45). Patients eligible for thrombolytic therapy may be considered for primary angioplasty as an alternative to thrombolysis if this is part of a concerted programme in an institution with a high volume of coronary angioplasties, ready availability of a catheterization laboratory, skilled team and high-volume operator.

In patients with progressive haemodynamic deterioration and likely progression to cardiogenic shock, thrombolytic therapy is unlikely to be helpful. Early coronary angiography and angioplasty of appropriate lesions may be helpful (see Ch. 57). Coronary artery bypass surgery may be considered but is a high risk procedure and should only be considered if haemodynamic status can be stabilized with intra-aortic balloon pumping.

'Rescue' angioplasty may be considered in the patient with clear-cut evidence of failure to reperfuse after thrombolytic therapy. This procedure carries a risk of haemorrhagic complications and re-occlusion and has a paucity of clinical trial data to support it.

Following reperfusion therapy subsequent management will depend on the patient's clinical status, particularly the presence or absence of continuing symptoms of myocardial ischaemia (see Chs 78–80).

Routine management and prevention of complications

Routine management of the MI patient is best conducted according to a set protocol which will vary with each patient but should serve as a guide for the coronary care staff as well as the patient and family (see information box). Monitoring of progress via a critical pathway is a helpful way of ensuring efficient passage through the CCU, enhancing communication with the patient and ensuring efficient use of post-CCU investigative facilities (see Ch. 2).

Bed-rest and activity

The patient with uncomplicated MI should initially be treated with bed-rest but can be sitting out of bed at 12 hours or the morning after the hospital admission. A bedside commode is usually less physical effort than using a bed pan and can be permitted the day following admission. Most patients can be walking in the room with a view to discharge from the CCU at 36–48 hours post admission. If the infarction has not been extensive and there has been no evidence of contining myocardial

Routine management and prevention of complications

- **Bed rest** for 12–24 hours, CCU stay 36–48 hours, hospital stay 5–6 days (dependent on severity)
- **Diet** light initially, then routine low fat and tailored diet based on serum lipids and blood glucose
- **Oxygen** routinely administered initially, but can cease if O_2 saturation satisfactory
- **Aspirin** in all patients unless contra-indicated
- **Heparin** as determined by reperfusion strategy and risk of thrombo-embolic complications (see separate information box)
- **Beta blockers** routinely unless contraindicated
- **Calcium channel blockers** if beta blocker contraindicated and no evidence of LV dysfunction (avoid sole use of nifedipine)
- **Nitrates** for continuing ischaemia, but not routinely
- **ACE inhibitors** in all patients with evidence of LV dysfunction and possibly in all patients

ischaemia, the risk of late arrhythmias is low and discharge to the open ward may be considered. If there is concern about the risk of arrhythmias or recurrence of ischaemia, the use of a step-down telemetry facility may be considered.[26]

Most patients with uncomplicated MI can be ready for hospital discharge on the fifth or sixth day after admission,[27] but it is important in the current era of shortened hospital stays not to overlook the needs of the patients who will benefit from longer hospital stays, such as those with extensive infarction, the elderly and those without adequate trial support.[28] To ensure efficient utilization of hospital facilities and investigative procedures, arrangements for investigation should be made as soon as the patient's condition on admission is clear and the likely rate of progression through the hospital course can be estimated. CCU staff have an important role in ensuring that procedures are booked as early as possible to avoid unnecessary delays in mobilization and early discharge.

Diet

In the early hours of hospital admission when the patient is apprehensive, there is the likelihood of nausea and vomiting from narcotics and there is a relatively high risk of high grade arrhythmias which may require resuscitation. There should be no solid foods, and only fluids as required to relieve thirst. As the patient settles, a light meal can be offered, usually returning to a normal but light diet the next day. It is important to establish the dietary principles of secondary coronary prevention at a time when the patient is aware of the need and receptive to advice. The CCU's diet should reflect the principles of fat reduction, adequate complex carbohydrates, fibre and anti-oxidants and avoidance of excess salt[29] (see Ch. 38).

Oxygen

Mild hypoxaemia is very frequent following AMI[30] (see Ch. 25). Although the benefits of oxygen in mild MI have not been clearly established, oxygen is routinely administered by intranasal prongs at 2–4 L/min or face mask at 4–6 L/min for the first 24 hours. If there is clinical evidence of cardiac failure, dyspnoea or hypotension, oxygen saturation should be monitored continuously. If more detailed information on oxygenation is required, arterial blood sampling and blood gas analysis will be necessary, but the need for this has become less in recent years with increased availability of O_2 saturation monitors and there are concerns about arterial bleeding complications with more aggressive use of antithrombotic and thrombolytic regimens.

Aspirin

Whether or not thrombolytic therapy is used, oral aspirin should be administered to every patient with AMI without contraindication to aspirin therapy[1–3,31–33] (see Ch. 36). In recent years in the Perth teaching hospital CCUs, aspirin has been administered to over 95% of patients with AMI, compared with less than 20% a decade before.[22]

The use of aspirin and other antithrombotic agents in the CCU has probably increased the risk of gastrointestinal and retroperitoneal bleeding, and regular checks on haemoglobin should be conducted throughout the hospital stay. Patients with a history of peptic ulcer disease should be prescribed an H2 antagonist to reduce the risk of gastrointestinal bleeding.

Heparin

Clinical trials have shown a clear-cut need for r-TPA to be accompanied and followed by IV heparin, continued for 24–48 hours[1–3,34] (see Ch. 35). The role of heparin with streptokinase therapy is still not clear.[34] Subcutaneous heparin with streptokinase achieves small improvement in survival but with an increased risk of haemorrhagic complications, and no evidence of an advantage of intravenous post SK heparin over subcutaneous SK heparin has been established. The prolonged systemic fibrinolytic effect of SK and a policy of universal aspirin administration may be adequate protection against post-thrombolysis rethrombosis. Increasing dissatisfaction with haemorrhagic complications with subcutaneous heparin and the unsightly and sometimes troublesome complications with subcutaneous heparin may justify abandoning routine use of heparin following streptokinase, particularly for patients who have a risk of bleeding from hypertension, peptic ulcer or oral anticoagulant therapy. In circumstances where warfarin anticoagulation should be considered—such as in patients with extensive anterior MI at risk of intracardiac thrombus, in patients with atrial fibrillation thought to be at risk of left atrial thrombus formation, or in patients with continuing myocardial ischaemia and presumed evidence of continuing subocclusive coronary thrombosis—full dose IV heparin should be continued until there is echocardiographic guidance about the need to change to warfarin (see Ch. 37). If cardiac catheterization is to be performed during the hospital stay, IV heparin should be continued.

In patients at high risk of deep vein thrombosis, subcutaneous heparin 12 500 units 12-hourly is the accepted regimen.

Recommendations for heparin in AMI are summarized in the information box.

Beta blocking drugs

The clinical trial data to support a policy of routine use of beta blockers post MI has been presented in Chapter 28. The large body of data derived from the prethrombolytic era has been supported by the results from the TIMI-II trial which demonstrated a benefit of beta blockade administered as early as possible.[35] Concerns about the benefits of IV beta blockers persist and IV administration is not routine. However the data in favour of oral administration is strong enough to regard this as routine and the proportion of patients receiving beta blockers can be researched as an indicator of quality of care in a CCU.[22]

Calcium channel blockers

On occasions the patient who is unable to take a beta blocker may need to be treated with a calcium channel blocker (see Ch. 29). The sole use of nifedipine is contraindicated; if used, it should be accompanied by a beta blocker. Diltiazem may prevent progression of non-Q wave infarction, and verapamil has some clinical trial evidence to support its use to prevent reinfarction in the presence of normal left ventricular function. However, both diltiazem and verapamil may have adverse effects in LV dysfunction and cause bradyarrhythmia in combination with beta blockers.[35] The newer dihydropyridines such as amlodipine have had limited use in AMI but have a satisfactory haemodynamic profile both for sole use and in combination with beta blockers.

AMI: recommendations for heparin in acute myocardial infarction

- **After r-TPA**
  — 5000 u IV bolus and 1000 u/h and then monitored to maintain APTT at 60–80 seconds. Continyue for 24–48 hours
- **After SK**
  — Optional IV (as above) *or* SC 12 500 u 12-hourly *or* nil
- **High risk intracardiac thrombus**
  — IV with need for coumarin determined by echocardiography
- **Continuing myocardial ischaemia**
  — IV heparin
- **High risk deep vein thrombosis**
  — SC 12 500 u 12-hourly until mobilized

Nitrates

Intravenous nitroglycerin has potent anti-ischaemic effects by producing coronary vasodilation and reduction of preload and is widely used in CCUs[36] (see Ch. 30) for control of unstable myocardial ischaemia. Meta-analysis of small trials has suggested a benefit in mortality but this is not proven.[37] The recent ISIS-IV[38] and GISSI-3[39] trial results were disappointing in showing no prognostic benefit for routine use of oral or transcutaneous nitrates and therefore these should not be routinely prescribed.

Angiotensin-converting enzyme (ACE) inhibitors

The large series of trials with ACE inhibitors have confirmed an important role for these drugs in the post-infarction patient[40] (see Ch. 33). ACE inhibitors should be considered in all patients with evidence of cardiac failure or echocardiographic evidence of LV dysfunction. The benefits are less in patients with small, haemodynamically stable infarction. Commencement within the first 24 hours is safe but it should be a routine precaution to avoid starting patients who are hypotensive (systolic BP less than 90 mmHg) or who are at risk of hypotension from aggressive diuretic therapy. Initial treatment can be with a low dose of a short-acting drug followed by conversion to a once per day ACE inhibitor 48 hours later, although initiation with low dose once per day therapy appears safe.

References

1. ACC/AHA Task Force report. Guidelines for the early manage-

ment of patients with acute myocardial infarction. J Am Coll Cardiol 1990; 16: 249–92

2. Weston CFM, Penny WJ, Julian DG, on behalf of the British Heart Foundation Working Group. Guidelines for the early management of patients with myocardial infarction. Br Med J 1994; 308: 767–71
3. Antman E. General hospital management. In: Julia D, Braunwald E (eds.) Management of acute myocardial infarction. London: Saunders, 1994: Ch. 2
4. Reinhart SI. Uncomplicated acute myocardial infarction: a critical path. Cardiovascular Nursing 1995; 31: 1–7
5. Chapman CR, Casey KL, Dubner R et al. Pain measurements: an overview. Pain 1985; 22: 1–31
6. Herlitz J. Analgesia in myocardial infarction. Drugs 1989; 37: 939–44
7. Jugdutt BI, Warnica JW. Intravenous nitroglycerin therapy to limit myocardial infarct size, expansion and its complications: effect of timing, dosage and infarct location. Circulation 1988; 78: 906–19
8. Flaherty JT. Role of nitrates in acute myocardial infarction. Am J Cardiol 1992; 73: 73B–81B
9. Lawrie DM, Higgins MR, Godman MJ et al. Ventricular fibrillation complicating acute myocardial infarction. Lancet 1968; 2: 523–8
10. Lown B, Fakhro AM, Hood WB, Thorn GW. The coronary care unit. New perspectives and directions. JAMA 1967; 199: 188–98
11. Hopper JL, Pathik B, Hunt D, Chan W. Improved prognosis since 1969 of myocardial infarction treated in a coronary care unit. Br Med J 1989; 299: 892–6
12. Antman EM, Berlin JA. Declining incidence of ventricular fibrillation in myocardial infarction: implications for the use of lidocaine. Circulation 1992; 84: 764–73
13. Adgey AAJ, Allen JD, Geddes JS et al. Acute phase of myocardial infarction. Lancet 1971; 2: 501–4
14. Solomon R. Ventricular arrhythmias in patients with myocardial infarction and ischaemia: the role of serum potassium. Drugs 1986; 31: 112–20
15. Nordrehaug JE, Von der Lippe G. Hypokalaemia and ventricular fibrillation in acute myocardial infarction. Br Heart J 1983; 50: 525–9
16. Johansson BW, Dziamski R. Malignant arrhythmias in acute myocardial infarction: relationship to serum potassium and effect of selective and non-selective beta blockade. Drugs 1984; 2 (Suppl. 2): 77–85
17. Norris RM, Barnaby PF, Brown MA et al. Prevention of ventricular fibrillation during acute myocardial infarction by intravenous propranolol. Lancet 1984; II: 883–6
18. Collins R, Julian D. British Heart Foundation surveys (1987 and 1989) of United Kingdom. Treatment policies for acute myocardial infarction. Br Heart J 1991; 66: 250–5
19. Rogers WJ, Bowlby LJ, Chandra NC, French WJ, Gore JM, Lambrew CJ et al. Treatment of myocardial infarction in the United States (1990–1993). Observations from the National Registry of Myocardial Infarction. Circulation 1994; 90: 2103–14
20. Robin E. Death by pulmonary artery flow-directed catheter. Chest 1987; 92: 727–31
21. MacMahon S, Collins R, Peto R et al. Effects of prophylactic lignocaine in suspected acute myocardial infarction. An overview of results from the randomized controlled trials. JAMA 1988; 260: 1910–6
22. Thompson PL, Parsons RW, Jamrozik K, Hockey RL, Hobbs MST, Broadhurst RJ. Changing patterns of medical treatment in acute myocardial infarction: observations from the Perth Monica Study 1984–1990. Med J Aust 1992; 157: 87–92
23. Ho DSW, Zecchin RP, Richards DAB, Uther JB, Ross DL. Double blind trial of lignocaine versus sotalol for acute termination of spontaneous sustained ventricular tachycardia. Lancet 1994; 344: 18–23
24. Gill J, Heel RC, Fitton A. Amiodarone. An overview of its pharmacological properties and review of its therapeutic use in cardiac arrhythmias. Drugs 1992; 43: 69–110
25. Thompson PL, Tonkin AM, Aylward P, White H. Thrombolysis 93—is there a consensus? Aust NZ J Med 1993; 23: 778
26. Weinberg SL. Intermediate coronary care—observations on the validity of the concept. Chest 1978; 73: 154
27. McNeer J, Wagner G, Ginsburg P et al. Hospital discharge one week after acute myocardial infarction. N Engl J Med 1978; 298: 229–32
28. Goldstein S. Early discharge after a myocardial infarction: what's the hurry? J Am Coll Cardiol 1993; 22: 1802–3
29. The management of hyperlipidaemia: a consensus statement. Med J Aust 1992; 156 (Suppl.): 51–58
30. Filmore SJ, Shapiro M, Killip T. Arterial oxygen tension in acute myocardial infarction. Am Heart J 1970; 79: 620–4
31. Conti CR. Conventional drug therapy of patients with acute myocardial infarction. Cardiovasc Clin 1989; 20: 259–81
32. Collaborative overview of randomized trials of active platelet therapy—I. Prevention of death, myocardial infarction and stroke by prolonged antiplatelet therapy in various categories of patients. Br Med J 1994; 308: 81–106
33. ISIS-2. Second International Study of Infarct Survival.

Randomised trial of intravenous streptokinase, oral aspirin, both or neither in 17 187 cases of suspected acute myocardial infarction: ISIS-2. Lancet 1988; 2: 349–60
34. White HD, Yusuf S. Heparin and thrombolysis therapy. J Thrombosis and Thrombolysis. Journal of thrombosis and thrombolysis 1995; 2: 5–10
35. Held PH, Yusuf S. Effects of beta blockers and calcium channel blockers in acute myocardial infarction. Eur Heart J 1993; 14(Suppl. F): 18–25
36. Jugdutt BI. Role of nitrates after acute myocardial infarction. Am J Cardiol 1992; 70:(Suppl. B): 82B–7B.
37. Yusuf S, Collins R, MacMahon S, Peto R. Effect of intravenous nitrates on mortality in acute myocardial infarction. An overview of randomised trials. Lancet 1988; I: 1088–92
38. ISIS Collaborative Group. ISIS-4: a randomised factorial trial assessing oral captopril, oral mononitrate and intravenous magnesium sulphate in 58 050 patients with suspected acute myocardial infarction. Lancet 1995; 345: 609–85
39. GISSI-3. Effects of lisinopril and transdermal glyceryl trinitrate singly and together on 6-week mortality and ventricular function after myocardial infarction. Lancet 1994; 343: 1115–22
40. Cleland JGF. ACE inhibitors for myocardial infarction: how should they be used? Eur Heart J 1995;16:153–9

55 AMI: Management of cardiac arrhythmias

Peter L Thompson

Introduction

Cardiac arrhythmias are extremely common in the early stages of acute myocardial infarction (AMI). With increasing coronary care experience, it is clear that not all arrhythmias require treatment. Current approaches to the management of arrhythmias in AMI are in contrast to the first two decades of coronary care where aggressive abolition of all arrhythmias was the mission of the coronary care unit (CCU).

In modern coronary care practice arrhythmias are treated actively only when they are symptomatic, life-threatening, or causing an increase in myocardial consumption.

Sinus node disturbances

Sinus bradycardia

Sinus bradycardia is common in inferior MI especially in the early stages[1,2] but rarely requires treatment. If the heart rate is persistently below 45 beats per minute or is causing symptoms or clinical signs of reduced cardiac output, it can be treated with a small dose (0.5 mg) of atropine intravenously. Higher doses of atropine may cause cholinergic side-effects including dry mouth, blurred vision, sinus tachycardia and rarely ventricular tachycardia (VT) or fibrillation (VF).[3,4] Repeated doses of atropine can cause non-cardiac-significant side-effects including urinary retention, acute glaucoma or bizarre or psychotic behaviour. If symptomatic sinus bradycardia is persistent despite repeated doses of atropine, atrial pacing should be considered.

Sinus arrest

Intermittent sinus arrest may occur in inferior MI due to right coronary artery occlusion with involvement of the sinus atrial node or as a vagal efferent response to the Bezold–Jarisch reflex during reperfusion of the right coronary artery[5] (see Fig. 55.1). It is usually self-limiting but may require a single dose of intravenous (IV) atropine.

Sinus tachycardia

Sinus tachycardia in MI is an adverse prognostic feature[6] as it is usually an indicator of extensive myocardial necrosis associated with excess catecholamine release. On occasions it may be a physiologic response to pain, and may settle with pain relief. If the sinus tachycardia is persistent, it can cause extension of myocardial necrosis by increasing myocardial oxygen consumption.

The use of IV beta blockers varies widely between CCUs, but there is strong physiologic and clinical trial[7,8] support for use of beta blockers to reduce myocardial oxygen consumption and improve prognosis. Although

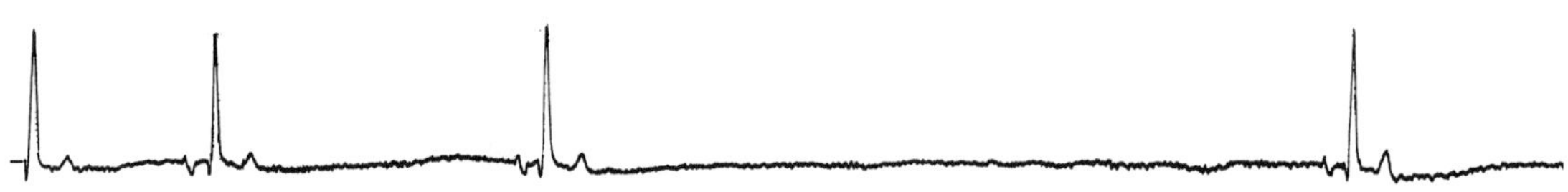

Fig. 55.1 Sinus arrest in a patient with inferior MI receiving IV streptokinase: the sinus arrest coincided with relief of chest pain and normalization of ST segment elevation typical of right coronary artery reperfusion and activation of the Bezold–Jarisch reflex.

there is no clear guidance from clinical trials on the optimum target heart rate, it seems reasonable to attempt to maintain the resting heart rate below 70 beats per minute unless the cardiac depressant (negative inotropic) effects of the beta blocker make this target unachievable.

Beta blocker treatment can be initiated with IV metoprolol[7] or atenolol.[8] Concern about negative inotropic effects may be an indication for a trial with IV esmolol.[9] Once treatment is initiated with IV beta blocker, it can be continued with oral beta blocker therapy, using a cardioselective beta blocker without intrinsic sympathomimetic activity (see Ch. 28).

Atrial arrhythmias

Atrial ectopic beats

Atrial ectopic beats require no therapy, but may herald the development of atrial fibrillation and be an indication for prophylaxis with a beta blocker. If beta blocker is contraindicated, verapamil can be used. Although digoxin prophylaxis is widely used in this situation, the evidence that it prevents or slows the rate of subsequent fibrillation is not convincing.

Atrial tachycardia and atrial flutter

Supraventricular arrhythmias other than atrial fibrillation are relatively uncommon in an AMI and are treated in a similar fashion to atrial fibrillation (see below).

Atrial fibrillation

The development of atrial fibrillation in AMI is an adverse prognostic indicator[10–12] (see Fig. 55.2). It occurs in 10–15% of patients following MI and is more frequently associated with extensive anterior infarction.[13]

The mechanism is thought to be increased atrial stretch with increased release of circulating catecholamines. Atrial fibrillation complicating anterior MI usually occurs after the first 24 hours, is preceded by minimal atrial ectopic activity, has a fast ventricular response, can cause significant haemodynamic compromise and usually responds well to heart rate slowing and antiarrhythmic therapy.[13] In contrast, the atrial fibrillation which is associated with inferior infarction may indicate sinus node and atrioventricular (AV) ischaemia and atrial infarction. This may occur early[14] and is associated with frequent bizarre atrial ectopic activity, with variants of atrial flutter and atrial tachycardia; it often does not have a fast ventricular response and is frequently resistant to antiarrhythmic therapy.

Until recently the choice of drugs available to delay atrioventricular conduction in atrial fibrillation complicating AMI was between digoxin,[15] which has a delayed effect, may be relatively ineffective in the setting of high circulating catecholamines, and may aggravate ventricular arrhythmias, versus beta blockers[16] or verapamil,[17] which effectively slow atrioventricular conduction but have negative inotropic effects. Because of these limitations there is now increasing use of IV amiodarone, which has heart rate-slowing effects as well as class III arrhythmic effect which encour-

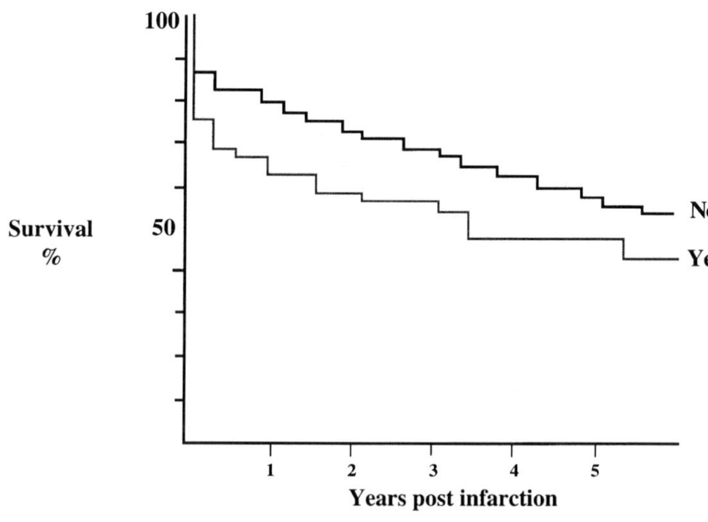

Fig. 55.2 Five year survival of patients with and without atrial fibrillation complicating AMI. 1000 patients treated in a CCU. Reproduced from Thompson PL. Prognosis of myocardial infarction with special reference to the role of infarct size. Perth: University of Western Australia, 1986.

ages return to sinus rhythm without negative inotropic properties.[18,19] Sometimes combined therapy is necessary using digoxin, beta blockers or verapamil to slow the ventricular rate and one of the class I or class III antiarrhythmic drugs to effect return to sinus rhythm. Cardioversion is a less preferred option in atrial fibrillation complicating MI because persistence of the factors which initiated the atrial fibrillation frequently encourage its relapse following reversion.

The route of administration of digoxin will depend on the rate of the atrial fibrillation and the haemodynamic response. If the rate is fast, for example in excess of 120 beats per minute, there will be an adverse effect on myocardial oxygen consumption and extension of the infarct size. In this situation, digoxin should be given intravenously. Oral therapy can be commenced at the same time as the IV administration. Return to sinus rhythm is relatively frequent and no further action is required. Digoxin therapy after AMI should be relatively short-term and could be considered for cessation prior to hospital discharge. If the atrial fibrillation persists, reversion to sinus rhythm by cardioversion prior to hospital discharge should be considered, recognizing the need for anticoagulant cover if the atrial fibrillation has persisted for longer than 24–36 hours.

Intravenous beta blocker therapy with atenolol and metoprolol may be effective in slowing the ventricular rate and encouraging return to sinus rhythm, and should be seriously considered as first line therapy unless there are contraindications or likelihood of cardiac decompensation from a negative inotropic effect. In the latter situation, a test dose of IV esmolol may be appropriate.[9]

Intravenous verapamil may be effective in slowing the ventricular rate and on occasions can encourage return to sinus rhythm.[17] The negative inotropic properties of verapamil can cause hypotension or accentuate cardiac failure. It should be used cautiously, with intermittent administration of 1–2 mg up to a maximum of 5–10 mg. Particular care should be taken in the CCU to ensure that the patient receiving IV verapamil is not already on a beta blocking drug.

Intravenous amiodarone is now the preferred form of therapy for atrial fibrillation complicating myocardial infarction because its potent class III antiarrhythmic property will frequently encourage return to sinus rhythm.[18,19] However, its atrioventricular blocking effect is relatively weak and it may need to be combined with digoxin if the ventricular response is very rapid. It is given in a bolus dose of 300 mg followed by an infusion of 0.7 mg/kg per 24 hours. Negative inotropic effects are rare with this regimen.

Following the slowing of the ventricular rate with digoxin, beta blocker or verapamil, reversion to sinus rhythm may be considered with the addition of an oral class I agent but there are concerns that these may be pro-arrhythmic in the post-infarction patient. Oral class III agents such as oral amiodarone may be preferable for this purpose. Sotalol has the benefit of combining beta blockade and class III activity, and for this reason it is being increasingly used for management of supraventricular arrhythmias following MI.[20]

Cardioversion shortly after the development of atrial fibrillation in myocardial infarction is of limited value, but when the ventricular rate has slowed and the patient has stabilized, reversion to sinus rhythm should be considered. The main factor encouraging a decision for predischarge reversion is to avoid the inconvenience of several weeks of oral anticoagulation.

Ventricular arrhythmias

Ventricular premature beats (VPBs)

Modern computer-based monitoring systems have shown that VPBs are universal following an acute myocardial infarction and their detection has no short- or long-term prognostic significance (see Fig. 55.3).

Their predictive value as harbingers of VF is less than previously thought and antiarrhythmic therapy to suppress VPBs is now far more selective than in previous decades of coronary care.[21] Recommendations for suppression of ventricular ectopic beats with intravenous antiarrhythmic drugs vary widely between CCUs. Detailed regimens based on the frequency, degree of prematurity, and presence or absence of repetitive beats have not been shown to be effective in preventing VF in controlled trials and are now less widely used than previously.[21,22] Prophylactic use of lignocaine in all cases of MI has no support from clinical trials.[23,24]

Although the authoritative ACC/AHA guidelines for early management of myocardial infarc-

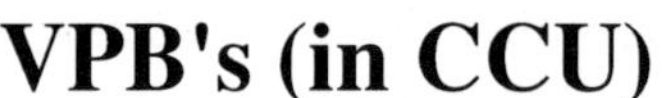

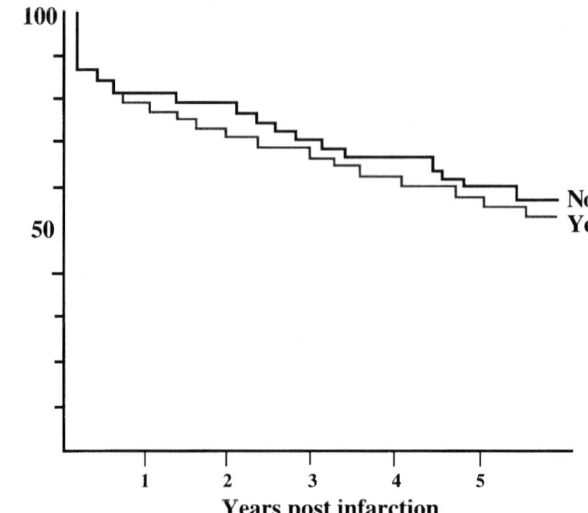

Fig. 55.3 Five year survival of patients with and without ventricular premature beats complicating AMI. 1000 patients treated in a CCU. Reproduced from Thompson PL. Prognosis of myocardial infarction with special reference to the role of infarct size. Perth: University of Western Australia, 1986.

tion still recommended intravenous antiarrhythmic therapy for frequent, R on T, multiform and repetitive VEBs as recently as 1990,[22] in most CCUs intravenous antiarrhythmic therapy is now reserved for prevention of recurrences of ventricular tachycardia, or attempting to prevent VF in patients with a crescendo pattern of frequent multi-focal salvos of ventricular tachycardia. The use of antiarrhythmic therapy in CCU patients declined from 60% to 33% in the Perth Monica project in the decade from 1984 (R Parsons, personal communication).

The most widely used IV antiarrhythmic drug remains lignocaine (lidocaine). Several loading dose regimens are in widespread use. Three commonly used loading regimens are:

- single bolus
  — bolus of 1mg/kg (50–100 mg)
- bolus/high dose infusion
  — bolus of 0.5 mg/kg (25–50 mg) followed by infusion of 100 mcg/kg/min (approximately 8 mg/min) for 20 minutes
- bolus/bolus
  — initial bolus dose of 1 mg/kg (50–100 mg) followed by bolus doses of 0.5 mg/kg (25–50 mg) every 10 minutes to a maximum of 4 mg/kg (approx 300 mg).

If the initial bolus dose is too high or given too rapidly, the patient can experience unpleasant neurologic side-effects of dizziness or confusion.

The loading dose is usually followed by an infusion of 25 mcg/kg/min (1–2 mg/min). Patients treated with a single initial bolus may experience subtherapeutic levels at 1–2 hours and therefore the bolus/high dose infusion or bolus/bolus regimens are preferable. Clearance is almost totally hepatic, and the maintenance (but not the loading doses) should be reduced in patients with persistent hypotension, or hepatic dysfunction, or in the elderly.

Toxic effects from lignocaine may be subtle, initially consisting of complaints of vagueness or dizziness, blurred vision, slurred speech or muscle twitching. It is important to cease lignocaine if these occur, to avoid major toxicity such as seizures.

If lignocaine is ineffective, IV amiodarone can be used in a loading dose of 3–5 mg/kg (approximately 300 mg) over 10 minutes followed by an infusion of 7 mg/kg (approximately 500 mg) over 24 hours.[19,25]

There is good clinical trial evidence that IV beta blockers can reduce the frequency of high grade ventricular arrhythmias,[7–8,26–27] and IV sotalol is being increasingly used for this purpose.[20] Correction of hypokalaemia[28,29] and hypomagnesaemia[30,31] are essential components of the management of ventricular arrhythmias in AMI.

Ventricular tachycardia

Short bursts of ventricular tachycardia from 3–10 beats are common in the first 24–36 hours after AMI. They have no prognostic significance and do not require any active therapy unless they are occurring frequently or causing symptoms or haemodynamic compromise.[32] If treatment is necessary, IV lignocaine, amiodarone or sotalol is usually effective and if the arrhythmia is rapidly controlled, maintenance therapy may not be necessary.

Rapid polymorphic ventricular tachycardia in the early stages of acute infarction can present a major diagnostic and management problem. In the patient with repetitive bursts of rapid polymorphic ventricular tachycardia and spontaneous reversion producing a torsades de pointes pattern of ventricular tachycardia, the possibility of proarrhythmia from antiarrhythmic therapy needs to be considered. This is especially likely to occur in the presence of hypokalaemia, hypomagnesaemia, phenothiazine, tricyclic antidepressant therapy, and combined erythromycin-antihistamine (terfenadine, astemizole) therapy. In these patients antiarrhythmic therapy, particularly class Ia or class III drugs, can perpetuate the arrhythmia and provoke uncontrollable repetitive bursts of torsades de pointes degenerating into ventricular fibrillation. Correction of the underlying abnormality, withdrawal of all antiarrhythmic drugs and sometimes rapid ventricular pacing will stabilize the arrhythmia.[3]

In contrast to the above scenario, polymorphic ventricular tachycardia (see Fig. 55.4) may be a direct result of MI and may respond well to antiarrhythmic therapy. If persistent, it can indicate severe ongoing myocardial ischaemia and may need aggressive anti-ischaemic treatment including intra-aortic balloon counterpulsation and revascularization. IV magnesium has been shown to be helpful in some cases.[31] Polymorphic ventricular tachycardia directly due to myocardial infarction is rarely associated with prolongation of the QT interval, in contrast to the situations which provoke torsades de pointes.[34]

Sustained monomorphic ventricular tachycardia usually occurs later after myocardial infarction, usually beginning on the third to tenth day post infarction. The management of this arrhythmia is dealt with in more detail in Chapter 63.

Accelerated idioventricular rhythm

Accelerated idioventricular rhythm (AIVR, 'slow ventricular tachycardia') is a frequent accompaniment of AMI.[35] It is often seen during coronary

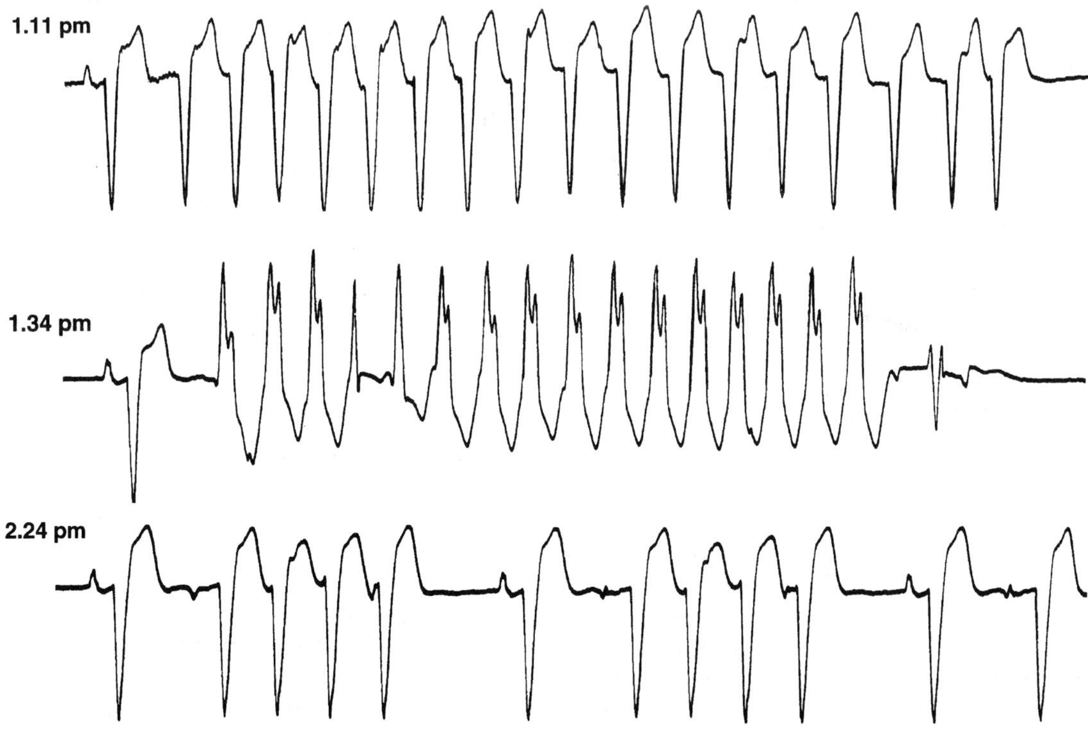

Fig. 55.4 Patient in the first 2 hours of AMI who had clinical and ECG features of polymorphic ventricular tachycardia without prolongation of the QT interval.

reperfusion following thrombolytic therapy.[36] In contrast to ventricular tachycardia in which the ventricular rate exceeds 100 per minute, there is competition between the sinus rate and accelerated ventricular rhythm. The accelerated ventricular rhythm may be sufficient to dominate the cardiac rhythm. If the ventricular rate is similar to the sinus rate there may be competition between the conducted and the idioventricular rhythm with fusion beats (see Fig. 55.5). AIVR does not degenerate into ventricular fibrillation. On occasions be associated with more rapid ventricular tachycardia[37] and does not usually require treatment. On occasions the sudden loss of atrial contribution to the cardiac output can cause symptomatic hypotension, and in this situation, it should be treated.

Treatment can be directed towards suppression of the ventricular ectopic focus with IV lignocaine or acceleration of the sinus rate with IV atropine. Atropine should be used sparingly and if repeated doses are required to prevent symptomatic hypotension, atrial pacing may be necessary. The rate of discharge of the ventricular focus usually settles gradually over 24 hours with spontaneous resolution of the arrhythmia.

Ventricular fibrillation

Prevention and early treatment of VF is one of the major aims of acute coronary care. The frequency of this arrhythmia has declined over the past 20 years, as noted by Antman et al, who demonstrated from the randomized trials of prevention of VF that the frequency in the 1970s was 5–10%, dropping through the 1980s to less than 2%.[38] The reasons for this include admission of lower risk patients to CCUs, wider use of beta blocking drugs and more effective treatment of ventricular dysfunction and electrolyte imbalances in the CCU.

The recognition that ventricular premature beats were unreliable warning arrhythmias for prediction of VF (see Fig. 55.6) led to a series of trials for prophylaxis of VF with non-selective use of IV lignocaine.

Results of individual trials with this approach were conflicting but meta-analysis of the clinical trials[23,24] has shown that prophylactic lignocaine can be effective in reducing the frequency of ventricular fibrillation (Fig. 55.7). Paradoxically, however, there was no improvement and a possible adverse effect on mortality. For this reason the use of IV lignocaine as prophylaxis against VF has been virtually abandoned.

Intravenous beta blockers have been shown to reduce mortality, particularly in high risk patients, with an apparent benefit in reduction of ventricular fibrillation[26,27] (see Ch. 28).

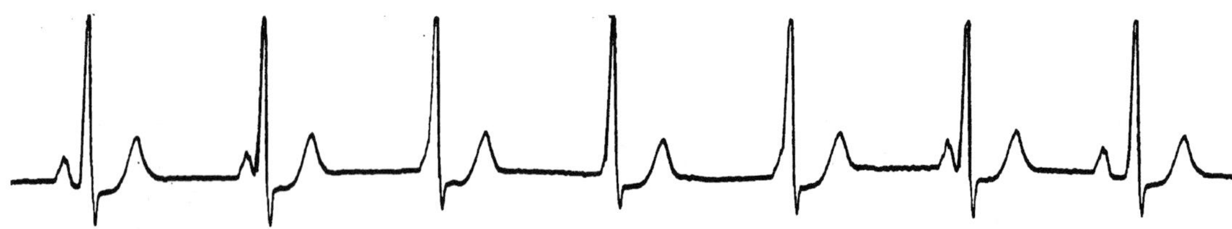

Fig. 55.5 Accelerated idioventricular rhythm (AIVR) occurring during right coronary artery reperfusion in acute inferior MI.

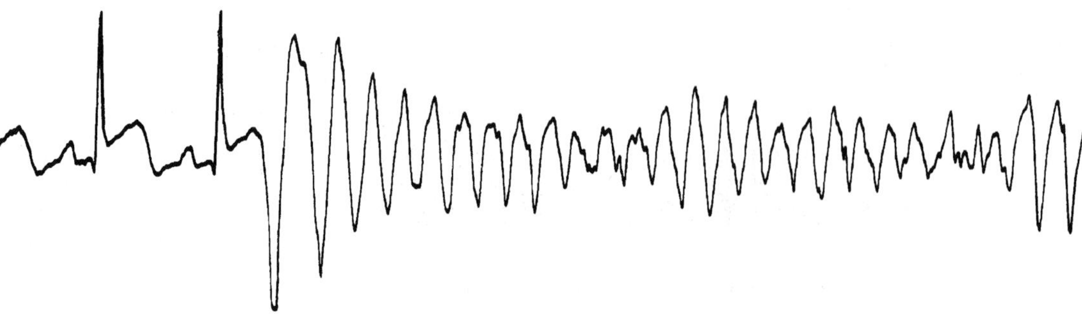

Fig. 55.6 Patient with acute inferior MI complicated by VF. Inpatient was on automated arrhythmia detection—there were no VPBs in the 15 minutes prior to the onset of VF.

Earlier and more widespread use of beta blockers in the CCU should be encouraged, particularly in high risk patients in the absence of contraindications.

Low serum potassium has been shown to indicate a higher risk of VF[28] (Fig. 55.8) especially in patients on diuretic therapy prior to their infarction.[29]

Correction of hypokalaemia with restoration of the serum potassium to above 4.5 mmol/L should be achievable in every patient. The use of IV magnesium may reduce the risk of VF. Clinical trials have demonstrated a benefit in selected patients, but widespread use in non-selected patients has been disappointing.[30]

If ventricular fibrillation occurs, the treatment is immediate defibrillation. In a well-conducted CCU, the delay between the onset of fibrillation and defibrillation should be no greater than 15–20 seconds.

The initial defibrillating shock should be 200 joules. This will usually restore sinus rhythm with rapid return of consciousness. If the initial shock is ineffective, 400 joules should be administered. If this is ineffective, cardiac pulmonary resuscitation (CPR) should be continued with intubation and oxygenation. Repeat shock of 400 joules should be administered. IV adrenaline followed by further defibrillation should be attempted. If this is ineffective a trial of anti-fibrillatory class III drugs such as amiodarone 300 mg[19,25] or bretylium tosylate[39,40] should be attempted, followed by a further shock of 400 joules.

Techniques of advanced life support are discussed in further detail in Chapter 42.

The prognosis of VF depends on the associated clinical state. Secondary VF occurring in the presence of haemodynamic compromise has a high hospital mortality of 80%.[41] Primary VF occurring in the absence of cardiogenic shock, severe heart failure or hypotension has a good short-term prognosis[42] although one major study showed a higher hospital mortality.[43] Following hospital discharge, there is no adverse effect on long-term survival.[44,45]

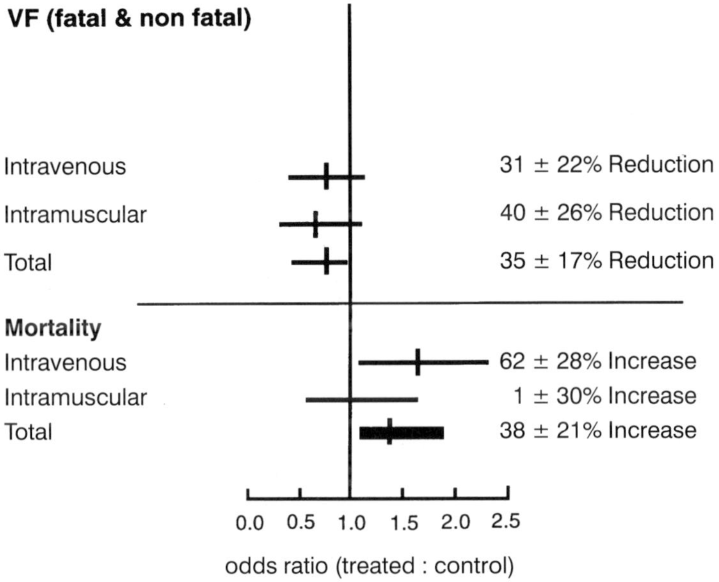

VF (fatal & non fatal)

Intravenous — 31 ± 22% Reduction
Intramuscular — 40 ± 26% Reduction
Total — 35 ± 17% Reduction

Mortality

Intravenous — 62 ± 28% Increase
Intramuscular — 1 ± 30% Increase
Total — 38 ± 21% Increase

0.0 0.5 1.0 1.5 2.0 2.5

odds ratio (treated : control)

Fig. 55.7 Meta-analysis of clinical trials of prophylactic lignocaine for prevention of VF. Adapted with permission from MacMahon S, Collins R, Peto R et al 1988.[23]

Hypokalaemia and Ventricular Fibrillation in Acute Myocardial Infarction

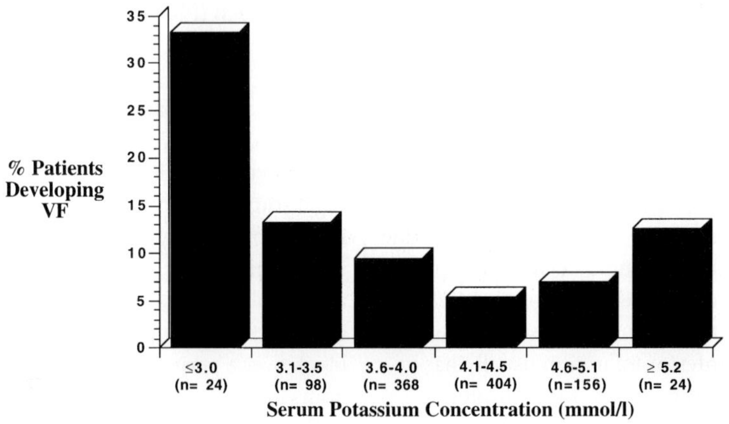

Fig. 55.8 Influence of serum potassium level on risk of developing ventricular fibrillation. Adapted with permission from Nordrehaug JE, Lippe GVD 1983.[28]

Conduction disturbances

Hemiblocks

Left anterior hemiblock may develop during MI, particularly with septal involvement in anterior MI. Apart from its association with extensive anteroseptal infarction, it is usually of no independent prognostic significance and does not require any treatment unless associated with a right bundle branch block indicating a bifascicular block and risk of high grade atrioventricular block.[46] Left posterior hemiblock occurs rarely during MI, and indicates posterior septal involvement.

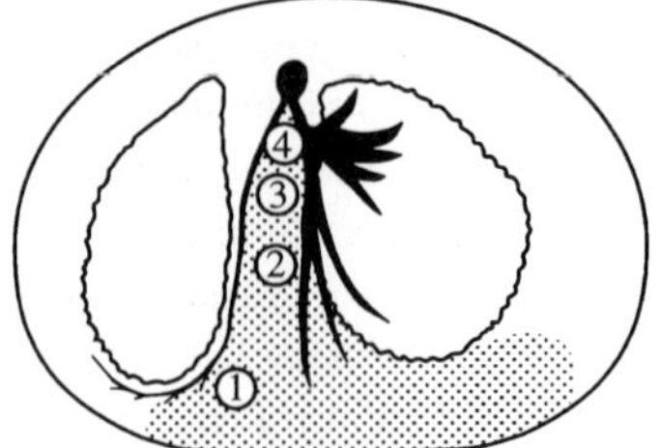

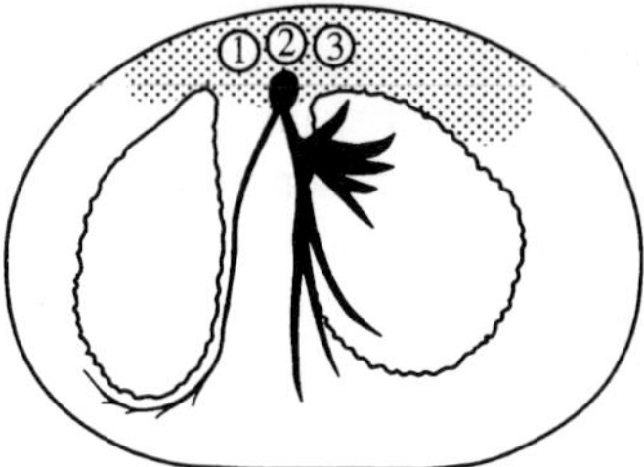

Fig. 55.9 A. Mechanism of 1° AV block, Wenckebach and complete AV block in infero-posterior MI. B. Development of progressive right bundle branch block, left anterior hemiblock Mobitz II and complete AV block in septal involvement in anteroseptal MI.

Bundle branch blocks

The development of a bundle branch block during an acute infarction is usually an indication of extensive septal involvement during anterior MI[47,48] (see Fig. 55.9A,B).

Bundle branch block is usually associated with extensive myocardial necrosis, significant left ventricular dysfunction and a poor prognosis. Right bundle branch block (RBBB) may occur with less extensive myocardial necrosis and septal involvement. It can be transient and self-limiting. It is frequently rate-dependent and becomes of particular significance when associated with left anterior hemiblock. RBBB may indicate increased risk of development of complete atrioventricular block, particularly if there are other indicators of delayed conductions such as a prolonged PR interval.[49] The combination of right bundle branch block, left axis deviation and prolonged PR interval is an indication for temporary pacing,[50] or standby external pacing.[51] There is ongoing controversy about the need for prophylactic permanent pacing in this situation.[52] There is no doubt that pacing is indicated if complete atrioventricular block should develop, but it remains uncertain whether this will improve the long-term prognosis, which is primarily determined by the degree of left ventricular dysfunction following the extensive infarction.

Atrioventricular blocks

First degree AV block may develop during infarction as a result of atrioventricular node involvement in inferior MI or due to His bundle delay with septal involvement in anterior MI. First degree AV block associated with inferior infarction usually has a benign prognosis, although it often progresses to self-terminating Wenckebach and complete atrioventricular block.[53,54] First degree AV block in anterior MI may be the final stage of extensive involvement of the conduction system in septal infarction.

In both types of first degree AV block, no active treatment is required, but drugs such as digoxin, verapamil and beta blockers which can prolong AV conduction should be avoided.

Second degree atrioventricular block

Wenckebach (Mobitz type I) block

Wenckebach block is usually the result of delayed AV node conduction due to AV node ischaemia or vagal stimulation of the AV node in inferior post myocardial infarction (see Fig. 55.9A). It is usually of gradual onset, progressing from first degree AV block over a period of several hours and often progressing to complete AV block, but reverting to normal conduction via a further period of Wenckebach block.[46,47] This gradual sequence may be accelerated following reperfusion of the right coronary artery with thrombolytic therapy as a result of activation of the Bezold–Jarisch reflex.[5] It is usually associated with a narrow QRS complex, a heart rate which is usually sufficient to maintain cardiac output and almost invariably a benign self-limiting course, although on occasions it can last for several days.

Wenckebach block can rarely occur as a result of delayed conduction through the intraventricular conduction system in anterior MI. In this situation it is often associated with a bundle branch block, as a result of septal infarction, and has a less benign course.

Mobitz type II—atrioventricular block

Mobitz type II block results from involvement of the septal infranodal conduction system in anterior MI (see Fig. 55.9B). The gradual prolongation of the PR interval is not seen and if third degree block develops, it often does so unpredictably with the development of a slow ventricular escape rhythm and sudden deterioration in haemodynamic status.[53]

Mobitz type II block can be associated with a narrow or wide QRS complex. Patients developing Mobitz type II block with anterior infarction and bundle branch block have a poor prognosis.[54]

Although controlled trials are not available to guide therapy, patients with Mobitz type II block are usually treated with temporary transvenous pacing or external pacing on standby.[50,51]

Third degree (complete) atrioventricular block

The pathophysiology, natural history and prognosis of complete AV block in acute myocardial infarction differs between anterior and inferior myocardial infarctions (Table 55.1).

In anterior infarction the pathophysiology is septal necrosis with progressive involvement of the right bundle or anterior superior division of the left bundle (Fig. 55.9B). There is usually extensive associated myocardial necrosis and left ventricular dysfunction. It can be of sudden onset following a period of Mobitz type II block, often with dramatic haemodynamic deterioration. Patients manifesting risk factors of 1° AV block, Mobitz II 2° block and bifascicular block are at high risk of complete AV block and should be treated with temporary transvenous or external pacing. A permanent pacemaker is usually implanted following this sequence of events.[52] To date there is no conclusive proof of benefit from this strategy, although clinical trials to answer this question are currently underway.

Complete AV block complicating inferior MI is the result of ischaemia or necrosis of the atrioventricular node, often with associated vagal activation. The development is slow, via a period of Wenckebach block. The ventricular rate is usually well-maintained and temporary pacing is not indicated unless there is marked bradycardia and haemodynamic compromise. This sometimes responds to atropine; if it does not, temporary pacing is indicated. Permanent pacing is rarely indicated, although on occasions the complete AV block with a slow ventricular rate is persistent and permanent pacing is necessary.[52] Although complete AV block in inferior MI has a high early mortality, patients who survive to leave hospital have a good long-term prognosis.[55]

Table 55.1 Third degree atrioventricular block complicating anterior and inferior myocardial infarction

	Anterior	Inferior
Pathophysiology	Extensive septal necrosis with damage to right and left bundle branches	Localized ischaemia or necrosis of the atrioventricular node ± vagotonia
Rapidity of onset	Sudden, following Mobitz II block	Gradual, following Wenckebach block
QRS	Wide	Narrow
Haemodynamic deterioration	Often dramatic	Normally minor
Prognosis	Poor	Excellent
Response to atropine	Poor	Good
Pacemaker	Urgent temporary, followed by permanent	Usually not necessary

References

1. Adgey AAJ, Geddes JS, Webb SW et al. Acute phase of myocardial infarction. Lancet 1971; 2: 501–4
2. Rotman M, Wagner GS, Wallace AG. Bradyarrythmias in acute myocardial infarction. Circulation 1972; 45: 703–18
3. Massumi RA, Mason DT, Amsterdam EA et al. Ventricular fibrillation and tachycardia after intravenous atropine for the treatment of bradycardia. N Engl J Med 1972; 287: 336–8
4. Cooper MJ, Abinader EG. Atropine induced ventricular fibrillation: case report and review of the literature. Am Heart J 1979; 97: 225–7
5. Koren G, Weiss AT, Ben-David Y, Hasin Y, Luria MH, Gotsman MS. Bradycardia and hypotension following reperfusion with streptokinase (Bezold–Jarisch reflex): a sign of coronary thrombolysis and myocardial salvage. Am Heart J 1986; 112: 468–71
6. Hjalmarson A, Gilpin E, Kjekshus J et al. Influence of heart rate on mortality after myocardial infarction. Am J Cardiol 1990; 65: 547–53
7. The MIAMI Trial Research Group—Metoprolol in acute myocardial infarction. A randomized placebo-controlled international trial. Eur Heart J 1985; 6: 199–266
8. ISIS-1 (First International Study of Infarct Survival) Collaborative Group. A randomised trial of intravenous atenolol among 16 027 cases of suspected myocardial infarction. Lancet 1986; 2: 57–66
9. Kirshenbaum JM, Klonn RA, Antman EM, Braunwald E. Use of an ultra-short acting beta blocker in patients with acute myocardial ischaemia. Circulation 1985; 72: 873–80
10. Hunt D, Sloman JG, Penington C. Effects of atrial fibrillation on prognosis of acute myocardial infarction. Br Heart J 1978; 40: 303–7
11. Thompson PL. Prognosis of myocardial infarction with special reference to the role of infarct size. Perth: University of Western Australia, 1986. Thesis
12. Goldberg RJ, Seely D, Becker RC et al. Impact of atrial fibrillation on the in-hospital and long-term survival of patients with acute myocardial infarction: a community-wide perspective. Am Heart J 1990; 119: 996–1001
13. Liberthson RR, Salisbury KW, Hutter AM, De Sanctis RW. Atrial tachyarrhythmias in acute myocardial infarction. Am J Med 1976; 60: 956–60
14. Hod H, Lew AS, Keltai M et al. Early atrial fibrillation during evolving myocardial infarction: a consequence of impaired left atrial perfusion. Circulation 1987; 75: 146–50
15. Marcus FI. Use of digitalis in acute myocardial infarction. Circulation 1980; 62: 17–9
16. Lemberg L, Castellanos A, Arcebal AG. The use of propranolol in arrhythmias complicating acute myocardial infarction. Am Heart J 1970; 80: 479–87
17. Hagermeijer F. Verapamil in the management of supraventricular arrhythmias occurring after a recent myocardial infarction. Circulation 1978; 57: 751–5
18. Krikler DM, McKenna WJ, Chamberlain D (eds). Amiodarone and arrhythmias. Oxford: Pergamon Press, 1983
19. Mason JW. Amiodarone. N Engl J Med 1987; 316: 455–65
20. Singh BN, Deedwania P, Nademanel K et al. Sotalol. A review of its pharmacodynamic and pharmacokinetic properties and therapeutic use. Drugs 1987; 34: 311–49
21. Lown B, Vassaux C. Lidocaine in acute myocardial infarction. Am Heart J 1968; 76: 586–7
22. Gunnar RM, Bourdillon PDV, Dixon DW et al. ACC/AHA guidelines for the early management of patients with acute myocardial infarction. Circulation 1990; 82: 664–707
23. MacMahon S, Collins R, Peto R et al. Effects of prophylactic lignocaine in suspected acute myocardial infarction. An overview of results from the randomized, controlled trials. JAMA 1988; 260: 1910–6. Copyright 1988, American Medical Association
24. Da Silva RA, Hennekens CH, Lown B, Cascells W. Lignocaine prophylaxis in acute myocardial infarction: an evaluation of the randomised trials. Lancet 1981; 2: 855–8
25. Mooss AN, Mohiuddin SM, Hee TT et al. Efficacy and tolerance of high dose intravenous amiodarone for recurrent refractory ventricular tachycardia. Am J Cardiol 1990; 65: 609–14
26. The MIAMI trial research group. Arrhythmias. Am J Cardiol 1985; 56: 35G–8G
27. Norris RM, Barnaby PF, Brown MA et al. Prevention of ventricular fibrillation during acute myocardial infarction with intravenous propranolol. Lancet 1984; 2: 883–6
28. Nordrehaug JE, Lippe GVD. Hypokalaemia and ventricular fibrillation in acute myocardial infarction. Br Heart J 1983; 50: 525–9
29. Stewart DE, Ikram H, Espiner EA, Nicholls MG. Arrhythmogenic potential of diuretic induced hypokalaemia in patients with mild hypertension and ischaemic heart disease. Br Heart J 1985; 54: 290–7
30. ISIS Collaboration Group. ISIS-4: a randomized factorial trial assessing oral captopril, oral mononitrate and intravenous magnesium sulphate in 58 080 patients with suspected acute myocardial infarction. Lancet 1995; 345: 669–85

31. Keren A, Tzivoni D. Magnesium therapy in ventricular arrhythmias. PACE 1990; 13: 937–45
32. Campbell RWF. Treatment and prophylaxis of ventricular arrhythmias in acute myocardial infarction. Am J Cardiol 1983; 52: 55C–9C
33. Keren A, Tzivoni D, Gavish D et al. Etiology, warning signs and therapy of torsades de pointes. Circulation 1981; 64: 1167–73
34. Tzivoni D, Keren A, Stern S. Torsades de pointes versus polymorphous ventricular tachycardia. Am J Cardiol 1983; 52: 639–40
35. Lichstein E, Ribas-Meneclier C, Gupta PK, Chadda AD. Incidence and descriptions of accelerated idioventricular rhythm complicating acute myocardial infarction. Am J Med 1975; 58: 192–8
36. Miller FC, Kruchoff MW, Satler LF et al. Ventricular arrhythmias during reperfusion. Am Heart J 1986; 112: 928–31
37. De Soyza N, Bisset JK, Kane JJ, Murphy ML, Doherty JE. Association of accelerated idioventricular rhythm and paroxysmal ventricular tachycardia in acute myocardial infarction. Am J Cardiol 1974; 34: 667–70
38. Antman EM, Berlin JA. Declining incidence of ventricular fibrillation in myocardial infarction. Implications for the prophylactic use of lidocaine. Circulation 1992; 86(3): 764–73
39. Chatterjee K, Mandel WJ, Vyden JK, Parmley WW, Forrester JS. Cardiovascular effects of bretylium tosylate in acute myocardial infarction. JAMA 1973; 223: 757–61
40. Koch-Weser J. Medical intelligence. Drug therapy. Bretylium. N Engl J Med 1979; 300: 473–7
41. Bigger JT, Dresdale RJ, Heissenbutter RH, Weld FM, Wit AL. Ventricular arrhythmias in ischemic heart disease: mechanism, prevalence, significance and management. Prog Cardiovasc Dis 1977; 19: 255–300
42. Tofler GH, Stone PH, Muller JE et al and the MILIS study group. Prognosis after cardiac arrest due to ventricular tachycardia or ventricular fibrillation associated with acute myocardial infarction. Am J Cardiol 1987; 60: 755–61
43. Volpi A, Maggioni A, Franzosi MG, Pampallona S, Mauri F, Tognoni G. In-hospital prognosis of patients with acute myocardial infarction complicated by primary ventricular fibrillation. N Engl J Med 1987; 317: 257–61
44. Nicod P, Gilpin E, Dittrich H et al. Late clinical outcome in patients with early ventricular fibrillation after myocardial infarction. J Am Coll Cardiol 1988; 11: 464–70
45. Volpi A, Cavalli A, Franzosi MG et al and the GISSI Investigators. One-year prognosis of primary ventricular fibrillation complicating acute myocardial infarction. Am J Cardiol 1989; 63: 1174–8
46. Scheinman MM, Gonzalez RP. Fascicular block and acute myocardial infarction. JAMA 1980; 244: 2646–9
47. Hindman MC, Wagner GS, Jaro M et al. The clinical significance of bundle branch block complicating acute myocardial infarction: clinical characterized hospital mortality and one year follow up. Circulation 1978; 58: 679–88
48. Mullins CB, Atkins JM. Prognoses and management of ventricular conduction blocks in acute myocardial infarction. Mod Concepts Cardiovasc Dis 1976; 45(10): 129–133
49. Lamas GA, Muller JE, Turi ZG et al and the MILIS study group. A simplified method to predict occurrence of complete heart block during acute myocardial infarction. Am J Cardiol 1986; 57: 1213–9
50. Hindman MC, Wagner GS, Jaro M et al. The clinical significance of bundle branch block complicating acute myocardial infarction: indications for temporary and permanent pacemaker insertion. Circulation 1978; 58: 689–99
51. Zoll PM, Zoll RH, Falk RH, Clinton JE, Eitel DR, Antman EM. External non-invasive temporary cardiac pacing: clinical trials. Circulation 1985; 71: 937–44
52. Guidelines for implantation of cardiac pacemakers and antiarrhythmia devices. A report of the ACC/AHA Task Force on assessment of diagnostic and therapeutic cardiovascular procedures (Committee on Pacemaker Implantation). JACC 1991; 18: 1–13
53. Brown RW, Hunt D, Sloman JG. The natural history of atrioventricular conduction defects in acute myocardial infarction. Am Heart J 1969; 78: 460–6
54. Rotman M, Wagner GS, Wallace AG. Bradyarrhythmias in acute myocardial infarction. Circulation 1972; 45: 703–22
55. Nicod P, Gilpin E, Dittrich H, Polikar R, Henning H, Ross J Jr. Long-term outcome in patients with inferior myocardial infarction and complete atrioventricular block. JACC 1988; 12: 589–94

56 AMI: Cardiac failure and pulmonary oedema

Peter L Thompson

The development of a mild degree of left ventricular (LV) failure following acute myocardial infarction (AMI) is very common. There is a close correlation (Fig. 56.1) between the degree of left ventricular failure and the prognosis.

This relationship has been recognized from the earliest days of treatment of MI[1] but has been formalized in several classification systems.

The most widely used of these is the Killip Classification first published in 1967.[2] It is based on simple clinical observations and is still widely used as a straightforward method of categorizing the extent of haemodynamic disturbance.[3] The Killip Classification is summarized in Table 56.1.

The Forrester Classification describes haemodynamic subsets based on pulmonary capillary wedge pressure and cardiac index.[4] It requires pulmonary artery pressure monitoring and for this reason has less wide application than the Killip Classification. The Forrester Classification is summarized in Table 56.2.

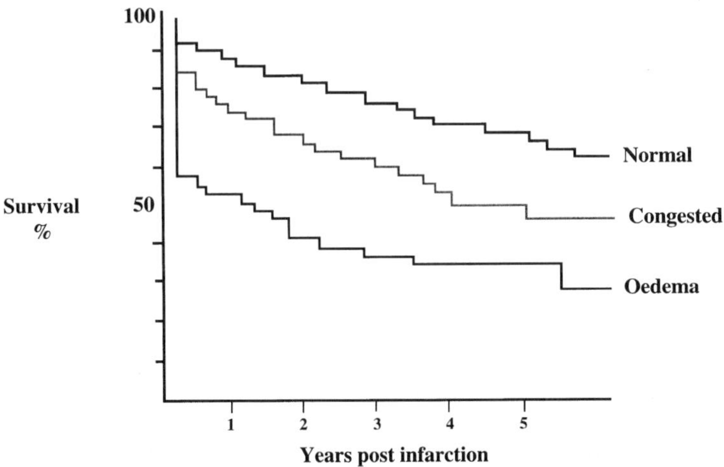

Fig. 56.1 Five year survival of patients without pulmonary congestion, with mild pulmonary congestion or with pulmonary oedema on the admission chest X-ray. 1000 patients admitted to a CCU. Adapted from Thompson PL Prognosis of myocardial infarction with special reference to the role of infarct size. Perth: University of Western Australia, 1986. Thesis.

In the modern CCU the degree of cardiac failure is still estimated with clinical assessment and a chest X-ray evaluation. The wider availability of echocardiography and continuous measurement of oxygen saturation allows rational decision making without the need for pulmonary artery pressure monitoring except in more advanced cases of pulmonary congestion and cardiac failure.

Terminology

The term 'pulmonary oedema' may refer to the full-blown clinical syndrome of acute pulmonary oedema or may be used to describe the disordered pathophysiology of increased lung volumes, interstitial oedema and alveolar oedema. For this reason the term 'pulmonary oedema' should be confined to the acute clinical syndrome and the term 'pulmonary congestion' should be used for lesser degrees of pulmonary oedema.

LV failure is the most common cause of pulmonary vascular congestion and pulmonary oedema, but it is important to recognize that there may be rare pulmonary vascular causes of pulmonary oedema and relatively common cardiac problems such as mitral valve disease where there is severe

Table 56.1 Killip classification of severity of infarction based on clinical assessment and its correlation with hospital mortality in 1967[2] and 30 day mortality in 1993[3]

		Case fatality Killip & Kimball (1967)	Gusto (1993)
Class 1	No failure	6%	5%
Class 2	Mild–moderate heart failure (S3, râles < 50% lung fields	17%	14%
Class 3	Severe heart failure (S3, râles >50% lung fields)	38%	32%
Class 4	Cardiogenic shock	81%	58%

Table 56.2 Forrester's haemodynamic subsets of myocardial infarction based on parameters measured via pulmonary artery pressure monitoring 4

	Cardiac index	Pulmonary capillary wedge pressure	Mortality (%)
1. No pulmonary congestion or peripheral hypoperfusion	2.7±0.5	12±7	2.2
2. Isolated pulmonary congestion	2.3±0.4	23±5	10.1
3. Isolated peripheral hypoperfusion	1.9±0.4	12±5	22.4
4. Both pulmonary congestion and hypoperfusion	1.6±0.6	27±8	55.5

pulmonary congestion without LV dysfunction. For this reason the preferable terminology is 'left heart failure' rather than 'left ventricular failure'.

In view of the difficulties in distinguishing the disordered pathophysiology of left heart failure and cardiogenic shock, many authorities consider the two conditions together under the heading of 'pump failure'. However, in most clinical situations the two conditions are separable in their disordered pathophysiology and management.

Discrepancies between assessments of cardiac failure and left ventricular dysfunction

Although in general there is an approximate correlation between clinical findings of left heart failure and objective assessment of LV dysfunction, there are frequently discrepancies between the clinical, radiographic and laboratory assessments. Reasons for this include:

1. Misinterpretation of clinical signs. Basal râles may be interpreted as evidence of pulmonary congestion and alveolar oedema but may be due to other causes such as dependency, small airway disease especially in smokers, concurrent infection or pulmonary fibrosis. Persistence of basal crackles after deep inspiration and coughing tends to favour alveolar oedema and pulmonary congestion as the cause but this is not totally reliable.
2. Variable rates of development and clearance of pulmonary congestion. On occasions basal crackles may be cleared following intravenous (IV) diuretic therapy but interstitial pulmonary oedema will remain and be detectable on chest X-ray and gas exchange parameters.[5] Occasionally, even without diuretic therapy, the lung fields may be clear to auscultation but still show clear-cut evidence of interstitial pulmonary oedema or signs of pulmonary congestion.
3. Misinterpretation of indices of ventricular dysfunction. Use of ejection fraction as the sole index of ventricular function can lead to apparent discrepancies, for the following reasons:
   - Hyperkinesis in the non-infarct zone may compensate for hypo- or akinesis in the infarct zone resulting in an apparently 'normal' global ejection fraction.[5]
   - Overemphasis on an index of systolic function may underestimate the importance of diastolic dysfunction; reduced ventricular compliance due to myocardial ischaemia or

pre-existing LV hypertrophy are important causes of diastolic dysfunction in acute myocardial infarction or ischaemia.

- There may be underestimation of the importance of infarct expansion and increased ventricular volumes in reducing cardiac efficiency, increasing wall tension and increasing myocardial oxygen consumption.
- The importance of loading conditions on the left ventricle as critical influences on ejection fraction measurement may not be appreciated.

For these reasons estimation of ejection fraction alone, either with radionuclide, echocardiographic or ventriculographic assessment, is an unreliable index of contractile function of the left ventricle. Better correlations with clinical severity and prognosis are obtained if the extent and localization of regional wall motion abnormality, as well as ventricular volumes, are evaluated.

4. Failure to recognize the evanescent nature of ventricular dysfunction in myocardial infarction/ischaemia. Catastrophic decompensation can result from transient LV dysfunction due to severe widespread myocardial ischaemia or from regional ischaemia and papillary muscle dysfunction resulting in disordered mitral valve function. On occasions, the therapy used for treatment of the pulmonary oedema (diuretics, nitrates) may also benefit the myocardial ischaemia. Assessments of LV function after recovery from the acute episode, may reveal only minimal abnormalities. For this reason a detailed assessment of the patient during an episode of LV failure can provide valuable diagnostic and management clues by detection of transient gallop rhythm or apical systolic bruit.
5. Iatrogenic fluid overload. Regrettably, on occasions miscalculations of the patient's fluid requirements can produce pulmonary congestion or pulmonary oedema during infusion of crystalloids, colloids or blood products even when there is only mild LV dysfunction. Therapeutic misadventure of this type usually becomes obvious on careful review of fluid administration orders over the previous 24 hours.

Diagnosis and assessment of left heart failure

The diagnosis of left heart failure is based on clinical assessment, chest X-ray and preferably evidence of impaired gas exchange and objective measure of LV dysfunction with echocardiography and occasionally pulmonary artery pressure monitoring. Clinical assessment should include an assessment of the severity of dyspnoea and measurement of respiratory rate, preferably including trends in respiratory rate and the pattern of breathing. A gradual increase in respiratory rate is often a valuable index of progressive pulmonary congestion. General observations including an appearance of apprehension, a desire to sit upright and possible use of accessory muscles are valuable clues. Detection of a third heart sound and basal crackles (râles) are the classic features of left heart failure but not necessarily present in milder cases. It is important to note the extent of basal crackles after deep inspiration and coughing to avoid over-diagnosing pulmonary congestion. Crackles which are asymmetrically distributed, fail to persist after coughing and are associated with known respiratory disease or smoking, are usually not indices of pulmonary congestion. The severity of pulmonary congestion can be graded by whether crackles are heard only below or below and above the mid-scapular level.

A chest X-ray should be carefully evaluated, looking for signs of upper lobe re-distribution and interstitial pulmonary oedema (see Ch. 15). The chest X-ray is also useful in excluding alternative causes of bilateral basal crackles due to lung disease.

Although arterial puncture and blood gas analysis usually is not necessary to document hypoxaemia due to pulmonary congestion, the detection of arterial desaturation on room air, using finger stall monitoring of oxygen saturation, is a useful adjunct to the assessment of the patient with suspected LV failure.

Patients with more obvious degrees of pulmonary congestion will have obvious clinical signs of respiratory distress, tachypnoea, cyanosis, gallop rhythm and widespread crackles.

Echocardiography has been a valuable adjunct to the assessment of left heart failure in the CCU (see Ch. 16). The detection of regional wall motion abnormality and overall systolic function as well as mitral valve function is extremely valuable information in planning the management of the patient with AMI. Insertion of a pulmonary artery catheter allows indirect measurement of LV pressure via pulmonary capillary wedge pressure; concurrent measurement of cardiac index can allow accurate physiologic assessment and categorization to a haemodynamic subset.[4]

The patient with acute pulmonary oedema has the typical syndrome of respiratory distress, pallor and cyanosis, profuse sweating, coughing, copious pink or frothy sputum, gallop rhythm and widespread crackles throughout all lung fields. Assessment of gas exchange may be helpful to assess the severity of the attack but should not delay treatment. Echocardiography and pulmonary artery pressure monitoring are usually not appropriate in this situation, but may be helpful when the acute crisis has passed.

Right heart failure

Surprisingly, clinical evidence of right heart failure complicating acute left heart failure and AMI is relatively uncommon. This is despite the knowledge derived from pulmonary artery pressure monitoring, that elevated end diastolic pressure is commonly elevated and transmitted readily through the left atrium via the pulmonary vasculature to the pulmonary artery. Presumably, pulmonary vascular and right heart compliance and insufficient time to develop the neurohumoral compensations of cardiac failure (see Ch. 10) prevent increased right heart pressures from developing. However, on occasions, elevation of the venous pressure and pulmonary congestion may be seen, particularly if left heart failure is prolonged or insufficiently treated. Usually right heart failure in myocardial infarction is a result of right ventricular infarction and requires specialized treatment. It is important to distinguish elevated right heart pressures secondary to left heart failure, which responds to vigorous diuretic therapy, and primary elevation of right heart pressures due to right ventricular infarction, which may respond adversely to diuretic therapy (see Ch. 59). Echocardiography or pulmonary artery pressure monitoring are sometimes necessary to make this distinction.

Management

Mild left heart failure

Although a mild degree of pulmonary congestion is common in AMI, it is not universal and diuretic therapy is not universally recommended. There is even controversy about the need for continuous intranasal oxygen (see Ch. 25) but most CCUs recommend intranasal or face-mask oxygen as a routine. Similarly, semi-recumbent posture and no added salt diet are standard routines directed towards prevention and management of left heart failure.

Low dose IV or oral diuretics

Evidence of pulmonary vascular congestion on clinical examination or chest X-ray is usually regarded as an indication for low dose diuretic therapy in the form of frusemide 20–40 mg intravenously or 40 mg orally. The response is monitored by measurement of urinary output, disappearance of basal crackles and improvement in chest X-ray appearances and if available, improvement in oxygen saturation levels on continuous oxygen saturation monitoring.

ACE inhibitors as an alternative to diuretics

With increasing experience of the use of ACE (angiotensin-converting enzyme) inhibitors in the early stages of myocardial infarction, a case can be made for avoiding IV diuretics in this situation and proceeding straight to an ACE inhibitor. Treatment may be initiated with a low-dose, rapidly cleared agent such as captopril 6.25 mg 8-hourly with careful monitoring of blood pressure response. Experience with the ACE inhibitor clinical trials post infarction (see Ch. 33) has suggested that this approach may be unnecessarily cautious when there is a low risk of hypotension. Treatment has been initiated in the clinical trials with longer acting agents; within the first 24 hours, in the GISSI study using lisinopril[8] and with intravenous enalaprilat, and oral enalapril within the first 24 hours in the CONSENSUS-2 study[9]. In patients with cardiac failure using ramipril, treatment was initiated a few days after the onset of the infarction in the AIRE study.[10] However, when the blood pressure is low (systolic < 100 mmHg) or there is a risk of producing hypotension as in patients with previous diuretic therapy or hyponatraemia, treatment should be initiated cautiously, e.g. with captopril at a very low dose, such as 1 mg (paediatric suspension) and gradually increased.

Nitrates in mild left heart failure

Although the careful studies of Jugdutt and colleagues have shown clear cut benefits on Killip Class and indices of left heart failure with low dose IV nitroglycerin,[11] and meta-analysis of small trials with nitroglycerin showed benefits on survival, there now seems little evidence to support the use of intravenous, oral or transcutaneous nitrates for mild heart failure in AMI, following the disappointing results from the recently completed large clinical trials which showed no effect on short- or long-term survival with the use of nitrates (see Ch. 30).

Digoxin

Digoxin has no place in the management of mild left heart failure in MI unless it is associated with rapid atrial fibrillation.

Special precautions

In patients with mild left heart failure complicating MI, special precautions include avoidance of unnecessary salt loading by minimizing salt intake in the diet, avoidance of excessive administration of saline infusions and minimizing the use of sodium-retaining medications such as non-steroidal anti-inflammatory drugs and oral steroids. Oral beta blocking drugs can be given to patients with mild cardiac failure; the benefits on stabilization of cardiac rhythm, limitation of cardiac size and improved survival outweigh any adverse effects on provocation of mild left heart failure. In contrast, calcium channel blockers appear to have adverse effects in post-infarction left heart failure, and should not be used. Most patients with mild left heart failure following infarction do not require long-term diuretic therapy and continuing degrees of left heart failure can usually be controlled with the use of ACE inhibitors.[10] If there is evidence of continuing pulmonary congestion, a small dose of oral frusemide or thiazide can be used for a short term but it is important to ensure that the need for these medications is reassessed after a few days' treatment to prevent longer-term metabolic disturbances and hypovolaemia.

Severe left heart failure

Patients with more severe degrees of left heart failure, manifest by widespread lung crackles, third heart sound, tachycardia, chest X-ray evidence of severe pulmonary congestion or interstitial pulmonary oedema, and evidence of reduced oxygen saturation require vigorous therapy.

Diuretics in severe heart failure

Treatment is usually initiated with IV frusemide in a dose of 40 mg. Response to frusemide is biphasic, with an initial improvement in pre-load due to its venodilating effect followed by a diuretic effect.[9] Response to treatment is monitored by the clinical response and if available, arterial oxygen saturations and urine output. The latter is best monitored by an indwelling urinary catheter with regular monitoring of urine flow. If there is no response to an initial dose of 40 mg of frusemide within 1 hour, a further dose of 80 mg can be administered. It is important to appreciate that frusemide will be ineffective if the renal blood flow is inadequate; if the left heart failure is associated with hypotension, no diuresis may be obtained. If the systolic blood pressure is persistently below 80 mmHg, elevation of the level above 100 mmHg with intravenous dopamine or dobutamine followed by a further dose of frusemide may initiate a satisfactory diuresis.

Many patients with severe cardiac failure following MI have had cardiac failure preceding their infarction and may have pre-infarction abnormalities due to diuretic therapy, such as hypokalaemia, hypomagnesaemia or hypovolaemia. Each of these will require careful attention and urgent correction before initiating aggressive diuretic therapy. Similarly, patients may have been on digitalis therapy and sudden electrolyte shifts with hypokalaemia following vigorous diuresis may unmask latent digitalis toxicity. Patients who have been on prior ACE inhibitors may be at risk of persisting hypotension or possibly at risk of renal dysfunction, particularly in elderly patients if there is the possibility of reduced renal blood flow. These patients require special attention to their electrolyte levels as well as to their serum creatinine.

ACE inhibitors in severe heart failure

Patients with severe post-infarction heart failure are most likely to benefit from ACE inhibitor therapy as demonstrated in the AIRE study,[10] and therefore treatment should be initiated as early as possible. However, there is a greater risk of provoking hypotension, and treatment should be initiated with low doses and with precautions for dealing with hypotension.

Can beta blockers be used in severe heart failure?

The intravenous beta blocker studies showed that patients with extensive infarction and evidence of cardiac failure have the most to benefit from beta blocker therapy.[12] This should also be administered as early as possible but with additional precautions using low dose therapy. Although the clinical trials have demonstrated that ACE inhibitors and beta blockers individually deliver survival benefits, the combination has not been studied in clinical trials and it is not known if the hypotensive effects of the combination will have a positive or negative benefit.

Intravenous nitrates

Intravenous nitrates are a valuable adjunct in stabilizing the patient with severe left heart failure. Nitroglycerin is now used more widely than nitroprusside for this purpose in AMI because its coronary vasodilating effect is more appropriate to the management of myocardial ischaemia.[11]

The patient with severe heart failure who does not respond rapidly to intravenous diuretic therapy should have a pulmonary artery catheter inserted to enable fluid requirements and drug therapy to be monitored closely.

Resistant left heart failure

The patient with severe left heart failure complicating MI who is resistant to the above measures for more than 24 hours has a poor prognosis. Resistance to therapy of left heart failure is a far more potent prognostic indicator than the severity of the initial cardiac failure.

Measurements for managing resistant left heart failure include:

- Increasing doses of frusemide up to 250 mg IV.
- The addition of an oral thiazide together with IV frusemide or substitution of an alternative IV diuretic such as ethacrynic acid or bumetamide.
- Use of inotropic agents may be helpful even in the absence of established cardiogenic shock using low dose dopamine for its dopaminergic renal effects, dobutamine for the combined inotropic and vasodilating effect, or milrinone.
- If dobutamine is ineffective, a combination of dopamine and nitroglycerin may be effective. Coronary revascularization should be seriously considered, but the decision to proceed with coronary angiography should be made as early as possible. The vicious circle of cardiac decompensation and resistance to high dose diuretics and inotropes increases the risk of the catheterization as well as reducing the likelihood of a successful result from revascularization.
- The possibility of temporarily stabilizing the left heart failure prior to cardiac catheterization by the insertion of an intra-aortic balloon pump.
- Ruling out a mechanical complication of the infarction such as septal rupture or mitral regurgitation as the cause of persistent left heart failure. An unexplained systolic murmur in a patient with persistent heart failure following infarction is an indication for urgent bedside echocardiographic and Doppler evaluation.

With aggressive therapy as outlined above, many patients with severe left heart failure following myocardial infarction can now be stabilized sufficiently to leave the CCU and be maintained on oral therapy. However, they face major post-coronary care problems including risk of renal dysfunction from the combined diuretic and ACE inhibitor therapy as well as high risk of ventricular arrhythmias and thrombotic complications, high rate of rehospitalization and high risk of death.

Acute pulmonary oedema

The full-blown syndrome (complicating AMI) of acute pulmonary oedema is a life-threatening emergency. However, frequently the prognosis seems to correlate better with the duration of the LV failure rather than the initial severity of the pulmonary oedema.

General measures

Patients will seek the most comfortable position for themselves. This will usually be sitting bolt upright, leaning forward, distressed and coughing. Oxygen should be administered by the route which is more comfortable for the patient, either by face mask or intranasal prongs. It is helpful for future management to document the extent of the pulmonary oedema and rule out other causes with a chest X-ray, but treatment should not be delayed whilst this is being obtained. Oxygen saturation monitoring should be initiated if possible. Arterial puncture with blood gas analysis is useful to document the degree of hypoxaemia, hypercarbia and acidosis. A venous sample should be obtained for urgent assessment of serum electrolytes. Pulmonary artery pressure monitoring and echocardiography provide useful information for assessment and subsequent management but the patient is usually too distressed to allow these procedures during the acute pulmonary oedema episode.

Morphine and frusemide

Initial treatment consists of intravenous morphine 2–5 mg and frusemide 40 mg. The mechanism of the action of morphine in acute pulmonary oedema has not been clearly established. It has been thought to act by venodilatation and reduction of pre-load, but direct study of its action has failed to confirm this and it is likely that the central relaxant effect is equally important.[14] The venodilating effect of frusemide often precedes the diuretic effect.[13] Therefore the response to frusemide is monitored by the patient's symptomatic response rather than a copious urine flow.

High dose diuretics

If there is no response after 15 minutes, a higher dose of frusemide is administered: 80 mg IV is given, followed by a further dose of 160–250 mg if necessary.

Vasodilators

Vasodilators may be attempted, starting with IV nitroglycerin 4–8 micrograms per minute. Because the administered dose may be variable according to the flow rate and may be limited by hypotension, nitrate treatment is initiated with sublingual nitroglycerin or nitroglycerin spray.

Reduced pre-load

Although phlebotomy of 500 ml has been used in the past, this is rarely necessary in current practice; however, rotating tourniquets may still be used with effect. Three of four limbs have a tourniquet applied with the cuff inflated above venous pressure, that is to 50–80 mmHg, and rotated each 5–10 minutes. Alternatively, rubber tourniquets fastened tightly can be utilized.

Assisted ventilation

In patients who fail to respond to these measures, assisted ventilation may be helpful and this can be administered as continuous positive airway pressure, or positive end expiratory pressure at 10 cm of water via an occlusive face mask,[15] or by intubation and assisted ventilation with muscle relaxation. Endotracheal intubation in acute pulmonary oedema is often compounded by the copious production of frothy sputum, and adequate suction may be necessary to keep the endotracheal tube patent.

Bronchodilators

Occasionally, cardiac pulmonary oedema can be associated with marked wheeze and bronchospasm which is best treated with administration of an inhaled bronchodilator such as salbutamol or terbutaline. Both agents are capable of producing cardiac arrhythmias and the minimum effective dose should be used. In the past, aminophylline has been recommended in this situation but unpredictable shunting and acute hypoxaemia may result. If aminophylline is used it should be done only with very careful administration and continuous monitoring of oxygen saturations.

Monitoring progress

Following stabilization after an episode of acute pulmonary oedema, urine flow should be monitored with an indwelling catheter. Depending on the patient's response and the underlying cause, monitoring of pulmonary artery pressure and wedge pressure may be helpful. Close monitoring and correction of electrolyte abnormalities is essential as sudden shifts in electrolytes can result from aggressive diuretic therapy.

References

1. Master AM, Dack S, Jaffe HL. Coronary thrombosis: an investigation of heart failure and other factors in its course and prognosis. Am Heart J 1936; 13: 330
2. Killip T, Kimball JT. Treatment of myocardial infarction in a coronary care unit; a two year experience with 250 patients. Am J Cardiol 1967; 20: 457–64
3. Lee KL, Woodlief LH, Topol EJ et al. Predictors of 30-day mortality in the era of reperfusion for acute myocardial infarction.

Results from an international trial of 41 021 patients. Circulation 1995; 91: 1659–68
4. Forrester JS, Diamond G, Chatterjee K, Swan HJC. Medical therapy of acute myocardial infarction by applications of haemodynamic subsets. N Engl J Med 1976: 295: 1356–62
5. Kostuk W, Barr JW, Simar AL, Ross J Jr. Correlations between the chest film and haemodynamics in acute myocardial infarction. Circulation 1973; 48: 629–32
6. Grines CL, Topol EJ, Califf RM et al and the TAMI study group. Prognostic implications and predicators of enhanced regional wall motions of non infarct zone after thrombolysis and angioplasty therapy of acute myocardial infarctions. Circulation 1989; 80: 245–53
7. White HD, Norris RM, Brown MA et al. Left ventricular end systolic volume as the major determinant of survival after recovery from myocardial infarction. Circulation 1987; 76: 44–51
8. GISSI-III. Effects of lisinopril and transdermal glyceryl trinitrate singly and together on 6 week mortality and ventricular function after myocardial infarction. Lancet 1993; 343: 1115–22
9. Swedberg K, Held P, Kjekshus J, Rasmussen K, Ryden L, Wedel H. Effects of the early administration of enalapril on mortality in patients with acute myocardial infarction. Results of the cooperative New Scandinavian Enalapril Survival Study II (Consensus II). N Engl J Med 327:678–84
10. The Acute Infarction Ramipril Efficacy (AIRE) study investigators. Effect of ramipril on mortality and morbidity in survivors of acute myocardial infarction with clinical evidence of cardiac failure. Lancet 1993;342:821–8
11. Jugdutt BI, Warnica JW. Intravenous nitroglycerine therapy to limit myocardial infarct size, expansion and complications: effect of timing, dosage and infarct location. Circulation 1988;78:907–19
12. Yusuf, S, Peto R, Lewis J, Collins R, Sleight P. Beta blockade during and after myocardial infarction. An overview of the randomised trials. Prog Cardiovasc Dis 1985;27:335–71
13. Dikshit K, Vyden JK, Forrester JS, Chatterjee K, Prakash R, Swan HJC. Renal and extra-renal haemodynamic effects of furosemide in congestive heart failure after acute myocardial infarction. N Engl J Med 1973;288:1087–90
14. Vismara LA, Leaman DM, Zelis R. The effects of morphine on venous tone in patients with acute pulmonary oedema. Circulation 1976;54:335–7
15. Raisanen J, Heikkila J, Downs J et al. Continuous positive airway pressure by face mask in acute cardiogenic pulmonary oedema. Am J Cardiol 1985;55:296–300

57 AMI: Cardiogenic shock

Mark E Hands

Definition

The condition of cardiogenic shock is characterized by significant persisting hypotension, despite adequate filling pressures, in association with abnormalities of peripheral circulation such as oliguria, impaired skin perfusion and altered sensorium. Haemodynamic findings include a systolic blood pressure less than 90 mmHg, a mean arterial pressure of less than 60–70 mmHg, a cardiac index less than 2 litres per minute[12] with a pulmonary capillary wedge pressure of greater than 18 mmHg. The condition may also be characterized by a need for vasopressors to maintain cardiac function above the aforementioned levels of arterial pressure and cardiac index.

Incidence

The overall incidence of cardiogenic shock complicating acute myocardial infarction (AMI) ranges from 5 to 15%.[1–6] There has been a suggestion that its incidence in recent years has declined, perhaps due to earlier hospitalization and the use of thrombolytic agents.[2] In the prethrombolytic era, 4.5% of patients with suspected myocardial infarction (MI) in the Multicenter Investigation of Limitation of Infarct Size (MILIS) Study[1] were in cardiogenic shock at the time of hospital admission. Of those randomized with definite infarction, 7.1% developed cardiogenic shock after hospitalization. In the thrombolytic trial GISSI-1,[3] 2.5% of patients were in cardiogenic shock on admission, while 6% subsequently developed cardiogenic shock during hospitalization.

Pathophysiology

Cardiogenic shock is usually secondary to AMI with associated significant left ventricular (LV) dysfunction. The latter may result from massive AMI, recent myocardial infarction superimposed on an old infarction, infarct extension, and/or ongoing myocardial ischaemia. Pathological studies have established that cardiogenic shock usually occurs when more than 40% of the left ventricle is damaged.[7,8] The condition occurs predominantly in those patients with extensive anterolateral MI, with nearly one half having three vessel coronary artery disease, and a third having had a prior infarction.[5] Occasionally, shock develops in patients with extensive inferior infarction involving the right ventricle.[9]

Cumulative damage to the left ventricle seems to be the most important factor in the development of cardiogenic shock, with previous myocardial infarction, acute infarct size and admission LV ejection fraction all being independent predictors.[1] Infarct extension undoubtedly contributes further to LV damage and dysfunction. Necropsy studies have confirmed the presence of infarct extension and re-infarction in a significant proportion of cases with cardiogenic shock,[7,8] while clinical studies have demonstrated enzymatic evidence of progressive myocardial necrosis in selected patients.[1,10] Among those developing cardiogenic shock after admission in the MILIS study, 23% had infarct extension by enzyme criteria.[1] This probably represents an underestimation, as patients whose infarct extension occurred within the first 48 hours of the initial event were excluded. In most cases, infarct extension or reinfarction was documented to have occurred before or at the time of cardiogenic shock.

In addition to damage to the LV myocardium, other possible contributing factors to the development of cardiogenic shock include ruptured interventricular septum, papillary muscle dysfunction or rupture, atrial and ventricular dysrhythmias, significant bradycardias including complete heart block, and pulmonary embolism.

Onset

Cardiogenic shock may evolve over hours or even days after the onset of symptoms of AMI. In the MILIS study,[1] more than half the patients who developed cardiogenic shock after admission did so more than 24 hours after hospitalization (see Fig. 57.1). This was the case for two-thirds of the SPRINT (Secondary Prevention Reinfarction Israeli Nifedipine Trial) registry patients developing cardiogenic shock after admission.[6] Notably, the SPRINT registry patients had no evidence of heart failure on admission. The delay in onset of cardiogenic shock presumably, in many cases, reflects the progressive nature of myocardial necrosis over time and the role of reinfarction in these patients.[1,8,10]

Treatment and prognosis

Cardiogenic shock remains the most common cause of in-hospital mortality following AMI. This mortality usually exceeds 80%.[4–6,11] Management of the patient with cardiogenic shock requires exclusion of possible extra-myocardial factors causing or contributing to hypotension and reduced cardiac output. These factors include hypovolaemia, sepsis, acidosis, hypoxaemia and arrhythmias. The administration of narcotics, vasodilators and negative inotropic drugs, such as beta blockers and certain calcium antagonists, needs to be excluded.

Two-dimensional echocardiography provides for rapid assessment of overall LV function, regional wall motion abnormalities and accompanying valve pathology, while enabling exclusion of mechanical lesions such as cardiac tamponade, ruptured ventricular septum or papillary muscle and pseudo-aneurysm formation. These complications are important to exclude, as they usually require immediate operative treatment. Haemodynamic monitoring with a Swan–Ganz catheter is appropriate to ensure adequate filling pressures, and haemodynamic stabilization is aided with vasopressors and frequently intra-aortic balloon pumping (IABP). In select cases, immediate angiography with a view to urgent revascularization is needed.

Inotropic agents

While inotropic agents such as dopamine and dobutamine usually improve the haemodynamics of patients with cardiogenic shock due to global impairment of left ventricular function, there is no convincing data that they improve survival. Low dose dopamine (3–5 micrograms/kg/min) may well enhance renal perfusion and preserve renal function. Higher doses may be needed to stabilize the patient and maintain coronary perfusion pending further interventions such as IABP and revascularization. However, a recent report suggests that high dose dobutamine prior to IABP insertion may adversely affect the survival of patients with cardiogenic shock.[12]

Systemic vascular resistance in patients with cardiogenic shock is usually elevated. However, vasodilators alone are usually contraindicated due to the signif-

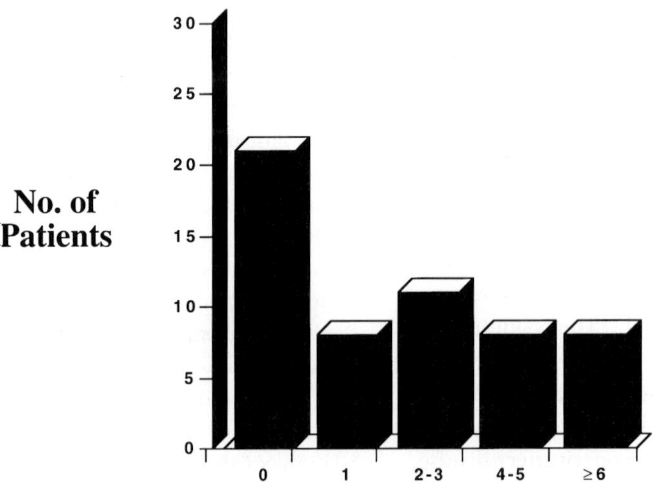

Fig. 57.1 Time from randomization into the MILIS Study to the onset of in-hospital cardiogenic shock. Adapted with permission from Hands ME, Rutherford JD, Muller JE et al 1989.[1]

icant hypotension present in these patients. In contrast, agents that have combined positive inotropic and peripheral vasodilating action, such as dobutamine and milrinone, may be well tolerated and assist in initial haemodynamic stabilization of the patient.[13] Alpha agents such as noradrenaline should only be used when adequate perfusion is unattainable by other means, including IABP.

Intra-aortic balloon counterpulsation

Intra-aortic balloon counterpulsation significantly augments cardiac output and diastolic coronary blood flow, providing a useful means of rapidly stabilizing and potentially relieving ischaemia in hypotensive patients with cardiogenic shock. However, survival rates among this group of patients where IABP is utilized vary considerably.[12,14,15] These differences probably reflect selection bias, timing of initiation of balloon pumping and the use of associated interventions such as thrombolysis and revascularization. Bengston et al[5] describe 99 out of 200 consecutive patients with cardiogenic shock who had intra-aortic balloon counterpulsation. In-hospital survival was 48% among those thus treated, and 50% among those not so treated ($P = 0.23$). Notably, the in-hospital mortality rate among the 56 patients treated with intra-aortic balloon counterpulsation and mechanical revascularization by percutaneous transluminal coronary angioplasty (PTCA) was 38%, versus 63% in the 43 patients treated with intra-aortic balloon counterpulsation alone ($P = 0.01$). Furthermore, results of a randomized trial by Ohman et al[16] indicate that aortic counterpulsation, after reperfusion is established by urgent PTCA, improves infarct-artery patency and reduces recurrent ischaemic events.

Thus, while there is no clear survival benefit conferred by IABP alone in patients with cardiogenic shock, it is important adjunct therapy in many patients, providing haemodynamic stabilization and reduced inotropic requirements and enabling more definitive revascularization procedures, such as PTCA, to be undertaken with improved patency rates and with less reocclusion. The contemporary practice of insertion of smaller sized catheters (8.5–10.5 French) with IABP has been associated with a reduced complication rate. However, major problems still occur in approximately 5% of patients, and these include local haemorrhage requiring arterial repair, septicaemia and limb ischaemia requiring surgery. Peripheral vascular disease and diabetes are significant predictors of limb ischaemia.

Thrombolytic therapy

While thrombolytic therapy has been demonstrated to limit infarct size, preserve LV function and improve survival in most patients treated early after AMI, many of the large randomized thrombolysis trials either excluded patients with cardiogenic shock or did not provide analysis of this sub-set. However, those studies examining the use of thrombolytic therapy in patients with established cardiogenic shock have all failed to show a clear survival benefit.[11,17,18] In the Society for Cardiac Angiographers Intracoronary Streptokinase Registry, 44 patients with cardiogenic shock were treated with thrombolytic therapy.[17] The overall in-hospital mortality remained high at 66%. In those with successful reperfusion, the mortality rate was 42%, while those in whom reperfusion was unsuccessful had a mortality rate of 84%. Notably, the overall infarct-related artery patency rate was only 44% in this group of patients. Others have reported similar low patency rates.[3,19] The reason for the lack of efficacy of thrombolytic agents in patients with established cardiogenic shock is not well defined, although a number of haemodynamic, mechanical and metabolic factors have been postulated.[20]

Revascularization

The poor outcome of cardiogenic shock with conventional therapy of haemodynamic monitoring and vasopressor agents with or without IABP has led to a number of small non-randomized, non-controlled trials of emergency coronary artery bypass surgery in select patients with this condition. The initial results were encouraging.[12,21–24]

However, the logistics of performing such surgery under these circumstances is, in many cases, prohibitive. In contrast, urgent balloon dilatation of the infarct-related artery is generally more feasible. There has been a recent reappraisal of immediate PTCA in acute infarction and, in particular, a number of small trials have examined the use of this procedure in patients with cardiogenic shock.[11] The overall results suggest a significant improvement of in-hospital and long-term survival for those patients receiving successful revascularization soon after the establishment of shock. However, the outcome remains poor for those patients in whom revascularization is unsuccessful, or is attempted late after the onset of cardiogenic shock.

Meta-analysis of 15 trials involving a total of 453 patients suggests an overall in-hospital or 30 day mortality of near 40%.[5,11,19,25–27] This rate was only 33% in those patients with successful reperfusion but over 80% in those with unsuccessful reperfusion (see Fig. 57.2). The latter is similar to the poor outcome of historical controls with cardiogenic shock.[1,4–6,12] The series by Gacioch et al[25] showed that the early benefits were maintained, with 48% of patients with a successful PTCA being alive at one year, whereas only 7% of patients with unsuccessful PTCA were alive at this stage. The timing of the PTCA is critical. Moosvi et al[27] found that successful revascularization within 24 hours of the onset of cardiogenic shock was associated with an in-hospital survival of 77%, compared with a low 10% survival when the procedure was performed successfully more than 24 hours after the diagnosis of shock ($P = 0.006$). Studies suggest that patients with single vessel disease have a better outcome than those with multi-vessel disease[19,25] while patients over 70 years of age tend to have a less favourable outcome with direct PTCA than their younger counterparts.[27]

The survival benefit of PTCA is presumably partly due to early interruption of the vicious cycle of progressive necrosis, reinfarction, compromised cardiac function and further ischaemia because of the reduced coronary perfusion found in cardiogenic shock patients. However, while the majority of patients in the studies underwent angioplasty within 4 hours of the onset of symptoms, improved survival was documented in patients undergoing angioplasty after this period.[19] Animal studies have demonstrated a beneficial effect of late reperfusion on limitation of infarct expansion and aneurysm formation, independent of myocardial salvage.[28] In addition, reperfusion may improve the rate and extent of infarct healing.

The role of urgent angioplasty in patients with cardiogenic shock continues to evolve. Studies have been limited by selection bias, non-randomization, retrospective analysis, and control groups being those with unsuccessful PTCA. Given the critical nature of cardiogenic shock, a randomized controlled clinical trial is difficult but is currently being attempted (Shock trial). Presently, urgent PTCA of the infarct-related artery, in combination with IABP, should be strongly considered in select patients with established cardiogenic shock. This may particularly be the case in younger patients who manifest the cardiogenic shock syndrome early in the course of their first infarction. The role of urgent bypass surgery in patients with cardiogenic shock, either as a primary procedure or in those with failed angioplasty, is less clear and needs to be dictated by the individual clinical circumstances.

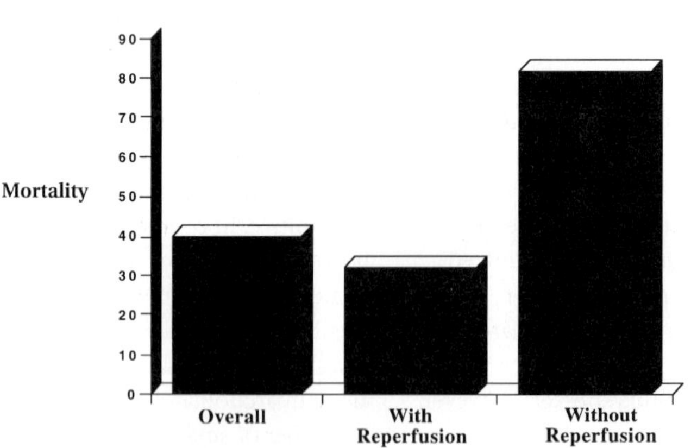

Fig. 57.2 Results of meta-analysis of trials of percutaneous transluminal coronary angioplasty (PTCA) in cardiogenic shock, complicating acute myocardial infarction (MI). Total number of patients = 453. Overall 74% patency rate achieved with PTCA. Based on data in reference.[5,11,19,25-27]

Predicting cardiogenic shock

Patients at high risk of developing cardiogenic shock following infarction should be considered for early aggressive therapy in the hope of preventing this condition and its accompanying high mortality. This is potentially feasible given the frequent delay between the onset of infarction and shock. Predictors of in-hospital development of cardiogenic shock include age greater than 65 years, admission LV ejection fraction < 35%, peak creatine kinase MB > 160 u/L, history of diabetes mellitus and previous myocardial infarction[1] (see Fig. 57.3). Leor et al[6] have identified predictive factors that are all available at the time of admission: age, female gender, history of angina, stroke, peripheral vascular disease and serum glucose > 180 mg/dl.

Support devices

New devices to support the systemic circulation, such as haemopump, percutaneous cardiopulmonary support and the ventricular assist device, have usually been reserved for patients in cardiogenic shock unresponsive to other modalities or as a bridge to cardiac transplantation. The experience, albeit limited, with these support devices has been disappointing in terms of their influence on ultimate outcome although this may reflect bias in the selection of more critically ill patients. Further studies with these devices in more stable patients with cardiogenic shock need to be undertaken before general recommendations can be made.

Prognostic indicators

Bengston et al[5] in a prospectively collected consecutive series of 200 patients with acute infarction complicated by cardiogenic shock, of whom one quarter had PTCA, demonstrated that patency of the infarct-related artery was the most important predictor of both in-hospital and long-term survival. The overall in-hospital mortality was 53%. Those with a patent infarct-related artery had only a 33% in-hospital mortality compared with 75% mortality in those with a closed infarct-related artery, and an 84% mortality in those of unknown status. Independent predictors of in-hospital mortality were patency of the infarct-related artery ($P = 0.00001$), lowest cardiac index ($P = 0.0002$), ejection fraction ($P = 0.002$), age ($P = 0.06$), and peak creatine kinase ($P = 0.08$). Patients discharged from hospital with an occluded infarct-related artery were nearly five times as likely to die during the following year compared with those discharged with a patent infarct-related artery. These data give further support to an aggressive interventional strategy in patients with cardiogenic shock.

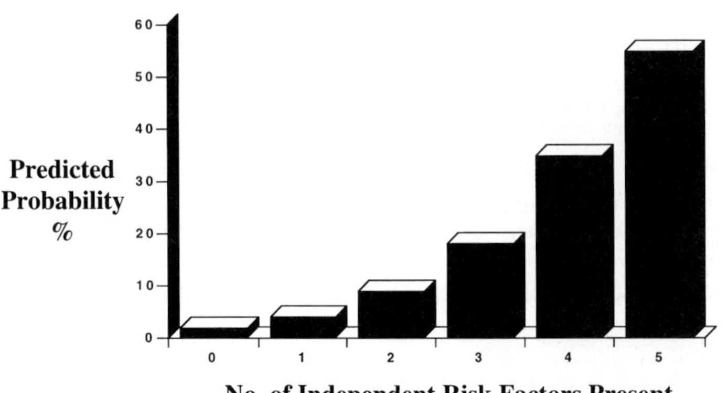

Fig. 57.3 Predicted probability for the in-hospital development of cardiogenic shock according to the number of independent risk factors present. Risk factors include age >65 years, LV ejection fraction on admission < 35%, peak CKMB > 160 i.u./L, history of diabetes mellitus and previous MI. CKMB = MB fraction of creatine kinase. Adapted with permission from Hands ME, Rutherford JD, Muller JE et al 1989.[1]

Conclusion

Cardiogenic shock remains a dreaded complication of AMI, accounting for the majority of in-hospital deaths. Its onset is frequently many hours or even days after the time of initial infarction, probably reflecting the progressive myocardial necrosis and re-infarction associated with this condition. Conventional therapy, including thrombolytic agents for established cardiogenic shock, continues to be associated with an extremely high mortality. Urgent angioplasty of the infarct-related artery, combined with haemodynamic support via IABP, appears to improve substantially both early and late survival in select cases. The use of emergency coronary artery bypass surgery in these patients is limited by logistics and is perhaps best reserved for those patients with failed PTCA or severe multi-vessel or left main disease. The role of new devices which assist systemic circulation is yet to be clearly defined in patients with cardiogenic shock.

References

1. Hands ME, Rutherford JD, Muller JE et al. The in-hospital development of cardiogenic shock after myocardial infarction: incidence, predictors of recurrence, outcome and prognostic factors. JACC 1989; 14: 40–6
2. Killip T. Cardiogenic shock complicating myocardial infarction. JACC 1989; 14: 47–8
3. GISSI-I trial. Effectiveness of intravenous thrombolytic treatment in acute myocardial infarction. Lancet 1986; 1: 397–401
4. Goldberg RJ, Gore JM, Albert JS et al. Cardiogenic shock after acute myocardial infarction. Incidence and mortality from community wide perspective, 1975–1988. N Engl J Med 1991; 325: 1117–22
5. Bengston JR, Kaplin AJ, Piper KS et al. Prognosis in cardiogenic shock after acute myocardial infarction in the interventional era. JACC 1992; 20(7): 1482–9
6. Leor J, Goldbourt U, Reicher-Reiss H et al and the SPRINT study group. Cardiogenic shock complicating acute myocardial infarction in patients without heart failure on admission: incidence, risk factors and outcome. Am J Med 1993; 94: 265–73
7. Page DL, Korfield JB, Kator JA et al. Myocardial changes associated with cardiogenic shock. N Engl J Med 1971; 285: 133–7
8. Alonso BR, Scheidt S, Post M et al. Pathophysiology of cardiogenic shock: quantitation of myocardial necrosis, clinical, pathological and electrocardiographic correlations. Circulation 1973; 48: 588–96
9. Roberts N, Harrison DG, Reimer KA et al. Right ventricular infarction with shock but without significant left ventricular function. A new clinical syndrome. Am Heart J 1985; 110: 1047–53
10. Gutovitz A, Sobel B, Roberts R. Progressive nature of myocardial injury in selected patients with cardiogenic shock. Am J Cardiol 1978; 41: 469–75
11. Bates ET, Topol EJ. Limitations of thrombolytic therapy in acute myocardial infarction, complicated by congestive heart failure and cardiogenic shock. JACC 1991; 18: 1077–84
12. Moulopoulos SD, Stamateolopoulos SF, Nanas JN et al. Effect of protracted dobutamine infusion on survival of patients in cardiogenic shock treated with an intra-aortic balloon pumping. Chest 1993; 103: 248–52
13. Klocke RK, Mager G, Kux A et al. Effects of twenty-four hour milrinone infusion in patients with severe heart failure in cardiogenic shock as a function of a haemodynamic initial condition. Am Heart J 1991; 121(6)(Pt II): 1965–73
14. Willerson JT, Frazier OH. Reducing mortality in patients with extensive myocardial infarction. N Engl J Med 1991; 325: 1166–8
15. O'Rourke M. Editorial. Eur Heart J 1986; 7: 400–3
16. Ohman EM, George BS, White CJ et al. Use of aortic counterpulsation to improve sustained coronary artery patency during acute myocardial infarction. Results of a randomised trial. Circulation 1994; 90(2); 792–9
17. Kennedy JW, Gensini GG, Timmus GC et al. Acute myocardial infarction treated with intracoronary streptokinase. A report of the Society for Cardiac Angiography. Am J Cardiol 1985; 55: 871
18. Garrahy PJ, Henzlova MJ, Foreman S et al. Has thrombolytic therapy improved survival from cardiogenic shock? Thrombolysis in myocardial infarction (TIMI-II results abstract). Circulation 1989: 80(Suppl. 2): 2–623
19. Lee L, Erbel R, Brown T et al. Multicentre registry of angioplasty therapy of cardiogenic shock: Initial and long-term survival. JACC 1991; 17(3): 599–603
20. Becker RC. Haemodynamic, mechanical and metabolic determinates of thrombolytic efficacy: A theoretic framework for assessing limitation of thrombolysis in patients with cardiogenic shock. Am Heart J 1993; 125: 919–29
21. Wood MA, Notske RH, Hensley GR et al. Intra-aortic balloon counterpulsation with and without reperfusion for myocardial infarction shock. Circulation 1980; 61: 1105–12
22. Dunkman WB, Leinbach RC, Buckley MJ et al. Clinical and hemodynamic results of intra-aortic balloon pumping and surgery for cardiogenic shock. Circulation 1972; 46: 465–77
23. Johnson SA, Scanlon PJ, Loeb HS et al. Treatment of cardiogenic shock in myocardial infarction by intra-aortic balloon counterpulsation and surgery. Am J Med 1977; 62: 687–92
24. Bordet J, Masquet C, Kahn J et al. Clinical and hemodynamic results of intra-aortic counterpulsation and surgery for cardiogenic shock. Am Heart J 1977; 93: 280–8
25. Gacioch GN, Ellis SG, Lee L et al. Cardiogenic shock complicating acute myocardial infarction: the use of coronary angioplasty in the integration of new support devices into patient management. JACC 1992; 19: 647–53
26. Moosvi RA, Villanueva L, Gheorghiadi M et al. Early revascularisation to improve survival in cardiogenic shock. Abst. Circulation 1990; 82(Suppl. 3): 308
27. Hibbard MD, Holmes DR, Bailey KR et al. Percutaneous transluminal coronary angioplasty in patients with cardiogenic shock. JACC 1992; 19(3): 639–46
28. Force T, Kemper A, Leavitt M et al. Acute reduction in functional infarct expansion with late coronary reperfusion: assessment with quantitative two-dimensional echocardiography. JACC 1988; 11: 192–200

58 AMI: Other complications

Peter L Thompson and Mark AJ Newman

Introduction

Chapters 55 to 58 have dealt with the arrhythmic and haemodynamic complications of acute myocardial infarction (AMI). This chapter deals with the mechanical and thromboembolic complications, the problems of infarct expansion and extension and pericarditis.

Mechanical complications

With improvement in the treatment of arrhythmias in heart failure after AMI, the significance of mechanical complications has increased as they now account for a greater proportion of deaths from AMI in the coronary care unit (CCU).[1–3]

The three main mechanical complications of AMI are:

- mitral valve dysfunction
- ventricular septal rupture
- rupture of the left ventricle.

Mitral valve dysfunction

Mitral regurgitation following AMI can be due to rupture or dysfunction of the papillary muscles, or from major wall motion abnormality with dyskinesis causing prolapse of the mitral valve leaflets in systole or to annular dilatation.[4,5] Severe mitral regurgitation due to papillary muscle rupture is usually seen in association with inferior MI and involvement of the posteromedial papillary muscle. It is thought that the anterolateral papillary muscle is less frequently involved because it has a dual blood supply from the left anterior descending and left circumflex coronary arteries.[6] The MI associated with papillary muscle rupture is often small, with postmortem studies showing that the infarction may be localized to the subendocardium.[6]

Diagnosis

Severe mitral regurgitation due to papillary muscle rupture usually presents 1–4 days after infarction. It may initially present simply as a new systolic murmur but is usually associated with significant deterioration in cardiac performance and sometimes with acute cardiogenic shock or pulmonary oedema.[7] The murmur may be soft or even absent because of the severity of the mitral regurgitation and the equalization of pressures between the left ventricle and left atrium.

The diagnosis is confirmed with echocardiography. Colour flow imaging reveals the severity of the mitral regurgitation, and direct visualization of the flail leaflet and on occasions the flail papillary muscle head are possible.[8,9] Bedside echocardiography can immediately exclude ventricular septal defect, the other major cause of a new systolic murmur and haemodynamic deterioration. Pulmonary artery pressure monitoring can also give valuable information by showing a prominent V wave on the wedge tracing and by excluding a left to right shunt at ventricular level. Image quality can be improved by trans-oesophageal echocardiography but this is usually not necessary as transthoracic echocardiography usually provides sufficient information and passage of the trans-oesophageal probe may delay definitive treatment. The chest X-ray may show acute pulmonary oedema.

Treatment

When mitral regurgitation is mild to moderate and thought to be due to papillary muscle dysfunction rather than rupture, medical therapy using afterload reduction with angiotensin-converting enzyme (ACE) inhibitors and nitrates with inotropic support for hypotension may be effective. However, when regurgitation is severe, as it is in papillary muscle rupture, and if there is severe haemodynamic impairment, urgent surgical intervention is required.

To stabilize the patient initially an intra-aortic balloon pump should be inserted. If possible, urgent coronary angiography should be obtained to assess the need for concomitant coronary bypass grafting. A ventriculogram will help confirm the severity of mitral regurgitation but is not essential if echocardiographic evidence is convincing. In the past, a policy of delayed surgery has been followed with urgent surgery limited to life-saving procedures. The Mayo Clinic has presented persuasive data in favour of early surgery in all patients because of the high risk of sudden death even in well-stabilized patients awaiting surgery.[6] Preparation for surgery should be made as soon as the diagnosis of papillary muscle rupture has been confirmed.

The surgical approach is to revascularize major coronary arteries with severe stenoses and to repair or replace the mitral valve. It is generally accepted that mitral valve replacement is indicated for papillary muscle rupture as reimplantation has uncertain results. Annuloplasty can be effective for some types of mitral insufficiency due to wall motion problems and annular dilatation, but again may not be as effective as mitral valve replacement. When the valve is replaced, preservation of annular mural connection by preserving the chordae tendineae results in better early and late ventricular function.[10]

The procedure of mitral valve surgery in the setting of AMI carries a high morbidity and mortality of about 30%.

Ventricular septal rupture

Acute rupture of the ventricular septum is a major complication of AMI. It occurs from 1–7 days after infarction when muscle softening occurs in a transmural infarction.[11,12] When the left anterior descending coronary artery is occluded the ventricular septal defect (VSD) occurs in the anterior septum or at the apex. The VSD is in the inferior septum and often extends up to the mitral annulus when associated with an inferior infarct due to right coronary artery or dominant circumflex coronary artery occlusion.[12] Frequently acute VSD is found to occur when there is single vessel disease as it is thought to be due to poor collateral supply to the infarcted territory. A decline in the incidence of acute infarction VSD in recent years may be due to wider use of thrombolytic therapy and afterload reduction.

Diagnosis

Acute haemodynamic deterioration with shock or pulmonary oedema and the development of a new murmur is seen in acute VSD. The differential diagnosis is acute mitral regurgitation, and they can occur together. Echocardiography can usually show the defect and colour Doppler imaging will detect the flow across the VSD.

A Swan–Ganz catheter with blood gas sampling from the right atrium and pulmonary artery, together with an arterial blood gas sample, will enable the calculation of the size of the VSD shunt.

The natural history of VSD is that 90% will die within 2 weeks and almost all within 2 months. Factors worsening prognosis are the presence of cardiogenic shock and associated right ventricular infarction in the presence of inferior infarction. It has been shown that the operative mortality is very high once multiple organ failure has commenced in acute VSD.[13,14] It is therefore essential that the diagnosis be made early and that operative intervention be performed urgently.[9]

Treatment

Once the diagnosis of acute VSD is made and it is determined that active management of the patient is indicated on the grounds of lack of concurrent medical problems or old age, then immediate notification of the cardiac surgical team and urgent treatment is essential. An intra-aortic balloon pump should be inserted to stabilize the patient and inotropes may be required. Usually coronary angiography is indicated but ventriculography is not performed. The patient is then prepared for urgent cardiac surgery and operated on as an emergency. Major coronary artery stenoses are bypassed and the VSD is repaired. The defect is approached via the infarcted LV wall and the defect patched from the left side of the septum. The repair can be very difficult due to the friability of the infarcted tissues and with inferior VSD the proximity to the mitral annulus is a complication.

The mortality is related to the size of the original infarct, and infarction of the right ventricle seems especially important. Technical improvements in the repair of acute post-infarction VSD have led to improvements in outcome;[15] however the mortality for an anterior VSD is 10–20%, while for an inferior VSD it is approximately 50%.

Following septal repair the patient should be anticoagulated for 6–8 weeks during the period of endothelialization of the prosthetic material used in the repair.

Left ventricular rupture

Left ventricular free wall rupture is usually rapidly fatal and is a common cause of death due to AMI. It accounts for approximately 10% of deaths from AMI. Most ruptures occur within the first 5 days of infarction. It is more common in women than men. The typical profile of the high risk patient is the elderly hypertensive female with initial myocardial infarction.[16] There have been concerns that thrombolytic therapy, particularly if given late after the onset of symptoms, may increase the risk of death in the first 24 hours.[17] Occasionally, pericardial adhesions will limit the extravasation of blood and allow survival of the patient, or there may be a slow leak with progressive pericardial tamponade without sudden death.[18]

Diagnosis

Acute cardiac rupture usually causes acute cardiovascular collapse with electromechanical dissociation, that is, sinus rhythm on ECG without cardiac output; however, electromechanical dissociation is not pathognomonic for cardiac rupture. In this situation urgent pericardiocentesis may confirm the diagnosis but it is usually not sufficient to relieve the acute tamponade, and death is the usual outcome despite vigorous resuscitation. 'Subacute' cardiac rupture[18] may result in progressive cardiogenic shock due to pericardial tamponade and can be confirmed on echocardiography.[19,20]

Treatment

The situation is obviously desperate and the only way to save the patient is with rapid thoracotomy and tamponade of the hole in the left ventricle. This should only be done by a cardiac surgeon. The patient is transferred urgently to an operating theatre and put on cardiopulmonary bypass to allow repair of the ruptured heart. This can prove difficult due to the friable tissues but successful long-term results have been obtained. Some benefit has been claimed by using GRF glue in this setting. The mortality is very high.

Left ventricular false aneurysm

On occasions a subacute cardiac rupture may organize and create a localized intrapericardial aneurysm with a narrow neck in contrast to a true LV aneurysm which has a broad neck. Recognition of false aneurysm is of some importance as pseudo-aneurysms have a tendency to rupture, in contrast to the behaviour of true aneurysms.[21]

Diagnosis

Echocardiography can distinguish true from false aneurysm by identification of the narrow neck of the pseudo-aneurysm.[22]

Treatment

Resection of the pseudo-aneurysm combined with coronary artery bypass grafting[23] can avoid the risk of rupture and improve long-term survival.

Left ventricular thrombus and systemic embolism

Thrombus formation within the left ventricle can occur after MI and may cause systemic embolism including embolic stroke. The overall risk of embolic stroke is 1–3%. The overwhelming evidence is that this risk is confined mainly to patients with extensive anterior infarction[24,25] although one recent study highlighted that inferior infarction may also be associated with a risk of embolic stroke.[26] The risk can be substantially reduced although not entirely abolished by anticoagulant therapy[24].

Echocardiography can detect LV thrombi in 30–40% of patients with anterior MI not treated with anticoagulants. The risk of cerebral embolism following detection of intraventricular thrombus in this situation is approximately 10%.[27] The notion that intraventricular thrombus necessarily predicts embolic stroke and therefore requires aggressive anticoagulant therapy has been questioned;[28] however, the weight of evidence favours an active approach when intraventricular thrombus is detected on echocardiography.[25,29] A protuberant mobile intraventricular thrombus detected on echocardiography is more likely to cause cerebral embolism than a sessile immobile thrombus.[30]

All patients with clinical evidence of extensive anterior MI should receive full dose anticoagulation with heparin. In patients who have not received thrombolytic therapy a peak creatine kinase (CK) or CKMB level in excess of 8–10 times normal is predictive of significant embolic risk; these patients should be continued on warfarin anticoagulant.[24] In patients who have received thrombolytic therapy in which the cardiac enzyme profile is an unreliable index of infarct size, echocardiography may be necessary to distinguish patients with well-preserved LV function from those with areas of extensive akinesis or dyskinesis who may be at risk of intra-ventricular thrombus formation and therefore in need of anticoagulant therapy.

Patients at lower risk of thromboembolic complications should have routine treatment with subcutaneous heparin 12 500 units 12-hourly until fully mobilized.[31]

Thrombolytic therapy appears to reduce the risk of LV thrombi after MI but the impact on cerebral embolism is not clear.[32,33]

Infarct expansion and remodelling

The clinicopathological consequences of infarct expansion, extension and reinfarction were clarified by a series of studies conducted in the mid 1980s.[34] The concept of infarct expansion extends earlier concepts of left ventricular aneurysm formation and highlights the importance of the thinning and increased surface area of the infarct. The non-infarcted tissue may undergo hypertrophy, resulting in extensive remodelling of the LV chamber.[35] Expansion of the infarct zone may increase the end systolic volume, thereby increasing oxygen demand on the non-infarcted and potentially ischaemic tissue, with adverse consequences for the later development of symptomatic ischaemia, cardiac failure and worsened survival (see Ch. 8).[36]

Clinical recognition

Infarct expansion and adverse remodelling of the left ventricle usually occur in patients with extensive anterior MI who have not been successfully treated with reperfusion therapy. It is less common with other infarct locations but may occur in extensive inferoposterior infarction. There may be few clinical features apart from persistent hypotension and dyspnoea due to pulmonary congestion. The ECG may show persistence of ST segment elevation indicative of dyskinesis. Serial echocardiography is the most reliable method of monitoring changes in LV remodelling and detected infarct expansion.[37]

Management

Current strategies for early reperfusion therapy with thrombolysis (see Ch. 34) or angioplasty (Ch. 45), afterload reduction with intravenous nitrates (Ch. 30) and early administration of ACE inhibitors (Ch. 33) are directed to preservation of LV function and prevention of infarct expansion.

The patient in whom these strategies appear to have failed and whose clinical ECG and echocardiographic features suggest a risk of infarct expansion should be considered for delayed mobilization. Clinical trials are not available for guidance but it is likely that current strategies of early mobilization and early hospital discharge may disadvantage this subgroup of patients. The benefits of delayed restoration of patency of the persistently occluded infarct-related artery remain controversial.[38] Revascularization of vessels supplying the non-infarcted tissue may improve prognosis by preventing the adverse effects of LV remodelling (see Ch. 78).

Infarct extension

Although pathological studies[34] have shown distinct differences between infarct extension and reinfarction, in the practical management of patients in the CCU it is sometimes difficult to distinguish between infarct extension, reinfarction and post-infarction angina.

Clinical recognition

The definition of infarct extension varies but it usually refers to the near-continuous persistence of ischaemia and extension of the original infarction in the patient with persistent or recurring chest pain, ST-T changes and progressive haemodynamic deterioration. Such patients may progress to cardiogenic shock and death. At post mortem the myocardial infarct will be surrounded by waves of necrosis of varying ages within the same vascular bed. It is important to realize that infarct extension may occur without obvious chest pain and may only be evident on serial estimation of biochemical markers.[38] Elderly women with non-Q wave infarction are at particular risk of developing this complication of infarction.

Management

Stabilization of myocardial ischaemia with intravenous beta blockers and nitrates may be helpful. Coronary thrombolysis is usually unhelpful and where facilities are available, early consideration of reperfusion with angioplasty should be considered.

Reinfarction

Reinfarction is a distinct phenomenon from infarct extension and is due to a recurrence of myocardial ischaemia after a delay of some hours or days from stabilization and relief of pain from the original infarction. It almost invariably indicates re-occlusion of the infarct-related artery.[39,40]

Clinical recognition

Clinical evidence of reinfarction occurs in 5–10% of patients in the first 10 days following MI and is substantially higher in patients who have received thrombolytic therapy or in patients with non-Q wave infarction. Silent re-occlusion of the infarct-related artery is a common phenomenon after coronary thrombolysis.

Management

Immediate management of reinfarction is similar to management of the initial infarction, including pain relief and electrocardiographic monitoring to reduce the risk of ventricular fibrillation. Restoration of blood flow through the infarct-related arteries should be a high priority. Initial treatment is with intravenous heparin and nitroglycerin and consideration of readministration of thrombolytic therapy or coronary angioplasty. TPA can be readministered without concern about immunological reactions. Streptokinase can be readministered within the first few days but after 5 days the likelihood of an antibody reaction and inactivation of the readministered streptokinase should be considered and TPA may be more appropriate. If intervention facilities are readily available, urgent angiography and angioplasty may be possible.

Post-infarction ischaemia

Post-infarction angina is common in patients treated in the CCU after acute myocardial infarction. These patients are at risk of reinfarction and require vigorous management. Natural history studies have shown a clear distinction between patients who suffer significant ST segment change during their post-infarction angina, compared with those who do not, particularly after non-Q wave infarction.[40,41]

Management

Patients with post-infarction ischaemia should have an ECG performed during their chest pain to document the location and severity of ST segment change. Medical therapy with beta blockers and nitrates should be maximized and if necessary the addition of a calcium channel blocker. Early angiography and revascularization should be considered. In institutions without on-site angiographic facilities, arrangements should be made for early transfer.

Pericarditis

A pericardial friction rub is detected in 10–15% of patients with AMI. Pericarditis can occur in anterior or inferior infarction, but a pericardial friction rub usually accompanies pericarditis only in anterior MI. In anterior infarction the pericardial pain is usually located in the precordial area. In pericarditis with inferior infarction, the pericardial friction rub is not usually heard and there may be unusual sites of radiation for the pericardial pain such as the left shoulder. Patients with pericarditis have a worse outcome than those without,[42] but this is probably due to the associated extensive infarction rather than the pericarditis per se. Post-infarction pericarditis may be associated with the development of pericardial tamponade. The progression of a pericardial rub to clinically significant tamponade following uncomplicated post-infarction pericarditis is extremely rare despite aggressive anticoagulant therapy. Thrombolytic therapy is associated with reduced frequency of pericardial rub and symptoms of pericarditis. It is not clear if this is due to reduction in the extent of myocardial damage or lysis of the fibrin in the fibrinous pericarditis.

Management

Differentiation of the pericardial pain from post-infarction ischaemia or reinfarction is essential to prevent unnecessary investigation or administration of anti-anginal therapy, and for relief of anxiety for the patient. In most cases, reassurance and simple analgesia is sufficient. If pericardial pain is distressing, a short course of higher dose of aspirin, for example 600–1200 mg per day, or non-steroidal anti-inflammatory drug, will relieve symptoms and shorten the duration of the pericardial friction rub. If the pericardial rub persists or if there is clinical evidence of pericardial compression, echocardiographic evaluation should be performed and appropriate action taken if there is evidence of pericardial tamponade.[43]

Dressler's syndrome

Dressler's syndrome differs from post-infarction pericarditis in occurring later, and can be associated with more generalized pericarditis and a loud pericardial friction rub together with fever and elevated ESR.[44] It may be associated with generalized serositis, including pleuritis with a pleural friction rub, and rarely, pulmonary infiltrates on chest X-ray. It is thought to be an immunological reaction to the myocardial necrosis.

For reasons that are not clear, Dressler's syndrome is now far less common than previously.[44]

Management

Dressler's syndrome will usually not settle spontaneously and requires a short course of non-steroidal anti-inflammatory drugs or oral corticosteroid such as prednisolone 50 mg, reducing over 10–14 days. In contrast to early post-infarction pericarditis, Dressler's syndrome is associated with a risk of pericardial haemorrhage and pericardial tamponade. For this reason anticoagulants should be ceased immediately and the patient should be monitored carefully for signs of pericardial compression.

References

1. Cohn, LH. Surgical management of acute and chronic cardiac complications due to myocardial infarction. Am Heart J 1981;1049–60
2. Miller DC, Stinson EB. Surgical management of acute mechanical defects secondary to myocardial infarction. Am J Surg 1981;141:677–83
3. Fox AC, Glassman E, Osom OW. Surgically remediable complications of myocardial infarctions. Prog Cardiovasc Dis 1979;21:461–84
4. Burch GE, De Pasquale NP, Phillips JH. Clinical manifestations of papillary muscle dysfunction. Arch Intern Med 1963;112:158
5. De Busk RF. The clinical spectrum of papillary muscle disease. N Engl J Med 281:1458–67
6. Nishimura RA, Schaff HV, Shub C et al. Papillary muscle rupture complicating acute myocardial infarction: analysis of 17 patients. Am J Cardiol 1983;51:373–7
7. Wei JY, Hutchins GM, Bulkley BH. Papillary muscle rupture in fatal acute myocardial infarction: a potentially treatable form of cardiogenic shock. Am Intern Med 1979;90:149–53
8. Smyllie JE, Sutherland GR, Geuskens R, Dawkins K, Conway N, Roelandt JRTC. Doppler color-flow mapping in the diagnosis of ventricular septal rupture and acute mitral regurgitation after myocardial infarction. J Am Coll Cardiol 1990;15:1449–55
9. Nishimura RA, Schaff HV, Gersh J et al. Early repair of mechanical complications after acute myocardial infarction. JAMA 1986;256:47–50
10. Hendren WG, Nemec JJ, Lytle BW et al. Mitral valve repair for ischaemic mitral insufficiency. Ann Thorac Surg 1991;52:1246–52
11. Sanders RJ, Kern WH, Blount SG. Perforation of the interventricular septum complicating myocardial infarction. Am Heart J 1956;51:736–48
12. Hutchins GM. Rupture of the interventricular septum complicating myocardial infarction. Pathological analysis of 10 patients with clinically diagnosed perforations. Am Heart J 1979;97:165–73
13. Radford MJ, Johnson RA, Daggett WM Jr et al. Ventricular septal rupture: a review of clinical physiologic features and an analysis of survival. Circulation 1991;64:545–53
14. Cummings RG, Reimer KA, Califf R et al. Quantitative analysis of right and left ventricular infarction in the presence of post-infarction ventricular septal defect. Circulation 1988;77:33–42
15. Alvarez JM, Brady PW, Ross DE. Technical improvements in the repair of acute post infarction ventricular septal rupture. J Cardiovasc Surg 1992;3:198
16. Bates RJ, Beutler S, Resnekov L et al. Cardiac rupture: challenge in diagnosis and management. Am J Cardiol 1977;42:429–37
17. Mauri F, De Biase AM, Franzosi MG et al. GISSI: analisi delle cause di morte intraospedaliera. G Ital Cardiol 1987;17:37–44
18. O'Rourke M. Subacute heart rupture following acute myocardial infarction. Lancet 1973;2:124–6
19. Hagemeijer F, Verbaan CJ, Sonke PC, de Rooij CH. Echocardiography and rupture of the heart. Br Heart J 1980;43:45–6
20. Feneley MP, Chang VP, O'Rourke MF. Myocardial rupture after acute myocardial infarction: ten year review. Br Heart J 1983;49:550–6

21. Vlodaver Z, Coe JI, Edwards JE. True and false left ventricular aneurysms: propensity for the latter to rupture. Circulation 1965;51:567–72
22. Gatewood RP Jr, Nanda NC. Differentiation of left ventricular pseudo-aneurysm from true aneurysm with two-dimensional echocardiography. Am J Cardiol 1980;46:869–78
23. Buehler DL, Stinson EB, Oyer PE, Shimway NE. Surgical treatment of aneurysms of the inferior left ventricular wall. J Thorac Cardiovasc Surg 1979;78:74–8
24. Thompson PL, Robinson JS. Stroke after acute myocardial infarction: relation to infarct size. Br Med J 1978;1:457–9
25. Halperin JL, Petersen P. Thrombosis in the cardiac chambers: ventricular dysfunction and atrial fibrillation. In: Fuster V, Verstraete M (eds). Thrombosis in cardiovascular disorders. Philadelphia: Saunders, 1992: Ch 12
26. Bodenheimer MM, Saver D, Shareef B, Brown MW, Fleiss JL, Moss AJ. Relation between myocardial infarct locations and stroke. J Am Coll Cardiol 1994;24:61–6
27. Vaitkus PT, Perlin JA, Schwartz JS, Barbathan ES. Stroke complicating acute myocardial infarction. A meta analysis of risk modification by anticoagulation and thrombolytic therapy. Arch Int Med 1992;152:2020–4
28. Nihoyannopoulos P, Smith GC, Maseri A, Foale RA. The natural history of left ventricular thrombus in myocardial infarction: a rationale in support of masterly inactivity. J Am Coll Cardiol 1989;14:903–11
29. Halperin JL, Fuster V. Left ventricular thrombus and stroke after myocardial infarctions: toward prevention or perplexity? J Am Coll Cardiol 1989;14:912–4
30. Visser CA, Kan G, Meltzer RS et al. Embolic potential of left ventricular thrombus after myocardial infarction: a two dimensional echocardiographic study of 119 patients. J Am Coll Cardiol 1985;5:1276–80
31. Turpie AGG, Robinson JG, Doyle DJ et al. Comparison of high dose with low dose subcutaneous heparin in the prevention of left ventricular mural thrombosis in patients with acute transmural anterior myocardial infarction. N Engl J Med 1989;320:352–7
32. Held AC, Gore JM, Paraskos J et al. Impact of thrombolytic therapy in left ventricular mural thrombi in acute myocardial infarction. Am J Cardiol 62:310–11
33. Vecchio C, Chiarella F, Lupi G, Bellotti P, Domenicucci S. Left ventricular thrombus in anterior acute myocardial infarction after thrombolysis—a GISSI-connected study. Circulation 1991;84:512–9
34. Weisman H, Healy B. Myocardial infarct expansion, infarct extension and reinfarction: pathophysiologic concepts. Prog Cardiovasc Dis 1987;30:73–110
35. Pfeffer MA, Braunwald E, Jugdutt BI. Ventricular remodelling after myocardial infarction. Experimental observations and clinical implications. Circulation 1990;81:1161–72
36. White HD, Norris RM, Brown MA. Left ventricular end-systolic volume as the major determinant of survival after recovering from myocardial infarction. Circulation 1987;76:44–51
37. St John Sutton M, Pfeffer MA, Plappert T et al for the SAVE investigators. Quantitative two dimensional echocardiographic measurements are major predictors of adverse cardiovascular events following acute myocardial infarction: the protective effects of captopril. Circulation 1994;89:68–75
38. Kim CB, Braunwald E. Potential benefits of late reperfusion of infarcted myocardium. The open artery hypothesis. Circulation 1993;88:2426–36
39. Schaer DH, Ross AM, Wasserman AG. Reinfarction, recurrent angina and re-occlusion after thrombolytic therapy. Circulation 1987;76(Suppl. II):57–62
40. Bosch X, Theroux P, Waters D, Pelletier GB, Roy D. Early postinfarction ischaemia. Clinical angiographic and prognostic significance. Circulation 1987;75:988–95
41. Boden WE, Gibson RS, Kleiger KE et al. Importance of early recurrent ischaemia on one year survival after non Q wave myocardial infarction. Am J Cardiol 1989;64:799–801
42. Thompson PL. Prognosis of acute myocardial infarction with special reference to infarct size. Thesis. Perth: University of Western Australia, 1988
43. Tofler GH, Muller JE, Stone PH et al. Pericarditis in acute myocardial infarction: characterization and clinical significance. Am Heart J 1989;117:86–92
44. Kossowsky W, Lyon AF, Spain DM. Reappraisal of the post myocardial infarction Dressler's syndrome. Am Heart J 1981;102:954–6

59 AMI: Right ventricular infarction

Peter L Thompson

Introduction

The significance of right ventricular (RV) infarction is that inappropriate management has the potential to seriously compound the disordered pathophysiology. Correct treatment can enable recovery of RV function and an excellent long-term prognosis.

Although right ventricular infarction was recognized at post mortem in the early literature on myocardial infarction (MI),[1] the clinical features of the condition were not recognized until the work of Cohn and co-workers in the early 1970s.[2] Since then there has been considerable progress in understanding the pathophysiology and clinical course of RV infarction.[3–5]

Pathophysiology

Right ventricular infarction occurs in association with infarction of the inferoposterior left ventricle following right coronary artery occlusion. Collateral blood flow from the left coronary circulation may limit the extent of RV infarction but this collateral support appears to be reduced in the presence of significant left anterior descending coronary artery disease.[4]

The clinical features of RV infarction are more readily understandable when the pathophysiologic importance of pericardial restriction is understood.[5] Detailed studies in canine MI have shown that right coronary artery occlusion with an intact pericardium produces the typical haemodynamics of RV infarction. There is an increase and equalization of right and left heart filling pressures, right ventricular dilatation and reduced left ventricular cardiac output.[6,7] Fluid loading improved cardiac output. After incising the pericardium, left ventricular volumes and cardiac output improved significantly.[6] These elegant experiments explain how many of the clinical features of RV infarction mimic those of pericardial constriction.

Clinical features

Cohn et al[2] described the typical clinical syndrome of RV infarction with hypotension, elevated jugular venous pressure (JVP) and clear lung fields. Testing these clinical features against the presence of RV infarction (confirmed on haemodynamic measurement) showed that this clinical triad was 96% specific for RV infarction but only 25% sensitive. An elevated JVP alone was less specific (69%) but more sensitive (88%) for RV infarction.

Other clinical features seen in more extreme cases of right ventricular infarction are those seen in right pericardial constriction including Kussmaul's sign and pulsus paradoxus.[8] On occasions the clinical features of significant tricuspid regurgitation may complicate RV infarction.[9]

It is clear from the above that regular and meticulous examination of the jugular venous pulse should be a routine part of management of inferior myocardial infarction in the CCU to allow early detection of right ventricular infarction.

Electrocardiographic features

Erhardt and co-workers[10] demonstrated the importance of right precordial leads in the diagnosis of RV infarction. ST segment elevation in V3 or V4 may be diagnostic of RV infarction even in the absence of clinically evident haemodynamic disturbance of right ventricular infarction. However, the ST segment change is evanescent and may not be present 24–48 hours after the onset of RV infarction. On occasions ST segment elevation in the standard precordial leads V1 and V2 may be a subtle indicator of RV infarction.[11,12]

Echocardiography

Bedside echocardiography can provide invaluable clues to the diagnosis of right ventricular infarction.[13] Subcostal views are of particular value in obtaining detailed evaluation of the right ventricle. Echocardiographic features of right ventricular infarction include right ventricular dilatation, wall motion abnormalities of the right ventricle and paradoxical septal motion.[14]

In addition, echo colour Doppler examination may help to clarify other causes of right heart failure in myocardial infarction such as ventricular septal defect or gross left ventricular dysfunction with pulmonary congestion.

Radionuclide studies

Myocardial uptake of Technetium-99m pyrophosphate may demonstrate RV uptake in inferior myocardial infarction,[15,16] but becomes positive at 48–72 hours, usually too late to be of value. Myocardial perfusion imaging with thallium does not have sufficient sensitivity to detect RV infarction.[15]

Radionuclide angiography

Studies have reported abnormalities of RV function in 40–50% of patients with inferior myocardial infarction.[17,18] These findings represent the upper limit of estimates of right ventricular involvement in inferoposterior infarction and suggest that radionuclide angiography may be over-sensitive for the detection of clinically or haemodynamically significant RV infarction.[19]

Pulmonary artery and right heart haemodynamic monitoring

The characteristic features of RV infarction on right heart haemodynamic monitoring are: disproportionate elevation of right ventricular filling pressure assessed by right atrial pressure, in comparison with left ventricular filling pressure as assessed by pulmonary artery capillary wedge pressure; and abnormalities of the right atrial and right ventricular pressure wave forms.[20]

Management of right ventricular infarction

The keys to correct management of RV infarction are:

- be aware of the possibility of RV involvement in inferoposterior myocardial infarction
- understand the pathophysiology and the importance of maintaining right heart filling pressures
- avoid manoeuvres which may reduce RV pre-load.

The common error in the management of RV infarction in the past has been to attribute the elevation of venous pressure to transmitted left heart pressures and left ventricular dysfunction, and to treat with aggressive diuretic therapy which will have an adverse effect by reducing right ventricular pre-load. Similar effects on right ventricular filling pressures will result from sharp reductions in pre-load by the administration of vasodilators. As a simple management rule of thumb, diuretic or vasodilator therapy should not be administered in inferior myocardial infarction until RV infarction has been considered and if appropriate, the necessary chest X-ray electrocardiographic and echocardiographic data can be obtained.[25]

The haemodynamic response to fluid loading in RV infarction is variable despite early encouraging reports.[2,21] Fluid infusion with normal saline or volume-expanding colloid is worth considering in the patient with established RV infarction and low cardiac output, particularly when there has been pre-infarction diuretic therapy and hypovolaemia is a strong possibility.

On occasions infusion of 1–2 litres of fluid over 4 hours can induce a dramatic improvement in the haemodynamic status; however, this must be done with considerable care, preferably with haemodynamic monitoring. If there is significant associated left ventricular dysfunction, pulmonary oedema may be provoked.[22] Nitroprusside in this situation may have a deleterious effect whereas dobutamine may produce significant improvement in cardiac output.[22] If response to fluid loading and dobutamine is ineffective and cardiac output remains low, intra-aortic balloon counterpulsation may be effective.[23]

Temporary atrioventricular (AV) sequential pacing has been reported to improve the haemodynamics in RV infarction.[24,25] If RV infarction is associated with high grade AV block, dual chamber rather than ventricular pacing should be the preferred mode of pacing.[25]

The contribution of reperfusion therapy to improving outcome in RV infarction is not clear, although there is evidence that thrombolytic therapy is associated with a lower incidence of RV infarction in inferior myocardial infarction[26] and early reports of direct angioplasty in RV infarction have been encouraging.[27]

Prognosis and natural history

The presence of RV infarction is an independent predictor of worse prognosis in inferior myocardial infarction.[28] However, in patients who survive the early phase of inferior infarction with RV involvement, the usual pattern is complete recovery, often with a dramatic improvement in haemodynamic status, with obvious signs of improved cardiac output occurring quite suddenly 1–2 weeks after the onset of infarction.[29] The long-term prognosis appears to be determined predominantly by the degree of left ventricular dysfunction rather than the degree of dominant right ventricular dysfunction.[30]

References

1. Laurie W, Woods JD. Infarction (ischaemic necrosis) of the right ventricle of the heart. Acta Cardiol 1963;18:399
2. Cohn JN, Guiha NH, Broder MI, Limas CJ. Right ventricular infarction: clinical and haemodynamic features. Am J Cardiol 1974;33:209–14
3. Backley CE, Russell RO. Right ventricular function in acute myocardial infarction. Am J Cardiol 1974;33:927–9
4. Isner JM, Roberts WE. Right ventricular infarction complicating left ventricular infarction secondary to coronary disease: frequency, location, associated findings and significance from analysis of 236 necropsy patients with acute or healed myocardial infarction. Am J Cardiol 1978;42:888–94
5. Kulbertus HE, Rigo P, Legrand V. Right ventricular infarction: pathophysiology, diagnosis, clinical course and treatment. Mod Concepts Cardiovasc Dis 1985;54:1–5
6. Goldstein JA, Vlahakes GJ, Verrier ED et al. The role of right ventricular systolic dysfunction and elevated intrapericardial pressure in the genesis of low output in experimental right ventricular infarction. Circulation 1982;65:513–22
7. Goldstein JA, Vlahakes GJ, Verrier ED et al. Volume loading improves low cardiac output in experimental right ventricular infarction. J Am Coll Cardiol 1983;2:270–8
8. Dell'Italia LJ, Starling MR, O'Rourke RA. Physical examination for exclusion of hemodynamically important right ventricular infarction. Ann Intern Med 1983;99:608–11
9. McAllister RG, Friesinger GC, Sinclair-Smith BC. Tricuspid regurgitation following inferior myocardial infarction. Arch Intern Med 1976;136:95–9
10. Erhardt LR, Sjogren A, Wahlberg I. Single right sided precordial load in the diagnosis of right ventricular involvement in inferior myocardial infarction. Am Heart J 1976;91:571–6
11. Chou T, Van der Bel-Khan J, Allen J et al. Electrocardiographic diagnosis of right ventricular infarction. Am J Med 1981;70:1175–80
12. Geft LL, Shah PK, Rodriguez L et al. ST elevations in leads V1 to V5 may be caused by right coronary artery occlusion and acute right ventricular infarction. Am J Cardiol 1984;53:991–6
13. Bellamy GR, Rasmussen HH, Nasser FN et al. Value of two-dimensional echocardiography, electrocardiography and clinical signs in detecting right ventricular infarction. Am Heart J 1986;112:304–9
14. D'Arcy B, Nanda NC. Two-dimensional echocardiographic features of right ventricular infarction. Circulation 1982;65:167–73
15. Wackers FJT, Lie KI, Sokole EB, van der Schoot JB, Durrer D. Prevalence of right ventricular involvement in inferior wall infarction assessed with myocardial imaging with thallium-201 and technetium-99m pyrophosphate. Am J Cardiol 1978;42:358–62
16. Legrand V, Rigo P, Smeets PJP et al. Right ventricular infarction diagnosed by 99m technetium pyrophosphate scintigraphy: clinical course and follow up. Eur Heart J 1983;4:9–19
17. Sharpe DN, Botvinick EH, Shames DM et al. The non invasive diagnosis of right ventricular infarction. Circulation 1978;57:1078–84
18. Starling MR, Dell'Italia LJ, Chaudhuri TK et al. First transit and equilibrium radionuclide angiography in patients with inferior transmural myocardial infarction: criteria for the diagnosis of associated hemodynamically significant right ventricular infarction. J Am Coll Cardiol 1984;4:923–30
19. Shak PK, Maddahi J, Berman DS et al. Scintigraphically detected predominant right ventricular dysfunction in acute myocardial infarction: clinical and hemodynamic correlates and implications for therapy and prognosis. J Am Coll Cardiol 1985;6:1264–72
20. Dell'Italia LJ, Starling MR, Crawford MH et al. Right ventricular infarction: identification by hemodynamic measurements before and after volume loading: correlation with non invasive techniques. J Am Coll Cardiol 1984;4:931–9
21. Lloyd EA, Gersh BJ, Kennelly BM. Hemodynamic spectrum of

'dominant' right ventricular infarction in 19 patients. Am J Cardiol 1981;48:1016–21
22. Dell-Italia LJ, Starling MR, Blumhardt R et al. Comparative effects of volume loading, dobutamine and nitroprusside in patients with predominant right ventricular infarction. Circulation 1985;72:1327–35
23. Iqbal MZ, Liebson PR. Counterpulsation and dobutamine: their use in treatment of cardiogenic shock due to right ventricular infarct. Arch Int Med 1981;141:247–9
24. Topol EJ, Goldschlager N, Ports TA et al. Hemodynamic benefit of atrial pacing in right ventricular myocardial infarction. Ann Intern Med 1982;96:594–7
25. Love JL, Haffajee CI, Gore JM, Alpert JS. Reversibility of hypotension and shock by atrial or atrioventricular sequential pacing in patients with right ventricular infarction. Am Heart J 1984;108:5–13
26. Berger PB, Ruocco NA, Timm TC. The impact of thrombolytic therapy on right ventricular infarction complicating inferior myocardial infarction; results from Thrombolysis in Myocardial Infarction (TIMI) II. Circulation 1989;80: II–313
27. Moreyra AE, Suh C, Porway MN, Kostis JB. Rapid haemodynamic improvement in right ventricular infarction after coronary angioplasty. Chest 1988;94:197–200
28. Zehender M, Kasper W, Kauder E et al. Right ventricular infarction as an independent predictor of prognosis after acute inferior myocardial infarction. N Engl J Med 1993;328:981–8
29. Steele P, Kirch D, Ellis J et al. Prompt return to normal of depressed right ventricular ejection fraction in acute inferior infarction. Br Heart J 1977;39:1319–23
30. Shah PK, Maddahi J, Staniloff HM et al. Variable spectrum and prognosis implications of left and right ventricular ejection fractions in patients with and without heart failure after acute myocardial infarction. Am J Cardiol 1986;58:387–98

Part 8
Other cardiac problems

60 Unstable angina pectoris

S Ben Freedman

Definition

Unstable angina pectoris is a clinically defined syndrome midway between stable angina pectoris and myocardial infarction. Historically, the term unstable angina supplants previous names for this syndrome such as 'acute coronary insufficiency', and 'intermediate coronary syndrome', and has gained widespread acceptance. There has been much confusion in the literature and in text-books about the definition of this syndrome because of the two different meanings of the word 'unstable': this can be taken to mean just a change in pattern of previous angina or new onset angina, or alternatively can be used in the sense implying a high risk of serious adverse events. A compromise is to define unstable angina as a change in pattern of pain, and within this definition to identify high and low risk subgroups.[1] This approach seems to have been widely adopted.

The three principal clinical presentations included in this definition of unstable angina are:

- prolonged rest pain, usually lasting >20 minutes
- new onset of exertional angina (particularly if Canadian class III or greater)
- crescendo effort angina (increasing severity or more easily provoked angina) to Canadian class III or greater.

Pathophysiology

Unstable angina is usually caused by fracture of an atherosclerotic plaque—frequently only minor—with intra-plaque and some intra-luminal thrombus.[2–4] The thrombus is usually not occlusive. At angioscopy, the thrombus appears white,[5] in keeping with the pathological findings of platelet-rich mural thrombi.[4] This appearance contrasts with acute coronary occlusion (myocardial infarction), where the thrombus appears red, and pathologically is rich in fibrin and red blood cells. This distinction may explain the different responses of the two conditions to thrombolytic drugs.[5]

The plaque underlying the thrombus is packed with activated macrophages suggesting an inflammatory process.[6] On their surface, these macrophages express tissue factor which is highly procoagulant.[7] At post mortem, the thrombus is multilayered, suggesting multiple episodes of thrombosis, and the thrombin between these layers acts as a continuing stimulus for platelet activation. Luminal encroachment by the lesion limits flow within the artery and increases shear stress, which together with systemic thrombotic factors plays a role in determining whether the lesion will stabilize and re-endothelialize or remain active with the potential for complete thrombosis and/or embolization.[4] This latter mechanism underlies myocardial infarction and cardiac death, the two major complications of unstable angina.

Initial management issues

When confronted with a patient with possible unstable angina pectoris—whether it be in the emergency department, surgery, or on the telephone—the most important decision facing the clinician is whether symptoms will require admission, and if so, what intensity of care will be required. Clarification of two questions will usually decide the issue: first, is the pain due to myocardial ischaemia, and second, are there any indicators of high risk?

Is pain ischaemic?

The most vital information here is an accurate history taken by a competent physician. The history should stress both the site of pain and its radiation, and the character of the pain—the two most important characteristics. In classification of the pain, physicians should attempt to assign one of three categories: a) definite ischaemic pain, b) possible ischaemic pain, and c) probably not ischaemic pain. This classification has important prognostic implications, with patients in the latter two categories having a much better prognosis.[8,9] After the history, a 12-lead electrocardiogram (ECG) is the most useful investigation.[10,11] Usually physicians do not take the history in isolation and will also use the ECG in categorizing the chest pain. Features on the 12-lead ECG suggesting that the pain is ischaemic are dynamic ST segment depression (≥ 1 mm planar or downsloping) or elevation, dynamic peaking of T waves or normalization of inverted T waves, or deep symmetrical T wave inversion in multiple leads following pain.[12] It should be noted that a normal ECG, even if recorded during chest pain, does not exclude the diagnosis, although the outlook of patients with a normal ECG, or an ECG with no new changes, is much better than for those in whom the ECG is abnormal.

A past history of coronary artery disease or the presence of coronary risk factors is somewhat helpful in making the discrimination between ischaemic and non-ischaemic pain, but even patients with documented coronary artery disease may have chest pain that is non-cardiac.[8] Age and gender are of limited assistance—the diagnosis is more likely in males over 60, and in females over 70.

In a patient with prior angina, sudden worsening of effort angina or even angina at rest may result from factors other than plaque rupture: for example, anaemia from gastrointestinal blood loss, hypoxaemia from chronic obstructive pulmonary disease, uncontrolled hypertension, tachy- and bradycardias, fever, hyperthyroidism, or poor compliance with anti-anginal medications. Such potential precipitants for increased angina should be sought in the history and physical examination, as their correction will usually stabilize symptoms.

Indicators of high risk

The risk of unstable angina pectoris relates to the instability of the ruptured plaque, which can lead to either myocardial infarction or cardiac death. The clinical pointers to a ruptured plaque with superimposed thrombosis are the occurrence of prolonged chest pain, usually at rest, particularly if pain is poorly relieved by sublingual nitroglycerin. The duration of pain usually taken as a cut-off is 20 minutes, although this is arbitrary. The most important indicator of high risk in patients with unstable angina is prolonged rest pain.[13] This presentation has a much worse prognosis than new onset of exertional angina or crescendo exertional angina. Prolonged pain following exertion probably has the same significance especially if pain is not relieved or only slightly relieved by sublingual nitroglycerin.

The risk of unstable angina declines exponentially following the onset of symptoms. The major risk is in the first 5 days, and the risk rapidly approaches that of stable angina pectoris by 4–6 weeks after onset of symptoms.[14] Patients who present during symptoms or within hours after symptom onset are at highest risk, while patients presenting after some weeks have probably passed through the time window of major increased risk of adverse outcome.

Other indicators of high risk include any manifestation of poor left ventricular function (for example a third heart sound), especially if associated with left heart failure (for example, crackles in the lung fields). Any evidence of haemodynamic embarrassment such as hypotension or new mitral regurgitation also indicates high risk. The ECG manifestations of high risk include dynamic ST depression of ≥ 1 mm, dynamic T wave normalization or peaking, and deep symmetrical T wave inversion in multiple leads (usually after pain. See Fig. 60.1).[11,15,16]

Patients at highest risk of events such as those with ongoing pain, dynamic ST segment shift, or any haemodynamic embarrassment, should be admitted to a CCU. Patients at low risk such as those with new onset effort angina or crescendo effort angina with a normal or unchanged ECG probably do not require admission and can be evaluated as outpatients. Those with intermediate risk, including patients in whom chest pain has resolved or with lesser degrees of ST change, can be treated in a step-down unit. The choice between management in a CCU

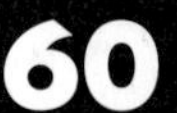

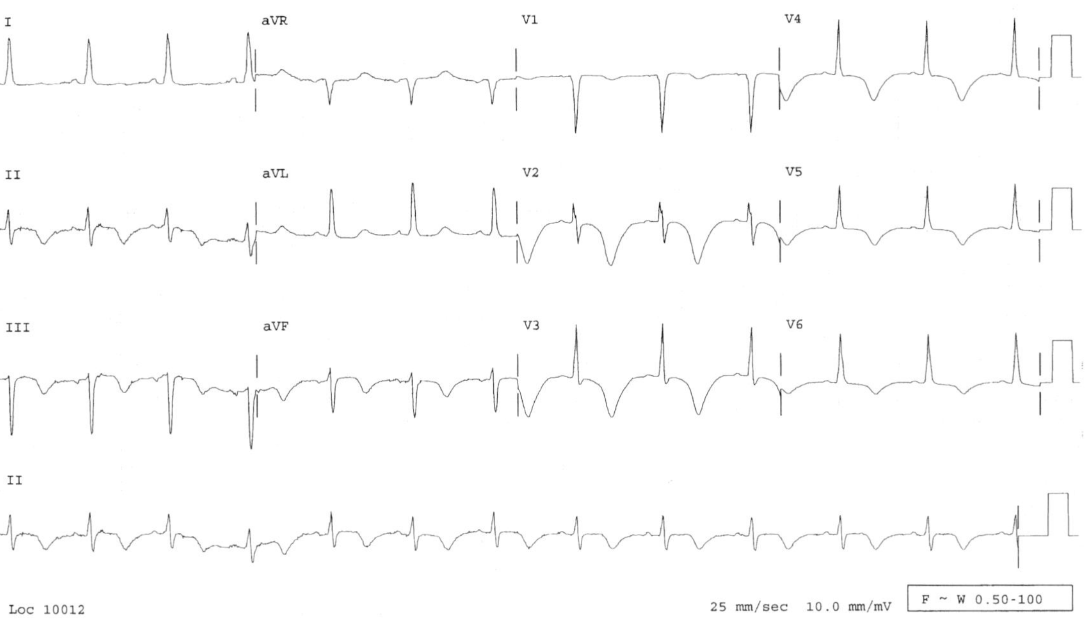

Fig. 60.1 Deep symmetrical T wave inversion in a patient with unstable angina. CKMB showed no evidence of myocardial necrosis.

or intermediate care unit is somewhat arbitrary, but there are certainly patients who do not require admission to a CCU. The following chapter will limit discussion to those patients in whom risk is considered high enough to warrant admission to hospital.

A number of predictive algorithms that can be implemented on small microprocessors or personal computers have been developed as an aid to clinical decision making.[11,17] Most of these have elements designed to indicate the likelihood that symptoms are due to myocardial ischaemia or infarction as well as elements that stratify the risk. The elements include most of the criteria listed above, and have been trialled with varying degrees of success, but have not become part of routine practice.

Management goals

There are three major goals of management in patients with unstable angina:

- Relieve current symptoms
- Prevent the major adverse events—myocardial infarction and cardiac death
- Prevent recurrent angina/ischaemia.

In achieving these goals, it must be remembered that angina is the main symptomatic manifestation of ischaemia and is therefore best treated by measures which reduce or abolish ischaemia, rather than with analgesics. Because many episodes of ischaemia are silent, it is also important to prevent silent ischaemia and not just angina, although abolition of angina is a clue that silent ischaemia has also been reduced.

Treatment of angina is facilitated by a knowledge of the pathophysiology of rest ischaemia. This is rarely preceded by a rise in heart rate or blood pressure, indicating that ischaemia is not caused by an increase in myocardial oxygen demand.[12] The heart rate and blood pressure may rise secondarily in response to ischaemia and may worsen ischaemia, so anti-anginal drugs which reduce oxygen demand by reducing heart rate, blood pressure, left ventricular volume and contractility, are worthwhile. This is not sufficient, however, as transient ischaemia is caused by reductions in coronary blood flow resulting from platelet-rich mural thrombi with superimposed distal embolization or vasoconstriction.[18] Treatment must therefore be directed towards preventing platelet aggregation, thrombosis, and vasoconstriction.

The major adverse outcomes are due to thrombotic occlusion at active thrombotic lesions which usually restrict flow. Prevention of events certainly requires antithrombotic and antiplatelet therapy, and in addition may require revascularization by angioplasty or bypass surgery. Revascularization is not required in all patients, and logistics and resources are too limited to perform angiography and revascularization universally. These constraints require some method of risk stratification after admission to select those patients at highest risk who are most likely to benefit. Such high risk patients require angiography during admission. If revascularization is required it should ideally be performed prior to discharge, because of the exquisite time-dependence of risk.

Initial evaluation and treatment

General measures

Rest and reassurance, with sedation if required, underpin general treatment. While taking a brief history and performing a brief physical examination to ensure haemodynamic stability, a secure IV line should be placed, and a 12-lead ECG performed, within 10–20 minutes after presentation. Oxygen is often given by nasal prongs using low inspired oxygen concentration. While there is little evidence to suggest that this has any beneficial effect in the majority of patients who are not hypoxic, it does not appear to do any harm.

A full history and physical examination can then be performed as appropriate to exclude the other serious differential diagnoses. These include acute coronary occlusion (myocardial infarction), aortic dissection, ruptured or leaking thoracic aortic aneurysm, acute pericarditis, acute pulmonary embolism, pneumothorax, and oesophageal or intra-abdominal disease. Blood should also be taken for creatine kinase (CK) and subfraction estimation.

Anti-ischaemic therapy

For patients who still have pain, particularly if accompanied by dynamic ECG changes, anti-ischaemic therapy should be commenced immediately.

Nitroglycerin

Nitroglycerin 300–600 micrograms should be given sublingually or by spray (400 micrograms) in two doses, 5 minutes apart, watching the blood pressure before the next dose. Isosorbide dinitrate 5 mg sublingually can be substituted for nitroglycerin. If pain and/or ischaemia are not relieved, patients may benefit from IV nitroglycerin 2.5–5 micrograms/min. Some recommend titrating this rapidly in steps of 5–10 micrograms/min to reduce systolic blood pressure by 10–20 mmHg, though not to below 100 mmHg. Such rapid increases in nitroglycerin dose, however, are likely to induce early tolerance, which is one of the major problems with continuous nitroglycerin administration.

Nitroglycerin works through both vascular and platelet mechanisms. It has a vasodilator effect on large and small coronary arteries, relaxing the major epicardial arteries, and also the resistance vessels. Collateral flow to ischaemic areas is also increased. Venodilatation reduces LV diastolic pressure and so enhances blood flow, particularly collateral flow, by widening the net driving pressure for coronary flow. This effect is in addition to reduction of LV dimension and thus myocardial oxygen demand through preload reduction. Afterload is reduced by relaxing the central arteries as well as by arteriolar dilatation. Nitroglycerin has an additional anti-aggregatory action on platelets, and more importantly promotes de-aggregation of platelets.[19]

Intravenous beta blockade

If pain or ischaemia persists after IV nitroglycerin and there are no contraindications to IV beta blocker (blood pressure < 100, heart rate < 60/minute, atrioventricular [AV] block, asthma or obstructive airways disease), then this should be given, particularly if there is tachycardia or hypertension. The beta blockers available are metoprolol, atenolol, and propranolol. Metoprolol is most commonly used and can be given as small IV bolus doses according to the following protocol: 5 mg over 2 minutes, followed at 5 minutes by 1 mg bolus doses every minute up to a maximum of 15 mg, stopping when the heart rate is < 60 or blood pressure is < 100 mmHg or if râles or bronchospasm develops.

Intravenous morphine

If chest pain is unrelieved by rapidly acting nitrates, morphine 2–5 mg can be given intravenously unless there is significant hypotension. If blood pressure is elevated or tachycardia is present, then beta blockers may be used first.

Anti-thrombotic therapy

Aspirin

Four randomized placebo-controlled studies have shown individually and in meta-analysis that aspirin is of major benefit in all patients with unstable angina.[20–23] Overall there is an approximate 50% reduction in both death and infarction at 3 months which is maintained at 1 and 2 years. By analogy with acute infarction studies, the aspirin should be started on admission. The first dose is usually 300 mg of a rapidly absorbed formulation such as glycine aspirin, which can be dissolved in the mouth. Subsequent doses vary between 75 and 300 mg per day and appear equally effective in trials. Practically speaking, the daily dose is usually given as a 100 mg tablet or half of a 300 mg tablet.

The main drawbacks are gastrointestinal intolerance and bleeding, again mainly from the gastrointestinal tract, although this is minimized with the low doses of aspirin given. There is also a higher incidence of perioperative bleeding and increased transfusion requirement if coronary artery bypass grafting is performed while patients are on aspirin. Some surgeons recommend cessation of aspirin with continuation of heparin prior to surgery. Otherwise aspirin should be continued indefinitely.

For patients intolerant of aspirin, ticlopidine can be substituted. This drug has also been shown effective in trials, but it takes 3–4 days to achieve a therapeutic effect.[24] During this time, patients should be covered by heparin.

Heparin

In hospitalized patients judged to be at intermediate or high risk, full intravenous heparin has been shown to reduce the combined endpoint of in-hospital infarction or death when compared to placebo.[22] A pooled analysis of trials suggests that heparin plus aspirin is more effective than aspirin alone,[25] and this was confirmed by extension of one of the studies used in the pooled analysis.[26]

Heparin should be given as a bolus dose plus infusion according to body weight, as shown in Table 60.1.

The activated partial thromboplastin time (APTT) should be checked 6-hourly for 24 hours and then daily, to keep it between 2 and 3 times baseline. A protocol for responding to APTT outside this range (approximately 60–90 seconds) is given in Table 60.2.

The heparin infusion should be continued for 3–5 days if there is no pain recurrence, or until revascularization. When heparin has been discontinued abruptly in the absence of concurrent aspirin therapy, rebound or reactivation of ischaemia has been observed with a peak at about 10 hours after cessation.[27] For this reason, heparin should not be ceased unless aspirin has been previously commenced.

The main adverse effect of heparin is haemorrhage, with intra-cerebral haemorrhage the most feared. Major bleeds, including retro-peritoneal haematoma and bleeds into the groin area, occur in about 3% of patients on combinations of heparin and aspirin. Another problem is heparin-induced thrombocytopenic syndrome (HITS),[28] which usually occurs with longer durations of heparin administration. The thrombocytopenia responds to cessation of heparin, although occasionally this may also produce a hypercoagulable state. Heparinoids can be substituted with no cross-sensitization in the majority of cases.

Thrombolytic agents

A number of small studies and one large study[29] of thrombolytic drugs in unstable angina have shown no benefit in meta-

Table 60.1 Adjustment of heparin therapy by body weight

Body weight	Bolus dose	Infusion rate
<63 kg	4000 u	900 u/hr
63–77 kg	5000 u	1000 u/hr
>77 kg	6000 u	1100 u/hr

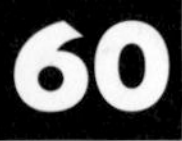

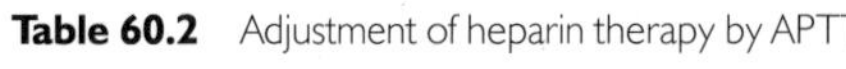

Table 60.2 Adjustment of heparin therapy by APTT

APTT	Bolus dose	Stop infusion for .... min	Change infusion rate	Repeat APTT
<50 sec	2500 u	nil	+200 u/hr	6 hr
50–59 sec	nil	nil	+100 u/hr	6 hr
60–90 sec	nil	nil	no change	next due
91–120 sec	nil	30 min	–100 u/hr	6 hr
>120 sec	nil	60 min	–200 u/hr	6 hr

analysis in reducing infarction or death.[14] One small study showed reduced ischaemic episodes in patients with frequent recurrence of angina. In general there is no place for thrombolytic therapy in patients with unstable angina.[30]

Invasive options

Patients with continuing pain despite nitrates, beta blockers and anti-thrombotic drugs may be considered for urgent angiography with a view to angioplasty, or may be improved by placement of a percutaneous intra-aortic balloon counterpulsation pump, particularly if there is haemodynamic decompensation. These options are required acutely for only a very small minority of patients.

Management after admission

General measures

Patients are kept at bed-rest initially with early active mobilization unless this is interrupted by recurrence of chest pain. 12-lead ECGs should be repeated on a daily basis, with regular CK measurements and MB subfractions over the first 48 hours, as T wave inversion may take some time to develop, and small enzyme leaks may be detected. Troponin-T is a much more sensitive guide to necrosis, and may have greater prognostic information than CK.[30a,30b]

When ST or T wave changes are noted on admission, particularly if there are transient ST or T wave changes during pain, then continuous monitoring of leads showing the most obvious changes is worthwhile for detection of silent ischaemia. In these selected high risk patients, recurrent ischaemia whether symptomatic or silent denotes a much higher risk and requires aggressive treatment.

Because of the important prognostic information contained in a measure of LV function, it is important to assess this non-invasively or invasively during admission. This can be done by echocardiography at the bedside or by gated heart pool scan, or by left ventricular angiography. Patients with reduced ventricular function should be considered for revascularization.

Anti-thrombotic drugs and nitrates

Oral aspirin and intravenous heparin should be continued throughout the admission, as detailed above under initial treatment. An alternative to full IV heparin therapy is subcutaneous low molecular weight heparin given twice daily, with studies confirming efficacy recently completed.[30] Other new products under investigation are the direct anti-thrombins such as hirudin and hirulog, and the platelet IIb/IIIa receptor antagonists. A role for the IIb/IIIa antagonists has now been demonstrated in reducing major cardiac events following angioplasty.[50] The major problem with use of these drugs is bleeding, particularly when combined with both aspirin and heparin.

Intravenous nitroglycerin should be continued for only 24–48 hours and then should be slowly weaned unless pain recurs. Abrupt cessation of nitroglycerin may produce rebound ischaemia, or even infarction, and must be avoided. The dose of nitroglycerin should be kept low—between 2.5 and 10 micrograms per minute—to avoid tolerance. One approach to reduce tolerance has been to co-administer n-acetylcysteine intravenously, and this has been reported to reduce myocardial infarction.[31,32]

Long-acting oral nitrates or cutaneous nitrates may be commenced before stopping IV nitroglycerin, or may be used in its place. The formulations used are isosorbide dinitrate 20 mg three times daily in eccentric dose, isosorbide mononitrate sustained action 60–120 mg once daily, or transcutaneous patches once daily. These medications are given with a nitrate-free or nitrate-low period to prevent tolerance, but patients are not covered during this time.

Rapidly acting nitrates should be given promptly for recurrent pain. When IV nitroglycerin is being used, a bolus of 600 micrograms given via the infusion pump over 1 minute can be very effective. Nursing staff should be able to respond quickly and record 12-lead ECGs during pain, particularly when there is some doubt about the diagnosis.

Beta blockers

These drugs should be given for interval therapy to prevent recurrent ischaemia unless there are contraindications, as listed above. The $beta_1$ selective blockers, metoprolol (25–100 mg three times daily) and atenolol (25–50 mg 12-hourly) are most commonly used. The dose should be titrated to achieve a resting heart rate of about 60 per minute. There is some evidence that they prevent infarction, although this is not conclusive.[33–35] Their use is also justified by analogy with the trials of myocardial infarction, where they reduce death and reinfarction.

Calcium antagonists

These drugs may be used to prevent ischaemia in patients who cannot take a beta blocker. Both verapamil (80–120 mg three times daily) and diltiazen (60–120 mg three times daily) are useful as single agents, and have been shown to reduce recurrent ischaemic episodes in unstable angina.[36] There is no convincing evidence to suggest any beneficial effect on death or infarction.[35,37] Nifedipine given alone has been shown to be deleterious as it appears to increase the risk of myocardial infarction.[34] However, when patients develop unstable angina or have recurrent pain while on a beta blocker, then nifedipine has been shown useful as an additional agent. The dose should be 10–20 mg twice daily of long acting tablets or 30–60 mg once daily of the sustained release formulation.

In the small subset of patients with 'variant angina' (or Prinzmetal angina), defined as recurrent ischaemic pain at rest accompanied by transient ST segment elevation, the calcium antagonists are particularly effective, because ischaemia in this case is due primarily to coronary artery spasm.[38] The main historical clue is recurrent nocturnal angina waking the patient in the early morning, frequently at the same time each day. Coronary spasm, however, can also occur during exertion,[39] may be accompanied by other ECG changes including ST depression and T wave peaking, and can occur in the setting of either minor coronary disease or more severe atheromatous narrowing.[38]

The major adverse effects of calcium antagonists are hypotension and heart failure (all drugs), and AV block or sinus bradycardia (verapamil and diltiazem).

Angiography and revascularization

Angiography

There are three broad indications for performing coronary angiography in patients with unstable angina:

- symptomatic—as a prelude to revascularization for recurrent symptoms despite medical therapy (this is the most frequent indication)
- prognostic—to detect high risk anatomy which would benefit from revascularization regardless of symptoms
- diagnostic—to confirm normal coronary arteries in patients presenting frequently but considered low risk or non-ischaemic.

Overall, studies utilizing coronary angiography show normal arteries or minor coronary artery disease in approximately 10–20% of patients, while 20–25% have 3-vessel or left main disease. Culprit lesions are often eccentric with irregular borders, and occasionally filling defects consistent with thrombus are seen, particularly if angiography is performed soon after pain.

Patients considered high risk should probably have angiography during admission unless there are co-morbid conditions or other patient-related considerations which preclude revascularization. Those at intermediate risk with a history of prior bypass surgery or angioplasty should also probably undergo angiography during admission.

The decision on whether to perform angiography on intermediate and low risk patients depends on the availability of facilities. Over the last 10 years, clinical practice has become increasingly aggressive, with early angiography and revascularization performed more frequently. There are no adequate comparisons of strategies using early aggressive investigation or early conservative approaches with the possible exception of the TIMI-IIIb study.[29] This was a large study comparing early invasive with early conservative therapy, although the 'conservative' approach still led to 64% of patients undergoing angiography and 49%, revascularization, which in many parts of the world would be considered relatively aggressive. In that study, there were no differences in mortality or infarction rates between the two strategies, although the 'conservative' group had longer hospital stays and more angina at follow-up.

The decision to perform angiography in intermediate and low risk patients can be based on non-invasive stress tests scheduled before discharge, as these appear helpful in stratifying risk. Testing is safe when patients have been free of angina for 72 hours, although some physicians will accept 48 hours. The most useful test is an exercise stress 12-lead ECG, usually performed using a sub-maximal protocol, stopping with the development of ischaemic ECG changes, chest pain, or attainment of 85% of predicted maximal heart rate.[15,40–45] Patients who develop ischaemia at low work levels (< 5 METS) should be referred for revascularization. Patients with no ischaemic changes but low work capacity, or ischaemia at high work levels, represent an intermediate risk group who can either be managed conservatively or referred for angiography. Patients with uninterpretable ECGs or with physical limitations to exercise can be referred for dipyridamole or adenosine stress thallium imaging.

Revascularization

Patients with pain unresponsive to medical therapy are usually referred for revascularization by percutaneous transluminal coronary angioplasty (PTCA) or bypass surgery. In very early studies before the advent of revascularization, these patients had a very high mortality, and it is likely that such patients are benefited prognostically by revascularization. In the remaining patients for whom revascularization is not required for symptoms, bypass surgery has been shown to improve prognosis in those with left main disease, and three vessel disease in association with left ventricular dysfunction.[46,47] Revascularization in patients with lesser disease has not been shown to be of prognostic benefit, although in stable angina, 2-vessel disease involving the left anterior descending artery probably benefits from surgery. Registry studies suggest the same benefit might be seen in unstable angina.[48]

For both PTCA and bypass surgery, unstable angina carries a slightly greater risk of peri-procedural events than stable angina. The risk of acute closure during PTCA is reduced by prior heparin therapy for 3–6 days, probably by reducing the amount of thrombus present, and this should be taken into consideration in decisions regarding the timing of PTCA.[49] Complications are also reduced by pre-treatment with platelet IIb/IIIa receptor antagonists.[50]

There have been no controlled studies comparing PTCA with medical therapy in unstable angina. In some studies comparing PTCA with bypass surgery, there appear to be similar infarction and death rates with both modalities,[51] although no studies have specifically examined unstable patients. A Duke database registry study suggests that both 3-vessel disease and 2-vessel disease may be improved by surgery,[48] although in non-randomized studies it is very difficult to control adequately for factors leading to medical rather than surgical decisions. This study found a slight advantage for bypass surgery in 3-vessel disease and severe 2-vessel disease, with a slight advantage for PTCA for less severe 2-vessel disease. No study has ever shown any prognostic benefit from revascularization in 1-vessel disease regardless of which artery is involved.

The current recommendation should therefore be to advise revascularization only when symptoms require it, or for high risk anatomy in patients whose symptoms have been controlled. The remaining patients can be managed conservatively without undue risk of adverse events using non-invasive testing to stratify risk. The alternative strategy of early angiography and revascularization might be justifiable on the basis of shorter hospital stay or less pain at follow-up if it can be demonstrated beneficial in a future cost-benefit analysis study.

Therapy at discharge

General measures such as counselling, risk factor reduction, and rehabilitation—particularly for anxious patients—should be undertaken in a fashion analogous to myocardial infarction. Cessation of smoking and reduction of cholesterol have both been shown to improve long-term survival.

All patients should be discharged on aspirin indefinitely, and most patients who have not been revascularized will also be on beta blockers and/or calcium antagonists with or without long acting nitrates. Patients should be instructed in the appropriate use of rapid acting nitrates and should be given a supply to take home. They should also be instructed in what to do in the event of recurrent chest pain.

Because of the significant increased risk of death or infarction or recurrent unstable angina requiring re-admission in the period following discharge, it has been suggested that additional anticoagulant therapy should be maintained for an extended period of up to 3 months following discharge.[25] A number of trials using low dose warfarin or self-injected low molecular weight heparin in addition to aspirin are currently in progress.

References

1. Braunwald E. Unstable angina. A classification. Circulation 1989; 80: 410–41
2. Davies M, Thomas A. Thrombosis and acute coronary-artery lesions in sudden cardiac ischemic death. N Engl J Med 1984; 310: 1137–40
3. Falk E. Morphologic features of unstable atherothrombotic plaques underlying acute coronary syndromes. Am J Cardiol 1989; 63: 114E–20E
4. Fuster V, Fuster V, Badimon L, Badimon JJ, Cheseboro JH. The pathogenesis of coronary artery disease and the acute coronary syndromes. 2. N Engl J Med 1992; 326: 242–50, 310–18
5. Mizuno K, Satomura K, Miyamoto A et al. Angioscopic evaluation of coronary-artery thrombi in acute coronary syndromes. N Engl J Med 1992; 326: 287–91
6. Fuster V, Stein B, Ambrose JA, Badimon L, Badimon JJ, Chesebro JH. Atherosclerotic plaque rupture and thrombosis. Evolving concepts. Circulation 1990; 82(Suppl. II): II47–59
7. Annex B, Denning S, Channon K et al. Differential expression of tissue factor protein in directional atherectomy specimens from patients with stable and unstable coronary syndromes. Circulation 1995; 91: 619–22
8. Wilcox I, Freedman SB, McCredie RJ, Carter GS, Kelly DT, Harris PJ. Risk of adverse outcome in patients admitted to the coronary care unit with suspected unstable angina pectoris. Am J Cardiol 1989; 64: 845–8
9. Pryor DB, Shaw L, McCants CB et al. Value of the history and physical in identifying patients at increased risk for coronary artery disease. Ann Intern Med 1993; 118: 81–90
10. Rouan GW, Lee TH, Cook EF, Brand DA, Weisberg MC, Goldman L. Clinical characteristics and outcome of acute myocardial infarction in patients with initially normal or nonspecific electrocardiograms (a report from the Multicenter Chest Pain study). Am J Cardiol 1989; 64: 1087–92
11. Jayes R Jr, Beshansky JR, D'Agostino RB, Selker HP. Do patients' coronary risk factor reports predict acute cardiac ischemia in the emergency department? A multicenter study. J Clin Epidemiol 1992; 45: 621–6
12. Chierchia S, Lazzari M, Freedman S, Brunelli C, Maseri A. Impairment of myocardial perfusion and function during painless myocardial ischaemia. J Am Coll Cardiol 1983; 1: 924–30
13. Califf RM, Mark DB, Harrell F Jr et al. Importance of clinical measures of ischemia in the prognosis of patients with documented coronary artery disease. J Am Coll Cardiol 1988; 11: 20–6
14. Braunwald E, Mark D, Jones D et al. Unstable angina: diagnosis and management. US Department of Health and Human Services. Clinical Practice Guideline 1994; 10
15. Wilcox I, Freedman SB, Allman KC et al. Prognostic significance of a predischarge exercise test in risk stratification after unstable angina pectoris. J Am Coll Cardiol 1991; 18: 677–83
16. Karlson BW, Herlitz J, Pettersson P, Hallgren P, Strombom U, Hjalmarson A. One-year prognosis in patients hospitalized with a history of unstable angina pectoris. Clin Cardiol 1993; 16: 397–402
17. Goldman L, Cook EF, Brand DA et al. A computer protocol to predict myocardial infarction in emergency department patients with chest pain. N Engl J Med 1988; 318: 797–803
18. Coller BS, Folts JD, Scudder LE, Smith SR. Antithrombotic effect of a monoclonal antibody to the platelet glycoprotein IIb/IIIa receptor in an experimental animal model. Blood 1986; 68: 783–6

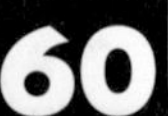

19. Chirkov YY, Naujalis JI, Sage RE, Horowitz JD. Antiplatelet effects of nitroglycerin in healthy subjects and in patients with stable angina pectoris. J Cardiovasc Pharmacol 1993; 21: 384–9
20. Lewis H, Davis J, Archibald D et al. Protective effects of aspirin against acute myocardial infarction and death in men with unstable angina. Results of a Veterans Administration Cooperative trial. N Engl J Med 1983; 309: 396–403
21. Cairns JA, Gent M, Singer J et al. Aspirin, sulfinpyrazone, or both in unstable angina. Results of a Canadian multicenter trial. N Engl J Med 1985; 313: 1369–75
22. Theroux P, Ouimet H, McCans J et al. Aspirin, heparin, or both to treat acute unstable angina. N Engl J Med 1988; 319: 1105–11
23. Risk of myocardial infarction and death during treatment with low dose aspirin and intravenous heparin in men with unstable coronary artery disease. The RISC group. Lancet 1990; 336: 827–30
24. Balsano F, Rizzon P, Violi F et al. Antiplatelet treatment with ticlopidine in unstable angina. A controlled multicenter clinical trial. The Studio della Ticlopidina nell'Angina Instabile group. Circulation 1990; 82: 17–26
25. Cohen M, Adams PC, Parry G et al. Combination antithrombotic therapy in unstable rest angina and non-Q-wave infarction in nonprior aspirin users. Primary end points analysis from the ATACS trial. Antithrombotic Therapy in Acute Coronary Syndromes research group. Circulation 1994; 89: 81–8
26. Theroux P, Waters D, Qiu S, McCans J, de Guise P, Juneau M. Aspirin versus heparin to prevent myocardial infarction during the acute phase of unstable angina. Circulation 1993; 88: 2045–8
27. Theroux P, Waters D, Lam J, Juneau M, McCans J. Reactivation of unstable angina after the discontinuation of heparin. N Engl J Med 1992; 327: 141–5
28. Aster R. Heparin-induced thrombocytopenia and thrombosis. N Engl J Med 1995; 332: 1374–6
29. The TIMI-IIIb Investigators. Effects of tissue plasminogen activator and a comparison of early invasive and conservative strategies in unstable angina and non-Q-wave myocardial infarction. Results of the TIMI-IIIb Trial. Thrombolysis in myocardial ischemia. Circulation 1994; 89: 1545–56
30. Saran RK, Bhandari K, Narain VS et al. Intravenous streptokinase in the management of a subset of patients with unstable angina: a randomized controlled trial. Int J Cardiol 1990; 28: 209–13
30a. Hamm CW, Ravkilde J, Gerhardt W et al. The prognostic value of serum traponin T in unstable angina. N Engl J Med 1992; 327: 146–50
30b. Lindahl B, Venge P, Wallentin L, and the FRISC study group. Relation between troponin T and the risk of subsequent cardiac events in unstable coronary artery disease. Circulation 1996; 93: 1651–57.
30c. See above
31. Horowitz JD, Henry CA, Syrjanen ML et al. Combined use of nitroglycerin and N-acetylcysteine in the management of unstable angina pectoris. Circulation 1988; 77: 787–94
32. Horowitz JD. Role of nitrates in unstable angina pectoris. Am J Cardiol 1992; 70: 64B–71B
33. Gottlieb SO, Weisfeldt ML, Ouyang P et al. Effect of the addition of propranolol to therapy with nifedipine for unstable angina pectoris: a randomized, double-blind, placebo-controlled trial. Circulation 1986; 73: 331–7
34. Lubsen J, Tijssen JG. Efficacy of nifedipine and metoprolol in the early treatment of unstable angina in the coronary care unit: findings from the Holland Interuniversity Nifedipine/metoprolol Trial (HINT). Am J Cardiol 1987; 60: 18A–25A
35. Yusuf S, Wittes J, Friedman L. Overview of results of randomized clinical trials in heart disease. II. Unstable angina, heart failure, primary prevention with aspirin, and risk factor modification. JAMA 1988; 260: 2259–63
36. Theroux P, Taeymans Y, Morissette D, Bosch X, Pelletier GB, Waters DD. A randomized study comparing propranolol and diltiazem in the treatment of unstable angina. J Am Coll Cardiol 1985; 5: 717–22
37. Held PH, Yusuf S, Furberg CD. Calcium channel blockers in acute myocardial infarction and unstable angina: an overview. Br Med J 1989; 299: 1187–92
38. Freedman S, Richmond D, Kelly D. Clinical studies of patients with coronary artery spasm. Am J Cardiol 1983; 52: 67
39. Freedman S, Dunn R, Richmond D, Kelly D. Coronary artery spasm on exercise: treatment with verapamil. Circulation 1981; 64: 68–75
40. Swahn E, Areskog M, Berglund U, Walfridsson H, Wallentin L. Predictive importance of clinical findings and a predischarge exercise test in patients with suspected unstable coronary artery disease. Am J Cardiol 1987; 59: 208–14
41. Severi S, Orsini E, Marraccini P, Michelassi C, L'Abbate A. The basal electrocardiogram and the exercise stress test in assessing prognosis in patients with unstable angina. Eur Heart J 1988; 9: 441–6
42. Madsen JK, Thomsen BL, Mellemgaard K, Hansen JF. Independent prognostic risk factors for patients referred because of suspected acute

myocardial infarction without confirmed diagnosis. Prognosis after discharge in relation to medical history and non-invasive investigations. Eur Heart J 1988; 9: 610–8

43. Krone RJ, Dwyer E Jr, Greenberg H, Miller JP, Gillespie JA. Risk stratification in patients with first non-Q wave infarction: limited value of the early low level exercise test after uncomplicated infarcts. The Multicenter Post-Infarction Research Group. J Am Coll Cardiol 1989; 14: 31–7
44. Nyman I, Wallentin L, Areskog M, Areskog NH, Swahn E. Risk stratification by early exercise testing after an episode of unstable coronary artery disease. The RISC study group. Int J Cardiol 1993; 39: 131–7
45. Moss AJ, Goldstein RE, Hall WJ et al. Detection and significance of myocardial ischemia in stable patients after recovery from an acute coronary event. Multicenter Myocardial Ischemia Research Group. JAMA 1993; 269: 2379–85
46. Luchi RJ, Scott SM, Deupree RH. Comparison of medical and surgical treatment for unstable angina pectoris. Results of a Veterans Administration Cooperative Study. N Engl J Med 1987; 316: 977–84
47. Sharma GV, Deupree RH, Khuri SF, Parisi AF, Luchi RJ, Scott SM. Coronary bypass surgery improves survival in high-risk unstable angina. Results of a Veterans Administration Cooperative study with an 8-year follow-up. Veterans Administration Unstable Angina Cooperative Study Group. Circulation 1991; 84(Suppl.): III260–7
48. Mark DB, Nelson CL, Califf RM et al. Continuing evolution of therapy for coronary artery disease. Initial results from the era of coronary angioplasty. Circulation 1994; 89: 2015–25
49. Topol EJ. Integration of anticoagulation, thrombolysis and coronary angioplasty for unstable angina pectoris. Am J Cardiol 1991; 68: 136B–44B
50. Use of a monoclonal antibody directed against the platelet glycoprotein IIb/IIIa receptor in high-risk coronary angioplasty. The EPIC Investigation. N Engl J Med 1994; 330: 956–61
51. Coronary angioplasty versus coronary artery bypass surgery: the Randomized Intervention Treatment of Angina (RITA) trial. Lancet 1993; 341: 573–80

61 Other causes of chest pain

John T Dowling

The coronary care unit serves an important role in the diagnosis and treatment of patients with chest pain which may simulate myocardial infarction or acute coronary syndromes.[1] A patient may use 'chest pain' to describe distressing sensations which other patients may refer to as tightness, pressure, numbness, emptiness, burning, choking, pin prick, nausea, indigestion or severe ache. The word 'chest' can also be very vague and encompass the epigastrium, hypochondrium, breast tissue, suprasternal notch, shoulders or axilla.

History taking, although time-consuming, should be precise (see Ch. 11) so that the cause of pain can be confidently managed initially as either 'SERIOUS/URGENT' or 'BENIGN/CHRONIC'. Life-threatening disorders are then treated promptly and the benign or chronic causes of pain do not lead to frightening, painful, dangerous or expensive investigations and treatment. In doubtful cases the serious alternative should be pursued.

The *context* of the chest pain (for example, the patient's age, sex and past social and family histories) may influence the significance of the pain markedly. Physical examination and simple tests can be invaluable in some instances.

Serious/urgent causes

Serious/urgent causes of chest pain can be intrathoracic or subdiaphragmatic, as listed in the information box.

Co-existing clinical features strongly favouring a serious cause include sweating, hypotension, severe pain, pallor and cyanosis.

Pulmonary embolism

There may be retrosternal pain of sudden onset with dyspnoea and often cyanosis, tachycardia, haemoptysis and hypotension. The context may be postpartum, post-operative state, presence of severe right heart failure or deep vein thrombosis (see Ch. 72). Simple tests include estimation of blood gases, chest X-ray and ventilation perfusion scan. The electrocardiogram (ECG) may be helpful if changes of acute cor pulmonale are present.

Acute aortic dissection

The pain is typically severe and may be described as tearing (see Ch. 76). It is characteristically very severe at the onset, in contrast to myocardial infarction where the pain may be mild at the onset and build up to more severe pain. The pain can be retrosternal but is more likely to be interscapular.

Pneumothorax

The pain may be unilateral but mediastinal pneumothorax can

Serious causes of chest pain other than myocardial infarction

Intrathoracic
- pulmonary embolism
- aortic dissection
- pneumothorax
- oesophageal rupture

Subdiaphragmatic
- perforation of peptic ulcer
- cholecystitis
- pancreatitis

produce retrosternal pain. The pain is of sudden onset and often pleuritic in nature. Physical signs are frequently absent in a small pneumothorax but in a larger or tension pneumothorax, hyper-resonance, diminished breath sounds and deviation of the trachea may be detected. Dyspnoea, cyanosis and hypotension may ensue. Often there is a history of previous pneumothorax, recent chest injury or known bullous emphysema. Sometimes pneumothorax follows procedures such as subclavian venepuncture. Simple tests include chest X-ray and blood gases. In most cases spontaneous resolution will occur and this should be documented with serial chest X-rays. Tension pneumothorax with respiratory distress and hypoxaemia will require urgent relief with an intercostal catheter.

Oesophageal rupture

Oesophageal rupture or perforation can produce severe central chest pain with sweating, cyanosis and shock developing. Dysphagia may have been present and rupture usually follows oesophageal instrumentation, carcinoma of the oesophagus or severe vomiting. If pain accompanies haematemesis without rupture of the oesophagus, a tear in the lower oesophagus may be present (Mallory–Weiss syndrome).

Oesophageal rupture with leakage of gastro-esophageal contents into the mediastimum can be rapidly lethal if untreated. As soon as the diagnosis is suspected, urgent thoracic surgery consultation should be obtained with a view to early oesophageal repair.

Perforated peptic ulcer, cholecystitis and pancreatitis

Upper abdominal injuries simulating myocardial infarction are usually accompanied by abdominal signs such as guarding and tenderness and generalized signs such as fever. The ECG in cholecystitis may show T wave inversion especially in the inferior leads.

Benign/chronic causes

The many benign causes of chest pain are often elusive and frustrating to treat especially if the patient is very anxious, is perceived to have a high likelihood of coronary artery disease or has an abnormal ECG. The major causes can be grouped into musculo-skeletal, neurological, oesophageal, pericardial and functional (psychiatric) categories.

Musculo-skeletal

Musculo-skeletal causes include cramps, ligamentous strain and inflammation of the costochondral or sternochondral junctions (Tietze's syndrome or costochondritis). Localized swelling and tenderness may be present and pain (often exacerbated by arm and chest movements) may quickly resolve with injection of local anaesthetic. Treatment is with oral analgesics and, occasionally, non-steroidal anti-inflammatory drugs.

Neurological

Neurological causes include compression of nerves at or near the cervical or upper thoracic vertebrae ('radicular syndromes') and inflammation of intercostal nerves (for example, herpes zoster, the pain preceding the rash by a few days). Post-herpetic pain can be severe and may require potent analgesics, carbemazapine, or occasionally the use of antidepressant drugs. Radicular syndromes may be from serious spinal column disease and produce severe arm pain.

Oesophageal

Oesophageal causes are probably most commonly confused with ischaemic cardiac pain because older patients tend to be affected and because pain can be severe, often at rest, relieved by nitrates and radiate to the jaw.[2] The relief with nitrates is sometimes more delayed, for example 15 minutes, in contrast to the near-immediate relief with angina. The difficulty in distinguishing angina from reflux oesophagitis is heightened by the lowering of the anginal threshold by oesophageal reflux.[3] Antecedent symptoms of dysphagia and oesophageal reflux are common and associated symptoms such as belching, regurgitation of stomach contents, epigastric pain and waterbrash may point to an oesophageal rather than cardiac cause. Endoscopy and measurement of oesophageal pressure may be required to establish the diagnosis[2] but if the clinical suspicion is strong, initial treatment should be commenced with antacids and H2 antagonists.[4] Endoscopy cannot be safely performed until myocardial ischaemia has been ruled out (see Ch. 74). Some drugs used for coronary heart disease, such as calcium channel blockers and aspirin, may exacerbate reflux oesophagitis, and their use may need to be reconsidered in patients with oesophageal symptoms.[5]

Pericarditis

Pericarditis may cause severe chest pain, especially if the neighbouring pleura is inflamed. Viruses, especially Coxsackie B group, are a well-recognized cause of pericarditis. Other causes of pericarditis are summarized in the information box.

Causes of pericarditis

- Idiopathic
- Viral
  - Coxsackie
  - Infectious mononucleosis
- Post-myocardial infarction
  - Early
  - Late (Dressler's)
- Uraemic
- Neoplastic
  - Lung
  - Mesothelioma
  - Breast
- Autoimmune
  - Acute rheumatic fever
  - Post-cardiotomy
  - Lupus
  - Rheumatoid
- Trauma
  - Post cardiac surgery
- Drugs
- Tuberculosis

Clinical features

A pericardial friction rub, with or without pleural component, is usual. The pain and rub are characteristically altered by change in posture and breathing. Pericardial pain may radiate to the arms, back, upper abdomen, tips of the shoulders or to the neck. The pericardial rub may be evanescent, varying from absent to loud from examination to examination and sometimes between observers. It is important to listen in different phases of respiration and in different postures, and to press firmly to hear the rub more clearly and to avoid artefacts from contact with the skin and stethoscope.[6] Because of the evanescence of the rub it is important to document the location, character and loudness of the rub when it is heard.

Causes

Viral pericarditis is the most common acute cause of pericarditis. There may be a history of non-specific viral type illness within the preceding few weeks. The pain of pericarditis following myocardial infarction may be the initial presentation of the patient with acute myocardial infarction. Other causes of pericarditis are usually readily identified by the associated clinical condition, although the possibility of tuberculosis should always be considered when the aetiology of pericarditis is not obvious. Pericarditis occurring weeks after myocardial infarction (Dressler's syndrome) or after cardiac surgery (post cardiotomy syndrome) is now very uncommon. It entails typical pain of pericarditis, leukocytosis, fever and ST segment elevation and may be associated with more generalized serositis including pleurisy.

Diagnosis

The ECG in acute pericarditis usually shows ST segment elevation (concave upwards like a saddle) in numerous leads. In some instances there is reciprocal depression in opposite leads. As the inflammation subsides ST segments return to baseline and T-waves become inverted. It may be difficult to distinguish ST segment elevation due to pericarditis from the normal variant of 'early repolarization'. A variety of criteria have been suggested to distinguish the two.[8] Of the various criteria, the most reliable is the variable nature of the ST segment deviation in pericarditis compared with the constancy of serial ECG tracings in early repolarization. The ECG monitor frequently shows atrial ectopic beats and occasionally atrial fibrillation. These do not necessarily coincide with myocardial involvement and are explained by the contiguity of the pericardium and the superficial location of the sinus node. Arrhythmias are rare in the absence of underlying heart disease.[9] Acute pericarditis is frequently accompanied by minor elevations of myocardial enzymes.[10] Significant elevation of CKMB indicating associated myocarditis which may be linked with left ventricular dysfunction can cause diagnostic difficulty in distinguishing the episode from myocardial infarction.

Management

Most patients with acute pericarditis settle with oral analgesics

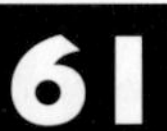

and bed-rest in 24–48 hours. Sometimes anti-inflammatory therapy is required with aspirin in moderately high doses of 900–1200 mg per day (in contrast to the low dose of 100–150 mg used for antithrombotic therapy) or a non-steroidal anti-inflammatory drug. There are no comparative studies of non-steroidal anti-inflammatory drugs (NSAIDS) for relief of pericarditis. Older drugs (indomethacin, ibuprofen) have been widely used but the newer NSAIDS are equally effective. If there is persistent pain and persistence of pericardial rub with evidence of fever and leukocytosis, oral corticosteroids may be necessary, i.e. prednisolone 50–60 mg per day for several days. A small proportion of patients with viral pericarditis may develop transient pericardial constriction or pericardial effusion.[7] Recurrence of pericardial pain in the weeks or months after an attack of viral pericarditis is relatively common. This can usually be controlled with the re-institution of non-steroidal anti-inflammatory drug therapy. It is important to warn patients that this may occur and that most cases are self-limiting and eventually settle within 6–12 months.[11,12]

'Functional' chest pain

'Functional' chest pain is common, often complicating anxiety, obsessive-compulsive disorders, depression, post-traumatic states or hyperventilation syndrome.[13,14] The diagnosis is by exclusion after careful history taking, examination of the chest and abdomen, chest X-ray and ECG. Symptoms of hyperventilation such as breathlessness, tingling, numbness or pins and needles in the fingers and around the mouth may be evident. If such symptoms had been present or are produced quickly during induced hyperventilation, hyperventilation syndrome may be the basis of the chest pain. Even 'functional' pains may have an organic cause for which no suitable diagnostic tests are yet available.[15] For instance, distension or spasm of the splenic flexure of the colon may produce a stabbing or prolonged ache or burning discomfort in the lower part of the left pectoral area. A patient with such symptoms can be provided with a positive explanation rather than being reassured unsatisfactorily by reference to a nebulous entity such as 'nerves' or 'imagination'.

References

1. Levine HJ. Difficult problems in the diagnosis of chest pain. Am Heart J 1980; 100: 406–18
2. Holloway RH, Orenstein SR. Gastro-oesophageal reflux disease in adults and children. Baillière's Clin Gastroenterol 1991; 5: 337–70
3. Davies HA, Rush EM, Lewis MJ et al. Oesophageal stimulation lowers angina thresholds. Lancet 1985; 1: 1011–4
4. Bell NJV, Hunt RH. Role of gastric acid suppression in the treatment of gastro-oesophageal reflux. Gut 1992; 33: 118–24
5. Richter JE, Castell DO. Drugs, foods and other substances in the causes and treatment of reflux oesophagitis. Med Clin Nth Amer 1981; 65: 1223–34
6. Spodick DH. Pericardial rub: prospective multiple observer investigations of pericardial friction rub in 100 patients. Am J Cardiol 1975; 35: 357–62
7. Permanyer-Miralda G, Sagrista-Sauleda J, Soler-Soler J. Primary acute pericardial disease: a prospective series of 231 consecutive patients. Am J Cardiol 1985; 56: 623–30
8. Ginzton LE, Laks MM. The differential diagnosis of acute pericarditis from the normal variant: new electrocardiographic criteria. Circulation 1982; 65: 1004–9
9. Spodick DH. Frequency of arrhythmias in acute pericarditis determined by Holter monitoring. Am J Cardiol 1984; 53: 842–5
10. Karjalainen J, Heikkila J. Acute pericarditis: myocardial enzyme release as evidence for myocarditis. Am Heart J 1986; 111: 546–52
11. Robinson T, Brigden W. Recurrent pericarditis. Br Med J 1968; 2: 272–5
12. Fowler NO, Harbin AD. Recurrent pericarditis: follow up of 31 patients. J Am Coll Cardiol 1986; 7: 300–5
13. Bass C, Chambers JB, Kiff P et al. Panic, anxiety and hyperventilation in patients with chest pain. Controlled Study. Quart J Med 1988; 69(260): 949–59
14. Beitman BD, Basha I, Flaker G et al. Atypical or non-anginal chest pain. Panic disorder or coronary artery disease? Arch Intern Med 1987; 147: 1548–52
15. Mayou R. Medically unexplained physical symptoms. Br Med J 1991; 303: 534–53

62 Atrial fibrillation

Eric G Whitford

Atrial fibrillation assessment and management

Atrial fibrillation is a disorganized and variable atrial rhythm. It is a very common cardiac arrhythmia. Its prevalence increases with age and it is present in more than 10% of patients aged 75 or more.[1]

Atrial fibrillation can occur in a wide variety of clinical settings and, although it is more likely to occur in patients with underlying heart disease, it can also occur in patients without any demonstrable cardiac disease.[2] Atrial fibrillation can be recurrent or paroxysmal or it can be present chronically. Any recommendations regarding the management of atrial fibrillation need to take into account the clinical setting in which the atrial fibrillation occurs.

Mechanism

Atrial fibrillation is thought to be due to multiple re-entrant circuits in the atrial myocardium occurring in a complex, variable and erratic manner.[3] Atrial fibrillation is more likely to occur if:

- conduction through the atrium is delayed
- the atrial myocardium is able to depolarize repeatedly at more rapid rates
- the atrial size is increased.[4]

Atrial fibrillation is usually triggered by a premature atrial depolarization which either arises from an atrial site or which has been conducted retrogradely from the ventricles through the atrioventricular (AV) node or over an accessory AV connection.[5]

ECG diagnosis

No P waves are visible and the baseline between successive QRS complexes is irregular. The ventricular response is usually irregular due to varying degrees of conduction of the atrial fibrillatory activity into the AV node.[6]

If there is a slow and regular ventricular response, complete heart block should be considered, particularly if the QRS complex is wide. If the baseline is irregular and the ventricular rate is regular, atrial flutter or re-entry within the atrioventricular node should be considered, particularly if the QRS complex is narrow.

Problems associated with atrial fibrillation

Atrial fibrillation may be a marker of significant underlying cardiac pathology. The increased heart rate and loss of atrial transport can lead to atrial congestion, cardiac ischaemia and decreased cardiac output in certain situations. This occurs more often if the ventricular rate is very rapid or if there is underlying structural heart disease.

There is a recognized increased risk of systemic thromboembolism[7] and the irregular and rapid heart rate often causes significant anxiety in the patient. In the elderly in particular there is a risk of significant pauses on reversion of the atrial fibrillation to sinus rhythm. There is also the possibility that the atrial fibrillation may organize into atrial flutter, which can then conduct to the ventricles more rapidly. This is more likely when class I and class III antiarrhythmic drugs are used.[8]

Precipitating factors

Atrial fibrillation can occur in the setting of infection and fever, pulmonary embolism, thyrotoxicosis, pericarditis and acute myocardial infarction as well as with toxins such as drugs and alcohol. Multivariate analysis has shown that increasing age, valvular heart disease, congestive heart failure, hypertension and diabetes are independent risk factors for the development of atrial fibrillation.[9] When treating a patient with atrial fibrillation any remediable factors should be addressed if possible.

Potentially useful drugs for the management of atrial fibrillation

The treatment of atrial fibrillation is directed at:

- slowing the ventricular response
- achieving reversion to normal sinus rhythm if possible
- either reducing the frequency and haemodynamic effects of subsequent atrial fibrillation or preventing further episodes altogether.

The ideal drug to prevent atrial fibrillation would increase atrial conduction velocity while lengthening the refractory period. No currently available antiarrhythmic drug achieves this and most are negatively inotropic, which may contribute to further ventricular dysfunction and subsequent atrial dilatation.

There is no data which carefully compares the effects of different antarrhythmic agents in the management of atrial fibrillation in the same patients.

Digoxin

Despite the traditional use of digoxin for management of atrial fibrillation, there is no good data to suggest that it increases the likelihood of reversion to sinus rhythm in paroxysmal atrial fibrillation. Spontaneous reversion to sinus rhythm is commonly seen in atrial fibrillation of recent onset and it has been suggested that the vagally mediated actions of digoxin may in fact perpetuate the tendency for atrial fibrillation to exist. There is not even convincing evidence that it significantly slows the ventricular response in patients with recent onset atrial fibrillation prior to reversion to normal sinus rhythm.[10]

Digoxin has been shown to reduce the rate of the ventricular response in chronic atrial fibrillation in the setting of cardiac failure but at this time its role in the management of paroxysmal atrial fibrillation is controversial. Nonetheless it has been used in this clinical setting for many years and is still felt to be a useful agent by many physicians.[1]

Class I antiarrhythmics

Procainamide, quinidine, disopyramide and flecainide have all been shown to be useful for slowing the ventricular rate and effecting acute reversion of paroxysmal atrial fibrillation (see Ch. 27). They are superior to placebo for maintaining normal sinus rhythm after cardioversion, but this is achieved at some increased risk of proarrhythmia, particularly in patients with underlying structural heart disease.[11] For example these drugs may allow the atrial fibrillation to organize into atrial flutter, which can then conduct to the ventricles more rapidly than the atrial fibrillation. If 1 : 1 AV conduction occurs this can result in dangerously rapid heart rates. For this reason a drug which slows AV node conduction, such as digoxin or a beta blocker, is often used in combination. Class I drugs can also predispose to a polymorphic ventricular tachycardia known as torsades de pointes in some patients.[12]

Proarrhythmia has been described as the provocation or exacerbation of an arrhythmia that is new or more severe than pre-existing baseline arrhythmias, in that it occurs after treatment with antiarrhythmic drugs. All antiarrhythmic drugs have this potential and the decision to initiate or continue maintenance therapy with antiarrhythmics to maintain sinus rhythm must involve a careful analysis of the risk/benefit ratio for each individual patient.

Beta blockers

Beta blockers (see Ch. 28) are useful for slowing the ventricular rate during atrial fibrillation but are negatively inotropic and may precipitate bronchospasm in some patients.

Sotalol is a unique beta blocker that at higher dosage has an effect of prolonging the action potential duration of myocardial cells (a class III effect). Sotalol has been shown to be as effective as quinidine in maintaining normal sinus rhythm post cardioversion[13] and further trials are necessary to establish more accurately its risk of proarrhythmia in various subgroups of patients.

Class III antiarrhythmics

Amiodarone (see Ch. 27) has complex electrophysiological effects on the action potential duration. It is the agent most likely to be successful for reverting paroxysmal atrial fibrillation and it is the agent most likely to be well-tolerated haemodynamically in the patient with atrial fibrillation associated with systemic illness such as sepsis. It possibly also has the least potential for proarrhythmia in patients with underlying structural heart disease, even though this question has not been specifically addressed in clinical trials.

Unfortunately amiodarone has a significant side-effect profile with chronic use, and its complex pharmacodynamics, particularly the long half-life, can interfere with subsequent investigation and management of arrhythmia patients.

There have been reports of torsades de pointes ventricular tachycardia with class Ia, class Ic and class III agents. Combination therapy with antiarrhythmic drugs such as the class Ia, class Ic and class III agents which prolong the QT interval should be avoided if possible.[11,14]

Calcium blockers

Both verapamil and diltiazem (see Ch. 29) will slow the ventricular rate but they are negatively inotropic and have no other beneficial effects in atrial fibrillation.[11]

Magnesium

There is some data that suggests magnesium sulphate (see Ch. 31) may be useful to control the ventricular rate,[15] and some contradictory data regarding the use of magnesium sulphate for prophylaxis of atrial fibrillation after coronary artery bypass surgery.[16,17] All of the in vitro data and most of the in vivo data suggest that magnesium supplementation suppresses myocardial irritability in the non-digitalized patient. The mechanism of this effect is uncertain.[18]

At this stage the use of magnesium for treatment of atrial fibrillation should be considered in patients likely to be magnesium deficient, such as alcoholics and patients receiving diuretics, but there is not enough data to recommend its routine use.

Anticoagulants

There is good evidence from randomized trials which demonstrate that chronic anticoagulation (see Ch. 37) can reduce the incidence of systemic thromboembolism in patients with chronic atrial fibrillation. Lower intensity regimens to maintain INR 1.8–2.5 are probably as effective as more intensive regimens, and safer. Aspirin has also been shown to be beneficial and more data is needed to answer which particular patients should receive warfarin and which should receive aspirin for prophylaxis against systemic thromboembolism.[11,19]

There is no adequate data regarding anticoagulation in recent onset atrial fibrillation.

Recent data from trans-oesophageal echocardiography has shown left atrial appendage thrombus, and the occurrence of new thrombotic events, are equally likely to occur in patients with acute atrial fibrillation (less than or equal to 4 days) as they are in patients with chronic atrial fibrillation. It has also been demonstrated that left atrial appendage function is further impaired and that blood flow in the atrial appendage is less following direct current (DC) cardioversion, which may mean that thrombus in the atrial appendage is more likely to occur early on after reversion to sinus rhythm. Echocardiography has also shown that it takes up to 3 weeks for atrial contraction to return to normal after cardioversion and there is data showing that thromboembolism can occur after reversion to sinus rhythm, so it is currently recommended that anticoagulation be continued for at least 3 weeks after DC cardioversion.[20]

A policy of anticoagulating all patients with atrial fibrillation of greater than 3 days' duration for 3 weeks before and 4 weeks after DC cardioversion has recently been endorsed by the American College of Chest Physicians[21] but earlier anticoagulation is likely to be beneficial in some patients with recent onset atrial fibrillation.

There is currently no good evidence regarding the appropriate use of anticoagulants in patients who revert spontaneously or who revert after antiarrhythmic drugs have been administered.

A suggested approach to the patient with recent onset atrial fibrillation

Given the current paucity of good data to guide the selection of appropriate therapy, and the myriad clinical settings where atrial fibrillation can occur, only general guidelines can be given.

First 24 hours

Staff must remember a significant number of patients will revert to sinus rhythm spontaneously.

If there is significant haemodynamic compromise, urgent DC cardioversion should be considered. However, it is usually preferable to control the ventricular rate and any atrial congestion by other means because of the risks associated with sedation, systemic thromboembolism or further impairment of left ventricular function that can be associated with DC cardioversion.

Potassium and magnesium levels must be checked. Anxiolytics, supplemental oxygen and the use of diuretics and vasodilators must be considered to reduce atrial congestion if this is present.

The ventricular rate can be slowed with beta blockers or calcium blockers if the increased cardiac rate is thought to be causing problems.

The role of digoxin is under review and further data is necessary to define its role accurately but it has been used for many years and is still felt to be a useful agent by many physicians despite the lack of data.

The patient must be clinically assessed, including if possible an echocardiograph as this helps to make an assessment of the risk of systemic thromboembolism and the need for anticoagulant prophylaxis for deep venous thrombosis. Thromboembolism is more likely in patients who have rheumatic mitral stenosis or a prosthetic mitral valve, or if there is evidence of cardiac failure or a history of a previous thromboembolic event.[22] An echocardiograph is extremely useful for assessing the function of the valves and the ventricles.

If the underlying cardiac function or the duration of the atrial fibrillation is uncertain, therapeutic anticoagulation should be considered. Aspirin may represent a useful compromise where formal anticoagulation is felt to be contraindicated or is difficult to arrange.

In the patient who has developed atrial fibrillation in the setting of systemic illness such as sepsis, the underlying cardiac function is often unknown. Antiarrhythmics at this stage may cause proarrhythmia if there is impaired cardiac function or significant associated metabolic disturbance, and it may be better to avoid their use at this stage. Intravenous amiodarone may also cause hypotension and predispose to proarrhythmia but is reasonable if acute antiarrhythmic drug use is felt to be necessary as amiodarone slows the ventricular rate and increases the likelihood of reversion to sinus rhythm. There is some evidence that amiodarone may be a more effective and safer agent than the class I agents in these patients.

After 24 hours

If it is felt that reversion to sinus rhythm is likely or desirable, elective cardioversion is reasonable if the atrial fibrillation has been present less than 2 days and there are no other risk factors for systemic thromboembolism.

An alternative approach is to commence warfarin at this stage and arrange elective DC cardioversion after at least 3 weeks of formal anticoagulation if late spontaneous reversion has not occurred. Both class I and class III antiarrhythmic drugs have been evaluated in this application and may be used in some patients to increase the likelihood of reversion after consideration of the risks and benefits.[11]

It is generally accepted that if there are no contraindications, patients with atrial fibrillation for more than 3 days should be anticoagulated for 3 weeks if cardioversion is contemplated. However some units recommend earlier anticoagulation because there is quite often uncertainty about the underlying cardiac substrate and the risks of thromboembolism. It is important to continue anticoagulation after the cardioversion for at least 3–4 weeks.

An alternative approach currently under investigation is to perform transoesophageal echocardiography and if there is no evidence of thrombus in the left atrium or left atrial appendage, to proceed directly to DC cardioversion. The relative risks and benefits of this approach are not established at this time.

Later management

As outlined above, the decision to use antiarrhythmic drugs chronically to attempt to maintain sinus rhythm after cardioversion also requires a careful and individualized analysis of the likely risk/benefit ratio for each patient.

The role of chronic anticoagulation in patients with atrial fibrillation and the role of aspirin is covered in more detail in Chapter 37.

Non-pharmacological management

There is some data that dual chamber atrial pacing in patients whose atrial fibrillation occurs in the setting of intermittent brady-arrhythmias may be beneficial in maintaining sinus rhythm.[23] His bundle ablation with implantation of a permanent ventricular pacemaker, and radiofrequency modification of the AV node, have both been performed to effect rate control of atrial fibrillation in patients who are intolerant of medications.[24,25]

This approach does not address all the haemodynamic effects of the atrial fibrillation or the risks of systemic thromboembolism but can give satisfactory control of ventricular rate in selected patients who are unable to tolerate medications or find them ineffective.

Various other experimental techniques such as implantable atrial defibrillators and surgical procedures are currently under investigation. One intriguing approach is the MAZE procedure where the atria are divided into small strips of tissue by extensive surgical incisions. The resulting scarring interferes with the ability of the multiple re-entrant pathways responsible for atrial fibrillation to be sustained, and has been effective in maintaining sinus rhythm in the short term in some patients.[26]

Conclusion

The management of atrial fibrillation remains problematic and is continuing to evolve. It seems likely that quite different approaches will be appropriate for different individual patients. Hopefully, further research in the next few years will more accurately define the appropriate management of this common and troublesome arrhythmia.

References

1. Lake FR, Thompson PL. Prevention of embolic complications in nonvalvular atrial fibrillation in the elderly. Drugs and Aging 1991; 1(6): 458–66
2. Kopecky SL, Gersh BJ, McGoon MD et al. The natural history of lone atrial fibrillation: a population based study over three decades. N Engl J Med 1987; 317: 669–74
3. Moe GK, Rheinboldt WC, Abildskov JA. A computer model of atrial fibrillation. Am Heart J 1964; 67: 200–203
4. Murgatroyd FD, Camm AJ. Current concepts in atrial fibrillation. Brit J Hospital Medicine 1993; 49: 544–60
5. Zipes DP. Genesis of cardiac arrhythmias: electrophysiological considerations. In: Braunwald E (ed). Heart disease: a textbook of cardiovascular medicine. 4th ed. Philadelphia: Saunders, 1992: 558–627
6. Josephson ME. Miscellaneous phenomena related to atrioventricular conduction. In: Josephson M (ed). Clinical cardiac electrophysiology. Techniques and interpretations. 2nd ed. Philadelphia: Lea & Febiger, 1993: 150–66
7. Wolf PA, Abbot R, Kannel W. Atrial fibrillation as an independent risk factor for stroke. The Framingham Study. Stroke 1991; 22: 983–8
8. Falk RH. Proarrhythmia in patients treated for atrial fibrillation or flutter. Ann Intern Med 1992; 117: 141–50
9. Kannel W, Abbot R, Savage D et al. Epidemiologic features of chronic atrial fibrillation: the Framingham Study. N Engl J Med 1982; 17: 1018–22
10. Falk RH, Knowlton AA, Bernard SA et al. Digoxin for converting recent onset atrial fibrillation to sinus rhythm. A randomised, double blind trial. Ann Intern Med 1987; 106: 503–6
11. Pritchett ELC. Drug therapy: management of atrial fibrillation. N Engl J Med 1992; 326: 1264–71
12. Bigger JT, Sahar DI. Clinical types of proarrhythmic response to antiarrhythmic drugs. Am J Cardiol 1987; 59: 2E–9E
13. Juul-Moller S, Edvardsson N, Rehnqvist-Ahlberg N. Sotalol versus quinidine for the maintenance of sinus rhythm after direct current conversion of atrial fibrillation. Circulation 1990; 82(6): 1932–9
14. Gill J, Heel RC, Fitton A. Amiodarone. An overview of its pharmacologic properties, and review of its therapeutic use in cardiac arrhythmias. Drugs 1992; 43(1): 69–110
15. Hays JV, Gilman JK, Rubal BJ. Effect of magnesium sulfate on ventricular rate control in atrial fibrillation. Ann Emerg Med 1994; 24(1): 61–4
16. Parikka H, Toivonen L, Pellinen T et al. The influence of intravenous magnesium sulphate on the occurrence of atrial fibrillation after coronary artery by-pass operation. Eur Heart J 1993; 14(2): 251–8
17. Fanning WJ, Thomas CS, Roach A et al. Prophylaxis of atrial fibrillation with magnesium sulfate after coronary artery bypass grafting. Eur Heart J 1993; 14(2): 251–8
18. Arsenian MA. Magnesium and cardiovascular disease. Prog Cardiovasc Dis 1993; 35: 271–310
19. Singer DE. Randomised trials of warfarin for atrial fibrillation. N Engl J Med 1992; 327: 1451–3
20. Grimm RA, Stewart WJ, Black IW et al. Should all patients undergo transoesophageal echocardiography before electrical

cardioversion of atrial fibrillation? J Am Coll Cardiol 1994; 23: 533–41
21. Dunn M, Alexander J, de Silva R et al. Antithrombotic therapy in atrial fibrillation; 2nd ACCP Conference on antithrombotic therapy. Chest 1989; 95(2)(Suppl.): 118S–28S
22. Halperin JL, Hart RG. Atrial fibrillation and stroke: new ideas, persisting dilemmas. Editorial. Stroke 1988; 19(8): 937–41
23. Lamas GA, Estes NM, Schneller S et al. Does dual chamber pacing or atrial pacing prevent atrial fibrillation? The need for a randomised controlled trial. PACE 1992; 15: 1109–13
24. Huang SK, Bharati S, Graham AR et al. Closed chest dessication of the atrioventricular junction using radiofrequency energy—a new method of catheter ablation. J Am Coll Cardiol 1987; 9: 349–58
25. Williamson BD, Ching Man K, Daoud E et al. Radiofrequency catheter modification of atrioventricular conduction to control the ventricular rate during atrial fibrillation. N Engl J Med 1994; 331: 910–17
26. Cox JL, Schnessler RB, D'Agostino HJJ et al. The surgical treatment of atrial fibrillation. Development of a definitive surgical procedure. J Thorac Cardiovasc Surg 1991; 101: 569–83

63 Ventricular tachycardia

David AB Richards, John B Uther and David Ross

Introduction

Ventricular tachycardia (VT) is a potentially lethal arrhythmia, for which carefully planned therapy is essential. It is always important to weigh the potential risks against the perceived benefits of any antiarrhythmic therapy. This principle was underscored by the publication of the Cardiac Arrhythmia Suppression Trial,[1] which demonstrated important proarrhythmic effects of antiarrhythmic drugs. As a result, long-term empiric usage of Vaughan Williams class I drugs, without ruling out a proarrhythmic effect in the individual patient, is now difficult to justify.

Definition of sustained ventricular tachycardia

Although there is no universally accepted definition of what is clinically important VT, most authorities agree that VT lasting more than 30 seconds is sustained, and generally should be treated.[2] Ventricular ectopic beats up to bigeminy, which may occur in normal individuals as well as in patients with organic heart disease, and rapid runs of consecutive ectopic beats (non-sustained ventricular tachycardia) lasting less than 10 seconds, have little prognostic significance and rarely require specific symptomatic therapy.

Diagnosis of ventricular tachycardia

VT should be suspected in any patient with tachycardia who has significant damage (acute or long-term) to the ventricular myocardium. It may also occur in the context of prior exposure to antiarrhythmic drugs, acute ischaemia or electrolyte imbalance. A rapid regular arterial pulse and irregular jugular venous cannon waves are the main physical findings, although regular cannon waves may occur if ventriculo-atrial conduction is present. On electrocardiogram (ECG) monitoring, the cardinal feature is a regular tachycardia with broad QRS complexes, often >0.16 seconds. The diagnosis should be confirmed on a 12-lead ECG whenever possible, before treatment is commenced. One can then more reliably determine QRS duration and timing of P waves than can be done on a rhythm strip alone.

Differential diagnosis

VT should be included in the differential diagnosis of any broad complex tachycardia. The main differential diagnosis is supraventricular or sinus tachycardia with aberrant His–Purkinje conduction. Misdiagnosis of VT as supraventricular tachycardia is one of the commonest important arrhythmia misclassifications in the CCU, and leads to inappropriate drug therapy. *If in doubt, treat as ventricular tachycardia.*

Ventricular muscle damage predating the first onset of arrhythmia strongly favours ventricular tachycardia. Ventricular rate and degree of haemodynamic disturbance are not reliable indicators of ventricular or supraventricular tachycardia. If the patient is haemodynamically stable, and if a supraventricular tachycardia of some sort is suspected, then reflex vagal stimulation by carotid sinus massage may be used to block atrioventricular nodal conduction. Intravenous adenosine, a short acting blocker of atrioventricular conduction, may also be helpful to distinguish between VT and other arrhythmias. If the tachycardia is unaffected by these manoeuvres, then clinicians should treat for ventricular tachycardia.

Electrocardiographic features

Electrocardiographic features which favour VT include:

- absence of 1:1 ventriculo-atrial association
- occasional fusion beats
- measured QRS complex duration in all precordial leads >0.14 seconds (that is, no iso-electric initial or terminal QRS segment in the chest leads)
- duration from the onset of R to the nadir of S in a precordial RS complex >0.10 seconds[2,3]
- a different broad QRS morphology during tachycardia from that seen during normal sinus rhythm in patients with bundle branch block in sinus rhythm.

Mechanisms of ventricular tachycardia

Periods of accelerated idioventricular rhythm occur in approximately 20% of patients after acute myocardial infarction, especially during sleep when the sinus node rate is slow. This arrhythmia, which is thought to be due to disturbed automaticity in damaged Purkinje fibres in the infarcted area, rarely requires specific antiarrhythmic therapy.

Rapid VT accompanying acute myocardial ischaemia or infarction is due to non-uniform conduction and refractoriness in the affected myocardium. This arrhythmia generally cannot be reproduced subsequently by programmed stimulation at electrophysiological study.[4]

When VT occurs in the context of healed myocardial infarction, the mechanism of tachycardia is usually re-entrant, and the arrhythmia may be induced and terminated by programmed electrical stimulation at electrophysiological study.[4] The re-entrant circuits are probably present in patchy scar at the interface between infarcted and normal myocardium.[5,6]

Re-entrant VT may occur around ventriculotomy scars in patients who have had surgical treatment for congenital heart disease, in patients with electrolyte disturbances such as hypokalaemia, hyperkalaemia and hypomagnesaemia, and in patients with a long QT interval. So-called antiarrhythmic therapy may actually induce VT (for example, ventricular fibrillation with quinidine, torsades de pointes with sotalol, ventricular tachycardia with flecainide), rather than prevent it in some patients.

Proarrhythmic drug action

Although agents that slow conduction without altering the refractory period are likely to slow the rate of a re-entrant tachycardia, such agents make ventricular tachycardia more likely to occur, and render the arrhythmia more stable and likely to continue once initiated (see Ch. 27). The relative effects on conduction velocity and refractory period determine whether a drug will increase or decrease the likelihood of VT occurring (see Fig. 27.2 in Chapter 27).

Torsades de pointes is well known to be an occasional idiosyncratic effect of quinidine and sotalol, while flecainide may precipitate ventricular tachycardia. Increased frequency of occurrence of VT, after initiation of antiarrhythmic therapy, may indicate a proarrhythmic action of the therapy.

Acute management of ventricular tachycardia

Cardiopulmonary resuscitation

If the patient with VT has no cardiac output, then cardiopulmonary resuscitation should begin immediately (See Ch. 40), including a thump on the chest, and an early attempt to terminate VT by direct current cardioversion. In an adult male the initial shock should be about 200 joules, and higher energy shocks should be employed in larger patients or when a lower energy shock has been unsuccessful.

Baseline observations

Intravenous access should be established promptly, and venous blood drawn to check electrolytes including potassium, calcium and magnesium, renal function, full blood count and liver function. Arterial blood gases must be measured, to facilitate acid-base management.

Specific antiarrhythmic therapy

Numerous antiarrhythmic agents are available which may alter acutely intraventricular conduction velocity and ventricular refractoriness and terminate tachycardia. On theoretical grounds, agents that prolong ventricular refractoriness without slowing intraventricular conduction velocity, or increase conduction velocity without shortening refractory period, should be most likely to terminate re-entrant VT and render it harder to induce. In practice there is a wide variation between patients in responses to specific therapy, and within patients on different occasions. In automatic VT, agents that slow the spontaneous diastolic depolarization of cells at the origin of the tachycardia are effective.

Avoid unnecessary polypharmacy

The ideal antiarrhythmic agent for acute termination of VT would exhibit rapid onset of effective antiarrhythmic action, minimal proarrhythmic and other side-effects, and be cleared promptly from the circulation. Since this ideal is rarely achieved, it is important to avoid unnecessary polypharmacy with multiple antiarrhythmic agents, especially in patients who are haemodynamically unstable with VT. The circulation must be supported with cardiopulmonary resuscitation while sufficient time is allowed for each agent to circulate and exert its action on the heart, before another agent is administered.

Sotalol

These authors recommend intravenous sotalol (1.5 mg/kg) as first line therapy for haemodynamically well-tolerated spontaneous ventricular tachycardia. This recommendation is based on a prospective double-blind controlled trial of sotalol versus lignocaine for acute termination of spontaneous sustained VT.[7] If VT recurs in the next few hours, and sotalol was initially successful, sotalol should be given (0.5–0.75 mg/kg).

- **Action**. Sotalol has two major electrophysiologic actions. Firstly it prolongs ventricular refractoriness (class III effect). Secondly, as a beta blocker it reduces the rate of spontaneous diastolic depolarization of myocardial cells. This beta blockade is competitive, and can be overcome if necessary by appropriate doses of beta agonists, such as adrenaline (up to 3.0 mg may be required) or isoprenaline. Sotalol is cleared by the kidney.
- **Side-effects.** Sotalol is contraindicated in torsades de pointes because QT interval is prolonged by sotalol. Reduce the dose of sotalol in renal failure. Clinically important side-effects of sotalol (hypotension and bronchospasm) occur infrequently.[7] The risk of hypotension is least when sotalol is administered alone, and greatest when it is given in combination with other agents that may depress myocardial contractility (for example lignocaine). Brochospasm is rarely a clinical problem with sotalol, unless severe life-threatening asthma is present.
- **Oral therapy.** Oral sotalol (40–160 mg twice daily) may be subsequently administered safely in most patients with VT, with only a minimal risk of proarrhythmia or torsades de pointes.[8,9] The beta blocking effect appears to be an important factor in improving the long-term outcome of patients with VT. This, in combination with the class III effects, makes sotalol one of the most effective antiarrhythmic agents available currently.

Lignocaine

Intravenous lignocaine (100 mg) may be used if sotalol has proven ineffective. If initially successful, lignocaine (50–100 mg) may be given subsequently if ventricular tachycardia recurs. Alternatively lignocaine may be continued as an infusion ≤ 4 mg/min.

- **Action.** Lignocaine blocks fast sodium channel current flow during the upstroke of the action potential (class I effect). Lignocaine is mostly metabolized in the liver.
- **Side-effects.** Common neurological side-effects include nausea, vomiting and convulsions.

Amiodarone

Intravenous amiodarone (5 mg/kg) over 5–10 minutes may be used instead of lignocaine if sotalol has been ineffective.

- **Action.** Given acutely, the predominant actions of this drug are those of a class I antiarrhythmic agent (slowed conduction velocity). Class III effects (prolonged action potential duration and refractoriness), and depressed automaticity are seen with chronic administration. Elimination from the body is very slow (half-life 1–2 months).
- **Side-effects.** Amiodarone contains iodine and may induce thyrotoxicosis.

However, since it is a competitive inhibitor of thyroid hormones at the nuclear receptor, it may also induce hypothyroidism. Other side-effects include photosensitivity, corneal deposits and pulmonary interstitial fibrosis.

Other agents

Intravenous verapamil (calcium channel blocker, 5–10 mg) is sometimes effective in automatic VT. However, it commonly causes hypotension and may induce heart block. There has been no reported prospective double-blind controlled study of amiodarone, procainamide (sodium channel blocker, 100 mg intravenously), phenytoin (depresses automaticity and improves conduction, 250 mg over 10–20 minutes) or bretylium (prolongs action potential duration and refractoriness, 5 mg/kg over 1–5 minutes), compared with other agents for the acute termination of ventricular tachycardia.

Pacing

Temporary transvenous right ventricular pacing can be used to terminate recurrent re-entrant ventricular tachycardia.[10] This may be done using a dedicated pacing wire, or an appropriate balloon flotation catheter with pacing wires incorporated in it. The pacing threshold of the catheter should be checked and should ideally be <1.0 mA. Pacing trains of 7–10 beats should be used, delivered at twice pacing threshold, commencing at approximately 80% of tachycardia cycle length. The coupling intervals of beats within the pacing train should be decremented, in successive bursts. Pacing rates >280/min are rarely effective, and often accelerate VT or induce ventricular fibrillation. Clinicians must remember to turn the pacing generator off before defibrillation, or when pacing is otherwise not required.

In patients who have anti-tachycardia pacing systems in situ, an external programmer may be utilized to allow customized anti-tachycardia pacing to be delivered by the device (see Chs 43, 50). If pacemaker-mediated tachycardia occurs in an individual with a ventricular pacemaker and intact ventriculo-atrial conduction, then the system should be reprogrammed to prevent further pacemaker-mediated tachycardia (for example, by increasing minimal interval between ventricular activations). If inappropriate pacing by a device has caused ventricular tachycardia, then check promptly the integrity of the sensing and pacing systems.

Other medical therapy

Whenever possible, specific medical therapy should be directed at any underlying pathology that may predispose to or precipitate ventricular tachycardia.

Treat ischaemia

If VT was precipitated by acute ischaemia, then the ischaemia must be treated. This should minimize the requirement for conventional antiarrhythmic therapy, and reduce the risk that unnecessary antiarrhythmic therapy may depress myocardial contractility and precipitate cardiac failure.

Electrolytes and acid-base

Significant electrolyte and acid-base abnormalities should be corrected.

Prevention of ventricular tachycardia

Since all so-called antiarrhythmic agents may have proarrhythmic and other side-effects, there is no indication for routine administration of prophylactic antiarrhythmic therapy (for example lignocaine) to patients who have not had ventricular tachycardia.[11] However, if VT is recurrent, and all treatable precipitating causes have been eliminated (such as ischaemia, proarrhythmic drugs, electrolyte abnormalities), then maintenance antiarrhythmic therapy with the agent that successfully terminated VT may be required.

Subsequent management

After the acute termination of ventricular tachycardia, it is important to complete the clinical examination in order to direct subsequent investigations and therapy to minimize the risk of recurrent ventricular tachycardia. Clinical examination and history (including chest pain, evidence of bleeding leading to anaemia and hypoxaemia, potentially proarrhythmic drug therapy, dyspnoea, obstructive sleep apnoea, respiratory infection, etc.) from relevant individuals should be obtained to identify potentially treatable precipitating causes for VT.

Prevent myocardial ischaemia

If ventricular tachycardia has occurred in the context of acute myocardial ischaemia within the preceding 48 hours, or has been associated with reperfusion induced by thrombolytic therapy after acute thrombotic coronary artery occlusion, then subsequent management should be directed towards prevention of further ischaemia (see Chs 54, 55) without specific antiarrhythmic therapy.

Antiarrhythmic drug therapy

In the authors' experience, sotalol is more effective than metoprolol, which in turn is more effective than amiodarone and sodium channel blockers.[8]

Drug testing

If spontaneous VT has occurred in the absence of acute myocardial ischaemia, proarrhythmic drug effect, metabolic disturbance or long QT interval syndrome, then it is probable that VT has been due to intraventricular re-entry. Oral sotalol may be used without electrophysiological testing, but is still associated with a 15% recurrence rate of spontaneous ventricular tachycardia.[8] If chronic oral class I antiarrhythmic drug therapy is contemplated, then the antiarrhythmic and proarrhythmic potential of such therapy should be checked at electrophysiological study.[8,12]

Radiofrequency ablation

In patients with recurrent unimorphic VT in whom there is a high chance that VT originates from a single localized focus within the heart, radiofrequency ablation directed by detailed mapping at electrophysiological study may eliminate ventricular tachycardia.[13]

This approach is very effective for VT occurring in otherwise normal hearts, where the origin of the tachycardia is usually in the right ventricular outflow tract, or in the left ventricular free wall. For ventricular tachycardia based on old myocardial infarction, where the origin of ventricular tachycardia is often in the septum, success rates are only moderate (30–60%), and frequently other morphologies of ventricular tachycardia remain inducible after radiofrequency ablation.

Automatic implanted cardioverter defibrillator (AICD)

In patients with recurrent VT in whom drug therapy or radiofrequency ablation are ineffective or not indicated, staff should consider implantation of an anti-tachycardia pacing system along with cardioverter defibrillator[14] (see Ch. 50). These devices do not prevent tachycardia. Rather, they promptly identify increased heart rate, and are programmed to deliver pacing trains to terminate tachycardia, or high energy shocks to terminate ventricular fibrillation. Low energy shocks to convert ventricular tachycardia to sinus rhythm are rarely used. Whereas these devices were initially large and cumbersome and required thoracotomy for deployment of defibrillator patches around the heart, modern systems are now smaller and utilize a single transvenous electrode with an 'active can'. Thus a thoracotomy is no longer required and the procedure is more akin to implantation of a complex pacemaker.

Surgical ablative procedures

In patients in whom the origin of ventricular tachycardia is localized, but in whom radiofrequency ablation is not indicated or is ineffective, clinicians should consider surgical ablative therapy using isolation techniques, resection, cryothermy and laser. However, such therapy is associated with at least 10–15% mortality[15] and is completely effective (that is, no need for antiarrhythmic drugs or implanted defibrillator) in only 70–85% of survivors.

Other investigations

In patients following myocardial infarction, the risk of developing spontaneous ventricular tachycardia is greatest amongst those with low ejection fraction, inducible VT at programmed stimulation, and delayed potentials detected at signal averaging (see Ch. 23). However, successful antiarrhythmic drug therapy usually does not abolish delayed potentials and signal averaging cannot be used to monitor drug therapy.

Summary

The management of ventricular tachycardia begins with establishing a firm diagnosis based on clinical features along with confirmatory 12-lead ECG findings. If VT is associated with haemodynamic collapse or cardiac arrest, then direct current cardioversion should be attempted immediately.

Intravenous sotalol is first line treatment for ventricular tachycardia, if urgent cardioversion is not required. Acute myocardial ischaemia and electrolyte disturbances, which may precipitate VT, should be treated without delay.

After initial termination of VT, the clinician should plan management to minimize the risk of further VT and to maximize the probability of survival should it recur.

References

1. Rogers WJ, Epstein AE, Arciniegas JG et al. The Cardiac Arrhythmia Suppression Trial (CAST) Investigators. Preliminary report: effect of encainide and flecainide on mortality in a randomized trial of arrhythmia suppression after myocardial infarction. CAST study. N Engl J Med 1989; 321:406–12
2. Josephson ME. Recurrent ventricular tachycardia. In: Josephson ME (ed). Clinical cardiac electrophysiology. Philadelphia: Lea & Febiger, 1993: 417–615
3. Brugada P, Brugada J, Mont L, Smeets J, Andries EW. A new approach to the differential diagnosis of a regular tachycardia with a wide QRS complex. Circulation 1991; 83:1649–59
4. Wellens HJ, Lie KI, Durrer D. Further observations on ventricular tachycardia as studied by electrical stimulation of the heart. Chronic recurrent ventricular tachycardia and ventricular tachycardia during acute myocardial infarction. Circulation 1974; 49:647–53
5. Denniss AR, Richards DA, Waywood JA et al. Electrophysiological and anatomic differences between canine hearts with inducible ventricular tachycardia and fibrillation associated with chronic myocardial infarction. Circ Research 1989; 64:155–66
6. Richards DA, Blake GJ, Spear JF, Moore EN. Electrophysiologic substrate for ventricular tachycardia: correlation of properties *in vivo* and *in vitro*. Circulation 1984; 69:369–81
7. Ho DSW, Zecchin RP, Richards DAB, Uther JB, Ross DL. Double-blind trial of lignocaine versus sotalol for acute termination of spontaneous sustained ventricular tachycardia. Lancet 1994; 344:18–23
8. Ross DL, Cooper MJ, Koo CC et al. Proarrhythmic effects of antiarrhythmic drugs. MJA 1990; 153:37–47
9. Mason J, for the Electrophysiologic Study Versus Electrocardiographic Monitoring Investigators. A comparison of electrophysiologic testing with Holter monitoring to predict antiarrhythmic-drug efficacy for ventricular tachyarrhythmias. N Engl J Med 1993;329:445–51
10. Josephson ME. Evaluation of electrical therapy for arrhythmias. In: Josephson ME (ed). Clinical cardiac electrophysiology. Philadelphia: Lea & Febiger, 1993:683–725
11. Antman EM, Berlin JA. Declining incidence of ventricular fibrillation in myocardial infarction: implications for the prophylactic use of lidocaine. Circulation 1992;86:764–73
12. Josephson ME. Evaluation of antiarrhythmic agents. In: Josephson ME (ed). Clinical cardiac electrophysiology. Philadelphia: Lea & Febiger, 1993:630–82
13. Morady F, Frank R, Kou WH et al. Identification and catheter ablation of a zone of slow conduction in the re-entrant circuit of ventricular tachycardia in humans. J Am Coll Cardiol 1988;12:262–7
14. Saksena S, for the Programmable Cardioverter Defibrillator (PCD) investigator group. Clinical outcome of patients with malignant ventricular tachyarrhythmias and a multiprogrammable implantable cardioverter-defibrillator implanted with or without thoracotomy: an international multicenter study. J Am Coll Cardiol 1994;23:15–21
15. Josephson ME. Surgical and non-surgical ablation in the therapy of arrhythmias. In: Josephson ME (ed). Clinical cardiac electrophysiology. Philadelphia: Lea & Febiger, 1993:726–821

64 Other arrhythmias

Peter L Thompson

Coronary care staff require a high level of skill in recognition and management of cardiac arrhythmias. Much of this skill is directed towards management of arrhythmias during myocardial infarction (see Ch. 55), but with the widening role of the coronary or cardiac care unit (CCU), patients with cardiac arrhythmias due to a wide spectrum of other cardiac conditions are treated in the CCU.

Sinus node disturbances

Sinus tachycardia

Sinus tachycardia is usually defined as normally conducted sinus rhythm at a rate in excess of 100 per minute. It can be a normal response to physiologic stimuli but persistent sinus tachycardia is usually an indication of disordered pathophysiology.[1] Rarely, paroxysmal or sustained sinus tachycardia can occur as a primary cardiac abnormality without apparent disordered cardiac pathophysiology. In this situation the tachycardia may have features of both sinus and atrial tachycardia and may be due to re-entry in the sino-atrial junction (sinus node re-entry tachycardia).[2] Sinus tachycardia is of particular significance in the presence of myocardial ischaemia, as it may increase myocardial oxygen consumption.

Recognition

The P wave is of normal contour. The PR interval usually shortens proportionate to the increase in heart rate. Distinction from supraventricular tachycardia or atrial flutter may, on occasions, require carotid sinus massage. The usual response in sinus tachycardia is a gradual slowing with rapid return to the prior heart rate. Sinus node re-entry tachycardia may show a normal P wave contour but can be reverted to a slower sinus rate with carotid sinus massage.[2] On occasions the factors causing the sinus tachycardia can be so overwhelming that no response is seen despite adequate vagal stimulus. In this situation review of the trends in the patient's vital signs or computer printout may be invaluable, showing a gradual increase in heart rate in sinus tachycardia versus a paroxsymal increase in other supraventricular arrhythmias.

Treatment

Treatment is directed towards correction of the underlying abnormality. On occasions this may be subtle and require careful enquiry to identify blood loss, hyperthyroidism, recent withdrawal of beta blocking drugs or recent withdrawal from alcohol. If there are distressing symptoms or if there is a likelihood of worsening myocardial ischaemia, intravenous (IV) or oral beta blockade may be necessary.

Sinus arrhythmia

Sinus arrhythmia is usually a normal physiologic response with slowing of the heart rate during inspiration. On occasions this can be so striking as to allow the expression of escape rhythms, such as junctional or ventricular escape beats. Loss of normal phasic variation with respiration has been recognized as an increased risk factor for sudden cardiac death.[3]

Recognition

There is phasic variation of the RR interval with preservation of normal P wave contour. This differs from atrial ectopic beats or wandering atrial pacemaker, which have variable P wave contours.

Treatment

Treatment is unnecessary.

Wandering atrial pacemaker

On occasions the P wave morphology can vary. This can occur in the healthy young but may also indicate atrial pathology.

Recognition

P wave morphology is variable with or without a variation in sinus rate.

Treatment

No treatment is necessary.

Sinus bradycardia

Sinus bradycardia is usually defined as a sinus rate below 50/min. It can be a normal variant and is often an indication of a high level of physical fitness. However, it can be a response to treatment with beta blockers or may occur as a result of vagal overactivity. A particularly exaggerated form of sinus bradycardia may occur from vagal overactivity during myocardial ischaemia and reperfusion as the efferent expression of the Bezold–Jarisch reflex.[4]

Sinus bradycardia may be a manifestation of the sick sinus syndrome.

Recognition

The P wave contour is normal but the rate is below 50/min.

Treatment

Sinus bradycardia usually requires no treatment. The patient's therapy should be checked for heart rate slowing medications such as beta blockers; occasionally beta blocking eye drops for glaucoma can cause a significant bradycardia.

Severe symptomatic sinus bradycardia may occasionally require intravenous atropine, 0.5–1.0 mg IV. Dopamine IV (2–5 μg/kg/min) can be used if associated with hypotension.[5] If it is persistent and affects cardiac output and causes symptoms it may require a pacemaker. An atrial pacemaker may be sufficient but as there is often associated conduction system disease a dual chamber pacemaker is usually used.[6]

Sinus arrest

Sinus arrest may occur as an isolated phenomenon in patients with sick sinus syndrome. It may occur as a reaction to the Bezold–Jarisch reflex in myocardial ischaemia or may be a response to pain or emotional stimuli. The haemodynamic effects are often self-limiting due to junctional or ventricular escape beats maintaining a cardiac rhythm, but may be severe enough to cause syncope.

Sinus arrest may be due to slowing or cessation of automaticity in the sinus node producing sudden slowing or arrest, or to sino-atrial block producing a sinus bradycardia whose rate is a fraction of the previous sinus rate (see Fig. 64.1).

It is important to distinguish sinus arrest from blocked atrial premature beats which may be difficult to recognize if the atrial complex is hidden in the preceding ECG complex's T wave (see Fig. 64.2).

Recognition

Sinus arrest is recognized by sudden slowing or absence of P waves often with a ventricular or junctional escape rhythm. On occasions there are no escape rhythms and a prolonged electrocardiographic pause is seen.

Sino-atrial block is recognized by the sudden development of bradycardia with P waves usually at half the rate of the preceding P waves. On careful analysis, more complex ratios of sino-atrial block, including Wenckebach phenomenon, can be recognized.[7]

Treatment

If recurrent and causing syncope, a permanent pacemaker may be necessary.

Sick sinus syndrome

Sick sinus syndrome is a term encompassing a variety of arrhythmias related to abnormal sinus node automaticity, sino-atrial block, atrial ectopic activity and atrial tachyarrhythmias.[8]

The following is a recommended classification of the sick sinus syndrome:

1. Intermittent sinus arrest
2. Stable sinus bradycardia
3. Brady-tachy syndrome.

The bradyarrhythmia may be sinus bradycardia or sinus arrest and this may precede intermittent tachycardia or may be a feature on sudden cessation of the tachyarrhythmia due to depression of

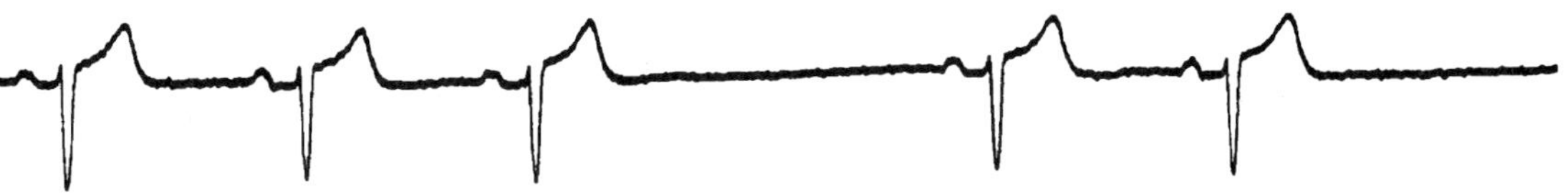

Fig. 64.1 Sinus arrest due to 2:1 sino-atrial block. Note the P–P interval is twice that of the preceding P–P interval. This phenomenon should be distinguished from apparent sinus arrest due to a hidden, non-conducted P wave (see Fig. 64.2).

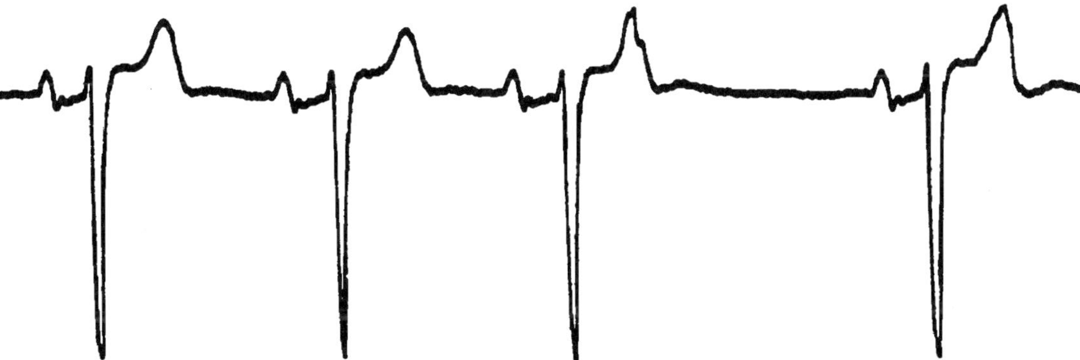

Fig. 64.2 Apparent sinus arrest due to a blocked atrial premature beat. The nearly hidden P wave is clearly discernible in the T wave of the third complex.

sinus node function. The tachyarrhythmia component is usually rapid atrial fibrillation.

Sick sinus syndrome does not respond well to antiarrhythmic drugs and is now the commonest indication for implantation of a permanent pacemaker. Previously VVI pacemakers were used to control the bradycardia component along with antiarrhythmic drugs. With the increasing use of DDD chamber pacemakers, sick sinus syndrome can often be controlled with pacemaker therapy alone (see Ch. 43).

Supraventricular tachyarrhythmias

Terminology

Although the abnormalities of the sinus node described in the preceding section are 'above the ventricle', the term 'supraventricular' usually refers to non-sinus node, non-ventricular arrhythmias, i.e. arrhythmias arising in the atrium and atrioventricular (AV) junction. The term 'supraventricular arrhythmia' is a generic descriptive term for atrial and junctional tachycardias, atrial flutter and atrial fibrillation.

The term 'supraventricular tachycardia' (SVT) is commonly used to describe atrial and junctional re-entrant tachycardias. The term is widely used because of the difficulties in distinguishing atrial from junctional tachycardias on the surface ECG. Although predominantly supraventricular in origin and associated with normal ventricular conduction, electrophysiological studies have shown that the ventricle may be involved in the re-entrant pathway.

The term 'paroxysmal atrial tachycardia' (PAT) is time-honoured and still used but it is an inappropriate description of an arrhythmia which is not usually 'atrial' in origin but predominantly due to re-entry in and around the AV junction.

The term 'PAT with block' was used when an atrial tachycardia with variable atrioventricular block was seen with digitalis toxicity. The term was always inappropriate because the arrhythmia was rarely paroxysmal.

Supraventricular ectopic beats

Ectopic beats can arise in the atrium or AV junction. They can be a normal variant and may be worsened with cardiac stimulants such as tobacco, caffeine and alcohol. They may indicate cardiac disease, particularly atrial enlargement, may be a predictor of atrial flutter or atrial fibrillation and can occasionally initiate paroxysmal supraventricular tachycardia.

Recognition

A typical atrial premature beat is initiated by a P wave of a different morphology from the sinus P wave, with a variable PR interval and a normal QRS complex. The PR interval is determined by the refractory period of the AV node and is longer if the premature beat occurs early or normal if it occurs later in the cardiac cycle. On occasions the atrial premature beat can occur when the intraventricular conduction pathways are partly refractory, producing a bizarre complex reminiscent of a ventricular ectopic beat. If the P wave is obscured by the preceding T wave, a ventricular ectopic may be incorrectly diagnosed. The atrial premature beat can occur when the AV node or intraventricular conduction pathways are totally refractory, producing a 'blocked' atrial premature beat which appears on the ECG as an isolated P wave. This is distinguished from sinus arrest by the finding of a premature, abnormal P wave (see Fig 64.2). On occasions these blocked atrial premature beats can initiate short runs of atrial flutter or without ventricular conduction, producing bizarre appearances on ECG monitoring.

Treatment

Normally no treatment is required. If symptoms are distressing, a small dose of beta blocker can be used, or a small dose of flecainide if there is no evidence of left ventricular dysfunction.

Supraventricular tachycardia

Paroxysmal supraventricular tachycardia (SVT) is now seen less frequently in the CCU, since increased availability of effective drugs to prevent and treat this common tachyarrhythmia has meant that most episodes can be managed in the emergency department and long-term management is becoming increasingly the focus of the electrophysiology laboratory and catheter ablation therapy.[9]

The mechanism of the arrhythmia has been defined with increasing accuracy with electrophysiology studies over the past decade.[10] The majority occur in patients who have a normal surface ECG between episodes of tachycardia. Most are due to entry within the atrioventricular node because of the coexistence of fast and slow pathways within the node, or due to re-entry through a concealed accessory pathway in which the antegrade limb of the pathway is the AV node and the retrograde limb is an accessory pathway.

Patients whose re-entrant circuit involves antegrade conduction through an accessory pathway will usually demonstrate features of the Wolff–Parkinson–White anomaly on the surface ECG.

Recognition

Supraventricular arrhythmias usually have a normal narrow QRS complex. The rate can vary from 130–250 beats per minute. The rate is usually constant throughout an episode but may slow down spontaneously or following drug therapy prior to reversion.

Frequently it is impossible to identify P wave on the surface ECG but when detectable, the finding of an inverted P wave immediately following the QRS complex argues for re-entry within the AV node; a P wave midway between the QRS complex argues for re-entry via a concealed pathway.

Carotid sinus massage may be ineffective, or may effect reversion to sinus rhythm, sometimes with a pause before re-establishing normal rhythm.

A supraventricular tachycardia may be associated with a wide QRS complex if there has been a pre-existing bundle branch block, or with the development of rate-dependent bundle branch block during the tachycardia or with conduction via an accessory pathway.

Treatment

The patient will frequently be aware of manoeuvres to terminate their tachycardia including breath holding, Valsalva manoeuvre, gagging or vomiting.

The most effective vagal manoeuvre is *carotid sinus massage*.[11,12] This should be performed with the patient semi-recumbent and with continuous ECG monitoring. It should not be used in patients with a history of recent transient cerebral ischaemia. Although carotid bruits are not a reliable sign of critical carotid stenosis, it would be unwise to perform vigorous carotid massage in a patient with a high-pitched carotid bruit.

With the patient's chin tilted upwards and away from the side to be massaged, the carotid bulb is palpated and pressed firmly posteromedially in a massaging motion for 3–5 seconds. If not initially successful, the procedure can be repeated on each side (separately, never together), if necessary with the addition of the Valsalva manoeuvre to achieve additional vagotonia. Alternative vagal manoeuvres such as gagging, eyeball pressure, facial immersion in cold water, etc., are unlikely to be effective if properly conducted carotid sinus massage is ineffective.

If carotid sinus massage is ineffective, the drug of choice is *intravenous adenosine*.[13] Although most experience has been with an initial dose of 6 mg, this can cause unpleasant flushing, apprehension and chest tightness.[14] To minimize this the current recommendation is for an initial dose of 3 mg bolus over 2 seconds.

If unsuccessful within 1–2 minutes, 6 mg should be given and if still unsuccessful, 12 mg. With this approach over 90% of supraventricular tachycardias can be reverted.

Adenosine can be given to patients on beta blockers; it has a faster effect than verapamil. It should be used with caution in patients with asthma as it can cause transient wheezing.

If the patient is not hypotensive (systolic BP below 90 mmHg) *intravenous verapamil* can be used in a total dose of 5–10 mg given in boluses of 1–2 mg at 1-minute intervals. In contrast to adenosine, verapamil should not be given as a single bolus.[15] It is essential to check that the patient receiving IV verapamil has not been treated with beta blocking drugs. Patients with significant left ventricular dysfunction should not be treated with verapamil. Intravenous diltiazem (20 mg over 2 minutes with repeat 25 mg over 2 minutes if required) has been used as a more rapidly acting alternative to verapamil.

Intravenous drug therapy can be followed by carotid sinus massage, often with good effect.

If there is haemodynamic compromise, particularly in the presence of myocardial ischaemia or pulmonary oedema, synchronized cardioversion may be necessary, starting with 50 joules. Before administering cardioversion it is important to check that the patient has not been receiving large doses of digitalis and especially that the arrhythmia is not an atrial tachycardia ('PAT with block') due to digitalis intoxication.

Maintenance therapy can be initiated with verapamil in a dose of 80 mg 8-hourly changing to 240 mg slow release once per day. In patients who are not able to take verapamil, oral digoxin is a suitable alternative. Some patients require long term therapy with class Ic drugs (flecainide) or class III drugs (amiodarone or sotalol). Patients refractory to drug therapy may be selected for electrophysiology study with a view to catheter ablation therapy (see Ch. 49).

Supraventricular arrhythmias associated with accessory pathways

In patients with known Wolff–Parkinson–White syndrome or known accessory pathways, emergency treatment of paroxysmal SVT can be treated in a similar manner as patients without an accessory pathway but digoxin should be avoided. Although verapamil, diltiazem and adenosine may block conduction through the AV node, they do not accentuate conduction through the accessory pathway and they have not been associated with any adverse effects in known SVT. However, in a broad complex tachycardia of unknown origin, verapamil should not be used.[5,16]

Class I drugs may affect conduction through the accessory pathway; for this reason response to IV lignocaine may not necessarily be diagnostic of ventricular tachycardia if there is a reciprocating tachycardia with a bundle branch block.

Non paroxysmal supraventricular tachycardias

Non paroxysmal tachycardias may be congenital, due to atrial infiltration, or atrial surgery, or atrial enlargement. They do not respond to vagal manoeuvres or AV junctional blocking drugs and may be resistant to cardioversion.

Non paroxysmal atrial tachycardia ('PAT with block') due to digitalis intoxication

This arrhythmia requires special attention because of the potential to cause harm with inappropriate treatment. The P waves are usually large and bizarre and may vary in rate as the degree of toxicity varies (increased P wave rates with greater degrees of toxicity) and there may be a Wenckebach block which can be enhanced with carotid sinus massage. In more advanced degrees of digitalis toxicity there is complete atrioventricular dissociation.

The degree of AV block and the rate of the atrial tachycardia gradually resolves as the digitalis toxicity resolves. Usually no active treatment apart from withdrawal of digoxin is required. Cardioversion must not be used in this arrhythmia as it may produce lethal ventricular fibrillation (VF) which does not respond to repeated defibrillating shocks.

Chaotic (multi-focal) atrial tachycardia

Chaotic (multi-focal) atrial tachycardia is usually seen in patients with respiratory disease, especially cor pulmonale or infiltrative disease of the atrium.[17] There are multiple foci of ectopic atrial activity with multi-focal P waves at varying rates and usually with 1:1 atrioventricular conduction. This arrhythmia is resistant to most antiarrhythmic drugs, may be worsened with digoxin and is sometimes worsened with sympathomimetic bronchodilators. It is not changed with cardioversion. It responds to improvement in the patient's respiratory status and reduction of sympathomimetic bronchodilators. Amiodarone may be helpful.[18]

Atrial flutter

Atrial flutter usually occurs in the presence of underlying cardiac disease associated with atrial enlargement such as ischaemic heart disease, cardiomyopathy or mitral valve disease. It rarely can occur in the apparently normal heart. The mechanism is thought to be re-entry within the atria.[19]

Recognition

The typical atrial flutter appearance is a saw-tooth (picket fence) atrial activity with normal QRS complexes. Frequently the saw-tooth pattern is obscured by the ST segment and T wave contour and may not be immediately obvious and may be confused with supraventricular tachycardia or sinus tachycardia. It is essential in assessing a patient with supraventricular tachyarrhythmia to consider the possibility of atrial flutter in every case and preferably examine a 12-lead ECG for the typical flutter pattern. The typical saw-tooth pattern can be frequently demonstrated by increasing the degree of atrioventricular block with carotid sinus massage (see Fig. 64.3).

Treatment

Management of atrial flutter depends on the clinical circumstances and the patient's symptoms. If it is likely that the atrial flutter is a transient phenomenon as part of a generalized illness, or the patient is asymptomatic and not haemodynamically affected by the arrhythmia, it may be preferable to manage the patient with medical therapy. In other circumstances it is usually preferable to achieve electrical reversion as soon as possible.

Synchronized cardioversion has a very high success rate in atrial flutter.[20] Although successful reversion can occur with low energy shocks such as 50 joules, this may produce atrial fibrillation which will then require higher energy shocks for reversion. For this reason it may be preferable to proceed immediately with a medium energy shock of 100–200 joules. Alternatively, reversion of atrial flutter can be achieved with rapid atrial pacing.[21] A J-tip wire is inserted via an antecubital or subclavian vein and advanced to the heart. Under fluoroscopic screening it is positioned at the right auricular appendage, observing a characteristic tail-wagging appearance of the tip of the pacing wire. Alternatively it can be positioned in the lateral mid-atrial wall to ensure atrial wall contact.

A clear signal should be recorded through the catheter. Atrial capture should be attempted at a stimulus level of 1–2 mA (milliamps) at a rate of 50 beats per minute in excess of the atrial flutter rate. Having ensured atrial capture, the atrium is paced at 400 per minute for 2 seconds, increasing the rate to 500 or 600 per minute in short bursts if unsuccessful. With each burst of rapid pacing, it is important to ensure that the pacing

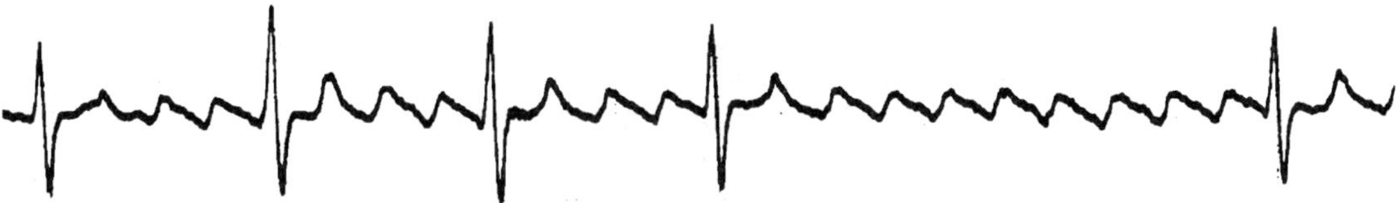

Fig. 64.3 Effect of carotid sinus massage on atrial flutter. The typical saw-tooth pattern may be obscured by QRS and T waves. Atrial flutter frequently masquerades as coarse atrial fibrillation (as in this example), sinus tachycardia or supraventricular tachycardia.

wire has remained in the atrium and not migrated into the ventricle. Rapid atrial pacing is effective in reverting to sinus rhythm in 60–70% of attempts. Sometimes atrial fibrillation is produced and this may later revert to sinus rhythm. Atrial thrombus formation does not appear to be a complication of atrial flutter and anticoagulation is not necessary unless there are other risk factors for atrial thrombus such as a marked left atrial enlargement or mitral stenosis.

Atrial fibrillation

Atrial fibrillation is dealt with in detail in Chapter 62.

Ventricular arrhythmias

Ventricular ectopic beats

There has been quite a dramatic change in clinical attitudes and guidelines for treatment of ventricular ectopic beats within the past few years. In early CCU practice, the use of antiarrhythmic drugs to attempt abolition of all ventricular ectopic beats was considered good practice. Detailed categorizations of ventricular ectopic beats based on morphology, frequency, occurrence in the cardiac cycle and repetitiveness were used as the basis of determining the likely hazard for ventricular fibrillation and the need for administration of antiarrhythmic therapy. The most widely used of these was the Lown classification based on synthesis of observations from the animal laboratory, coronary care and Holter monitor experience.[22]

The major reasons for disaffection with the aggressive approach to the management of ventricular ectopic beats have been:

- In the coronary care setting, the use of ventricular premature beats (VPBs) as warning arrhythmias to predict ventricular fibrillation has been generally unsatisfactory, with many patients experiencing frequent high grade arrhythmias without developing fibrillation and many developing fibrillation without any warning arrhythmias.[23]
- Increasing evidence that ventricular arrhythmias are predominantly markers of left ventricular dysfunction rather than predictors of risk in their own right[24,25] and that risk is determined by other factors such as the extent of instability of coronary atherosclerosis.[26]
- The major determinant against the 'VPB hypothesis' has been the observation from clinical trials in the CCU that prophylactic lignocaine can suppress the arrhythmia but does not improve or may worsen mortality[27] and, most persuasively, the findings of the CAST study in ambulatory patients[28] indicating that currently available antiarrhythmic drugs, whilst effective in suppressing VPBs, have an adverse effect on mortality via a propensity to proarrhythmia.

For these reasons, coronary care practice in the 1990s has become less focused on the management of ventricular arrhythmias at the lower end of risk, such as ventricular ectopic beats, and more focussed on the management of the malignant and life-threatening ventricular tachycardias (see Ch. 63). Nevertheless, an understanding of the terminology and significance of ventricular ectopic beats remains an integral component of coronary care management.

Terminology

Whilst there are subtle reasons for some of the differences in terminology, most of the terms—ventricular extra systoles (VEs), ventricular ectopic beats (VEBs), ventricular premature beats (VPBs), ventricular premature depolizarizations (VPDs) —are used interchangeably.

VEBs may be:

- **Unifocal vs bifocal vs multi-focal**. Unifocal (uniform) VEBs remain constant from beat to beat. Bifocal refers to two different morphologies and multi-focal (multi-form) to multiple morphologies.
- **Frequent**. May refer to the number of VEBs per minute (e.g. 20 per minute) or the number of VEBs per normal beat (e.g. 1:10).
- **Repetitive**. More than one VEB together, as a couplet (2 VEBs together), or triplet (3 VEBs together). Runs of more than three repetitive beats constitute ventricular tachycardia. A salvo of VEBs refers to a run of two, three or four. The term coupling is used loosely and refers to repeated coupling of VEBs and a normal beat (as in bigeminal rhythm) or can refer to occurrence of 2 VEBs together in a couplet.
- **R/T**. R/T ectopic beats interrupt the preceding T wave by the ectopic beat. They may ini-

tiate ventricular tachycardia or ventricular fibrillation.

Other terms describing VEBs include:

- **Fusion beats**. On occasions a VEB may be so delayed as to interfere with the subsequent QRS complex producing a fusion beat. These may be seen in any arrhythmia when ventricular and supraventricular beats occur together—accelerated idioventricular rhythm, ventricular tachycardia or pacing rhythm.
- **Escape beats**. Escape rhythms are those which occur as a result of suppression of the normal cardiac pacemaker and reflect automaticity in the ventricular muscle or Purkinje fibres.
- **Bigeminy**. Bigeminy refers to a VEB after every sinus beat, trigeminy after every second, quadrigeminy after every third, etc.

Treatment

The 'search and destroy' approach to the management of ventricular ectopic beats is no longer favoured.[29,30] However, many CCUs still prefer to treat VEBs which occur early in the cardiac cycle in multi focal salvos of two or three in an attempt to stabilize the cardiac rhythm and reduce the risk of ventricular tachycardia and fibrillation. Correction of hypokalaemia and hypomagnesaemia may avert the need for specific antiarrhythmic drug therapy.[31] Intravenous lignocaine in bolus followed by infusion remains the standard first line of therapy but increasingly, amiodarone or sotalol are being favoured.

Intravenous beta blockers may be sufficient to stabilize the cardiac rhythm.

In patients who are troubled with symptomatic ventricular ectopic beats, administration of oral beta blocking drugs may be effective in reducing the frequency and the patient's awareness of the irregular heart rhythm, especially when there is associated anxiety or evidence of excess circulating catecholamines.

Sometimes beta blocking drugs will be ineffective and an oral antiarrhythmic drug needs to be considered. Oral sotalol (80–160 mg 8-hourly) is being used increasingly for this purpose as it combines both class III antiarrhythmic and beta blocking properties.

On occasions a patient who is seriously distressed and unable to take antiarrhythmic drugs can have their symptoms controlled with a pacemaker. This strategy is particularly useful in patients who are suffering symptoms of poor cardiac output due to a persistent pseudo-bradycardia resulting from bigeminal rhythm.

Ventricular tachycardia

The management of ventricular tachycardia is dealt with in detail in Chapter 63.

Ventricular fibrillation

Ventricular fibrillation is the usual cause of sudden death in ischaemic heart disease. It is often preceded by rapid ventricular tachycaradia or ventricular flutter which, on occasions, can be self-reverting but ventricular fibrillation is almost never self-terminating in the human heart. If left untreated it will be fatal within 3–5 minutes.

Recognition

The ECG shows coarse irregular rhythm, sometimes with a phasic organized pattern. The patient with VF will rapidly lose consciousness. 'Pseudo VF' patterns due to artefact, tremor, displaced electrode, etc., should not be confused with VF and are usually not associated with any change in conscious state (see Ch. 22).

Treatment

The only effective management is immediate, unsynchronized defibrillation[5,32] with a shock of 200 joules.[33] If the first shock is not effective, a second shock of 200–300 joules is administered, followed by a third shock of 360 joules if necessary. The shocks should be delivered in rapid sequence, without delay for cardiopulmonary resuscitation (CPR) or drug administration. If VF persists after three shocks delivered in this fashion, CPR should be continued, followed by 1 mg of adrenaline (epinephrine) by IV push and then defibrillation again at 360 joules. Cardiopulmonary resuscitation will not achieve reversion but can maintain the circulation if a defibrillator is not immediately available.

In patients with a prolonged episode of VF, higher doses of intravenous adrenaline (epinephrine) (2–5 mg) or rarely, anti-fibrillatory drugs such as lignocaine (lidocaine) (1.5 mg/kg IV) or bretylium tosylate

(5 mg/kg IV) may be needed to achieve reversion. It is essential to maintain adequate external cardiac massage and ventilation between defibrillation attempts. Sodium bicarbonate 1 mg/kg IV may help reversion of VF if the resuscitation has been protracted. Known hypokalaemia or hypomagnesaemia should be corrected. Following correction of VF, antiarrhythmic therapy with lignocaine (lidocaine) is frequently used, although there is no convincing evidence to support this practice.[34]

Conduction defects

Bundle branch block

Right and left bundle branch blocks[35] are due to delayed conduction through the bundle branches or more rarely, the distal radicles of the conduction system. Electrocardiographically they are characterized by slurring and notching of the QRS complex with QRS duration in excess of 0.12 seconds (3 small squares) at the widest point. It is sometimes necessary to examine several different ECG leads to determine the maximum width of the QRS complex.

Terminology

QRS notching and widening less than 0.12 seconds is referred to as a partial or incomplete bundle branch block if the electrocardiographic pattern is typical of right or left bundle branch block. Nonspecific widening of the QRS complex is referred to as an intraventricular conduction defect. Notching of the QRS without widening may be within normal limits.

Right bundle branch block

The right bundle branch[35] may be damaged or disturbed anywhere along its length by congenital defect, fibrosis, ischaemia or right ventricular dilatation.

The right bundle branch may conduct abnormally only under certain circumstances which increase its refractoriness: for example, supraventricular ectopic beats or supraventricular tachycardia. Right bundle branch block usually has no prognostic significance unless associated with left axis deviation indicating left anterior hemiblock and bifascicular block.[36]

Recognition

Right bundle branch block shows slurring and notching of the QRS, with widening greater than 0.12 seconds, a typical RSR pattern in lead V1 and slurred S wave in the lateral leads.

Treatment

No management is necessary except in the presence of bifascicular block. Patients with bifascicular block with syncope warrant further investigation and consideration of pacemaker implantation.[35]

Left bundle branch block

Left bundle branch block[35] is usually associated with diffuse disease involving the left ventricle such as cardiomyopathy, ischaemic heart disease, myocardial infarction or left ventricular hypertrophy. On occasions it can be due to localized calcific or fibrotic disease in the conduction system and like right bundle branch block can be intermittent.

Recognition

The QRS is slurred, notched, measures greater than 0.12 seconds, there is no tall R wave in lead V1 and there is the characteristic M shape in the lateral ECG leads.

Treatment

Management is directed towards the underlying cardiac problem.

Fascicular blocks (hemiblocks)[35]

The intraventricular conduction system consists of three fascicles:[35] the right bundle branch, the anterior/superior division of the left bundle branch and the posterior/inferior division of the left bundle branch. The right bundle is a long, thin tract of conduction tissue running on the endocardial surface of the right ventricular septum; the fascicles of the left bundle are a more diffuse, fan-shaped collection of conduction fibres.

Involvement of the anterior/superior division of the left bundle will produce left anterior fascicular block (hemiblock) and involvement of the posterior/inferior division will produce a left posterior fascicular block (hemiblock).

Involvement of the anterior/superior division will cause delayed depolarization of the anterior/superior portion of the left ventricle. Depolarization will initially be via the posterior/inferior division resulting in unopposed anterior/superior activity and therefore left axis deviation. Conversely, involvement of the posterior/inferior division will produce right axis deviation.

Left anterior fascicular block (left anterior hemiblock)

Recognition

The QRS complex may not be widened but the main frontal axis will be directed leftwards to greater than −30°, that is, the QRS complex will be positive in lead I, negative in lead III and predominantly negative in lead II.

Treatment

Left anterior hemiblock by itself requires no treatment but may indicate a risk of atrioventricular block if associated with right bundle branch block indicating bifascicular block (see below).[35]

Left posterior fascicular block (left posterior hemiblock)

In the left posterior hemiblock[35] the conduction through the posterior/inferior division of the left bundle is affected. Depolarization of the left ventricle is via the anterior/superior division resulting in unopposed rightward forces and a right axis deviation on the mean frontal axis. Left posterior hemiblock is far less common than left anterior hemiblock.

Recognition

The ECG shows marked right axis deviation. Left posterior hemiblock can only be diagnosed in the absence of other causes of right axis deviation such as right ventricular hypertrophy but can be confidently diagnosed if sudden right axis deviation occurs.

Treatment

No special action is required but management of higher grades of conduction blocks should be anticipated.

Bifascicular block

The combination of right bundle branch block with left anterior hemiblock is referred to as bifascicular block.[35] In this situation depolarization of the left ventricle is solely via the left posterior/inferior division of the left bundle and cardiac conduction becomes tenuous. There is a low risk of developing high grade AV block in a stable patient with bifascicular block, but in circumstances where further stresses on the cardiac conduction system are possible, such as myocardial ischaemia, infarction, general anaesthesia or surgery, cardiac pacing may be necessary.[36] Drug therapy is ineffective.

Atrioventricular blocks

Atrioventricular block[37] can occur as a result of conduction delay in the atrioventricular node, the bundle of His, or in the bundle branches. Usually AV block with a narrow QRS complex indicates delay in the AV node, whereas AV block with associated bundle branch block indicates disease in the ventricular conduction system.

First degree AV block

First degree AV block can occur as a congenital normal variant, as a result of vagal influences on the AV node due to disease in the AV node or ventricular conduction system, or as a result of drugs which slow AV conduction such as digitalis, beta blockers and verapamil.

Recognition

Prolongation of the PR interval greater than 0.2 seconds (5 small squares) constitutes first degree AV block.

Treatment

If the first degree AV block is drug-induced, withdrawal of the drug causing AV conduction delay is the only management necessary. Administration of these drugs should be avoided. Careful observation of first degree AV block is essential in establishing whether the PR interval is lengthening, indicating a likelihood of second degree AV block of Wenckebach type.

Second degree atrioventricular block

Second degree atrioventricular block can occur as a result of delay through the atrioventricular node or in the His-Purkinje system. Delays in the AV node characteristically show the Wenckebach phenomenon, whereas second degree block in the His-Purkinje system characteristically does not. Rarely the Wenckebach phenomenon can occur in the distal conduction system that is usually preceded by other conduction abnormalities. Wenckebach block may result from degenerative disease, or infiltration of the AV node, or be a transient result of digitalis, beta blocker, verapamil or diltiazem excess.

Recognition

The two types of second degree AV block are referred to as Mobitz types I and II. Mobitz I is more commonly referred to as Wenckebach AV block.

Wenckebach block (Mobitz type I block)

There is gradual prolongation of the PR interval leading eventually to a dropped beat before the cycle re-starts. The QRS complex is usually narrow, although when the Wenckebach phenomenon affects the distal conduction system (rarely) the QRS complex may be widened.

Mobitz type II block

In Mobitz type II block there is no lengthening of the PR interval prior to the sudden drop of conduction leading to 2:1, 3:1, or even higher grades of atrioventricular block.

Treatment

The two types of AV block have different natural histories and clinical significance. Wenckebach block due to drugs affecting AV node function may be self-limiting or require a temporary pacemaker.[38] Degenerative disease of the conduction system causing persistent second degree block may require a permanent pacemaker. The management of these abnormalities complicating myocardial infarction is described in more detail in Chapter 55.

Third degree (complete) atrioventricular block

In the third degree AV block there is no conduction of atrial impulses to the ventricle, which maintains its rhythm by a junctional or ventricular escape rhythm. This conduction abnormality is a common abnormality in degenerative or infiltrative cardiac disease, and can occur as a result of intoxication with drugs which affect the atrioventricular node. On occasions it can be a congenital anomaly which may remain asymptomatic throughout life.

The clinical features depend primarily on the rate of the ventricular escape rhythm. Rates below 40 per minute are frequently associated with syncope or near syncope, rates 40–60 per minute associated with symptoms of weakness, faintness and lethargy. Often the rate of ventricular firing will be intermittent, producing intermittent loss of consciousness (the Stokes–Adams syndrome).

Recognition

The ECG abnormality is readily recognized, with total dissociation of the P waves and QRS complexes. On occasions there may be partial atrioventricular conduction producing fusion beats between the conducted QRS and the ventricular escape beat.

Electrocardiographic AV dissociation is not necessarily synonymous with AV block, as some persons with intermittent sinus bradycardia may have junctional or ventricular escape rhythms which exceed the rate of the sinus rhythm.

Treatment

Patients with symptomatic atrioventricular block will require cardiac pacing.[38] The type of pacemaker will depend on the clinical circumstances if there is longstanding infiltrative or degenerative heart disease. A permanent pacemaker will be necessary if there is a correctable cause such as myocardial infarction or drug intoxication. Temporary pacemaking may suffice. Transcutaneous pacing can be used in the emergency situation. For some patients who are asymptomatic from their atrioventricular block, particularly those with a well-maintained ventricular rate or those with congenital atrioventricular block, no action may be necessary.

Some patients with AV block may respond temporarily to drug therapy but this will depend on the site of the block. When the AV block is at the site of the AV node, atropine 0.5–1.0 mg intravenously may restore atrioventricular conduction. When the site of AV block is distal to the AV node and due to increased refractoriness in the His-Purkinje system, acceleration of the atrial rate may accentuate rather than reverse the block. Alternatively sympathomimetic amines may be used.[5] Intravenous isoprenaline has been widely used for this purpose but frequently causes ventricular arrhythmias. Intravenous dopamine 2–5 μg/kg/min is also effective, with less propensity for arrhythmias. If there is associated severe hypotension, IV adrenaline (epinephrine) in a dose of 2–10 mg/min can be used.

References

1. Randall WC, Ardell JL. Nervous control of the heart: anatomy and pathophysiology. In: Zipes DP, Jalife J (eds). Cardiac electrophysiology: from cell to bedside. Philadelphia: Saunders, 1990: 291
2. Bonke FIM, Kirchoff CJHS, Allesie MA. Sinus node re entry. In: Zipes DP, Jalife J (eds). Cardiac electrophysiology: from cell to bedside. Philadelphia: Saunders, 1990: 526
3. Kleiger RE, Miller JP, Bigger JT Jr, Moss AJ. The Multicenter Post Infarction research group. Decreased heart rate variability and its association with increased mortality after acute myocardial infarction. Am J Cardiol 1987; 59: 256–62
4. Mark AL. The Bezold–Jarisch reflex revisited. Clinical implication of inhibitory reflexes originating in the heart. J Am Coll Cardiol 1983; 1: 90–102
5. American Heart Association Emergency Cardiac Care Committee and Subcommittees. Guidelines for cardiopulmonary resuscitation and emergency cardiac care. JAMA 1992; 268: 2171–302
6. Rosenqvist M, Brandt J, Schuller H. Long-term pacing in sinus node disease: effects of stimulation node on cardiovascular morbidity and mortality. Am Heart J 1988; 116: 16–22
7. Fisch C. Electrocardiographic manifestations of exit block. In: Zipes DP, Jalife J (eds). Cardiac electrophysiology: from cell to bedside. Philadelphia: Saunders, 1990: 628
8. Ferrer MI. The sick sinus syndrome. Circulation 1973; 47: 635–41
9. Roskin J. Catheter ablation for supraventricular tachycardia. N Engl J Med 1991; 324: 1160–2
10. Josephson ME. Paroxysmal supraventricular tachycardia: an electrophysiologic approach. Am J Cardiol 1978; 41: 1123–6
11. Waxman MB, Wald RW, Sharma AD, Huerta F, Cameron DA. Vagal techniques for termination of paroxysmal supraventricular tachycardia. Am J Cardiol 1980; 46: 655–64
12. Mehta D, Wafa S, Ward DE, Camm AJ. Reactive efficacy of various physical manoeuvres in termination of junctional tachycardia. Lancet 1988; 1: 1181–5
13. Camm AJ, Garratt CJ. Adenosine and supraventricular tachycardia. N Engl J Med 1991; 325: 1621–9
14. Sylven C, Beerman B, Jonzon B, Brandt Z. Angina pectoris-like pain provoked by intravenous adenosine in healthy volunteers. Br Med J 1986; 293: 227–30
15. Garratt C, Linker N, Griffith M, Ward D, Camm AJ. Comparison of adenosine and verapamil for termination of paroxysmal junctional tachycardia. Am J Cardiol 1989; 64: 1310–6
16. Rankin AC, Rae AP, Cobbe SM. Misuse of intravenous verapamil in patients with ventricular tachycardia. Lancet 1987; 2: 472–4
17. Scher DL, Asura EL. Multifocal atrial tachycardia: mechanisms, clinical correlates and treatment. Am Heart J 1989; 118: 574–80
18. Kouvaras G, Cokkinos DV, Halal G et al. The effective treatment of multifocal atrial tachycardia with amiodarone. Jpn Heart J 1989; 30: 301
19. Waldo AL. Mechanisms of atrial fibrillation, atrial flutter and ectopic atrial tachycardia: a brief review. Circulation 1987; 75 (Suppl. III): 73–80
20. De Silva RA, Graboys TB, Podrid PJ, Lown B. Cardioversion and defibrillation. Am Heart J 1980; 100: 881–95
21. Haft JI, Kowosky BD, Lau SH et al. Termination of atrial flutter by rapid electrical pacing of the atrium. Am J Cardiol 1967; 20: 239–44
22. Lown B, Wolf M. Approaches to sudden death from coronary heart disease. Circulation 1971; 44: 30–42
23. Campbell RWF, Murray A, Julian DG. Ventricular arrhythmias in first 12 hours of acute myocardial infarction. Natural History Study. Br Heart J 1981; 46: 351–7
24. Kjekshus J. Arrhythmias and mortality in congestive heart failure. Am J Cardiol 1990; 65: 42I–48I
25. Marchlinski FE, Buxton AE, Waxman HL, Josephson ME. Identifying patients at risk of sudden death after myocardial infarction: value of the response to programmed stimulation, degree of ventricular ectopic activity and severity of ventricular dysfunction. Am J Cardiol 1983; 52: 1190–6
26. Davies MJ, Thomas A. Thrombosis and acute coronary lesions in sudden cardiac ischaemic death. N Engl J Med 1984; 310: 1137–40
27. MacMahon S, Collins R, Peto R et al. Effects of prophylactic lidocaine in suspected acute myocardial infarction. An overview of results from the randomized controlled trials. JAMA 1988; 2601: 1910–6
28. The Cardiac Arrhythmia Suppression Trial (CAST) investigators: preliminary report. Effect of flecainide and encainide on mortality in a randomized trial of arrhythmia suppression after

myocardial infarction. N Engl J Med 1989; 321: 406–12
29. Roden DM. Risks and benefits of anti-arrhythmic therapy. N Engl J Med 1994; 331: 785–91
30. Ward DE, Camm AJ. Dangerous ventricular arrhythmias—can we predict drug efficacy? N Engl J Med 1993; 329: 498–9
31. Gettes LS. Electrolyte abnormalities underlying lethal and ventricular arrhythmias. Circulation 1992; 85 (Suppl. I): I-70–I-76
32. Martin TG, Hawkins NS, Weigel JA, Rider DE, Buckingham BD. Initial treatment of ventricular fibrillation: defibrillation or drug therapy. Am J Emerg Med 1988; 6: 113–9
33. Weaver WD, Cobb LA, Copass MK, Hallstrom AP. Ventricular defibrillation: a comparative trial using 175-J and 320-J shocks. N Engl J Med 1982; 307: 1101–6
34. Kertes P, Hunt D. Prophylaxis of primary ventricular fibrillation in acute myocardial infarction. The case against lignocaine. Br Heart J 1984; 52: 241–7
35. Fisch C. Electrocardiography and vector cardiography. In: Braunwald E (ed). Heart disease. A textbook of cardiovascular medicine. 4th ed. Philadelphia: Saunders, 1992: Ch 5
36. McAnulty JH, Rahimtoola SH, Murphy E et al. Natural history of 'high-risk' bundle branch block: final report of a prospective study. N Engl J Med 1982; 307: 137–143
37. Zipes DP. Specific arrhythmias: diagnosis and treatment. In: Braunwald E (ed). Heart disease. A textbook of cardiovascular medicine. 4th ed. Philadelphia: Saunders, 1992: Ch 24
38. Dreifus LS, Fisch C, Griffin JC et al. Guidelines for implantation of cardiac pacemakers and anti-arrhythmia devices: a report of the ACC/AHA task force on assessment of diagnostic and therapeutic cardiovascular procedures (Committee on Pacemaker Implantation). Circulation 1991; 84: 455–67

65 The cardiac surgery patient

Bradley M Power

Introduction

Care of the adult post-operative cardiac surgical patient is enhanced if they and their relatives have realistic expectations of surgery and some understanding of its associated morbidity and mortality. Educational booklets and pre-operative visits to the post-operative area, with explanations of common procedures, may assist patient preparation.

Most post-operative care is predictable with low mortality and morbidity. Common complications and therapies allow unit protocols and critical pathways of management to be developed for the efficient resolution of problems.

Clinicians should be able to identify those patients at increased risk following surgery so that resources may be appropriately prescribed.[1,2] Table 65.1 and Figure 65.1 outline one method of estimating operative mortality and morbidity. Units should subject themselves to audit so that problems in management may be rapidly addressed.

Table 65.1 Simplified clinical risk scoring system. Reproduced with permission from Tuman KJ et al 1992[1]

Pre-operative factors	Score
Emergency surgery	4
Age 65–74 yr	1
≥ 75 yr	2
Renal dysfunction	2
Age of previous MI	
3–36 mo	1
<3 mo	2
Female gender	2
Reoperation	2
Pulmonary hypertension	2
Cerebrovascular disease	2
Multivalve or CABG + valve surgery	2
Mitral or aortic valve surgery	1
Congestive heart failure	1
LV dysfunction	1

MI = myocardial infarction. CABG = coronary artery bypass graft. LV = left ventricular.

Return from theatre

The post-surgical patient is returned from theatre to the intensive monitoring area accompanied by an anaesthetist, with continuation of cardiac monitoring and support systems. Initial handover information should include:

- medical history
- cardiac history
- assessment of left ventricular (LV) function
- quantification of risk factors (see Table 65.1)
- medications and date of aspirin or other anticoagulant cessation
- surgical procedure
- specific problems during surgery
- duration of bypass and cross-clamping and difficulties with separation
- medications, e.g. inotropes, antihypertensives, diuretics and antibiotics
- haemostasis and renal function
- lines, and drains in situ
- specific surgical problems or instructions
- pacemaker settings and electrode placement

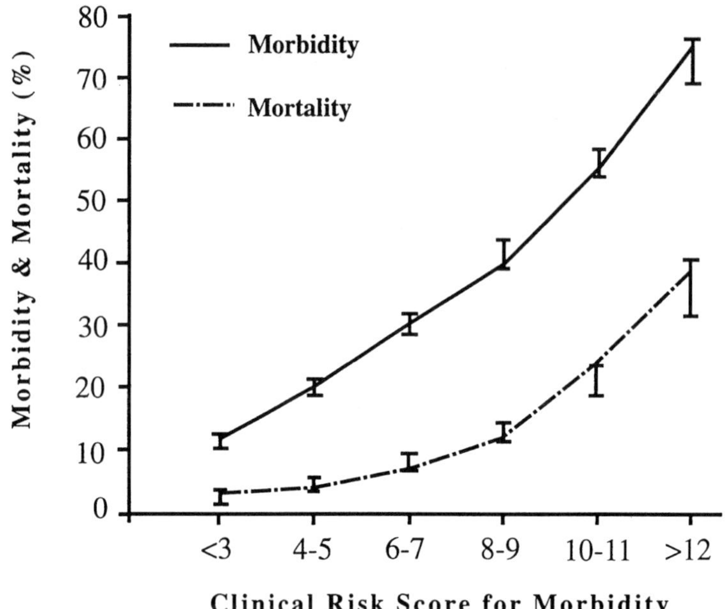

Fig. 65.1 Predictions of mortality and morbidity from the preoperative clinical factors detailed in Table 65.1. Observed morbidity and mortality in reference sample (n = 3156). 95% confidence intervals predicted from logistic regression model denoted by vertical bars. Observed outcomes not significantly different from predicted values (p >0.05) at all levels of clinical risk score. Reproduced with permission from Tuman KJ et al., 1994.[1]

Initial examination and assessment

Initial examination is based on a systems approach and includes patient examination, documentation of lines in situ, of fluids medications and of ventilatory and pacemaker settings together with assessment of preliminary laboratory data. Investigations as shown in Table 65.2 (below) are performed.

Management in the first 6 hours: rewarming and haemodynamic stabilization

Respiratory

Continued ventilation beyond the immediate operative period has generally become the norm for cardiothoracic care. It is believed that this allows more controlled emergence from surgery and anaesthesia. Ventilation is generally continued until the patient is warm and haemodynamically stable, with adequate ventilation and airway reflexes. Aims at this point are:

- pO_2 80–100 mmHg
- O_2 saturation >95%
- normocarbia, i.e. pCO_2 35–45 mmHg

To achieve these ends:

- Initially controlled mandatory ventilation (CMV) mode should be used.
- Minute volume is adjusted to maintain normocarbia
  — tidal volume (V_T) 10–12 ml/kg
  — ventilator rate 8–10 per minute
- Fractional inspired oxygen concentration is set (FIO_2).
- Positive expiratory end pressure (PEEP) is added where FIO_2 >0.6.
- Chest X-ray is reviewed (see Table 65.2).

Haemodynamic and fluid therapy

Myocardial contractility, peripheral resistance and intravascular volume all change throughout the immediate post-operative period. Frequent examination and assessment are necessary to plan therapy. While broad recommendations can be made, patient variation requires that titration of therapy and the assessment of response must accompany any empirical guidelines.

Aims include:

- **Cardiac Index (L/min/m²)**
  <2.5 —requires frequent assessment. Usually needs intervention
  2.5–3.5 —may need intervention if poor clinical progress
  >3.5 —desirable
- **Blood pressure**. Modify desired levels according to surgical procedure, presence of vascular disease and pre-operative blood pressure. Goals in the uncomplicated patient are:
  — Mean blood pressure 70–80 mmHg
  — Avoid systolic hypertension (SBP > 140 mmHg) as may stress suture lines
  — Avoid diastolic hypotension (DBP < 50 mmHg) as low BP may aggravate myocardial ischaemia.

Table 65.2 Routine and special investigations for the post-cardiac surgery patient

Routine investigations	Purpose
Arterial blood gases	Exclude hypoxaemia, check pH & pCO_2. Review BE for unexplained metabolic acidosis
Full blood picture	Assess need for transfusion of blood or platelets
Potassium	Monitor and avoid hypokalaemia
Chest radiology	Check position of ETT, NGT, CVC and pulmonary flotation catheter. Exclude pneumothorax, pleural effusion, lobar collapse and interstitial infiltrate
Coagulation studies (ACT, INR, APTT ± fibrinogen)	Check adequacy of heparin reversal Exclude factor deficiency
Electrocardiogram (without ventricular pacing if feasible)	Consider perioperative infarction. Note new conduction disturbance
Other investigations	**Purpose**
Magnesium	Avoid hypomagnesaemia
Lactate & mixed venous oxygen saturation (SvO_2)	May be useful as markers of adequacy of tissue perfusion
Thromboelastogram (TEG)	May help differentiate fibrinolysis from platelet defect or factor deficiency

- **Volume status**
  If cardiac index and blood pressure adequate:
  - accept pulmonary artery wedge pressure (PAWP) 5–15 mmHg
  - accept central venous pressure (CVP) 8–15 mmHg (if no pulmonary catheter).

  If cardiac index clinically inadequate, consider:
  - raise PAWP to 15 mmHg or higher, assessing response
  - raise CVP to > 15 mmHg closely assessing response, or insert pulmonary flotation catheter.
- **Haemoglobin (g/dl)**
  - >10 —transfusion seldom indicated
  - 7–10 —consider transfusion if other risk factors
  - <7 —transfusion usually indicated
- **Fluids**
  - Replace drain losses with colloid or packed cells.
  - Crystalloid or colloid for other requirements.
  - 5% Dextrose in water, 20–50 ml per hour for IV drugs.
- **Assess adequacy of cardiovascular status by:**
  clinical examination
  - basic haemodynamic parameters
  - peripheral perfusion and rewarming
  - urine output

  invasive monitoring
  - cardiac output studies
  - invasive vascular pressures

  special tests
  - base deficit and lactate
  - mixed venous oxygen saturation.

Haemostasis

Bleeding represents a major threat to a smooth post-operative course. Policies are essential for the recognition and treatment of excessive bleeding. Establishment and audit of a blood conservation protocol results in reduced homologous blood transfusion.[3]

Strategies for control of bleeding begin pre-operatively with timed cessation of aspirin (preferably 10 days pre-operation) and warfarin (preferably 1 week pre-operation with heparin cover), and continue into the operative period. Surgical technique and meticulous attention to control of bleeding are important determinants of bleeding.[4] Prophylactic use of anti-fibrinolytic agents in the bypass period may have a favourable effect on blood loss and this benefit is most marked in high risk cases[5] (see Complications).

Investigations useful in assessing coagulopathy after cardiopulmonary bypass (CPB) include:

- platelet count
- activated clotting time (ACT)
- coagulation profile (INR, APTT, TCT and fibrinogen level)
- thromboelastography (TEG)

Most adult patients require consideration for return to theatre for re exploration where in the absence of an overt coagulopathy there is:

- rapid blood loss (> 500 ml in any 1 hour)
- continuing blood loss (> 200 ml/hr for 3–4 hours)
- total loss > 1000–1500 ml.

Such scales are empirical and patients with bleeding who have been 'dry' at the completion of surgery and have no coagulopathy may require earlier return to theatre. Sudden haemorrhage with extreme hypotension unresponsive to volume therapy and inotropes requires immediate sternotomy. In the rapidly deteriorating patient, this may need to be performed in the surgical recovery area.

Sedation and analgesia

Intravenous narcotics remain the mainstay of analgesia. Minimal analgesia may be required where high doses of opioids have been used during anaesthesia. The presence of pain should be established if possible prior to administration.

Agents useful for sedation include:

- propofol (bolus 10–50 mg then infusion 10–100 mg/hr)
- midazolam (bolus 1–5 mg then infusion 2–5 mg/hr)
- higher doses can be used but analgesia should be reviewed.

Patients with poor LV function may be sensitive to even small doses of sedation.

Other

- **Renal function**
  - A large diuresis is expected immediately on return from theatre and its absence requires attention. Urine output should be at least 0.5–1.0 mg/kg in the steady state if no previous diuretics.
  - major determinant is haemodynamic stability.[6]
  - 'Low dose dopamine' is used by many units but its benefit is uncertain.[7]
- **Shivering**
  - common, and results in excessive VO_2.
  - rewarm until ceases, usually this is above 37°C.
  - pethidine may abolish visible shivering but paralysis[8] for example, vecuronium 4–8 mg IV) with sedation and controlled ventilation is needed to reduce excessive VO_2 and DO_2.
  - adjust ventilator to remove excess CO_2.
- **Electrolyte disturbance**
  - electrolyte shifts are common and can be dramatic (e.g. hypokalaemia).
  - unit policies need to be in place to monitor and correct hypokalaemia, hypomagnesaemia and hypocalcaemia.
  - disturbance can depend upon anaesthetic bypass technique and the cardiac/intensive care unit should be made aware, should bypass practice change.

Management hours 6–24: extubation and decannulation

Progression to extubation

Extubation is usually possible 6–18 hours following surgery. Weaning is accomplished using a method with low work of breathing (± PEEP), this being especially important where there is poor LV function or a history of pulmonary oedema. Some units have suggested earlier extubation (0–6 hours) may be possible with low morbidity in selected groups of patients.[9,10]

Supplemental oxygen is provided post extubation and is required for at least a further 24–48 hours. Early mobilization is encouraged and a physiotherapy regimen implemented to minimize post-operative atelectasis.

Management of drains & lines

Invasive monitoring is de-escalated following extubation in the uncomplicated patient. Mediastinal and pleural drains are removed on the day after surgery if losses are negligible. Chest X-ray is performed to exclude pneumothorax and to assess lung re-expansion.

Pacemaker leads may be capped, dependent upon the nature of the surgery and the likely need for pacing. Continuous ECG monitoring is usually continued for 24–48 hours post-operatively.

Initiation of ongoing therapy

Therapy which may be initiated before ward transfer includes:

- short-term diuretic therapy—salt and water retention is common in the post-bypass period
- potassium supplementation
- heparin (subcutaneous) to decrease risk of venous thrombosis
- aspirin introduced as early as possible to minimize chances of graft occlusion
- analgesia

The following additional tests are reviewed:

- urea and electrolytes
- serial ECGs and cardiac enzyme studies—unit definitions are required to exclude the presence of peri-operative myocardial infarction
- haemoglobin

Complications of cardiothoracic surgery

Despite the uncomplicated course of most patients, significant complications can rapidly occur. A clear knowledge and experience of their presentation and treatment is necessary.

Haemodynamic

Low cardiac output syndrome

Inadequate cardiac output is one of the commonest problems following surgery. It has a strong correlation with pre-operative risk score[1] and is most likely to arise in patients with poor pre-operative LV function.

Pre-operative assessment should be available including angiography, echocardiography or gated scanning. Cardiopulmonary bypass is associated with graded injury to myocardium. Post-operatively there is evolving myocardial oedema with variation in myocardial contractility and function. Injury varies with the surgery, and the duration and type of cardioplegia.

Reasons for low cardiac output include:

- tamponade
- poor pre-operative LV function
- myocardial 'stunning' post cardiopulmonary bypass
- acute myocardial ischaemia or infarction
- negative inotropic effect of drugs, e.g. sedatives
- acid-base imbalance.

Invasive monitoring with flow-directed pulmonary artery catheters is generally advised for optimal therapy of the patient with low cardiac output (see Ch. 24). Left atrial lines may be used in some patients and trans-oesophageal echocardiography shows increasing promise in continuous monitoring of selected patients.

The goal of therapy is to minimize myocardial oxygen demands while maintaining optimal oxygen delivery to peripheral tissues. Peripheral oxygen requirement is minimized by sedation and avoidance of shivering and hyperpyrexia. Determinants of DO_2 are cardiac output and blood oxygen content (haemoglobin and haemoglobin saturation). Effective treatment of patients with poor LV function requires meticulous assessment and treatment of the determinants of cardiac output.

Important steps in the optimization of cardiac output include:

- **Maintain cardiac rhythm**
  - —Revert atrial fibrillation if possible (electrical, pharmacological)
  - —Maintain AV synchrony[11] (use of atrial and ventricular pacing electrodes). Consider insertion of transvenous atrial pacemaker where 'atrial kick' of demonstrated importance and no atrial electrode in situ.
- **Optimize cardiac rate**
  - —Serial cardiac output studies may indicate optimal rate[12] and AV interval[13] where AV sequential pacing is used.
  - —More advanced modes of pacing (e.g. DDD) may offer beneficial increments in patients with marginal function.[14]
- **Maintain cardiac preload and exclude volume deficit**
  - —Increase PAWP to 15 mmHg if cardiac index is inadequate. Assess

response to volume challenge.
- — Consider higher PAWP depending upon response to volume but recognize risk of increased interstitial pulmonary fluid. Assess pulmonary artery and CVP waveforms for 'v waves'.
- — While bypass is usually associated with the retention of excess body water, large temperature shifts, bleeding, capillary leak and the evolution of myocardial oedema may produce dramatic changes in volume status.

- **Optimize contractility and afterload**
  - — titrate inotropes to obtain cardiac output desired, with secondary adjustment then to maintain perfusion pressure.
  - — Response to inotropes varies in individuals and in the same person over time because of evolving myocardial changes.
- **Cardiac support may be provided with**:
  - — inotropes (e.g. dopexamine, dobutamine)
  - — 'inodilators' (e.g. amrinone, milrinone)
  - — 'inoconstrictors' (e.g. dopamine, adrenaline)
  - — vasodilators (e.g. nitroprusside)
  - — vasoconstrictors (e.g. noradrenaline)
  - — combinations of these agents (see Chapter 32).
- **Counterpulsation (IABP) or left ventricular assist device (LVAD)**
  - — In the patient with poor LV function, these may have been inserted in order to separate from bypass.
  - — Some patients demonstrate acute LV failure or may require gradually increasing inotropic support in the post bypass period. These patients may benefit from early IABP insertion both to assist haemodynamic function and to salvage myocardium at risk of infarction. Tamponade should be excluded.
  - — In the patient progressing poorly following return from theatre, insertion of a balloon pump may be more efficacious than serial increases in inotropic therapy. LVAD may be indicated on the basis of set indications.

Tamponade

Post cardiothoracic surgery tamponade does not present with the classical signs of tamponade. Thus Kussmaul's sign, arterial paradox and equalization of right- and left-sided diastolic pressures may not be present. The essential sign is a low cardiac output. Falling cardiac output with rising filling pressures is the commonest presenting sign but the latter is neither sensitive nor specific.

Tamponade should be considered when there is one or more of:

- unexplained low cardiac output, or falling cardiac output with rising filling pressures (increasing inotropes may mask falling cardiac index)
- unexplained oliguria or tissue acidosis
- large drain losses, especially when these suddenly cease.

The diagnosis of tamponade is a clinical one. It should be strongly considered in any patient who shows poor progression following bypass in the absence of an obvious cause. Special investigations may delay return to theatre in patients who have significant tamponade. Echocardiography is often unhelpful or misleading in diagnosis.

The treatment of tamponade is always surgical. Needle drainage is not suitable. Clot may often be localized, impairing filling to one cardiac chamber, and a thorough inspection is necessary upon return to theatre.

Late re-exploration (24–96 hours) with removal of localized thrombus has frequently dramatically reversed the downward spiral of many patients. Unrecognized tamponade can be a cause of progressive renal dysfunction and multiple organ dysfunction 24–72 hours following surgery. Tamponade may still be present, even when another cause for poor output has been demonstrated, and patients with known poor LV function tolerate any degree of tamponade poorly.

Tamponade should always be considered in a patient with poor cardiac output who in the absence of an obvious explanation has not been progressing as planned.

Myocardial ischaemia

Acute coronary ischaemia may result from mechanical graft occlusion (kinking or thrombus), spasm in graft or native circulation, or from unrecognized disease in ungrafted vessels. Inadequate perfusion pressure, especially where mammary artery grafts have been used, should be considered.

Ischaemia may be suspected on the basis of:

- ECG changes
- clinical evidence of abnormal cardiac function
- new regional wall motion abnormality on echocardiogram.

Treatment strategies after correction of inadequate perfusion pressure depend on the clinical situation but options include:

- return to theatre with review of graft
- cardiac catheterization with therapy according to findings (that is antispasm agents, angioplasty, return to theatre)
- supportive and empiric therapy with intravenous nitrates, calcium antagonists and if necessary balloon counterpulsation.

Arrhythmias

Supraventricular arrhythmias

Supraventricular arrhythmias are common following cardiopulmonary bypass. Classification of these into atrial fibrillation, supraventricular tachycardia and atrial flutter should be done on the basis of surface ECG. Atrial ECGs (where atrial leads present) can confirm the diagnosis.

Therapeutic options are determined by the rhythm, patient stability and likelihood of recurrence. Such options include:

- atrial overdrive pacing (not atrial fibrillation)
- synchronized DC cardioversion
- pharmacological therapy
- observation alone.

Common to all therapy is the need to maintain normal electrolytes, rewarm the patient and avoid atrial overdistension.

Atrial fibrillation is the commonest atrial dysrrhythmia requiring treatment, occurring in 15–40% of post-operative patients. Pharmacological therapeutic options include:

- magnesium and potassium supplements
- amiodarone (intravenous) 3–5 mg/kg over 30–60 minutes (infusion up to 1200 mg per day if necessary)
- digoxin (intravenous).

Ventricular arrhythmias

Ventricular ectopy is common following cardiopulmonary bypass. Hypokalaemia and hypomagnesaemia should be strictly avoided. Such ectopy may in many instances be observed and where not haemodynamically disabling, does not require treatment. Ventricular pacing or atrioventricular pacing may be adjusted in many cases to suppress ectopy. The possibility that arrhythmias may be iatrogenic, secondary to invasive lines or inappropriate pacemaker sensing, should always be considered.

Sustained ventricular tachycardia is treated with cardioversion or standard pharmacological regimens (see Ch. 63). In the patient with extreme ventricular irritability poorly responsive to conventional antiarrhythmics, or where there is known poor LV function, amiodarone infusion may be the preferred drug. Overdrive pacing and counterpulsation will occasionally have a role.

Post perfusion syndrome (low systemic vascular resistance syndrome)

Some patients develop significant vasodilatation and low systemic vascular resistance (SVR) following cardiopulmonary bypass, with the classical appearance of the 'Sepsis Syndrome'. Such a syndrome[15,16] is usually marked by systemic vasodilatation, elevated cardiac output, leukocytosis, a bleeding diathesis, metabolic acidosis, shivering and temperature overshoot.

Hypotension in the setting of high cardiac output may be observed if graft perfusion is not compromised but may require treatment with fluids and vasoconstrictors. The syndrome is usually self-limiting, resolving within 12–24 hours of surgery.

On occasion the syndrome may be fulminant, with marked respiratory infiltrates and multiple organ dysfunction. The therapeutic role of steroids and NSAIDS has not been proven. The differential diagnosis will include drug reaction (e.g. protamine), pancreatitis and gut ischaemia.

Hypertension

Surgeons require close blood pressure control as part of post-operative care. Adequate analgesia and anxiolysis are necessary prerequisites. Short-acting agents such as intravenous nitroglycerine or sodium nitroprusside may be rapidly titrated. The short-acting intravenous beta blocker esmolol may be used but longer-acting beta blockers should be used cautiously in the immediate post-operative period, especially where there is poor LV function or conduction defect but no pace-

maker. Nifedipine given sublingually or via the nasogastric tube may be effective, and may also minimize graft spasm, although reflex tachycardia can be troublesome especially in the setting of myocardial ischaemia. (For more detailed discussion of hypertensive crises, see Ch. 69.)

Left ventricular failure

LV failure is treated according to standard protocols similar to those used for myocardial infarction (see Ch. 56).

Post-operative bleeding

The risk of post-operative bleeding can often be anticipated pre-operatively.

High risk:[4]

- emergency surgery receiving aspirin
- combination valve and aortocoronary bypass (initial or re-do operation)
- re-do valve replacement
- endocarditis.

Intermediate risk:[4]

- re-do coronary artery bypass grafting
- arterial conduit
- valvular surgery.

The most common causes of bleeding after cardiopulmonary bypass are:

- inadequate surgical haemostasis
- pre-existing disease or drug treatment
- heparin-protamine interaction
- disordered platelet quality or thrombocytopenia
- fibrinolysis
- hypertension.

Of patients who return to theatre for control of bleeding, in perhaps 50% generalized oozing seems to be the sole or major contributor to the bleeding.[17] This coagulopathy is often multifactorial and many therapies have been tried to treat it.

Platelet shortage or defect in function is the commonest non-surgical cause of bleeding. Hypothermia and bypass are associated with a reversible defect in platelet function that may persist for 2–4 hours post bypass. In some patients this defect is severe and prolonged, resulting in bleeding. A mild fall in coagulation factors can be demonstrated after CPB due to dilutional change. It may be more severe in patients on pre-operative warfarin therapy. Moderate thrombocytopenia (100 000) is usually due to haemodilution and adherence to bypass circuitry but is not usually associated with bleeding.

Some patients demonstrate significant fibrinolysis following CPB. Lambert[18] found hyperfibrinolytic haemorrhage was responsible for bleeding in 20% of patients with excessive bleeding post CPB. Antifibrinolytic agents[5,18–20] (for example, aprotinin, Σ-aminocaproic acid [EACA], tranexamic acid [TA]) given prophylactically have been demonstrated to reduce post-operative blood loss. This effect is most marked when given before CPB and is less marked when given prophylactically after CPB. The cost, the marginal effect of these agents in patients with low blood loss and concern about producing a procoagulable state has seen their use reserved for patients at risk of high blood loss.[5,20] Reliable studies on efficacy and safety of these agents for the *post bypass* treatment of excessive bleeding are not available.

Common factors in the control of bleeding are:

- rewarming
- control of blood pressure and avoidance of hypertension.

More specific treatments will depend upon the results of clinical observation (oozing suggestive of coagulopathy) and laboratory tests. Treatment includes:

- **Reversal of heparin**
  - — need for additional protamine is assessed by ACT or APTT. ACT can have false negatives and empiric protamine may be indicated. APTT is less specific but more sensitive.
  - — while protamine excess may be associated theoretically with coagulopathy, the dose required is very large.
- **Reversal of factor VII deficiency**
  Empirical fresh frozen plasma (FFP)[21,22] does not appear to reduce 24 hours blood loss nor does it reduce the need for re-sternotomy. FFP is probably indicated[23] where:
  - — PT > 1.5 × normal
  - — APTT > 1.5 × normal
  - — blood loss > 100% of estimated blood volume.
- **Reversal of platelet deficiency or qualitative defect**
  Platelet transfusion is generally indicated[24] where:
  - — platelet count < 50 000

— transfused RBCs > 100% of estimated blood volume.

Platelet transfusion (4–8 units) is also usually indicated in the bleeding patient where:

— tests display platelet dysfunction, e.g. prolonged bleeding time or thromboelastograph (TEG) with poor α takeoff

— tests for platelet dysfunction are not available but dysfunction is likely, e.g. pre-operative aspirin therapy, bleeding in absence of other overt cause.

Other strategies for treatment of platelet dysfunction include:

— desmopressin acetate (DDAVP) (0.3–0.4 μg/kg intravenously). Studies have not shown a universal role for DDAVP, but Mongan[25] has suggested it may reduce blood loss by 30% when the early stage of the TEG shows poor α takeoff.

— aprotinin[5] (500 000 KIU IV followed by 100 000 KIU hourly). While beneficial to platelet function when given pre-bypass, its effect on platelet function when given after CPB has not been adequately studied.

- **Control of hyperfibrinolysis**[5,18,26]
  There is little data available on the effectiveness of antifibrinolytic agents given in the post-operative period. Some would recommend their administration where excessive bleeding secondary to fibrinolysis has been demonstrated. Agents suggested have included:
  — Σ-aminocaproic acid (EACA) (up to 15 g over 2 hours)
  — tranexamic acid (TA)
  — aprotinin (up to 1 million KIU/24 hours post-operatively).[5] Aprotinin has been suggested to control significant post-CPB bleeding[26] but is expensive. The use of TA and EACA has been advocated on the basis of their lower cost and from extrapolation of their effectiveness when given prophylactically.[5] Theoretical objections that these agents may enhance graft occlusion have not been proven in small trials, but large trials are not yet available.[20]

The TEG has gained increasing prominence in patients with post-bypass bleeding and may help differentiate between the presence of poor platelet function, factor insufficiency and secondary fibrinolysis.[27] The art is then to tailor the therapy to the demonstrated abnormality.

Pulmonary complications

Post-operative pulmonary problems include:

- **Hypoxaemic respiratory failure**
  — Cardiogenic pulmonary oedema (LV failure)
  — Ventilation perfusion (V/Q) mismatch due to segmental or lobar atelectasis or vasodilator therapy, e.g. GTN, nitroprusside, nifedipine.
  — Low pressure pulmonary oedema ('pump lung' or ARDS).
- **Ventilatory failure**
  — Residual paralysis or opioid effect
  — Mechanical defects due to pleural effusion (especially if mammary grafts) or pneumothorax.
  — Diaphragmatic palsy (unilateral or bilateral).

Diaphragmatic palsy may complicate surgery, especially where mammary artery grafts have been used and can produce significant orthopnoea. Bilateral palsy can lead to prolonged ventilator dependence. Fluoroscopy is useful in confirmation of diagnosis.

Renal

Renal dysfunction is a cause of prolonged intensive care unit stay but is seldom an isolated event.[28] It usually occurs in the patient with pre-operative renal impairment or poor LV function. The major determinant of the return of normal renal function is the re-establishment of normal haemodynamic function.[6] Major steps in the treatment or avoidance of renal dysfunction are:

- optimize cardiac output
- ensure adequate renal perfusing pressure
- avoid further renal insults, e.g. aminoglycosides, NSAIDS
- consider early veno-venous haemofiltration where significant cardiorespiratory failure.

Treatment is otherwise standard ICU care for renal failure. In the

patient with marginal renal function, cardiac output and mean blood pressure should be optimized before recourse to diuretics.

Cardiac tamponade should always be considered in the patient with unexplained progressive deterioration in renal function.

Neurological

Neurologic defects (incidence 1–6%):[29,30,31]

- stroke
- impaired conscious level or confusional state
- seizures
- spinal cord injury
- peripheral nerve injury.

Neuropsychologic defects (incidence 50–70%):[29]

- defects of concentration, memory and learning—60–80% 1 week post surgery, 20–40% 8 weeks post surgery.

Stroke is probably the most common source of morbidity in the post-cardiac surgical population.[29,30] Rankin has found it to be due to vascular embolism in 57% of cases and to a border zone infarction in 43% of cases.[30] Clinically it may manifest as delayed awakening or as a focal neurological deficit. In some, stroke develops in the post-operative period and may follow post-operative supraventricular arrhythmia.[31]

The presence of a severe focal neurological defect in the immediate post-operative period represents a difficult problem for management. Treatable causes such as cerebral haemorrhage or air embolism are uncommon and the likelihood of a treatable problem should be balanced against the risks of moving patients for CT scanning or hyperbaric therapy. The possibility of cerebral haemorrhage should be considered in the patient with focal defect who has had coagulopathy or hypertension, or concomitant carotid surgery, and who is suitable for surgery should a haemorrhage be proven. The presence of air embolism is difficult to confirm but may be considered[32] where such embolism has been seen or thought possible during CPB and where focal defect is present. Such a defect may respond to hyperbaric oxygen therapy, but this may not be readily safely available. Delayed computed tomography (CT) scanning may best demonstrate the defect of cerebral infarction.

References

1. Tuman KJ, McCarthy JR, March HR, Najafi H, Ivankovich AD. Morbidity and duration of ICU stay after cardiac surgery—a model for preoperative risk assessment. Chest 1992; 102: 36–44
2. Tu JV, Jaglal SB, Naylor CD. Multicenter validation of a risk index for mortality, intensive care unit stay, and overall hospital length of stay after cardiac surgery. Circulation 1995; 91: 677–84
3. Rosen NR, Bates IH, Herod G. Transfusion therapy: improved patient care and resource utilisation. Transfusion 1993; 33: 341–7
4. Hardy J-F, Perrault J, Tremblay N, Robitaille D, Blain R, Carrier M. The stratification of cardiac surgical procedures according to use of blood products: a retrospective analysis of 1480 cases. Can J Anaesth 1991; 38: 511–7
5. Hardy J-F, Desroches J. Natural and synthetic antifibrinolytics in cardiac surgery. Can J Anaesth 1992; 39: 353–65
6. Hilberman M, Derby GC, Spencer RJ, Stinson EB. Sequential pathophysiological changes characterizing the progression from renal dysfunction to acute renal failure following cardiac operation. J Thorac Cardiovasc Surg 1980; 79: 838–44
7. Myles PS, Buckland MR, Schenk NJ, Cannon GB, Langley M, Davis BB, Weeks AM. Effect of 'Renal-Dose' dopamine on renal function following cardiac surgery. Anaesth Intens Care 1993; 21: 56–61
8. Cruise C, MacKinnon J, Tough J, Houston P. Comparison of meperidine and pancuronium for the treatment of shivering after cardiac surgery. Can J Anaesth 1992; 39: 563–8
9. Chong JL, Grebenik C, Sinclair M, Fisher A, Pillai R, Westaby S. The effect of a cardiac surgical recovery area on the timing of extubation. J Cardiothorac Vasc Anesth 1993; 7: 137–41
10. Shapiro BA, Lichtenthal PR. Inhalation-based anesthetic techniques are the key to early extubation of the cardiac surgical patient. Editorial. J Cardiothorac Vasc Anesth 1993; 7: 135–6
11. Donovan KD, Dobb GJ, Lee KY. Hemodynamic benefit of maintaining atrioventricular synchrony during cardiac pacing in critically ill patients. Crit Care Med 1991; 19: 320–6
12. Watkins DN, Donovan KD, Dobb GJ, Lee KY, Murdock C. Heart rate determines cardiac output in critically ill, pacemaker dependent patients. Anaesth Intens Care 1994; 22: 221–2
13. Ferguson TB Jr, Cox JL. Temporary external DDD pacing after cardiac operations. Ann Thorac Surg 1991; 51: 723–732

14. Durbin CG Jr, Kopel RF. Optimal atrioventricular (AV) pacing interval during temporary AV sequential pacing after cardiac surgery. J Cardiothorac Vasc Anesth 1993; 7: 316–20
15. Westaby S. Organ dysfunction after cardiopulmonary bypass. A systemic inflammatory reaction initiated by the extracorporeal circuit. Intensive Care Med 1987; 13: 89–95
16. Casey LC. Role of cytokines in the pathogenesis of cardiopulmonary-induced multisystem organ failure. Ann Thorac Surg 1993; 56: S92-S96
17. Karski JM, Teasdale SJ, Norman P, Carroll J, Glynn M. Mechanisms of excessive bleeding after cardiopulmonary bypass. Can J Anaesth 1992; 39: A140
18. Lambert CJ, Marengo-Rowe AJ, Leveson JE et al. The treatment of postperfusion bleeding using Σ-aminocaproic acid, cryoprecipitate, fresh-frozen plasma, and protamine sulfate. Ann Thorac Surg 1979; 28: 440–4
19. Royston D. Aprotinin therapy. Editorial. Br J Anaesth 1994; 73: 734–7
20. Royston D. Intraoperative coronary thrombosis: can aprotinin be incriminated? Editorial. J Cardiothorac Vasc Anesth 1994; 8: 137–41
21. Kaplan JA, Cannarella C, Jones EL, Kutner MH, Hatcher CR, Dunbar RW. Autologous blood transfusion during cardiac surgery. J Thorac Cardiovasc Surg 1977; 74: 4–10
22. Roy RC, Stafford MA, Hudspeth AS, Meredith JW. Failure of prophylaxis with fresh frozen plasma after cardiopulmonary bypass. Anesthesiology 1988; 69: 254–7
23. Consensus Conference: fresh frozen plasma. indications and risks. JAMA 1985; 253: 551–3
24. Consensus Conference: platelet transfusion therapy. JAMA 1987; 257: 1777–80
25. Mongan PD, Hosking MP. The role of desmopressin acetate in patients undergoing coronary artery bypass surgery—a controlled clinical trial with thromboelastographic risk of stratification. Anaesthesiology 1992; 77: 38–46
26. Angelini GD, Cooper GJ, Lamarra M, Bryan AJ. Unorthodox use of aprotinin to control life-threatening bleeding after cardiopulmonary bypass. Lancet 1990; 335: 799–800
27. Essell JH, Martin TJ, Salinas J, Thompson JM, Smith VC. Comparison of thromboelastography to bleeding time and standard coagulation tests in patients after cardiopulmonary bypass. J Cardiothorac Vasc Anesth 1993; 7: 410–5
28. Zanardo G, Michielon P, Paccagnella A, Rosi P, Calo M, Salandin V et al. Acute renal failure in the patient undergoing cardiac operation. J Thorac Cardiovasc Surg 1994; 107: 1489–95
29. Mills SA. Cerebral injury and cardiac operations. Ann Thorac Surg 1993; 56: S86–91
30. Rankin JM, Silbert PL, Yadava OP, Hankey GJ, Stewart-Wynne EG. Mechanism of stroke complicating cardiopulmonary bypass surgery. Aust NZ J Med 1994; 24: 154–60
31. Johansson T, Aren C, Fransson S-G, Uhre P. Intra and postoperative cerebral complications of open-heart surgery. Scand J Thor Cardiovasc Surg 1995; 29: 17–22
32. Tuxen DV, Scheinkestel CD, Salamonson R. Air embolism—a neglected cause of stroke complicating cardiopulmonary bypass (CPB) surgery. Aust NZ J Med 1994; 24: 732–3

66 The cardiac catheterization patient

Barry E Hopkins

Staff in the coronary care unit will frequently be involved in the pre- and post-procedural management of patients having cardiac catheterization and coronary angioplasty. There should be a clear understanding of the technique and its benefits and limitations, as well as its potential complications[1] (see Ch. 21).

The following outlines the practical management of the patient undergoing cardiac catheterization.

Vascular access

The majority of patients are catheterized through the right femoral artery using a 6 French sheath and catheters. Problems may arise if the patient has had previous vascular graft surgery to the femoral arteries or has an abdominal aortic aneurysm. In the case of diminished or absent femoral pulses the right brachial artery may be employed but it should be ensured that this vessel is easily accessible, that the elbow can be straightened and that there is no contraindication to access via this site. If the brachial approach is likely to be needed, intravenous (IV) access drip sites should be in the left arm.

Complicating medical conditions

There are several of these which make cardiac catheterization more difficult or possibly more hazardous and requiring further precaution.

Diabetes mellitus

Patients with diabetes should be catheterized first thing in the morning with omission of their morning dose of oral hypoglycaemics or insulin. An IV access must always be in situ. Adequate pre-operative hydration and post-operative hydration is essential to diminish the effects of contrast media on the kidneys. This is especially important if there is any renal insufficiency.

Pre-existing allergy or reaction to contrast media

Although there is doubt whether a previous contrast reaction predicts a subsequent contrast reaction, all precaution is necessary. Such patients are warned a further reaction may occur, are pre-medicated with oral prednisone or prednisolone (a total of 60 mg) over the previous 24 hours and are given intravenous hydrocortisone 100 mg pre-catheter and promethazine 25 mg orally at least 1 hour before catheterization.

Renal insufficiency

A serum creatinine between 100 and 200 mmol/L does not usually produce any problems, providing an IV access is in situ and the patient is adequately hydrated pre-operatively and post-operatively. Patients with a higher creatinine should be discussed in detail with one of the catheterizing cardiologists before the patient is booked for catheterization. Acute renal failure can ensue in these individuals.

Previous cerebrovascular accident

Patients who previously have had a cerebrovascular accident (CVA) may experience transient return of symptoms (due possibly to contrast sludging) in the immediate post-operative period. Transient aphasia or weakness is not uncommon in such patients. Adequate hydration and patience over 4–5 hours usually means a return to normal. If a defect persists for more than 4–5 hours, CVA complicating the procedure must be entertained.

Anticoagulation

Patients on long-term warfarin will need to have the drug stopped and anticoagulation continued with heparin. It is usually safe to proceed with an INR level of 1.5–2.0. These patients are given a heparin infusion which is stopped 4 hours before the procedure. If the patient has unstable angina, however, the heparin may be continued right up to the procedure, depending on the operator's discretion.

Patient education and preparation

Written and illustrated material which clearly outlines the procedure of cardiac catheterization should be given to all patients at least 2 or 3 hours before the catheterizing cardiologist sees the patient, and time should be allowed for discussion with nursing staff for education. At the time of the visit by the operator the patient should be well-informed and can ask questions. The operator will usually reinforce several points. If coronary care staff are in doubt how to answer the patient's questions, they should refer them to the operator. It is important that the patient realize that the passage of the catheter through the arteries is not felt at all and there is no pain associated with such a procedure.

Risk

It is imperative that all patients have explained to them that there is some risk in the procedure, but that the risk is small. Quantifying the risk is indeed difficult, although the best guide is from the Society of Cardiac Angiography and Intervention in the United States where a registry based on 60 000 catheterizations showed the following:[2]

- The risk of death in patients with NYHA functional class 1 or 2 is 1 in 5000.
- Patients with more severe cardiac failure or left main disease may have risks approaching 1 in 200. On the other hand the risk of disease untreated is much greater and this should be explained to the patient. If they are not seriously ill and do not have severe heart failure or unstable angina, their risk is small.
- The risk of myocardial infarction is about 1 in 1000.
- The risk of vascular complications such as haematoma is around 1 in 50.
- The risk of more serious complications such as vascular occlusion is less than 1 in 200.
- The risk of stroke is less than 1 in 1000.

Discussion of these risks with the patient should be placed within the context of the general health of the patient. If they have unstable angina the risk of continuing without catheterization is probably much greater than the procedure itself. An empathetic manner in discussing these risks can greatly allay the patient's fears.

Pre-medication

Opinions on the use of pre-medication differ from operator to operator. In general, 10 mg of diazepam given at least 1 hour before the procedure is good pre-medication for most patients. Some operators use 25 mg of promethazine in addition, to provide greater relaxation and reduce the risk of allergies. The use of steroids has been discussed above.

IV access

In general, IV access in the left arm is very useful during the procedure and should be encouraged. In some patients it is mandatory. This is particularly so in patients with a prior history of syncope associated with needle stick, with recent unstable angina and with other complicating medical features such as renal failure or diabetes. If in doubt, IV access should be in situ, preferably with IV saline running slowly on the patient transported from the ward or CCU.

Post-procedure care

General

In the case of femoral catheterization the patient should lie for at least 6 hours with the leg straight and unmoving. After 2–3 hours the patient's head can be elevated 10–20 degrees but the patient should not be allowed to reach above the bed or roll over unassisted. The use of smaller calibre catheters (e.g. 5 French) can shorten these periods of immobilization. In the case of back pain, intravenous diazepam may be useful; in severe cases the patient can be log-rolled on to their side by expert nursing/medical staff after 2–3 hours.

Bleeding

If the femoral or brachial arteriotomy sites bleed, the immediate treatment is *manual compression*. The use of pressure bandages is useless. Compression should be applied sufficient to stop any bleeding but not to completely obliterate peripheral pulses. An air of confidence and quiet is maintained with the patient. The emergency is over once manual compression is applied and the situation will *always* come under control given patience. Most post-operative bleeds, particularly from femoral sites, will subside within 10–15 minutes of compression. In the interim the operator can be notified to review the patient.

Localized swelling

Swelling over the femoral puncture site or at the brachial arteriotomy site is usually due to a localised haematoma. Most are self-limiting. A pulsatile swelling may indicate a false aneurysm (i.e. localised arterial wall dissection). This can be identified by ultrasound; in many cases the false lumen can be obliterated by local pressure with the ultrasound transducer.

Peripheral limb ischaemia

The loss of previously palpable peripheral pulses, or signs of pallor or cyanosis peripherally in the limb, is a medical emergency. The operator should be notified immediately and the patient given a bolus of heparin determined by the operator. *The operator must be notified immediately in all cases*. Urgent vascular surgical intervention may be necessary in some cases.

Infection

Infection of the wound site is rarely a problem with femoral punctures but sometimes with brachial arteriotomy this can occur and usually will not be evident for several days post-catheterization. Brachial arteriotomy wound infection is an emergency and *requires hospitalization*. The operator must be notified, the wound swabbed and cultured and several blood cultures taken. Intravenous antibiotics must then be administered in high doses. The causative organism is usually staphylococcus which has a lytic toxin and can result in mycotic aneurysms of the brachial artery unless treated vigorously. There is no place for the use of oral antibiotics in such patients.

Follow-up

Results of the coronary angiogram should be discussed with the patient by the cardiologist caring for the patient. The coronary care staff should not form an opinion based on the operation record or on their own assessment of the coronary angiogram, since this may be incorrect and does not take full cognisance of all of the facts.

Conclusions

Cardiac catheterization is a safe and effective diagnostic procedure in good hands. Attention to detail in the pre-operative assessment and preparation of the patient and in their post-operative care will minimize risk.

References

1. Grossman W, Baim DS. Cardiac catheterization, angiography and intervention. 4th edition. Philadelphia: Lea & Febiger, 1991
2. Johnson LW, Lozner EC, Johnson S et al. Coronary angiography 1984–1987. A report of the Registry of the Society for Cardiac Angiography and Interventions. 1. Results and comparisons. Cath Cardiovasc Diagn 1989; 17: 5

67 The coronary angioplasty patient

Mark E Hands and Eric G Whitford

The management of the patient before and after coronary angioplasty is usually conducted in the coronary care unit (CCU). Coronary care staff should have a clear concept of the technique, as well as its application to the patient with myocardial infarction and unstable angina pectoris[1] (see Ch. 45).

The following outlines the current practical management of the patient undergoing coronary angioplasty in our unit.

Pre-angioplasty

Medication

For at least 24 hours before, and on the day of the operation, the patient is prescribed the following:

- aspirin 100 mg daily (if the patient is *not* on aspirin, the operator should be notified)
- if the patient is likely to receive a stent at the time of angioplasty, additional antithrombotic therapy—for example, ticlopidine—should be considered
- other anti-anginal drugs as pre-admission
- topical, oral or IV nitroglycerin at the discretion of the operator.

Informed consent

Informed consent is obtained for:

- cardiac catheterization and coronary angiography
- coronary angioplasty
- possible intracoronary stent insertion
- possible coronary bypass surgery in the event of its being required in an emergency.

The consent for the procedures is obtained in writing.

Explanation

Ideally, written and illustrated material is given to patients to read at their leisure. The points to be emphasized include the potential risks of the procedure and the possible need for emergency coronary artery bypass surgery, the risks of early re-occlusion and late stenosis and the possible need for intracoronary stent insertion and post-operative anticoagulation.

Fasting

The patient is usually fasted for solids for at least 8 hours pre-angioplasty and for fluids for at least 4 hours.

Intravenous line

An IV line should be inserted in the left arm, using a 16 or 18 gauge cannula, as an access for drugs and so that the patient may receive fluids. The patient is kept well hydrated and normal saline should be running on transfer to the catheter laboratory.

Pre-procedure

- 12-lead ECG is taken.
- Blood is taken for full blood examination and baseline cardiac enzymes and electrolytes are checked.
- The patient is premedicated with oral sedation, e.g. 10–15 mg diazepam. Promethazine and steroids are only given if directed by the operator.

Post angioplasty care

On arrival in CCU

The arterial sheath is kept in situ post percutanous transluminal coronary angioplasty (PTCA),

and pressure is monitored through the side arm of the sheath.

- *Arterial* sheath—5 ml is aspirated prior to connecting to arterial pressure transducer line continuous flush with 5000 u heparin in 500 ml n/saline at 3 ml/hr). The obturator must remain in and locked in the sheath.
- *Venous* sheath (if present) should also be flushed continuously with heparinized saline (5000 u heparin in 500 ml n/saline) at 3 ml/hr via infusion pump.
- 12-lead ECG is taken.
- Peripheral IV heparin is given as directed by post-operative orders and the directions given by the operator.
- IV hydration line remains in situ until the sheath is removed, as it may be utilized for fluid and drug administration.
- Blood is drawn for cardiac enzymes including creatine kinase (CK) total and CKMB.

Care of the sheath

- The sheath site is inspected for haematoma/ooze. Foot pulses and vital signs are recorded at least every 15 minutes for the first 2 hours, then if satisfactory, hourly whilst the sheath is in situ.
- The patient must not sit up more than 30° with the sheath in situ. If a flexible sheath is in situ, the patient may sit up no more than 60° but *any* patient with a sheath in situ must NOT flex the affected leg.
- The time of sheath removal will be notified by the operator. Peripheral IV heparin should be stopped at least 4 hours before the time of predicted sheath removal. The measured ACT will determine the exact time of removal of the sheath, e.g. ACT < 150. The heparin/saline continuous flush infusion through the sheath(s) MUST NOT stop until the time of removal.

Fluid intake and output

The patient should take soup and sandwiches or light diet only, and oral fluids are encouraged.

Medication

- Aspirin 100 mg daily continues.
- Antithrombotic therapy as charted
- Anti-anginal therapy as charted
- IV fluids for hypotension and dehydration
- IV relaxants (e.g. benzodiazepines) may be required for back discomfort
- Occasionally narcotics and a local anaesthetic may be used for sheath removal.

Electrocardiogram and bloods

ECG and bloods for cardiac enzymes should be carried out the following morning.

Back pain

During the post-angioplasty period in the CCU, many patients have back pain and muscle spasm due to their restricted mobility. The principles of management should be:

- Explain the problem to the patient.
- Perform log roll and back rub.
- Move the head of the bed up and down (to a maximum of 30°, or 60° if hemaflex sheath) to relieve back muscle spasm.
- Use IV sedative and relaxants, e.g. diazemuls 2–5 mg 3-hourly prn for spasm.
- Use IV narcotics if the above is ineffective.
- Ensure that some other cause of back pain (such as dissection or retroperitoneal haemorrhage) is not responsible.

Post-operative complications

Any troublesome complications should be reported immediately to the operator. Of particular importance are:

- chest pain
- new ECG changes of ischaemia
- new arrhythmias
- bleeding from wound sites
- excessive haematoma
- changes in foot pulses
- unexplained hypotension
- neurological symptoms.

Angioplasty sheath removal

- Requires trolley and angioplasty tray contents.
- Prior to sheath removal the following may be required:
  - —local anaesthesia (1% lignocaine); and/or
  - —IV narcotics.
- Reflex bradycardia and/or hypotension may occur during

sheath removal and subsequent pressure, therefore:
- — ensure adequate volume, i.e. IV hydration fluid bag is available
- — have atropine available
- — continually monitor heart rate (HR) and blood pressure (BP) during and immediately after removal.

- Patient must NOT be left unattended when groin clamp is in use.
- Observation (after removal) of vital signs and limb pulses should be done at least:
  - — every 15 minutes for two hours
  - — hourly for four hours
  - — two hourly while at bedrest.
- A SANDBAG may be placed on the groin or as directed.
- Rest in bed for 8–12 hours, but may sit up to 30°–40° provided that the hip is not flexed.
- The dressing is normally removed and the transparent adhesive dressing applied before mobilizing the patient. After 20–30 minutes of mobilization, the site should be checked for any secondary haematoma.

Intracoronary stents

General

Since stents are constructed of metal they are thrombogenic. The technique of post-dilatation of the stent insertion site has reduced the need for anticoagulation and most patients are now managed with anti-platelet agents, permitting early discharge and reduced risk of haemorrhage.[2,3]

All angioplasty patients should already be receiving aspirin. Ticlopidine is added if a stent has been placed.[4]

Post-stent protocol

When a stent is placed in a coronary artery the principal complications are:

- subacute thrombosis at the stent site
- bleeding, particularly when aggressive anticoagulant regimes are utilized
- local vascular problems such as false aneurysm formation at the site of arterial access.

On return to the CCU

If the standard post-stent antithrombotic regimen is being used, special precautions are required to minimize the risk of bleeding:

- The sheath insertion site should be observed for swelling and/or bruising, and where appropriate the extent of the bruising should be delineated with a marker pen. The patient is to be log rolled at all times and not moved more often than is absolutely necessary up until 12 hours after the sheath is removed.
- Observations of the femoral artery puncture site, the presence of foot pulses and the vital signs are to be performed at least every 15 minutes for the first 2 hours after return from the catheter laboratory and then at least hourly while the sheath is in situ.
- Heparin is stopped for sheath removal. The sheath is removed when the ACT is less than 150 seconds.

Sheath removal

This is to be performed as per the angioplasty sheath removal protocol.

- Aspirin 100 mg daily should be continued.
- 2 hours post clamp removal the patient may sit up 30° in bed provided that the hip is not flexed.
- Observations of vital signs and limb pulses are performed at least every 15 minutes for 2 hours post clamp removal, then hourly for 4 hours, then 2-hourly for 24 hours.
- A sandbag may be placed at the groin as directed by the operator.
- The dressing is normally removed and 'Op Site' applied before mobilizing the patient. After 20–30 minutes of mobilization, the site is checked for any secondary haematoma.

Discharge plan for stent patients

- Aspirin is continued, as well as ticlopidine 250 mg bd for 3–4 weeks post procedure.
- The patient is advised not to do any heavy manual labour or lifting in the week after discharge.
- The full blood picture is checked 10–14 days post-procedure due to the risk (1–2%) of neutropenia or thrombocytopenia with the use of ticlopidine.

With stenting there is still a risk of re-stenosis of the angioplasty site, and prior to discharge all patients are instructed what to do if there is any recurrence of ischaemic chest pain post angioplasty.

References

1. Topol EJ. Textbook of Interventional Cardiology 2nd Ed 1995 Philadelphia WB Saunders
2. Goods CM, Al-Shaibi KF, Yadav SS et al. Utilization of coronary balloon-expandable coil stent without anti-coagulation or intravascular ultrasound. Circulation 1996; 93: 1803–8
3. Colombo A, Hall P, Nakamuta S et al. Intracoronary stenting without anti-ultrasound guidance. Circulation 1995; 91: 1676–88
4. Hall P, Nakamura S, Maiello L et al. A randomized comparison of combined ticlopidine and aspirin therapy versus aspirin therapy alone after successful ultrasound-guided stent implantation. Circulation 1996; 93: 215–22

68 The cardiac transplant patient

Anne M Keogh

The background to cardiac transplantation as an option for treatment of advanced cardiac disease has been discussed in Chapter 48. Coronary care staff may be involved in the management of the cardiac transplant recipient. This chapter presents practical advice for coronary care unit (CCU) staff managing the patient before and after transplant.

Support to the time of transplant

General measures

When the patient has been accepted for transplantation, general measures include an active structured rhythmic exercise programme where possible, avoidance of blood transfusion (risk of pre-sensitizing recipient to potential donors), routine methicillin-resistant *Staphylococcus aureus* (MRSA) line swabs, and minimal use of indwelling lines. A no-added salt diet should be followed; salt allowed in the cooking, but not added at mealtimes. Total salt restriction is not desirable.

All patients should be receiving maximal tolerated doses of angiotension II-converting enzyme (ACE) inhibitors,[1–3] diuretics and vasodilators (whether infused, topical or oral). Chronic right heart failure patients may benefit from spironolactone until creatinine ≥ 18 mmol/L (180 μmol/L). If ACE inhibitors are not tolerated due to cough or hypotension, hydralazine and isosorbide dinitrate combination should be used instead.[4] Intravenous nitroglycerin infusion is extremely useful unless the patient is hypovolaemic or severely hypotensive.

Heart failure patients (especially if chronic) will fare better with systolic blood pressure around 85–110 mmHg.

The information box outlines the tests for assessing a patient for cardiac transplantation.

Inotropic drugs

Dopamine (2–4.5 mcg/kg/min)

Use should be considered where there is resistant fluid overload (especially with renal dysfunction), relative hypotension with reduced peripheral perfusion, evidence of moderately severe hepatic or renal dysfunction, or hyponatraemia resistant to fluid restriction. Dopamine should be used with care, however, where there is angina, aortic stenosis, atrial fibrillation or tachycardia. Doses greater than 4.5 mcg/kg/min will cause peripheral vasoconstriction and increase myocardial oxygen consumption, and hence should be avoided.[5,6]

If creatinine ≥ 0.18 mmol/L, a trial of dopamine should be considered (3–7 days) to assess reversibility of renal dysfunction.

Dobutamine (5–10 mcg/kg/min)

Dobutamine may be better tolerated in patients with ischaemic heart disease due to its effect of increasing coronary blood flow via coronary vasodilatation.

Combination inotropes (dopamine and dobutamine) often give optimal control. The optimal dosage combination is dopamine 3–4.5 mg/kg/min and with dobutamine, 7–9 mcg/kg/min.

Antiarrhythmic agents

In general, the only agents which will be tolerated are amiodarone and quinidine. Amiodarone will control ventricular arrhythmias and rate of response to atrial fibrillation, and is certainly the drug of choice.

Precipitation of heart failure is rare with amiodarone, as its negative inotropic effect is almost always offset by vasodilatation

Assessment of a potential cardiac transplant recipient

Tests:
Echocardiogram ± radionuclide ventriculography
Right heart catheter ± vasodilator challenge if transpulmonary gradient ≥ 12

Full blood count, differential white cell count, sedimentation rate, platelets
ABO group and ABO antibody screen
Serum sodium, potassium, magnesium, urea, creatinine, and liver function tests
Glucose, lipids
HIV, Hep A, and C, Hep B_s Ag
Serum electrophoretogram, antinuclear antigen
Cytomegalovirus titre

Computed Tomography (CT) scan head, chest and abdomen for occult malignancy (over 55 years only)
Haemoccult (over 45 years), rectal examination
Infection control swabs
Tissue typing and cell panel (cytotoxicity screen)—Blood Bank

Consults:
Dentist
Social worker
Dietician
Physiotherapist (structured exercise programme)

Special:
Digital Subtraction Angiography (DSA) if claudication
Gastroscopy if symptoms or iron deficient
Colonoscopy if haemoccult positive
Patient education
Carotid Doppler (if over 55 years with IHD)

with resultant fall in LV end-diastolic dimension and rise in ejection fraction.[7] Routine use may reduce medium-term mortality from both sudden death and cardiac failure.[8,9] Digoxin dosage should be halved. Torsades de pointes occurs in < 1% of those on amiodarone. Thyrotoxicosis is a common side-effect of amiodarone therapy, but often responds to neomercazole or propylthiouracil without ceasing amiodarone, if its continuation is important. Low dose maintenance therapy (100–200 mg per day, or less) is well tolerated.

NYHA class III patients may tolerate metoprotol 2.5–25 mg 12-hourly or carvedilol up to 25 mg 12-hourly, but may experience an initial deterioration when starting the medication.

Anticoagulants

Warfarin is more effective than aspirin in preventing ventricular thrombi. The INR should be kept between 1.8 and 2.5. Aspirin is difficult to reverse at the time of transplantation, so should be ceased when the patient is listed for transplant.

Diuretics

Frusemide is the mainstay diuretic. If unresponsive, ethacrynic acid 50–100 mg IV or orally, or metolazone 1.25–2.5 mg orally as needed can be used as alternatives. In general, daily metolazone will lead to severe hyponatraemia and renal impairment. Regular usage should be avoided, and electrolytes closely monitored.

Advanced support

Intra-aortic balloon pump

For heart failure unresponsive to these measures, intra-aortic balloon pumping (see Ch. 47) may be required. The insertion point should be kept as high as possible (just below the inguinal ligament) to avoid cannulating the superficial femoral artery (leg ischaemia) and a 30 ml balloon should be considered in patients under 168 cm in height, to avoid balloon impaction in the sheath.[10] A halving of platelet count can be expected because of mechanical trauma. If on heparin, however, the patient should be monitored for thrombocytopenia due to heparin-induced antibody syndrome (HITS). If HITS is suspected, Rheomacrodex or low molecular weight heparin should be substituted immediately. Heparin antibodies can prevent use of heparin during cardiopulmonary bypass but organon may still be able to be used, depending on the cross-reactivity of antibodies.

Left ventricular assist device

The Heart Mate, Novacor or Thoratec LV assist devices are now available but should be reserved for patients who are responding poorly to the intra-aortic balloon pump (IABP—see Ch. 47) or considered electively after 14 days of IABP. Food and Drug Administration (FDA) suggested criteria for use currently are: pulmonary capillary wedge pressure ≥ 20 mmHg with (a) systolic pressure ≤ 80 mmHg or (b) cardiac index ≤ 2.0 L/min/m^2. Transplantation should not be performed at the earliest possible opportunity, but clinicians should wait instead for maximal improvement in other organ function (usually in excess of 1 month).

Criteria for long-term usage have not yet been clearly defined.[11,12]

A patient who is to be considered for a transplant, and their family, will need considerable psychological support and explanation. Support groups and meeting with other recipients do more to encourage such patients than protracted medical explanations. A social worker should be involved early on.

Some patients (once heart failure is controlled) may be suited to revascularization (see Ch. 46) or to cardiomyoplasty (criteria are given in the information box).

Care of the cardiac transplant recipient

Immediate post-operative care will occur in a specialized critical care unit, but the patient may be transferred to the CCU for continuing management.

Heart failure in the cardiac transplant recipient

The most common reason for a cardiac transplant recipient to be admitted to coronary care is heart failure due to either (a) cardiac rejection or (b) transplant coronary artery disease. Signs of early rejection are malaise, fever, atrial arrhythmias (almost always atrial flutter with 2:1 block) and elevated jugular venous pressure (diastolic dysfunction). Signs of advanced rejection are systolic heart failure (right or left), hypoperfusion, hypotension and cardiomegaly. Subtle signs should be noted. ECG and chest X-ray are mandatory and echocardiography may show thick walls (rejection or hypertrophy), systolic dysfunction or regional dysfunction and will exclude significant pericardial effusion.

When a patient is admitted to CCU it is important to contact the transplanting centre as soon as possible for guidance.

Cardiac biopsy (≥ 5 samples) is the only way to exclude acute cellular rejection and must be performed immediately.

Where there is systolic dysfunction, dobutamine (5–10 mcg/kg/min) is the most effective agent and should be used early.[13] Renal dose dopamine may be needed for renal impairment due to hypoperfusion on the background of cyclosporin nephrotoxicity.

If International Society of Heart and Lung Transplantation grade 3a or worse cellular rejection is diagnosed, treatment will be with 0.5–1 g of methylprednisolone intravenously for three consecutive days.[14] Where there is haemodynamic compromise, OKT_3 or ATG (antithymocyte globulin) may be used in addition. Side-effects of OKT_3 are pulmonary capillary leak syndrome (pulmonary oedema), aseptic meningitis and propensity to opportunistic infections.[15] A schedule for administration is detailed in the information box. If necessary, a diuretic is given before administration to avoid pulmonary oedema.

If the cardiac biopsy shows no acute rejection, transplant coronary artery disease should be considered. This is a form of chronic rejection compounded by hyperlipidaemia, characterized by diffuse intimal thickening due to smooth muscle cell proliferation.[16] When advanced, it may result in

Criteria for cardiomyoplasty

For inclusion:

- Dilated cardiomyopathy due to ischaemic, idiopathic or other heart disease with class III symptoms

For exclusion:

- Class IV symptoms
- Valvular heart disease
- Atrial fibrillation (with uncontrolled ventricular response rate)
- Significant pulmonary hypertension
- Ischaemic heart disease (IHD) with unstable lesion
- Right ventricular failure
- Left ventricular ejection fraction (LVEF) < 0.15
- Unstable heart failure

Administration of OKT_3

Premedication
- Methylprednisolone 500–1000 mg IV daily for 3 days, then hydrocortisone 100 mg IV daily
- Promethazine 12.5 mg IV
- Ranitidine 100 mg IV

One hour later
- OKT_3 5 mg by IV push bolus

One hour later
- Ranitidine 100 mg IV

acute infarction, shock, heart failure or sudden death.[17] Because 50% of patients remain denervated at 12 months post transplant,[18] infarction may be painless and detected electrocardiographically or by cardiac enzyme rise.

Use of thrombolysis should be considered according to usual indications. Heparin and nitrate infusions should be used where angina or ischaemia is apparently unstable. Transplanted coronary arteries dilate with nitrates, and heparin may reduce smooth muscle cell proliferation.

In the long term, percutaneous transluminal coronary angioplasty (PTCA) or, less commonly, coronary artery bypass surgery may have a role.[19] All recipients with coronary disease should be on diltiazem and pravastatin or simvastatin because of their anti-atherogenic effects.[20,21] HMG CoA reductase inhibitors reduce serum cholesterol but also reduce natural killer cell activity, reducing rejection rates and improving survival post transplant. Lovastatin should be avoided because of increased risk of rhabdomyolysis.

General management

If oral immunosuppressants have to be discontinued for any reason, switch to intravenous formulation observing the following dosing rules:

- cyclosporin as a 24 hour IV continuous infusion in normal saline at one third of the usual total oral daily dose
- azathioprine IV once daily (same as oral dose)
- hydrocortisone IV at 4 times the daily milligram dose of oral prednisolone
- antibiotic coverage as for non-transplant patients
- oral immunosuppression should resume as soon as possible

Staff should be alert to a possible fall in cyclosporin levels due to ceasing cyclosporin-sparing agents such as diltiazem or ketoconazole.[22]

References

1. CONSENSUS trial study group. Effects of enalapril on mortality in severe congestive heart failure. N Engl J Med 1987; 316: 1429–35
2. SOLVD investigators. Effect of enalapril on survival in patients with reduced left ventricular ejection fractions and congestive heart failure. N Engl J Med 1991; 325:293–302
3. Cohn J, Archibald D, Phil M et al. Effect of vasodilator therapy on mortality in chronic congestive heart failure—results of Veterans Administration Cooperative study. N Engl J Med 1986;314:1547–52
4. Cohn J, Archibald D, Ziesche S et al. A comparison of enalapril with hydralazine—isosorbide dinitrate in the treatment of chronic congestive heart failure. N Engl J Med 1991; 325:303–10
5. Richard C, Ricome J, Rimailho A et al. Combined hemodynamic effects of dopamine and dobutamine in cardiogenic shock. Circulation 1983; 67: 620–6
6. DiSesa V. Pharmacologic support for post-operative low cardiac output. Seminars in Thoracic and Cardiovascular Surgery 1991; 3; 1:13–23
7. Hamer A, Arkles B, Johns J. Beneficial effects of low dose amiodarone in patients with congestive cardiac failure: a placebo-controlled trial. J Am Coll Cardiol 1989; 14:1768–74
8. Doval H, Nul D, Grancelli H, Perrone S, Bortman G, Curiel R. Randomised trial of low-dose amiodarone in severe congestive heart failure. Lancet 1994; 344: 493–8
9. Gargiuchevich J, Ramos J, Gambarte A et al. Argentine pilot study of sudden death and amiodarone. Circulation 1993; 88(Suppl 1): 447
10. O'Rourke M, Johnston R, Keogh A. Sheath impaction as a cause of defective intra-aortic balloon pump action in man. Aust NZ J Med 1985; 15:33–7
11. Frasier O, Duncan M, Radovancevic B et al. Successful bridge to heart transplantation with a new left ventricular assist device. J Heart Lung Transplant 1992; 11:530–7
12. Radovancevic B, Frasier O, Duncan J. Implantation technique for the Heart Mate left

ventricular assist device. J Cardiac Surgery 1992; 7; 3: 203–7
13. DeBroux E, Lagace G, Dumont L, Chartrand C. Efficacy of dobutamine in the failing transplanted heart. J Heart Lung Transplant 1992; 11:1133–9
14. Billingham M, Cary N, Hammond E et al. A working formulation for the standardisation of nomenclature in the diagnosis of heart and lung rejection: heart rejection study group. J Heart Transplant 1990; 9; 6: 587–93
15. Bristow M, Gilbert E, Renlund D, Dewitt C, Burton N, O'Connell J. Use of OKT_3 monoclonal antibody in heart transplantation—review of the initial experience. J Heart Transplant 1988; 7:1–11
16. Libby P, Tanaka H. The pathogenesis of coronary arteriosclerosis ('chronic rejection') in transplanted hearts. Clin Transplantation 1994; 8:313–8
17. Keogh A, Valatine H, Hunt S et al. Impact of proximal or midvessel discrete coronary artery stenoses on survival after heart transplantation. J Heart Lung Transplant 1992; 11: 892–901
18. Stark R, McGinn A, Wilson R. Chest pains in cardiac transplant recipients—evidence of sensory reinnervation after cardiac transplantation. N Engl J Med 1991; 324:179–4
19. Halle A, DiSciascio G, Wilson R et al. Coronary angioplasty in cardiac transplant recipients: results of a multicentre study. Abst. J Heart Lung Transplant 1991; 10:173
20. Schroeder J, Gao S, Aldema E et al. A preliminary study of diltiazem in the prevention of coronary artery disease in heart transplant recipients. N Engl J Med 1993; 328:164–70
21. Kobashigawa J, Gleeson M, Stevenson L et al. Pravastatin lowers cholesterol and may prevent severe cardiac transplant rejection: a randomised trial. N Engl J Med 1995; 333: 621–7
22. Keogh A, Spratt P, McCosker C, Macdonald P, Mundy J, Kaan A. Ketoconazole to reduce the need for cyclosporine after cardiac transplantation. N Engl J Med 1995; 333: 628–33

69 Hypertensive crises

P Vernon van Heerden

Introduction

Hypertensive states requiring acute care (hypertensive crises)[1,2] may be divided into *hypertensive emergencies*, where the blood pressure (BP) elevation is life-threatening and needs to be lowered in minutes to hours, and *hypertensive urgencies*, where the BP needs to be lowered in hours to days (see the information box).

Aetiology

With better control of elevated blood pressure, hypertensive crises are now relatively infrequent in the coronary care unit (CCU). However, markedly elevated blood pressure complicating acute myocardial infarction may still occur in the hours following the onset of symptoms. Aortic dissection may be accompanied by severe hypertension requiring urgent treatment. Paroxysmal hypertension may be a feature of phaeochromocytoma.

Malignant hypertension is a relatively rare condition in developed countries.[2,3,4] It is defined as severe hypertension associated with rapid and severe end-organ damage to the heart, central nervous system (CNS) and kidneys.[2] Malignant and accelerated hypertension appear to

Hypertensive emergencies—require BP control in minutes to hours

Severe hypertension with evidence of end-organ dysfunction (malignant hypertension)
- left ventricular failure
- acute renal failure
- acute on chronic renal failure
- hypertensive encephalopathy.

Aim is to prevent worsening of the end-organ damage.

Severe hypertension associated with:
- acute aortic dissection
- acute myocardial infarction
- recent open-heart surgery
- acute closed head injury
- raised intracranial pressure
- uncontrolled surgical bleeding
- severe burns

Aim is to prevent impact of the hypertension on the associated pathology

Severe hypertension secondary to excess circulating catecholamines
- phaeochromocytoma
- monoamine oxidase inhibitor crisis

Pregnancy-induced hypertension with impending eclampsia

Hypertensive urgencies—required BP control in hours to days

- Severe benign hypertension
  - — asymptomatic, with laboratory evidence of subacute end-organ dysfunction
  - — symptomatic, with clinical evidence of subacute end-organ dysfunction
- Pregnancy-induced hypertension—asymptomatic
- Hypertension secondary to acute renal failure (acute glomerulonephritis)
- Rebound hypertension following discontinuation of antihypertensive therapy
- Severe hypertension in the peri-operative period—e.g. post renal transplantation, post cardiac surgery
- Severe hypertension due to illicit drug ingestion, e.g. cocaine

behave similarly when treated,[5,6] but malignant hypertension is more rapidly fatal (90% mortality in one year[7] when left untreated).[3]

Pathophysiology

The major pathophysiological changes seen in patients with *malignant hypertension* are:

- disordered autoregulation in various vascular beds; in particular the renal and cerebral circulations.[1,3] Flow within these vascular beds becomes pressure-dependent within the 'normal' range of BP. The effect of this may be seen when renal or neurological function deteriorates if BP is too rapidly normalized in these patients.
- arteritis, including the hallmark fibrinoid necrosis, with the changes essentially those of thrombotic microangiopathy.[1,3] Whether the vascular lesions are a cause of or an effect of malignant hypertension is not known. What is known is that the vascular lesions become evident when severe hypertension becomes 'malignant' and that there are no real differences between severe benign hypertension and malignant hypertension on the basis of BP alone.[3]

The vasculitic lesion is thought to be associated with relative ischaemia in the affected area.[1] In the *kidney* this may result in an elevation of renin production and release, with subsequent increases in BP via its effect on angiotensin II.[2] Hyper-reninaemia is also responsible for relative hypovolaemia and a contracted intravascular space in the patient with malignant hypertension.[3,8] In the *brain* hypertensive encephalopathy, a serious and potentially fatal complication, may be associated with fibrinoid necrosis and cerebral infarction. These changes can result in focal neurological signs or coma.

The hypertension accompanying *acute myocardial infarction* is usually transient due to pain and transient catecholamine release. The hypertension may persist where there is ongoing high sympathetic outflow, or where there is preceding hypertensive disease, in particular when antihypertensive medication has been acutely ceased. A hypertensive response to myocardial infarction can increase myocardial oxygen demand and potentiate myocardial ischaemia and necrosis. Hypertension in the early stages of myocardial infarction increases the risk of intracranial haemorrhage when thrombolytic therapy is used and has an adverse effect on long-term survival. Catecholamine levels in plasma and serum during the early postinfarction period correlate well with short- and long-term prognoses.

In the case of *aortic dissection*, systolic pressures are a key factor in the shear forces which initiate and extend the separation of the aortic wall interfaces. On occasion the dissection may extend to involve the renal arteries. This can create a situation of uni- or bilateral renal artery stenosis, further potentiating the hypertension. Mesenteric artery involvement can result in gut ischaemia and infarction, a potentially lethal condition.

The hypertension of *phaeochromocytoma* results from catecholamine excess produced by tumours of chromaffin origin in the adrenal medulla. Occasionally these tumours may be extra-adrenal or involve both adrenal glands. In common with other forms of hypertension where an increased sympathetic outflow exists there is a decrease in circulating volume. Volume expansion should occur at the same time that the hypertension is treated. The direct effect of the circulating catecholamines on the myocardium can result in focal necrosis and T wave changes on the ECG.

Assessment of the patient with severe hypertension

Malignant hypertension is diagnosed by the association of a very high BP and clinical and/or laboratory evidence of acute end-organ dysfunction.[1,2] The clinical history will be useful in determining symptoms due to the high BP, as well as excluding possible causes of a high BP, for example phaeochromocytoma, recent cessation of antihypertensive medication, or oral contraceptive usage. The classical features of episodic hypertension associated with profuse sweating seen in patients with phaeochromocytoma should be sought if this diagnosis is suspected.

It is extremely important to enquire after the symptoms of cardiac, renal and CNS dysfunction. In particular, the signs and symptoms of hypertensive encephalopathy should be avidly sought. They include headache, nausea, vomiting, visual disturbances, confusion, focal or generalized weakness, focal neurological signs, nystagmus and seizures.[2] Diagnostic difficulties in determining cause and effect may arise when a patient presents with hypertension following an intracranial event, such as subarachnoid haemorrhage (SAH). A similar problem occurs in the hypertensive patient with acute renal failure due to glomerulonephritis.

Clinical examination attempts to elicit all the signs of end-organ damage associated with the severe hypertension, as well as search for signs of a possible cause for the hypertension. In particular, the fundi are carefully examined for evidence of high grade retinopathy, including papilloedema. Signs of cardiac and renal failure are also sought. It is important to measure the BP carefully, comparing BP in both upper limbs in the recumbent patient who is well rested, especially if aortic dissection with involvement of the subclavian arteries is suspected. Radio-femoral delay and renal arterial bruits should be excluded in the hypertensive patient.

Most patients with a hypertensive response to myocardial infarction will revert to a normotensive state on relief of pain and anxiety. When hypertension persists a more detailed assessment is necessary, including obtaining a history of prior anti-hypertensive therapy and particularly whether such therapy has recently been withdrawn.

Principles of management

Hypertensive emergencies

In these conditions, listed in the information box, rapid control of BP is required, usually with a parenteral agent, to avoid the associated high levels of morbidity and mortality. The potent drugs used for BP control require careful and often invasive monitoring (that is, indwelling arterial cannula). The lack of invasive monitoring should however not delay the rapid institution of therapy in this group of patients.

Too rapid reduction in BP may have adverse renal and neurological effects. In general the mean arterial pressure (MAP) should only be reduced by 15% in the first hour, followed by a more gradual reduction to a DBP of 100–110 mmHg.[1,9] Oral medications are administered as soon as the emergency has been dealt with by the parenteral agents described below—usually after a period of stability at the target BP lasting 6–48 hours.[1,2] The parenteral agents are 'tailed off' once the oral medications have been successfully instituted.

Treatment can often be initiated with oral or sublingual nifedipine (5–10 mg 6-hourly). Although use of this agent may avoid the need for parenteral therapy it has the disadvantage of variable patient response, especially in the presence of hypovolaemia, with occasional profound hypotension. There is also a lack of fine titration, which is possible with parenteral agents.

Useful parenteral antihypertensive agents include the following:[1–3,11,12]

- *Sodium nitroprusside* (SNP) is a potent arterial and venous vasodilator when administered in a dose of 0.25–10 micrograms per kilogram per minute (mcg/kg/min) by constant IV infusion. The short duration of action of the drug allows rapid titration against effect. Its use is limited by tachyphylaxis and cyanide and thiocyanate toxicity when administered in high dose or for prolonged periods. For these reasons SNP should rarely be used for periods exceeding 24 hours.
- *Glyceryl trinitrate* (GTN) by infusion at a rate of 5–20 mcg/min is a very useful agent for hypertension where SNP is contraindicated or when there is evidence of myocardial ischaemia.
- *Beta blockers* such as metoprolol or atenolol (in 5 mg boluses; up to 15 mg over 10 minutes) are frequently used to control hypertension associated with acute myocardial infarction. The dose is titrated to effect and is limited by the effect on heart rate. Beta blockers such as esmolol, which have a short duration of action, are readily titratable, and therefore are useful in the setting of poor response to SNP or GTN, or when hypertension occurs with aortic dissection. Esmolol is administered intravenously as a loading dose (0.5–1.0 mg/kg), followed by an infusion at 100–300 mcg/kg/min.
- Other short-acting agents from the *calcium channel blocking* group of drugs are showing promise in the treatment of hypertensive emergencies. One such drug is nicardipine,

which is supplied in a 25 mg in 10 ml ampoule and is diluted with 240 ml of normal saline (to a 0.1 mg/ml solution) and then infused intravenously to effect.

- When the expertise or equipment are lacking to provide IV infusions, then intermittent intravenous (IV) bolus doses of *hydralazine* (10–20 mg) or one of the newer agents (e.g. enalaprilat) may be considered. Bolus (IV) dosing, in common with enteral administration of drugs, is not readily titratable and therefore not ideal. This is all the more so in this group of patients in whom a large proportion of inappropriate side-effects to antihypertensive therapy are seen when treatment commences.[1] For this reason diazoxide is less utilized now than previously, but it remains a potent agent to use if other agents are unavailable, or if hypertensive encephalopathy is developing and rapid BP control is required. The dose of diazoxide is 2.5–5 mg/kg IV.

Special precautions are necessary if a phaeochromocytoma is suspected. The temptation to initiate treatment with a beta blocker alone must be resisted, as this will leave the alpha effects of circulating catecholamines unopposed with resultant vasoconstriction and exacerbation of the hypertension. Treatment should be initiated with intravenous alpha antagonists such as phentolamine in 2.5 mg IV boluses. An oral agent like phenoxybenzamine (10 mg 12-hourly) can be substituted once adequate control is obtained. Other facets of management include careful intra-arterial BP monitoring, plasma volume expansion and judicious use of beta blockers for the treatment of tachycardia, arrhythmias and palpitations. Labetolol, a combined alpha and beta blocker, may be useful in this setting.

Hypertensive urgencies

Hypertensive urgencies, examples of which are listed in the information box above, are usually treated with oral antihypertensive agents. The BP is reduced over a period of 2–3 days, thereby avoiding ischaemic renal and neurological changes.

Useful drugs, given by the oral route, include:[1–3,11,12]

- *calcium channel antagonists*, for example nifedipine 5–10 mg 6-hourly. Nifedipine is rapidly absorbed from the gut, but for an even more rapid response the liquid contents of a nifedipine capsule may be administered sublingually. The disadvantage of this method is that the patient response is variable and, particularly where there is a circulating volume deficit, the resultant hypotension may be severe.
- *angiotensin-converting enzyme (ACE) inhibitors*, for example captopril 6.25–25 mg, 6–12-hourly. Renal artery stenosis should be excluded prior to the use of this group of drugs.
- other *vasodilators* such as prazosin and minoxidil are still used to good effect.

Combination of the above with loop or thiazide *diuretics* and/or *beta blocker* therapy may be required for long-term control of hypertension.

Although controlled trials are lacking, it is suggested that the diastolic blood pressure (DBP) should not be reduced below 100 mmHg for the first 3 days.[2]

Prognosis

The 10–22% survival rate for untreated malignant hypertension is markedly improved by effective therapy.[1,3] The eventual outcome depends largely on the underlying cause and the subsequent renal function. With good long-term BP control a large proportion of patients with hypertensive nephropathy will recover adequate renal function.[10] In acute myocardial infarction complicated by hypertension, the risk of thrombolytic therapy can be reduced by adequate BP control. In aortic dissection, the progression of the condition can be controlled if the elevated BP is stabilized.

References

1. Elliott WJ. Malignant hypertension. In: Hall JB, Schmidt GA, Wood LDH (eds). Principles of critical care. New York: McGraw-Hill, 1992: 1563–71
2. Veriava Y, Milne FJ. Hypertensive crisis—the South African perspective. South African Medical Journal 1993; 83: 166–7
3. Kincaid-Smith P. Malignant hypertension. Journal of Hypertension 1991; 9: 893–9
4. Kincaid-Smith P. What has happened to malignant hypertension? In: Bulpitt CJ, Birkenhager WH, Reid JL (eds). Handbook of hypertension. Vol 6. Epidemiology of hypertension. Amsterdam: Elsevier, 1985: 255–65

5. Ahmed MEK, Walker JM, Beevers DG, Beevers M. Lack of difference between malignant and accelerated hypertension. Br Med J 1986; 292: 235–7
6. McGregor E, Isles CG, Jay JL et al. Retinal changes in malignant hypertension. Br Med J 1986; 292: 233–4
7. Keith NM, Wagener HP, Barker NW. Some different types of essential hypertension: their course and prognosis. Am J Med Sci 1939; 196: 332–43
8. Barraclough MA. Sodium and water depletion with acute malignant hypertension. Am J Med 1966; 40: 265–72
9. Ferguson RK, Vlasses PH. Hypertensive emergencies and urgencies. JAMA 1986; 255: 1607–13
10. Bakir AA, Bazilinski N, Dunea G. Transient and sustained recovery from renal shutdown in accelerated hypertension. Am J Med 1986; 80: 172–5
11. Chobanian AV, Alderman MH, DeQuattro V et al. The 1988 Report of the Joint National Committee on Detection, Evaluation, and Treatment of High Blood Pressure. Arch Intern Med 1988; 148: 1023–38
12. Kaplan N. Management of hypertensive emergencies. Lancet 1994; 344: 1335–8

70 Aortic dissection

Peter L Thompson

Introduction

Although acute aortic dissection has become relatively less frequent in recent years because of better treatment of hypertension in the community, it is a condition of major importance in the coronary care unit (CCU) for several reasons.

Firstly, it is a highly lethal condition in which misdiagnosis and inappropriate management can have catastrophic consequences.[1] Secondly, the clinical features of chest pain and shock may mimic acute myocardial infarction (MI).[2] Thirdly, dissection into a coronary artery may cause acute coronary occlusion so that a patient with acute aortic dissection may have co-existent MI with the typical electrocardiographic features.[3] Finally, in the current thrombolytic era of treatment of MI, inappropriate thrombolysis in aortic dissection can have fatal consequences.[4]

Clinical presentation

Pathogenesis

Dissection follows a rupture of the intima with passage of blood into the wall of the aorta. The most usual entry sites are just above the aortic valve and just distal to the left subclavian artery. In most cases there is some underlying process which affects the aortic media, usually Marfan's disease causing cystic medial necrosis in younger patients and hypertensive vascular disease in older patients. In addition there are some congenital anomalies such as bicuspid aortic valve and aortic coarctation which predispose to dissection. The condition is more common in men but can occur in the last trimester of pregnancy.

Classification

There are several classification systems based on the location and extent of the dissection in the aorta. The classification systems are of relevance in identifying patients with *proximal* dissection—who are at high risk from aortic root and cerebrovascular involvement and will require a median stenotomy approach for operative repair—from patients with *distal* involvement who are at lower risk may be best managed medically, and if operative repair is needed, will require a thoracotomy approach.

DeBakey classification[5]

- **type 1** involving the whole aorta
- **type 2** involving only the ascending aorta
- **type 3** involving the thoracic aorta distal to the left subclavian artery (type 3A involving the thoracic aorta and type 3B extending into the abdominal aorta).

Stanford classification[6]

- **type A**—proximal dissection and distal dissection which extends proximally
- **type B**—distal dissection without proximal extension.

Mass. General classification[3]

- **proximal** involving the ascending aorta
- **distal** involving the descending aorta distal to the left subclavian.

European classification[7]

- A new classification of distal dissection has been proposed based on the presence of a communication between the true and false lumen and whether the dissection extends anterograde or retrograde. Best survival is observed in patients with non-communicating dissections and worst in those with communicating dissections which spread retrograde to the aortic root. This classification depends on findings on transoesophageal echocardiography.

The most readily comprehensible and widely used is the Stanford classification.

Natural history

Proximal (type A) dissections have a far worse survival than distal (type B) dissections because of involvement of the aortic root, coronary arteries and major cerebral vessels (see Fig. 70.1).

In untreated proximal (type A) dissection there is less than 50% survival within the first few days, 40% at 1 year and 33% at 5 years. In contrast, distal (type B) dissection has an over 90% survival in the first month with 80% survival at 5 years.[8] The prognosis is further determined in distal dissection by the presence of a communicating channel and proximal dissection. The presence of these features carries an ominous prognosis, with 50% early mortality for the combination and only 10% early mortality for non-communicating localized dissection.[7] Surgical repair substantially improves survival in proximal dissection. In distal dissection the benefits of surgery are less clear-cut.

Clinical features

The chest pain which accompanies aortic dissection may be described as tearing. It is characteristically very severe at the onset, in contrast to MI in which the pain may build up slowly. The pain is typically located in the interscapular area but may be felt in the retrosternal area and radiate to both arms and throat in the identical distribution of the chest pain of MI. Initial presentation may be with hemiplegia due to dissection of the head and neck vessels or features of cardiac tamponade or pleural effusion due to aortic leakage. More subtle physical signs which may be present are inequality of blood pressure or pulse amplitude in the upper limbs or detection of a new aortic regurgitant murmur due to aortic root involvement. In a recent study, over half the cases were misdiagnosed on initial presentation.[9]

The ECG may be normal or may show evidence of acute myocardial infarction if there is coronary artery dissection.

The chest X-ray may show widening of the mediastinum but this is a difficult radiographic sign to interpret because the aortic root is frequently widened in hypertension or Marfan's syndrome. A useful sign is a separation of the line of aortic calcification from the outline of the aorta at the aortic arch. If this measures greater than 0.5 cm, dissection of the aortic arch is likely.

CCU staff should have a low threshold for considering the diagnosis of aortic dissection in any patient who presents with chest pain atypical for MI. This is particularly true if there is a history of hypertension or clinical features to suggest Marfan's syndrome.

Survival curves for medically treated patients with aortic dissections

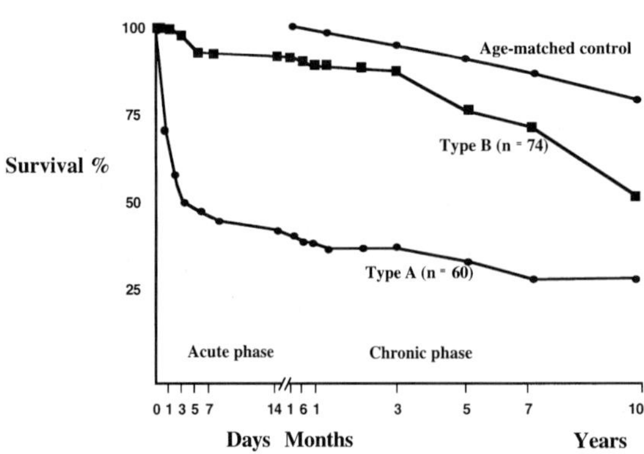

Fig. 70.1 Natural history of type A (proximal with potential for involvement of coronary and cerebral vessels) versus type B (distal) aortic dissection. Adapted with permission from Masuda Y, Yamada Z, Morooka N, Watanabe S, Inagaki Y 1991.[8]

Diagnostic tests

Aortography

Contrast aortography has until recently been regarded as the gold standard for diagnosis of aortic dissection. It has the advantage of imaging the whole of the intra-thoracic aorta, may identify the intimal flap and can identify aortic valve involvement with aortic regurgitation. In addition coronary angiography can be performed at the same time.

However, there has recently been a swing away from aortography because there are frequently delays in obtaining access to a vascular radiography suite and passage of the catheter through the aorta can potentially cause further dissection. Increased availability and sophistication of alternative imaging modalities has diminished the role of aortography in the diagnosis of aortic dissection, although it is still used when the diagnosis is unclear from other methods.[10]

Computed tomography

Thoracic computed tomography (CT) scan enhanced with intravenous contrast gives excellent definition with a diagnostic accuracy equivalent to aortography (see Fig. 15.10).[11]

Magnetic resonance imaging

Magnetic resonance imaging (MRI) scanning can also provide excellent imaging of the aorta and major blood vessels;[12] however, considerable expertise is required for accurate interpretation (see Fig. 15.11).[13]

Intravenous digital subtraction angiography

This has been claimed to be as accurate as aortography[14] but there is not a large experience with this technique in aortic dissection.

Echocardiography—transthoracic

Routine transthoracic echocardiography can provide excellent imaging of the aortic root and aortic valve but many dissections do not involve this region. Imaging from the suprasternal notch can provide images of the ascending aorta but views of the aortic arch and descending aorta are limited.[15]

Echocardiography—trans-oesophageal

Trans-oesophageal echocardiography can provide high quality images of the aortic valve, aortic root and ascending aorta and much of the descending aorta.[16] There is some limitation in imaging the aortic arch. Additional information about left ventricular function and the presence of pericardial tamponade can be obtained and by the use of colour flow Doppler imaging the degree of aortic regurgitation can be assessed.

In addition, information about the presence of prognostically significant communications between the true and false lumen can be obtained by colour flow Doppler imaging.[7]

Biplane and multiplane trans-oesophageal probes have improved the visualization of the aorta particularly in the aortic arch area.

Selection of imaging technique

All of the radiologic imaging techniques and MRI scanning require removal of the patient to a radiologic facility where continuous monitoring may be difficult. This is particularly the case with computed tomography and magnetic resonance imaging. Trans-oesophageal echocardiography is readily available. In skilled hands it can be done at the bedside in the CCU and can provide sufficiently accurate information to determine management in most cases. For this reason it now has a strong claim as the method of choice in the investigation of aortic dissection.[17]

Medical management

An important component of the medical management of aortic dissection is to consider the diagnosis in any patient presenting with chest pain, particularly when thrombolytic or aggressive anticoagulant therapy is being contemplated.[4]

Medical management should be commenced immediately, even before confirmation by diagnostic imaging, if there is a strong clinical suspicion such as atypical or interscapular chest pain, Marfan's syndrome or severe hypertension or diagnostic clues such as newly developed aortic regurgitation or inequality of upper limb pulses.

Initial management consists of pain relief as for acute myocardial infarction and reduction of systolic blood pressure to reduce aortic wall shear stresses and reduce the chance of extension of the dissection. Initial therapy should be directed to reducing blood pressure, reducing the rate of rise of systolic pulsation and reducing heart rate.

Intravenous beta blockers are capable of achieving this and are the mainstay of initial management. The traditional medication has been propranolol in doses of 1 mg repeated each 5 minutes but the cardio-selective beta blockers more widely used for MI are equally effective in a dose of metoprolol 5 mg in three separate doses at 5-minute intervals up to 15 mg or atenolol 5 mg in two separate doses 5 minutes apart up to 10 mg. Intravenous labetalol can be given in repeated doses of 10 mg.[18] The indicators of effective beta blockade are a reduction in systolic blood pressure to 100–120 mmHg and a reduction in heart rate to 55–60 beats per minute. Intravenous beta blockers are continued, with booster doses as required in the first 24 hours followed by oral beta blockade.

If the blood pressure cannot be adequately controlled with beta blockers, infusion of nitroprusside or nitroglycerin can be employed but these should not be used as first line therapy for control of blood pressure because the nitrate-induced vasodilatation may cause an increase in the rate of rise of the arterial pressure and increase rather than reduce shear stresses in the aortic wall.

In patients who are unable to take beta blockers because of asthma or bradycardia, calcium channel blockers can be substituted.[19]

Surgical therapy

When the ascending aorta is involved, immediate surgery is essential to prevent the catastrophic complications of pericardial tamponade, coronary dissection, aortic rupture or stroke from dissection into the cerebral vessels. There are a variety of surgical approaches, the aim being removal of the dissected aorta and replacement with a Dacron graft and/or obliteration of a false channel.

Resection of the diseased aorta and replacement of the resected aorta by an end-to-end graft has been superseded in most units by the inter-position technique in which a tube graft is placed within the aorta thus creating a new lumen.[20,21] When the aortic valve has been disrupted it is normally re-suspended to restore function, except in Marfan's syndrome when repair of the ascending aorta is combined with aortic valve prosthesis (Bentall's procedure).[22]

In dissection of the descending aorta, surgical therapy is performed only if there is evidence of rupture from proximal extension or ischaemic complications. Patients with Marfan's syndrome usually have surgical repair even in distal dissection. Detection of aortic leakage on trans-oesophageal echocardiography may be an additional indication for repair of distal dissection.[7,23]

Post-acute management

Patients who have survived aortic dissection need careful follow-up with control of blood pressure, continuation of beta blockers and regular echocardiographic monitoring to detect re-dissection or aneurysm formation, particularly in patients with Marfan's syndrome.[24]

References

1. Chirillo F, Marchiori MC, Andriold L et al. Outcome of 209 patients with aortic dissections: a 12 year multicentre experience. Eur Heart J 1990; 11:311–9
2. Hirst AE, Johns VJ, Kime SW Jr. Dissecting aneurysm of the aorta. A review of 505 cases. Medicine 1958; 37:217–79
3. De Sanctis RW, Doroghazi RM, Austen WG, Buckley MJ. Aortic dissection. N Engl J Med 1987; 317:1060–7
4. Butler J, Davies AH, Westaby S. Streptokinase in acute aortic dissection. Br Med J 1990; 30:517–9
5. DeBakey ME, McCollum CH, Crawford ES et al. Dissection and dissecting aneurysms of the aorta: 20 year follow up of 527 patients treated surgically. Surgery 1982; 92:1118–34
6. Daily PO, Trueblood HW, Stinson EB, Weurflein RD, Shumway NE. Management of acute aortic dissections. Am Thorac Surg 1970; 10:237–47
7. Erbel R, Oelert H, Meyer J et al. Effect of medical and surgical therapy on aortic dissection evaluated by trans-oesophageal echocardiography. Implications for prognosis and therapy. Circulation 1993; 87:1604–15
8. Masuda Y, Yamada Z, Morooka N, Watanabe S, Inagaki Y. Prognosis of patients with medically treated aortic dissections. Circulation 1991; 84(Suppl. III): III-7–III-19
9. Butler J, Ormerod OJM, Giannopoulos N et al. Diagnostic delay and outcome in surgery for type A aortic dissection. Quart J Med 1991; 289:391–6
10. Cigarros JE, Isselbacher EM, De Sanctis RW, Eagle KA. Diagnostic imaging in the evaluation of suspected thoracic aortic dissection. N Engl J Med 1993; 328: 35–43
11. Nienaber CA, Vonkodolitsch Y, Nicolas V et al. The diagnosis of thoracic aortic dissection by non-invasive imaging procedures. N Engl J Med 1993; 328: 1–9
12. Nienaber CA, Spielmann RP, Von Kodolitsch V et al. Diagnosis of thoracic aortic dissection: magnetic resonance imaging versus transesophageal echocardiography. Circulation 1992; 85: 434–37
13. Kersting-Sommerhoff B, Higgins CB et al. Aortic dissection: sensitivity and specificity of MR imaging. Radiology 1988; 166: 651–5
14. Lyons J, Gershlick A, Norell M et al. Intravenous digital subtraction angiography in the diagnosis and management of acute aortic dissection. Eur Heart J 1987; 8: 186–9
15. Erbel R, Engberding ER, Darvel W et al. Echocardiography in diagnosis of aortic dissection. Lancet 1989; 1: 457–61

16. Ballal RS, Nanda NC, Gatewood R et al. Usefulness of trans-esophageal echocardiography in assessment of aortic dissection. Circulation 1991; 84: 1903–14
17. Banning AP, Ruttley MST, Musumeu F, Fraser AG. Acute dissection of the thoracic aorta: trans-oesophageal echocardiography is the investigation of choice. Br Med J 1995; 310: 72–3
18. Grubb BP, Sirio C, Zelis R. Intravenous labetalol in acute aortic dissection. JAMA 1987; 258: 78–9
19. White SR, Hall JB. Control of hypertension with nifedipine in the setting of aortic dissection. Chest 1985; 88: 780–1
20. DaGama AD. The surgical management of aortic dissection: from uniformity to diversity, a continuous challenge. J Cardiovasc Surgery 1991; 32: 141–53
21. Kirklin JW, Barrett-Boyes BG. Acute aortic dissection. In: Kirklin JW, Barrett-Boyes BG. Cardiac surgery. New York: Churchill Livingstone: Ch 54
22. Bentall H, De Bond A. A technique for complete replacement of the ascending aorta. Thorax 1968; 23: 338–9
23. Khandheria BK. Aortic dissection: the last frontier. Circulation 1993; 87: 1765–7
24. Dapunt OE, Galla JD, Sadegift AM et al. The natural history of thoracic aortic aneurysms. J Thoracic Cardiovasc Surg 1994; 107: 1323–33

71 Pericardial effusion and tamponade

Peter L Thompson

Introduction

With the expanding role of the coronary care unit (CCU), patients with pericardial effusion or tamponade may be transferred into the unit for management, which may include pericardiocentesis.

Causes of pericardial effusion

The commonest cause of pericardial effusion is malignant effusion in patients with secondary neoplastic deposits in the pericardium. Other causes include viral or idiopathic pericarditis, uraemic pericarditis and post-infarction Dressler's syndrome. Rare causes include myxoedema, tuberculosis and rheumatic diseases, such as systemic or rheumatoid arthritis. Haemorrhagic pericardial compression may occur from perforation of a cardiac chamber during cardiac catheterization or penetrating chest injury. It may also occur from a myocardial infarction (MI), with acute compression occurring with cardiac rupture or subacute compression, or if post-infarction pericarditis is complicated by intrapericardial bleeding due to thrombolytic or anticoagulant therapy. Intrapericardial bleeding following cardiac surgery may cause the typical syndrome of pericardial effusion or tamponade, or may be localized, causing bizarre, diagnostically challenging syndromes if the bleeding causes localized compression of a cardiac chamber.

CCUs in hospitals with oncology, renal and cardiac surgical services will frequently be called on to manage pericardial effusion and tamponade. Units dealing primarily with MI will face the diagnostic challenge and need for emergency treatment less frequently, and will need to be even more vigilant to ensure that facilities and staff training are directed towards the management and emergency treatment of the infrequent case of pericardial tamponade.

Pathophysiology[2,3]

The haemodynamic consequences of pericardial effusion are determined by the intrapericardial pressure. This in turn is determined not only by the volume of fluid in the pericardium, but also by the rate of accumulation. In circumstances of rapid accumulation of fluids, such as cardiac rupture following myocardial infarction, intrapericardial pressure can rise rapidly and cause severe haemodynamic compromise with only 250 ml of fluid. A slowly developing pericardial effusion may not cause haemodynamic embarrassment with an effusion of one litre or more. However, the gradual stretching of the pericardium cannot accommodate an indefinite build-up of fluid and it will reach a point where the addition of only a small volume will cause the intrapericardial pressure to rise and cause haemodynamic embarrassment (see Fig. 71.1).

As the pericardial pressure rises, it may reach the level of the diastolic pressure in the right atrium and right ventricle. When this occurs, right atrial and ventricular filling are compromised. As the intrapericardial pressure rises further, the right ventricular diastolic pressure rises to the level of the left ventricular diastolic pressure, affecting left ventricular filling and causing a drop in stroke volume. The falling stroke volume is initially compensated by an increase in adrenergic tone resulting in an increase in contractility, and activation of other neurohumoral mechanisms which increase systemic vascular resistance and retain sodium. This pre-shock state may then rapidly progress to declining output, generalized hypoperfusion and cardiogenic shock.

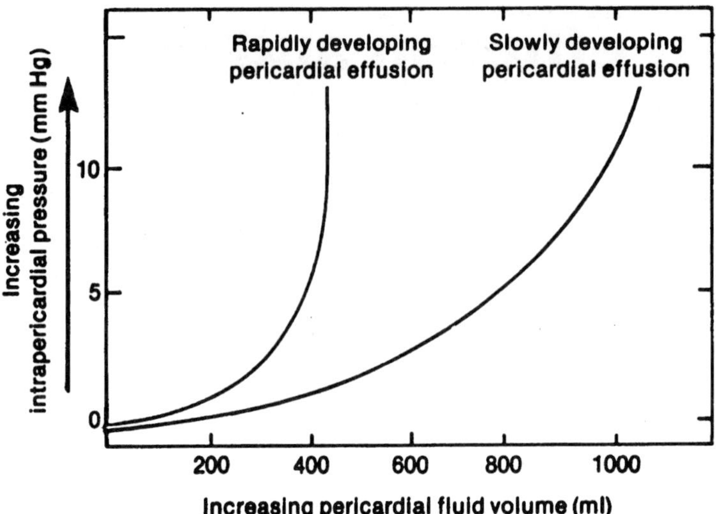

Fig. 71.1 Relationship between pericardial volume and pressure: the pericardium can accommodate a slowly developing pericardial effusion with only gradual rise in pressure, but in a rapidly developing effusion, the pericardial pressure may rise rapidly with minimal increase in volume.

Diagnosis

Symptoms

Patients with quite large pericardial effusions may complain of no symptoms at all, or may complain of a sensation of fullness or oppression in the chest and dyspnoea. There may be symptoms due to compression of intrathoracic structures, such as dysphagia from oesophageal compression, cough from tracheal or bronchial compression, hiccoughs from phrenic nerve compression or hoarseness from recurrent laryngeal nerve compression. Patients with pericardial tamponade may be agitated, or in more advanced cases, stuporous and confused.

Physical signs

The physical signs of pericardial effusion may include:

- dullness to percussion may be noted over the lower sternum or right parasternal intercostal spaces. On occasion there may be bronchial breathing detected below and medial to the left scapula (Ewart's sign).
- Elevation of the venous pressure is usually the first sign of acute pericardial compression, although this sign may be delayed in the presence of hypovolaemia, as in the patient who has received aggressive diuretic therapy. In the usual case of pericardial tamponade, the venous pressure is tense and it may be difficult or impossible to detect the classical signs of prominent X descent and absent Y descent.
  Apart from the usual causes of severe biventricular cardiac failure, predominant right heart abnormalities such as right ventricular infarction or massive pulmonary embolism may pose problems with the differential diagnosis of pericardial tamponade, and it is not possible to make the diagnosis from the jugular venous pulse alone.
  There is usually a sinus tachycardia and lowered pulse volume, but in the terminal stages of pericardial compression, there may be a profound bradycardia.
- Pulsus paradoxus is the classical sign of pericardial tamponade.[2] This is an exaggeration of the normal respiratory variation in systolic blood pressure. In the normal state, systolic pressure drops slightly during inspiration due to reduction in left ventricular filling. The normal limit for this drop is 10 mmHg or less. In pericardial tamponade this drop may be 20 mmHg or greater and may be detectable on palpation of the brachial or radial pulse. However, it usually needs to be checked with a sphygmomanometer cuff. The cuff is inflated and the systolic blood pressure is checked by auscultation. The cuff is then reinflated to just above systolic pressure and gradually deflated to detect the systolic pressure during expiration. At this point, the Korotkoff sounds will disappear during inspiration. The cuff is then gradually deflated until sounds are heard equally well during inspiration and expiration. The difference in pressure between the first detection of sounds during expiration and the point at which sounds are heard clearly during inspiration represents the difference between inspiratory and expiratory pressures. When this difference is greater than

10 mmHg, pulsus paradoxus is present. It is important to distinguish pulsus paradoxus from pulsus alternans, in which the systolic pressure of alternate beats varies, and from pulsus bigeminus, in which the premature beat generates a lower pressure than the normal sinus beat. Other causes of pulsus paradoxus include severe asthma, or chronic airways limitation, massive pulmonary embolism and positive pressure ventilation.

Progressive hypotension is a sign of critical pericardial compression. A falling blood pressure in a patient with a documented pericardial effusion may be a sign of impending cardiac arrest indicating a need for immediate pericardiocentesis.

Electrocardiogram

The typical electrocardiographic finding is diffuse small voltages. This is not a particularly reliable sign unless there is a clear reduction in voltages compared with those of previous tracings. Critical pericardial tamponade may be present without any abnormality of the surface ECG. Electrical alternans, an alternating variation in the height of the QRS complex, may be seen in large pericardial effusions with or without tamponade.[4]

Echocardiography

The availability of bedside echocardiography has revolutionized the diagnosis and management of pericardial effusion and tamponade.[5] In addition to distinguishing an effusion from a tamponade causing haemodynamic embarrassment, other causes of right heart abnormality such as right ventricular infarction, pulmonary hypertension, or associated severe left ventricular dysfunctions, may be identified. An effusion is readily identified as a large echo-free space around the heart usually readily identified from parasternal views (see Ch. 16). On occasions, particularly in the post-operative cardiac surgical patient, specialized subcostal and/or other views may be necessary to identify localized collections.

Right atrial compression is an early sign of haemodynamic embarrassment. On occasions, clear-cut invagination of the right atrial wall may be seen, but this is not necessarily a sign of pericardial tamponade requiring pericardiocentesis. On the other hand, compression of the right ventricular chamber is a clear-cut sign that the intrapericardial pressure has exceeded the right ventricular filling pressure and pericardiocentesis is indicated.

Echocardiography is useful in guiding pericardiocentesis by identifying the position in which the largest and most accessible pool of pericardial fluid is sitting. It is also used to check the extent of residual fluid following the pericardiocentesis.[5]

Pericardiocentesis

Although a variety of approaches have been described, the subxiphoid approach is the most widely used.[7,8] On occasions, two-dimensional echocardiography may demonstrate a localized effusion which is best approached from other sites.[5] With the introduction of echocardiography-guided pericardiocentesis[5] and the use of the modified Seldinger technique and flexible pericardial catheters,[5,9] the risk of pericardiocentesis has been greatly reduced. However, the technique still carries a significant risk, particularly in patients with localized effusions or in patients who have suffered significant haemodynamic embarrassment with small collections which have accumulated rapidly.[10] Elective pericardiocentesis should not be considered in patients who have a significant bleeding tendency, such as a patient on anticoagulant therapy or with thrombocytopenia below 50 000 per mm^3. Ideally the procedure should take place in a cardiac catheterization laboratory with fluoroscopic facilities and echocardiography on standby. In the absence of a catheterization laboratory, however, the technique can be performed as an echo-guided technique at the bedside in the CCU. Except in the presence of life-threatening tamponade, pericardiocentesis should not be attempted without echocardiographic confirmation.

The patient should be sitting comfortably at an angle of 30–45 degrees from the horizontal. If necessary, mild sedation with intravenous diazepam or midazolam may be necessary. Pre-medication with atropine may reduce the risk of bradycardias associated with entry into the pericardium.

After careful shaving, skin preparation and isolation of the area with sterile drapes, the skin is entered at the angle between the xiphisternum and the left rib margin, and the area is infiltrated with 1% lignocaine. The local anaesthetic entry site is enlarged with a small scalpel cut. The pericardiocentesis kit should contain a short bevelled needle with guide wire introducer dilator and flexible pigtail catheter. The short bevelled needle is attached to a 5 ml syringe containing 1% lignocaine and the needle is carefully advanced at a 30-degree angle to the skin surface, aiming towards the left shoulder.

The needle is advanced gently past the costal margin with small injections of lignocaine along the needle track. The pericardium is felt as a firm resistance. A further injection of lignocaine is made, and after a short delay, the needle is gently advanced into the pericardial space. The needle is gently advanced a further 1 mm until a free flow of pericardial fluid is obtained on aspiration. If the fluid is bloody, the possibility of entry into a cardiac chamber or pericardial vessel should be considered, but this is unlikely if the effusion has been documented as large on echocardiography and cardiac pulsations have not been transmitted through the needle. An alligator clip attached to the needle and the V (chest) lead of an ECG has been used in the past to identify epicardial contact by detecting ST segment elevation.[11] In this author's experience, however, this complicates the procedure and is not necessary in the presence of a relatively large effusion. Pericardiocentesis in malignant effusion or post cardiac surgery frequently produces bloody pericardial fluid. If doubt persists as to the origin of the bloody fluid, the following procedure should be followed:

- An urgent haemoglobin level should be obtained on the sample. If the haemoglobin is substantially less than the patient's haemoglobin, bloody pericardial fluid, rather than blood, is likely.
- A drop should be spread on a gauze pad. A homogeneous deep red spot is indicative of blood, whereas a central red spot with a pale periphery is more likely to be pericardial fluid.
- Blood will clot (unless anticoagulated) whereas blood-stained pericardial fluid will not.
- If in doubt, bedside echocardiography after injection of agitated saline through the pericardiocentesis needle will demonstrate bubbles appearing in the pericardial sac or in a cardiac chamber.[12]
- If fluoroscopy is available, injection of contrast media into the pericardial sac will show sluggish pooling, whereas injection into a cardiac chamber will show brisk disappearance.

Whether clear or bloody pericardial fluid is aspirated, the time the needle remains within the pericardial sac must be minimized. When clear pericardial fluid is detected, time should not be wasted in further sampling. The floppy end of a flexible guide wire is rapidly passed through the needle and advanced without resistance into the pericardial sac, and the needle is immediately removed from the pericardial sac. The firm dilator is used to clear the track into the pericardium. On removal of the dilator, the soft pigtail catheter is advanced over the guide wire and advanced about 10 cm into the pericardium. The guide wire is then removed. A large syringe is used to aspirate 50–100 ml of fluid for cytology, biochemistry and bacteriology. In the patient with pericardial tamponade, immediate haemodynamic improvement will follow the removal of 100 ml of fluid.

The remainder of the fluid is then aspirated using a syringe. When the free flow of fluid on aspiration slows, the catheter is attached to a sterile closed drainage bag and left in the pericardial space for the drainage to continue over the next 12–24 hours. The bag is then secured for drainage below the patient's chest.

At the time of removal of the catheter, the sutures are removed under sterile conditions, the catheter is withdrawn gently, and the puncture site is sealed with a sterile dressing.

Adjunctive resuscitation measures for pericardial tamponade

In the patient who is in severe haemodynamic distress with falling blood pressure prior to pericardiocentesis, rapid infusion with 500 ml saline or a plasma expander may be necessary.[13] Inotropic support with dopamine may be necessary. The use of vasodilators should be avoided as this may further lower right ventricular filling pressures.

Haemodynamic monitoring

With the use of echocardiography-guided pericardiocentesis and the use of flexible pericardial catheters and slow drainage, haemodynamic monitoring is not usually necessary. It may however be helpful, if the cause of the right heart disturbance has not been clearly established.

Follow-up

Echocardiography should be performed following the pericardiocentesis[5] and repeated several days later if there is a likelihood of recurrence. Recurrent pericardial effusion or tamponade may require surgical drainage of the pericardium with pericardial window drainage into the left pleural space either by direct surgical or by percutaneous fibreoptic approach,[14] or by use of a balloon dilating technique.

References

1. Guberman B, Fowler NO, Engel PJ, Gveron M, Allen JM. Cardiac tamponade in medical patients. Circulation 1981;64:633–40
2. Spodick DH. The normal and diseased pericardium: current concepts of pericardial physiology, diagnosis and treatment. J Am Coll Cardiol 1983;1:240–51
3. Shabetai R. Changing concepts of cardiac tamponade. Mod Concepts Cardiovasc Dis 1983;52:19–23
4. Spodick DH. Electrical alternans of the heart. Its relation to the kinetics and physiology of the heart during cardiac tamponade. Am J Cardiol 1962;10:155–65
5. Callahan JA, Seward JB, Nishimura RA et al. Two-dimensional echocardiographically guided pericardiocentesis: experience in 117 consecutive patients. Am J Cardiol 1985; 55: 476–84
6. Armstrong WF, Schilt BF, Helper DJ, Dillon JC, Feigenbaum H. Diastolic collapse of the right ventricle with cardiac tamponade. Circulation 1982; 65: 1491–6
7. Hancock EW. Management of pericardial disease. Mod Concepts Cardiovasc Dis 1979; 48: 1–6
8. Krikorian JG, Hancock EW. Pericardiocentesis. Am J Med 1978; 65: 808–14
9. Lock JE, Bass JL, Kulik TJ, Fuhrman BP. Chronic percutaneous pericardial drainage with modified pigtail catheters in children. Am J Cardiol 1984; 53: 1179–82
10. Wong B, Murphy J, Chang CJ, Hassenein K, Dunn M. The risk of pericardiocentesis. Am J Cardiol 1979; 44: 1110–4
11. Bishop LH, Estes EH Jr, McIntosh HD. The ECG as a safeguard in pericardiocentesis. JAMA 1956; 162: 264–5
12. Chandaratna P, First J, Langevin E, O'Dell R. Application of 2-dimensional contrast studies during pericardiocentesis. Am J Cardiol 1983; 52: 1120–2
13. Kerber RE, Jascho JA, Litchfield R, Wolfson P, Ott D, Pandian N. Hemodynamic effects of volume expansion and nitroprusside compared with pericardiocentesis in patients with acute cardiac tamponade. N Engl J Med 1982; 307: 929–33
14. Little AG, Ferguson MK. Pericardioscopy as adjunct to pericardial window. Chest 1986; 89: 53–5

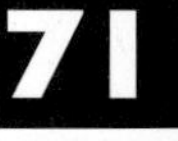

72 Pulmonary embolism

Peter L Thompson

Introduction

Although reliable data is not available, clinical experience suggests that early mobilization and anticoagulant regimens have reduced the frequency of pulmonary embolism after surgical procedures and medical conditions such as myocardial infarction. However, the condition remains relatively common and has been estimated to have been the cause of 250 000 hospitalizations and 50 000 deaths in the United States each year.[1] The fatality rate following pulmonary embolism does not seem to have declined over the past 30 years.[2] Coronary care staff are most likely to be involved in the management of pulmonary embolism in a patient who presents with cardiovascular collapse due to massive embolism; however, the multifarious clinical manifestations of pulmonary embolism may bring staff into contact with the condition in a variety of clinical circumstances including pulmonary infarction and chronic pulmonary hypertension.

Diagnosis

Symptoms

Dyspnoea of sudden onset is the most common symptom of pulmonary embolism but retrosternal chest pain may be present and on occasions may simulate myocardial infarction. Presentation with syncope or collapse is usually an indication of massive pulmonary embolism.

Physical signs

Tachypnoea and tachycardia and signs of apprehension may be present in moderate or massive pulmonary embolism. Signs of right heart failure with elevated venous pressure may be present, raising the differential diagnosis of right ventricular infarction. Accentuation of the pulmonary component of the second heart sound may distinguish the pulmonary hypertension resulting from pulmonary embolism from the venous congestion resulting from right ventricular infarction. However, this is a subtle sign and not detected easily in the apprehensive tachypnoeic patient.

Electrocardiogram

The classical $S_I Q_{II} T_{III}$ pattern is only seen with gross right heart strain and massive pulmonary embolism. More commonly ST depression or T wave inversion in the anterior precordial leads, indicative of right heart strain, may be seen. This can be confused with anterior myocardial ischaemia.[4]

Chest X-ray

Occlusion of a lobar or segmental artery resulting in relative hyperlucency and diminished vascular markings, a 'plump' pulmonary artery or localized infiltrates may be of diagnostic value especially if detected on serial chest X-rays.[3]

Blood gases

Arterial blood gases have been used to screen for pulmonary embolism. The characteristic feature is hypoxaemia due to reduced gas exchange and hypocarbia due to the associated tachypnoea. However, hypoxaemia is a non-specific finding and in particular may be present in conditions being considered in the differential diagnosis, such as myocardial infarction or pulmonary oedema due to other causes. Because of difficulties in interpretation and risk of bleeding with anticoagulant and thrombolytic therapy, the use of arterial blood gases for diagnosis of pulmonary embolism should be discouraged. O_2 saturation monitoring may be helpful to assess response to therapy.

Echocardiography

Marked dilatation and hypokinesis of the right ventricle with bulging of the septum towards the left ventricle may be seen on parasternal views.[6]

Ventilation perfusion scanning

A perfusion lung scan using intravenous (IV) technetium 99m-labelled albumin can detect lobar segmental or subsegmental perfusion defects. However, these can be due to a variety of causes besides pulmonary embolism including obstructive airways disease, atelectasis, pulmonary oedema or pulmonary fibrosis. Specificity is improved markedly by concurrent ventilation scanning using inhalation of Xenon 133. Mismatches between ventilation and perfusion (V/Q mismatch) can identify pulmonary embolism with high, intermediate or low probability (see the information box).

The accuracy of abnormal ventilation perfusion lung scans to identify pulmonary embolism detected on pulmonary angiography has been studied in detail.[7,8] In the Prospective Investigation of Pulmonary Embolism (PIOPED) study, only 41% of those shown to have pulmonary embolism on angiography had high probability lung scans. However, when clinical suspicion of pulmonary embolism was added to the probability of the lung scan the accuracy improved. In patients with a high clinical and scan probability of pulmonary embolism the positive predictive value was 96%. At the other end of the scale, patients with a low probability both clinically and on lung scan had a likelihood of pulmonary embolism of only 4%. In patients in these categories the high or low clinical and lung scan probabilities are satisfactory for therapeutic decision-making such as the need for thrombolytic therapy. Patients with intermediate clinical and lung scan probabilities may be considered for pulmonary angiography to make an accurate diagnosis which may determine therapy.

Pulmonary angiography

Pulmonary angiography can be used in patients with intermediate probability of pulmonary embolism, particularly if there is the possibility of major pulmonary embolism which may benefit from aggressive anticoagulant or thrombolytic therapy. The most common clinical situation is in the patient with haemodynamic compromise in whom pre-existing lung disease reduces the chances of accurate interpretation of the V/Q scan. However, pulmonary angiography carries a mortality and morbidity and presents difficulties in interpretation especially in centres where the technique is not performed routinely. The diagnostic sign of pulmonary embolism on pulmonary angiography is significant filling defects in two or more lobar arteries. An advantage of pulmonary angiography is that the catheter can be used to measure pulmonary artery pressure and as an infusion catheter for thrombolytic therapy and repeat angiography.

Angioscopy

A fibreoptic pulmonary angioscope can be passed into the pulmonary arteries to inspect vessels as small as 3.5 mm diameter.[9]

Ventilation/perfusion (V/Q) lung scans—probability of pulmonary embolism. From Biello DR 1987, reference 6

High probability
- Two or more medium or large V/Q mismatches
- Perfusion defect considerably larger than radiological density

Intermediate probability
- Perfusion defect with severe obstructive airways disease
- Perfusion defect of similar size as radiological density
- Single medium or large V/Q mismatches

Low probability
- Small V/Q mismatches
- V/Q mismatches without corresponding radiological change
- Perfusion defect considerably smaller than radiological density
- Normal lung
- No perfusion defects

Management of pulmonary embolism

Oxygen

High flow oxygen should be administered in severe hypoxaemia and cardiovascular collapse. Intubation and mechanical ventilation may be necessary.

Inotropic support

In the presence of poor cardiac output, inotropic support with dobutamine or a phosphodiesterase inhibitor such as milrinone may be necessary. Right heart filling pressure should be maintained with fluid infusions.

Heparin

Immediately on diagnosis of pulmonary embolism, IV heparin should be initiated with 5000 to 10 000 units bolus followed by 1000 units per hour. Patients with pulmonary embolism clear heparin more rapidly than other patients and have higher heparin requirements than patients without pulmonary embolism.[10] Therefore, meticulous monitoring of the activated partial thromboplastin time (APTT) is necessary, with target range 1.5–2.5 times the upper limit of the control value with a check on the APTT each 4–6 hours until the target range is achieved.

If heparin is the sole antithrombotic therapy it should be continued for 7–10 days before continuing anticoagulation with oral warfarin.

Thrombolytic therapy

There have now been well documented reports from clinical trials that each of streptokinase, urokinase and r-TPA can produce improvement in right ventricular haemodynamics and speed the resolution of pulmonary angiographic appearances.[11] The currently recommended thrombolytic regimens are for shorter durations of therapy than the early experiences, which were characterized by extremely high rates of haemorrhage.[12] The recommended regimes for each of the agents is shown in Table 72.1.

Table 72.1 Recommended thrombolytic regimens for pulmonary embolism (based on reference 12a) Copyright 1987. Adapted from JAMA 1987; 257: 3257–9 copyright 1987, American Medical Association

Streptokinase	250 000 units IV loading dose over 30 minutes followed by 100 000 u/h IV for 24 hours
Urokinase	4400 u/kg IV loading dose over 10 minutes followed by 4400 u/h IV for 12–24 hours
r-TPA	100 mg as a peripheral IV infusion over 2 hours

It is worth noting that these dosage regimens differ from those recommended for myocardial infarction.

These infusions can be administered by a peripheral IV line and do not necessarily require a pulmonary artery catheter, although if this has been left in situ following pulmonary angiography it can be used for the administration of the thrombolytic agent followed by repeat angiography if thought necessary. As in the treatment of myocardial infarction, haemostatic monitoring is not essential although this may be necessary if bleeding complications occur.

The same contraindications to thrombolytic therapy as for myocardial infarction should be observed (see Ch. 34). Wider use of thrombolytic therapy in pulmonary embolism has led to discouragement of the use of arterial blood gases in the diagnosis of pulmonary embolism.

Heparin therapy should be ceased prior to administration of a thrombolytic agent and recommenced immediately on cessation of it.

Despite the demonstration of short-term haemodynamic benefits and angiographic appearances, the long-term benefits of thrombolytic therapy for pulmonary embolism have not been established, and further clinical trials are necessary.[13]

References

1. Anderson FA Jr, Wheeler HB, Goldberg RJ et al. A population-based perspective of the hospital incidence and case fatality rates of venous thrombosis and pulmonary embolism: the Worcester DVT Study. Arch Intern Med 1991;151:933–8
2. Lilienfeld DE, Chan E, Ehland J et al. Mortality from pulmonary embolism in the United States. 1962 to 1984. Chest 1990;98:1067–72
3. Sasahara AA, Sharma GVRT, Barsamiam EM, Schoolman M, Cella G. Pulmonary thromboembolism. Diagnosis and treatment. JAMA 1983;249:2945–50
4. Stein PD, Dalen JR, McIntyre KM, Sasahara AA, Wenger NK, Willis PW. The electrocardiogram in acute pulmonary embolism. Cardiovasc Dis 1975;17:247–57
5. Come PC. Echocardiographic evaluation of pulmonary embolism and its response to therapeutic interventions. Chest 1992;101:151s–62s
6. Biello DR. Radiological (scintigraphic) evaluation of patients with suspected pulmonary thromboembolism. JAMA 1987;257:3257–9
7. Hull RD, Hirsh J, Carter CJ et al. Pulmonary angiography, ventilation lung scanning, and venography for clinically suspected pulmonary embolism with abnormal perfusion lung scan. Ann Intern Med 1983;98:891–8

8. The PIOPED Investigators. Value of the ventilation/perfusion scan in acute pulmonary embolism: results of the Prospective Investigation of Pulmonary Embolism Diagnosis (PIOPED). JAMA 1990;263:2753–9
9. Simmons K. Angioscope 'sees' chronic pulmonary emboli. JAMA 1984;251:695–9
10. Hirsh J, Van Aken WG, Gallus AS, Dollery CT, Cade JF, Yung WL. Heparin kinetics in venous thrombosis and pulmonary embolism. Circulation 1976;53:691–5
11. Goldhaber SZ. Thrombolysis for pulmonary embolism. Prog Cardiovasc Dis 1991;34:113–34
12. The Urokinase Pulmonary Embolism Trial. A national co-operative study. Circulation 1973;47:108
12a. Goldhaber SZ. Thrombolytic therapy for pulmonary embolism. Thrombolysis Yearbook 1993 p 144–162. Amsterdam. Excerpta Medica
13. Goldhaber SZ. Pulmonary embolism thrombolysis: a clarion call for international collaboration. J Am Coll Cardiol 1992;19:246–7

Part 9
Special problems in the CCU patient

73 Diabetes in the coronary care unit

Timothy A Welborn

Patients admitted to coronary care who have diabetes are in a high-risk category and require focused management. They have an increased risk of myocardial infarction (MI) through accelerated atherosclerosis and an increased tendency to thrombosis. The prognosis after MI is less favourable. There is a trend to have larger infarcts and an increased frequency of serious arrhythmias.[1] There is an increased risk of acute and long-term mortality.[2] Diabetic patients may have had previously unrecognized silent MI, which is a common cause of diabetic ischaemic cardiomyopathy.[3] The outcome after revascularization surgery is worse, especially for those on insulin therapy.[4] As with any critically ill patient, marked hyperglycaemia can occur, and is due to increased insulin resistance secondary to the stress-related counter-regulatory hormones, especially catecholamines.[5]

Types of diabetes

Type 2 or non-insulin-dependent diabetes (NIDDM) is the most common form of diabetes, characterized usually by obesity and mature age onset (over 40 years). The pathophysiology involves insulin resistance. Newly diagnosed diabetes has to be distinguished from stress hyperglycaemia by the clinical course over 24–48 hours. Persistence of high blood sugar levels is most likely due to unrecognized NIDDM and should be treated accordingly. Glycated haemoglobin (HbA_{1C}) provides a measure of hyperglycaemia over the preceding 6 weeks and can be used to distinguish established diabetes in those who give no previous history of the condition.

Type 1 or insulin-dependent diabetes (IDDM) is recognized by young age of onset (under 30 years), lean build and absolute insulin deficiency. These patients are prone to ketoacidosis and are likely to have increased insulin requirements with stress.

Diabetic patients who present with cardiac problems may have uncommon syndromes including haemochromatosis, Cushing's syndrome, phaeochromocytoma, and pancreatic or alcohol-related diabetes. These specific conditions should be identified and treated.

Clinical presentation

A history of prior diabetes or high blood sugar levels should be sought in patients with hyperglycaemia, together with details of any oral therapy or daily insulin requirement. Myocardial infarction in diabetic patients requires an added dimension of care. Post-infarction blood glucose levels are of prognostic significance: profound hyperglycaemia can have adverse influences on myocardial function.[6] Heart failure in diabetes may be associated with previously unrecognized ischaemic infarcts. Early invasive assessment (Swan–Ganz catheter) will facilitate management. Angina symptoms also may be obscured and additional diagnostic measures including thallium perfusion scanning should be considered.

Principles of management

With the lack of published data on clinical trials in diabetic subjects, the following empirical guidelines are provided. Careful monitoring of blood glucose levels, electrolytes (especially potassium levels, urinary ketones and fluid balance) is mandatory. It should be noted that renal impairment due to diabetic nephropathy is common in long-duration diabetes.

Management of hyperglycaemia clearly will depend on individual circumstances and in particular on the severity of the critical illness. In general blood glucose levels should be maintained in the range 5–15 mmol/L. It is better to accept moderate hyperglycaemia (10–15 mmol/L) than to allow the risk of hypoglycaemia (< 5 mmol/L) with the attendant adrenergic response and increased myocardial oxygen needs. The use of accurate blood glucose meters on the ward, in experienced hands, greatly facilitates adjustment of insulin dosage.

In IDDM, intermittent subcutaneous insulin therapy should be continued if the patient is able to take food, with at least the normal total daily insulin requirement being given. Where fasting is necessary prior to surgery or investigation, monitoring for hypoglycaemia is essential. There are advantages in using a basal-bolus regime where about 40% of the daily insulin requirement is long-acting insulin, and the remainder is divided into short-acting insulin doses before the meals. (For example, a 70 kg man requiring 50 units of insulin daily would have regular insulin 10/10/10 units before meals and intermediate or long-acting insulin 20 units before bed.)

In IDDM with more severe hyperglycaemia (< 15 mmol/L), IV insulin infusion may be necessary to prevent ketoacidosis. As a general rule, a sliding scale for IV insulin infusion is effective: soluble insulin at the rate of 1 unit per hour is used for plasma glucose levels in the range 4–8 mmol/L; 2 units per hour for plasma glucose levels 8–12 mmol/L; 4 units per hour if plasma glucose levels exceed 12 mmol/L. Blood glucose levels should be monitored every 1–2 hours.

Where short-term (8–24 hour) fasting is necessary for investigational procedures or surgery, and with a patient who is in a stable metabolic and haemodynamic state, insulin infusion with glucose and potassium (Alberti regime) is useful.[7] (Note: Alberti regime = 10 units of regular/soluble insulin in 1000 ml of 10% dextrose with 10 mmol KCl, infused at 100 ml/hour).

The transfer from continuous insulin infusion to subcutaneous injections can be made when the patient is able to tolerate oral feeding. Long acting or 'basal' insulin should be commenced preferably overnight, and boluses of short-acting insulin given before each meal. In this situation a sliding scale 4- to 6-hourly subcutaneous insulin should never be used since it predisposes to wide swings in plasma glucose and the risk of hypoglycaemia.

NIDDM patients in the CCU showing short-term hyperglycaemia can usually continue oral therapy while monitoring blood glucose levels. Metformin however should be ceased temporarily because of the potential risk of lactic acidosis in patients with poor central perfusion. Chlorpropamide also is best ceased since this long-acting sulfonylurea has a very long half-life and carries an increased risk of hypoglycaemia.

In NIDDM with sustained fasting, plasma glucose greater than 15 mmol/L overnight, intermediate or long-acting insulin can be used, or an insulin infusion.[8] An increased dose of insulin may be necessary in NIDDM because of insulin resistance.

Special considerations

The increased tendency to coagulopathy in diabetic patients implies that thrombolytic therapy will require careful titration. Thrombolytic therapy does confer a major benefit on diabetic patients with myocardial infarction.[9] However, in diabetic patients with manifest proliferative retinopathy, the need for anticoagulation and/or thrombolysis should be balanced against the risk of vitreous haemorrhage.

In the long-term management of diabetic patients, loop diuretics and calcium channel antagonists are preferred to thiazide diuretics and beta blockers unless the latter are essential. Thiazide diuretics and beta blockers can compound insulin resistance, leading to impaired glycaemic control, and they can exacerbate dyslipidaemia. Angiotensin-converting enzyme (ACE) inhibitors have a particularly valuable role in diabetes therapy because of their established benefits in retarding progression of diabetic nephropathy.[10]

It is useful to consult diabetic physicians early in the course of management, so that the long-term and discharge care can be planned. This should include appropriate patient education, and specific instructions concerning anti-diabetic, lipid-lowering, and anti-hypertensive medications.

A recently reported controlled trial tested the hypothesis that in diabetic patients with blood glucose levels ≥ 11.0 mmol/l, rapid metabolic control in the acute phase of myocardial infarction and in the early post infarction period, followed by extended intensive blood glucose control. Prognosis improved significantly. Insulin glucose infusion followed by an intensive insulin regime resulted in a 29% reduction of mortality at one year.[11]

References

1. Gwilt DJ. Why do diabetics die after myocardial infarction? Practical Diabetes 1984; 1: 36–9
2. Orlander PR, Goff DC, Morrissey M et al. The relation of diabetes to the severity of acute myocardial infarction and post myocardial infarction survival. Diabetes 1994; 43: 897–902
3. Shapiro LM. A prospective study of heart disease in diabetes mellitus. Quarterly J Med 1984; 209: 55–68
4. Lawrie GM, Morris GC, Glaeser DM. Influence of diabetes mellitus on the results of coronary bypass surgery. J Amer Med Ass 1986; 256: 2967–71
5. Miles JM. Alterations in insulin action in the critically ill patient. J Critical Care Nutrition 1994; 2: 30–4
6. Yudkin JS, Oswald GA. Determinants of hospital admission and case fatality in diabetic patients with myocardial infarction. Diabetes Care 1988; 11: 351–8
7. Alberti KGMM. Low-dose insulin in the treatment of diabetic ketoacidosis. Arch Intern Med 1977; 137: 1367–76
8. Gwilt DJ, Petri M, Lamb P, Nattrass M, Pentecost BL. Effect of intravenous insulin infusion on mortality among diabetic patients after myocardial infarction. Br Heart J 1984; 51: 626–31
9. Lynch M, Gammage MD, Lamb P, Nattrass M, Pentecost BL. Acute myocardial infarction in diabetic patients in the thrombolytic era. Diab Med 1994; 11: 162–5
10. Lewis EJ, Hunsicker LG, Bain RP, Rohde RD. The effects of angiotensin-converting enzyme inhibition on diabetic nephropathy. The Collaborative Study Group. N Engl J Med 1993; 329: 1456–62
11. Malmberg K, Ryden L, Efendic S et al. Randomised trial of insulin-glucose infusion followed by subcutaneous insulin treatment in diabetic patients with acute myocardial infarction (Digami study): Effects on mortality at one year. J Am Coll Cardiol 1995; 26: 56–65

74 Gastrointestinal haemorrhage

Bernard H Laurence

Gastrointestinal (GI) bleeding is a serious and potentially life-threatening illness, particularly in the elderly and high risk patients. Over the age of 60 years, the risk of death from upper gastrointestinal bleeding increases two- to fourfold, and the mortality rate rises substantially in patients with underlying heart disease (12.5%), congestive cardiac failure (28%), or respiratory failure (57%).[1]

The incidence of haematemesis and/or melaena following myocardial infarction is not well documented, but the widespread use of aspirin, anticoagulants and thrombolytic agents in the peri-infarct period is likely to be an important causative factor. In Capell's studies, bleeding considered to be of upper or lower gastrointestinal origin occurred in 1.2% and 0.4% of all myocardial infarcts respectively.[2,3] The mean age of the patients was 72 years; in those with the most severe bleeding who underwent gastroscopy, one third had been taking aspirin or other non-steroidal anti-inflammatory drugs and 12% were on anticoagulants.

Uncommonly, myocardial infarction may also be a consequence of massive gastrointestinal bleeding.

Prevention

The occurrence of upper gastrointestinal mucosal inflammation, ulceration and bleeding are significantly increased by the long-term use of aspirin or other non-steroidal anti-inflammatory drugs (NSAIDs) (important in the older, infarct risk age group).[4,5] Although these effects tend to be dose-dependent, NSAID type-dependent and with bleeding, combination-dependent (aspirin plus NSAID), even low dose aspirin may cause significant mucosal damage and may be asymptomatic until overt bleeding ensues.[6] Use of enteric coated aspirin reduces but does not eliminate this problem. Concomitant administration of H2 antagonists or misoprostol provides some protection from duodenal and gastric lesions respectively; omeprazole seems to protect against both. Most gastric and duodenal ulcers heal on H2 antagonists and omeprazole, even though aspirin or other NSAIDs are continued, but are likely to heal faster if all anti-inflammatory drugs are ceased.[7]

Resuscitation

Adequate resuscitation, with stabilization of the patient's cardiovascular and general medical condition if possible, is essential before undertaking endoscopy. Serious complications during endoscopy may occur in 40% of patients with a recent infarct if they are critically ill (with two or more of the conditions listed in the information box). Blood replacement may be difficult to assess accurately in patients with cardiac failure, and pulmonary capillary wedge pressure measurements may be necessary. Coagulation defects should be excluded early and corrected if clinically significant (see Chs 32–35).

Diagnosis

Endoscopy

In upper gastrointestinal haemorrhage, the source and nature of the bleeding are important determinants of outcome and have a critical influence on management. The site of bleeding can be identified by endoscopy[8] and approximately half the patients (with or without a recent myocardial infarct) have duodenal or gastric ulceration. Haemorrhagic gastritis, secondary to stress or medication (aspirin, NSAIDs), occurs in less than 10% of post-infarct patients;

Major medical problems after MI which may contribute to critical illness at time of endoscopy. Adapted from Capell MS 1993[2]

- Congestive cardiac failure or pneumonia requiring assisted ventilation due to respiratory decompensation
- Hypotension or syncope in the 12 hours before endoscopy
- Life-threatening arrhythmia in the 24 hours before endoscopy
- Massive bleeding requiring transfusion of more than 8 units of packed red blood cells
- Severe uncorrected coagulopathy
- Recurrent angina in the 12 hours before endoscopy
- Acute renal failure
- Severe sepsis (apart from pneumonia[1])
- Cerebrovascular accident in the 24 hours before endoscopy

in this setting, variceal bleeding is comparatively rare.[2]

Although ulcer bleeding stops spontaneously in the majority of patients, in 20–25% the bleeding continues or recurs. These 'high risk lesions' can be determined endoscopically by the appearance of the ulcer base. Spurting, arterial bleeding has a re-bleeding rate of 85–90%; in ulcers not bleeding at endoscopy, re-bleeding occurs in 50% of those with a visible vessel but in less than 2% with a clear ulcer base.[9] Because of the dangers of recurrent, large-volume arterial (or variceal) bleeding in post-infarct patients, these 'high risk lesions' should be treated at the time of the initial endoscopy.

In Capell's patients with overt bleeding after myocardial infarction, endoscopy confirmed the site of bleeding in 79% and was clinically useful in a further 12%. Serious complications—fatal ventricular tachycardia, respiratory arrest and hypotension—occurred in 9.5% of the procedures, but only in patients who were critically ill at the time of endoscopy; 10 patients—eight with active bleeding and one with a non-bleeding visible vessel—were treated endoscopically by diathermy or a heater probe; permanent control of bleeding was achieved in four.[2]

Risks

Diagnostic upper gastrointestinal endoscopy in good risk patients is a relatively safe procedure. Nevertheless, half the major complications are cardio-pulmonary in origin and these contribute to half the procedure-related deaths. In a survey of 21 000 endoscopies, serious cardiac or respiratory complications occurred in 114 (0.54%) and resulted in seven deaths (0.03%).[10] Not surprisingly, the risk of these complications is increased in patients with cardiac or chronic obstructive pulmonary disease or with upper gastrointestinal bleeding.

Cardiac complications[11]

Sinus tachycardia with a rise in blood pressure (BP) is common during insertion of the endoscope, particularly in the unsedated patient. Electrocardiogram (ECG) changes—sinus tachycardia, ST depression, supraventricular tachycardia and ventricular ectopics—occur in 7–50% of patients, but are usually transient and seldom result in myocardial infarction (0.02%) or cardiac arrest (0.04%). The risk of an arrhythmia in a patient with cardiac disease is increased about threefold. Drugs with anticholinergic effects such as Buscopan (hyoscine-N-butylbromide) which are given to reduce peristalsis during endoscopy, cause or accentuate tachycardia and should not be used.

Pulmonary complications[12]

Hypoxaemia with a fall in SpO_2 below 90% occurs in 40% of otherwise normal patients undergoing endoscopy under sedation, and is probably the most important preventable factor contributing to arrhythmias in patients with cardiac disease. It is usually transient and mild but with deep sedation, chronic obstructive pulmonary disease or cardiac failure, it may be profound and last long after the procedure is completed.

The use of supplemental oxygen (2–3 litres per minute) by the nasal route will abolish hypoxaemia during endoscopy and the recovery period in most, but not all, patients. It does not however correct hypoventilation which, with too heavy sedation or with chronic obstructive pulmonary disease, may lead to severe CO_2 retention, arrhythmias or respiratory arrest. In patients with pulmonary oedema complicating myocardial infarction, endotracheal intubation with assisted ventilation may be necessary to carry out endoscopy safely.

Aspiration of blood is an ever-present threat during endoscopy for GI bleeding and may cause serious pulmonary complications in up to 20% of cases.[13] Although the risk can be lessened by aspiration of stomach contents before the procedure, in the unsedated patient with a recent infarct, this may be unduly stressful. The use of heavy sedation and pharyngeal anaesthesia should be avoided and a decision to protect the airway with an endotracheal tube should not be delayed if there is large volume regurgitation or vomiting, or continued heavy bleeding.

Risk management

Risk management during endoscopy after a recent myocardial infarction can be facilitated by the following:

- The decision to carry out upper gastrointestinal endoscopy should be made early, preferably while the patient's cardio-pulmonary state is stable and before bleeding recurs.
- Since the most serious complications during endoscopy are likely to be cardio-pulmonary, the procedure should be carried out in the CCU, with a cardiologist available.
- Because of the dangers of inadequate or excessive sedation, the possible need for endotracheal intubation and the overall reduced margin of safety in 'high risk patients', sedation should, if possible, be supervised by an anaesthetist.
- The procedure should be performed by an endoscopist with extensive experience in the treatment of GI bleeding and there should be at least two skilled assistants trained in cardio-pulmonary resuscitation.
- Pulse oximetry, continuous ECG and intermittent BP monitoring should be available if the procedure is performed outside a CCU, with resuscitation equipment including a defibrillator at hand.

Radiology

Barium meal

A barium meal examination is an inadequate substitute for endoscopy in this clinical situation—it is less accurate, gives little information on 'high risk lesions', cannot be performed at the bedside and has no therapeutic capability.

Angiography

Mesenteric angiography[14] may be useful in massive bleeding where diagnostic endoscopy has failed or endoscopic therapy is unsuccessful. Embolization of a bleeding vessel is sometimes possible; and the risks may be justified if surgery is contraindicated. Intra-arterial vasopressin can control ulcer bleeding, but its use, even with the simultaneous administration of nitrates, is contraindicated in patients with ischaemic heart disease.

Treatment

Drug therapy

Acid suppression[15,16]

Patients bleeding from peptic ulceration, oesophagitis or haemorrhagic gastritis should be commenced on an H2 antagonist (cimetidine, ranitidine, famotidine, nizatidine) or a proton-pump inhibitor (omeprazole, lansoprazole) once the diagnosis has been established. These initiate healing but have no effect on active bleeding or the incidence of re-bleeding from peptic ulceration; they may control bleeding in stress-related mucosal damage. Oral administration is effective in most patients and intravenous use should be reserved for patients with vomiting, delayed gastric emptying or an ileus.

Others

Somatostatin or its analogue octreotide, which reduce acid secretion and splanchnic blood flow, may control ulcer bleeding and should be considered after unsuccessful endoscopic therapy in patients unsuitable for surgery.[17]

Control of bleeding

Endoscopic methods[8,18]

Sclerotherapy

Injection of 1:10 000 adrenalin or a sclerosant such as absolute alcohol into the base of an ulcer will control arterial bleeding in 80–90% of cases and reduce the risk of re-bleeding to 15–20%. This is a relatively simple and safe technique which is readily applicable outside the endoscopy unit and can be repeated safely if necessary. The absorption of adrenalin (up to 10 ml) is a potential hazard after myocardial infarction and this should be remembered if more than one lesion is treated.

Bicap, laser, heater probe

Bipolar diathermy with a Bicap, laser photocoagulation or the direct application of thermal energy with a heater probe are all equally effective in immediate and long-term control of ulcer bleeding. They are, however, more difficult to apply and have a higher perforation rate than sclerotherapy (0.4–1.5% versus 0%).

Surgery

Although major, non-cardiac surgery[19] soon after myocardial infarction has a substantial re-infarction and mortality rate, this is usually outweighed by the dangers of continuing conservative treatment too long when endoscopic and other therapies have obviously failed. This is particularly so when massive exsanguinating haemorrhage precludes effective endoscopy. Nevertheless, in the elderly and frail, even in the absence of severe coronary artery disease, emergency surgery to control bleeding carries a high mortality (25–50%); every endeavour should be made to stabilize the patient's cardiovascular and general medical condition prior to operation. The shortest possible procedure compatible with permanent control of bleeding (for example, undersewing the vessel, truncal vagotomy and drainage) should be considered in the high risk patient with cardiac disease.

References

1. Silverstein FE, Gilbert DA, Tedesco FJ et al. The national ASGE survey on upper gastrointestinal bleeding. II. Clinical prognostic factors. Gastro Intest Endosc 1981; 27: 80–93
2. Cappell MS. The safety and clinical utility of oesophagogastroduodenoscopy for acute gastrointestinal bleeding after myocardial infarction: a six-year study of 42 endoscopies in 34 consecutive patients at two university teaching hospitals. Am J Gastro 1993; 88: 344–9
3. Cappell MS. Safety and clinical efficiency of flexible sigmoidoscopy and colonoscopy for gastrointestinal bleeding after myocardial infarction: a six-year study of 15 consecutive lower endoscopies at two university teaching hospitals. Dig Dis Sci 1994; 39: 473–80
4. Aabakken L. Non steroidal anti-inflammatory drugs—the extending scope of gastrointestinal side-effects. Aliment Pharmacol Ther 1992; 6: 143–62
5. Langman MJ, Weil J, Wainwright PE et al. Risks of bleeding peptic ulcer associated with individual non-steroidal anti-inflammatory drugs. Lancet 1994; 343: 1075–8
6. Leivenen M, Sipponen F, Kivilaakso E. Gastric changes in coronary-operated patients with low-dose aspirin. Scand J Gastroenterol 1992; 27: 912–6
7. Scheiman JM, Behler EM, Loeffler KM, Elta GH. Omeprazole ameliorates aspirin-induced gastroduodenal injury. Dig Dis Sci 1994; 39: 97–103
8. Zuccaro G. Bleeding peptic ulcer: pathogenesis and endoscopic therapy. In: Friedman LS (ed.) Gastroenterology clinics of North America: gastrointestinal bleeding I. Philadelphia: Saunders, 1993: 737–50
9. Laurence BH, Cotton PB. Bleeding gastroduodenal ulcers: non-operative treatment. World J Surg 1987; 11: 295–303
10. Arrowsmith JB, Gerstman BB, Fleischer DE et al. Results from the American Society for Gastrointestinal Endoscopy/US Food & Drug Administration Collaborative Study on complication rates and drug use during gastrointestinal endoscopy. Gastro Intest Endos 1991; 37: 421
11. Newcomer MK, Brazer SR. Complications of upper gastrointestinal endoscopy and their management. In: Blades EW, Chak A (eds). Gastrointestinal endoscopy clinics of North America: upper gastrointestinal endoscopy. Philadelphia: Saunders, 1994: 551–70
12. Freeman ML. Sedation and monitoring for gastrointestinal endoscopy. In: Blades EW, Chak A (eds). Gastrointestinal endoscopy clinics of North America: upper gastrointestinal endoscopy. Philadelphia: Saunders, 1994: 475–99
13. Lipper B, Simon D, Cerrone F. Pulmonary aspiration during emergency endoscopy in patients with upper gastrointestinal haemorrhage. Crit Care Med 1991; 19: 330
14. Keller FS, Routh WD. Angiographic diagnosis and management. Hepato Gastroenterol 1991; 38: 207–15
15. Daneshmend TK, Hawkey CJ, Langman MJ et al. Omeprazole versus placebo for acute upper gastrointestinal bleeding: randomised double blind controlled trial. Br Med J 1992; 304: 143–7
16. Chamberlain CE. Acute haemorrhagic gastritis. In: Friedman LS (ed). Gastroenterology clinics of North America: gastrointestinal bleeding I. Philadelphia: Saunders, 1993: 843–73
17. Jenkins SA, Taylor BA, Nott DM et al. Management of upper massive gastrointestinal haemorrhage from multiple sites of peptic ulceration with somatostatin and octreotide: a report of five cases. Gut 1992; 33: 404–7
18. Cook DJ, Guyatt GH, Salena BJ, Laine LA. Endoscopic therapy for acute non-variceal upper

gastrointestinal haemorrhage: a meta-analysis. Gastroenterol 1992; 102: 139–48
19. Cochran TA. Bleeding peptic ulcer: surgical therapy. In: Friedman LS (ed). Gastroenterology clinics of North America: gastrointestinal bleeding I. Philadelphia: Saunders, 1993: 751–78

75 Stroke

Timothy J Day

Introduction

Stroke is the third most common cause of death in our community and patients with cerebrovascular disease share many of the same risk factors as those with coronary artery disease (see the first information box).[1–3] Patients with acute myocardial infarction, cardiac arrhythmias or congestive heart failure are at increased risk of developing a cardioembolic stroke, while the risk of cerebral bleeding is increased with thrombolytic therapy (see the second box).[4–6]

Stroke is defined as a sudden, nonconvulsive focal neurological deficit due to vascular disease, and may vary widely in duration and severity. The hallmark of a stroke is its relatively abrupt onset while the constellation of signs often conforms to a particular vascular territory. Most strokes are ischaemic (due to embolism, thrombosis or reduced perfusion); roughly 15% are haemorrhagic (see the information box).[3,7,8] In all types, a variable degree of recovery can be expected due to resolution of oedema and/or recovery of injured but still viable tissue in the 'ischaemic penumbra'. For this reason, prompt recognition and diagnosis of stroke is essential to maximize the degree of recovery through acute reperfusion and neuroprotective strategies, prevention of complications and structured rehabilitation measures.

Risk factors for ischaemic stroke

- Cigarette smoking
- Hypertension
- Diabetes
- Hypercholesterolaemia
- Ischaemic heart disease
- Atrial fibrillation
- Structural heart disease
  - — mitral valve disease
  - — congestive cardiomyopathy
  - — recent myocardial infarction
  - — left ventricular thrombus
  - — right to left shunts
- Intravascular procedures—cardiac catheter, angiography, angioplasty

Risk factors for cerebral haemorrhage

- Hypertension
- Embolic stroke, especially septic embolism
- Thrombolytic therapy
- Anticoagulant therapy
- Coagulation disorders
- Vascular malformations
- Brain tumour
- Amyloid angiopathy

Recognition—is it a stroke?

Embolic stroke typically has an abrupt onset; a carotid or cardiac bruit or atrial fibrillation may provide clues to the source. Thrombotic stroke may be more gradual or progressive in onset, although some start suddenly. Cerebral haemorrhage may present abruptly or evolve over minutes to hours. Clinical features of stroke include unilateral weakness, loss of sensation or loss of vision, while apparent 'confusion' can reflect dysphasia in dominant

Types of stroke

- **Ischaemia**
  large vessel thrombosis
  — carotid artery
  — intracranial arteries
  lacunar infarct (small vessel thrombosis)
  embolic infarction
  — artery to artery
  — cardioembolism
  borderzone (watershed) infarction
- **Haemorrhage**
  parenchymal haemorrhage
  subarachnoid haemorrhage

hemisphere events, or neglect in non-dominant hemisphere strokes. The most common stroke syndrome is unilateral weakness, while altered sensation, dysphasia, hemianopia, diplopia or hemi-ataxia may occur in different combinations.[3] Often mild weakness or ataxia is not recognized because the patient is confined to bed, sensory loss is overlooked or disturbed speech or vision is wrongly attributed to medication. In particular, confusion and slurred speech can be attributed to lignocaine toxicity. The lignocaine infusion should be ceased immediately to help clarify the clinical picture. Coronary care unit (CCU) staff need to be able to quickly assess alertness, speech, vision, power, reflexes and sensation in patients with neurological complaints. Loss of consciousness without focal neurological signs is almost never due to stroke, although in some cases acute ischaemic or haemorrhagic lesions may be complicated by seizures.

CT scans

Widespread use of CT (computed tomography) scanning has taught us that there are no reliable clinical signs which predict whether an acute focal deficit is due to haemorrhage or ischaemia; all patients will therefore need to have a CT head scan to define accurately the type (and site) of pathology. Although stroke with prominent headache, drowsiness and vomiting is classically due to cerebral haemorrhage, similar symptoms and signs may be observed following a large ischaemic infarct. Similar degrees of hemiparesis may be produced by large cortical lesions and by small deep white matter (lacunar) infarcts, although the former usually demonstrate cortical signs such as dysphasia, neglect or dyspraxia. Unfortunately, small capsular haemorrhages are indistinguishable clinically from lacunar infarcts, and even moderate sized lobar haemorrhages may not develop significant headache, drowsiness or vomiting. CT scans will show cerebral bleeding immediately, whereas some ischaemic infarcts may not show changes on CT scans for several days.[9,10]

Examples of the typical CT scan appearance of cerebral infarction (Fig. 75.1) and cerebral haemorrhage (Fig. 75.2) are shown below.

Acute management

Acute management of stroke includes prompt diagnosis, anticipation and prevention of early complications, and institution of specific treatment for thrombosis or raised intracranial pressure if necessary. Venous access and adequate oxygenation should be ensured. The earliest assessments should focus on mental state and level of communication, moni toring vital functions including blood pressure, heart rate and rhythm, and respiration, and documenting the neurological symptoms and signs, which may well alter in the first few hours. Patients with stroke may deteriorate for a number of reasons (see the information box), not all of which are due to further ischaemia.[11]

The mainstays of nursing management include assessment and recording of mental state, limb power, pupil reactions and other vital signs, with notification of medical staff if there is significant decline in any parameter. Patients should be kept at bed-rest and if the mental state is significantly impaired, be nursed on their sides. Oral intake should be withheld until adequate protection of the airway is demonstrated. Paralysed limbs should be supported on pillows to avoid compression neuropathies or excessive ligamentous strain. These precautions may be continued or relaxed depending on the degree of recovery in limb power, speech or swallowing

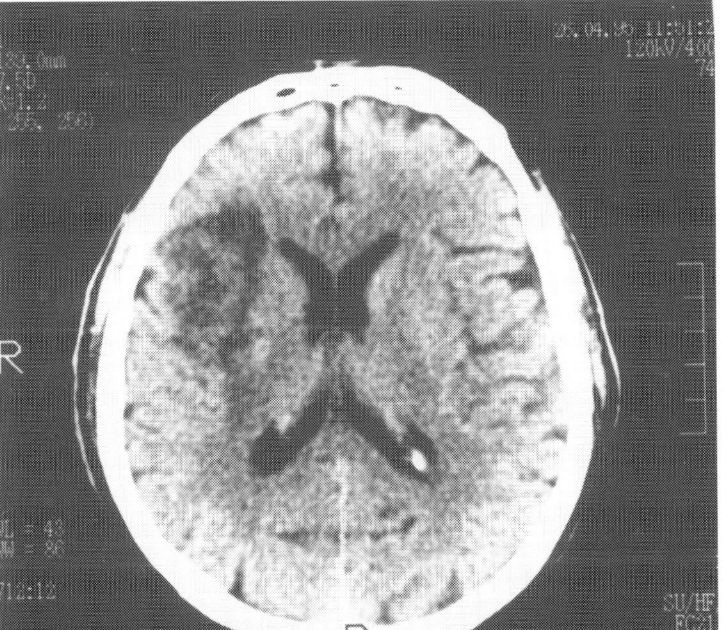

Fig. 75.1 Large area of cerebral infarction with surrounding oedema in the parieto-frontal area in a patient with stroke complicating acute myocardial infarction.

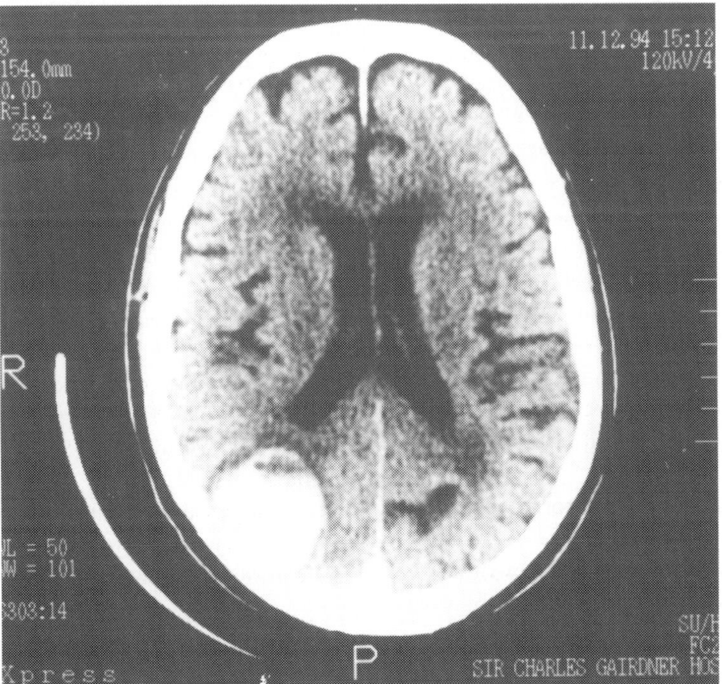

Fig. 75.2 Cerebral haemorrhage in the right occipital lobe complicating acute myocardial infarction treated with thrombolytic therapy.

functions, or conscious level in each individual case.

Early management

Early management of the patient with stroke depends greatly on the underlying pathology.

Cerebral ischaemia

Cerebral ischaemia may be due to thromboembolism from carotid or vertebro-basilar artery disease, from the heart or, as increasingly recognized, from aortic atheroma.[12] Thrombosis of extra- or intra-cranial large vessels, or of small perforating vessels, may each produce a similar stroke syndrome.[3] Invasive vascular procedures including coronary angiography also carry a small risk of systemic embolism (including stroke), as thrombus or atheroma may be dislodged by manipulation of the catheter.

As yet there is no proven strategy to improve recovery of 'stunned' tissue in the 'ischaemic penumbra' but clinical trials are in progress with antithrombotic drugs (heparin, aspirin), thrombolytic agents (streptokinase, tissue plasminogen activator [TPA]) and neuroprotective drugs (N-methyl D-aspartate receptor [NMDA] antagonists, calcium channel blockers, free radical scavengers), aiming to maximize the degree of possible recovery. (See references for overviews.)[6,13–15] The major acute priority is to prevent recurrence of embolism and prevent progression of thrombosis—although controversial, many centres would anticoagulate acutely with heparin following transient ischaemic attack (TIA)

Causes of deterioration after stroke

- Progressive thrombosis
- Recurrent embolism
- Hypotension (causing secondary ischaemia)
  - low cardiac output
  - postural hypotension
  - inappropriate medication
- Cerebral oedema with brain herniation
- Haemorrhagic transformation with haematoma formation
- Metabolic disturbance—hypoxia, hypoglycaemia, hyponatraemia
- Seizures
- Sepsis—pneumonia, urinary tract infection, septicaemia
- Psychological factors—depression, anxiety

or submaximal stroke, particularly if there were a known cardiac source of embolism. The risk of haemorrhagic transformation appears greatest with large-volume infarcts treated within the first week, particularly if these are embolic in origin[16,17] but a previous ischaemic stroke, whether large or small, does not necessarily contraindicate use of anticoagulants.[18] Provided that haemorrhage is excluded on CT scan, IV heparinization can be commenced in most patients, although caution is advised in patients with large cerebral infarcts. A common practice is to initiate treatment with a loading dose of 5000 u heparin intravenously followed by infusion initially at 1000 u/hour, the infusion rate to be adjusted according to at least daily measurements of heparin activity or activated partial thromboplastin time (APTT). Intravenous anticoagulation should be continued until a decision is made about long-term therapy depending on age, general condition and other medical factors. Some patients will be converted to platelet antiaggregant therapy (such as aspirin) while others will be transferred to oral anticoagulants (such as warfarin). Warfarin should be withheld if further invasive procedures such as angiography, carotid endarterectomy or cardiac surgery are contemplated in the near future.

Important supportive care of ischaemic stroke also includes strict avoidance of hypotension, supplemental oxygen and maintenance of normoglycaemia. Massive life-threatening cerebral oedema may occur (usually in younger patients) causing impaired consciousness and worsening neurological signs; in such cases, aggressive anti-oedema therapy with fluid restriction, IV mannitol, assisted hyperventilation and even hemicraniectomy may be contemplated in individual cases.

Cerebral haemorrhage

Thrombolytic therapy carries a 0.1–0.6% risk of cerebral haemorrhage,[19–21] while chronic anticoagulant therapy also increases the risk of bleeding.[4,5] Most spontaneous cerebral parenchymal haemorrhages are related to hypertension and are attributed to rupture of Charcot–Bouchard microaneurysms.[3,4] Less commonly, bleeding from amyloid angiopathy, arterio-venous malformation, brain tumour or vasculitis is the cause.[5]

The stroke syndromes may be similar to those seen with ischaemic stroke, although headache and drowsiness are more likely, but a CT scan is essential to accurate diagnosis. Once haemorrhage is identified, the treatment comprises control of hypertension, reversal of anticoagulant therapy and close monitoring of the patient. Early neurological consultation is advisable to optimize acute management and subsequent rehabilitation. In most cases bedrest and control of hypertension are sufficient to offset deterioration due to brain swelling; stabilization and recovery occur in most cases after the first few days. In large hemispheric bleeds and cerebellar haematomas, progressive life-threatening deterioration may occur rapidly and in these circumstances neurosurgical intervention with evacuation of the haematoma is indicated.

Difficult management decisions arise when cerebral bleeding occurs secondary to cardioembolism (for example, with atrial fibrillation [AF] or rheumatic valvular disease) and in such cases careful evaluation must be made of the risks and benefits of continuing with anticoagulant therapy once the haematoma has resolved. In the acute period, anticoagulation is contraindicated but where there is a high risk of further embolism, it may be reasonable to resume anticoagulant therapy at lower levels.

Secondary prevention of ischaemic stroke

Early investigation should help to:

- determine the mechanism of the stroke
- devise a rational plan for long-term medication and/or surgical treatment
- identify modifiable cardiac or other vascular risk factors.

Coexistent carotid artery disease needs to be identified; if carotid Doppler duplex ultrasound suggests a significant stenosis, formal angiography with a view to carotid endarterectomy should be considered.[22,23] The timing of such surgery depends on the degree of recovery from the stroke syndrome and the patient's fitness for general anaesthesia.

Standard haematology, biochemistry, blood glucose, fasting lipids, chest X-ray and ECG will usually have been performed on patients in the CCU.

Echocardiography can be useful in identifying a cardiac source for embolism where this is not clear from the clinical setting. The duration of anticoagulant therapy or the choice between platelet anti-aggregants and anticoagulants may be influenced by knowledge of a cardio-embolic source. Trans-thoracic techniques detect some relevant abnormalities but it is clear that trans-oesophageal echocardiography provides superior information.[24,25]

General care

Whether stroke is caused by haemorrhage or infarction, the level of nursing and medical care will depend on the clinical status of the patient. Patients with significant limb weakness should have at least daily passive limb exercises under the supervision of a physiotherapist, while the limbs should be supported to avoid pressure palsies and excessive distraction at the shoulder joint. Chest physiotherapy and deep breathing exercises may forestall hypostatic or aspiration pneumonia and thus prevent secondary deterioration. Patients who are drowsy, dyspraxic or demonstrate significant neglect are likely to have swallowing problems and should have oral intake withheld until they can safely tolerate this. Medications and feeding should be continued by nasogastric tube if pharyngeal dysfunction is likely to be prolonged for more than several days. Speech, swallowing and communication impairments may require assessment and treatment by a speech pathologist. Unless there is substantial early recovery, patients should be kept rested in bed with appropriate care to prevent deep venous thrombosis in the legs and skin pressure areas. Problems with bowel and bladder function should be anticipated.

Depending on the degree and rate of recovery, plans may be made for more intensive rehabilitation once the patient's cardiac and general condition permits. Attention to the potential sources of deterioration in a stroke patient, many of which are avoidable or treatable, will prevent the patient carrying an additional legacy during the period of recovery.

Summary

Stroke is a relatively common problem, both in the community and in cardiac patients in particular. Patients in a CCU share common risk factors for cerebrovascular disease while their underlying cardiac conditions and treatments may predispose them to cerebral embolism or haemorrhage. It is important for CCU staff to be aware of the possibility of stroke in patients with atrial fibrillation, congestive cardiac failure and myocardial infarction, and to be able to assess them with a brief screening neurological examination. Following exclusion of haemorrhage by CT scan, many patients will be treated with intravenous anticoagulation, with further investigation of cardiac status and carotid arteries prior to a decision on long-term management. Treatment of cerebral haemorrhage is supportive, but both ischaemia and haemorrhage may cause acute deterioration requiring more aggressive treatment. With patient monitoring, dedicated nursing care and early involvement of physiotherapists and speech pathologists, many stroke complications can be avoided, providing the best long-term outcome for these patients.

References

1. Wolf PA, Kannel WB, McGee DL. Prevention of ischemic stroke: risk factors. In: Barnett HJM, Stein BM, Mohr JP, Yatsu FM (eds). Stroke—pathophysiology, diagnosis and management. New York: Churchill Livingstone, 1986; Vol 2: 967–88
2. Dyken M. Stroke risk factors. In: Norris JW, Hachinski VC (eds).

Prevention of stroke. New York: Springer Verlag, 1991: 83–101
3. Adams RD, Victor M. Cerebrovascular disease. In: Principles of neurology. 5th ed. New York: McGraw-Hill, 1993: 669–748
4. Kase CS, Mohr JP. General features of intracerebral hemorrhage. In: Barnett HJM, Stein BM, Mohr JP, Yatsu FM (eds). Stroke—pathophysiology, diagnosis and management. New York: Churchill Livingstone, 1986; Vol 1: 497–524
5. Kase CS. Intracerebral hemorrhage—non-hypertensive causes. Stroke 1986;17:590–5
6. Wardlaw JM, Warlow CP. Thrombolysis in acute ischemic stroke. Does it work? Stroke 1992;23:1826–39
7. Ward G, Jamrozik K, Stewart-Wynne EG. Incidence and outcome of cerebrovascular disease in Perth, Western Australia. Stroke 1988;19:1501–6
8. Bamford J, Sandercock PAG, Dennis M, Burn J, Warlow CP. A prospective study of acute cerebrovascular disease in the community: the Oxfordshire Community Stroke Project—1981–1986. 2. Incidence, case fatality rates and overall outcome at one year of cerebral infarction, primary intracerebral and subarachnoid haemorrhage. J Neurol Neurosurg Psychiat 1990;53:16–22
9. Tatemichi TK, Mohr JP, Rubinstein LV et al. CT findings and clinical course in acute stroke: the NINCDS Stroke Data Bank. Presented at the Tenth International Joint Conference on Stroke and Cerebral Circulation, 22 February 1985, New Orleans
10. Savoiardo M. CT scanning. In: Barnett HJM, Stein BM, Mohr JP, Yatsu FM (eds). Stroke—pathophysiology, diagnosis and management. New York: Churchill Livingstone, 1986; Vol 1:189–219
11. Price TR. Progressing ischemic stroke. In: Barnett HJM, Stein BM, Mohr JP, Yatsu FM (eds). Stroke—pathophysiology, diagnosis and management. New York: Churchill Livingstone, 1986;Vol 2:1059–68
12. Amarenco P, Cohen A, Tzourio C et al. Atherosclerotic disease of the aortic arch and the risk of ischemic stroke. N Engl J Med 1994;331:1474–9
13. Donnan G. Therapy in cerebrovascular disease: current status and future directions. Med J Aust 1991;155:563–71
14. Sandercock PAG, van den Belt AGM, Lindley RI, Slattery J. Antithrombotic therapy in acute ischaemic stroke: an overview of the completed randomised trials. J Neurol Neurosurg Psychiat 1993;56:17–25
15. Marshall RS, Mohr JP. Current management of ischaemic stroke. J Neurol Neurosurg Psychiat 1993; 56: 6–16
16. Hart RG, Easton JD. Hemorrhagic infarcts. Stroke 1992;23:586–9
17. Ott BR, Zamani A, Kleefield J, Funkenstein HH. The clinical spectrum of hemorrhagic infarction. Stroke 1986;17: 630–7
18. Lodder J. CT detected hemorrhagic infarction: relation with the size of the infarct and the presence of midline shift. Acta Neurol Scand 1984;70:329–35
19. Maggioni AP, Franzosi MG, Santoro E et al. The risk of stroke in patients with acute myocardial infarction after thrombolytic and antithrombotic treatment. N Engl J Med 1992; 327: 1–6
20. ISIS-2 (2nd International Study of Infarct Survival) Collaborative Group. A randomised trial of intravenous streptokinase, oral aspirin, both or neither among 7187 cases of suspected acute myocardial infarction. Lancet 1988; 2: 349–60
21. ISIS-3 (3rd International Study of Infarct Survival) Collaborative Group. ISIS-3: a randomised comparison of streptokinase vs tissue plasminogen activator vs anistreplase and of aspirin and heparin vs aspirin alone among 41 299 cases of suspected acute myocardial infarction. Lancet 1992; 339: 753–70
22. North American Symptomatic Carotid Endarterectomy Trial Collaborators. Beneficial effect of carotid endarterectomy in symptomatic patients with high-grade carotid stenosis. N Engl J Med 1991; 325: 445–53
23. European Carotid Surgery Trialists Collaborative Group. MRC European Carotid Surgery Trial: interim results for symptomatic patients with severe (70–99%) or with mild (0–29%) carotid stenosis. Lancet 1991; 337: 1235–43
24. Comess KA, DeRook FA, Beach KW, Lytle NJ, Golby AJ, Albers GW. Transesophageal echocardiography and carotid ultrasound in patients with cerebral ischemia: prevalence of findings and recurrent stroke risk. J Am Coll Cardiol 1994; 23: 1598–1603
25. Pearson AC. Transthoracic echocardiography versus transesophageal echocardiography in detecting cardiac sources of embolism. Echocardiography 1993; 10: 397–403

Part 10
Post-CCU management

76 Discharge planning and rehabilitation

Donna M O'Shannessy and Tom G Briffa

The overall goals of cardiac rehabilitation are to assist the patient in resuming a satisfying and productive life, decrease risky health behaviours, maximize physical potential without endangering life, and reduce morbidity and mortality. Rehabilitation is a continuous process that begins in the coronary care unit (CCU) (in-patient) and extends to a lifelong programme of prudent life style adaptation.[1–4] Cardiac rehabilitation, using a comprehensive and multi-disciplinary approach, is essential to obtain optimum patient outcomes.

The rehabilitation team

The patient admitted to the CCU has a range of needs which require the expertise of a diverse team in addition to medical and nursing staff. The team members and their responsibilities are summarized in Table 76.1. The responsibilities of each team member should be clear. The group should meet regularly to clarify responsibilities and the process ideally should be coordinated by a cardiac rehabilitation coordinator.

Table 76.1 The cardiac rehabilitation team and responsibilities

Team member	Responsibility
Nurse	First line education
Physiotherapist	Planning mobilization and management of mobility problems
Exercise physiologist	Exercise policies and individual prescription
Occupational therapist	Assessing special work and home needs
Diet therapist	Individual dietary therapy and dietary policy for the Cardiac Unit
Social worker	Assessing and managing specialized social and financial needs
Pharmacist	Advice on medications and specialized advice (e.g. on anticoagulants)
Rehabilitation coordinator	Rehabilitation and patient education policies, coordination of team, liaison with community services

Responsibilities will differ between units, but should be clarified to avoid duplication. Initial contact should be made as early as possible, preferably while the patient is still in the CCU.

Discharge planning

Abbreviated hospital stays are now a reality in most medical care systems.[5] The challenge to deliver seamless hospital and post-hospital care demands detailed discharge planning. The physical, psychosocial, financial and emotional needs of the patient should be established at the time of admission to the CCU, and integrated with the medical requirements for treatment and investigations. The 'critical pathway' the patient is likely to follow should be established as early as possible, and explained to the patient and family. Bookings for investigations must be made early, and the involvement of members of the rehabilitation team should begin in the first 24 hours of admission to the CCU. Special needs which may require attention from members of the rehabilitation team should be recognized early. External agencies who may be required, such as community nursing and voluntary support groups, should be contacted early in the hospital course. It is imperative that the family doctor be made aware of the services with which the patient and family have been provided in hospital, and those planned for on discharge. Planning for discharge for any patient must include the education of that patient and their family with regard to their cardiac condition and their life thereafter.

Patient education

There has been an increased emphasis on patient education in the last 15 years. The reasons are many, and include an increased demand for knowledge from patients, legal pressure for 'informed' consent, promotion of self-care and preventive measures, earlier hospital discharge, higher incidence of chronic diseases, and a belief on the part of health professionals that patient education improves compliance and thus health and well-being.[3,4,6]

The educational process

The process of patient education includes the steps of assessment, planning, implementation, and evaluation and documentation. Prior to their involvement in the education process it is imperative that the patient educator and preferably all members of the CCU staff have a basic understanding of the principles of learning and teaching.

• Assessment of readiness to learn

Before education begins the patient must be physically and mentally ready for learning. This includes being alert and free from pain and anxiety, or excessive denial of the coronary event. Prior to this only simple explanations should be offered to both patient and family in order to eliminate immediate anxieties.

Readiness to learn is often signalled by the patient, usually by asking questions. When the patient is comfortable and indicates interest or receptiveness to learning, formal education can begin. Although patients have the right to refuse education and not to participate in a teaching programme, distinguishing obstinate but logical refusal from inappropriate denial may be difficult. In some resource-intensive areas such as cardiac transplantation it is usual for the patient entering the transplant programme, and their support person, to be involved in the educational programme.

The patient educator needs to assess that the patient has the mental capacity to learn, and an adequate attention span, and is psychologically ready.

Patients or their families who have problems in communication related to hearing, speech, sight, or literacy, should be catered for with the appropriate services. One difficulty in a country like Australia is the lack of multilingual information for cardiac patients of non-English speaking backgrounds. Involving the family is often beneficial but it is important to recognize that family may at times dilute information in an effort to protect the patient. Interpreter services should be engaged for all issues requiring consent.

Learning needs are influenced by educational and cultural backgrounds and by the values and beliefs of patients and their families. They are also affected by the current concerns of the patient; for instance, it is not appropriate to pursue detailed descriptions of heart anatomy when the patient is preoccupied with job security or sexual ability.

• Planning

The planning of patient education should be a cooperative process between the patient and the educator which includes defining mutual objectives for the outcome, selecting the teaching tool and the time frame for the completion of teaching. When planning an education session, staff should give consideration to the support person, who may be working, or caring for a young family. For example, those working will be more likely to be involved in the education process if some of the sessions are scheduled after work hours.

• Implementation

Patient teaching can be implemented by any one of a combination of methods: informal or formal teaching, individualized or group teaching. Patient education, to some degree, is the responsibility of all members of the health team. The primary nurse or cardiac rehabilitation coordinator plays the most important role in coordinating the education efforts.[6] A holistic approach to patient education by the cardiac rehabilitation team is essential for success of the programme.

Group sessions have the benefit of providing patient interaction, sharing of experiences, and a level of camaraderie. However it is essential that an experienced facilitator controls the direction of the group discussion to avoid the pitfall of an individual monopolizing the discussion.

Along with verbal instructions, teaching tools – such as flip charts, heart models, audiovisual tapes, close-circuit television, posters, notice board displays, written pamphlets and handouts – enhance learning. Such teaching aids can be obtained from various avenues, for example: National Heart Foundations, Nutrition Foundations, Health Department Health Promotion divisions, pharmaceutical companies, and in-house information packages.

A referral to an out-patient cardiac rehabilitation programme and post-discharge, follow-up phone calls by a cardiac rehabilitation coordinator, help to reinforce discharge instructions, answer questions and alleviate patient and family anxieties. There is a growing body of evidence supporting the cost-benefit of such measures.[7–9]

• Evaluation

Evaluation of learning is an ongoing process. It is accomplished by measuring whether the objectives have been met and by observing behavioural changes. An effective means of measuring objective criteria is the use of pre- and post-tests. Pretesting is done before teaching is initiated and provides the baseline for knowledge assessment.

Post-testing is done upon completion of the teaching programme; it documents learning and subjective perception of well-being[10] and identifies areas that need further clarification. Mention of behavioural objectives includes demonstration of manual skills such as the utilization of sublingual nitroglycerin medication.

It is equally important to evaluate the programmes themselves, which can be done by the utilization of quality assurance tools. This evaluation allows for feedback from patients and families that will help the programme to keep up with the demands of an ever changing society.

• Documentation

Patient education should be documented either on a special record designed for this purpose or on a permanent part of the patient's chart. Documentation communicates to each member of the team where the patient is in the learning process and records the learning accomplished. It would be helpful at the time of discharge for a summary of the content of the rehabilitation programme, and the patient's progress with symptom management and risk factor modification, to be sent to the general practitioner.

• The educational content

Patients who experience heart disease have unique learning needs. They need to understand what caused their coronary event, how to manage symptoms or disability after the event and how to prevent reinfarction or other complications in the future. The core content of patient and family teaching programmes should be decided by each CCU but should address the following issues:

- **Anatomy and physiology**. This includes anatomy of the heart and pathogenesis of atherosclerosis and myocardial infarction. The healing stage of myocardial infarction and cardiac surgery can be related to the levels of activity restriction, thereby aiding the patient in understanding the importance of activity limitation. Similarly for cardiomyopathy and transplant patients, such core knowledge is important.
- **Survival strategies**. A major cause of death from myocardial infarction, cardiac failure or cardiac transplant rejection is delay in obtaining medical assistance. Patients should be able to recognize signs and symptoms of heart attack, cardiac failure, cardiac rejection or opportunistic infection, and know the appropriate action to take. For example, chest pain that is not relieved by two sublingual nitroglycerin doses taken 5 minutes apart requires immediate ambulance transfer to the nearest emergency department. Patients and their families should also understand the appropriate management of pain, dyspnoea, palpitations and dizziness.

Throughout their hospital stay and particularly upon discharge, attention should be given to the education of patients with regard to their prescribed medications. Information such as the name, the dose, the purpose and effect of taking the medication, any side-effects from taking or consequences of not taking the medication, the importance of compliance, and the reporting of any undue side-effects, should be given to the patient and their support person.

- **Risk factors**. The patient should be encouraged to identify his or her own risk factors and how they can be modified to reduce the potential for progression of heart disease. Modifiable risk factors include smoking, hypertension, obesity, diabetes, diet high in saturated fat, cholesterol and sodium, sedentary living and stress.

The patient's adherence to prescribed lifestyle changes depends on his or her perception of the benefits versus the risk and the degree of inconvenience incurred – a variety of motivational strategies should be tried.

Even the most thorough patient education programme meets with compliance problems. Studies show that among major risk factor change prescriptions, cessation of smoking has the highest level of compliance (60–80%), followed by special diet and exercise (40–60%); adherence to stress management has the lowest level (< 40%). Predictors of low compliance include lack of spouse support, poor self-motivation and mood disturbance. When it is not realistic to attempt modification of several risk factors, those that impinge most heavily on future health should be emphasized, with selective intervention by members of the rehabilitation team on a case-by-case basis.[11]

- **Dietary advice**. Any modification in diet should include explanation of the benefits of adherence to the diet and list the foods that are recommended or to be avoided. Typically, a low fat, low cholesterol diet, modified sodium intake and close diabetic control are prescribed.[12,13] It is of equal importance for patients to appreciate that alcohol consumption should be limited to the recommended daily maximum allowance – that is, two standard glasses. Increased consumption of fish is encouraged. While simplified food labelling in supermarkets is very helpful (such as the National Heart Foundation of Australia's 'pick the tick' guidelines), it is important to remember that cheaper products of equal dietary value are also available, making them more accessible to low income cardiac patients. Equally of importance when discussing a patient's dietary history is to remember the anxiety of the spouse. It is essential that one does not make the spouse feel guilty ('My God, I have poisoned my husband ...') about the meals that have been cooked in the past.
- **Hypertension**. The benefits of weight reduction, exercise, limited alcohol and sodium intake should be highlighted to the hypertensive patient.
- **Stress management and relaxation**. The health professionals most equipped to offer education and practical sessions on these topics are the social worker or occupational therapist. Referral to community services ranging from psychology counselling to tai chi or yoga can also be offered.
- **Smoking**. Numerous studies indicate that permanent cessation of smoking often follows from the recommendation of the medical staff at the bedside. Occupational therapists, social workers or nurse educators are often utilized to run QUIT programmes within the hospital setting.[14] The value of medical advice informing patients to stop smoking, given at the bedside or in the primary health care setting, should not be underestimated. It is also important to offer QUIT programme services to a smoking partner as a patient returning to a smoking environment will be less likely to maintain their abstinence than one returning to a household in which no one smokes.

Mobilization and exercise

Once the patient is clinically stable, mobilization should begin. The aim of this is to prevent the deconditioning effects of bedrest. Patients with a complicated post-operative course or post-myocardial infarction who continue to experience symptoms of angina, heart failure or uncontrolled arrhythmia may have their mobilization delayed and will start at a lower level and progress more slowly.

Exercise after an acute myocardial infarction (AMI) or cardiac surgery should be compatible with the function of the cardiovascular system and in the early phases patients should be closely monitored for any signs and symptoms of cardiovascular insufficiency.

To prevent deleterious effects of bed-rest, breathing exercises and a simple range of arm and leg movement exercises may be given to bed-bound patients. The earlier that patients can be permitted to sit up and start such exercises, the less potential for physiological deterioration. These exercises should be done to a set routine, for example repeated five times each, several times per day, and should be continued until normal ambulation about the ward is allowed. Cardiac rehabilitation professionals refer to this in-hospital phase of rehabilitation as phase I (leading into phase II early post discharge and phase III maintenance).[15]

Mobilization begins by sitting the patient out of bed and walking around the bed area, gradually progressing to self care activities, functional exercises and an in-patient walking programme. The actual physical activity programme should be individualized so that the exercises cover movements and activities used in normal life, and the person is aware that such movements are safe. Surgical patients should perform a range of neck, shoulder and trunk exercises, avoiding excessive discomfort to the sternal wound. Patients who experience sternal movement or have post-surgical sternal wound complications should not start these exercises.

A walking programme can be started in hospital with initial ambulation in wards and corridors supervised. Encourage a normal gait pattern, arm swing and posture from the start. Any symptoms should be noted and acted upon accordingly. Before discharge the inclusion of stairs and some outdoor walking is desirable. Walking should be continued at a steady comfortable pace which allows the patient to talk at the same time. Clear guidelines should be given for increase of activity and/or reporting of progress or problems after discharge. Progress should be checked prior to hospital discharge by demonstrating satisfactory cardiovascular performance in a supervised bicycle ergometer or treadmill for about 5 METS.[17]

The education and mobilization components of the rehabilitation programme should be coordinated and follow a set schedule. An example is shown in Table 76.2.

Home activity programme

Home activity guidelines should be given individually, based upon the rate of progress and amount of exercise achieved as an in-patient. If an out-patient (phase II) rehabilitation programme is available, attendance at this should be encouraged. Patients following coronary artery bypass graft (CABG) surgery usually progress at a faster rate than post-MI patients through the 4–8 week convalescent phase, during which permitting adequate development of scar tissue and healing of the sternum takes place.[18]

After discharge, walk time or distance should be increased every few days until a 3 or 4 kilometre distance can be covered in 40–60 minutes. This level of walking should be continued three to five times per week (see Table 76.3). Patients should be encouraged to resume activities of daily living within the convalescent phase.

Any symptoms such as excessive breathlessness, lightheadedness or angina should be noted and acted upon appropriately. A diary may be used to record the frequency, time or distance walked, at what pace, perceived rate of exertion and any symptoms.[11]

Activity limitations

Another core component of the education programme for cardiac patients is the level of activity one may undertake in the first weeks and months post myocardial infarction, coronary artery bypass and transplant surgery. Three of the main areas of concern are: the issue of sexual function, resumption of driving, and return to work.

- **Sexual function**. Many patients and their partners will share concerns regarding sexual function. It is essential that the educators themselves are comfortable with discussing this issue before attempting to offer advice – the embarrassment of the educator will send definite signals to a patient which usually cause any discussion to be stifled or completely avoided. Transplant patients and their partners should be counselled to practice 'safe sex' for the first 6 months post transplant, at which time repeat serology will be undertaken to ensure the recipient has not contracted a latent

Table 76.2 Integration of educational and mobilization programme

Stage	1	2	3	4	5	6	7
Activity and rest	RIB. Deep breathing & leg exercises	RIB. Deep breathing & leg exercises	Sit out 30 min twice daily. Deep breathing & leg exercises	Ambulation programme: ambulant in room and to bathroom	Walk in corridor	Walk in corridor	As desired
Physiotherapy				Ambulation programme		Home programme	
Teaching and discharge preparation		Cause of MI/ angina. Information manual	Risk factor assessment and review strategies	Test dose GTN. Medications and home care angina	Diagnostic test information		
Other, e.g. (allied health)			Consult as indicated by risk factor assessment	Attend cardiac rehabilitation programme	Continue	Continue	Continue
Diet therapy				Dietary assessment for risk factor	Counselling with patient and care giver	Arrange follow-up appointment	Diet sheets with patient

The role of progression through each stage is determined by a 'critical pathway' or by clinical need. Steps do not necessarily correspond to hospital days. A patient with uncomplicated MI may progress through the seven stages in 4–5 days.
RIB = rest in bed; GTN = glyceryl trinitrate

Table 76.3 Post hospital/convalescent walking programme

Week	Time (min)	Minimum distance (metres)	Times per day	Speed
1	5–10	250	2	Stroll
2	10–15	500	2	Comfortable
3	15–20	1000	2	Comfortable
4	20–25	1500	1–2	Stride out
5	25–30	1500	1–2	Stride out
6	30	2000	1–2	Stride out

donor HIV or hepatitis C virus. As a general rule of thumb, patients are advised that two flights (floors) of stairs closely equate to the energy expenditure required to partake in heterosexual vaginal intercourse. Anal intercourse requires a larger energy expenditure. All patients are recommended to take a more passive role when initially resuming sexual intercourse after their cardiac event.

- **Driving**. It is important to be aware of local regulations with regard to resumption of driving post infarct or cardiac surgery (see Ch. 82). It is most important that any patient suffering a cardiac arrest understand the necessity of total driving restriction until the underlying cause and treatment for the same is established. Those implanted with an AICD pacemaker will be required not to drive again.
- **Return to work**. 'When can I return to work?' is a major concern for most people. Generally those working in office environments can expect to return to work around 4 weeks post hospital discharge. Those with more physically demanding jobs will require a longer convalescence period. Sometimes the suitability for return to work

cannot be judged until a supervised exercise test at a MET level equivalent to their working conditions has been completed. Some may not be able to return to work (for example, airline pilots), and support must be provided to assist these patients in accepting such a situation and provide an avenue for retraining.

Out-patient rehabilitation programme

Although supervised programmes have not been shown convincingly to affect prognosis (see Ch. 51), their value in providing support and coordinated return to normal activity, and motivation for control of risk factors, should not be overlooked.[1,2] Programmes should provide group exercise and education, allowing for individual needs. The exercise component should include at least six sessions of light to moderate exercise. Activities should involve walking or an equivalent exercise and low level resistance training. Each session should last about 45 minutes, including a warm-up and cool-down period, and cater for the individual needs and capacities of each patient. Individual review of the home activity programme should be undertaken each week with particular attention to the walking routine. Written guidelines for all exercises prescribed should be provided.

One health professional may supervise as many as 10–15 patients in a group session, or as few as five if exercise is individually supervised.[2] For high intensity exercise, medical clearance and supervision is necessary and emergency equipment should be available in the exercise area.

An exercise test is not essential for admission to a cardiac rehabilitation programme with a light to moderate exercise component. It is optional for assessment of physical capacity at any time or for assessment of progress. It may be useful for patient and family reassurance.

An alternative to supervised group programmes is an individually prescribed home programme, especially for well-motivated patients unable to attend a group.

Maintenance

A maintenance level of exercise is usually achieved after 4–8 weeks, at which time no further increases in exercise are necessary, having attained an adequate functional capacity of 6–8 METs. One MET is defined as the energy expenditure for sitting quietly, which for the average adult is approximately 3.5 ml of oxygen per kilogram of body weight per minute. Patients should try to maintain about 30 minutes of walking at a normal pace, five times per week, and perform all activities of daily living. Higher levels of physical fitness may be achieved by some patients but this should be discussed with the patient's cardiologist.

References

1. American Heart Association medical/scientific statement. Cardiac rehabilitation programs. A statement for health care professionals from the American Heart Association. Circulation 1994; 90: 1602–10
2. American Association of Cardiovascular and Pulmonary Rehabilitation. Guidelines for cardiac rehabilitation programs. Champaign, Illinois: Human Kinetics Books, 1991: 1–4
3. Pashkow FJ. Issues in contemporary cardiac rehabilitation. A historical perspective. J Am Coll Cardiol 1993; 21: 822–34
4. World Health Organization. Rehabilitation after cardiovascular diseases, with special emphasis on developing countries: report of a WHO committee. Tech Rep Ser 1993; 831: 1–122
5. Hlatky MA, Cotugno HE, Mark DB, O'Connor C, Califf RM, Pryor DB. Trends in physician management of uncomplicated acute myocardial infarction 1970–1987. Am J Cardiol 1988; 61: 515–8
6. Pozen M, Stechmiller J, Harris W, Smith S, Fried D, Voight G. A nurse rehabilitator's impact on patients with myocardial infarction. Med Care 1977; 15: 830–7
7. DeBusk RF, Haskell WL, Miller NH et al. Medically directed at-home rehabilitation soon after clinically uncomplicated acute myocardial infarctions. A new model for patient care. Am J Cardiol 1985; 55: 251–7
8. Ades PA. Decreased medical costs after cardiac rehabilitation. A case for universal reimbursement. J Cardiopulm Rehab 1993; 13: 75–7
9. Miller NH, Taylor CB, Davidson DM, Hill MN, Krantz DS. The efficacy of risk factor interventions and psychosocial aspects of cardiac rehabilitation. J Cardiopulm Rehab 1990; 10: 198–209
10. Ott CR, Sivarajan ES, Newton KM et al. A controlled randomized study of early cardiac rehabilitation: the Sickness Impact Profile

as an assessment tool. Heart Lung 1983; 12: 162–170
11. DeBusk RF, Miller NH, Superko R et al. A case-management system for coronary risk factor modification after acute myocardial infarction. Ann Intern Med 1994; 120: 721–9
12. Gotto AM Jr, Bierman EL, Connor WE et al. Recommendations for treatment of hyperlipidaemia in adults: a joint statement of the Nutrition Committee and the Council on Arteriosclerosis. Circulation 1984; 69: 1065A–90A
13. The management of hyperlipidaemia: a consensus statement. Med J Aust 1992; 156: 52–8
14. Taylor CB, Houston-Miller N, Killen JD, DeBusk RF. Smoking cessation after acute myocardial infarction: effects of a nurse-managed intervention. Ann Int Med 1990; 113: 118–23
15. Wenger NK, Gilbert C, Skoropa M. Cardiac conditioning after myocardial infarction. An early intervention program. J Cardiac Rehab 1971; 2: 17–22
16. Borg G. Perceived exertion as an indicator of somatic stress. Scand J Rehab Med 1970; 2: 92
17. Fletcher GF, Froelicher VF, Hartley LH, Haskett WL, Pollock ML. Exercise standards: a statement for health professionals from the American Heart Association. Circulation 1992; 82: 2286–322
18. Pollock ML, Foster C, Ward A. Exercise prescriptions for rehabilitation of the cardiac patient. In: Pollock ML, Schmidt DH (eds). Heart disease and rehabilitation. New York: John Wiley, 1979: 413

77 Assessment of prognosis and risk stratification

Peter L Thompson

Introduction

'There are few diseases in which the prognosis in any individual case is more difficult to predict than in coronary thrombosis. It is striking that there is hardly any specific criterion that is decisive or indicative of probable recovery or of the reverse.'[1] Samuel A. Levine's assessment 65 years ago remains true today. Intensive study of the natural history and improved understanding of the interactions between myocardial infarct size, left ventricular dysfunction, myocardial ischaemia and cardiac arrhythmias allows patient groups at high and low risk to be identified,[2–7] but the clinical course in the individual patient is determined by multiple factors which are not clearly understood.

This chapter will not attempt to provide an exhaustive overview of the copious literature on post-coronary prognosis and risk stratification.[2–7] It will attempt to summarize the main determinants of prognosis, the importance of maximizing the predictive value of routine observations in the CCU and the selective use of post-coronary investigations, and will briefly review factors determining the prognosis in other coronary syndromes, such as unstable angina pectoris and resuscitated sudden cardiac death.

Acute myocardial infarction

Trends in post-MI prognosis

A meta-analysis of studies published from the early 1960s to the late 1980s have shown 28 day case fatalities dropping from 31% in the 1960s to 25% in the 1970s and 18% in the 1980s.[8] Studies from the Perth MONICA community-wide study in the decade from 1984 in patients under the age of 65 have shown a decline in 28 day case fatality from 8% to 4.5%, a highly significant improvement.[9] The precise reasons for this improvement in case fatality in the past two decades are not clear. It appears to be a real phenomenon and independent of casemix and length of stay in hospital. The impact of new forms of therapy, such as beta blockers, aspirin and thrombolytic therapy, versus a change in the natural history of AMI, has not been determined.

Factors determining prognosis

The main factors determining prognosis in AMI are summarized in the information box.

Age

All studies have shown a strong relationship between age and prognosis, with approximate doubling of risk for each decade of increase in age for short-term survival, with possibly a less striking effect on long-term survival.[2–7] The mechanism of the worsening prognosis with increasing age is not entirely

Factors determining prognosis in acute myocardial infarction

- Age
- Sex (gender)
- Prior history
  - previous infarction
  - diabetes
  - smoking
  - hypertension
  - hypercholesterolaemia
- Infarct size
- Infarct location
- LV dysfunction
- Residual myocardial ischaemia
- Extent of coronary artery disease
- Patency of infarct-related artery
- Ventricular electrical instability

clear. Many studies using sophisticated multivariate techniques have demonstrated an effect of age which is statistically independent of other indices of the extent of atherosclerotic disease. It is conceivable that the ageing myocardium, irrespective of the associated conditions, is less able to withstand AMI.

Sex (gender)

Females have a higher mortality from AMI than males, with many studies showing a two-fold increase in 28 day case fatality after hospital admission. Earlier studies of this phenomenon tended to show an interaction between age and sex with the difference partly explained by women having their MI at an age approximately 10 years older than males.[2–5] More detailed studies have shown that the relationship is more complex,[10] with women tending to have a greater prevalence of associated metabolic and vascular diseases contributing to their worse prognosis.[11] However, several very carefully conducted multi-variate analyses have shown that gender remains a significant factor in prognosis independent of age and associated conditions.[12] A recent community wide study has shown that women have equivalent rates of death, lower rate of early sudden death but a delayed pattern of mortality compared with men.[12a]

Pre-infarction characteristics

Prior myocardial infarction

A previous episode of MI has a highly adverse effect on survival after an AMI. This is consistent with current concepts that prognosis is determined by the cumulative extent of left ventricular (LV) damage.[4] In some patients prior infarction may not have been extensive but may be a marker of extensive coronary disease, and it is this which determines the prognosis rather than the extent of myocardial damage.[13]

Previous angina

Pre-infarction angina usually indicates extensive pre-infarction coronary artery disease with an adverse prognosis.[2–7] There have been some suggestions recently that previous angina may in some cases indicate ischaemic pre-conditioning with a protective effect during myocardial infarction.[14] There have been some difficulties in evaluating the effect of angina because of problems in differentiating the effect of long-established angina, indicating diffuse coronary artery disease, from short-term pre-infarction angina, indicating localized unstable coronary atherosclerosis and localized myocardial ischaemia.

Diabetes

Diabetic patients with myocardial infarction have a worse prognosis than non-diabetics after MI.[15] The effect is more striking on long-term than short-term survival.[16]

Smoking

The effect of smoking on survival after myocardial infarction has been paradoxical and difficult to interpret.[17] Continuing smoking post-infarction has a highly adverse effect, with the increased risk of re-infarction and death.[18] However, a history of smoking prior to infarction in several reported series has indicated a better short term outcome.[5,19] This puzzling observation has been studied in considerable detail. Smokers tend to have the onset of their AMI approximately 10 years earlier than non-smokers, and the apparent benefit of smoking may be due to the relative youth of the smokers at the time of their infarction. However, some studies have shown an apparent better outcome even when corrected for age.[7] Further angiographic studies are needed to evaluate the possibility that smoking may induce a localized thrombotic coronary occlusion in a relatively mildly diseased coronary vasculature.

Other coronary risk factors

Prior hypertension has an adverse effect on survival from AMI, particularly in patients treated with thrombolytic therapy where it is associated with an increased risk of cerebral haemorrhage.[7]

Hyperlipidaemia has no effect on short-term survival, but it is now recognized to have a significant effect on long-term survival after AMI.[20] There is some evidence that the adverse effect of hypercholesterolaemia may be mediated by contributing to instability of the intracoronary lipid plaque, thus predisposing to thrombosis and re-infarction, as well as its role in progression of atherosclerosis.[21]

Myocardial infarct size

Clinical, electrocardiographic, enzymatic, echocardiographic and radionuclide studies all confirm the importance of myocardial infarct size in determining the outcome of acute myocardial infarction.[5,22] Unfortunately, no single index of infarct size is sufficiently reliable to predict prognosis with accuracy.

Clinical indicators of the extent of haemodynamic embarrassment correlate broadly with the extent of myocardial necrosis during the acute insult, but may be determined by other factors which determine LV dysfunction, such as pre-existent myocardial damage from prior infarction and associated myocardial ischaemia.[5]

The extent and area of ST segment elevation on the surface ECG may predict the area of myocardium at risk of myocardial necrosis and prognosis in the early stages.[23,24] If reperfusion does not occur, it may reflect with reasonable accuracy the extent of myocardial damage. However, with widespread use of reperfusion therapy, the lability of ST segment elevation is now well recognized. While Q waves are generally taken to indicate permanent myocardial damage, this is not necessarily a reliable index of the extent of myocardial necrosis. There have been many attempts to relate the extent of myocardium at risk (ST elevation) to the extent of myocardial damage (Q waves) but with varying success because of the many factors which affect both ST segments and Q wave development.[24]

Biochemical indicators have been widely used to estimate the extent of myocardial necrosis and prognosis. The earliest studies on cardiac enzymes showed a correlation between the peak enzyme levels and prognosis,[26] and these observations have been repeatedly confirmed for creatine kinase (CK) and aspartate aminotransferase (AST).[5,27] In the coronary care era prior to the widespread use of reperfusion therapy, sequential estimation of CK and CK-MB, with results expressed either as units per litre of creatine kinase released or gram equivalents of myocardial necrosis, the central role of myocardial infarct size in determining prognosis was confirmed.[28] With reperfusion therapy, however, the assumptions underlying plasma enzyme kinetics are no longer tenable (see Ch. 14) and estimation of infarct size from cardiac enzymes is no longer widely used. However, peak cardiac enzyme levels in patients who have not been treated with thrombolytic therapy or shown clinical evidence of reperfusion may still be used as an approximate index of myocardial infarct size and prognosis.[27] The role of other biochemical markers of myocardial necrosis in estimating infarct size has not been studied in the same detail as CK and CK-MB. It remains to be established whether infarct size can be accurately measured from the serum profile of troponin release after myocardial infarction.[29]

Echocardiographic assessment of myocardial infarct size has proven to be a useful technique as it is readily available at the bedside and can provide immediate useful information (see Ch. 16).

In the patient with a completed initial infarction, prognosis is accurately predicted from the wall motion abnormality, which reflects infarct size.[30] In patients with old as well as new infarctions, or in patients who have had reperfusion therapy, the wall motion abnormality may reflect old scar, new myocardial injury or transient stunning of viable myocardium, and prediction of prognosis is less precise.

Radionuclide studies have been widely used in attempts to measure myocardial infarct size and correlate it with prognosis (see Ch. 18). Wall motion abnormalities can be identified in gated blood pool studies using technetium, but the definition is less reliable than with more direct visualisation of the myocardial tissue available with echocardiography. Myocardial perfusion studies with thallium have been shown to correlate with infarct size and to be a useful predictor of both early[31] and late[32] prognosis. More recently, serial studies using technetium Sestamibi have confirmed that final as well as threatened infarct size predicts mortality in patients undergoing reperfusion.[22] However, the high-grade resolution required for reliable estimates of infarct size is usually not available in mobile equipment and studies need to be done on nuclear medicine equipment which may be some distance from the CCU.

Imaging of the necrotic tissue with technetium pyrophosphate is now not used routinely for assessment of infarct size, but is reserved for special cases, and has also been shown to predict prognosis.[33]

The use of more advanced imaging techniques such as **magnetic resonance imaging (MRI), positron emission tomography (PET), and ultra-fast computed tomography (CT)** have all been used to study infarct size, but there are more readily available techniques which can measure infarct size with sufficient accuracy to predict prognosis.

Q vs non-Q wave infarction

It is particularly important to utilize clinical, electrocardiographic, biochemical and imaging techniques to distinguish the patient who has suffered a small but completed MI from the patient whose small infarct is due to incomplete or aborted myocardial necrosis.[34] Numerous studies have shown that the patient with non-Q wave infarction had a better short-term but equivalent or worse long-term prognosis to the patient with Q wave infarction.[35,36] The worse prognosis in the non-Q wave infarction group is generally thought to be due to the persistence of residual myocardial ischaemia with risk of later infarction or lethal arrhythmias.[37] Since the wide use of reperfusion therapy, aborted MI is now relatively common and careful assessment of the extent of residual myocardial ischaemia may be required to define the prognosis acurately.

Infarct location

Patients with anterior MI generally have a worse prognosis than those with infarctions in other locations.[7,38,39] There have been some confusing reports which fail to show any difference,[24] sometimes because of variable criteria for identifying the ECG location and sometimes due to the inclusion of large numbers of non-Q wave infarctions where the prognostic significance of infarct site is less important.[40] It is not clear from these reports whether the worse prognosis of anterior infarction is due to the location of the myocardial damage or because anterior infarctions tend to be more extensive. This question has been analysed in detail by Stone et al[38] and Hands et al.[39] When patients were matched for infarct size with peak CK levels, the mortality was higher for anterior infarctions in each sub-group of peak CK. Recent detailed analysis of patients treated with thrombolytic therapy has confirmed the statistically independent significance of infarct location with an adjusted odds ratio for 28 day case fatality of 1.5 for anterior versus inferior myocardial infarctions.[7]

Left ventricular dysfunction

It has been recognized from the earliest descriptions of prognosis in AMI that the degree of haemodynamic disturbance is predictive of the risk of dying from the myocardial infarction.[2,3] Killip and Kimball in the 1960s[41] recommended a classification based on haemodynamic severity which has subsequently been referred to as the Killip Classification, showing a clear gradient of risk for early mortality, both in the original description in the 1960s and still relevant in the 1990s.[7] (See Table 56.1.)

The Norris coronary prognostic indices for short[3] and long-term[42] survival included a variety of variables,[5] but predominantly clinical and chest X-ray indicators of LV dysfunction. The clinical indicators of extent of LV dysfunction in the acute episode continue to determine prognosis for at least the next decade.[43,44]

The subsets identified by Forrester in the mid 1970s[45] (Table 56.2) confirmed with haemodynamic monitoring that LV dysfunction, as evidenced by elevated pulmonary artery pressure and reduced cardiac output, is the primary determinant of the degree of haemodynamic distress and the risk of dying from myocardial infarction. Cardiac catheterization and radionuclide studies allow more direct measurement of LV function, expressed as ejection fraction. These studies have shown a steady increase in risk with reduction in LV ejection fraction and a sharp increase in risk when ejection fraction falls below 20%.[4] However, global ejection fraction is determined not only by the behaviour of the infarcted tissue but also by hyperkinesis of the non-infarcted tissue, which may over-estimate the global ejection fraction and under-estimate the prognostic significance of the LV damage.[46] Indices of regional wall function can be derived non-invasively using radionuclide studies[31,32] and echocardiography[30] and show an excellent correlation with prognosis after recovery from infarction.

Since the wider use of reperfusion therapy, it has been recognized that reperfused myocardium may remain 'stunned' for a variable time after successful reperfusion.[47] The importance of follow-up studies to provide a more accurate index of ventricular function is widely recognized.

More recently, the importance of the adverse effects of remodelling after MI has been recognized,[48] and systolic volume has been identified as a key indicator of prognosis independent of the degree of systolic dysfunction.[49] Progressive dilatation, especially after anterior infarction, has been shown to have an adverse outcome.

Residual myocardial ischaemia

Prognosis will be adversely affected by residual myocardial ischaemia, resulting from incomplete reperfusion within the infarcted tissue or from imbalances in the coronary circulation creating ischaemia at a distance from the infarcted tissue. The risk is potentially modifiable by coronary revascularization, particularly if there is associated left ventricular dysfunction. The identification of viable myocardium after myocardial infarction and selection of patients for revascularization is a topic of major interest which is dealt with in more detail in Chapter 78.

Extent of coronary artery disease

Most reports indicate that the extent of coronary artery disease on coronary angiography is an important indicator of prognosis, especially long-term,[50,51] but demonstrate a relationship between the extent of coronary disease and prognosis.[52] In general, studies which have used complex coronary angiographic scoring systems have failed to relate to prognosis, whereas studies which use simpler scoring systems such as grading single, double, triple vessel, left main or left main equivalent disease have shown clear-cut relationships.

Coronary angiography is unable to predict the physiologic status of myocardium distal to an obstruction, and needs to be combined with a test of myocardial viability to maximize its prognostic value.[53] Furthermore, the detection of minor lesions which may be the site of future coronary thrombosis has proven to be beyond the scope of contrast angiography.[54]

Patency of the infarct related artery

Detailed angiographic studies and clinical trials of thrombolytic therapy over the past decade have clearly demonstrated that the patient who comes through MI with a patent infarct-related artery will have a better short- and long-term prognosis than the patient whose infarct-related artery remains occluded.[55] Studies from the angiographic substudy of the GUSTO I trial of thrombolytic therapy clearly showed the importance of re-establishing normal coronary blood flow. Patients with TIMI grade 3 (normal) flow at 90 minutes had half the 30 day mortality of patients with persistent occlusion (TIMI grade 0) or only partial restoration of coronary blood flow (TIMI grades 1 and 2).[56] Identification of infarct patency with non-invasive monitoring such as ST segment monitoring may provide useful prognostic information.[57] It remains controversial whether restoration of coronary blood flow after a delay of hours or even days after the myocardial infarction will improve prognosis.[58] There is some evidence that this may be the case, particularly in preventing adverse effects from late remodelling and enhancing electrical stability[58a] reducing the likelihood of ischaemia at a distance from the infarction and improving the likelihood of survival in the event of a subsequent coronary occlusion.[59] This controversy will not be clarified until a clinical trial has been conducted to study the effect of establishing late patency.

Electrical instability

Ventricular arrhythmias during the acute stages of acute myocardial infarction have no prognostic significance.[60] Ventricular fibrillation may be more common in the early stages of extensive infarction and for this reason may in some cases be a predictor of a poor outcome.[61] Persistent ventricular tachycardia similarly indicates an extensive infarction with a poor prognosis. While the presence of high-grade ventricular ectopic beats on Holter monitoring prior to hospital discharge is a predictor of poor outcome, this has been shown to be associated with significant LV dysfunction.[62]

Electrophysiology testing has been used to stratify risk of sudden death or recurrence of ventricular arrhythmia.[63] Patients who have readily inducible ventricular arrhythmias are more likely to suffer a major cardiac arrhythmia or death on long-term follow-up (see Ch. 23). Non-invasive evaluation of electrical instability with the signal-averaged ECG has prognostic value,[64] somewhat limited by a high false-positive rate.[65]

A cost-effective approach to risk stratification after myocardial infarction

Table 77.1 gives an indication of the relative value of tests versus the indices of prognosis.

In selecting investigations to stratify the risk of the post-infarction patient, the following four principles should be considered:

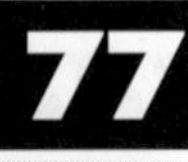

Table 77.1 Selection of the most appropriate test for assessing indices of prognosis after acute myocardial infarction. Code: – test of no value; + some information; ++ helpful information; +++ test of choice.

INDICES OF PROGNOSIS

	CHD risk factors	Previous MI	Infarct size	Infarct location	LV dysfunction	Residual myocardial ischaemia	Extent of CAD	Patency of IRA	Electrical instability
Clinical assessment									
Admission	+++	+++	–	–	++	–	–	–	–
CCU	+	–	++	–	++	++	–	–	+
Post-CCU	+	–	–	–	–	–	–	–	–
Electrocardiogram	–	++	++	+++	–	+	–	+	–
Biochemical markers	–	–	++	–	–	+	–	++	–
Echocardiography									
Resting	–	–	++	–	+++	–	–	–	–
Stress	–	–	++	–	+	+++	–	–	–
Exercise test	–	–	+	–	+	++	+	–	–
Radionuclide									
RNVG	–	–	++	+	++	–	–	–	–
Perfusion studies									
Resting	–	–	++	+	–	+	–	–	–
Stress	–	–	++	+	++	+++	–	–	–
Cardiac catheter									
Angiogram	–	–	–	–	–	–	+++	+++	–
LV gram	–	–	–	–	+++	–	–	–	–
Holter	–	–	–	–	–	–	–	–	+
Signal averaged ECG	–	–	–	–	–	–	–	–	++
E-P studies	–	–	–	–	–	–	–	–	+++

CHD = Coronary heart disease; CAD = Coronary artery disease; IRA = Infarct related artery; RNVG = Radionuclide ventriculogram; E-P = Electro-physiology

- **Maximum use should be made of data which is collected routinely in the coronary care unit**. Risk stratification by considering age and sex, past history (previous infarction, angina, diabetes, hypertension and smoking), physical examination (blood pressure, heart rate and signs of pulmonary congestion), ECG findings (the degree of ST segment elevation, location of infarction), chest X-ray abnormalities (cardiomegaly and pulmonary congestion) and the extent and pattern of biochemical markers of myocardial necrosis can frequently give a very accurate estimate of short- and long-term risk after infarction.

  It is possible with this data to identify groups of patients with a short- and long-term risk of death ranging from 1% to over 50%.[66–68] One recent large study showed that 90% of the prognostic information in the clinical data was contained in five simple observations of increasing age, low blood pressure, high Killip class, elevated heart rate and anterior ECG location.[68a]
- **A post-infarction investigation should be selected only if its prognostic value is additive to information already available**. While most of the post-infarction tests available can stratify risk, several studies have shown that some complex tests add only marginally to the risk stratification when the results of clinical evaluation and a pre-discharge exercise test are available.
- **The selection of a post-infarction test will depend on the time interval post-infarction**. The major determinants of *early death in hospital* are the degree of LV dysfunction and the infarct size. Risk *early after recovery* will

be determined also by the extent of residual myocardial ischaemia. *Long term*, the above factors are still of importance but other factors, such as the extent of coronary artery disease and its rate of progression, may be more relevant. Each time interval will require a different strategy for investigation.

- **The cost of a post-infarction investigation can only be justified if an improved outcome is likely from knowing the result.**

Since economical risk stratification can be obtained from routinely collected coronary care information and a pre-discharge sub-maximal exercise test, this level of investigation may be appropriate for the many patients who have experienced an uncomplicated MI. When more detailed risk stratification is required, a quantitative estimate of the degree of LV dysfunction will provide the most useful information, and echocardiography is the most cost-effective option. When further information is required, it is often most economical to proceed directly to coronary angiography to evaluate the coronary anatomy, reserving the use of other investigations for selected cases who may be considered suitable for revascularization.

The choice of radionuclide myocardial perfusion studies versus stress echocardiography to evaluate myocardial viability will often depend on the availability of equipment and local expertise (see Ch. 78). A variety of strategies has been recommended for stratification of risk post myocardial infarction, but risk stratification for its own sake is rarely cost-effective and is of less importance than targeting investigations to identify patients who require specific management strategies.

Specialised risk stratification strategies in AMI

Selection of patients for thrombolytic therapy

The patients most likely to benefit from thrombolytic therapy have been well defined, with some sub-groups of patients able to achieve a reduction in the relative risk of death by up to 30–40%. However, the absolute risk reduction will be minimal when baseline risk is low. Defining the baseline risk has been studied in detail by Nidorf et al,[66] using data from the Perth MONICA Study. In patients under the age of 60, groups of patients have been identified with a baseline risk of dying within 30 days of less than 1%. Clearly the administration of thrombolytic therapy to patients at very low risk will save few lives. A similar approach has been recommended by other authors.[67]

Selection of patients suitable for early hospital discharge

Data from soon after admission to the CCU have been used to identify parameters which on review of the first 3 days of hospital treatment can be used to stratify risk of dying within the subsequent 28 days. Patients at very low risk have been identified and may well be suitable for early hospital discharge.[68] A similar approach can be used for thrombolytic-treated patients.[68a]

Other studies using more complex identifiers such as a pre-discharge exercise-thallium study have confirmed that this may well be a cost-effective strategy for management of low-risk patients after myocardial infarction.[69]

Selection of patients for revascularization
(See Ch. 78)

Stratification of risk in unstable angina

The prognosis of unstable angina depends largely on the clinical presentation. Patients with new-onset angina rather than chronic stable angina have a worse prognosis.[69a,70,71] The development of angina after MI also carries a very high risk, 28% 1 year mortality compared with 2% in the absence of post-infarction angina.[72]

The pattern of angina shortly after hospital admission is an important determinant. Patients who settle rapidly have a good prognosis compared with patients with recurrent persistent angina who have a three-fold risk of infarction or death during hospitalization.[73] The combination of ischaemic ECG changes and ongoing angina was associated with a very high risk of complications.[74] Patients with fluctuating ST segment and T wave changes have a far worse prognosis than patients with normal ECG or stable T wave change.

Angiographic findings of eccentric and irregular plaques with intra-coronary thrombus have a worse prognosis, and these patients are often considered for early revascularization.[75]

The development of minor degrees of myocardial necrosis, short of classic myocardial infarction, appears to confer an adverse outcome. Patients who have an elevated troponin T in unstable angina have a higher frequency of in hospital MI than those without this evidence of myocardial necrosis.[76]

Prognosis after aborted sudden death

The aetiology of the underlying heart disease is the major determinant of prognosis in a patient who has suffered an episode of cardiac arrest with resuscitation. Patients with previous myocardial infarction have a far worse prognosis than those with ventricular tachycardia or VF from other aetiologies.[77] Within the group of patients with MI the major determinants are the presence of associated cardiac failure, increased age, onset of VT or VF within 6 weeks after MI or multiple previous infarctions, anterior infarction and Q wave infarction.[78]

In contrast to the adverse effect of VF occurring remote from a myocardial infarction, the development of VF during the acute episode carries limited prognostic significance.[60,61] Patients who suffer this complication of acute infarction usually have their prognosis determined by factors other than the development of the arrhythmia.

References

1. Levine SA, Brown CL. Coronary thrombosis: its various clinical features. Medicine 1929; 8: 245
2. Honey GR, Truelove SC. Prognostic factors in myocardial infarction. Lancet 1957; 1: 1155
3. Norris RM, Brandt DWT, Caughey DE, Lee AJ, Scott PJ. A new coronary prognostic index. Lancet 1969; 1: 274–8
4. The Multicenter Post Infarction Research Group. Risk stratification after myocardial infarction from the Multicenter Post Infarction Research Group. N Engl J Med 1983; 309: 331–6
5. Thompson PL. Prognosis of myocardial infarction with special reference to the role of infarct size. Perth: University of Western Australia, 1989. Thesis
6. The International Study Group. In-hospital mortality and clinical course of 20 891 patients with suspected acute myocardial infarction randomised between alteplase and streptokinase with or without heparin. Lancet 1990; 336: 71–9
7. Lee KL, Woodlieff LH, Topol EJ et al. Predictors of 30 day mortality in the era of reperfusion for acute myocardial infarction. Results from an international trial of 41 021 patients. Circulation 1995; 91: 1659–68
8. De Vreede JJM, Gorgels AP, Verstraaten GMP, Vermeer F, Dassen WRM, Wellens HJ. Did prognosis after acute myocardial infarction change during the past 30 years? J Am Coll Cardiol 1991; 18: 698–706
9. Jamrozik KD, Broadhurst R, Parsons R, Hobbs MST, Thompson PL. Ten year trends in medical management and case fatality in acute myocardial infarction (Abit). J Am Coll Cardiol 1996; in press
10. Tofler GH, Stone PH, Muller JE et al. Effects of gender and race on prognosis after myocardial infarction: adverse prognosis for women, particularly black women. J Am Coll Cardiol 1987; 9: 473–82
11. White HD, Barbash GI, Modan M et al. After correcting for worse baseline characteristics, women treated with thrombolytic therapy for acute myocardial infarction have the same mortality and morbidity as men except for a higher incidence of hemorrhage stroke. Circulation 1993; 88: 2097–103
12. Ridolfo B, Jamrozik KD, Hobbs MST, Parsons RJ, Broadhurst RJ, Thompson PL et al. A higher rate of prior cardiovascular disease contributes to the higher case fatality of women after myocardial infarction. J Am Coll Cardiol 1993; 21: 237A

12a. Tunstall-Pedoe H, Morrison C, Woodward M, Fitzpatrick B, Watt G. Sex differences in myocardial infarctions and coronary deaths in the Scottish MONICA population of Glasgow 1985 to 1991. Circulation 1996; 93: 1981–92

13. Miller RR, De Maria AN, Vismara LA. Chronic stable inferior myocardial infarction: unsuspected harbinger of high-risk proximal left coronary arterial obstruction amenable to surgical revascularization. Am J Cardiol 1977; 39: 954–60
14. Kloner RA, Shook T, Przyklenk K et al. Previous angina alters in-hospital outcome in TIMI-4: a clinical correlate to preconditioning? Circulation 1995; 91: 37–47
15. Barbash GI, White HD, Modan M, Van de Werf F. Significance of diabetes mellitus in patients with acute myocardial infarction receiving thrombolytic therapy. J Am Coll Cardiol 1993; 22: 707–13
16. Granger CB, Califf RM, Young S et al. Outcome of patients with diabetes mellitus and acute myocardial infarction treated with thrombolytic agents. J Am Coll Cardiol 1993; 21: 290–5

17. Ockene IS, Ockene JK. Smoking after acute myocardial infarction: a good thing? Circulation 1993; 87: 297–9
18. Rivers JT, White HD, Cross DB et al. Reinfarction after thrombolytic therapy for acute myocardial infarction followed by conservative management: incidence and effect of smoking. J Am Coll Cardiol 1990; 16: 340–8
19. Barbash GI, White HD, Modan M et al. Significance of smoking in patients receiving thrombolytic therapy for acute myocardial infarction. J Am Coll Cardiol 1993; 87: 53–8
20. Rossouw JE, Lewis B, Rifkind BM. The value of lowering cholesterol after myocardial infarction. N Engl J Med 1990; 323: 1112–19
21. Byington RP, Jukema JW, Salonen JT et al. Reduction in cardiovascular events during pravastatin therapy. Pooled analysis of clinical events of the pravastatin atherosclerosis intervention program. Circulation 1995; 92: 2419–25
22. Miller TD, Christian TF, Hopfenspirger RN et al. Infarct size after acute myocardial infarction measured by quantitative tomographic 99^{m}TC sestamibi imaging predicts subsequent mortality. Circulation 1995; 92: 334–41
23. Yusuf S, Lopez R, Maddison A et al. Value of electrocardiogram in predicting and estimating infarct size in man. Br Heart J 1979; 42: 286–93
24. Mauri F, Gasparini M, Barbonaglia L et al. Prognostic significance of the extent of myocardial injury in acute myocardial infarction treated by streptokinase (the GISSI trial). Am J Cardiol 1989; 63: 1291–5
25. Christian TF, Clements IP, Behrenbeck T et al. Limitations of the electrocardiogram in estimating infarction size after acute reperfusion therapy for myocardial infarction. Am Intern Med 1991; 114: 264–70
26. Kibe O, Nilsson NJ. Observations in the diagnostic and prognostic value of some enzyme tests in myocardial infarctions. Acta Med Icond 1967; 182: 577
27. Thompson PL, Fletcher EE, Katavatis V. Enzymatic indices of myocardial necrosis: influence on short and long-term prognosis after myocardial infarction. Circulation 1979; 59: 113–19
28. Sobel BE, Bresvahan GF, Shell WE, Yoder RD. Estimation of infarct size in man and its relation to prognosis. Circulation 1972; 46: 640–8
29. Editorial. Troponin T and myocardial damage. Lancet 1991; 338: 23–4
30. Bhatnagar SK, Moussa MAA, Al-Yusuf AR. The role of pre-discharge two-dimensional echocardiography in determining the prognosis of survivors of acute myocardial infarction. Am Heart J 1985; 109: 472–7
31. Ong L, Green S, Reiser P, Morrison J. Early prediction of mortality in patients with acute myocardial infarction: a prospective study of clinical and radionuclide risk factors. Am J Cardiol 1986; 57: 33–8
32. Botvinick EH, Perez-Gonzalez JF, Dunn R et al. Late prognostic value of scintigraphic parameters of acute myocardial infarction size in complicated myocardial infarction without heart failure. Am J Cardiol 1983; 51: 1045–51
33. Corbett JR, Lewis SE, Wolfe CL et al. Measurement of myocardial infarct size by technetium pyrophosphate single-photonography. Am J Cardiol 1984; 54: 1232–36
34. Carpeggiani C, L'Abbate A, Marzullo P et al. Multiparametric approach to diagnosis of non Q wave acute myocardial infarction. Am J Cardiol 1989; 63: 404–8
35. Hutter AM Jr, De Sanctis RW, Flynn T, Yeatman LA. Non-transmural myocardial infarction: a comparison of hospital and late clinical course of patients with that of matched patients with transmural anterior and transmural inferior myocardial infarction. Am J Cardiol 1981; 48: 595–602
36. Thanavaro S, Krone RJ, Kleiger RE. In-hospital prognosis with non transmural and transmural infarctions. Circulation 1980; 61: 29–33
37. Gibson RS, Beller GA, Gheorgiade M et al. The prevalence and clinical significance of residual myocardial ischaemia 2 weeks after uncomplicated non-Q wave infarction: a prospective natural history study. Circulation 1986; 73: 1186–98
38. Stone PH, Raabe DS, Jaffe AS. Prognostic significance of location and type of myocardial infarctions: independent adverse outcome associated with anterior locations. J Am Coll Cardiol 1988; 11: 453–63
39. Hands ME, Lloyd BL, Robinson JS, Thompson PL. Prognostic significance of electrocardiographic site of infarction after correction for enzymatic size of infarction. Circulation 1986; 73: 885–91
40. Kao W, Khaja F, Foldstein S, Gheorgiade M. Cardiac event-rate after non-Q wave acute myocardial infarction and the significance of its anterior location. Am J Cardiol 1989; 64: 1236–42
41. Killip T, Kimball JT. Treatment of myocardial infarction in a coronary care unit: a two year experience with 250 patients. Am J Cardiol 1967; 20: 457–64
42. Norris RM, Caughey DE, Deeming LW et al. Coronary prognostic index for predicting survival after recovery from acute myocardial infarction. Lancet 1970; 1: 485–8
43. Martin CA, Thompson PL, Armstrong BK, Hobbs MST, De

Klerk N. Long-term prognosis after recovery from myocardial infarction: a nine-year follow up of the Perth Coronary Register. Circulation 1983; 68: 961–9.
44. Merilees MA, Scott PJ, Norris RM. Prognosis after myocardial infarction: results of 15 year follow up. Br Med J 1984; 228: 355–9
45. Forrester JS, Diamond G, Chatterjee K, Swan HJC. Medical therapy of acute myocardial infarction by applications of haemodynamic subsets. N Engl J Med 1976; 295: 1356–62
46. Sheehan FH, Stewart DK, Dodge HT et al. Variability in the measurement of regional left ventricular wall motion from contrast angiograms. Circulation 1983; 68: 550–9
47. Braunwald E, Kloner RA. The stunned myocardium: prolonged post-ischaemic ventricular dysfunction. Circulation 1982; 66: 1146–9
48. Gaudron P, Ellis C, Kugler I, Ertl G. Progressive left ventricular dysfunction and remodelling after myocardial infarction. Potential mechanisms and early predictors. Circulation 1993; 87: 755–63
49. White HD, Norris RM, Brown MA et al. Left ventricular end systolic volume as the major determinant of survival after recovery from myocardial infarction. Circulation 1987; 76: 44–51
50. Ganz G, Castaner A, Betriu et al. Determinants of prognosis in survivors of myocardial infarction. A prospective clinical angiographic study. N Engl J Med 1982; 306: 1065–70
51. Roubin GS, Harris PJ, Bernstein L, Kelly DT. Coronary anatomy and prognosis after myocardial infarction in patients 60 years and younger. Circulation 1983; 67: 743–9
52. Norris RM, Barnaby PF, Brandt PWT et al. Prognosis after recovery from first acute myocardial infarction: determinants of reinfarction and sudden death. Am J Cardiol 1984; 53: 408–13
53. Abraham RD, Freedman SB, Dunn RF et al. Prediction of multivessel coronary artery disease and prognosis early after acute myocardial infarction by exercise echocardiography and thallium 201 myocardial perfusion scintigraphy. Am J Cardiol 1986; 58: 423–7
54. Ambrose JA, Tannenbaum MA, Alexopoulos D et al. Angiographic progression of coronary disease and the development of myocardial infarction. J Am Coll Cardiol 1988; 12: 56–62
55. Lamas GA, Flaker GC, Mitchell G et al. Effect of infarct artery patency on prognosis after acute myocardial infarction. Circulation 1995; 92: 1101–9
56. The Gusto I Angiographic Investigators. The effects of tissue plasminogen activator, streptokinase, or both, on coronary artery patency, ventricular function and survival after acute myocardial infarction. N Engl J Med 1993; 329: 1615–22
57. Krucoff MW, Green CE, Satler LF et al. Non-invasive detection of coronary patency using continuous ST segment monitoring. Am J Cardiol 1986; 57: 916–22
58. Tiefenbrun AJ, Sobel BE. Timing of coronary recanalization. Paradigm, paradoxes and pertinence. Circulation 1992; 85: 2311–5
58a. Boehrer JD, Glamann DB, Lange KA et al. Effect of coronary angioplasty on late potentials one to two weeks after acute myocardial infarction. Am J Cardiol 1992; 70: 1515–9
59. Gersh BJ, Anderson JL. Thrombolysis and myocardial salvage: results of clinical trials and the animal paradigm: paradoxic or predictable? Circulation 1993; 88: 296–306
60. Nicod P, Gilpon E, Dittrich H et al. Late clinical outcome in patients with early ventricular fibrillation after myocardial infarction. J Am Coll Cardiol 1988; 11: 464–70
61. Volpi A, Cavalli A, Franzosi MG et al and the GISSI investigators. One year prognosis of primary ventricular fibrillation complicating acute myocardial infarction. Am J Cardiol 1989; 63: 1174–8
62. Bigger JT Jr, Fleiss JL, Kleiger R et al. The relationship among ventricular arrhythmias, left ventricular dysfunction and mortality in the 2 years after myocardial infarctions. Circulation 1984; 69: 250–8
63. Bourke JP, Richards DA, Ross DL et al. Routine programmed electrical stimulation in survivors of acute myocardial infarction for prediction of spontaneous tachyarrhythmias during follow-up: results, official stimulation protocol and cost-effective screening. J Am Coll Cardiol 1991; 18: 780–8
64. Steinberg JS, Regan A, Sciacca RR et al. Predicting arrhythmic events after acute myocardial infarction using the signal-averaged echocardiogram. Am J Cardiol 1992; 69: 13–21
65. Gomes JA, Winters SL, IP J. Post-myocardial infarction stratification and the signal-averaged electrocardiogram. Prog Cardiovasc Dis 1993; 35: 263–70
66. Nidorf SM, Parsons R, Jamrozik K, Hobbs MST, Thompson PL. Immediate assessment of the baseline risk of death following acute myocardial infarction: implications in the thrombolytic era. Submitted for publication
67. Simoons ML, Arnold AER. Tailored thrombolytic therapy. A perspective. Circulation 1993; 88: 2556–64
68. Parsons RW, Jamrozik KD, Hobbs MST, Thompson PL. Early identification of patients at low risk of

death after myocardial infarction and potentially suitable for early hospital discharge. Br Med J 1994; 308: 1006–10
68a. Newby LK, Califf RM, Guerci A et al. Early discharge in the thrombolytic era: an analysis of criteria for uncomplicated infarction from the Global Utilization of Streptokinase and t-PA for Occluded Coronary Arteries (GUSTO) trial. J Am Coll Cardiol 1996; 27: 625–32
69. Topol EJ, Burek K, O'Neill WW et al. A randomised controlled trial of hospital discharge three days after myocardial infarction in the era of reperfusion. N Engl J Med 1988; 318: 1083–8
69a. Unstable angina: diagnosis and management. Clinical Practice Guideline Number 10. AHCPR publication No 94-0602. US Dept of Health and Human Services
70. Mulcahy R, Daly L, Graham L et al. Unstable angina: natural history and determinants of prognosis. Am J Cardiol 1981; 48: 525
71. Duncan B, Fulton M, Morrison SL et al. Prognosis of new and worsening angina pectoris. Br Med J 1976; 1: 98
72. Bosch X, Theroux P, Waters D, Pelletier GB, Roy D. Early post-infarction ischemia: clinical, angiographic and diagnostic significance. Circulation 1987; 75: 988–95
73. Heng MK, Norris RM, Singh BN et al. Prognosis in unstable angina pectoris. Br Heart J 1976; 38: 921
74. Olson HG, Lyons KP, Aronow WS, Stinson PJ, Kuperus T, Waters HJ. The high risk angina patient. Identification by clinical features, hospital course, electrocardiography and technetium 99 stannous pyrophosphate scintigraphy. Circulation 1981; 64: 674–84
75. Bugiardini R, Pozzati A, Borghi A et al. Angiographic morphology in unstable angina and its relation to transient myocardial ischaemia and hospital outcome. Am J Cardiol 1991; 67: 460–4
76. Hamm C-W, Ravkilde J, Gerhardt W et al. The prognostic value of serum troponin-T in unstable angina. N Engl J Med 1992; 327: 146–50
77. Trappe HJ, Brugada P, Talajic M et al. Prognosis of patients with ventricular tachycardia and ventricular fibrillation; role of underlying etiology. J Am Coll Cardiol 1988; 12: 166–74
78. Willems AR, Tijssen JGP, Van Capelle FJC et al. Determinants of prognosis in symptomatic ventricular tachycardia or ventricular fibrillation late after myocardial infarction. J Am Coll Cardiol 1990; 16: 521–32

78 Selection of patients for revascularization after myocardial infarction

Phillip J Harris and Peter L Thompson

Introduction

Selecting infarct patients who will benefit from revascularization is one of the most important responsibilities of the physician managing patients with myocardial infarction. Management policies vary widely between individual clinicians and centres. Comparison of the rates of post-infarction revascularization following thrombolytic therapy in an Australian study showed a sevenfold difference in the rates of revascularization between states.[1] The range of management policies varies from the conservative, in which revascularization is performed only for incapacitating symptoms of angina, through to the aggressive revascularization policy in full pursuit of the open artery hypothesis. In most centres a middle course is followed with wide individual variation.

The selection of a management strategy and judicious use of the diagnostic procedures available is a challenging exercise for the clinician. In comparison with the relatively clear guidance available from clinical trials in pharmacologic management post infarction, selection of a management pathway for revascularization must be based on anticipated rather than proven benefits. Frequently the management decisions will be influenced significantly by patient convenience and clinical status as well as facilities available.

Intervention in the acute phase

The results of the angiographic sub-study of the GUSTO study[2] and further analysis of the total study[3] have confirmed the hypothesis that rapid reperfusion of the infarcting myocardium is the major determinant of improved outcome following myocardial infarction. However, to achieve maximum survival benefit, TIMI grade 3 or near normal flow[4] must be achieved within 90 minutes of administration of thrombolytic therapy. Unfortunately, even the currently used aggressive thrombolytic regimes achieve TIMI-3 flow in only 54% of patients at 90 minutes.[2] Immediate angioplasty without thrombolytic therapy, which is discussed in chapter 45, is an alternative approach.[5–7] For the majority of patients, however, thrombolytic therapy is and will remain the economically and logistically most appropriate method of trying to achieve myocardial reperfusion (see Ch. 34).

Rescue angioplasty

The question which then arises is whether those who fail to reperfuse rapidly with thrombolytic therapy should undergo early cardiac catheterization with a view to angioplasty—so-called 'rescue' angioplasty. Such a strategy depends on having a method for recognizing failed reperfusion. An economical and non-invasive method of recognizing reperfusion is unfortunately not available.[8] The methods which have been studied include:

- Resolution of chest pain
  This has been shown to correlate reasonably well with coronary reperfusion.[8,9]
- Resolution of ST segment elevation
  Complete resolution of ST segment elevation correlates strongly with successful coronary reperfusion[9] but only a few patients will show this phenomenon.

  Continuous 12-lead ST segment monitoring and graphical superimposition of the ST segment contour can be achieved with a portable 12-lead ECG (see Fig. 22.10). This technique has proven to be quite effective in monitoring coronary reperfusion.

- Bedside nuclear imaging techniques
  Combinations of various radionuclide agents such as thallium 201 and technetium 99m have been attempted but have been disappointing in detecting reperfusion, and of course bedside radionuclide studies are not routinely available (see Ch. 18).
- Serum enzyme patterns
  Reperfusion of myocardium is associated with rapid release of creatine kinase (CK) into the plasma. Early peaking of the CKMB correlates closely with early reperfusion. Regular sampling of plasma and a rapid assay is required for clinical decision-making. Alternative serum markers such as myoglobin and troponine T have not been widely used (see Ch. 14).

Rescue angioplasty has been studied in a series of small trials in which coronary angiography was performed after thrombolysis (see Ch. 45). If reperfusion had not occurred, immediate angioplasty was performed. A high rate of primary success has been reported but with a disappointingly high rate of re-occlusion.[11] The TAMI-5 study[12] compared a strategy of catheterization with rescue angioplasty if thrombolysis was unsuccessful, versus delayed catheterization, and showed only marginal differences in outcome.

In centres which have access to facilities for angioplasty, early intervention in patients who remain in pain with ST segment elevation despite thrombolytic therapy is a compelling option. Further clinical trial evidence is needed to justify this course of action as a routine. In the meantime it is important to take note of the fact that the previous studies indicate that patients who undergo attempted rescue angioplasty which fails have an extremely poor prognosis.

Patients with recurrent ischaemia

There is little controversy that the post-infarction patient who is experiencing symptoms of angina at rest or with minimal exertion should have coronary revascularization. The main issue is the timing of the revascularization. There is a preference to stabilize the patient with medical therapy prior to revascularization.

The revascularization strategy will be determined by the coronary anatomy and the extent of left ventricular dysfunction. When there is left main coronary artery disease or multiple vessel disease with left ventricular dysfunction, coronary artery bypass surgery is the preferred revascularization strategy. When there is localized single vessel disease, angioplasty is the preferred strategy. Between these two extremes there is a wide range of individual variation. Ongoing trials comparing angioplasty with bypass surgery should help clarify the indications for angioplasty versus surgery in the large overlap group.

Close liaison between the coronary care, cardiac catheterization and cardiac surgical teams, with careful review and discussion of the clinical and angiographic features, will enhance the decision-making process.

When coronary artery bypass surgery is the preferred revascularization strategy, every attempt should be made to stabilize the patient's angina and haemodynamic status prior to undertaking surgery. Up to eightfold differences in mortality and post-operative complications have been observed when stable versus unstable patients have been compared.[13,14] Even when the degree of ischaemia and haemodynamic status have been stabilized, the extent of left ventricular dysfunction is a major determinant of outcome.[14]

There are no prospective data available to determine the optimum time of surgical revascularization for the symptomatic post-infarction patient; however, a detailed retrospective study by Hochberg et al[15] showed that for patients with well-preserved left ventricular function who had surgery within 4 weeks following myocardial infarction, no operative deaths were observed. However, for patients with depressed left ventricular function (ejection fraction less than 50%) there was a progressively increasing risk with much higher mortalities when surgery was undertaken within the first 2 weeks. However, these studies were undertaken in the pre-thrombolysis area.

Data from patients treated with thrombolytic therapy

Review of published studies on operative mortality and blood loss in patients undergoing bypass surgery following thrombolytic therapy with streptokinase showed no increase in mortality when surgery was performed from 3 to 16 days post infarction.[16] However, there was an increased bleeding risk and need for transfusion when the operation was undertaken within 12 hours following streptokinase. Reports of the operative experience in patients in the TAMI trials[16] showed a tendency for greater blood loss when surgery was performed early after thrombolysis, as well as a tendency for the surgical procedure to be performed with saphenous vein grafting rather than internal mammary artery conduits when surgery was performed early after the thrombolytic therapy.

Therefore current recommendations for the post-infarction patient who is undergoing bypass surgery primarily for post-infarction angina are:

- Attempt to stabilize the angina with medical therapy prior to undertaking surgery.
- For patients with well-preserved LV function, surgery can be undertaken during the initial hospital admission.
- Patients with poor LV function may benefit from a closely supervised period of several weeks' delay prior to undertaking surgery.
- Surgery should be delayed for several days after streptokinase to prevent bleeding complications from the lytic agent.

The timing of the procedure is equally important when angioplasty is the preferred procedure for the post-infarction patient with angina. Increasing experience with early angiography in coronary thrombosis has shown that a single angiogram is merely a snapshot in the dynamic process of coronary thrombosis, lysis and re-thrombosis. Despite the characteristic appearance of typical thrombus it is frequently difficult to distinguish thrombus from atherosclerosis.

In addition, the surprisingly adverse results of early angioplasty as an adjunct to thrombolysis in the TIMI[18], TAMI[19] and ECSG[19] studies highlighted the fact that balloon angioplasty after thrombolytic therapy has the potential to encourage thrombosis and coronary re-occlusion. There is some evidence that the lytic agent will expose a greater number of thrombin binding sites and that the disruption following balloon angioplasty will create a milieu which actively encourages intracoronary thrombosis. This phenomenon may be more obvious with recombinant tissue plasminogen activator (r-TPA) than with streptokinase or urokinase. The clinical trial data is consonant with the clinical experience, that attempts at coronary angioplasty early after coronary thrombosis are associated with a high rate of re-thrombosis despite a high dose of heparin therapy.

For these reasons it is preferable not to proceed with immediate angioplasty at the time of cardiac catheterization but to treat with aggressive heparin therapy for several days prior to repeating the angiogram to assess the appearance of the coronary obstruction and then proceed if it is still indicated and there is evidence of continuing ischaemia distal to the coronary stenosis.

Current recommendations for treatment of the post-infarction patient with unstable angina with angioplasty are as follows:

- Avoid angioplasty at the time of the initial catheterization unless compelled to proceed by the instability of the symptoms.
- Encourage continuing clot lysis with aspirin and full-dose, adequately monitored IV heparin.
- Schedule re-catheterization prior to hospital discharge while on continuous heparin, and proceed with angioplasty if there is still evidence of significant stenosis of the infarct-related artery.

Asymptomatic patients

Identification of the asymptomatic post-infarct patient who will benefit from coronary revascularization requires a perspective on a number of issues, including the open artery hypothesis, the clinical trials of conservative versus aggressive post-infarction revascularization, and the principles of preserving myocardium.

The open artery hypothesis

The open artery hypothesis proposes that a patent infarct artery confers prognostic benefits independent of the benefits conferred by the immediate myocardial salvage.[21] The hypothesis evolved from retrospective non-randomized comparisons of the post-infarction survival of patients who had an open versus a closed infarct-related artery on cardiac catheterization in hospital after thrombolytic therapy. Published studies on approximately 1900 patients have confirmed that the subsequent mortality in patients with a closed infarct artery is 2–3 times that of patients with an open infarct artery. While the benefit of early recanalization of the infarct artery is established, some proponents of the open artery hypothesis have also argued that there is a long-term benefit from late opening of the infarct artery.[21,22] The theoretical benefits of late opening include a reduction in ventricular arrhythmias[23] and prevention of left ventricular dilatation and infarct expansion.[24] Clinical trial evidence is not yet available and in the absence of this information the usual approach is to base the revascularization decision on the viability of the myocardium as discussed below.

Clinical trials of conservative versus aggressive revascularization strategies

The TIMI-IIb[18] and SWIFT[25] trials compared a strategy of routine catheterization within 24–48 hours after thrombolysis, followed by angioplasty, with an alternative strategy of performing catheterization and angioplasty if there was evidence of myocardial ischaemia.

In the TIMI-IIb study, 3262 patients were studied after TPA. Angioplasty was performed in 60% of the elective catheterization group. Cardiac catheterization was performed in 33% of the conservative management group, of whom 13% underwent angioplasty. The in-hospital reinfarction rate was 5.9 versus 5.4% and the mortality was 5.2 versus 4.6%. In the conservative arm, one in three patients received catheterization and one in six received angioplasty in hospital. In many countries of the world this approach would not be regarded as conservative.

The SWIFT trial[25] studied 800 patients with a similar design. The re-infarction rate was slightly higher in the conservative group (12.1 versus 8.2%) but there was no difference in mortality (2.7 versus 3.3%).

Neither study provides any support for the practice of routine catheterization and angioplasty based solely on the coronary anatomy. The question then becomes how best to select patients who will benefit optimally from late revascularization.

New concepts of the post-MI myocardium

New concepts about the state of the post-infarct myocardium are still being developed (see Ch. 8). Understanding what happens to myocardium after infarction is critical to the approach to post-infarct revascularization. The concept of 'myocardium at risk' is fundamental. It is the myocardium which would die if a coronary artery were permanently occluded at a particular site. A guide to the amount of myocardium at risk can be obtained from extent and severity of ST segment elevation at its peak.[26] It can also be identified by technetium-99m Sestamibi imaging if the radionuclide is injected when the artery is occluded.[27]

The earlier reperfusion occurs, the larger the proportion of myocardium at risk which will be salvaged. Salvaged myocardium remains at risk if re-occlusion occurs. Although salvaged myocardium usually has intact metabolism, it may not contract normally. If its perfusion is normal and its contraction is impaired, it is said to be 'stunned'. If its blood flow is sub-optimal and its contraction is impaired, it is said to be 'hibernating'. It has been demonstrated in several studies[27–29] that restoration of blood supply to 'hibernating' myocardium will restore myocardial function.

If reperfusion fails to occur, all the myocardium at risk will die. However, in addition to the myocardium at risk, there is likely to be some myocardium which is underperfused but is maintained alive by collateral perfusion. If coronary recanalization occurs but flow is sub-optimal because of residual stenosis in the infarct artery, the salvaged myocardium may remain underperfused. In this situation, the total amount underperfused is made up of salvaged myocardium at risk and myocardium sustained by collaterals but underperfused. The underperfused, or ischaemic, myocardium may be within the area at risk, adjacent to it or at some distance, depending on the location of the infarct-related artery and the pre-infarction status of potential collaterals.

The term 'viable myocardium' is usually used to refer to the total amount of underperfused myocardium which may benefit from revascularization.

Clinically, the viability of the abnormally functioning myocardium is investigated by one of a variety of techniques described in Chapters 16–20. If viability is demonstrated and angiography reveals a severe coronary lesion, revascularization is usually recommended. Alternatively, radionuclide imaging or stress echocardiography identifies a significant amount of myocardium which is underperfused and coronary angiography identifies significant residual stenosis. Again revascularization is usually recommended.

Rationales for revascularization

The decision to advise revascularization in an asymptomatic post-infarct patient can be based on a number of different rationales. They are not necessarily mutually exclusive and the clinical decision to revascularize may be based on more than one rationale. While all of the rationales have some scientific basis, most have not been tested in clinical trials and in this era of evidence-based medicine there is great need to do so.

Protection of myocardium at risk

Revascularization is usually advocated when a significant amount of myocardium remains at risk. This can be determined by relating the final infarct size to the amount of myocardium at risk. The extreme example is when there is extensive ST segment elevation but only a small CK rise or limited Q wave development, the so-called aborted infarct. The real issue in this situation is whether the artery is likely to re-occlude, an event which remains unpredictable. However, it occurs with sufficient frequency to justify revascularization if the amount of myocardium at risk is large. Further research should be directed at better predicting and preventing reocclusion.

Reduction of underperfused myocardium

Revascularization of underperfused myocardium adjacent to or distant from the infarcted tissue and myocardium at risk from the infarct related artery, will reduce the likelihood of symptomatic ischaemia. It also reduces the substrate for ventricular arrhythmia formation. By investing resources to identify viable myocardium and revascularize early after myocardial infarction, the patient's subsequent clinical course should be less complicated and the need for re-hospitalization reduced.

Improving left ventricular function

When there is a significant post-infarct contraction abnormality and the myocardium is viable, revascularization can improve left ventricular function. It is assumed that this also improves prognosis. However there is no general agreement about how much poorly contracting viable myocardium has to be reperfused to improve prognosis.

Prevention of remodelling

Under this rationale, revascularization is performed to prevent the remodelling processes which continue to affect the myocardium for several months after the initiating coronary occlusion. It is assumed that if myocardium remains chronically underperfused its viability and ultimately its function is likely to deteriorate and this may be the basis of continuing infarct expansion and remodelling.

Role of coronary angiography

Coronary angiography provides valuable information on coronary anatomy relevant to prognosis and differentiation of coronary arterial patterns suitable for medical management, angioplasty or surgical revascularization. While this information is invaluable, it is incapable of predicting the benefits of revascularization without accompanying evidence of viability of the myocardium distal to a significant coronary stenosis or in another vascular distribution. Therefore the use of the invasive angiographic assessment cannot be a substitute for the non-invasive assessment of myocardial viability.

Strategies for selection of the post-infarction patient suitable for revascularization

From the above it is clear that there is a range of approaches and techniques available for selecting the patient who will benefit from revascularization. There is clear-cut guidance from the clinical trials to indicate that a policy of routine revascularization after infarction is not justified.[18] The diagnostic techniques chosen for non-invasive testing will depend on availability and local experience. It is clear that a single algorithm for a revascularization strategy is not possible for all patients. We therefore propose three separate algorithms as follows:

- symptomatic patient
- asymptomatic patient—angiographic approach

- asymptomatic patient—non-invasive approach.

The symptomatic patient

In the symptomatic patient the primary purpose of revascularization is symptom relief and the issue is to select the most appropriate revascularization strategy. Coronary angiography is the definitive procedure. The revascularization strategy will depend on the coronary anatomy. If there is doubt about the significance of a coronary stenosis, an evaluation of the localization and extent of myocardial ischaemia can be undertaken usually with stress thallium imaging stress echocardiography, or positron emission tomography (PET) scanning if available.

Asymptomatic patient—angiographic approach

In the angiographic approach (see Fig. 78.1) the initial investigation is coronary angiography which can be performed at any stage after the myocardial infarction. Patients at high risk because they have had a complication or have had a previous infarction, those who are young, live remote from medical care or are responsible for public transport, are managed by the angiographic approach. There may be a limitation in using a very early angiogram in a patient receiving thrombolytic therapy as the angiographic appearances may change with resolution of the thrombus and restoration of blood flow. The most suitable time for angiography is to schedule the procedure prior to discharge from the CCU, for the second or third day post infarction.

When left main or three vessel disease is identified, the decision in favour of revascularization is easy. When one or two vessel disease is identified, the rationale for revascularization is based on identifying either significant myocardium at risk or viable myocardium.

Asymptomatic patient—non-invasive approach

In the non-invasive approach the use of coronary angiography is more selective (see Fig. 78.2). Patients not in high-risk categories undergo a protocol of non-invasive testing to select those who have a large quantity of myocardium at risk or have evidence of potentially viable myocardium. Left ventricular function is assessed initially. All patients should, if possible, have a non-invasive measurement of left ventricular function by echocardiography or radionuclide techniques. Those with left ventricular dysfunction or a significant contraction abnormality should undergo angiography.

In patients with normal LV function, the issue is the potential for the development of myocardial ischaemia. Those who are suitable for exercise testing should have an exercise test. Depending on the local experience and facilities available this can be an electrocardiographic symptom-limited stress test, an exercise thallium or exercise echo study. If there is evidence of myocardial ischaemia on these tests, angiography is performed. In patients unsuitable for exercise testing, evidence of myocardial ischaemia is sought with dipyridamole thallium if the nuclear medicine laboratory is experienced in perfusion imaging, or with dobutamine echocardiography if the echo laboratory is experienced in stress echo interpretation. If there is evidence of myocardial ischaemia, the patient proceeds with coronary angiography as described.

Recommendations for revascularization

Patients with left main coronary artery disease are referred for bypass surgery, which is best performed prior to hospital discharge. Patients with triple vessel disease and left ventricular dysfunction are also referred for surgery, with several weeks of recovery post-infarction before operation. When the coronary angiogram reveals single or double vessel disease, further action depends on the degree of coronary stenosis. If there is no stenosis greater than 50%, medical therapy is recommended. If stenosis is greater than 70% and the vessel supplies a significant quantity of viable myocardium, coronary angioplasty is performed prior to hospital discharge. If 50–70% stenosis is present, the issue is the risk of re-occlusion. The judgement of whether or not to revascularize is based on the amount of myocardium at risk and indications from the morphology of the lesion that it is likely to re-occlude.

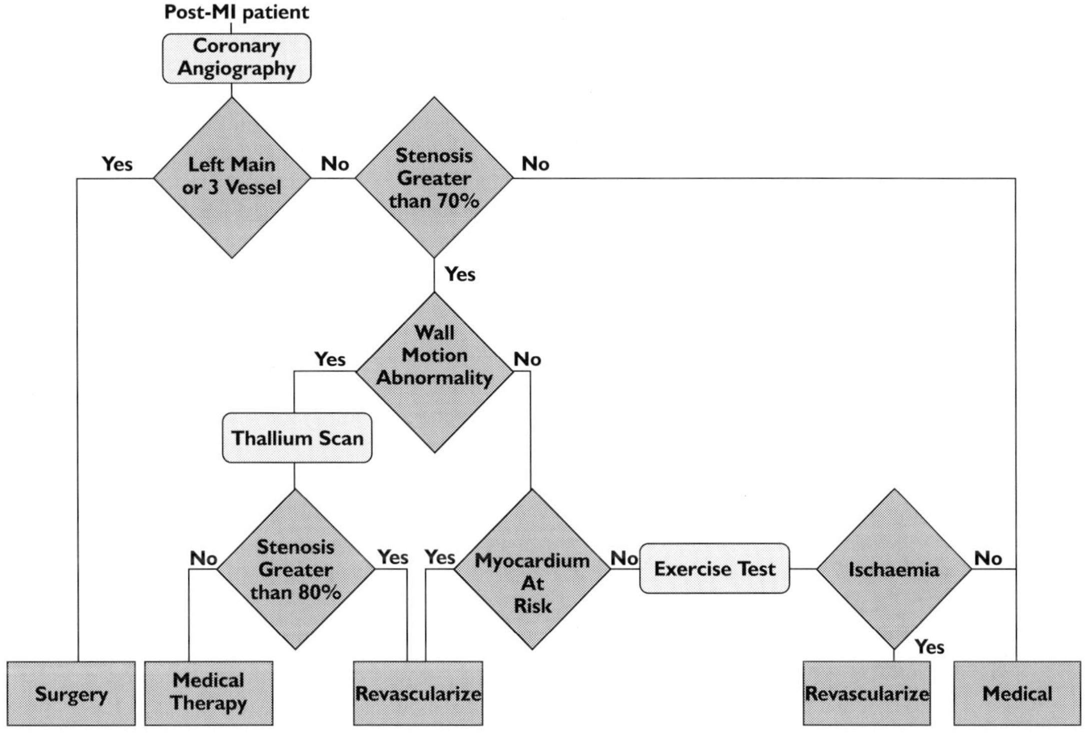

Fig. 78.1 The *angiographic* approach to selection of the asymptomatic post-infarction patient for revascularization.

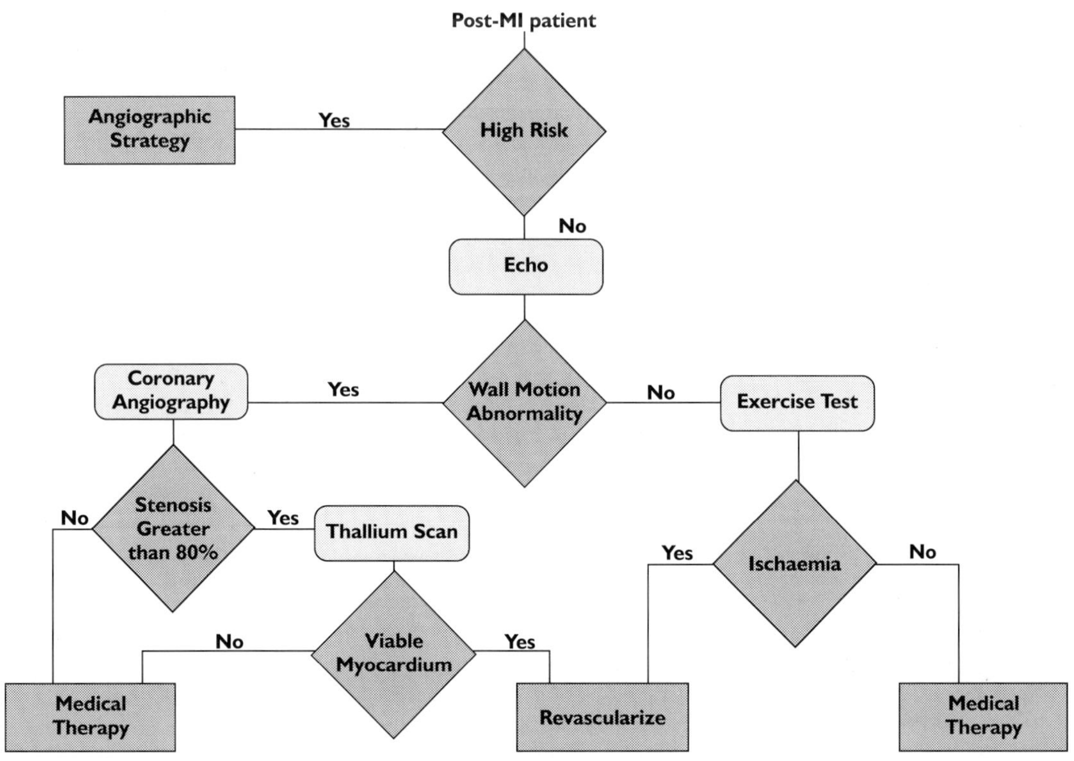

Fig. 78.2 The *non-invasive* approach to selection of the asymptomatic post-infarction patient for revascularization.

References

1. Aylward P, Margrie S, Simes RJ for the AUS-TASK Investigators. Intervention post myocardial infarction. Abst. Aust NZ J Med 1993; (Suppl.): 589
2. The GUSTO Angiographic Investigators. The effects of tissue plasminogen activator, streptokinase, or both on coronary artery patency, ventricular function, and survival after acute myocardial infarction. N Engl J Med 1993; 329: 1615–22
3. The GUSTO Investigators. An international randomized trial comparing four thrombolytic strategies for acute myocardial infarction. N Engl J Med 1993; 329: 673–82
4. The TIMI study group. The thrombolysis in myocardial infarction (TIMI) trial, phase I findings. N Engl J Med 1985; 312: 932–6
5. Grines CL, Browne KF, Marco J et al for the Primary Angioplasty In Myocardial Infarction Study Group. A comparison of immediate angioplasty with thrombolytic therapy for acute myocardial infarction. N Engl J Med 1993; 328: 673–9
6. Zijstra F, Jan de Boer M, Hoorntje JCA, Reiffers S, Reiber JHC, Suryapranata H. A comparison of immediate coronary angioplasty with intravenous streptokinase in acute myocardial infarction. N Engl J Med 1993; 328: 680–4
7. Gibbons RJ, Holmes DR, Reeder GS, Bailey KR, Hopfenspirger MR, Gersh BJ for the Mayo Coronary Care Unit and Catheterization Laboratory groups. Immediate angioplasty compared with the administration of a thrombolytic agent followed by conservative treatment for myocardial infarction. N Engl J Med 1993; 328: 685–91
8. Kircher BJ, Topol EJ, O'Neill WW, Pitt B. Prediction of infarct coronary artery recanalization after intravenous thrombolytic therapy. Am J Cardiol 1987; 59: 513–5
9. Califf RM, O'Neill W, Stack RS et al and the TAMI study group. Failure of simple clinical measurements to predict perfusion status after intravenous thrombolysis. Ann Intern Med 1988; 108: 658–62
10. Krucoff MW, Wagner NB, Pope JE et al. The portable programmable microprocessor-driven real-time 12-lead electrocardiographic monitor: A preliminary report of a new device for the noninvasive detection of successful reperfusion or silent coronary reocclusion. Am J Cardiol 1990; 65: 143–8
11. Ellis SG, Van de Werf F, Ribeiro-da Silva E, Topol EJ. Present status of rescue coronary angioplasty: Current polarization of opinion and randomized trials. J Am Coll Cardiol 1992; 19: 681–6
12. Califf RM, Topol EJ, Stack RS et al and the TAMI study group. Evaluation of combination thrombolytic therapy and timing of cardiac catheterization in acute myocardial infarction: results of thrombolysis and angioplasty in myocardial infarction-phase 5 randomized trial. Circulation 1991; 83(5): 1543–56
13. Naunheim KS, Kesler KA, Kanter KR et al. Coronary artery bypass for recent infarction. Predictors of mortality. Circulation 1988; Sep; 78 (3 pt 2): I 122–8
14. Katz NM, Kubanick TE, Ahmed SW et al. Determinants of cardiac failure after coronary bypass surgery within 30 days of acute myocardial infarction. Ann J Thorac Surg 1986; 42: 658–63
15. Hochberg MS, Parsonnet V, Gielchinsky I, Hussain SM, Fisch DA, Norman JC. Timing of coronary revascularization after acute myocardial infarction. J Thorac Cardiovasc Surg 1984; 88: 914–21
16. Lee KF, Mandell J, Rankin JS et al. Immediate versus delayed coronary grafting after streptokinase treatment: post operative blood loss and clinical results. J Thorac Cardiovasc Surg 1988; 95: 216–22
17. Kereiakes DJ, Topol EJ, George BS et al and the TAMI study group. Favorable early and long term prognosis following coronary bypass surgery therapy for myocardial infarction: results of a multicentre trial. Am Heart J 1989; 118(2): 199–207
18. TIMI Research Group. Comparison of invasive and conservative strategies after treatment with intravenous tissue plasminogen activator in acute myocardial infarction: results of the thrombolysis in myocardial ischaemia TIMI-II trial. N Engl J Med 1989; 320: 618–27
19. Topol EJ, Califf RM, George BS et al. Myocardial infarction study group. A randomized trial of immediate versus delayed elective angioplasty after intravenous tissue plasminogen activator in acute myocardial infarction. N Engl J Med 1987; 317: 581–8
20. Simoons ML, Arnold AE, Betriu A et al. Thrombolysis with tissue plasminogen activator in acute myocardial infarction: no additional benefit from immediate percutaneous coronary angioplasty. Lancet 1988; 1(8579): 197–203
21. Kim CB, Braunwald E. Potential benefits of late reperfusion of infarcted myocardium. The open artery hypothesis. Circulation 1993; 88: 2426–36
22. Hillis LD, Lange RA. Time for a prospective, randomized trial of the 'open artery hypothesis' in survivors of acute myocardial infarction. Am J Cardiol 1992; 69: 1359–60
23. Hohnloser SH, Frank P, Klingenheben T, Zabel M, Just H. Open infarct artery, late potentials, and other prognostic factors in patients after acute myocardial

infarction in the thrombolytic era. A prospective trial. Circulation 1994; 901: 747–56
24. Bates ER. Is survival in acute myocardial infarction related to thrombolytic efficacy or the open-artery hypothesis? A controversy to be investigated with GUSTO. Chest 1992; 101: 140–50
25. SWIFT Trial study group. SWIFT trial of delayed elective intervention vs conservative treatment after thrombolysis with anistreplase in acute myocardial infarction. Br Med J 1991; 302: 555–60
26. Hasche ET, Fernandes C, Freedman SB, Jeremy RW. Relation between ischaemia time, infarct size, and left ventricular function in humans. Circulation 1995; 92. In press
27. Sinusas AJ, Trautman KA, Bergin JD et al. Quantification of area at risk during coronary occlusion and myocardial salvage after reperfusion with technetium-99m methoxyisobutyl isonitrile. Circulation 1990; 82: 1424–37
28. Tillisch J, Brunken R, Marshall R et al. Reversibility of cardiac wall-motion abnormalities predicted by positron tomography. N Engl J Med 1986; 314: 884–8
29. Gibson RS, Watson DD, Taylor GJ et al. Prospective assessment of regional myocardial perfusion before and after coronary revascularization surgery by quantitative thallium-201 scintigraphy. J Am Coll Cardiol 1983; 1: 804–15
30. Ohtani H, Tamaki N, Yonekura Y et al. Value of thallium-201 reinjection after delayed SPECT imaging for predicting reversible ischaemia after coronary artery bypass grafting. Am J Cardiol 1990; 66: 394–9

79 Management of the symptomatic post-MI patient

Andrew Thomson

Introduction

Patients who have survived the acute stages of myocardial infarction (MI) may suffer symptoms from angina or cardiac failure.

Post-infarction angina

Angina continuing after MI is known to be the harbinger of a worse prognosis in the short and long term.[1–3] Early ischaemia after MI implies the existence of further 'at risk' myocardium and is associated with more severe coronary disease, non-Q wave infarction and a previous history of angina.[2] This group of patients is at high risk of infarct extension and ischaemic events during follow-up.[2] Extension of infarction occurs in about 10% of patients[4] and probably double this number in those patients treated with thrombolytic therapy.[5,6] Due consideration of the possibility of revascularization should be undertaken as outlined in Chapter 78.

Correct diagnosis

Before considering drug therapy, the correct diagnosis of chest pain must be established. Angina early after infarction can never be considered stable. True angina in this situation is either unstable angina or represents reinfarction or infarct expansion. The differential diagnosis of chest pain after MI includes pericarditis which is usually experienced day 2 to 3 post infarct, and beginning 10 days after the infarct, Dressler's syndrome, characterized by pericardial chest pain, fever and general malaise. Other diagnoses worthy of exclusion are pulmonary embolism and gastrointestinal discomfort secondary to aspirin therapy. In general, chest pain after MI should be regarded as and treated as angina until shown otherwise.

Post-infarct angina in the coronary care unit

The typical patient has already been treated with thrombolytic agents and is being treated with intravenous (IV) heparin and nitrates. Beta blocker therapy has been commenced and the commencement of angiotensin-converting enzyme inhibitors is being considered. IV nitrate therapy should be continued for 48 hours after thrombolysis.[7,8] Heparin may be ceased 48 hours after r-TPA without increased risk of reinfarction.[21]

Angina may not be accompanied by ECG changes and conversely ST segment changes may not be associated with angina in the early post-infarction period.[9] While patients with 'silent ischaemia' may have a worse prognosis, there is no convincing evidence that treatment of silent ischaemia will alter the prognosis. Pathophysiologically, these transient silent ischaemic episodes probably represent either reocclusion at the original site of thrombosis or distal embolization of thrombus from this site. Patients with non-Q wave infarction, previous angina and more severe coronary disease are more at risk for developing post-infarct angina.[2] Angiographically, the more severe the residual stenosis after thrombolysis, the greater the likelihood of post-infarct angina.[6]

Post-infarct angina in the post-CCU patient

Angina occurring at rest following discharge from the coronary care unit (CCU) in the post-infarct patient has a similar pathophysiology to that described above and is an indication for re-admission to the CCU.

Angina which manifests with increasing mobilization probably represents different pathophysiological mechanisms, either the symptomatic manifestation of new ischaemia in a portion of the myocardium at a distance from the infarct or ischaemia resulting from established three vessel coronary artery disease. Such angina may appear late in the hospital course or following hospital discharge because of the increased myocardial oxygen demands of aggressive mobilization or left ventricular dilatation due to ventricular remodelling.

These patients should preferably be managed by documentation of coronary anatomy with coronary angiography and consideration of coronary revascularization. If this approach is not possible by virtue of the patient's general condition or unsuitable coronary anatomy, medical therapy becomes the prime mode of management.

General measures

When post-infarct angina occurs in the CCU, intranasal oxygen, sublingual nitroglycerin or increase in the flow rate of intravenous GTN should be instituted immediately. The patient should be asked to rank the severity of their chest pain on a scale of ten, and a 12-lead ECG should be performed to document the severity and localize the myocardial ischaemia. If the chest pain is persistent, IV morphine may be necessary and serial ECGs and cardiac enzymes should be performed to document possible re-infarction.

In the patient who has been discharged from the CCU, the onset of angina at rest should be treated with similar measures as well as considering re-admission to the CCU if the angina persists for more than a few minutes.

In the post-CCU patient being prepared for hospital discharge, it is important to ensure that the patient understands the use of sublingual nitrates and has a clear-cut 'emergency drill' if angina should occur post discharge. Routine advice prior to discharge should include the following or similar 'drill':

- Assume that chest pain is angina until proven otherwise.
- Adminster sublingual nitroglycerine tablet or spray or sublingual isosorbide dinitrate.
- Wait 5 minutes and if there is no relief, repeat the dose
- If there is no relief after a further 5 minutes assume that myocardial reinfarction is occurring and contact an ambulance immediately for hospital re-admission.

To ensure that this 'drill' is followed and to provide confidence in the use of sublingual nitrates, a test dose should be administered prior to hospital discharge.

Apart from general measures, the basis of medical management of the patient with symptomatic angina post infarction are nitrates, beta blockers and calcium channel blockers. The clinical variables to consider in choosing each of these forms of treatment are summarized in Table 79.1.

Nitrates

Indications

Glyceryl trinitrate and the longer acting dinitrates and mononitrates have been the mainstay of anti-anginal therapy for many years. Nitrates are the appropriate first line therapy for most patients both as useful therapeutic agents for a treatment of anginal episodes and for prophylaxis. Although nitrates have been shown to be useful in the acute treatment of myocardial infarction,[7,8] there does not appear to be any sustained prognostic benefit (see Ch. 30).

Dosage

In the post-infarct phase, if IV nitrate is still running, this is clearly the most efficacious mode of delivery. If IV therapy has ceased, the choice is between cutaneous or oral nitrates. Conventional doses after MI for the treatment of anginal symptoms are isosorbide dinitrate 10–20 mg 8-hourly to 6-hourly or isosorbide mononitrate 60 mg daily or transdermal patches containing 5–10 mg of glyceryl trinitrate.

Problems

The common problem of nitrate tolerance can be overcome by using a conventional nitrate-free period of 6–8 hours to maintain efficacy. If clinically indicated by continuing angina, efficacy can be maintained by increasing dosage, often to very high levels. Headache usually subsides within 48–72 hours and should be treated with analgesics rather than a reduction in nitrate dose.

Patients being prescribed sublingual nitrates should understand their use. It is important to emphasize that these are not analgesics which 'cover over' the pain but have a beneficial physiological effect and that the potentially unpleasant side-effects such as hypotension and headache can be

Table 79.1 Clinical variables to be considered in the choice of anti-anginal medication in the post-infarction patient

	Clinical variable	Nitrates	Beta blockers	Calcium channel blockers
Infarct related	LV dysfunction	Safe to use; may temporarily benefit LV dysfunction Nil benefit on survival in clinical trials	Negative inotropic effect but can be used with caution;	Negative inotropic effect; adverse effect in clinical trials Diltiazem and verapamil should be avoided; nifedipine may be used with caution
	Arrhythmias	Safe to use, preferred agents	May cause bradyarrhythmias	Diltiazem and verapamil may cause bradyarrhythmias
Other cardiac diseases	Valvular disease	Acute hypotension may cause collapse	Use with caution because of negative inotropic effect	Use with caution because of negative inotropic effect
	Hypertension	No antihypertensive effect	Antihypertensive effect	Antihypertensive effect
Other medical history	Pulmonary disease	No effect	May cause bronchospasm	No effect
	Peripheral vascular disease	No effect	May reduce peripheral blood flow and increase claudication	No effect
	Diabetes mellitus	No effect	May mask hypoglycaemia in insulin-dependent diabetes	May increase insulin requirements
	Hyperlipidaemia	No effect	May increase LDL and educe HDL in long term treatment	No effect
	Depression	No effect	May worsen depression	No effect

identified with a test dose prior to hospital discharge.

It is important to emphasize that nitroglycerin tablets can lose their potency if exposed to the air or to plastic containers and should be carried in a metal or glass container. Even with this care nitroglycerin tablets will lose their potency after several months and it is important to obtain new supplies of the tablets at intervals of approximately 3 months. For these reasons it may be preferable to consider the use of a nitroglycerin spray or sublingual isosorbide dinitrate.

Beta blockers

Indications

Beta blocker therapy in the acute phase of MI may decrease infarct size and improve mortality. (See Ch. 28)[10,11] Beta blockers are effective in stable angina and unstable angina, and there is some evidence that beta blockade may reduce the frequency of silent ischaemia.[12,13] Not only are beta blockers useful in the treatment of angina post MI, but there is evidence that beta blockers provide a survival benefit for up to 6 years post MI[14,15] (see Ch. 28). Beta blockers with intrinsic sympathomimetic activity are probably not effective and may be detrimental.[16,17] The benefit from beta blocker therapy is greatest in those patients at highest risk, whereas those patients with small uncomplicated infarctions probably derive little benefit from beta blocker therapy.[18]

Virtually all beta blockers, including selective and non-selective agents, decrease the frequency of anginal attacks and improve exercise tolerance. Despite having different pharmacological modes of action including different degrees of cardioselectivity, intrinsic sympathomimetic activity and alpha blocking activity, the overall major mechanism of action is a decrease in the heart rate blood pressure product, reducing myocardial oxygen consumption at any given cardiac workload.

Dosage

The most commonly used beta blocker in Australia is atenolol, followed closely by metoprolol, both of which are cardioselective, water soluble, lacking both intrinsic sympathomimetic activity and alpha blocking activity. Standard dosage of atenolol is 50–100 mg once daily, while metoprolol dosage is 50–100 mg 12-hourly. Variable gastrointestinal absorption may require higher doses to achieve the desired therapeutic effect.

The addition of a calcium antagonist to a beta blocker is not necessarily superior to a single agent alone, as long as the agent is administered in maximally tolerated doses.[19] The addition of a beta blocker to verapamil or diltiazem does not appear to enhance the anti-anginal efficacy of these agents and may cause bradyarrhythmias. Some benefit can be gained by adding a beta blocker to nifedipine,[19] and co-administration of a beta blocker and amlodipine appears safe and efficacious.[20]

Problems

Beta blockade is not without problems in post-infarction patients. The negative inotropic effects of beta blockers are well recognized and there is a tendency not to prescribe beta blockers to patients with left ventricular failure. Although some trials have reported a slight excess of heart failure, there is good evidence that those patients with the larger infarcts and more left ventricular function derive the greatest benefit from beta blockade.[18]

Chronic therapy with beta blockers without intrinsic sympathomimetic activity tends to increase triglycerides and reduce high density lipoprotein (HDL).[21]

Calcium channel blockers

Indications

The mechanism of the beneficial effect of calcium channel antagonists in treating angina pectoris is uncertain, but probably is due to multiple actions including coronary vasodilatation, peripheral arteriolar dilatation reducing afterload, and negative inotropic effects. Calcium antagonists are primarily vasodilators of both the coronary and peripheral circulation but differ in their electrophysiological affects.

Although calcium antagonists are theoretically beneficial in the treatment of acute myocardial infarction due to their ability to prevent calcium overload at the cellular level, they have not been shown to be effective in reducing mortality in clinical trials (see Ch. 29). Verapamil and nifedipine[23,24] have failed to show clinical benefit. Diltiazem may reduce mortality in certain subsets of patients after myocardial infarction.[25] Those patients with evidence of pulmonary congestion or an ejection fraction of less than 40% have a worse outcome with diltiazem use, as opposed to those without these changes, where diltiazem reduced the risk of death or non-fatal infarction. Benefit was also observed in patients with non-Q wave infarction where after a year, diltiazem reduced recurrent cardiac events.[26]

A meta-analysis of the effect of moderate to high doses of short-acting nifedipine on outcome after myocardial infarction or with unstable angina suggested an increase in total mortality in those patients taking on the drug.[26a] Despite the findings being somewhat controversial, short-acting nifedipine cannot be regarded as appropriate monotherapy in the symptomatic patient after infarction. Its role in combination with a beta blocker remains unclear.

Dosage

Diltiazem would appear to be useful in symptomatic patients post MI with well-preserved left ventricular function, but should be used with caution in those with impaired systolic function. Conventional dosages are 60–120 mg 8-hourly before food. Slow-release preparations are well tolerated. A case cannot be made for the use of either nifedipine or verapamil to treat post-infarction angina,[27] but some of these reservations may be overcome by the use of the second generation dihydropyridines or longer acting preparations.[20]

Post-infarction cardiac failure

Although some degree of left ventricular dysfunction is very common in the early stages of acute myocardial infarction, persisting symptoms due to left heart failure are relatively infrequent and occur only in 10–15% of post-infarction survivors. In the Perth MONICA study of all coronary care patients in 1993, 14% were discharged from hospital on diuretic therapy (personal communication, Richard Parsons, 1995).

Post-infarction cardiac failure may be due to extensive irreversible left ventricular dysfunction and will need to be controlled with long-term administration of medical anti-failure therapy. Before committing a patient to this long-term course, however, it is important to rule out correctable causes such as continuing myocardial ischaemia[28] (see Ch. 78) or mechanical complications such as mitral regurgitation[29] (see Ch. 58). Echocardiographic evaluation of left ventricular and mitral valve function and other investigations as appropriate for detection of viable myocardium should be an integral part of the management of the post-infarction patient with cardiac failure.

As in all patients with cardiac failure, patient compliance with medications, reduced dietary salt intake and avoidance of sodium-retaining medications such as non-steroidal anti-inflammatory drugs need to be addressed.

Choice of therapy

Recent clinical trial results and changed attitudes to therapy have resulted in dramatic shifts in the usage of anti-failure therapy for post-infarction patients with a dramatic decline in the use of diuretics, a steady decline in the use of digoxin and a dramatic increase in the use of angiotensin-converting enzyme (ACE) inhibitors at the time of hospital discharge (Perth MONICA study, personal communication Richard Parsons).

Diuretics

Oral frusemide 40 mg per day is usually sufficient to control symptoms of pulmonary congestion in most patients with post-infarction cardiac failure. Potassium supplementation is not essential for short-term use of loop diuretics. It is important to reassess the patient's need for continuing diuretic therapy prior to discharge, to ensure that diuretics are not continued indiscriminately.

If there is symptomatic evidence of continuing pulmonary congestion a higher dose of frusemide may be necessary, and this can be continued post discharge, but again with plans to ensure that it is stopped if the symptoms of cardiac failure stabilize.

On occasions cardiac failure post MI is more refractory and requires more aggressive diuretic therapy with combined high-dose loop diuretic and thiazide.[30] Spironolactone remains a valuable diuretic as adjunct to a loop diuretic or a thiazide. Its propensity to hyperkalaemia requires special attention when used in conjunction with an ACE inhibitor, although with careful monitoring the combination can be used in selected cases.[31]

Particular care is required with diuretic therapy in the post-infarction patient to avoid hypotension when used in conjunction with other potent blood pressure lowering drugs such as ACE inhibitors and beta blockers, and to avoid hypokalaemia with associated cardiac arrhythmias or digoxin therapy.

Oral inotropes

Despite the demonstration that digoxin has clinically relevant inotropic effect in selected patients,[32,33] controversy about the role of digoxin therapy in cardiac failure persists.[34] In the post-infarction patient with cardiac failure the controversy is compounded by observations from post-infarction databases which suggest that digoxin therapy may have an adverse effect on outcome. However, critical review of these studies has shown that the conclusion is unreliable and cannot be resolved until large randomized trials have been completed.[35] Despite the uncertainty about the role of digoxin from randomized clinical trial data, the addition of digoxin can sometimes effect an improvement in the post-infarction patient with dilated heart and cardiac failure resistant to combined ACE inhibitor and diuretic therapy.

Other inotropic agents such as milrinone, xamoterol and flosequenan have produced disappointing results in randomized clinical trials despite apparent beneficial haemodynamic effects[36,37] and cannot be recommended for the post-infarction patient.

ACE inhibitors

The role of ACE inhibitors in improving survival in patients with left ventricular dysfunction[38] and cardiac failure[39] is now well established (see Ch. 33). Furthermore the ACE inhibitors have proven to be a major addition to the treatment of patients symptomatic with dyspnoea or oedema from cardiac failure post MI. Apart from occasional acute hypotensive reactions with the initiation of therapy and the rare case of angioneurotic oedema, the only significant side-effect with the ACE inhibitors is the dry irritating cough which can develop in about 5% of patients on continued therapy. This may present a diagnostic challenge in distinguishing whether the cough is due to persistence of pulmonary congestion or to the ACE inhibitor. On occasions change to an alternative ACE inhibitor agent or reduction of the dosage may be helpful but usually the ACE inhibitor has to be stopped if the cough is persistent. Sometimes the cough responds to inhaled disodium cromoglycate.

References

1. Schuster EH, Bulkley BH. Early postinfarction angina. Ischemia at a distance and ischemia in the infarct zone. N Engl J Med 1981;305:1101–5
2. Bosch X, Theroux P, Waters DD, Pelletier GB, Roy D. Early post infarction ischemia: clinical, angiographic, and prognostic significance. Circulation 1987; 75: 988–95
3. Benhorin J, Andrews ML, Carleen ED, Moss AJ and the Multicentre Postinfarction Research Group. Occurrence, characteristics, and prognostic significance of early postacute myocardial infarction angina pectoris. Am J Cardiol 1988; 62: 679–85
4. Muller JE, Rude RE, Braunwald E et al for the MILIS study group. Myocardial infarct extension: occurrence, outcome, and risk factors in the Multicenter Investigation of Limitation of Infarct Size. Ann Int Med 1988; 108: 1–6
5. Ellis SG, Topol EJ, George BS et al. Recurrent ischemia without warning. Analysis of risk factors for in-hospital ischemic events following successful thrombolysis with intravenous tissue plasminogen activator. Circulation 1989; 80: 1159–65
6. Harrison DG, Ferguson DW, Collins SM et al. Rethrombosis after reperfusion with streptokinase: Importance of geometry of residual lesions. Circulation 1984; 69: 991–9
7. Jugdutt BI, Warnica JW. Intravenous nitroglycerin therapy to limit myocardial infarct size, expansion and complications. Effect of timing, dosage and infarct location. Circulation 1988; 78: 906–19
8. Flaherty JT, Becker LC, Bulkley BH et al. A randomized prospective trial of intravenous nitroglycerin in patients with acute myocardial infarction. Circulation 1983; 68: 576–88
9. Kwon K, Freedman B, Wilcox I et al. The unstable ST segment early after thrombolysis for acute infarction and its usefulness as a marker of recurrent coronary occlusion. Am J Cardiol 1991; 67: 109–15
10. Hjalmarson A, Elmfeldt D, Herlitz J et al. Effect on mortality of metoprolol in acute myocardial infarction. Lancet 1981; 2: 823–7
11. MIAMI Trial Research Group. Metoprolol in acute myocardial infarction. A randomised placebo-controlled international trial. Eur Heart J 1985; 6: 199
12. Imperi GA, Lambert CR, Coy K, Lopez L, Pepine CJ, Shephard C. Effects of titrated beta blockade (metoprolol) on silent myocardial ischemia in ambulatory patients with coronary disease. Am J Cardiol 1987; 60: 519–24
13. Deanfield JE, Shea M, Ribeiro P et al. Transient ST segment depression as a marker of myocardial ischemia during daily life: a physiological validation in patients with angina and coronary disease. Am J Cardiol 1984; 54: 1195–200
14. The Norwegian Multicenter Study Group. Timolol induced reduction in mortality and reinfarction in patients surviving acute myocardial infarction. N Engl J Med 1981; 304: 801–7
15. Beta Blocker Heart Attack Trial Research Group. A randomised trial of propranolol in patients with acute myocardial infarction. I. Mortality results. JAMA 1981; 247: 1707
16. European Infarction Study Group. A secondary prevention study with slow-release oxprenolol after myocardial infarction: morbidity and mortality. Eur Heart J 1984; 5: 189
17. Australian and Swedish Pindolol Study Group. The effect of pindolol on the 2-year mortality after complicated myocardial infarction. Eur Heart J 1983; 4: 367–75
18. Furberg CD, Hawkins CM, Lichstein E for the Beta Blocker Heart Attack Trial Study Group. Effect of propranolol in post-infarction patients with

mechanical or electrical complications. Circulation 1984; 69: 761–5

19. Packer M. Combined beta-adrenergic and calcium entry blockade in angina pectoris. N Eng J Med 1989; 320: 709–18
20. Taylor SH. Usefulness of amlodipine for angina pectoris. Am J Cardiol 1994; 73: 28A–33A
21. Lehtonen A. Effect of beta-blockers on blood lipid profile. Am Heart J 1985; 109: 1192–6
22. Thompson PL, Aylward PE, Federman J et al. A randomised comparison of intravenous heparin versus oral aspirin and dipyridamole commenced at 24 hours after recombinant tissue plasminogen activator for acute myocardial infarction. Circulation 1991; 83(5): 1534–42
23. The Danish Study Group on Verapamil in Myocardial Infarction. Verapamil in acute myocardial infarction. Eur Heart J 1984; 5(7): 516–28
24. Muller JE, Morrison J, Stone PH et al Nifedipine therapy for patients with threatened and acute myocardial infarction: a randomised, double blind, placebo-controlled comparison. Circulation 1984; 69: 740–7
25. The Multicenter Diltiazem Post-Infarction Trial Research Group. The effect of diltiazem on mortality and reinfarction after myocardial infarction. N Engl J Med 1988; 319: 385–92
26. Gibson RS, Boden WE, Theroux P et al and the Diltiazem Reinfarction Study Group. Diltiazem and reinfarction in patients with non-Q wave myocardial infarction: results of a double blind, randomised multicenter trial. N Engl J Med 1986; 315: 423–9

26a. Furberg CD, Psaty BM, Meyer JV. Nifedipine dose-related increase in mortality in patients with coronary heart disease. Circulation 1995; 92: 1326–31
27. Held PH, Yusuf S, Furberg CD. Calcium channel blockers in acute myocardial infarction and unstable angina: an overview. Br Med J 1989; 299: 1187–92
28. Braunwald E, Rutherford JD. Reversible ischaemic left ventricular dysfunction: evidence for the hibernating myocardium. J Am Coll Cardiol 1988; 12: 1193–8
29. Schreiber TL, Fisher J, Mangla A, Miller D. Severe 'silent' mitral regurgitation. A potentially reversible cause of refractory heart failure. Chest 1989; 96: 242–6
30. Brater C. Resistance to loop diuretics. Why it happens and what to do about it. Drugs 1985; 30: 427–33
31. Ikram H, Webster WI, Nicholls MG, Lewis GRJ, Richards AM, Crozier IG. Combined spironolactone and angiotensine-converting enzyme inhibitor therapy for refractory heart failure. Aust NZ J Med 1986; 83: 43–8
32. Arnold B, Byrd RC, Meister W et al. Long-term digitalis therapy improves left ventricular function in heart failure. N Engl J Med 1980; 303: 1443–8
33. Lee DL, Johnson RA, Bingham JB et al. Heart failure in outpatients: a randomized trial of digoxin versus placebo. N Engl J Med 1982; 306: 699–705
34. Jaeschke R, Oxman AD, Guyatt GH. To what extent do congestive heart failure patients in sinus rhythm benefit from digoxin therapy? Asymptomatic overview and meta-analysis. Am J Med 1990; 88: 279–86
35. Yusuf S, Wittes J, Bailey K, Furberg C. Digitalis—a new controversy regarding an old drug. The pitfalls of inappropriate methods. Circulation 1986; 73: 14–8
36. Yusuf S, Teo KK. Inotropic agents increase mortality in patients with congestive heart failure. Abst. Circulation 1990; 82: III–197
37. Packer M, Carter JR, Rodeheffer RJ et al for PROMISE Study Research Group. Effects of oral milrinone on mortality in severe chronic heart failure. N Engl J Med 1991; 325: 1468–75
38. Pfeffer MA, Braunwald E, Moye LA et al. Effect of captopril on mortality and morbidity in patients with left ventricular dysfunction after myocardial infarction. Results of the survival and ventricular enlargement trial. N Engl J Med 1992; 327: 669–77
39. The Acute Infarction Ramipril Efficacy (AIRE) Study Investigations. Effect of ramipril on mortality and morbidity of survivors of acute myocardial infarction with clinical evidence of heart failure. Lancet 1993; 342: 821–8

80 Management of the asymptomatic post-MI patient

David Hunt

This chapter will exclude any rehabilitation or exercise programmes, treatment of coronary risk factors and consideration of investigations with a view to prognosis stratification or revascularization. It will deal only with the medications that asymptomatic patients may require.

Aspirin

The great majority of patients with myocardial infarction without contraindications to aspirin are commenced on aspirin (see also Ch. 36) in the acute phase of infarction following the landmark ISIS-2 study[1] and the many long-term studies on the use of antiplatelet agents. The Antiplatelet Trialists Collaboration Group[2] published their first review in 1988 and updated it in 1994.[2a] Aspirin is now prescribed in over 90% of patients leaving hospital, with the use rising dramatically in the past decade (see Fig. 80.1). There was no significant difference between the effects of aspirin 300–325 mg per day or higher doses of up to 1500 mg per day in the long-term studies. The best dose of aspirin has not been clarified but the ISIS-2 Study achieved major benefit with 160 mg. There appears to be no benefit to use

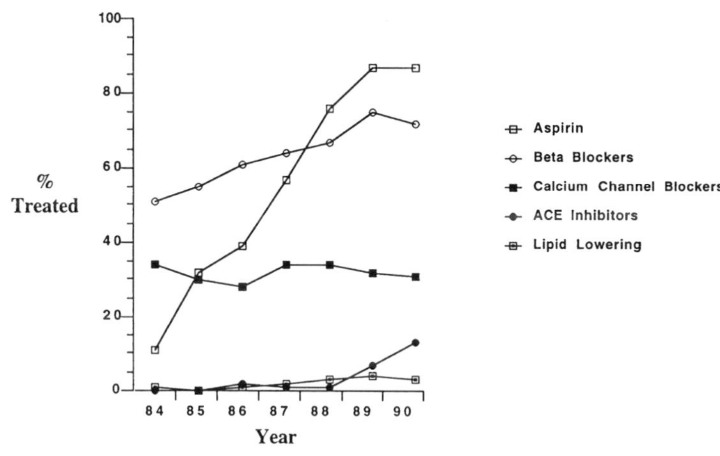

Fig. 80.1 Trends in prescribing post-infarction medications at the time of hospital discharge 1984–1990. Data from the Perth MONICA Project.

more than 300–325 mg per day and the higher doses are associated with an increase in gastrointestinal side-effects including stomach pain, heartburn and nausea as well as gastrointestinal blood loss.[3] More recent studies have tended to use lower doses of aspirin, in the 50–300 mg per day range, as such doses result in virtually complete suppression of platelet thromboxane synthesis. The results of these clinical studies are eagerly awaited. In the meantime however it would seem reasonable to use a dose of 150–325 mg per day in patients in whom there are no contraindications. As the risk of reinfarction is greatest early after a myocardial infarction, early treatment is essential.

The optimal duration of aspirin therapy has not been determined. Most of the studies reviewed in the Antiplatelet Trialists Collaboration had follow-ups of only 2–3 years. As the risk of death and reinfarction decreases with time after myocardial infarction there must be a diminishing benefit of aspirin. However as the drug in commonly used doses is tolerated so well, it would seem prudent to continue therapy on a permanent basis and it is unlikely that there will be trials of longer-term therapy.

Contraindications to aspirin include aspirin sensitivity, which is uncommon but important. Patients with known peptic ulcers, active indigestion or oesophagitis or who are concurrently receiving non-steroidal anti-inflammatory drugs (NSAIDs) should not be given aspirin. In such patients the use of ticlopidine should be considered. The use of aspirin in patients on warfarin is generally contraindicated, although there is some encouraging data on patients receiving aspirin and small doses of warfarin.

Beta adrenergic blocking drugs

Most studies to assess the place of beta blockers after myocardial infarction were conducted before the thrombolytic era[4] (see Ch. 28). The early onset trials such as the ISIS-I and MIAMI Trials were of short duration, but they showed a 15% reduction in mortality over 35 days follow-up. In the longer-term trials, treatment was started several days after the infarction and continued for up to 2 years. Many different drugs were used, and probably all the beta blocking drugs are effective.

The dose of beta blocker that should be used is not clear, as in some trials the dose was adjusted to have a demonstrable effect on heart rate whilst in other trials the dose was given in a standard dosage. Again, the optimal duration of therapy is not clear and most of the trials have only gone for 2 years after the index myocardial infarction. As the risk of death of infarction decreases after a year, especially in the uncomplicated patient, perhaps the use of these drugs in these patients beyond 1 year should be confined to those who have hypertension or angina, providing of course that the beta blocking drug does not cause side-effects. In patients who do not have severe heart failure the use of beta blockers gives more benefit in patients at higher risk of recurrent infarct or ischaemia. Such patients however might be investigated with a view to revascularization. In patients who would be unsuitable for revascularization (on grounds such as other medical conditions or patient refusal), beta blocking drugs may be particularly valuable.

Remember that the side-effects, especially tiredness and lethargy, can interfere with the physical and intellectual life of the patient and that there are also possibilities of worsening left ventricular systolic function, bradycardia or bronchospasm. Some data suggest that the beneficial effects of beta blocking drugs depend on the degree of heart rate slowing induced—if this is so, then drugs with intrinsic stimulating activity should be avoided. In general the side-effects of the so-called 'relatively cardioselective' beta blocking drugs (no agent is truly cardioselective) are less than those of the non-selective group (that is, those which block both $beta_1$ and $beta_2$ receptors)—especially less bronchospasm and Raynaud's phenomenon. Non-selective drugs however may be the agents of choice on the grounds that if recurrent myocardial infarction occurs there is a marked release of catecholamines which lowers serum potassium by forcing potassium into cells—a fall of serum potassium 0.5 mmol/L would be quite common in this situation. Hypokalaemia is a major risk factor for ventricular fibrillation and sudden death. Non-selective beta blockers tend to block this movement of potassium into cells by a $beta_2$ effect, whereas the relative cardioselective agents would not have this action.

There have been no trials to compare non-selective and 'relatively cardioselective' beta blockers after myocardial infarction. It is unlikely that such trials would be conducted, as the numbers involved would be huge even by ISIS standards.

In general, therefore, it would be reasonable to use a 'relatively cardioselective' beta blocking drug without intrinsic stimulating activity in doses that cause some heart rate slowing for a year or so after an uncomplicated myocardial infarction, provided the drug is well tolerated. Long-term use should be considered in higher risk patients in whom revascularization is not being considered and in patients with hypertension or angina.

Antiarrhythmic drugs

Sudden death, nearly always due to ventricular fibrillation, is the major cause of death after myocardial infarction, so it is not surprising that many trials of antiarrhythmic treatment (see also Ch. 27) have been performed. These have been well reviewed recently.[5] None of the Class I antiarrhythmic drugs has been shown to be effective, with the majority of the evidence showing an adverse effect. The only group of drugs clearly shown to reduce mortality are beta blockers, although there are strong suggestions that amiodarone may be effective.[6] Amiodarone has a number of unusual properties, which include a very long half-life, anti-adrenergic action (beta blocking effect), little or no negative inotropic effect in contrast to most antiarrhythmic drugs and finally, a low incidence of pro-arrhythmic effects. Approximately 1000 post-infarction patients have been randomized in four major clinical studies.[6] The odds ratio reduction of total mortality was 0.70, cardiac death 0.54 and sudden death 0.42 respectively, with the latter two figures reaching conventional statistical significance. At least three other major trials are in progress, involving over 3400 patients. It has been suggested that as most deaths after infarction occur in the first year, amiodarone may need only to be given for the first year, and some data points to a persistence of the beneficial effects of one year's treatment over many years of follow-up. It is important to note that the data on the use of amiodarone in patients with reduced ejection fraction, the group with the highest mortality, are scanty. Trials in progress are addressing this issue. One recently reported trial[7] randomized 516 patients with heart failure to amiodarone (300 mg per day) or placebo. The patients were a high risk group with a 2-year mortality of 41% on placebo and 34% on amiodarone. There was a reduction in sudden death and death from progressive heart failure. These initial data look encouraging, but until the results of other trials are available it would probably be unwise to use amiodarone routinely in post-infarction patients, particularly with the high rate of adverse effects with this drug.

It is important to remember the lessons from the CAST study[8] where mortality was actually increased by therapy (encainide or flecainide) despite good logic that such therapy would be helpful. This shows the importance of adequate clinical trials of any new therapy.

Calcium channel blocking drugs

Despite impressive data from animal studies, the results of human trials with calcium channel blockers have been very disappointing (see also Ch. 29). In an overview published in 1989 the authors concluded that these drugs did not reduce the risk of recurrent infarction or death when given routinely to patients with myocardial infarction or unstable angina.[9] Data on the use of calcium channel blocking drugs in non Q wave infarction were considered incomplete even for the diltiazem trials, which had shown some encouraging trends. Since then the second Danish verapamil study (DAVIT 2) showed a marginal benefit on mortality with some benefit in reinfarction rates with verapamil therapy.[10] A later editorial review of calcium channel blocker trials after myocardial infarction, however, concluded that the evidence of benefit of verapamil on mortality was weak and evidence of benefit on non-fatal myocardial infarction was only modest.[11] Such data therefore are far less compelling than the data for beta blockers. If however beta blockers are contraindicated or non-tolerated then perhaps verapamil might be used as an alternative in selected patients. As far as the dihydropyridine drugs are concerned (of which most data relates to nifedipine), newer trials have strengthened the conclusions on adverse trends on mortality and reinfarction and these drugs currently have no routine place in secondary prevention.

Oral anticoagulant therapy

Many trials of the routine use of anticoagulant therapy (see also Ch. 37) were conducted in the 1950s and 1960s, but most do not meet present day standards for adequate trial design and conduct. The only major randomized trial in recent years, WARIS, randomized 1214 patients less than 75 years of age to warfarin (INR 2.8–4.8) or placebo for an average follow-up of 37 months.[12] In the warfarin group, 15% died compared to 20% in the placebo group, recurrent myocardial infarction was reduced and there was a 55% reduction in cerebrovascular accidents. The incidence of intracerebral haemorrhage was 0.2% per patient year in the warfarin group, and 16% of these were fatal. The overall incidence of major bleeding, therefore, including intracerebral haemorrhage, was 0.6% per patient year. Apart from the WARIS Trial there have been three other major randomized, controlled trials.[13] The British Medical Research Council Trial of 1964 showed an odds ratio reduction of death of 0.65 and reinfarction of 0.28; the

Veterans Administration Trial (1969) showed figures of 0.94 and 0.58 respectively and the Dutch 60 Plus Trial (1980) showed odds ratio reduction of death of 0.70 and of reinfarction of 0.41. A review of these trials (Smith 1993) 'strongly support the concept of a beneficial effect of anticoagulation on mortality and reinfarction after myocardial infarction'.[13] Two trials have compared aspirin with warfarin (with a total patient number of only 1700). Neither found a significant difference between the groups but the numbers were small. Data from the Antiplatelet Trialists' Collaboration Group of 1988[2,2a] showed that after myocardial infarction aspirin reduced mortality by 13% and reinfarction by 25%. These benefits appear considerably less than those seen in patients with warfarin, so further trials are still needed in this area. Warfarin therapy may therefore have a place in patients after myocardial infarction for those with large anterior infarcts, but until further trials are done, most cardiologists will probably not use it widely on a routine basis. Warfarin, however, is used regularly in patients who have had systemic emboli, a left ventricular apical thrombus, persistent atrial fibrillation, or in clinical situations where the clinical trial data is inconclusive but generally in favour of anticoagulation.[14]

Digoxin

Digoxin (see also Ch. 31) is usually started in hospital for atrial fibrillation, which is nearly always self-limiting within 3–7 days. Treatment is often continued at discharge, especially if pulmonary venous congestion persists. Digoxin can nearly always be stopped 4–6 weeks after the infarction. The only indications to continue this drug long-term would be persistent atrial fibrillation with a rapid ventricular rate, or persistent pulmonary venous congestion. Serum levels do not usually need to be measured unless significant renal impairment is present. Studies to assess whether digoxin affects survival in post-infarction left ventricular dysfunction are currently underway.

Angiotensin-converting enzyme inhibitors

There are a number of important questions of timing, selection of patients, selection of drug, dose and duration of treatment that relate to the use of angiotensin-converting enzyme (ACE) inhibitors after myocardial infarction (see also Ch. 33).

The sicker patients receive more absolute benefit following treatment with ACE inhibitors. The SAVE Study,[15] which included only patients with left ventricular dysfunction, and the AIRE Study,[16] which included only patients with clinical heart failure, showed relative reductions in mortality of 25% or more while GISSI-I[17] and ISIS-4,[18] which included patients with or without heart failure, showed lesser but still significant reductions in mortality. Some physicians would advocate the use of ACE inhibitors in all post-infarction patients but most would restrict their use to those with anterior or large infarcts or those with heart failure or who have ejection fractions of less than 40%.

Starting time for treatment varied, with benefits seen in both early and late commencement. GISSI-III and ISIS-4 entered patients within 24 hours, AIRE 3–10 days and SAVE 3–16 days after infarction. It would seem sensible to start oral therapy in the first 24 hours providing the patient is not hypotensive and has no contraindications to ACE inhibitors, on the grounds that the process of remodelling does start very early indeed.

Captopril, ramipril and lisinopril have all been shown to be effective and there are no good data to suggest that any one agent is better than any other. It is probably best for the physician to use the drug with which he or she has had the most clinical experience.

There are no clear data on dose. It would seem reasonable to use the agent in doses up to the maximum clinically recommended doses, providing that no significant postural hypotension or other side-effects develop.

Treatments in the trials have ranged from 35 days to 42 months. It would seem prudent to continue the drugs on a long-term basis in high-risk patients, especially those with heart failure or with ejection fractions below 40%.

Other medications and post-hospital management

Patients are often discharged from hospital on medications which are appropriate for early post-coronary management, but which may no longer be needed at a later stage. It is always worthwhile looking at a patient's tablets at the time of hospital discharge to see what can safely be stopped later, and provide specific advice to the patient and the primary care physician on when they can be stopped. In general, it is better to stop one medicine at a time rather than stopping a number of different medicines at the same time. Again it may be better to wean the patient off the medicine rather than stopping it suddenly. This is particularly important for beta blocking drugs, which on sudden withdrawal may cause unpleasant 'rebound' symptoms of palpitation or tachycardia and on occasions, significant symptoms of angina requiring hospital re-admission. Sleeping tablets may be useful in hospital but can usually be discontinued once the patient has settled in at home. Digoxin in most patients can be stopped a month or so after discharge, unless atrial arrhythmias persist with a rapid ventricular response or the patient remains in heart failure. Warfarin when given to patients with large anterior infarcts can often be stopped at 3 months unless the patient has a persisting left ventricular clot, has had a systemic embolus or has some other long-term indication present. Often echocardiography is needed to assist this decision.

Many patients go home on nitrates, either a patch or sustained release tablet. In the absence of ongoing pain or heart failure there is no evidence that nitrates are required. It is very reasonable however for patients to carry tablets or a spray of nitroglycerin for use in the treatment or prophylaxis of angina and to be carefully instructed in their correct use. Diuretics are widely used in hospital, and again their continued use should be carefully assessed, particularly in elderly patients where hypovolaemia may lead to orthostatic hypotension and risk of falls.

Conversely, it is important to emphasize to the patient that some medications, such as aspirin and lipid-lowering drugs, require life-time therapy and are not a short-term curative treatment.

The need for effective communications between the coronary care team and the primary care physician cannot be over-emphasized.

References

1. ISIS-2 Collaborative Group. Randomised trial of intravenous streptokinase, oral aspirin, both, or neither among 17 187 cases of suspected acute myocardial infarction: ISIS-2. Lancet 1988; 2:349–60
2. Antiplatelet Trialists Collaboration. Secondary prevention of vascular disease by prolonged antiplatelet treatment. Br Med J 1988; 296:320–31

2a. Collaborative overview of randomized trials of antiplatelet therapy. Antiplatelet triality collaboration Brit Med J 1994; 308: 81–106

3. Patrono C. Aspirin as an antiplatelet drug. N Engl J Med 1994; 330:1287–94
4. Yusuf S, Wittes J, Friedman L. Overview of results of randomised clinical trials in heart disease. (Pt 1.) Treatments following myocardial infarction. JAMA 1988; 260: 2088–93
5. Teo KK, Yusuf S, Furberg CD. Effects of prophylactic antiarrhythmic drug therapy in acute myocardial infarction. JAMA 1993; 270:1589–95
6. Nademanee K, Singh BN, Stevenson WG, Weiss JN. Amiodarone and post-MI patients. Circ 1993; 88:764–74
7. Duval HC, Nui DR, Grancelli HO, Perrone SV, Bortman GR, Curiel R. Randomised trial of low dose amiodarone in severe congestive heart failure. Lancet 1994; 344:493–8
8. Echt DS, Liebson PR, Mitchell LB et al. Mortality and morbidity in patients receiving encainide, flecainide or placebo. The Cardiac Arrhythmia Suppression Trial. N Engl J Med 1991; 324:781–8
9. Held PH, Yusuf S, Furberg CD. Calcium channel blockers in acute myocardial infarction and unstable angina: an overview. Br Med J 1989; 299:1187–92
10. The Danish Study Group on Verapamil in Myocardial Infarction. Effect of verapamil on mortality and major events after acute myocardial infarction. The Danish Verapamil Infarction Trial II (DAVIT II). Am J Cardiol 1990; 66:779–85
11. Yusuf S, Held PH, Furberg C. Update of effects of calcium antagonists in myocardial infarction or angina in light of the Second Danish Verapamil Infarction Trial (DAVIT II) and other recent studies. Amer J Cardiol 1991; 67:1295–97
12. Smith P, Arnesen H, Holme I. The effect of warfarin on mortality and reinfarction after myocardial infarction. N Engl J Med 1990; 323:147–52
13. Smith P. Oral anticoagulant therapy in the chronic phase of myocardial infarction. Arch Pathol Lab Med 1993; 117: 97–101
14. Halperin JL, Peterson P. Thrombosis in the cardiac chambers. In: Fuster V, Verstraete M (eds). Thrombosis in cardiovascular disorders. Philadelphia: Saunders, 1992: Chapter 12
15. Pfeffer MA, Braunwald E, Moye LA et al. Effect of captopril on mortality and morbidity in patients with left ventricular dysfunction after myocardial

infarction. Results of the Survival and Ventricular Enlargement Trial. N Engl J Med 1992; 327: 669–77

16. The Acute Infarction Ramipril Efficacy (AIRE) Study Investigators. Effect of ramipril on mortality and morbidity of survivors of acute myocardial infarction with clinical evidence of heart failure. Lancet 1993; 342: 821–8
17. Gruppo Italiano Per Lo Studio Della Sopravvivenza Nell'Infarto Miocardico. GISSI-III: effects of lisinopril and transdermal glyceryl trinitrate singly and together on six week mortality and ventricular function after acute myocardial infarction. Lancet 1994; 343: 1115–22
18. ISIS Collaborative Group. ISIS-4: a randomised factorial trial assessing oral captopril, oral mononitrate and intravenous magnesium sulphate in 58 050 patients with suspected acute myocardial infarction. Lancet 1995; 345: 669–85

81 Insurability after a coronary event

JG (Dick) Richards

Background

In most countries the insurance industry offers products which cover death, temporary disability (income protection) and total and permanent disability. More recently a product was marketed termed 'dread diseases cover', 'crisis cover' or similar names, in which a lump sum payment is made should any of the nominated medical conditions arise—sometimes numbering up to thirty separate disorders. This latter product was introduced as an attachment to a death cover policy designed to allow early payment of a significant amount of the death cover before the claimant dies or is stricken by a severe illness, to assist in the financial problems which often arise in such a period. However in many insurance markets it is now sold as a stand-alone product.

Many individual employees are covered under group superannuation policies provided by their employers, to provide for payment of lump sums or salary continuance or total and permanent disability benefits; however there are many employees for whom this cover is inadequate. The self-employed are responsible for providing their own benefits.

It is therefore not uncommon, in the recovery phase from an acute myocardial infarction, an episode of unstable angina or revascularization procedures, for the individual concerned, or their family, to realize that insurance cover other than health cost cover may be inadequate or non-existent. Enquiries are often made as to future insurability knowing that once manifest, coronary artery disease has a tendency to recur and progress, necessitating further hospitalization, absence from work, early retirement or premature death. Although an experienced insurance agent is the most helpful source of information, it is prudent for medical, nursing and paramedic staff to have some knowledge of the likely implication of the diagnosis on future insurability. For those wishing to enquire in greater depth, *Medical selection of life risk*[1] offers a satisfactory text.

Principles of medical underwriting

The principle of medical underwriting is to offer cover to as large a group as possible for a given premium. More than 85–90% of persons applying are taken at standard rates. The remaining substandard cases are covered, if possible, by appropriately increased premium rates in order to establish fairness of the process. These rates are determined by actuaries who in each country produce tables known as Medically Examined Mortality Rates for both men and women, based on a large amount of pooled data from a number of insurance companies.[2]

These data differ significantly from the mortality rates of the general population supplied by government statistical services; in all cases the mortality of the medically examined groups is less—in some age groups markedly so.

This fact is not often realised when follow-up data following a medical procedure is compared to actuarial survival curves, which are from the general population. This comparison often leads to some physicians and surgeons suggesting that such cases should be accepted at standard rates if the mortality curve followed that of the general population curve. Such cases however would, depending on the age group, have in most instances at least twice the mortality rate, that is +100% mortality when compared to medically examined insurance company data. If cover were offered it would therefore be at a substantially increased premium in those cases whose follow-up mortality data is similar to that of the general population.

As a general rule, primary insurance companies offer death cover up to an excess mortality of +450%. However, some reinsurers may offer up to +600% at markedly increased premium rates.

Insurance after a myocardial infarction

In the circumstances of coronary artery disease complicated by an acute myocardial infarction from which recovery has occurred, any offer of insurance, and premium applicable for such cover, would depend as far as life cover is concerned on the prognosis of each individual case.

Medically we know that post-infarct prognosis depends on the severity of myocardial damage, the extent of the coronary disease, the presence of late arrhythmias and the nature and degree of risk factors, especially smoking, hypertension, diabetes and hyperlipidaemia. Medically these cases, after appropriate investigations, are divided into low-risk cases, where annual mortality may be 1–2% per year, and high-risk, where they may rise above 8% per year.

The estimated risk of death in the year after examination for Australian 'insured lives' compared with a 'low risk' post-infarction patient is shown in Table 81.1. For the young post-infarct patient, the multiples of risk over the non-coronary subject are extremely high.

This is due to the extra mortality in the first year and knowing that once manifest, coronary artery disease is, up to the present time, usually a progressive disease. The excess mortality in subsequent years is likely to escalate in comparison to the gradually increasing mortality in the standard groups as age advances.

Table 81.1 Comparison of risks for 'insured lives' versus low- and high-risk post-coronary patients. From Brackenridge RDC, Elder WJ, 1992, 3rd ed

Estimated risk in year post-examination	Age 40	45	50	55	60
Australian insured lives	0.067%	0.069%	0.13%	0.19%	0.31%
Post-coronary patient					
Low-risk risk	1%	1%	1%	1%	1%
Multiple of risk*	15	14.5	7.5	5.3	3.2
Moderate-risk risk	4%	4%	4%	4%	4%
Multiple of risk*	60	58	31	21	13

* VI non-coronary subject

However, if we take a post-infarct case with a moderate risk of 4–5% mortality per year, it is not too difficult to see the marked difference between standard cases and extra mortality multiples this group would attract as far as premium rates are concerned.

Unfortunately for the patient, comparative risk is highest in the younger patients, who usually have a greater need for insurance cover.

Having said that, companies do offer cover if they consider it financially prudent to do so as far as death cover is concerned. Very few, if any, would consider cover for future temporary or permanent disability. This risk cannot be appropriately covered by exclusion clauses for cardiovascular disorders. In particular psychosomatic disorders and depression are not uncommon when a return to work is made, and premature retirement is often sought on these grounds.

Similarly, cover under the new policies for 'crisis cover' or 'dread disease' would not be available.

Defining the risk after a myocardial infarction

In relation to death cover, it is known that progress of survivors of myocardial infarction and those known to have coronary artery disease depends on a number of parameters: left ventricular function, extent of the coronary disease and presence of late ventricular arrhythmias, hypertension, diabetes, smoking habits, lipid profile, physical inactivity and obesity.

Most post-infarct survivors have at least modified exercise stress tests after recovery, and many have gated heart blood pool scans, echocardiography or angiography in order to more accurately define their risk status and allow decisions to be made regarding intervention on a symptomatic or prognostic basis.

As a general rule, to consider an application for death cover requires at least a 3–6 month interval, from the time of the event. Applicants under 40 years at the time of the event are often not acceptable or at a very high extra premium since their risk even in most favourable cases is so much higher than standard.

Other cases are considered after the 3–6 month period with full details of the result of post-infarction investigations made available, together with a current full medical examination and electrocardiogram (ECG). Sometimes further investigations, such as thallium perfusion exercise scan or stress echocardiography, are required if the sum at risk is very large.

We know that coronary disease, once present, tends to be progressive, the rate varying from case to case, and although we have some evidence of therapeutically induced regression of coronary atheroma, knowledge of this field and its effect is not complete.

Premium calculation based on risk

Companies have adopted premium calculation in different ways, some simply adding on additional extra mortality to the standard premium—for example, +400%. Most, however, add a temporary extra to a basic sub-standard premium, for example +150% +$20 per thousand dollars sum insured, indicating that in addition to the basic extra mortality there is an additional 2% mortality per year expected. This extra premium may be for 10 years and sometimes longer. The standard premium rates for death cover are very low and in the younger age group even a +600% extra risk of mortality would attract a premium rate 6 times that of standard rates. We know that even with the very low mortality rate of 1% one year in best risk groups is at age 45 years, fourteen and a half times standard mortality rate which is clearly not covered by a +600% mortality rating. Therefore the use of a lower basic extra mortality +10–$20 per thousand sum insured gives a much fairer determination of the risk.

Naturally therefore age, ejection fraction (EF), angiographic findings, echo studies, history of late arrhythmias or an exercise study are most important in arriving at an underwriting decision. Those with normal EF, single vessel disease, good exercise performances and currently stable ECG after 6 months would be assessed probably at 150% + $15 per thousand sum insured for a period of 10 or more years.

Those with EF of 45–50%, two vessel disease, and mild reversible ischaemia on thallium study would attract +200% + $20 per thousand sum insured for 10 or more years. Those with EF of 35–39%, three vessel disease, moderate reversible ischaemia on thallium scan or a positive exercise test would be declined for a period of 5–6 years and then if stable, considered at a premium of +400% + $40 per thousand sum insured for ten or more years. Those with more serious findings, especially EF of <35% or strongly positive tests, would be declined for cover indefinitely.

Factors such as hypertension, diabetes, smoking habits and lipid profile would all be taken into account when considering insurability.

Insurance after other coronary events

The methods described above and the parameters used enable cover to be considered in forms of presentation other than post-infarction, such as following presentation with stable angina, unstable angina or following angioplasty or coronary bypass grafting.

These premiums are very high but the small mortality experiences of companies offering this type of cover suggests that the above outlines may be too generous. It may be that with further experience and future medical and surgical therapeutic regimes, the mortality rates will be markedly altered—in which case premium calculation would be actuarially reviewed.

Currently it would be prudent however to suggest that cover in the best cases may be available after a period of 3–6 months at a significantly increased premium rating, but that disability benefits are rarely, if ever, available.

References

1. Brackenridge RDC, Elder WJ. Medical selection of life risks. 3rd ed. 1992.
2. Institute of Actuaries of Australia. Mortality investigation 1A: 90–2.

82 Driving, flying, sport after a coronary event

Michael V Jelinek

The patient who is recovering from an acute coronary event frequently intends to resume driving and often wishes to fly as a passenger or resume sporting activity. Less common needs include the resumption of professional driving, piloting an aeroplane, or the wish to resume higher intensity aerobic sports. This chapter will discuss the clinical, physiological and epidemiological factors which should be considered in advising the patient. Such advice must be adjusted to the law wherever the patient lives—such laws varying from place to place and usually considering the safety of people other than the individual patient.

Driving a motor vehicle

Private car

There is little cardiovascular stress in driving a private car near home or to and from work. After recovering from an uncomplicated myocardial infarction (MI) or after uncomplicated coronary artery angioplasty (PTCA) the patient is fit to resume private driving soon after leaving hospital. This may be as soon as 1–2 weeks after the acute event.[1]

Angina is not a reason for advising against driving unless the angina is unstable or easily provoked by driving. Very high levels of blood pressure should be controlled before the patient resumes driving after a coronary event.

Patients with cardiac failure should not drive until this condition is controlled medically. Cardiac failure complicating acute myocardial infarction (AMI) reflects severe underlying myocardial damage and represents a substantially increased risk of sudden cardiac death. Such patients often spend longer in hospital in order to control their symptoms, signs and arrhythmias and may require up to a month after the acute event before they are fit to resume driving.

A cardiac arrest early in the course of an otherwise uncomplicated AMI is almost invariably due to ventricular fibrillation resulting from the acute event and should not influence the timing of resumption of private driving. However, if the cardiac arrest or an episode of ventricular tachycardia occurs as a result of extensive cardiovascular damage, often with heart failure, then the patient should be free of these symptomatic arrhythmias for at least 1 month before commencing driving. Cardiac arrest occurring outside the context of acute ischaemia or infarction has a high risk of recurrence and would normally preclude the patient from driving.

The pain from the median sternotomy performed as part of open heart surgery delays resumption of driving for at least 1 month after the operation. Factors to be considered in advising resumption of private driving in such cases include the patient's concentration, field of vision, neck mobility, the degree of sternal pain, the presence of power steering in the vehicle or, if power steering is absent, how heavy the car is to turn. Some patients are not fit to resume driving for up to 2–3 months after heart surgery.

Patients who have undergone percutaneous transluminal coronary angioplasty (PTCA) can normally resume driving within a few days of the procedure. This may occasionally be delayed if there is a large haematoma with discomfort in the groin.

Driving of taxis, buses, trucks and semi trailers

Permission to drive these large, heavy vehicles will be under legislative control. The time spent by professional drivers on the road is much greater than that of private drivers and the consequences of driver failure are potentially much greater considering the weight of the vehicle being driven. However, an autopsy report on sudden death in drivers indicated that only one driver death in 30 resulted in major damage to a vehicle other than that driven by the deceased.

In perhaps 10 cases, the deceased had either stopped the car or had not driven it, presumably as a result of symptoms of the terminal disease.[2] It may be therefore that the fears engendered by the possibilities of sudden driver failure are excessive.

Nevertheless, most licensing bodies demand a much greater period from the acute event to the commencement of professional driving. Times such as 6 weeks after uncomplicated AMI or unstable angina, 3 months after coronary artery bypass graft (CABG), and 2 weeks after successful PTCA are typical. Patients with a history of congestive heart failure, even if under medical control, are normally excluded from professional driving. There are no clear guidelines on the permission to drive in patients with asymptomatic untreated left ventricular dysfunction but such patients have probably a much lower risk of sudden death than their symptomatic counterparts.[3,4] Of course, patients with poor ventricular function and symptomatic ventricular arrhythmias or a history of unexpected cardiac arrest are not fit to drive.

Flying

As passenger

Many a coronary event takes place in a patient who is many miles from home. Most airlines will permit the patient to travel by air when the attending doctor issues a medical certificate of fitness to fly. Short flights of up to 3 hours may be permissible within 2 weeks of an uncomplicated acute event. However, it may be wise to delay permission to fly in patients who have experienced AMI complicated by heart failure or major arrhythmias, or if the proposed journey involves intercontinental travel. The prospect of the patient having to seek out medical care in unfamiliar surroundings on arrival at their destination may be as important a consideration as the risk of an in-flight medical crisis.

As pilot

No situation illustrates the importance of accurate assessment of the risk of sudden incapacity more than licensing a pilot to fly after a coronary event. While most potential harm could occur with sudden incapacity of a pilot of a large commercial airliner, the presence in the cockpit of a co-pilot reduces the consequences of sudden incapacity to the few seconds during takeoff or landing—when control of the plane is in the hands of one pilot who may be unable to communicate sudden incapacity to the co-pilot. On the other hand, lighter aircraft usually have a single pilot and sudden incapacity may have grave consequences for the passengers and the public on the ground.

By and large, pilots who are not responsible for large commercial aircraft may be re-licensed 1 year after their last coronary event if formal testing reveals good left ventricular function, no evidence of myocardial ischaemia on effort using ECG and isotope perfusion criteria, and after viewing of a coronary angiogram.[5] The actual requirements will vary from country to country and be under legislative control. It should be recognized, however, that acute non-fatal myocardial infarction is poorly predicted by the coronary angiogram and tests of myocardial ischaemia,[6] and that such infarction may seriously reduce the performance of a solo pilot.

Sport

The physically active and physically fit are less likely to die of cardiovascular disease, and have a better cardiovascular risk profile than the habitually inactive.[7] Better aerobic capacity is associated with better survival in patients with coronary heart disease[8] and congestive heart failure.[9] Hence the performance of physical activity such as sport is usually encouraged in patients surviving a coronary event. There are many caveats.

Many of the patients, particularly the elderly, have previously been totally inactive. These patients should be encouraged to take up regular, moderate exercise such as a walking programme or sports such as bowls or golf. Attempts to encourage patients to be more active than this are not supported by studies of survival or quality of life, and actually may be hazardous.[10–12]

There is a recovery period of at least 3 months after a myocardial infarction during which exercise tolerance continues to improve independent of formal exercise training.[13] The average patient can be expected to improve their exercise tolerance around 50% during this phase. Thus, the convalescent patient should be informed of this and encouraged to continue with exercise considerably below their eventual capacity. The rate of resumption of activity should be slower in patients with extensive myocardial infarction, when early mobilization could conceivably weaken the developing scar and result in excessive cardiac dilatation. Nevertheless, even patients with controlled cardiac failure benefit from physical activity programmes and these should be encouraged even in such patients, with due regard to convalescence, over 6–8 weeks after myocardial infarction.

High intensity aerobic activity is a risk factor for ventricular fibrillation and cardiac arrest. The incidence of cardiac arrest vastly exceeds the incidence of fatal myocardial infarction in cardiac rehabilitation programmes based on aerobic exercise.[14] In order to reduce such risks, patients are only permitted to undergo higher levels of exercise if they have been screened by a cardiologist, have undergone a maximal exercise test, and have had a formal exercise prescription written. This best limits exercise levels below that required to raise the pulse to 85% of the pulse at maximum exercise, or the onset of ECG ischaemia.[15] In addition, cardiac rehabilitation programmes involving exercise should be equipped with defibrillators to cope with the occasional cardiac arrest.

Patients who have recovered from an acute coronary event should not undertake high intensity sport unless in an environment with a defibrillator and a team skilled in cardiopulmonary resuscitation. Such sports include long distance running, squash and probably singles tennis. Furthermore, performance of such sports should be guided by the stage of convalescence and the satisfactory performance of a maximal exercise test.

Conclusion

Where such activities are not governed by law, permission for the patient to drive, fly or play sport should be governed by their clinical status, duration of convalescence, level of activity desired and the estimate of cardiovascular risk of the task involved. On occasions, detailed cardiac investigation may be required to assess this risk more precisely.

References

1. Fitness of cardiac patients to hold driving licences. Cardiac Society of Australia and New Zealand, Sydney, 1993.
2. Antecol DH, Roberts WC. Sudden death behind the wheel from natural disease in drivers of four-wheeled motorised vehicles. Am J Cardiol 1990; 66: 1329–35
3. The SOLVD Investigators. Effect of enalapril on survival in patients with reduced left ventricular ejection fractions and congestive heart failure. N Engl J Med 1991; 325: 293–302
4. The SOLVD Investigators. Effect of enalapril on mortality and the development of heart failure in asymptomatic patients with reduced left ventricular ejection fractions. N Engl J Med 1992; 327: 685–91
5. Vohra J, Plowright R. An appraisal of cardiovascular standards for Australian Civilian Flying Licences. Aust NZ J Med 1989; 19: 76–82
6. Ambrose JA, Tannenbaum MA, Alexopoulos D et al. Angiographic progression of coronary artery disease and development of myocardial infarction. JACC 1988; 12: 56–62
7. Jelinek VM. Exercise to prevent heart disease. How much should we advise? Ann Acad Med (Singapore) 1992; 21: 101–5
8. Morris CK, Ueshima K, Kawaguchi T, Hideg A, Frolicher V. The prognostic value of exercise capacity: a review of the literature. Am Heart J 1991; 122: 1423–1431
9. Van den Broek SAJ, Van Veldhuisen DJ, De Graeff PA, Landsman MLJ, Hillege H, Lie KI. Comparison between New York Heart Association classification and peak oxygen consumption in the assessment of functional status and prognosis in patients with mild to moderate chronic congestive heart failure secondary to either ischaemic or idiopathic dilated cardiomyopathy. Am J Cardiol 1992; 70: 359–63
10. Rechnitzer PA, Cunningham DA, Andrew GM et al. Relation of exercise to the recurrence rate of myocardial infarction in men. Ontario Exercise Heart Collaborative Study. Am J Cardiol 1983; 51: 65–9
11. Worcester MC, Hare DL, Oliver RG, Reid MA, Goble AJ. Early programmes of high and low intensity exercise and quality of life after acute myocardial infarction. Br Med J 1993; 307: 1294–7
12. Willich SN, Lewis M, Lowel H et al. Physical exertion as a trigger of acute myocardial infarction. N Engl J Med 1993; 329: 1684–90
13. Haskell WL, Debusk R. Cardiovascular responses to

repeated treadmill exercise testing soon after myocardial infarction. Circulation 1979; 60: 1247–51

14. Van Camp SP, Peterson RA. Cardiovascular complications of outpatient rehabilitation programs. JAMA 1986; 256: 1160–3
15. Fox SM III, Naughton JP, Haskell WL. Physical activity in the prevention of coronary heart disease. Ann Clin Res 1971; 3: 404–32

Part 11
Other CCU issues

83 Infection control in the CCU

Clay Golledge

The importance of hospital acquired infection

Prevalence surveys of hospital infection in many countries have shown that about one in 10 patients in hospital have acquired an infection.[1] The main acquired infections are of the urinary tract, of surgical wounds, lower respiratory tract and skin. The frequency and severity varies with the age of the patient, type of operation in surgical cases, length of time of urinary or intravenous catheterization, immunosuppressive treatment and other factors.

The importance of hospital infection can be considered both in terms of the patients' illness, and of the prolonged occupancy of hospital beds. The cost of a prolonged stay is a convenient measure of the cost of infection, although it represents a reduction in the number of beds available from the waiting list rather than an actual increased cost to the hospital. This estimated cost was about £120 million per year in England and Wales in 1987, but was likely to have been a very conservative underestimate of the true costs. A figure over 20 times this magnitude has been quoted from the United States.[2] Accurate Australian figures are not available but nosocomial infection rates of 5–10% are quoted for many Australian hospitals, with an estimated average prolongation of bed stay of 5.5 days.

A large number of nosocomial infections are preventable, and the principles of control of infection fall under three headings:

- To remove the sources or potential sources of infection—this includes treatment of infected patients as well as sterilizing, disinfection and cleaning of contaminated materials and surfaces.
- To block the routes of transfer of bacteria from those potential sources and reservoirs to uninfected patients, which include isolation of infected or susceptible patients, embracing the principles of body substance isolation, aseptic operations, 'no touch' dressing techniques and particularly handwashing.
- To enhance the patient's resistance to infection (e.g. by good surgical technique, rational antibiotic use, control of diabetes, immunization, etc.).

In a number of hospitals worldwide there has been a decline in the incidence of staphylococcal cross-infection but to offset that there has been the emergence of methicillin-resistant *Staphylococcus aureus* (MRSA). In developing countries *Pseudomonas aeruginosa* is still a common cause of death in patients with burns. Outbreaks of infection with other antibiotic-resistant Gram-negative bacilli (such as *Klebsiella* spp., *Enterobacter* spp., *Acinetobacter* spp.) are commonly reported, particularly in intensive care units and urological wards. There has been a general reduction in cross-infection, however. The focus of attention is shifting to the control of endogenous infection in colorectal surgery and in patients with diminished antimicrobial resistance, to problems of sterilization of difficult pieces of equipment, and to containment of dangerous communicable disease. The spread of hepatitis B and HIV is prevented by care in taking blood from infected persons, safe disposal of sharps, screening of blood and blood products and reliable processing of equipment.

There is an increasing awareness of the importance of the personal factor in preventing hospital infection, and of the need of a proper understanding of the facts by all members of the hospital staff. The basic ideas and practices are simple and many of the details of asepsis can be made easier by forms of standardization based on evidence of effectiveness and practicability.

The infection control team

Every hospital, no matter how small, should have at least one person experienced in, and responsible for, infection control. In a teaching hospital situation, a team approach is usually employed with at least one and possibly two or three infection control nurses occupying dedicated positions. A clinical microbiologist or infectious disease physician usually provides medical support with laboratory back-up.

The role of the team is made considerably more efficient if there is close liaison between the team members and the nursing and medical staff. The art and science of infection control has improved considerably over the years and a lot of the unproven rituals have disappeared from clinical practice. It is vitally important that medical and nursing staff believe in their infection control practitioners, and equally important that the infection control team follow accepted standard practice and remain current with the scientific literature.

The coronary care unit

Although the coronary care unit (CCU) is a high-dependency unit containing patients with severe, potentially life-threatening illness, there is no evidence that these units pose a higher infection risk to patients than do general medical wards.[3] Nevertheless there are specific and important issues relevant to the CCU.

- Every patient will have some form of intravenous (IV) access and the principles of IV line management need to be thoroughly understood.
- Because of intravascular procedures such as coronary angiography and angioplasty, blood-borne viruses become an important issue both for patients and staff.
- The re-use of expensive single-use equipment such as cardiac catheters needs to be considered and a formal hospital procedure adopted and adhered to considering all the technical and medico-legal facts.

The remainder of this brief chapter will look at issues relevant to the CCU: namely the principles of body substance isolation, the management of peripheral and central IV lines, routine screening for blood-borne viruses and re-use of cardiac catheters.

Body substance isolation

All medical and nursing staff, as well as all other staff with patient contact, need to be aware of the principle of body substance isolation (BSI). BSI is designed to remove diagnosis-driven infection control practices by regarding all patients as potentially infectious. The protocol for BSI includes the following:

1. wearing of gloves for anticipated contact with all moist body substances.
2. handwashing before and after all patient contact.
3. gowns, plastic aprons, masks, or goggles are worn when secretions, blood or body fluids are likely to splash on clothing, skin, or the face
4. soiled reusable items, linen and waste are contained to prevent leaking. Double bagging is not necessary unless the outside of the bag is visibly soiled.
5. safe disposal of sharps: non-recapping (or recapping using an appropriate device) and disposal into a rigid, puncture-proof container.
6. additional precautions for infections transmitted by the airborne route, such as single room and wearing of masks.

In addition to the above, all staff with patient contact should be immune to hepatitis B and ideally should be immune, or know their immune status, to measles, mumps, rubella and varicella.

The BSI protocol as noted in point 6 does not cover all isolation categories and disease-specific isolation precautions. Additional isolation precautions are required for infectious diseases transmitted by aerosol and droplet spread, examples being smear-positive tuberculosis and varicella.

The BSI protocol has been modified to emphasize the importance of handwashing even after the wearing of gloves. Handwashing is the single most important means of preventing the spread of infection, and soap and water will effectively remove transient flora without the routine need for antiseptic solutions.

Among the advantages of BSI are that it is a simple system that is easy to learn and administer, that it avoids the assumptions that persons without known or suspected diagnosis of transmissible infectious diseases are free of risk, and that only body fluids containing visible blood are associated with risk of infection.

The disadvantages of BSI include the added cost of increased use of barrier equipment, particularly gloves, the perceived difficulty in maintaining routine application of the protocol for all patients, and the potential for misapplication of the protocol to overprotect the health-care worker at the expense of the patient.

Overall, however, BSI has been shown to work in many centres and the advantages of this system outweigh the disadvantages when properly practised and followed.

Intravenous lines

Peripheral and central venous catheters carry small but significant risks of infection and have the ability, because of their intravascular site, to be directly associated with bacteraemia with potentially disastrous consequences. The pathogenesis of catheter-associated infection is shown in Figure 83.1, and it can be seen that the skin is the most important portal of entry.

Most infectious complications associated with peripheral IV lines are related to phlebitis, and this is primarily a physicochemical phenomenon. True infections usually occur in fewer than 10% of patients. Infections can be minimized by adopting a strict IV control policy, and the following approach is suggested:

- Insert IV lines only when absolutely necessary and review the need for continued use daily.
- Record the date and time of the IV line insertion in both the medical and nursing notes.
- Prepare the skin for IV line insertion with a suitable antiseptic (an alcohol swab is probably inadequate and best results are obtained with a chlorhexidine-based solution[4]).
- Allow at least 30 seconds for the antiseptic solution to act.
- Wash hands prior to the procedure and insert the line using a 'no-touch' technique.
- Inspect the site daily for signs of redness, swelling, pus or streaking. Ask the patient about pain related to the IV site.

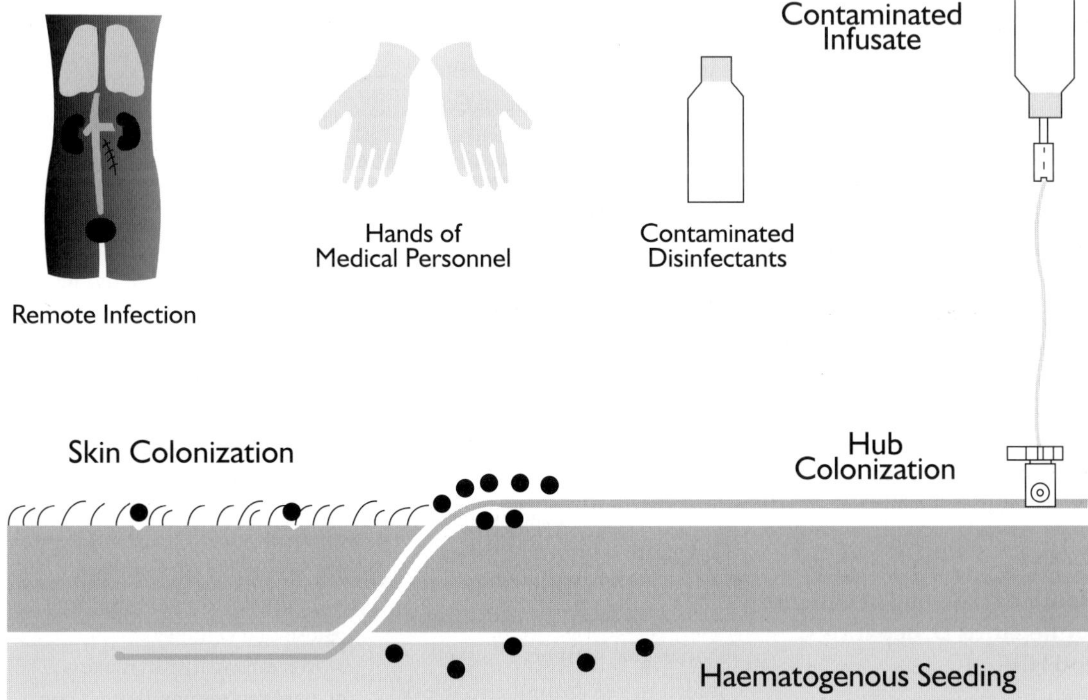

Fig. 83.1 Pathogenesis of catheter-associated infection. Sources of bacterial entry in order of importance: (1) skin colonization; (2) hub colonization; (3) contaminated infusate or transducer domes; (4) haematogenous seeding from remote infection; and (5) skin colonization by remote infection.

- Remove the IV line at the first sign of sepsis.
- Electively rotate peripheral lines every 72 hours *maximum*.

Central venous lines carry a greater risk of infection and they should be rigorously inspected daily and again removed as soon as possible or at the first signs of sepsis or unexplained fever. If longer-term IV access (4 weeks or more) is planned it may be better to contemplate the use of a cuffed catheter such as the Groshong® or Hickman® catheter.

Central lines should ideally not be left in place longer than 14 days. Frequently they need to be removed much earlier than this and if lines are removed for suspected sepsis they should be removed aseptically and the tip sent to the laboratory for microbiological culture.

The routine use of antibiotic or antiseptic ointments for dressing peripheral or central lines is not recommended. Controversy exists as to the most suitable dressing materials for IV lines. A recent trial[5] showed that sterile gauze dressings were superior to transparent dressings for peripheral catheters. If a transparent dressing is to be used for central or peripheral lines then employing a dressing with a high moisture vapour transmission ratio such as Op-Site 3000® may decrease the accumulation of organisms under the transparent dressing.

Routine screening of patients for hepatitis B, hepatitis C and HIV

Some units still screen patients for HBV, HCV and HIV prior to elective or emergency procedures. The adoption of BSI negates the need for screening and avoids a 'two-tier' approach. The use of adequate equipment, sterilization and the safe handling of sharps, coupled with staff immunity to hepatitis B, should minimize risks to all concerned. Thus routine screening for blood-borne viruses prior to procedures is not recommended.

Re-use of cardiac catheters

Any reprocessing of a disposable or single-use item must attain a standard which is appropriate for the intended use of the item. Careful consideration should be given to the difficulties associated with the recycling of these items.

Standard of sterility

The Therapeutic Goods Administration (TGA) in Australia has developed a Code of Good Manufacturing Practice for the preparation of all sterile articles used in hospitals. When reprocessing used items for re-use, institutions should adhere to the quality assurance controls required by the TGA Code of Good Manufacturing Practice. Institutions reprocessing cardiac catheters must be able to demonstrate that these catheters are adequately sterilized at all times. The narrow lumen of the catheter theoretically makes it difficult to do this, although there are no studies that support a higher infection risk from the re-use of catheters; however, no good comparative trials have been undertaken to date.

Durability of materials

A Canadian paper[6] found no degradation of the physical properties of cardiac catheters re-used up to 10 times. Further, the group also stated that biological debris was minimal, that what was present in the catheter lumen was firmly fixed to the lumen and that new catheters exhibited a substantially higher loose particle count than those that had been adequately cleaned and sterilized.

Economics

Some institutions have agreed that there is a considerable cost saving in reprocessing sterile items. In calculating reprocessing costs, it is important to distinguish between the marginal cost of resterilization and the true cost when allowance is made for labour, plant, equipment, maintenance and all consumables. It is usually possible, however, after considering all these variables, to demonstrate cost-savings after reprocessing.

Legal issues

This topic is complex and needs to be considered under four areas: manufacturers' liability, institutional liability, physician liability and informed consent. It is beyond the scope of this chapter to address these issues but each institution should have guidelines that ensure maximum protection for itself and staff, should a legal issue arise from the re-use of a catheter.

It is impossible to make a blanket recommendation about the re-use of single-use items as there clearly are some items capable of being safely reprocessed. National and international guidelines need to be developed to aid institutions in coming to a responsible, reasonable and scientific conclusion about whether any item of equipment should be processed after use, no matter whether it is labelled 'single use only' or not.

References

1. Meers PD, Ayliffe GAJ, Emmerson AM et al. Report on the national survey of infection in hospitals 1980. J Hosp Infect 1981; 2: 136–42
2. Dixon RE. Costs of nosocomial infections and benefits of infection control programmes. In: Wenzel RP (ed). Prevention and control of nosocomial infections. Baltimore: Williams & Wilkins, 1987: 19–25
3. Schendorf WA, Brown RB, Sands M, Hosman D. Infections in a coronary care unit. Am J Cardiol 1985; 56: 757–9
4. Maki DG, Ringer M, Alvarado CJ. Prospective randomised trial of povidone-iodine, alcohol, and chlorhexidine for prevention of infection associated with central venous and arterial catheters. Lancet 1991; 328: 339–43
5. Conly JM, Grieves K, Peters B. A prospective, randomised study comparing transparent and dry gauze dressings for central venous catheters. J Infect Dis 1989; 159: 310–19
6. Bentolilan P, Jacob R, Robenge F. Effects of re-use on the physical characteristics of angiographic catheters. J Med Eng Tech 1990; 14: 254–9

84 Coronary care database

JH Nick Bett

Reasons for having a database

A coronary care database is essential to undertake any form of quality assurance or 'housekeeping' and is invaluable for research. It will enable reports and summaries of events during coronary care admissions to be generated and patients to be flagged for follow-up.[1] Some form of coronary care database is now essential to monitor outcomes and benchmark against other institutions for accreditation with insurers and hospital licencing authorities.

Equipment and software

If there is no local experience or interest in setting up a database application, software such as that developed by Summit Medical Systems for the American College of Cardiology can be used. On the other hand a simple database can be set up on an IBM-compatible or Macintosh personal computer using one of the standard commercial packages (Oracle, Paradox, Access, dBase for Windows, Clinical Report System, Cardiobase) from which data can be exported into statistical analysis programs (SPSS, SAS, S-Plus) or spreadsheets (Lotus 123, Excel). It may be convenient to install it on a network so that it can be used at more than one site and interfaced with other clinical or administrative databases. The choice of packages may depend on local experience, but there are advantages in selecting one that can be accessed from Microsoft Windows.

Confidentiality

As with any clinical information, there is a need to restrict access to those who are authorized to read, write or analyse the data. At the same time the data and the structure of the database must be protected against accidental or malicious damage. This is generally done by requiring users to enter a password in order to log onto the database. A hierarchy of users will need to be established and access restricted, particularly if the database is installed on a network. Some will be licensed only to read data, others to enter or edit information, and only a few to modify the structure of the database. From the outset there must be a reliable routine for the regular backup of data. It may be convenient to store the files on the hard disk of a network fileserver which is backed up each day.

Structure

The database must be able to store records of multiple admissions for one patient. Demographic data (name, date of birth, sex and hospital record number) is therefore entered in a 'root' table, with one record for each patient. This has a *one-to-many* relationship with the coronary care data table and is linked to it by a primary key which is always present but is unique for each patient. This may be the hospital record number. Each coronary care data record contains the information relating to one admission—date, diagnosis, treatment and outcome (see Fig. 84.1). Each patient therefore has one record in the 'root' table, and a record in the coronary care table on each occasion he or she is admitted. At the same time the 'root' table may be linked to others containing administrative information (address, cardiologist, etc.) or recording other clinical events such as catheterization or surgery.

Data fields

Data fields are of different types. Character, text or string fields are used for alphanumerical entries (for example, name), but are better avoided for clinical information, as subsequent analysis is much simpler for data recorded as numbers (including dates and times) or in logical (yes/no) fields. Some free text fields must be allowed for information that

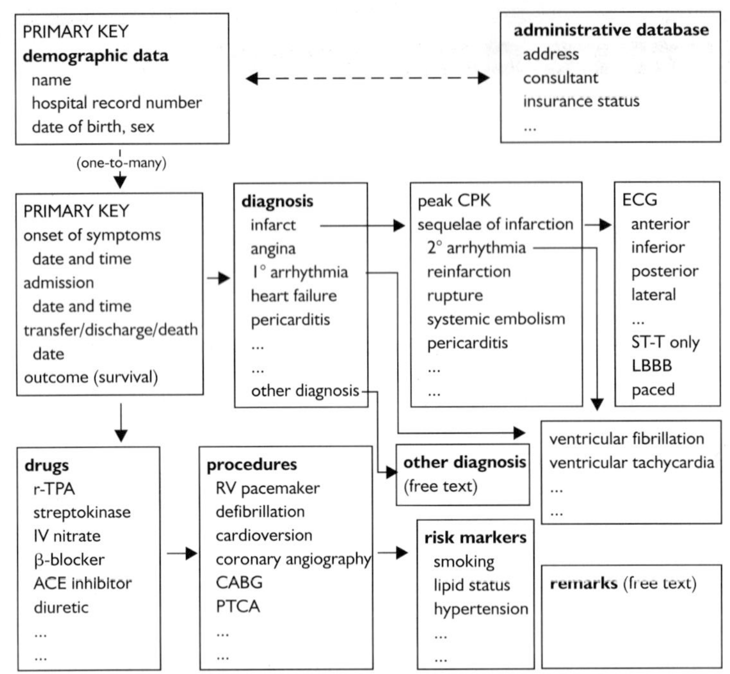

Fig. 84.1 The demographic table (name, sex, date of birth, etc.) has a *one-to-many* relationship to the coronary care table, to which it is linked by a primary key, allowing multiple records (admissions) for each patient. It may be linked to the main hospital administrative table. The first of the coronary care screen forms contains fields for date and time of symptom onset, admission to coronary care and separation (discharge, transfer or death) and outcome. The next form allows the principal diagnosis to be chosen. If this is *myocardial infarction*, other forms are presented to record enzyme data and major sequelae (rupture, systemic embolism, etc.) and ECG diagnosis (e.g. anterior infarction). The diagnosis of *primary arrhythmia* or the recording of a *secondary arrhythmia* as a sequel to MI brings up a screen form to note these arrhythmias. The choice of *other diagnosis* allows this to be described with free text. Other forms are to document drugs given, procedures undertaken and risk markers (smoking, hypertension, etc.). The final screen form is for free text remarks.

cannot readily be coded. It is probable that the fields will need to be modified or additional fields added from time to time.

Data entry

Much effort is needed in setting up a database to ensure that it is easy to enter data, particularly by those who are not familiar with computers or whose typing skills are limited. Screen form design is important and it is worth testing the ease of data entry with several users before introducing the 'definitive' version of the database in practice. Most database packages will allow data verification so that inappropriate values and dates are flagged (for example, date of admission after date of discharge) and may be corrected as soon as they are entered. 'Double entry' (i.e. requiring all data to be entered twice) improves accuracy but is too tedious for routine use. Current PC-based packages require data to be entered by keyboard or mouse, but other methods will become available. These will include entering demographic information from barcodes with a scanner and voice-operated data entry programs.[2]

Content

Perhaps the most important and difficult decisions are to determine what data are essential and what may be omitted. It is unrealistic to expect to record reliably more than several hundred separate data items (fields) for each admission. The data to be collected should satisfy the unit's requirements for monitoring trends in casemix, treatment and outcomes, for quality improvement activities and for identifying patient subgroups for research or special follow-up. Information about a patient's progress after discharge from the CCU may be of interest but collecting it requires a great deal of time and effort if it is to be useful. It is preferable, unless generous resources are available, to restrict data to that readily available in the CCU except for major outcomes, such as death, readmission, cardiac arrest or revascularization. The more value the doctors and nurses in the unit see in the database, and the easier it is to use, the more they will be committed to maintaining accurate and up-to-date records. Regular reporting and feedback from the database is essential.

References

1. Hlatky MA, Lee KL Harrell Fe Jr et al. Tying clinical research to patient care by use of an observational database Stat Med 1984; 3: 375–87
2. Fortin DF, Califf RM, Pryor DB, Mark DB. The way of the future redux. Am J Cardiol 1995; 76: 1177–82

85 Clinical trial management in the CCU

Pamela J Bradshaw

Benefits of participating in clinical trials

Both patients and staff can benefit from involvement in research studies carried out in the coronary care unit (CCU). Clinical trials provide access to drugs and technology which may be otherwise unavailable for months or years. Patients on trials may directly benefit from new therapies, and subsequent patients also benefit if effective treatments are adopted early. CCUs which participate in studies are more likely to use new drugs or technologies with which they have become familiar.

Staff who participate in research projects are at the forefront of cardiovascular medicine and can hone clinical skills and critical thinking as they adhere to the requirements of a protocol. The research process engenders an awareness of ethical issues and an emphasis on human rights.

Opportunities for participation in clinical trials

Given the large number of people suffering ischaemic heart disease, even moderate effects of a new treatment may have worthwhile benefits to humanity. These effects are difficult to detect. A risk reduction in mortality of as much as 20% requires at least 1000 *deaths* among the treatment and control groups.[1] A smaller treatment effect would require much greater numbers. Thus as the expected gains of new treatments become more modest, the size of clinical trials grows.

The GUSTO study, which compared thrombolysis with r-TPA versus streptokinase, enrolled over 41 000 participants with deaths of 2800. An absolute reduction in 30-day mortality of 1% (10 per 1000 patients treated) for r-TPA over streptokinase was demonstrated. This translated to a 14% risk reduction.

Without such a large number of participants, GUSTO would have been unable to demonstrate the benefit of accelerated r-TPA.[2]

Large, simple, randomized clinical trials are the best means of reliably answering clinical questions. Such large numbers are required that it is only through collaborative, multicentre and generally international efforts that the number of subjects can be recruited within a reasonable time. Trial centres and sponsors actively seek sites to contribute to the large studies.

CCUs may also take part in local or national studies. These smaller clinical trials also have their place. Although some may not have sufficient power to demonstrate reliably a statistically significant result, if they are conducted so that the results are not open to confounding, then they can be incorporated into an overview or meta-analysis. Studies utilizing a randomized, unbiased study design with a commonly used endpoint such as death from all causes, cardiac death or events such as stroke or reinfarction (as long as the definitions are comparable) can be combined for analysis with other similar trials. The increase in power obtained from the combined studies allows for meaningful results.[3,4] Meta-analyses can provide directions for further research and are valuable when it is improbable that any further randomized trials will be undertaken due to costs, ethical considerations or feasibility. Further clinical trials of aspirin in acute myocardial infarction (AMI) are not likely but the use of overviews produces medically useful results, such as the determination of the optimum dose and the groups likely to benefit from aspirin therapy.[5]

Selection of sites

The cost to the sponsor of funding very large trials means

that centres must demonstrate their ability to meet the requirements of the protocol, and to recruit sufficient patients to warrant the expenditure in their unit.

The need for reliable data extends to all departments having input into the study. Laboratories require certification from a standards authority and all departments will have to demonstrate that they have quality control mechanisms. Centres participating in clinical trials must be prepared to meet the requirements of a protocol into which they may have had little or no input. Conduct of a clinical trial in the CCU requires cooperation at all levels of the institution in order to meet the regulatory requirements attendant upon research studies.

Good clinical research practice

Clinical trials have to meet the regulations of authorities in the country in which the sponsor is seeking approval to market the drug or device, as well as those of participant countries. National bodies such as the US Food and Drug Administration (FDA) control the introduction of new medical therapies to the market. Most study protocols are designed to meet FDA requirements.

Additionally, international bodies such as the World Health Organization and the European Union have developed guidelines for Good Clinical Research Practice (GCRP). These incorporate the ethical rules contained in the current version of the World Medical Association's 1964 Declaration of Helsinki (amended Tokyo 1975, Venice 1983 and Hong Kong 1989). The World Health Organization, in recognizing the need for biomedical research involving human subjects 'to improve diagnostic, therapeutic and prophylactic procedures' and to understand the aetiology and pathogenesis of disease, has set out recommendations for physicians engaged in research.[6] The protection of the patient's/subject's rights is given priority and the individual's well-being takes precedence over the interests of science and society. The keys to GCRP such as the importance of informed consent, the requirements to undertake research in which the objective is proportionately important to the inherent risks and the need for accurate data, are stated in the Declaration.

The Therapeutic Goods Administration (TGA) in Australia states that the intent of GCRP guidelines is to 'provide the basis for ensuring that clinical studies are not only designed to scientific and ethical standards but are also meticulously conducted, recorded, terminated and reported, according to pre-established criteria detailed in the study protocol.'[7] Contained are detailed instructions for the conduct of clinical trials including the responsibilities of sponsors, ethics committees and the investigator. The elements of informed consent are given which are the basis for the patient information and consent forms. All staff involved in clinical trials should have some knowledge of the codes of practice, which are designed to protect patients and staff as well as to further scientific knowledge.

Clinical trial management

In order to meet GCRP standards the investigator must provide the resources to meet the regulatory as well as the clinical demands of the study. Many of the responsibilities for the conduct of a study may be undertaken by a study coordinator, and this is often a CCU nurse with an interest in research. Study coordination requires appropriate clinical experience and administrative skills so that the work of the CCU is not disrupted. Further education in research methodology and data management is needed so that the conduct of the study meets the requirements of the regulatory and ethical bodies and the sponsor.

CCU staff education

The staff in the CCU, the 'step-down' and general wards and, increasingly, the emergency department, need in-service education in the background to the study, the requirements of the protocol, patient selection using inclusion and exclusion criteria, randomization procedures, drug handling, clinical care, documentation, adverse events and emergency measures. Staff must be familiar with study documents which they are to use.

Consent

As they will be caring for patients, rather than 'study subjects', the staff members particularly need an opportunity to discuss the consent procedures. There is an ethical dilemma inherent in many CCU trials when patients admitted with conditions requiring rapid treatment are asked to participate. The patients often are in pain, ill and frightened, have received drugs such as morphine, and may have been brought in alone by ambulance. Consent procedures must be expedited so that study treatment, such as thrombolysis, can be instituted. The need for urgent action and rapid decision-making contrasts with the process of obtaining an informed consent in a less acute situation, such as before elective surgery. Investigators must ensure that patients are not deprived of their right to duly consider their decision. An understanding of the elements of informed consent, and of the benefits to patient care which have accrued because of clinical trials, will help staff overcome any conflict that they may feel with their role in the study.

Consensus

In order to conduct research successfully in the CCU it is important that the medical and nursing staff are committed to the project. Joint discussion of proposed studies allows staff to gauge the likely impact on the unit and to plan ahead to meet any special needs for equipment, training or personnel placement. Clinical trials have special requirements for the handling and accounting of study drugs. Departments such as the pharmacy and laboratories will need to be involved in the discussions.

Other research opportunities

The CCU is also a valuable resource for research other than clinical trials. The patient population, in general, recovers quickly during hospitalization and is thus accessible as a source of research subjects. The chronic nature of cardiovascular disease also allows for in-hospital recruitment in more extended post-hospital projects. As 'lifestyle' factors are contributors to cardiovascular disease, research projects can be undertaken which examine socio-economic and psychological as well as physical variables. This provides an opportunity for health research which encompasses theories from other disciplines, leading to interesting collaborative projects. The sponsors of a clinical trial may fund sub-studies related to the major study.

Quality improvement (QI) projects require research skills. Staff who have participated in clinical trials are better prepared to undertake the design of projects and to collect and analyse data.

Conclusion

Large, randomized trials have been central to cardiovascular clinical research for over a decade and are unchallenged as a reliable method of investigation. Coronary care units which participate in clinical trials are in the best position to ensure the currency of their clinical care. Opportunities for innovative sub-studies of major trials or independent single-unit projects should not be overlooked.

References

1. Peto R. Why do we need systematic overviews of randomized trials? Statistics in Medicine 1987; 6: 233–40
2. The GUSTO Investigators. An international randomized trial comparing four thrombolytic strategies for acute myocardial infarction. N Engl J Med 1993; 329: 673–82
3. Yusuf S. Obtaining medically meaningful answers from an overview of randomized clinical trials. Statistics in Medicine 1987; 6: 281–6
4. Flather MD, Farkouh ME, Yusuf S. Meta-analysis in the evaluation of therapies. In: Julian D, Braunwald E (eds). Management of acute myocardial infarction. Philadelphia: Saunders, 1994
5. Antiplatelet Trialists' Collaboration. Collaborative overview of randomized clinical trials of antiplatelet therapy. (Pt 1.) Prevention of death, myocardial infarction, and stroke by prolonged antiplatelet therapy in various categories of patient. Br Med J 1994; 308: 81–106
6. World Health Organization Division of Drug Management and Policies. WHO guidelines for good clinical practice (GCP) for trials on pharmaceutical products. Canberra, 1993
7. Guidelines for good clinical research practice (GCRP) in Australia. Canberra: Commonwealth Department of Health, Housing and Community Services Therapeutic Goods Administration. 1991.

Appendices

Appendix I

IV doses for single use drugs in adult patients

NOTE: Dosage should be double checked and package insert should be read before administration.

Drug	Recommended formulation for CCU	Dose and method of use
Adenosine	Ampoules 6 mg adenosine in 2 mL.	3 mg over 2 seconds. If no response in 2 minutes, 6 mg over 2 seconds. If no response in 2 minutes, 12 mg over 2 seconds.
Adrenaline (Epinephrine)	Ampoules 1 mg adrenaline acid tartrate in 1 mL (1:1000) NB. Ampoules of 0.1 μg/mL 1:10,000 also available.	0.5–1.0 mg bolus: May be repeated.
Alteplase (See TPA)		
Amiodarone	Ampoules 150 mg amiodarone hydrochloride in 3 mL.	5 mg/kg (300 mg for average patient) over 30–60 minutes.
Atenolol	Ampoules 5 mg atenolol in 10mL.	2.5 mg over 2.5 minutes i.e. 1mg/min. Repeat at 5 minute intervals to a maximum of 10 mg.
Atropine	Ampoules 0.6 mg atropine sulphate in 1 mL NB. 0.4, 0.6, 1,0 and 1.2 mg in 1 mL, 0.5 mg in 5 mL and 1.0 mg in 10 mL also available.	0.3–1.2 mg bolus. May be repeated to a maximum of 2.4 mg.
Bretylium* *Discontinued in many countries in 1996	Ampoules 500 mg Bretylium tosylate in 10 mL.	5 mg/kg bolus (350–400 mg for average patient) 5–15 mg/kg bolus in refractory VF (unconscious patient). 5–10 mg/kg dilute in 100 m/L 5% dextrose over 15 mins for VT/VF prophylaxis (conscious patient).
Digoxin	Ampoules 0.5 mg digoxin in 2 mL.	0.5 mg in 50 mL normal saline or 5% dextrose in 15–20 minutes.
Diltiazem	25 mg diltiazem hydrochloride in 2 mL.	0.25 mg/kg (20 mg for average patient) over 2 minutes. Repeat if necessary with 0.35 mg/kg (25 mg for average patient) over 2 minutes.
Epinephrine (See adrenaline)		

Drug	Recommended formulation for CCU	Dose and method of use
Esmolol	Ampoules 100 mg esmolol hydrochloride in 10 mL. NB. Ampoules of 2.5 grams in 10 mL also available.	0.5 mg/kg (35 mg for average patient) over 1 minute followed by a further 0.05 mg/kg/min over 4 minutes, i.e. 0.2 mg/kg (15 mg for average patient), a total of 50 mg for the average patient. If no response, repeat the 0.5 mg/kg bolus followed by a further 0.1 mg/kg/min over 4 minutes, i.e. 0.4 mg/kg, a total of 65 mg for the average patient.
Flecainide	Ampoules 150 mg flecainide acetate in 15 mL.	2 mg/kg (150 mg for average patient) in 50 mL 5% dextrose over 15 minutes.
Lidocaine (See Lignocaine)		
Lignocaine (Lidocaine)	Ampoules 100 mg lignocaine hydrochloride in 10 mL (1%) or 100 mg in 5 mL (2%). NB. A wide range of ampoule sizes from 50 mg (5 mL of 1%) to 1000 mg (50 mL of 2%) available.	1.0–1.5 mg/kg (80-120 for the average patient) over 1–2 minutes. Smaller dose for elderly or patients with liver disease.
Magnesium sulphate	Ampoules 10 mmol or 20 mEq of magnesium in 5 mL.	8 mmol in 50 mL of normal saline over 8 minutes.
Metoprolol	Ampoules 5 mg metoprolol tartrate in in 5 mL.	5 mg at 1–2 mg/min. Repeat at 5 minute intervals to a maximum of 15 mg.
Procainamide	Ampoules 1 G procainamide hydrochloride in 10 mL	25–50 mg/min (with monitoring of blood pressure after each 100 mg) to a maximum of 500 mg.
r-TPA (See TPA)		
Sotalol	Ampoules 80 mg sotalol in 8 mL.	1.0–1.5 mg/kg (80-120 mg for the average patient) in 5% dextrose over 10-20 minutes.
Streptokinase	Vials of 250,000 IU, 750,000 IU or 1,500,000 streptokinase lyophylized powder reconstituted with 5 mL 5% dextrose or normal saline.	1.5 million units in 100 mL 5% dextrose or normal saline over 30–60 minutes.
TPA (alteplase)	Vials 50 mg alteplase lyophylized powder reconstituted with 50 mLs sterile water.	15 mg bolus then 0.75 mg/kg over 30 minutes (up to 50 mg) then 0.5 mg/kg over 60 minutes (up to 35 mg) to a maximum dose of 100 mg.
Verapamil	Ampoules 5 mg verapamil hydrochloride in 2 mL.	1 mg/min up to 5 mg monitoring blood pressure and response to carotid sinus massage. Repeat injection of 5 mg at 1 mg/min if necessary.

Appendix 2

Loading and maintenance doses for infusion

Note: Dosage and flow rate should be double checked and package insert should be read before administration.

Adrenaline (epinephrine)

IV loading dose:
None

Standard solution:
6 mg/100 mL 5% dextrose

Infusion dose:
1–15 µg/min

Rate: In mL/hour of Standard solution. (0.06 mg/mL = 60 µg/ mL of **adrenaline**). (See App2.1).

App 2.1: adrenaline

Dose µg/min	1	2	3	5	10	15
Rate mL/hr	1	2	3	5	10	15

Note
- Infuse via central line.
- Titrate cautiously.

Amiodarone

IV loading dose:
150–300 mg in 100 mLs dextrose 5% over 30–60 minutes
150–300 mg with 10–20 mL 5% dextrose over 1–2 min
(In extreme clinical emergency)

Standard solution:
300 mg/100 mL 5% dextrose

Infusion dose:
5–15 mg/kg/24 hours (Up to max dose of 1200 mg/24 hours) according to clinical response.

Rate: In mL/hour of Standard Solution (3 mg/mL) of **amiodarone**. (See App2.2).

App 2.2: amiodarone

Wt (kg)	Dose mg/kg/24 hours	5	10	15
50		3	7	10
60	Rate	4	8	12
70	mL/hour	5	10	14
80		5	11	16

Note
- *Amiodarone is incompatible with saline* and must be infused with 5% dextrose (glass bottles and non PVC sets preferred).
- Amiodarone is incompatible with most drugs, therefore infuse via separate cannula or double lumen cannula.
- Check QTc on ECG daily.

Bretylium*

IV loading dose:
In refractory VF (patient unconscious) 5–15 mg/kg rapidly undiluted (500 mg for average patient)

For VT/VF prophylaxis (conscious patient) infuse 5–10 mg/kg (dilute in 100 mL 5% dextrose over 15 min).

Standard solution:
2 gm in 500 mL 5% dextrose.

Infusion dose:
1 mg/min

Rate: In mL/hour of Standard solution (4 mg/mL) of **bretylium**. (See App2.3).

App 2.3: bretylium

Dose mg/min	1	1.5	2
Rate mL/hr	15	22	30

Note
- Profound hypotension may occur.
- Check QTc on ECG daily.

* Deleted by manufacturer in many countries in 1996.

Dobutamine

IV loading dose:
None

Standard solution:
500 mg/100 mL 5% dextrose

Infusion dose:
2.5–10 µg/kg/min

Rate: In mL/hour of Standard solution (5 mg/mL) of **dobutamine.** (See App2.4).

App 2.4: dobutamine

Weight (kg)	Dose (mg/kg/min)	2.5	5	10	20
50		2	3	6	12
60	Rate	2	3	7	14
70	mL/hour	2	4	8	17
80		2	5	10	19

Note

- Titrate dosage as per clinical status.
- Preferably infused via central line.
- Weaning. Usually at 1 mL/hour, with consideration of haemodynamic parameters (e.g. HR, BP, PAWP, CO studies).

Dopamine

IV loading dose:
None.

Standard solution:
400 mg/100 mL 5% dextrose

Infusion dose:
2.5–20 μg/kg/min

Rate: 1 mL of Standard solution (4 mg/mL) of **dopamine**. (See App2.5).

Note

- Renal dose: 2.5 μg/kg/min
- Inotropic dose > 2.5 μg/kg/min
- Infuse via central line.

Epinephrine—see Adrenaline

Flecainide

IV loading dose:
2 mg/kg over 30 min

Standard solution:
300 mg/100 mL 5% dextrose

Infusion dose:
After loading dose, 1.5 mg/kg over the next 60 min, then 0.25 mg/kg/hr and maintain

Rate: In mL/hour of Standard solution (3 mg/mL) of **flecainide.**
(See App 2.6).

Note
Contraindication in presence of significant left ventricular dysfunction.

Glyceryl trinitrate (GTN)

IV Loading dose:
None.

Standard solution:
50 mg/100 mL 5% dextrose
Glass bottles and non PVC sets to be used only (PVC absorbs GTN)

Infusion dose:
Increments of 8 μg/min at 2–5 minute intervals until required result achieved

Rate: In mL/hour of Standard solution (0.5 mg/mL = 500 μg/mL) of **glyceryl trinitrate** (GTN). (See App2.7).

Note

- Commence at 1 mL/hr titrate in 1 mL/hr increments 2–5 minutely as tolerated, i.e. BP maintained and no significant increase in heart rate noted.
- Weaning. Decrease infusion rate by 1 mL/hour.
- When priming the IV line ensure GTN fully primed.

Heparin

IV Loading dose:
5000 IU

Standard solution:
25 000 IU in 500 mL 5% dextrose

Infusion dose:
Commence at 1000 IU/hour. Adjust to maintain APTT 60–80 seconds or 2–2.5 times the mean of the reference range.

Rate: In mL/hour of Standard solution (50 IU/mL) of **heparin.**
(See App 2.8)

App 2.5: dopamine

Weight (kg)	Dose μg/kg/min	2.5	5	10	15	20
50		2	4	8	12	16
60	Rate	2	4	9	12	18
70	mL/hour	3	5	10	16	20
80		3	6	12	18	24

App 2.6: flecainide

Weight (kg)	Dose mg/kg/hour	2 mg/kg over 30 min	1.5 mg/kg over 60 min	0.25 mg/kg/hr
50		66	25	4
60	Rate	74	30	5
70	mL/hour	86	35	6
80		106	40	7

App 2.7: glyceryl trinitrate (GTN)

Dose mcg/min	8	16	24	32	40	48	56	64
Rate mL/hr	1	2	3	4	5	6	7	8

App 2.8 heparin

Dose IU/hour	800	1000	1200
Rate mL/hr	16	20	24

Note
APTT should be checked at 6 hours after 5000 IU bolus and infusion at 1000 IU/hour, and adjusted according to the APTT level. If APTT is < 35, an additional bolus of 5000 units should be administered. If APTT is 35–45, an additional bolus of 2500 IU should be administered. When dosage has been adjusted, an APTT should be obtained 6 hours later, and when APTT is therapeutic, APTT should be measured daily.

Isoprenaline (Isoproterenol)

IV Loading dose:
None.

Standard solution:
2 mg (i.e. 10 mL of 1:5000 solution) in 500 mL 5% dextrose

Infusion dose:
0.5–5 µg/min

Rate: In mL/hour of Standard solution (0.004 mg/mL or 4 µg/mL) of **isoprenaline**. (See App2.9).

App 2.9: isoprenaline

Dose µg/min	0.5	1	2	3	4	5
Rate mL/hr	8	15	30	45	60	75

Note
- Observe for tachycardia arrhythmias and fluctuating BP.
- Observe cardiac rhythm and rate when weaning.

Lignocaine (Lidocaine)

IV Loading dose:
1.5 mg/kg at rate of 25–50 mg/min
½ dose may be repeated at 5 min and at 15 min if necessary. No more than 200 mg–300 mg in one hour.

Standard solution:
2 gm i.e. 100 mL of 2% Lignocaine in 500 mL 5% dextrose

Infusion dose:
4 mg/min for 1 hour
3 mg/min for 1 hour
Maintain at 1–2 mg/min (lower if elderly, hypotensive or evidence of liver disease)

Rate: In mL/hour of Standard solution (4 mg/mL) of **lignocaine**. (See App2.10).

App 2.10: standard lignocaine

Dose mg/min	4	3	2	1
Rate mL/hr	60	45	30	15

Note
- Watch carefully for lignocaine toxicity—drowsiness, slurred speech, twitching.
- **If fluid restriction applies** make up infusion bag with 4 gms (i.e. 40 mL of 10%) Lignocaine/500 mL 5% dextrose and use the following regime:

Rate: In mL/hour of **Non**-Standard solution (8 mg/mL) of **lignocaine**. (See App 2.11).

App 2.11: non-standard lignocaine

Dose mcg/min	4	3	2	1
Rate mL/hr	30	22	15	7

Magnesium sulphate

IV Loading dose:
8 mmol in 50 mL normal saline over 30 minutes

Standard solution:
65 mmol mg/100 mL N/saline.

Infusion dose:
65 mmol over 24 hours

Rate: In mL/hour of Standard solution of **magnesium sulphate.** (See App 2.12).

App 2.12: magnesium sulphate

Dose mmol/hour	2–7
Rate mL/hour	4

Note
- Contra-indicated if bradyarrhythmias or serum creatinine above 150 µmol/L.
- 65 mmol Mg equals 32.5 mL volume.
- Remove 30 mL of N/saline from bag prior to adding Mg therefore total volume = 102.5 mL.

Milrinone

IV Loading dose:
50 µg/kg over 10 mins

50 kg = 2.5 mg
60 kg = 3.0 mg
70 kg = 3.5 mg
80 kg = 4.0 mg
90 kg = 4.5 mg
100 kg = 5.0 mg
} in 5% dextrose 50ml over 10 min

Standard solution:
30 mg/100 mL 5% dextrose

Infusion dose:
0.375–0.75 µg/kg/min

Rate: In mL/hour of Standard solution (0.3 mg/mL = 300 µg/mL) of **milrinone.** (See App 2.13).

Note
SVT and ventricular arrhythmias have been observed.
Patients with atrial fibrillation/flutter may have enhanced atrioventricular conduction as Milrinone slightly shortens AV conduction.

Nitroglycerine—*see glyceryl trinitrate*

Nitroprusside—*see sodium nitroprusside*

App 2.13: milrinone

Weight (kg)	Dose µg/min	Min = 0.375 µg/kg/min	Standard = 0.5 µg/kg/min	Max = 0.75 µg/kg/min
60	Rate mL/hour	4–5 mL/hr	6 mL/hr	9 mL/hr
70		5–6 mL/hr	7–8 mL/hr	10–11 mL/hr
80		6 mL/hr	8 mL/hr	12 mL/hr
90		7 mL/hr	9 mL/hr	14 mL/hr

Procainamide

IV loading dose:
Up to 10 mg/kg at rate of 25–50 mg/min

Standard solution:
4 gm/500 mL

Infusion dose:
4 mg/min for 1 hour
3 mg/min for 1 hour
2 mg/min–maintain

Rate: In mL/hour of Standard solution (8 mg/mL) of **procainamide.** (See App2.14).

App 2.14: procainamide

Dose mg/min	4 mg	3 mg	2 mg	1 mg
Rate mL/hr	30	21	15	7

Note
- Observe for hypotension and/or widening of QRS during loading dose.
- Check QTc on ECG daily.

Sodium nitroprusside

IV loading dose:
None.

Standard solution:
50 mg/100 mL 5% dextrose

Infusion dose:
Commence at 0.5 µg/kg/min
Increase in 0.5 µg/kg increments every 5 minutes until desired blood pressure is attained
Recommended dose = 0.5– 10 µg/kg/min

Rate: In mL/hour Standard solution (0.6 mg/mL = 600 µg/mL) of sodium nitroprusside. (See App 2.15).

App 2.15: sodium nitroprusside

Weight (kg)	**Dose µg/min**	**0.5 µg**	**2 µg**	**5 µg**
50		3	12	30
60	Rate	4	14	36
70	mL/hour	4	17	42
80		5	19	48

Note
- Never add these drugs into line.
- If administration exceeds 48 hours at high rates, thiocyanate level should be obtained.
- Dilute only in 5% dextrose.
  Change infusion every 24 hours.
  Protect bag and tubing from light.
  Monitor blood pressure every 5 minutes (minimum) when titrating.

Calculation of flow rate via volumetric pumps

$$\frac{\text{Volume in flask (mL) and dose required per minute} \times 60}{\text{Dose in flask}} = \text{FLOW RATE/hour}$$

Example 1
2 mg lignocaine in 500 mL 5% dextrose
Dose ordered is 4 mg/min

$$\frac{500 \text{ (vol in flask in mL)} \times 4 \text{ mg (dose required/min)} \times 60}{2000 \text{ mg (2G = dose in flask)}}$$

$$= \frac{500 \times 4 \times 60}{2000}$$

= 60 mL/hour

Example 2
500 mg dobutamine in 100 mL 5% dextrose
Dose ordered is 5 µg/kg/min
Weight is 70 kg

$$\frac{100 \text{ (vol in flask in mL)} \times 5\ \mu\text{g/kg (dose required/min)} \times 70 \text{ (weight in kg)} \times 60}{500\,000\ \mu\text{g (500 mg = dose in flask)}}$$

$$= \frac{100 \times 5 \times 70 \times 60}{500\,000}$$

= 3 mL/hour

Index